Robert Hart.

TEXTBOOK OF MEDICAL TREATMENT

Textbook of
Medical Treatment

By Various Authors

Edited by

Stanley Alstead

C.B.E., M.D., F.R.S.E., F.R.C.P.Ed., F.R.C.P.Glasg., F.R.C.P.Lond.

Emeritus Professor of Materia Medica, University of Glasgow;
Physician, Stobhill General Hospital, Glasgow 1948-1970

Alastair G. Macgregor

B.Sc., M.D., F.R.C.P.Ed., F.R.C.P.Glasg., F.R.C.P.Lond.

Regius Professor of Materia Medica, Department of Therapeutics and Clinical
Pharmacology, University of Aberdeen;
Physician, Royal Infirmary, Aberdeen

Ronald H. Girdwood

M.D., Ph.D., F.R.C.P.Ed., F.R.C.P.Lond., F.R.C.Path.

Professor of Therapeutics, University of Edinburgh;
Physician, Royal Infirmary, Edinburgh

Twelfth Edition

CHURCHILL LIVINGSTONE, EDINBURGH & LONDON, 1971

First Edition	.	.	.	*1939*
Reprint	.	.	.	*1940*
Second Edition	.	.	.	*1942*
Reprint	.	.	.	*1943*
Third Edition	.	.	.	*1944*
Fourth Edition	.	.	.	*1946*
Reprint	.	.	.	*1946*
Reprint	.	.	.	*1947*
Fifth Edition	.	.	.	*1949*
Reprint	.	.	.	*1950*
Sixth Edition	.	.	.	*1953*
Reprint	.	.	.	*1955*
Seventh Edition	.	.	.	*1958*
Reprint	.	.	.	*1959*
Eighth Edition	.	.	.	*1961*
Ninth Edition	.	.	.	*1964*
Tenth Edition	.	.	.	*1966*
Eleventh Edition	.	.	.	*1968*
Twelfth Edition	.	.	.	*1971*

ISBN 0 443 00779 9

PRINTED IN GREAT BRITAIN

Preface to the Twelfth Edition

THIS edition of the *Textbook of Medical Treatment* differs from all of the preceding eleven editions: it records the retirement of Sir Derrick Dunlop from the editorial board in 1968. His wide knowledge of medicine and therapeutics, his well-known capacity for lucid exposition and his exceptional skill as an editor are qualities that have sustained his colleagues and established standards for future editors and contributors. Sir Derrick's salutary influence on the content and style of the book, exerted over a period of thirty years, will undoubtedly persist for as long as this book is published.

The vacancy on the editorial board has been filled by Sir Derrick's successor in the Chair of Therapeutics in the University of Edinburgh, Professor Ronald H. Girdwood.

The textbook lost one of its most distinguished contributors by the death of Professor H. W. Fullerton. In consequence of this, Professor Girdwood has assumed responsibility for the whole section on Disorders of the Blood; the editors are grateful to Professor Stuart Douglas for re-drafting much of that part of the chapter which deals with haemorrhagic disorders. With the retirement of Professor Thomas Anderson as a contributor, Dr J. McC. Murdoch has conveniently extended his writing on chemotherapy to undertake the revision of the chapter on Infectious Diseases, but few changes in Professor Anderson's authoritative essay have been required. Professor W. I. Card, now occupying the Chair of Medicine in relation to Mathematics in the University of Glasgow, suggested to the Editors that he should cease to contribute the section on Alimentary Diseases and, accordingly, this chapter has been rewritten by Mr W. P. Small and Dr D. J. C. Shearman of the Edinburgh Medical School. Dr E. G. Collins' retirement affected editorial policy regarding the place of diseases of the ear, nose and throat in a textbook of general therapeutics. It was decided to assimilate much of this material into other parts of the book, especially the chapters on Infectious Diseases and the Respiratory System. Miss Catherine Burt has also retired and the chapter on the Effects of Cold is now written by Professor D. M. Douglas. In similar circumstances Dr Arnold Klopper has taken over the section on Female Sex Endocrinology which was previously the responsibility of Dr T. N. Macgregor. In Sir Ian Hill's chapter on Diseases of the Heart and Circulation the sections on the treatment of systemic hypertension and the cardiac arrhythmias have been rewritten by Dr D. Emslie-Smith. Professor Girdwood has collaborated with Sir Stanley Davidson in writing the section on Nutritional Disorders. Finally, Diseases of the Eye, contributed for many years by Professor G. I. Scott, has been rewritten by Professor W. S. Foulds. With one or two exceptions noted above, new contributors have elected to adopt a fresh presentation of their subject matter and seven sections have been completely rewritten. In the remaining twenty-three chapters the writers have again carefully revised their material, taking note of new developments when these have achieved an established place in practical therapeutics.

Dr Iain W. Dymock has continued the compilation of the Glossary, showing proprietary equivalents of the drugs mentioned in the text by their Official or Approved names. We are indebted to Dr Norman MacKay for compiling the Index, to Dr Brian Whiting and Dr Thomas Ward for help with proof reading, and to Miss Eleanor Newell and Miss Elspeth Shields for their assistance in preparing manuscript for the press.

In this edition it is hoped that the use of bolder type for headings will make the book more acceptable for reference purposes. In this and many other matters we have enjoyed the expert guidance of the Publishers, Messrs. E. & S. Livingstone, and we are accordingly grateful to them.

STANLEY ALSTEAD
ALASTAIR G. MACGREGOR
RONALD H. GIRDWOOD

1971

Extract from Preface to the First Edition

THIS book has been written for students and practitioners in the hope that it may fill the therapeutic gap left by the majority of textbooks on general medicine in which, owing to exigencies of space, the section devoted to treatment is often inadequate. In addition, the information given is not infrequently couched in such indefinite terms as to be of little value in helping the practitioner to determine whether a particular line of treatment is worthy of trial and, if so, how it can be put into practice. The following statements, for instance, are frequently made: 'vaccines may be of value', 'arsenic may be tried', 'a well-balanced diet should be given', 'the general health should receive attention'. Further, it is not uncommon for many drugs and measures recommended by our forefathers to continue to be included in such works year after year in spite of the fact that some of them have been shown to be useless and others are known to be less efficacious than modern substitutes.

An attempt has, therefore, been made by the authors of this book to be extremely explicit in regard to the treatment recommended, in the hope that the directions given will suffice to enable a doctor without much previous experience to carry out the measures which have been described. As far as possible the indications, contraindications and dangers of each recommended method or drug are fully discussed.

Further, an attempt has been made to indicate why and when certain drugs and methods formerly widely used should no longer be employed for the particular purpose under discussion. From this it follows that the number of drugs advised are considerably fewer than in some books of therapeutics, but this we believe to be wise, for undue reliance on the 'bottle of medicine' has tended in the past to obscure and diminish the importance of certain general measures of paramount importance which may be included under the heading 'General Management of the Patient', i.e. diet, rest, exercise, nursing, etc., which in the past have received too little attention in medical teaching and textbooks. In addition, the general problem of handling patients and relations under the various circumstances which continually confront the young doctor is dealt with. This entails a consideration of what information should or should not be given to the relatives and patient in certain circumstances, and general advice on where and when to send patients to sanatoria, spas or for a change of air and climate. Lastly, the good management of a case frequently requires a knowledge of common-sense psychological principles which are so important in the art of medicine.

The work is not a small handbook of treatment, nor yet a vast encyclopædia, since there are already a number of such books. Neither is it a textbook of pharmacology, since a large portion of the book deals not with drugs but with the 'Management of the Case' in the widest sense of the term. It is not concerned with surgery, but includes sections on the treatment of venereal diseases, tropical medicine, some diseases peculiar to infants, common diseases of the skin, industrial diseases and the neuroses. There is, in addition, a section which describes in detail the technique of certain essential medical procedures—such as lumbar puncture, venesection, paracentesis, blood transfusion, oxygen therapy, etc.

It is a pleasure to acknowledge the help received from Mr T. H. Graham and Miss Margaret P. Russell, M.A.—Librarian and Assistant Librarian in the Royal College of Physicians, Edinburgh—for their help in proof-reading and in the compilation of the index; to various editors and publishers who have given us permission to use certain plates and diagrams appearing in their journals, and in particular to Messrs Lippincott, of Philadelphia, the publishers of 'Body Mechanics', and to Messrs Oliver & Boyd, publishers of the *Edinburgh Medical Journal*; and, lastly to Mr McDonald Walker, of Messrs E. & S. Livingstone, who on all occasions has assisted us in every possible way.

D. M. DUNLOP
L. S. P. DAVIDSON
1939　　　J. W. MCNEE

Contributors

Antibiotics and Chemotherapy

J.McC. MURDOCH, F.R.C.P.Ed., F.R.C.P.Glasg., Hon. Senior Lecturer in Infectious Diseases, University of Edinburgh.

Infectious Diseases

J. McC. MURDOCH

Tuberculosis

J. W. CROFTON, M.A., M.D., F.R.C.P.Ed., F.R.C.P.Lond., Professor of Respiratory Diseases and Tuberculosis, University of Edinburgh.

Diseases of the Heart and Circulation

SIR IAN HILL, *C.B.E.*, *T.D.*, M.B., Ch.B., Hon. LL.D., F.R.S.E., F.R.C.P.Ed., F.R.C.P.Lond., Hon. F.R.A.C.P., Hon. F.A.C.P., Emeritus Professor of Medicine, University of Dundee.

Diseases of the Blood Vessels of the Limbs and the Effects of Cold

D. M. DOUGLAS, *M.B.E.*, M.S., Ch.M., P.R.C.S.Ed., F.R.C.S.Eng., Professor of Surgery, University of Dundee.

Disorders of the Blood

R. H. GIRDWOOD, M.D., Ph.D., F.R.C.P.Ed., F.R.C.P.Lond, F.R.C.Path., Professor of Therapeutics, University of Edinburgh.

Anticoagulant Therapy

A. S. DOUGLAS, B.Sc., M.D., F.R.C.P.Ed., F.R.C.P.Glasg., F.R.C.P.Lond., F.R.C.Path., Regius Professor of Medicine, University of Aberdeen.

Disease of the Respiratory System

I. GORDON, *O.B.E.*, B.Sc., M.B., Ch.B., F.R.C.P. Ed., F.R.C.P.Lond., Physician, Royal Infirmary, Aberdeen.

I. W. B. GRANT, M.B., Ch.B., F.R.C.P.Ed., Physician, Respiratory Diseases Unit, Northern General Hospital, Edinburgh.

Diseases of the Alimentary System

W. P. SMALL, *V.R.D.*, M.B., Ch.M., F.R.C.S.Ed., F.R.C.P.Ed., Surgeon, Western General Hospital, Edinburgh.

D. J. C. SHEARMAN, B.Sc., Ph.D., M.B., Ch.B., F.R.C.P.Ed., Physician, Royal Infirmary, Edinburgh.

Disturbance in Water and Electrolyte Balance and in Acid-base Equilibrium

J. S. ROBSON, M.D., F.R.C.P.Ed., Reader in Medicine, University of Edinburgh.

Renal Diseases

J. S. ROBSON.

Hormone Therapy and Diseases of the Endocrine Glands

A. G. MACGREGOR, B.Sc., M.D., F.R.C.P.Ed., F.R.C.P.Glasg., F.R.C.P.Lond., Regius Professor of Materia Medica, University of Aberdeen.

J. A. STRONG, *M.B.E.*, M.A., M.D., F.R.S.E., F.R.C.P.Ed., F.R.C.P.Lond., Professor in the University Department of Medicine, Western General Hospital, Edinburgh.

Female Sex Endocrinology

A. J. KLOPPER, Ph.D., M.D., F.R.C.O.G., Reader in Obstetrics and Gynaecology, University of Aberdeen.

Metabolic Diseases—Diabetes Mellitus, Obesity

L. J. P. DUNCAN, B.Sc., M.B., Ch.B., F.R.C.P.Ed., Physician, Royal Infirmary, Edinburgh.

Nutritional Disorders

SIR STANLEY DAVIDSON, B.A., M.D., F.R.S.E., F.R.C.P.Ed., F.R.C.P.Lond., Hon. M.D.Oslo, Hon. LL.D. (Edin. and Aberd.), Emeritus Professor of Medicine, University of Edinburgh.

R. H. GIRDWOOD.

Diseases of the Nervous System

J. A. SIMPSON, M.D., F.R.S.E., F.R.C.P.Ed., F.R.C.P.Glasg., F.R.C.P.Lond., Professor of Neurology, University of Glasgow.

Psychiatry in General Practice

T. F. RODGER, *C.B.E.*, B.Sc., M.B., Ch.B., D.P.M., F.R.C.P.Ed., F.R.C.P.Glasg., Professor of Psychological Medicine, University of Glasgow.

Analgesics and Hypnotics

S. ALSTEAD, *C.B.E.*, M.D., F.R.S.E., F.R.C.P. Ed., F.R.C.P.Glasg., F.R.C.P.Lond., Emeritus Professor of Materia Medica, University of Glasgow.

T. J. THOMSON, M.B., Ch.B., F.R.C.P.Glasg., F.R.C.P.Lond., Hon. Lecturer in Materia Medica University of Glasgow.

Chronic Rheumatic Diseases

J. J. R. DUTHIE, M.B., Ch.B., F.R.C.P.Ed., Professor (Rheumatology) in the Department of Medicine, University of Edinburgh.

Common Disorders in Infancy and Early Childhood

J. H. HUTCHINSON, *C.B.E.*, M.D., F.R.S.E., F.R.C.P.Ed., F.R.C.P.Glasg., F.R.C.P.Lond., Hon. F.A.C.P., Professor of Child Health, University of Glasgow.

The Care of Old People

S. ALSTEAD.

W. F. ANDERSON, *O.B.E.*, M.D., F.R.C.P.Ed., F.R.C.P.Glasg., F.R.C.P.Lond., Professor of Geriatric Medicine, University of Glasgow.

Common Tropical Diseases and Helminthic Infections

F. J. WRIGHT, M.A., M.D., D.T.M. & H., F.R.C.P.Ed., F.R.C.P.Lond., Senior Lecturer in Diseases of Tropical Climates, University of Edinburgh.

Pesticides and Repellents

A. R. MILLS, Ph.D., M.R.C.S., L.R.C.P., D.P.H., D.T.M. & H., Formerly Senior Lecturer in Social Medicine, University of Edinburgh.

Acute Poisoning

H. J. S. MATTHEW, M.D., F.R.C.P.Ed., Physician, Poisoning Treatment Centre, Royal Infirmary, Edinburgh.

Ill-health due to Drugs

G. M. WILSON, M.D., D.Sc., F.R.C.P.Ed., F.R.C.P.Glasg., F.R.C.P.Lond., Regius Professor of the Practice of Medicine, University of Glasgow.

Industrial Diseases

A. T. DOIG, M.D., F.R.S.E., D.P.H., F.R.C.P. Ed., F.R.C.P.Glasg., H.M. Deputy Senior Medical Inspector of Factories.

S. ALSTEAD.

Common Diseases of the Skin

A. LYELL, M.D., F.R.C.P.Ed., F.R.C.P.Glasg., Physician in charge of Department of Dermatology, Royal Infirmary, Glasgow.

Venereal Diseases

R. LEES, M.D., F.R.C.P.Ed., Formerly Senior Lecturer in Venereal Diseases, University of Edinburgh.

Diseases of the Eye

W. S. FOULDS, M.D., Ch.M., F.R.C.S.Eng., D.O., Tennent Professor of Ophthalmology, University of Glasgow.

Principles of Prescribing

A. G. MACGREGOR.

Technical Procedures

SIR JAMES FRASER, Bart., B.A., Ch.M., F.R.C.S. Ed., Professor of Clinical Science in Surgery, University of Southampton.

Oxygen Therapy—Artificial Respiration

I. W. B. GRANT.

Contents

A*

ix

1. Antibiotics and Chemotherapy

J. McC. Murdoch

INTRODUCTION

The work of Pasteur in microbiology followed by Lister's practical application of this new knowledge led to the researches of Ehrlich during the late nineteenth and early twentieth centuries. Ehrlich conceived the idea of chemotherapy—the eradication of bacteria from the tissues of an infected animal by the infusion into the blood stream of chemical substances having a bactericidal effect. The subsequent treatment of syphilis with organic arsenical compounds was the beginning of a new chapter in medical history. It soon became apparent, however, that chemotherapeutic substances, besides destroying micro-organisms in tissues, were also potentially toxic to the host. Since Ehrlich's time many attempts have been made to find substances with antibacterial effects *in vivo*, the most notable of which has been the discovery of the sulphonamides by Domagk in 1935 and the subsequent clinical application of the antibiotics initiated by Fleming in 1928. Since that time many new antibiotics have been developed, mainly from screening samples of soil for fungi producing chemical substances which have the effect of inhibiting the growth of other micro-organisms or even of totally destroying them. Literally thousands of such samples have now been screened from which only a few therapeutically effective and relatively non-toxic antibiotics have been found suitable for the treatment of infections in man.

Despite the development of the sulphonamides and the subsequent antibiotics, it is important to remember that there are still many infections, notably those caused by most viruses, which remain insusceptible to antibiotics or chemotherapy. Further, the widespread introduction of these drugs has led, not unnaturally, to the development of bacterial resistance to some of the earlier forms of treatment. This is especially true of the *Staphylococcus aureus* and of certain gram-negative bacteria. It is, therefore, possible that a patient may be infected with micro-organisms which are naturally resistant to present forms of treatment, or that the infection may be caused by bacteria which have acquired resistance to therapy which was effective in the past. Before deciding to treat a patient, the doctor should consider these points, and he should also be aware of the possible side-effects of antibiotic drugs. Their administration inevitably disturbs the bacterial flora in the human host so that micro-organisms, insensitive to the particular drug being given, will colonize and sometimes infect him. Similarly the patient's environment will be considerably altered as he will be excreting antibiotic in his urine, faeces, saliva, sputum and sweat. In a hospital ward this may be of importance, as an accumulation of antibiotic contamination will result in a parallel rise of resistant organisms in such a closed environment.

Obviously there are also many febrile conditions which are not due to infection and the administration of an antibiotic in a 'blind' way to patients simply because they have a fever is to be deplored. Ideally the infecting organism should be identified and its susceptibility to antibacterial drugs ascertained before treatment is given. This is usually possible in large urban centres and in hospital practice, but may be impracticable if the patient is seriously ill or in areas where no bacteriological services are available. In such circumstances a knowledge of the clinical features of the known bacterial infections and their prevalence in that area at any given time should give a reasonable clue to the choice of antibiotic. 'Blunderbuss' treatment with so-called wide-spectrum antibiotics or the use of two or more antibiotics is, in general, bad practice. Antibiotics are present in trace amounts in some of our foodstuffs and in certain vaccines such as the injectable form of poliomyelitis vaccine. This is not a great menace, but an occasional serious reaction may arise if hypersensitive humans are exposed to even minute amounts.

It is wise to administer an antibiotic only when the diagnosis is certain or reasonably certain and to use the best one available in terms of its antibacterial activity and its lack of toxicity. Adequate doses should be given for a sufficient time to ensure total eradication of the infection. If these principles are observed, the widespread and indiscriminate use of

1

antibiotics will not occur and the risk of producing a large population of antibiotic-resistant micro-organisms will be reduced. The incidence of serious and sometimes fatal side-effects of treatment will also be diminished.

THE SULPHONAMIDES

While it cannot be doubted that the sulphonamides must have saved countless lives since their introduction in 1935, it is important to evaluate their place in antibacterial therapy at the present time. Many different types of sulphonamide compound have been developed in an attempt to avoid serious toxicity. Perhaps the most popular soluble sulphonamide is now sulphadimidine, but there are also the recently developed long-acting sulphonamides which can be given at much longer intervals varying from one administration per day to one every five days. Nevertheless, there are now serious objections to the use of any form of sulphonamide as the primary treatment for any infection. First, there are many strains of micro-organism which have become resistant to the action of sulphonamide. Good examples are *Neisseria gonorrhoeae, Staphylococcus aureus, Shigella sonnei* and many coliform strains. It is worth recording that in certain parts of the world a significant percentage of *Neisseria meningitidis* are now sulphonamide-resistant. Second, all forms of sulphonamide are capable of affecting the bone marrow by depression of all or some of its elements. Thrombocytopenia, agranulocytosis and marrow aplasia have been recorded. Third, sensitization phenomena have arisen and the administration of sulphonamides has been implicated in the aetiology of connective-tissue disorders such as disseminated lupus and polyarteritis nodosa. In this context the long-acting sulphonamides have also been further implicated in the aetiology of the Stevens–Johnson syndrome which can be very dangerous and even fatal for young children. Fourth, the sulphonamide compounds may cause serious skin rashes, especially if applied topically.

An interesting development is the combination of trimethoprim, 80 mg., with sulphamethoxazole, 400 mg., sold under the trade names Bactrim or Septrin. For paediatric use the compound is also available as trimethoprim, 20 mg., with sulphamethoxazole, 100 mg., in tablet form or trimethoprim, 40 mg., with sulphamethoxazole, 200 mg., in 5 ml. suspension. Trimethoprim inhibits dihydrofolic acid reductase while sulphonamides derive their bacteriostatic activity by competitive inhibition of the enzyme involved in the incorporation of para-aminobenzoic acid into the dihydrofolic acid molecule. The combination thus deranges purine synthesis and ultimately that of DNA by bacteria. It is therefore bactericidal to a wide range of common pathogens even if an organism is partially resistant to one or other of the drugs *in vitro*. Clinical effectiveness has been shown in many common infections, particularly acute and chronic bacteriuria, chronic bronchitis, and salmonellosis, even, it is claimed, in chronic typhoid carriers. It is too early to assess the possible long-term toxicity of trimethoprim and there is always the possibility of sulphonamide toxicity, especially if the combination is used for prolonged treatment as in chronic bacteriuria. At present, bacterial resistance is not a problem, but this may well emerge with widespread and indiscriminate use of new and effective combination of drugs.

THE NITROFURANS

Nitrofurantoin—a synthetic chemical—is bacteriostatic in action but when given by mouth fails to reach adequate levels in the blood though effective levels can be achieved in the urine. Thus, the only therapeutic indication for the use of this drug is for the treatment of susceptible urinary tract infections. For acute infections, 200 mg. or 400 mg. in divided doses by mouth should be given for 10 days. In patients suffering from chronic bacteriuria, nitrofurantoin may be given suppressively for long periods of time in a dose of 100 mg. at night. The drug is expensive and potentially toxic, especially when administered for a long time. Nausea and heartburn are common side-effects, but these can be lessened by taking the drug with or immediately after a meal. Peripheral neuropathies have been reported following prolonged administration in patients with impaired renal function.

ANTIBIOTICS MAINLY ACTIVE AGAINST GRAM-POSITIVE ORGANISMS

BENZYLPENICILLIN

Benzylpenicillin is still the most widely used antibiotic in the world and remains pre-eminent over its successors in terms of activity, weight for weight, against micro-organisms susceptible to its action. The mortality and morbidity of certain gram-positive infections have been dramatically reduced since its commercial development in 1942. Resistance to benzylpenicillin has not become a problem with some bacterial species, notably *Streptococcus pneumoniae*, *Streptococcus pyogenes* and the treponemes, but has risen to serious proportions with the *Staphylococcus aureus* and, to a limited extent, with the gonococcus. Benzylpenicillin has the great merit of almost total absence of pharmacological toxicity which can only be caused by the administration of really massive doses or by intrathecal use in an excessive dose. Despite this, benzylpenicillin is the antibiotic most likely to produce sensitization, and a significant percentage of the population is now allergic to penicillin. Serious anaphylactoid reactions, occasionally fatal, have been increasing in recent years. A history of sensitivity to penicillin should always be sought before any penicillin is given to a patient.

Pharmacology. Benzylpenicillin is usually administered by the intramuscular route and after a single injection blood levels rise steeply to attain an optimal bactericidal effect after 30 to 60 minutes. Thereafter the antibiotic level falls steadily and in six hours little can be detected in the blood. Benzylpenicillin diffuses into most body tissues and fluids with the exception of the cerebrospinal fluid, as the healthy blood–brain barrier does not allow of much permeation. It is active in the presence of pus. Renal excretion is rapid so that intramuscular injections must be given six-hourly or more often in severe infections in order to maintain satisfactory blood and tissue levels. If the meninges are inflamed, effective penicillin levels can be achieved in the cerebrospinal fluid by giving relatively big doses intramuscularly. Gastric acid will largely destroy benzylpenicillin, allowing only small and ineffective quantities to be absorbed from the upper intestine. This drawback has been overcome by the development of synthetic oral penicillin preparations which will be discussed later. Benzylpenicillin may also be injected into infected cavities such as the pleura, pericardium or a joint space, and thus bring about a high concentration at the site of infection.

Administration and dosage. The dose of intramuscular benzylpenicillin will vary in quantity and frequency of injection according to the type of infection to be treated. Certain common gram-positive organisms remain highly susceptible to its action—for example, *Str. pneumoniae* and *Str.*

pyogenes are inhibited by very small amounts of benzylpenicillin both *in vitro* and *in vivo*. For most infections caused by these pathogens the dose need not be very high. There has been a continual tendency to increase the dose of benzylpenicillin in the belief that the bigger the dose the better the result. This is unnecessary and, indeed, undesirable as large amounts of penicillin given intramuscularly are painful. For pneumococcal infections, apart from pneumococcal meningitis, the adult dose should be about 100,000 units (60 mg.) six-hourly which, in uncomplicated cases, should be effective in five to seven days. For a haemolytic streptococcal infection, even with septicaemia, a similar regimen will be satisfactory. An infection caused by a penicillin-sensitive strain of *Staphylococcus aureus* can be treated in the same way but the duration of treatment may require to be longer, depending upon the site of the infection. Thus, several weeks may be necessary in the treatment of a susceptible staphylococcal osteomyelitis. High doses and additional routes of administration will be required even when sensitive organisms are located in differing anatomical sites. Adult patients suffering from pneumococcal meningitis should be given 500,000 units (300 mg.) four-hourly intramuscularly until the cerebrospinal fluid has returned to normal. If infection of a serous membrane occurs, up to 100,000 units (60 mg.) diluted in 20 ml. of saline should be injected into the cavity. In the event of osteomyelitis due to these organisms, 100,000 units (60 mg.) intramuscularly will be insufficient if the infection is chronic. The presence of osteosclerotic bone with a poor blood supply will necessitate the giving of up to 1,000,000 units (600 mg.) six-hourly. Staphylococcal infection of the urinary tract will respond to a relatively small dose if the organism is sensitive to penicillin, such as 100,000 units (60 mg.) six-hourly for five days. Meningococcal septicaemia will respond to a dose of 100,000 units (60 mg.) six-hourly as the meningococcus is extremely sensitive to the action of benzylpenicillin (p. 43).

Certain micro-organisms are relatively insensitive to the action of penicillin, notably *Streptococcus viridans*. Bacterial endocarditis caused by this organism necessitates the administration of frequent large doses of benzylpenicillin (p. 109). The patient may require 500,000 units (300 mg.) four-hourly or even three-hourly for up to six weeks before this infection is overcome. It is possible to reduce the number of injections by the use of probenecid—a renal tubular blocking agent—which delays the excretion of benzylpenicillin by the kidneys. A dose of 2 g. daily by mouth will help to achieve this and, where possible, estimations of the blood levels of penicillin should be made to ensure that these do not fall at any time below the minimum inhibitory concentration for the patient's own organism *in vitro*. Very large intramuscular doses are required in the treatment of actinomycosis. One million units (600 mg.) six-hourly for several weeks are usually necessary in this type of infection. The treponemal diseases—syphilis and yaws—are treated with long-acting penicillins such as procaine benzylpenicillin or benzathine penicillin. Treatment for these diseases varies according to the stage of the infection (p. 597).

The use of benzylpenicillin as a topical antibiotic has been abandoned except in the management of burns which have become infected with *Str. pyogenes*. The incorporation of benzylpenicillin in throat lozenges, chewing-gum, eye-drops, ear-drops or ointments should be condemned, not only because of the ineffectiveness of these preparations but also because of the risk of producing sensitization.

Indications. Benzylpenicillin remains the antibiotic of first choice in the treatment of acute systemic infections caused by pyogenic gram-positive cocci with the notable exception of the *Staphylococcus aureus.* Almost 100 per cent. of hospital strains of the latter are now penicillin-resistant and 10 to 20 per cent. of strains outside hospitals have been shown to be so. The practitioner should elect to use benzylpenicillin for the treatment of pneumococcal and haemolytic streptococcal infections in preference to the sulphonamides as the antibiotic is bactericidal and gives over-all better results in seriously ill patients, especially those at the extremes of life. Benzylpenicillin is the drug of choice in the treatment of syphilis, yaws and gonococcal infections, although the gonococcus is not so sensitive to its action as the meningococcus and in recent years much larger doses have proved necessary to produce successful results in comparison to the doses originally required.

Benzylpenicillin should also be used to prevent bacteraemia following dental extraction or tonsillectomy in subjects suffering from valvular heart disease (p. 109). If bacterial endocarditis has developed and the organism responsible is sensitive to benzylpenicillin, it may be given alone in large doses or in combination with streptomycin (p. 109).

The prophylactic use of benzylpenicillin is also defensible when there is a risk of tetanus or gas gangrene. Severely traumatized patients with much damage to their muscles, especially troops wounded in the field, should be given large intramuscular doses of benzylpenicillin, since this form of treatment has been shown greatly to reduce the incidence of tetanus and gas gangrene. Penicillin prophylaxis is, however, usually undesirable and may be positively dangerous in the unconscious patient, since this inevitably alters the flora of the bronchi which could be colonized from the surrounding environment by resistant pathogens commonly found in hospitals. Finally, to give benzylpenicillin to a febrile patient when the diagnosis has not been firmly established is an act of panic which, for similar reasons, may be dangerous to the patient, especially in hospital.

Toxicity, side-effects and contraindications. Benzylpenicillin has a remarkably low toxicity except when given in large doses by the intrathecal route as this may produce a meningo-encephalopathy. The most important side-effect is the production of urticarial skin rashes in hypersensitive subjects. This is especially true of topical applications but may occur when the drug has been administered by any route. The incidence of such reactions in the United States has been put as high as 4 per cent. of the population. This seems high by British standards, but there is no doubt that severe and sometimes fatal anaphylactoid reactions to penicillin do occur. If a patient collapses following the injection of benzylpenicillin, the prompt administration of hydrocortisone hemisuccinate in a dose of 100 mg. intravenously will usually prevent death and, if this substance is not immediately available, adrenaline hydrochloride, 0·5 ml. of 1 in 1,000 solution, should be given intramuscularly as an alternative. Penicillinase is now commercially available and has been used for the treatment of sensitization reactions with some success. Being a protein, penicillinase may itself provoke antigenicity if a patient has previously received it. He should be skin tested for sensitivity before the drug is given.

Benzylpenicillin and, indeed, all penicillins should not be administered when there is a clear-cut history of previous reactions to penicillin, however mild. They should be given only in a small initial dose to patients with a history of allergy to other chemical substances or drugs. One potential allergen is common to all the penicillins—the so-called nucleus, 6-amino-penicillanic acid. Cross allergenicity is, therefore, possible between the penicillins. It is still not known whether a patient who has developed sensitization to 6-amino-penicillanic acid remains sensitive to it for the rest of his life. What is now known, however, is that there is a wide variation in the incidence of allergic skin rashes to the different forms of penicillin now available. It is possible, therefore, that allergens other than the penicillin nucleus can cause such clinical reactions as skin rashes. Further, the underlying disease process may affect the frequency of such reactions. This is especially true for ampicillin which will be discussed later.

THE SYNTHETIC PENICILLINS

The most important practical disadvantage of benzylpenicillin is the fact that it must be given by intramuscular injection at frequent intervals, and for many years efforts were made to produce preparations which could be given by mouth. These must be unaffected by the acid of the gastric juice and must reach the upper intestine in a form capable of satisfactory absorption, thus resulting in effective concentrations in the blood and tissues. The first form of penicillin to satisfy these requirements was phenoxymethylpenicillin, or penicillin V, and this

has remained a popular form of oral penicillin in general practice, especially for the treatment of infants and young children. In 1959 Batchelor and his co-workers were able to synthesize the penicillin nucleus—6-amino-penicillanic acid—and since then many new chemical penicillins have been derived from the nucleus. It is understandable that these synthetic penicillins are expensive, and when they are prescribed the question of cost will have to be carefully considered. Preparations for oral administration should be given about half an hour before a meal.

Table 1 summarizes the important differences between the penicillins of proven therapeutic usefulness at the present time.

Phenoxymethylpenicillin

500,000 u = 300 mgm.

The potassium salt of phenoxymethylpenicillin is given orally as a tablet in a dose of 125 mg. or 250 mg., depending upon the severity of the infection. The tablets are taken six-hourly. Effective blood levels are obtained and the rate of excretion by the kidneys is somewhat less than that for benzylpenicillin. The antibiotic activity of this penicillin given orally is slightly less than that of benzylpenicillin given intramuscularly and it is not resistant

TABLE 1
Comparison of Actions and Cost of the different Penicillins

	Antibacterial Activity (Streptococci)	Antibacterial Activity		Absorption from Jejunum	Stability to Penicillinase	Rate of Excretion	Cost
		Gram +ve	Gram −ve				
Benzylpenicillin . .	++++++	++++	+	Poor	−	Very rapid	Very low
Phenoxymethylpenicillin .	++++	+++	−	+	±	Rapid	Low
Phenethicillin . . .	+++	+++	−	++	±	Slower	Moderate
Propicillin . . .	+++	+++	−	+++	±	Slower	Moderate
Phenbenicillin . . .	+++	+++	−	++++	±	Slower	Moderate
Penamecillin . .	+++	+++	−	+++	±	Slower	Low
Ampicillin . . .	+++	+++	+++	+++	−	Moderate	Moderate
Cloxacillin . . .	+++	+++	−	+++	+++	Rapid	High
Methicillin . . .	++	+++	−	−	++++	Very rapid	Very high
Carbenicillin . . .	+	+	++	−	+++	Very rapid	Very high

to the action of penicillinase. Flavoured suspensions, suitable for administration to young children and infants are available, each 5 ml. containing 62·5 or 125 mg. Treatment should extend over a period of seven to ten days. Such diseases as pneumococcal or streptococcal infections of the respiratory tract and also of the middle ear are common in young patients, for whom this form of penicillin will have a wide application in general practice. It can also be recommended for the prevention of recurrent attacks of rheumatic fever or acute glomerulonephritis in children who give a past history of those disorders and are susceptible to streptococcal infections of the tonsils. A dose of 125 mg. daily will be effective for this purpose.

Overgrowth of *Monilia albicans* in the oro-pharynx and ano-vulvar regions may sometimes occur when an oral penicillin has been given. The appearance of a red 'beefy' tongue with thrush-like flecks on the mucosa is usually obvious, while the development of pruritus ani or pruritus vulvae indicates monilial overgrowth in these areas. Allergic reactions can also occur to any oral penicillin.

Phenethicillin, Propicillin and Phenbenicillin

These are all orally active derivatives of 6-amino-penicillanic acid with similar ranges of activity to that of benzylpenicillin. Reference to Table 1 summarizes their absorption and activity. There is no real therapeutic advantage in using these drugs in preference to phenoxymethylpenicillin, and they are more expensive.

Methicillin and Cloxacillins

These synthetic penicillins are important because they are unaffected by staphylococcal penicillinase, and cloxacillin has the further advantage that it is resistant to acid and can be given by mouth. Methicillin, when tested *in vitro*, is slightly more active, weight for weight, than cloxacillin. For severe staphylococcal infections acquired in hospital, either drug may be given and it is preferable in the initial stages of treatment to give the antibiotic by the intramuscular route. For methicillin the dose is 1 g. four-hourly and for cloxacillin 500 mg. four- or six-hourly. Cloxacillin will probably supersede methicillin and has already done so where treatment can be given by mouth to patients who are less severely ill. Recently the preparation flucloxacillin has been introduced; it is claimed that it is more readily absorbed than cloxacillin.

For adults the usual dose is 250 mg. six-hourly by mouth. Flucloxacillin can also be given by injection.

These penicillins are much less active than benzylpenicillin and should be reserved *exclusively* for the treatment of *serious* systemic infections caused by penicillinase-producing *Staphylococcus aureus* species. These are usually hospital acquired. Some strains of staphyloccocci have already been shown to be methicillin and/or cloxacillin-resistant, but it is very doubtful whether such strains have ever caused a serious infection in hospital practice. These penicillins, therefore, remain the antibiotics of first choice for the treatment of systemic staphylococcal infections acquired in hospital, and it is a wise policy to treat the patients in strict isolation.

Ampicillin

This is a very interesting synthetic oral penicillin because it is the first to show activity against certain gram-negative bacteria. It is described with the other anti-gram-negative antibiotics (p. 15).

THE ERYTHROMYCIN GROUP
(THE MACROLIDES)

Erythromycin, the first of the macrolide antibiotics, was isolated in 1952 and since then oleandomycin and spiramycin have been produced. These two antibiotics are weaker in activity and show cross-resistance with the erythromycins. Their use is not recommended.

Erythromycin

Several different forms of erythromycin are now available. These include erythromycin base, erythromycin stearate, erythromycin ethylcarbonate and erythromycin estolate, all of which are given orally, and for parenteral administration the lactobionate is used. Their range of activity is very similar to that of benzylpenicillin and they are mainly active against gram-positive bacteria. Their mode of action is bacteriostatic, although occasionally bactericidal action may be achieved with the estolate.

Pharmacology. The oral preparations are readily absorbed from the upper intestinal tract although there are definite differences in the rates of absorption and variations in the serum levels obtained, depending on which preparation is given. The estolate has the advantage over the base or stearate that it gives higher and more predictable blood levels with increased bacteriostatic or even bactericidal activity; in addition, these desirable results can be produced by a lower dose, thus reducing the incidence of side-effects. Peak serum concentrations are found between two and six hours after the administration of the estolate. There is a marked diminution in the antibacterial activity of the serum six hours after an oral dose. Tissue levels can be related to serum levels. Thus, concentration in ascitic fluid is 50 per cent. of that found in the serum. The antibiotic also enters pleural effusions or empyemata but does not pass across the blood–brain barrier in effective concentrations. Concentration in the liver and in bile is high. About 20 per cent. of the administered dose appears in the urine, in which the antibiotic is usually concentrated many times. Detectable amounts of erythromycin are also excreted in the faeces. The only advantage that erythromycin lactobionate has over the estolate is that it can be given by the intramuscular or intravenous routes.

Administration and dosage. The various preparations of erythromycin are made up in tablet or capsule form for adults and in suspensions for children. For adults the estolate is preferable for oral use in a dose of 250 mg. six-hourly or 500 mg. 12-hourly for most infections. For fulminating infections, 500 mg. six-hourly can be given. For infants and children the usual oral dose is 4 to 11 mg. per kg. six-hourly.

The normal single intravenous dose of the lactobionate for adults is 300 mg., but larger doses can be used for fulminating infections, a total of 2 g. being given by continuous intravenous drip over a 24-hour period. For intramuscular injection the dose can be calculated as 2 to 5 mg. per kg. three times daily.

Indications. For many years erythromycin was held in reserve exclusively for the treatment of penicillin-resistant infections with *Staphylococcus aureus* and its widespread use was discouraged. This wise precaution was taken because resistance to erythromycin is rapidly acquired by staphylococci. Nevertheless, the development of more powerful antistaphylococcal antibiotics (e.g. cloxacillin, fucidin, cephaloridine and lincomycin) has led to some relaxation of the restrictions imposed upon the use of erythromycin. It has the great merit of remarkably low toxicity and is very well tolerated by children. For the treatment of common gram-positive coccal infections in patients known to be allergic to penicillin it should be preferred. Further, some strains of *Staphylococcus*

aureus in general practice will be resistant to benzylpenicillin, in which case erythromycin will be the antibiotic of first choice. Again, provided the patient can be nursed in conditions of strict isolation, even adults with staphylococcal disease acquired in hospital can be treated safely with erythromycin. Some strains of *Staphylococcus aureus* are capable of existing in an erythromycin-resistant form and the establishment and spread of such strains in a hospital is encouraged by the widespread use of this antibiotic. Full measures to combat cross-infection, including careful bacteriological surveys in hospital, should prevent this. Under these conditions erythromycin is an extremely safe and effective antistaphylococcal antibiotic. In general practice the risk of dissemination of erythromycin-resistant organisms is not nearly so great, and if the use of benzylpenicillin is contraindicated for one reason or another erythromycin should be chosen as the first alternative antibiotic where gram-positive coccal infection is diagnosed. Because of the necessity for frequent intramuscular injections, methicillin is unsuitable for use in general practice. Cloxacillin is a better alternative but it is, of course, contraindicated in the patient with a history of penicillin sensitization and is more expensive than erythromycin. The development of cloxacillin-resistance is a theoretical possibility which might militate against its use as the drug of first choice in mild or moderate gram-positive coccal infections. It is probably best reserved for the oral treatment of *severe* infections.

The use of erythromycin in combination with other antibiotics has been suggested in an attempt to delay or prevent the emergence of resistant strains. The evidence in favour of this procedure is slight and will be discussed later (p. 21). Cross-resistance with other members of the macrolide group is complete.

Toxicity, side-effects and contraindications. Toxicity is not a serious problem with any erythromycin preparation, but jaundice has been reported when the estolate has been given for periods of more than 14 days. Since most infections will respond to shorter courses this potential risk is minimal and should not preclude its use. Heartburn, nausea and looseness of the bowels are more often produced with the base or stearate than with the estolate and are probably due to direct chemical irritation of the gut. They very rarely necessitate stopping the treatment. Sensitization phenomena are extremely uncommon, but can develop if erythromycin is used topically, and this method of administration must, therefore, be avoided

Lincomycin Hydrochloride

Lincomycin was isolated from *Streptomyces lincolnesis* in 1955 but did not reach the stage of clinical evaluation until 1962. The hydrochloride is used therapeutically, being very soluble in water, methanol and ethanol. The antibiotic has comparable activity *in vitro* against the same range of gram-positive organisms as erythromycin. Its action is bacteriostatic, but bactericidal activity can sometimes be achieved when the drug is given by the intravenous route.

Pharmacology. As it is acid-stable, the drug can be given by mouth and absorption from the upper intestine is satisfactory. Peak serum levels are reached after four hours. It can be given parenterally, and peak levels are then achieved very rapidly. Renal excretion is rather slow and irregular. About one-third of the antibiotic can be recovered from the stool. An important route of excretion is in the bile. Concentration of the antibiotic in most body tissues is adequate. Penetration into the cerebrospinal fluid is usually poor unless large doses are given intravenously. An interesting property of this antibiotic is that, *in vivo*, it readily penetrates into bone, either healthy or diseased. This penetration is not permanent and the drug cannot be found in bone samples 48 hours after an administered dose.

Administration and dosage. Lincomycin is given orally in capsules containing 500 mg. of the hydrochloride. By this route the usual dose is 500 mg. six-hourly, which can be given for indefinite periods, depending upon the type of infection under treatment. For parenteral administration lincomycin is available in ampoules of the hydrochloride containing 600 mg. in 2 ml. The intramuscular dose is 600 mg. eight-hourly and the intravenous dose is 600 mg. in 250 ml. of saline given over a period of 15 minutes. For children the oral dose is 4 to 11 mg. per kg. six-hourly and the parenteral dose 2 to 5 mg. per kg. eight-hourly.

Indications. Lincomycin has no chemical similarity to the erythromycins, but it has already been suggested that dissociated cross-resistance between erythromycin and lincomycin can arise in relation to certain strains of *Staphylococcus aureus*. This *in vitro* finding has yet to be confirmed *in vivo*. From a therapeutic point of view, therefore, lincomycin should not be considered as merely

another erythromycin-like substance with the same indications and contraindications. Because of its ability to penetrate into bone, lincomycin has proved to be a very useful drug in the treatment of acute or chronic suppurative bone and joint disease caused by penicillin-resistant strains of *Staphylococcus aureus*. In these circumstances it has the advantage that it can be given by mouth for prolonged periods, with no evidence of toxicity. It is also relatively inexpensive. Many patients suffering from chronic suppurative osteomyelitis, who have failed to respond to all previous forms of antistaphylococcal therapy, have been successfully treated with lincomycin. For the acute case, 500 mg. six-hourly by mouth for 6 to 12 weeks is recommended; and for the chronic case, initially 500 mg. six-hourly for four to six weeks and thereafter 500 mg. eight-hourly for periods ranging up to one year, depending upon the severity and chronicity of the disease. A further possible indication for the use of lincomycin is in the management of pneumococcal meningitis when penicillin is contraindicated or has failed to affect the course of the disease. Here the drug should be given intravenously in high doses to ensure an adequate concentration in the cerebrospinal fluid. Lincomycin is also useful in the management of gram-positive septicaemias, especially those due to staphylococci, pneumococci and haemolytic streptococci, and it has also proved to be effective in the treatment of bacteroides septicaemia. Recent work has shown that this antibiotic penetrates well into the aqueous humour of the eye and has had a good effect in the management of certain gram-positive infections affecting its anterior chamber.

Toxicity, side-effects and contraindications. No serious toxic properties have been reported. When given by mouth some looseness of the bowels occurs in a few patients. This is probably a direct effect of lincomycin on the gut and disappears upon withdrawal of the drug—or even if therapy is continued in some patients. Sensitization skin rashes rarely arise following its use. Acquired resistance to lincomycin by strains of *Staphylococcus aureus* has not yet assumed clinical importance. Naturally-resistant strains have been isolated *in vitro* in a few instances, but in the laboratory induced resistance is slow to develop.

Clindamycin

This is a semi-synthetic modification of lincomycin produced by the chemical substitution of a chloro-moiety for the hydroxyl group in the 7 position. Absorption after oral administration is almost complete even if food is taken at the same time. The range of activity of this antibiotic is similar to that of lincomycin hydrochloride and the indications for its use are the same. The drug is available as clindamycin in 150 mg. capsules. In most infections 150 mg. to 300 mg. every six hours is recommended, the higher dose being indicated if the infection is severe. For children, 8 to 16 mg. per kg. per day—divided into three or four equal doses—is suggested.

Toxicity and side-effects. Raised serum transaminase levels have occasionally been seen during treatment, but serious liver or bone marrow damage has not been reported. Skin rashes have been attributed to clindamycin but they are uncommon. In a small number of patients mild gastro-intestinal side-effects have been attributed to clindamycin. This antibiotic should not be confused with Clinimycin which is the proprietary name for an oxytetracycline preparation.

THE TETRACYCLINES

This group comprises tetracycline, oxytetracycline, chlortetracycline, demethylchlortetracycline (DMCT) and the more recently developed methacycline, lymecycline, chlormethylencycline and tetracycline-phosphate complex. From the point of view of antibacterial activity they are virtually identical, being bacteriostatic against both gram-positive and gram-negative organisms, certain rickettsiae and *Entamoeba histolytica*. These preparations differ considerably in cost. Absolute cross-resistance exists within this group; if a micro-organism is resistant to one it can be assumed to be resistant to all eight analogues.

Pharmacology. The tetracyclines are usually given by mouth. Absorption from the upper intestine is variable and depends partly on the preparation used. After absorption it is transported to the liver where a proportion of the ingested dose will be inactivated by protein-binding and metabolic breakdown. Thereafter active tetracycline is absorbed into the systemic circulation, giving effective blood levels for up to six hours with the three original analogues. Good absorption from the jejunum and the slower renal excretion of DMCT gives more prolonged antibacterial concentrations for up to 12 hours. Tetracyclines are also concentrated and excreted in the bile. They diffuse well into most body tissues, but transmission across the blood–brain barrier is poor and only very small quantities enter the cerebrospinal fluid. Active tetracycline is excreted by the kidneys in appreciable amounts.

Tetracycline may be administered either intravenously or intramuscularly but the hydrochloride is not very soluble and may be irritant to muscle. A new derivative rolitetracycline, which is N-(pyrrolidinomethyl) tetracycline, is two thousand times more soluble in water than tetracycline itself, is much less irritant to tissues and is, therefore, the most satisfactory preparation for parenteral administration.

Administration and dosage. *Tetracycline, oxytetracycline and chlortetracycline* are usually made up in capsules or tablets containing 250 mg. of antibiotic. For the oral treatment of moderately severe infections a dose of 250 mg. six-hourly is indicated. For fulminating infections, 500 mg. six-hourly should be given. The duration of treatment varies with the infection, but in most cases should not be more than 14 days. For children, various suitably flavoured suspensions are available and the dose is calculated on the basis of 30 mg. per kg. of body weight per day.

DMCT differs slightly from the other tetracyclines, having the advantage of lower dosage and less frequent administration. It is made up in capsules, each containing 150 mg. of antibiotic. The usual dose is 300 mg. twice daily.

Methacycline is more rapidly excreted than DMCT; this applies to both oral and intravenous administration. The degree of protein-binding is similar for the two drugs. In order to avoid gastro-intestinal side-effects, the oral dose should not exceed 150 mg. six-hourly. With oral doses of 300 mg. four times daily, *lymecycline* produces higher blood levels than any other tetracycline and these are achieved more rapidly. The results of controlled clinical trials show that lymecycline is absorbed more rapidly from the intestine than tetracycline, but there is no significant difference in their therapeutic value.

Chlormethylencycline is also well absorbed and gives good blood levels, somewhat higher than those obtained following the administration of chlortetracycline itself.

Rolitetracycline. For parenteral administration by the intramuscular or intravenous routes, rolitetracycline is available. It should be injected slowly over a period of one to three minutes in a dose equivalent to 250 mg. of tetracycline hydrochloride.

This avoids pain at the site of injection and the possibility of flushings which occur if the antibiotic is injected too rapidly. Effective blood levels are maintained for 12 hours and injections should, therefore, be given at 12-hourly intervals.

The only advantage that can as yet be claimed for the newer tetracyclines is that they are less apt to cause gastro-intestinal upset, and this is probably because they are effective in relatively small doses.

Topical preparations are available for the treatment of tetracycline-sensitive superficial dermatological lesions, conjunctival infections, infected burns and some forms of infective otitis.

Indications. Because certain micro-organisms readily develop resistance to the tetracyclines, especially when they have been widely used in hospital practice, a considerable percentage of resistant strains are encountered in such environments. The use of the tetracyclines in hospitals and in general practice will, therefore, be considered separately.

During the past few years there has been an increasing appreciation that the widespread use of a tetracycline in hospitals has led to the development of a resident tetracycline-resistant population of micro-organisms, notably strains of *Staphylococcus aureus* and gram-negative species. Cross-infection with these organisms has been common, creating serious morbidity and mortality, and some authorities have advocated that the tetracyclines be withdrawn altogether from hospital practice until such times as these resident organisms have been eradicated. These antibiotics, having a so-called wide-spectrum activity, will inevitably create in the patient's own body a large bacterial 'vacuum' which will be filled from his surrounding environment by potentially resistant pathogens which may cause very serious disease. The tetracyclines should be used in hospital only under certain well-defined conditions, namely: when an infection is susceptible *only* to tetracycline therapy; when a patient can be nursed under conditions of strict isolation so as to reduce the risk of cross-infection; and when accurate bacteriological data are available from day to day, indicating the patient's progress while under treatment. If these conditions are accepted, the indications for the use of a tetracycline in hospital at the present time will be very few.

Conditions outside hospital are fortunately entirely different and here the indications for the use of a tetracycline are numerous. They are active against most gram-positive and some gram-negative organisms, and in North America and tropical countries they are of great value in the treatment of rickettsial diseases and amoebiasis. In Britain, important infections caused by *Haemophilus influenzae* and *Streptococcus pneumoniae* frequently cause acute exacerbations of chronic bronchitis. There is much evidence in favour of treating such exacerbations with a tetracycline, and some authorities have advocated the continuous administration of a tetracycline throughout the winter months to patients with moderately severe or advanced chronic bronchitis. This is expensive as the dose of tetracycline should be 1 g. daily for up to six months. If DMCT is employed, 300 mg. twice daily may be used for a similar period. If, however, the total cost of treatment is compared with the cost of recurrent invalidism with consequent loss of work, it is relatively cheap. As chronic bronchitis is one of the most common diseases in the United Kingdom, the tetracyclines have a wide application either as short-term treatment for acute exacerbations when they arise, or for continuous treatment in the patient with a permanently purulent sputum. Nevertheless, the frequent administration of a tetracycline or its continuous administration to bronchitic patients has led to the finding of tetracycline-resistant *H. influenzae* strains in sputum cultures. In such patients ampicillin would be the alternative therapy. A tetracycline given to a patient with whooping-cough may shorten the course of the disease provided the antibiotic is given in the early stages. Although the tetracyclines are active against some gram-negative bacteria, especially *Escherichia coli*, they should not be regarded as the drugs of first choice for treating *E. coli* infections of the urinary tract since they are only bacteriostatic and hence resistance often develops. The tetracyclines are the most effective form of treatment for brucellosis. This infection often relapses and it is, therefore, advisable to give full doses for at least 14 days. Topical preparations are effective if a surface infection is caused by a tetracycline-sensitive organism. Chlortetracycline ointment is widely used, for example, in the treatment of streptococcal impetigo or sycosis barbae.

Toxicity, side-effects and contraindications. The tetracyclines as a group possess remarkably few truly toxic properties. Allergy, neurotoxicity and marrow dyscrasias are very rarely encountered after their use. Recently, however, some alarm has been created by reports that the tetracyclines are deposited in bones and in teeth which are actively growing. Because of this there has been a natural concern that these drugs may be teratogenic. So far, however, there is no evidence that they can cause malformations in human subjects. Nevertheless, it is prudent to avoid their administration to pregnant women—especially during the active period of bone formation in the foetus—and in the growing child.

On the other hand, side-effects during tetracycline treatment are common. The main danger is the overgrowth of potential pathogens in the gastro-intestinal, respiratory and genito-urinary tracts. *Candida albicans* is common to all patients, while the *Staphylococcus aureus* is largely confined to patients in hospital. Overgrowth of *C. albicans* is usually mild, causing glossitis, stomatitis, black hairy tongue and pruritus ani or pruritus vulvae. This form of the oro-genital syndrome is not due to the impairment of vitamin B production in the intestine because of depression of the coliform organisms by the antibiotic, and there is, therefore, no need to administer tablets of vitamin B complex with the tetracyclines. More serious invasion of the mucous membranes of the alimentary, respiratory and genito-urinary tracts, progressing to fatal septicaemia with *C. albicans*, is fortunately rare. Staphylococcal pneumonia with the development of multiple lung abscesses and septicaemia has occurred in hospitals and especially in surgical wards where tetracyclines have been given to combat gram-negative infection of the peritoneum. For the reasons already stated it is to be hoped that this practice will cease. Staphylococcal entero-colitis is a fulminating cholera-like illness and may arise under similar conditions.

The passage of soft, bulky, odourless stools not infrequently occurs during the early stages of treatment with the tetracyclines. Alteration in the colonic flora has been suggested as the cause, but this is not the full explanation and tetracycline diarrhoea is more probably due to a direct chemical action on the wall of the gut. This side-effect is common to all the tetracyclines. To avoid serious side-effects, there must be attention to oral and ano-genital hygiene during treatment. Obviously, it is far better for a patient to have tetracycline treatment in his own home than in a hospital where there is the ever-present menace of infection with tetracycline-resistant organisms. In countries where sunlight is prolonged, phototoxicity can arise in patients taking DMCT, but this is exceptional in Western Europe.

The intravenous administration of large doses of tetracycline, especially in pregnancy, is absolutely contraindicated as fatal or very serious hepatic damage has been reported in these circumstances. The pathological finding is acute, diffuse necrosis, but the exact mechanism of its production is not fully understood. It has been stated that tetracycline degradation products may have deleterious effects. For instance it has been said that they may cause renal tubular damage and give rise to features of the Fanconi syndrome (p. 286). No such reports have been made from the United Kingdom, and it has been suggested that tetracycline degradation does not occur in this area because of the absence of acidic excipients in the capsules manufactured in the British Isles.

CHLORAMPHENICOL

This was the first of the wide-spectrum antibiotics to be discovered and for a few years after its production it was extensively used. Its clinical usefulness has now been much curtailed because chloramphenicol can cause serious and even fatal bone marrow depression and pancytopenia (p. 159). Indeed, some advise that its use should be entirely discontinued, but this is an extreme view.

Pharmacology. This antibiotic has been chemically identified and is now prepared synthetically. Given orally it is well absorbed, and in the liver a significant proportion is metabolized to glucuronic acid and a further amount becomes protein-bound. Active blood levels will be present for up to six hours. Chloramphenicol reaches high concentrations in the tissues and body fluids because of ready diffusibility, the highest concentrations being found in the kidney and liver, and it has the additional advantage of good penetration into the cerebrospinal fluid. Only a small amount is excreted by the kidneys, about 15 per cent. of the oral dose being present in the urine in an active state.

Administration and dosage. Chloramphenicol is usually given by mouth in capsules containing 250 mg. The usual adult dose is 250 mg. six-hourly, but in severe infections 500 mg. six-hourly may be required. For children a suspension of the palmitate ester is available to mask its bitter taste. Each 5 ml. contains the equivalent of 125 mg. chloramphenicol. To reduce the risk of toxicity to a minimum, chloramphenicol should never be given for long nor in repeated courses to the same patient. For most infections in this country five to seven days should suffice. Ready diffusibility makes it useful as a topical preparation in ophthalmic practice for the treatment of conjunctival and other anterior ocular infections. Ointments containing it are also available. For intravenous or intramuscular administration chloramphenicol succinate is used, the dose being 250 mg. to 1 g. eight-hourly.

Indications. Chloramphenicol has a similar range of activity to the tetracyclines, but its use may be justified only if its greater diffusibility into the tissues is likely to give an improved clinical response. This is particularly true in the treatment of infections caused by *Salmonella typhi* and *Salmonella paratyphi* for which it is highly effective and has markedly reduced the morbidity and mortality from these serious infections. In fulminating enteric fever, chloramphenicol remains the antibiotic of first choice. Ampicillin is a useful alternative in the milder cases or in paratyphoid fever and it has been shown to be more effective in the eradication of the 'carrier' state. In the enteric fevers, chloramphenicol should be given in full doses for 14 days. Apart from this indication, there is controversy as to whether it should ever be used. *H. influenzae* meningitis in young children is a serious infection, and chloramphenicol gives very good results because of its excellent diffusion into the cerebrospinal fluid. A short course of treatment for five to seven days should overcome this form of meningitis without sequelae and the risk of aplasia of the bone marrow is outweighed by the danger of the disease. Chloramphenicol may be employed for the treatment of a severe exacerbation of chronic bronchitis caused by *H. influenzae* and *Str. pneumoniae* and is probably superior to the tetracyclines, but it has the great disadvantage that repeated short courses cannot be recommended. If it is restricted to the treatment of one particularly severe episode which has not responded to less toxic forms of antibiotic treatment, its use may be justified. Chloramphenicol is not a good antistaphylococcal antibiotic and should never be employed for the treatment of hospital-acquired infections caused by this organism.

Toxicity, side-effects and contraindications. Chloramphenicol causes side-effects similar to the tetracyclines, but these are not so common. Allergic skin reactions, urticarial in type, can occur and the Jarisch–Herxheimer reaction has been encountered in patients with syphilis, brucellosis and typhoid fever. Blood dyscrasias, ranging from leucopenia to severe thrombocytopenic purpura

and pancytopenia have been the most notable toxic effects attributed to chloramphenicol. The number of affected patients has been estimated at between one in 10,000 and one in 100,000. The administration of chloramphenicol to neonates, especially in high doses, is also contraindicated because the infant liver cannot metabolize the drug and this leads to the so-called 'grey syndrome'. If the drug is to be used at all, the total dose should be limited to 10 g. in adults, except in the treatment of typhoid fever. Repeated courses should be avoided. Despite the obvious dangers of chloramphenicol therapy, the antibiotic continues to be widely prescribed in this country. Casual use is reprehensible, and except for the treatment of the diseases mentioned above, chloramphenicol is not recommended.

NOVOBIOCIN

This was discovered in 1955. Its range of antibacterial activity is similar to that of benzylpenicillin or erythromycin, but novobiocin is not inhibited by penicillinase, and was primarily intended as an antistaphylococcal antibiotic. Given by mouth, absorption from the intestine gives maximum serum levels in two to three hours which remain high up to 12 hours; thus 12-hourly doses of 500 mg. are indicated. Novobiocin has the serious disadvantage that it is only bacteriostatic and not bactericidal in staphylococcal disease. Its efficacy is still further reduced because a large amount of the drug becomes bound to the plasma proteins. Toxicity is a further disadvantage since the drug can cause urticaria, gastro-intestinal upsets, agranulocytosis and serious thrombocytopenia. The development of resistance to it by *Staphylococcus aureus* species is rapid. The disadvantages of novobiocin are so obvious that it is doubtful if it has any place in the treatment of infections whether it is given alone or in combination with other antibiotics.

FUCIDIN

The recently developed crystalline sodium salt of fusidic acid—fucidin—has been found to be highly active against gram-positive micro-organisms, especially the *Staphylococcus aureus*. Fucidin is well absorbed after oral administration and tends to accumulate in the blood after repeated doses. It is excreted in the faeces but not in the urine. Cross-resistance with other antibiotics has not been demonstrated. Fucidin is an antistaphylococcal antibiotic which is bactericidal. Serious toxic effects have not been reported, but mild gastro-intestinal upsets—nausea, heartburn and diarrhoea—may occur. Promising reports of its effectiveness in the treatment of serious staphylococcal infections caused by penicillin-resistant strains have appeared. The use of fucidin may also be considered for a patient with severe staphylococcal infection who is hypersensitive to penicillins. As it is excreted by the liver it should be used with caution in severe hepatic disease. The antibiotic is also useful in the treatment of staphylococcal infections of the eye as it passes the blood-aqueous barrier in thera-peutic concentrations; and penetration of the drug is enhanced in the presence of inflammation. Fuci-din is available in capsules of 250 mg. and for adults the dose is 500 mg. three times daily, given with meals or, preferably, immediately before a meal. Treatment is continued until the infection is overcome and the course will vary from a week to three weeks according to severity.

Fucidin is now available for intravenous in-fusion. It is supplied in packs of two ampoules: one contains 580 mg. of diethanolamine fusidate B.P.C. (equivalent to 500 mg. sodium fusidate B.P.); in the other there is 50 ml. of sterile phos-phate/citrate buffer. The dry powder is dissolved in the buffer, which is then diluted to 250 to 500 ml. with sodium chloride injection, B.P. The intra-venous infusion should be given slowly over a period of two to four hours, the smaller the volume the longer the infusion period. In adults the infusion will be repeated three or four times in 24 hours.

BACITRACIN

Early preparations of bacitracin contained a mix-ture of bacitracins A, B, C and F. The more modern preparations contain only bacitracin A in appreciable amounts. The bacitracins are unsuit-able for parenteral administration on account of severe nephrotoxicity. Hence they cannot be recommended for parenteral treatment; there are other antibiotics which are safer and more effective against gram-positive organisms. Topical appli-cation and oral administration are free from toxicity. It may be given by mouth in a dose of 20,000 units in 10 ml. of saline six-hourly to remove *Staphylo-coccus aureus* from the intestinal flora. In combination with other antibiotics such as poly-myxin B, topical preparations for spraying or irrigating wounds, burns, abscess cavities and the like are sometimes used. For these purposes an effective dose would be 25,000 units of bacitracin in

25 ml. of saline. Bacitracin has also been incor-porated in ointments for the treatment of minor staphylococcal skin disease.

ANTIBIOTICS MAINLY ACTIVE AGAINST GRAM-NEGATIVE ORGANISMS

The Amino-Hexose Group

This group comprises five antibiotics having very similar chemical characteristics and comparable antibacterial activity, but each has a distinctively different therapeutic application.

STREPTOMYCIN

Streptomycin is active against certain gram-negative bacteria, and especially against *M. tuberculosis*—its most important therapeutic indica-tion.

Pharmacology. Streptomycin is not absorbed from the intact intestine. For a systemic effect intramuscular injection is necessary after which maximum blood concentration is reached in one to two hours, falling to low values in about six hours. The antibiotic does not penetrate well into cells but is distributed in the extracellular fluids with the notable exception of the cerebrospinal fluid. The liver concentrates and excretes it in bile and a sig-nificant proportion of the injected dose is excreted in the urine as active streptomycin. Penetration into necrotic tuberculous lesions is good, but little passes into thick-walled non-tuberculous abscesses. Streptomycin can be given intrathecally in tuber-culous meningitis although this form of treatment is now less frequently required.

Administration and dosage. Streptomycin sul-phate is the usual preparation. Full details of antituberculous therapy are given elsewhere (p. 68). For the treatment of non-tuberculous infections, streptomycin is given intramuscularly in a dose of 250 mg. six-hourly. In severe infections 500 mg. may be given. Acute infections will be overcome by short courses lasting from five to ten days if they are caused by sensitive organisms.

Streptomycin may also be given orally in liquid form for the treatment of intestinal infections in a dose of 250 mg. six-hourly or as 500 mg. tablets. The solution of the sulphate is practically tasteless and needs no flavouring. The powdered antibiotic, made up in ampoules, can be diluted in the same way as for intramuscular injection. Commercial preparations containing proportions of strepto-mycin and penicillin in one ampoule are also available for combined parenteral therapy.

Indications. In spite of the early promise of streptomycin as an anti-gram-negative and anti-tuberculous antibiotic it soon became apparent that bacterial resistance to it developed very rapidly. Streptomycin is an effective drug for the treatment of certain gram-negative urinary tract infections, but many of the common causative pathogens have now become resistant to it. Further this antibiotic is only effective when the urine is kept alkaline, and this may be difficult to achieve in general practice. For these reasons streptomycin should no longer be considered as the antibiotic of first choice for urinary tract infections. Bacterial endocarditis caused by certain strains of *Streptococcus viridans* will sometimes respond to a combination of penicillin and streptomycin when this is indicated (p. 109). Despite its undoubted activity against *H. influenzae*, more modern antibiotics have supplanted it owing to the rapidity with which bacterial resistance is acquired and because of its poor penetration across the blood–brain barrier.

Streptomycin by mouth, 250 mg. six-hourly for five days, has a wide therapeutic application in the treatment of infections of the bowel with organisms of the dysentery group and with certain pathogenic types of *E. coli*. A similar course of streptomycin combined with oral sulphonamides is standard therapy in the treatment of plague.

Toxicity, side-effects and contraindications. These are fully discussed in the section on the treatment of tuberculosis (p. 68).

In summary, streptomycin, given parenterally, should be reserved for the treatment of tuberculous disease in combination with isoniazid and PAS, and it is also indicated for the oral treatment of the bacillary dysenteries. It is absolutely contra-indicated as a topical preparation in eye-drops, ointments and sprays because of the danger of producing sensitization.

KANAMYCIN

Developed in 1957, kanamycin has certain material advantages over streptomycin in the treatment of *serious* gram-negative infections, while it has virtually the same pharmacological properties and similar toxicity.

Pharmacology. Kanamycin sulphate must be given parenterally for systemic effect because its absorption from the intestine is so poor. Peak

serum levels are achieved in about one hour after an intramuscular injection and the antibiotic cannot be detected after six hours. Appreciable quantities are excreted in the urine and its antibacterial activity is unaffected by the urinary pH.

Many micro-organisms, including *M. tuberculosis*, are affected *in vitro* by the bactericidal action of kanamycin, but because of its toxicity and because staphylococci rapidly develop resistance to it, kanamycin should be reserved exclusively for the treatment of certain gram-negative infections. *In vitro* almost all strains of *E. coli* and *Proteus* are inhibited by 8 mcg. per ml. or less of kanamycin. *In vivo* these levels can be readily achieved in the blood and are greatly exceeded in the urine by non-toxic therapeutic doses.

Administration and dosage. The standard adult dose is 250 mg. intramuscularly six-hourly. Treat-ment should be effective within 14 days for almost all infections. For children the dose should range from 12·5 to 15 mg. per kg. per day, depending upon the severity of the infection. Kanamycin may also be given intrathecally, well diluted, in a dose of 25 to 50 mg. daily. The intravenous route can be employed in fulminating infections with septicaemia and the doses are the same as for the intramuscular route. In severe peritoneal infections intramuscular treatment can be augmented by the intraperitoneal injection of 250 mg. of kanamycin in 500 ml. of saline twice daily for three days. Kanamycin can be given by mouth when it will greatly reduce the intestinal flora.

Indications. If it is appreciated that kanamycin sulphate is actively bactericidal against common gram-negative pathogens, its use should be con-sidered for the treatment of *serious* infections caused by these organisms. For example, ful-minating urinary tract infections in young women are by no means uncommon and these may be complicated by septicaemia. Sudden septicaemic illnesses with grave constitutional upset may com-plicate pyelonephritis of pregnancy or the puer-perium. Kanamycin should be the antibiotic of first choice in treating such infections in an emer-gency when accurate bacteriology is not available or until such time as it becomes so. The mortality from *Proteus* septicaemia was extremely high until the advent of kanamycin which is life-saving in this condition. It is also the first line of attack in the treatment of newly born infants with *E. coli* menin-gitis, when it should be given intrathecally as well as intramuscularly. Gram-negative infections of the peritoneum or biliary tract, with or without septi-caemia, are further indications for the use of kanamycin, and when the peritoneum is involved the intraperitoneal route should be used in addition to intramuscular therapy.

Toxicity, side-effects and contraindications. Kana-mycin is capable of producing 8th nerve damage in the same way as streptomycin. Hence the total dose of this antibiotic should never exceed 40 g. This limits its usefulness in the treatment of tuberculosis. The same precaution applies to kanamycin when it is prescribed for a patient with impaired renal function. Nephrotoxicity arises if high doses are administered or if the drug is allowed to accumulate in the blood in the presence of advanced renal disease. Rashes and blood dys-crasias are exceedingly rare with this member of the amino-hexose group. The use of this drug for so-called sterilization of the bowel or as a topical antibiotic should be actively discouraged so as to avoid the risk of creating a kanamycin-resistant population of gram-negative organisms.

NEOMYCIN

Neomycin sulphate is the most toxic member of this group to both the 8th nerve and the kidney. Hence its parenteral administration for the treat-ment of systemic infections is absolutely contra-indicated. As a topical antibiotic incorporated in eye-drops, ear-drops, ointments and aerosol sprays it has a limited value. In surgical practice neo-mycin may be combined with bacitracin and poly-myxin in sprays or fine powders for the insufflation of wounds or operation sites such as the brain.

Neomycin is available in tablet form, each con-taining 250 mg. or 500 mg., or as a liquid containing 500 mg. per 30 ml. It may be used in the treatment of bacillary dysentery, *E. coli* enteritis caused by specific sero-types, and for so-called bowel steriliza-tion in colonic surgery. For adults, a five-day course of 500 mg. six-hourly should suffice for alimentary infections and a three-day course as a pre-operative procedure. For infants and young children, the daily dose is 50 mg. per kg. body weight, given as Neomycin Mixture B.P.C. which contains about 20 mg. per ml. in divided doses. One to two teaspoonfuls for younger children and three to four teaspoonfuls for older children four times daily for up to five days is the usual course of treatment. Oral neomycin therapy is much more expensive than oral streptomycin, which should be preferred in the first instance unless streptomycin-

resistance has been demonstrated. Neomycin should not be given to patients with hepatic failure to reduce the bacterial flora of the small intestine as in these circumstances appreciable and potentially toxic amounts are absorbed from the damaged bowel.

PAROMOMYCIN

This antibiotic is also severely oto- and nephro-toxic if given parenterally and its use is almost exclusively limited to the oral treatment of bacillary dysentery. It is given in comparable doses and preparations to neomycin but at present the cost prohibits widespread use, even for a five-day course, and it should be reserved for patients in whom the infection is known to be resistant to standard forms of treatment.

GENTAMICIN

This is derived from a species of the genus *micro-monospora*. It is a broad-spectrum bactericidal antibiotic with a range of activity which includes *Escherichia coli*, *Proteus* spp., *Klebsiella aerogenes* and *Pseudomonas pyocyanea*. Some strains of *Staphylococcus aureus* are also susceptible to its action.

Absorption from the intestine is poor and the drug must be given intramuscularly or, initially, intravenously. Following an intramuscular injec-tion, absorption is rapid and the drug is excreted almost entirely in active form by glomerular filtra-tion. It is made up in 2 ml. ampoules con-taining 80 mg. of gentamicin base. Provided renal function is normal the standard adult dose is 1 ml. twice daily. If there is impairment of glomerular filtration cumulation of the drug will result and this will lead to ototoxicity and labyrinthine disturbance.

At present gentamicin sulphate is a suitable alternative therapy against serious infections with gram-negative bacilli provided that sensitivity tests have shown that the organisms are sensitive to its action and that renal function is normal. *Pseudo-monas pyocyanea* infections have been successfully treated with this drug when no other therapy has been effective because of resistance.

The Semi-synthetic Penicillins

AMPICILLIN

This acid-stable derivative of 6-amino-penicillanic acid is bactericidal not only to some gram-positive but also to some gram-negative bacteria, especially the *Proteus* spp., some strains of *E. coli*, salmonellae and *H. influenzae*. As it is usually well absorbed from the intestine, the concentration of the drug in the blood is adequate; it is higher and better sustained than the blood levels of earlier penicillins. Concentrations of ampicillin in bile and urine are very high. Nevertheless, this antibiotic is rapidly destroyed by penicillinase—an enzyme produced by most strains of *Staphylococcus aureus* in hospital and by some strains of *Aerobacter aerogenes* and *Proteus*.

The drug is given by mouth in capsules containing 250 mg. For urinary tract infections with susceptible gram-negative bacteria, the usual dose is 500 mg. six-hourly for 10 to 14 days. For the treatment of acute exacerbations of chronic bronchitis caused by *H. influenzae*, ampicillin may also be given in a dose of 500 mg. six-hourly. Although this antibiotic is highly active *in vitro* against many salmonella strains, including *S. typhi* and *S. paratyphi*, under clinical conditions substantial doses are required to produce bactericidal concentrations in the tissues. For the typhoid and paratyphoid group, an oral dose of at least 1 g. six-hourly for 14 to 28 days is recommended. For the other salmonelloses a similar regimen will be required to reduce the risk of relapse. Ampicillin is often effective in the treatment of carriers of *S. typhi* and *S. paratyphi*; the same dose regimen is recommended. To a large extent ampicillin has replaced chloramphenicol for the treatment of acute exacerbations of chronic bronchitis. It is also useful in the management of certain infections of the urinary tract, especially those caused by sensitive strains of *Escherichia coli* and *Proteus mirabilis*. Some forms of systemic salmonellosis other than the enteric fevers will also respond to ampicillin treatment. Here again, however, the dose must be high and prolonged.

Nausea, heartburn and looseness of the bowels sometimes occur with ampicillin therapy. Sensitization rashes have unfortunately arisen more frequently with this form of penicillin therapy than with others. The incidence of such rashes approaches 100 per cent. if ampicillin is given to a patient suffering from infectious mononucleosis. Indeed sensitization to ampicillin in these patients can be so severe as to lead to laryngeal oedema and obstruction, and they may require not only intramuscular hydrocortisone but even tracheostomy may be called for. It follows that in a young patient with an undiagnosed sore throat, ampicillin is absolutely contraindicated. Otherwise ampicillin is free from serious toxicity. A further disturbing development in our knowledge of this semi-synthetic penicillin is its variability of absorption after oral administration and, for serious infections, therefore, the intramuscular route is to be preferred to guarantee consistently effective blood levels.

The Cephalosporins

CEPHALORIDINE

The cephalosporins are a large and interesting group of antibiotics derived from *Cephalosporium*, a fungus first isolated from sewage outfall near Sardinia in 1945. Most of them are, as yet, of only theoretical interest. From the clinical standpoint cephalosporin C and its chemical analogues are probably the most important at present. Cephaloridine is derived from cephalosporin C, of which 7-amino-cephalosporanic acid is the nucleus. This resembles the penicillin nucleus, 6-amino-penicillanic acid, and can be manipulated synthetically in a similar manner to the penicillin nucleus. Cephaloridine is one of the synthetic analogues produced in recent years in the United Kingdom. The range of activity of this antibiotic is very wide and it is bactericidal against many common gram-positive and gram-negative pathogens. It has no activity against *M. tuberculosis*, *Pseudomonas pyocyanea*, fungi, protozoa or helminths.

Pharmacology. Cephaloridine is not absorbed from the upper intestinal tract and parenteral administration is, therefore, necessary. Following intramuscular injection, peak serum levels are reached within 30 minutes, and adequate levels can be maintained for up to eight hours. Protein-binding in the serum is insignificant and the drug is largely excreted unchanged in the urine. High concentrations are, therefore, achieved in urine and also in renal tissue. Penetration into inflamed muscular tissue is satisfactory, but only a little appears in the biliary tract or in the cerebrospinal fluid.

Administration and dosage. Cephaloridine can be given by the intramuscular and intrathecal routes. The standard intramuscular dose for severe infections is 500 mg. six-hourly. The course lasts between 5 and 14 days, depending upon the type and severity of the infection. For less severe infections the intramuscular dose can be reduced to

250 mg. six-hourly. Intravenously the drug can be given into a drip at six-hourly intervals in a dose of 250 mg. The intrathecal dose is 25 mg. in 10 ml. of saline once daily.

Indications. Although this antibiotic is highly active against such common pathogens as *Streptococcus pneumoniae, Streptococcus pyogenes, Streptococcus viridans* and *Staphylococcus aureus*—even when the last mentioned is penicillin-resistant—it is not suggested that all infections caused by these organisms should be treated at the outset with cephaloridine. The site and type of infection will determine the choice of antibiotic, and the doctor should decide whether older and equally effective methods of treatment might be employed. Certain gram-positive infections should respond well to cephaloridine treatment; a good example is the patient suffering from pneumococcal meningitis which has not responded to 48 hours of intensive benzylpenicillin therapy. Here a change to both intramuscular and intrathecal cephaloridine is highly effective. If *Streptococcus viridans* endocarditis is shown to be either relatively resistant to benzylpenicillin *in vitro* or if there is no clinical response to intensive treatment with that drug, cephaloridine should be considered as an alternative, especially when the organism is highly sensitive to its action *in vitro*. Because cephaloridine is excreted in high concentrations in the urine a staphylococcal urinary tract infection caused by a penicillin-resistant organism will respond rapidly to it. Minor gram-positive infections caused by other sensitive bacteria should not at present be treated with cephaloridine.

Cephaloridine also shows bactericidal activity *in vitro* against many strains of salmonella, *Escherichia coli, Proteus mirabilis* and some *Shigella* spp. Obviously it would not be suitable for the treatment of salmonella infections of the gut or shigella infections. The drug might be useful if there is salmonella septicaemia where the organism is shown to be highly sensitive to its action. Cephaloridine should be considered for the treatment of fulminating *Escherichia coli* or *Proteus mirabilis* pyelonephritis, especially if there is an associated septicaemia. In areas where there are no facilities for estimating blood levels of antibiotic, cephaloridine is preferable to kanamycin because of its low toxicity. In obstetric practice, cephaloridine is safe and during pregnancy should be considered for the treatment of infections sensitive to it.

Debilitated patients are particularly liable to multiple or mixed infections in hospital. Such patients may be receiving prolonged corticosteroid therapy, antimetabolites or radiotherapy, or they may be under treatment by dialysis or extensive surgical operations. Septicaemias caused by different pathogens can arise from day to day, and bacteriological diagnosis then lags behind the clinical indications for appropriate antibiotic treatment. If such patients are obviously septicaemic, cephaloridine might now be considered as the emergency antibiotic of first choice before an accurate bacteriological diagnosis is established.

Toxicity, side-effects and contraindications. Cephaloridine in the usual therapeutic doses is non-toxic, but excessive intrathecal doses may cause drowsiness and mental change. Intramuscular injection is almost painless. Erythematous skin rashes may occur; and this suggests that sensitization to the cephaloridine nucleus may develop—similar in type to that produced by the penicillin nucleus. Fortunately there is no evidence of cross-sensitization between the two antibiotics.

In summary, cephaloridine is a powerful bactericide suitable for treating severe and fulminating infections. It is of special value when such infections have failed to respond to conventional therapy or when the causative organisms are resistant to standard antibiotics.

CEPHALOTHIN

This cephalosporin C derivative is similar pharmacologically to cephaloridine and must also be given by the systemic route. Its range of activity is very similar to that of cephaloridine. It is available in ampoules equivalent to 1 g. cephalothin in 10 ml. solution. The usual dose in adults is 0·5 to 1 g. of cephalothin every four or six hours, depending on the severity of the infection. In infants and young children daily administration of 40 to 80 mg. per kg. in divided doses is effective. As for cephaloridine the drug may be given by the intramuscular or intravenous route.

Indications. This antibiotic has been widely used in the United States and more recently it has also been studied in Britain. It would appear to have the same clinical effectiveness as cephaloridine in the treatment of moderate or severe gram-negative infections. Only comparative trials between the two antibiotics will eventually determine which is the more effective preparation.

Toxicity, side-effects and contraindications.

Cephalothin may also produce skin rashes and it should not be given to patients with a strong history of allergy or to anyone who has developed a rash following treatment with cephaloridine. Claims have been made that renal tubular damage may result from treatment with either of these cephalosporins. Such damage will be minimal, however, if the doses do not exceed 6 g. per day; and there can be very few infections which require a higher dose than this.

CEPHALEXIN

Much research has been directed to producing an oral cephalosporin C derivative which would be predictably absorbed and produce effective blood and tissue levels. Cephalexin appears to satisfy these criteria. It is available in capsules, each containing either 250 mg. or 500 mg., as tablets containing 500 mg., and as a syrup. For most infections the adult dose is 250 to 500 mg. six-hourly. In severe infections the dose may be raised to 1 g. six-hourly.

Indications. This cephalosporin is active against the same range of bacteria as the intramuscular analogues, but clinical evaluation has been undertaken on a large scale only in the past few years. It is not suggested that it should be used as the antibiotic of first choice in all infections, caused by susceptible organisms. Nevertheless it will be effective in treating susceptible urinary tract infections, respiratory tract infections and in infections in patients who show penicillin allergy.

Cephalexin should not be given to patients with a known history of skin rashes following prior treatment with any other cephalosporin.

The Polypeptides

POLYMYXIN

The commercial preparations of polymyxin are polymyxin B and the sodium salt—sulphomyxin. Despite their wide range of activity against gram-negative bacteria, pain at the site of intramuscular injection and neurotoxicity—glove-and-stocking paraesthesia, vertigo, ataxia and even encephalopathy—are toxic properties which reduce their efficacy. Both can be given by the intramuscular, intravenous or intrathecal routes, but the patient must be warned to inform his attendants at the first sign of tingling in the mouth, hands or feet, when the drug should be immediately withdrawn.

COLISTIN

This antibiotic is chemically identical with polymyxin E and has the same antibacterial activity. It is available as colistin sulphomethate sodium for parenteral use and as colistin sulphate for oral use. For systemic effect colistin must be given by the intramuscular route as it is poorly absorbed from the intestine. Peak serum concentrations are reached in two hours after an intramuscular injection, receding to ineffective therapeutic levels at eight hours. Large amounts of active colistin are excreted in the urine. This antibiotic is bactericidal against *Pseudomonas pyocyanea*. Urinary tract and systemic infections by this organism have been increasing and carry a high mortality unless promptly and effectively dealt with.

The antibiotic is administered intramuscularly in a minimum dose of 1·5 million units eight-hourly until the infection is overcome. Patients weighing 140 lb. or more should be given up to 3 million units eight-hourly.

The toxic effects include digital and circumoral paraesthesia and urticarial skin rashes. The alleged differences in toxicity between colistin and polymyxin B were due to comparing different salts of the two substances. The sulphates are more toxic than the methanesulphonates and also more active therapeutically.

CYCLOSERINE

This antibiotic is particularly active against most strains of *Escherichia coli* and also *Mycobacterium tuberculosis*. Oral administration is followed by rapid absorption from the intestine. Thereafter the drug diffuses well into most body fluids and, if renal function is normal, active cycloserine is excreted in the urine in much higher concentrations than in plasma. Urinary tract infections, especially those of a refractory nature, caused by *E. coli* are very common and cycloserine has an important part to play in their management. In the treatment of tuberculosis it has a very small place (p. 72).

The antibiotic is available in capsules containing 125 mg. and 250 mg. *E. coli* urinary tract infections will often respond to an adult dose of 250 mg. twice daily for 14 days. Where advanced structural defects are present and there is a history of frequent recurrence in the past, the initial eradication of the organisms can be followed by effective suppression by the long-term administration of 250 mg. on alternate nights for periods ranging up to many years. If the patient weighs less than 60 kg. the suppressive dose can be reduced to 125 mg. on alternate nights. For very young children the dose is further reduced to 62·5 mg. on alternate nights. If the blood urea level is raised, a therapeutic concentration of the drug may not be obtained in the urine.

The toxic effects of cycloserine are alarming; they occur if blood levels are allowed to rise excessively by giving large doses or even with standard doses when renal function is impaired, or if the patient is very old. Initial drowsiness and headache may be followed by psychotic disturbances and epileptiform seizures. These effects, however, are completely reversible when the drug is withdrawn and no deaths have been reported.

NALIDIXIC ACID

Nalidixic acid is not an antibiotic, being a chemotherapeutic agent first described in 1962 as a 1-8 naphthymidine. The drug is effective *in vitro* against a wide range of gram-negative organisms including *Escherichia coli*, *Aerobacter aerogenes*, *Klebsiella pneumoniae* and *Proteus* spp., but it has no significant activity against the gram-positive organisms or *Pseudomonas pyocyanea*.

Pharmacology. The drug is well absorbed from the upper intestine after oral administration. Its fate thereafter is not yet fully known but it is highly concentrated in renal tissue and in urine.

Administration and dosage. Nalidixic acid is given by mouth in tablet form, each tablet containing 500 mg. For adults suffering from acute uncomplicated urinary tract infection, 4 g. daily in divided dose for 7 to 14 days is recommended. In a chronic refractory infection treatment can be continued for many weeks in a dose of 2 g. daily in divided doses. For children, 60 mg. per kg. in divided doses is recommended. Nalidixic acid should not be given to children under one year.

Indications. As nalidixic acid is effective against certain gram-negative organisms which commonly cause urinary tract infections, it should be considered for use if the evidence *in vitro* shows that the infecting organism is highly sensitive to its action and resistant to the standard forms of treatment. In acute uncomplicated urinary tract infections, provided the organism is sensitive, nalidixic acid is just as effective as any other form of treatment. Prolonged suppressive therapy with nalidixic acid is

theoretically possible but extensive and long-term neurotoxic effects may well arise, especially if there is impaired renal function.

Toxicity, side-effects and contraindications. Gastro-intestinal upset occurs in about 10 per cent. of patients. The usual symptoms are heartburn, nausea, occasional vomiting and diarrhoea, which may be severe enough to warrant withdrawal of the drug. Nalidixic acid causes toxic effects in the central nervous system—visual disturbances, sensory hallucinations and migrainous headaches. Skin reactions have also been attributed to the drug, possibly associated with photosensitization. No permanent ill-effects have so far been reported; all the disturbances mentioned have subsided on withdrawing treatment.

CARBENICILLIN   *PYOPEN*

This is a further semi-synthetic penicillin with activity *in vitro* against many gram-negative pathogens but most importantly against *Pseudomonas pyocyanea*. It is not absorbed from the intestine and must, therefore, be administered by the intramuscular or intravenous route. As with most penicillins, peak serum levels are reached within one hour of injection and this is followed by high urinary excretion. For this reason, to achieve effective serum levels for the treatment of systemic pseudomonas infections, a dose of 1 g. four-hourly intramuscularly is required. Some strains of *Pseudomonas pyocyanea* require high concentrations to inhibit them in the laboratory and, if this is so, to achieve equivalent serum concentrations it may be necessary to give carbenicillin intravenously as frequently as 1 g. hourly. Even with such high doses toxicity has not been shown to be a problem. Nevertheless it should not be given to patients known to be sensitive to penicillins. As it is excreted in high concentration in the urine it will often eradicate pseudomonas species from the renal tract. Pseudomonas meningitis is occasionally seen, especially in debilitated infants. Here carbenicillin can be injected intrathecally: a single daily dose is given—up to 2 years, 10 mg.; from 2 to 12 years, 20 mg.; and over 12 years, 40 mg. daily, well diluted. Laboratory guidance is of great value in assessing whether carbenicillin will be the antibiotic of choice against pseudomonas infections which are often serious and may well be fatal.

RIFAMPICIN

Derived from rifamycin B, rifampicin was found to be highly active *in vitro* against many mycobacteria. After oral administration predictable blood levels result. In treating human tuberculosis, conversion of the sputum to negative takes place within months but reconversion with rifampicin-resistant bacilli occurs. Controlled trials of this drug in the treatment of tuberculosis are continuing and it remains to be seen whether it will prove to be an effective addition to antituberculous treatment. Rifampicin is also active *in vitro* against most common urinary pathogens. Here, however, results are disappointing; even with high oral doses and high urine concentrations of the drug, sterility of the urine is not adequately maintained and urine cultures become positive while treatment is continuing. Rifampicin-resistant strains of gram-negative urinary pathogens emerge rapidly and the drug is, therefore, of little or no value in this field of therapy. Occasional reports of mild liver damage due to rifampicin have appeared, and this antibiotic should be avoided in the presence of hepatic disease.

ANTIBIOTICS ACTIVE AGAINST FUNGI

GRISEOFULVIN

The development of this antibiotic is a significant advance in the systemic treatment of superficial dermatomycoses (p. 581). Griseofulvin is well absorbed from the upper intestine and is thought to be concentrated thereafter in keratin-forming tissues so that an increasing proportion of newly formed keratin will contain this fungicide over a period of several weeks. Gradual eradication of the infection will then take place. Human ringworm infection of the finger or toe nails is eradicated when griseofulvin has been given for a period long enough for a new nail to grow. It is also successful in the treatment of tinea corporis due to *Tinea rubrum*, tinea capitis due to *M. audouini* and *T. tonsurans* and tinea cruris due to *Epidermophyton flocculosum*.

The usual daily adult dose is 500 mg. given as one 125 mg. tablet four times daily. For severe cases, up to 1 g. may be given in the first few days of treatment. One or two tablets daily should suffice for children. The minimum period of treatment is four weeks, but more prolonged courses up to six months may be necessary, depending on the nature, site and chronicity of the fungal infection.

Occasionally mild headache, diarrhoea and skin rashes occur during treatment. Griseofulvin should not be given to patients with established porphyria as it has been shown to interfere with porphyrin metabolism in experimental animals; and it must be avoided in pregnancy.

NYSTATIN

Although this antibiotic is active against a wide range of pathogenic fungi *in vitro*, it is poorly absorbed from the intestine and cannot be given parenterally because of marked toxicity. It is most useful for the local treatment of *C. albicans* infections of the mouth, ano-rectal and genital tracts. Taken in tablets containing 500,000 units three times daily for up to three weeks, it is effective and non-toxic. Diabetic and pregnant women are particularly susceptible to vulvo-vaginitis, and in these patients nystatin is especially useful. One tablet may be taken four times daily by mouth and at the same time two vaginal tablets each containing 100,000 units may be inserted daily high into the vagina.

AMPHOTERICIN B

This is an effective antibiotic in the treatment of deep systemic mycoses and is particularly useful in the treatment of coccidioidomycosis and sometimes of blastomycosis, histoplasmosis and sporotrichosis. Severe toxic effects are not infrequent and limit its usefulness. Nausea, headache, fever and nitrogen-retention may occur while severe renal damage, cardiac arrhythmias and anaphylactoid reactions have also been encountered. Amphotericin B should be given by slow intravenous injection in dilute solution, starting with 5 to 10 mg. daily and increasing by daily increments of 5 mg. to the level of tolerance. Because of toxicity it should be reserved for *serious* systemic mycoses which carry a high mortality, when it may well be life saving.

NATAMYCIN (*Pimaricin*)

Natamycin is a fungicidal antibiotic related chemically to nystatin and other heptaenes such as amphotericin. It is active against a wide range of fungi including *Aspergillus fumigatus* and *Candida albicans*. The drug is said to have no serious toxic effects after oral administration of doses up to 400 mg. daily. It is non-irritant to human mucous membranes and can be administered as an inhalation of an aerosol suspension in alkaline solution. Pulmonary aspergillosis will sometimes respond favourably to inhalations of a 2·5 per cent. suspension diluted in an alkaline medium in doses of 2·5 mg. two or three times daily.

A non-toxic antibiotic for dangerous systemic mycoses has yet to be found.

COMBINATIONS OF ANTIBIOTICS

The development of microbial resistance to a single antibiotic can be induced artificially or it may arise in the course of clinical practice. By combining an antibiotic with other antibacterial substances, as in the treatment of tuberculosis, bacterial resistance can be avoided. The theoretical advantage of using combinations of antibiotics in the treatment of other infections, in which bacterial resistance is known to develop, is an appealing one. Synergism between antibiotics can be demonstrated in the laboratory but is very difficult to prove in the treatment of human infections. Any beneficial action resulting from a combination of antibiotics is probably due to a simple additive effect, the result of widening the antibacterial spectrum. The risk of super-infection with already resistant pathogens in the patient's environment then increases, especially if he is in hospital.

Penicillin combined with streptomycin remains a common form of treatment for acute exacerbations of chronic bronchitis because of the twofold attack of these antibiotics against *S. pneumoniae* and *H. influenzae* respectively. There is no convincing evidence, however, that this combination is synergistic rather than merely additive in effect. Obvious disadvantages are the necessity for injections and the risk of ototoxicity in subjects over 50 years— the very age-group in which chronic bronchitis is common. Oral therapy with a tetracycline seems preferable, especially in general practice. The combination is of proven value in the treatment of *Streptococcus viridans* endocarditis.

Treatment with an oral sulphonamide-penicillin combination has been suggested for infections with gram-positive organisms. Clear-cut evidence of synergism is again lacking while the risk of causing sensitization phenomena with two rather than one potential allergen is increased, and the cost of treatment is higher. Sulphonamides have been prescribed with streptomycin for the systemic treatment of brucellosis, but this therapy has been superseded by the tetracyclines. Oral preparations of these two drugs are still widely advocated for the treatment of bacillary dysentery. As there is now a very high sulphonamide-resistance rate in *Shigella* species in Britain and North America there is no advantage to be gained by combining sulphonamide drugs with streptomycin.

Although the tetracyclines have no direct antituberculous action *in vitro*, they have been clearly shown to delay the emergence of resistant strains of tubercle bacilli to streptomycin, viomycin and isoniazid. For this purpose they must be given in very large doses and the indications for such combinations will arise very infrequently. A combination of tetracycline with oleandomycin in a proportion of two to one has been claimed to be synergistic and to delay the emergence of bacterial resistance to oxytetracycline. This has been disproved and the prescription of this expensive preparation should be abandoned.

Novobiocin has been advocated in combination with erythromycin in an attempt to delay the emergence of resistance in staphylococci. There is no evidence to substantiate this claim and novobiocin toxicity is a further drawback.

More recently a combination of ampicillin and cloxacillin has been advocated, especially for the treatment of neonatal mixed infections caused by penicillinase-producing *Staphylococcus aureus* and various gram-negative pathogens. It has even been suggested that this combination might be given prophylactically to neonates. Until convincing evidence is produced that this is a rational form of prophylaxis or treatment it would be better to avoid this combination.

In summary, the dangers and disadvantages of antibiotic combinations are not offset by proven advantages. In general this type of treatment should not be employed except in antituberculous therapy, *S. viridans* endocarditis, and in the topical preparations previously mentioned.

ANTIVIRAL AGENTS

Clinical interest in the discovery of new antiviral substances has been stimulated by their application to certain virus infections in man. Research in this field is in its early stages and only brief mention is made here of results which may have important clinical applications.

Methisazone

This is a thiosemicarbazone derivative which has been shown in tissue culture to affect the synthesis of proteins in the late growth-cycle of pox virus. It is noteworthy that on account of their toxicity the thiosemicarbazones were abandoned some years ago as antituberculous drugs. Methisazone is no exception to this; it causes severe nausea and vomiting. However, this drug has been given prophylactically to large numbers of patients in contact with smallpox in an attempt to prevent the development of florid disease, and the results have been encouraging. Methisazone is also valuable in preventing vaccinia gangrenosa—a serious complication of infant vaccination.

1-Adamanatadine Hydrochloride

This drug has now been marketed in the United States as a prophylactic in humans during epidemics caused by influenza viruses. The evidence so far is that in this situation it may be helpful in reducing mortality but it has no place in the therapy of individual attacks of infection caused by influenza viruses.

Idoxuridine

This substance, 5-iodo-2-deoxyridine, and chemically kindred products became incorporated in the DNA of the virus and of the cell of the host. This accounts for their potential toxicity when they are given systemically. Idoxuridine has been used *locally* in the treatment of herpes simplex infections of the eye. Early studies suggested that this was an advance in the treatment of this locally serious virus infection, but further controlled studies have failed to prove its therapeutic value.

Interferon

Interferon differs from the above substances in that its antiviral action in blocking virus multiplication takes place entirely within cells and not on extracellular virus. A single cell produces one type of interferon in response to different viruses, but different interferons will be produced against the same virus by different cell systems. These substances are of great theoretical interest, but they have not yet reached a stage of development which secures for them a place in the therapy of virus diseases.

A note of cautious optimism regarding the future of antiviral chemotherapy now seems to be warranted, but there are many problems to be solved before efficient antiviral therapy can become established. Accurate virological diagnosis of clinical disease syndromes often lags far behind the

stage of therapy. In many of the virus diseases the patient has usually recovered completely from his illness before the nature of the infection is diagnosed in the laboratory. Even when early diagnosis is possible, some doubt remains regarding the wisdom of interference with virus multiplication within living cells by means of chemical substances which are obviously toxic to the cells as well as to the virus. At present it is clear that the use of these drugs is inadvisable. Only in very serious virus diseases such as smallpox does it seem ethical to resort to potentially toxic chemotherapy on a large scale. Experience in this field, if carefully documented, may well provide invaluable guidance for the application of chemotherapy in the management of other viral infections.

GENERAL CONCLUSIONS

Many of the older and well-established antibiotics remain highly effective in the treatment of certain infections, but their widespread and often indiscriminate use has tended to bring them into discredit. Accurate bacteriological data as well as a working knowledge of the pharmacology of the antibiotic to be used is the keystone of rational treatment. New antibiotics must be subjected to careful laboratory and clinical study before being prescribed. The doctor has a responsibility to adopt a critical attitude towards each new drug and to decide whether it is an advance in treatment over well-established remedies. He should hesitate before prescribing an antibiotic for a febrile patient when the diagnosis is not clearly established and, if the patient is not critically ill, bacteriological information should be sought before specific therapy is begun. This branch of therapeutics is rapidly expanding and confusion results from conflicting views about the choice of antibiotic. This is largely because sufficient time has not elapsed between the production of an antibiotic and a long-term assessment of its advantages and disadvantages from the point of view of bacterial resistance and human toxicity.

Antibiotics are not simple, harmless remedies which can be prescribed in a haphazard way, changed from day to day or given in massive combinations. They should be prescribed in full doses for a sufficient length of time and preferably after the infecting organism has been properly identified so that the most effective bactericidal drug can be selected. If these principles were adopted, antibiotic therapy would become more rational and, as a result, more beneficial to the community.

References

MURDOCH, J. McC. (1965). Cephaloridine. *Practitioner*, **195**, 109.

MURDOCH, J. McC. (1969). Recent advances in antibacterial therapy. *Scot. med. J.*, **14**, 441.

Post-graduate Medical Journal (1964). Therapy with the new penicillins. **40**, Suppl.

Post-graduate Medical Journal (1967). Cephaloridine. **43**, Suppl.

Post-graduate Medical Journal (1969). The synergy of trimethoprim and sulphonamides. **45**, Suppl.

Post-graduate Medical Journal (1970). Cephalosporins. **46**, Suppl.

WATT, P. J. (1970). *The Control of Chemotherapy*. Edinburgh: Livingstone.

2. Infectious Diseases

J. M. MURDOCH

INTRODUCTION

The presence of fever in a patient does not necessarily prove that he is suffering from an infection. An accurate clinical diagnosis will depend on several important factors—the age and sex of the patient, the clinical history, and any physical signs which point to a focus of infection. In general, a diagnosis of infection is more likely to be made at the extremes of life; or it may be strongly suspected in adult patients who are debilitated for other reasons—after severe trauma, in the cachexia of malignant disease or during therapy with corticosteroids or antimetabolites.

Whatever may be the underlying cause of fever the symptomatic management of the febrile state is important for the patient's comfort; and if he is hyperthermic, reduction in the body temperature may well be life-saving, especially in young children. Traditionally good nursing in clean surroundings with frequent bed bathing and tepid sponging will greatly add to the patient's well-being. The giving of antipyretics such as aspirin perhaps combined with an analgesic such as codeine (p. 444) may again be symptomatically beneficial in the febrile state. This is especially true for patients suffering from acute viral diseases for which there is no specific therapy. Body temperature is most accurately measured in the rectum, and in young children there is no practical alternative to this method. In states of hyperthermia the rectal temperature in a baby may greatly differ from the skin temperature. For example, infantile convulsions may be associated with a rectal temperature as high as 41·1° C. and yet the skin temperature may be normal or even sub-normal. Hyperthermia can be rapidly relieved by the administration of chlorpromazine intravenously; a small dose is given slowly—2·5 mg. in 5 ml. of solution. The dose can be repeated while the rectal temperature is monitored. This procedure can be life-saving in infancy and early childhood.

In the febrile state there may be considerable loss of fluid by sweating, and this may be aggravated by losses from the bowel—as in infective diarrhoeas. In these circumstances it will often be necessary to correct dehydration and imbalance of electro-lytes by the use of fluids given intravenously. In hot climates few, if any, bed-clothes should be placed over the patient and then preferably over a protective cage. If possible a fan should be used over the patient's bed. The giving of fluids by mouth may not always be possible because of nausea or vomiting. Rigors in the adult, if repeated, are very exhausting and reduction in body temperature must be quickly achieved to avoid this. This may be done by the procedures mentioned above. Better still, if the nature of the infection is diagnosed and specific therapy is given the rigors cease as the patient responds to treatment.

Many patients with high fever suffer from cerebral disturbances. Nightmares are common in children and may be very distressing. In the adult, delirium may occur. Here again reduction in the body temperature is the best method of relieving these alarming disorders. Thus, every effort should be made in a febrile patient to achieve symptomatic relief. At the same time a comprehensive diagnosis should be arrived at as early as possible so that specific therapy can be applied when it is available. The choice of an antibacterial drug will depend in the first place on the clinician's acumen, but his plan of treatment may call for modification in the light of accurate bacteriological diagnosis. Specific drug therapy should not be given until the appropriate specimens have been sent to the laboratory. Unfortunately, this ideal cannot always be achieved, since many febrile patients are given antibiotics blindly before any attempt at an accurate diagnosis has been made (p. 1). None the less it must be emphasized that not all infections are susceptible to specific therapy, and that many febrile patients are suffering from non-infective conditions.

GENERAL MANAGEMENT OF THE FEBRILE STATE

Although pyrexia, arising from interference with the function of the heat-regulating centre, is usually a cardinal sign of an infection, in some of the most toxic cases the temperature may not rise above normal. Wasting, due to increased catabolism; dry hot skin, acceleration of the pulse and respiration; coated tongue, anorexia, vomiting and constipation or diarrhoea; headache, restlessness, insomnia and delirium; quantitative and qualitative changes in the urine; all these manifestations are a result of the reactions of the tissues of the host to the effects of the pathogen or its products.

In the general management of the febrile patient the essential needs are (a) rest; (b) efficient nursing; (c) a suitable diet with adequate intake of water; and (d) relief of symptoms.

Rest. Confinement to bed is essential as long as the temperature remains elevated, and should be continued for a few days in convalescence. Strict rest in bed should never be regarded as an end in itself. When there is no obvious contraindication, early activity should be encouraged. The young patient is better to be up and properly dressed than to be continually in and out of bed without adequate clothing. In the elderly the real risks of a long period in bed far outweigh the potential risks of allowing a fair degree of activity.

A single bed and firm mattress are preferable for nursing purposes. Careful bed-making contributes greatly to the patient's comfort. A length of plastic across the bed covered by a taut drawsheet will prevent extensive soiling and save linen. The bed should be made twice daily—oftener if the patient is perspiring profusely. An adequate supply of pillows will make for comfort. Bedclothes should be light and not tucked in tightly. A cage at the foot is often desirable. Quietness in the sickroom and its environment is essential; traffic in and out should be cut down to a minimum.

Ideally the sickroom should be bright and adequately ventilated and heated. Proximity to a bathroom, which should if possible be reserved for the patient's use, is advantageous. The temperature should be kept around 15° C.

Nursing. In diseases where there is scope for precise bacteriological diagnosis and specific therapy based on sensitivity tests, the patient should be admitted to hospital. Apart from this—and with the obvious exception of patients whose infections are unusually severe or complicated—the great majority should be treated at home. The mother will as a rule prove the best nurse. With modern therapy the period of heavy infectivity is comparatively short, so that the risk of spread of infection is slight. The mother should be given instructions in simple home nursing. Supervision by the district nurse is invaluable. Emphasis should be placed on the following points.

An overall should be worn when attending to the patient and should be hung conveniently near the door. A bowl of chloroxylenol or even plain water, with soap and towels, should also be adjacent to the door and the mother should be instructed to use this frequently for hand-washing. The practitioner should be careful to practise what he teaches. A simple temperature chart should be constructed; the thermometer should be placed in the groin or the axilla and left in position for two minutes. All treatment ordered should be entered on the chart and precise instructions given regarding administration.

The patient's *skin* should be kept clean by sponging with soap and warm water daily, especial care being paid to areas liable to soiling. These should be freely dusted with talcum powder. The body should be washed and dried limb by limb. The windows, of course, must be kept closed during the bathing process. The refreshing and soothing effect of a 'blanket bath' of this nature is of inestimable value in any febrile condition. The seriously ill patient must have his position changed every two or three hours; areas subject to pressure should be massaged with spirit and dried with talcum powder twice daily.

Food should be given at the usual meal times, but the individual patient's likes and dislikes must be noted. Any remaining scraps of food should be removed from the sickroom and burnt. Cold water, plain or with various flavourings, must be given freely. In young children the *mouth* should be gently cleansed after each meal by inserting the index finger enveloped in cotton-wool soaked in warm water or warm solution of bicarbonate of soda containing 2 g. to 600 ml. (1 pint). In older children the teeth should be brushed and the mouth rinsed with warm water or mild antiseptic solution. The lips may be smeared with petroleum jelly.

Nasal discharge must be promptly removed preferably on paper handkerchiefs, and the nostrils gently cleaned with a cotton-wool swab soaked in warm saline or bicarbonate solution. Older children should be encouraged to clear the nose by gentle blowing. Petroleum jelly applied to the nostrils and upper lips prevents crusting and excoriation.

The *eyes* may require regular cleansing, and saline swabbing is usually best. The very toxic or comatose patient often lies for long periods with the eyelids partially separated so that the cornea dries, and may become ulcerated. This can be prevented by instilling a drop of castor oil into the conjunctival sac.

All *excreta* should be removed from the sickroom and consigned to the closet as quickly as possible. Care must be taken to avoid contamination of water-closet seats. Specimens required for the physician's inspection should be placed in covered fly-proof receptacles. Bed-linen, towels, etc., which may have been soiled with excreta should be left soaking in weak lysol solution overnight before being thoroughly washed with soap and water. Swabs used for wiping away discharges from the mouth, nose, ears, eyes and other organs must be burnt.

Flies must be excluded from the sickroom and, in summer, spraying with dicophane or some similar material is an important measure.

Diet. In the pyrexial state there is a considerable increase in the metabolism of the tissue proteins. Instead of trying to make good this loss by giving a high protein diet, carbohydrates are ordered because they act as 'protein sparers' and incidentally are more acceptable. Febrile patients do not tolerate fatty foods. Theoretically, during fever a high caloric intake is indicated, but in practice, owing to loss of appetite and actual distaste for food, this is impossible to attain during the height of the fever.

When the febrile period does not exceed four or five days (and, it may be noted, this is now usual with specific therapy), the diet should be restricted to fluids; 'feeding up' is to be deprecated. One and a half to three pints of milk daily usually form the basis of the diet. Not more than 150 to 180 ml. (5 to 6 fl. oz.) should be given at a feed. Glucose is a most valuable and easily assimilated food, which should be given freely in the form of sweetened lemon or orange juice drinks; but many patients tire of too much glucose and may ask for occasional unsweetened fruit juice. From 150 to 300 g. of glucose can readily be administered in the 24 hours. Jellies, clear soups, eggs and custards are useful additions to the diet, and varying flavouring agents can add spice to an otherwise monotonous round. Because of their low nutritive value and relative cost, the various commercial beef-juice preparations have little to commend them apart from novelty.

A dehydrated patient suffers excessively from the constitutional effects of toxaemia and infection. He should, therefore, be encouraged to drink cold or hot water freely between feeds. Including glucose lemonade, the water intake should amount to at least 2 to 3 litres in the 24 hours. The best indication of an adequate fluid intake is the excretion of

1·5 to 2 litres of urine daily. Alcohol should not be administered as a routine.

Relief of symptoms. *Pyrexia.* A raised body temperature is in itself not harmful but the effects of sustained pyrexia such as dehydration, general discomfort and restlessness are very disagreeable and warrant symptomatic relief.

When the temperature exceeds 39·5° C., the skin of the whole body should be sponged with warm (37° C.), tepid (27° C.), or even cold water. Apart from any effect in reducing temperature, the application of tepid or cold water to the skin is conducive to relaxation and sleep.

Headache and ill-defined pains in the limbs are common accompaniments of the pyrexial state. Aspirin (600 mg.) or paracetamol (1 g.) administered at intervals of six hours usually give relief.

Insomnia may be abolished after the use of an antipyretic-analgesic drug such as aspirin. Distension of the bladder or intractable thirst may keep the patient awake and demand corrective measures. The use of hypnotics is described elsewhere (p. 445). In febrile states accompanied by toxaemia care should be taken to avoid using sedatives which depress the respiratory centre. Alcohol (brandy or whisky 30 ml. diluted with water) is often highly effective and especially if followed by a dose of chloral hydrate (1 g. in water well diluted and flavoured).

Nausea and vomiting. These symptoms are common at the onset of many infectious diseases but are seldom sufficiently severe or persistent to cause anxiety once specific therapy has been started. Vomiting may interfere with the oral administration of drugs; parenteral therapy is then necessary.

When vomiting is persistent and severe, the electrolyte disturbance may require to be rectified by intravenous infusions. This demands the closest co-operation between biochemist and clinician and is in general beyond the scope of domiciliary practice (p. 253).

Constipation. Constipation is present during the course of many infectious fevers. It is seldom a matter of much importance though it may cause the patient great concern. During a severe illness it is usually better to empty the bowel by an enema or suppositories (p. 501) than by the administration of purgatives.

In convalescence from a severe fever a patient may become excessively anxious about constipation. He should be reassured that his normal bowel habit will be regained. One of the anthracene purgatives may be given temporarily such as a teaspoonful of the elixir of cascara at night.

Disinfection. Disinfectants are intended to destroy the micro-organisms released from the patient in his various discharges and excretions, but in practice they are not very effective. Many spores resist their action, viruses vary considerably in their susceptibility to them and the physical properties of the excretions themselves usually impair their lethal effect. Nevertheless in the home, disinfectants have a limited place in reducing the contamination of objects surrounding the patient. As a rule the aim is to destroy the vegetative forms of bacteria; spores do not constitute a serious problem.

The most useful disinfectants are: *Chloroxylenol* (B.P.C.), a phenol-related substance which makes a pleasant disinfectant for hand-washing and damp-dusting and which is particularly effective against gram-positive but not against most gram-negative organisms; *lysol* and its allied preparations which are valuable general-purpose disinfectants for bed linen, etc., but which must not be brought into contact with the skin; *hypochlorites* which are useful in dealing with dishes and glassware, but to be effective must be mixed with a detergent; and *chlorhexidine* or *hexachlorophane* which have gained a wide popularity and are often contained in soaps, handcreams and dusting powders. They are specially effective against gram-positive organisms and, since *Staph. aureus* can be so dangerous in nurseries, they are of value in the care of the new-born. To be of greatest benefit they must be used repeatedly. Unfortunately they are ineffective against some gram-negative organisms, in particular *Ps. pyocyanea*—a species of increasing importance in hospital infection. The most important point to realize is that no disinfectant can be regarded as serving all purposes and that none is a sterilizing agent. Sunlight, fresh air and soap and water are equally important.

The attendant. The attendant must be instructed in the importance of observing some simple rules. The hands will become grossly contaminated by bed-manipulations, cleansing of discharges, etc., and the importance of washing the hands after any attention to the patient must be emphasized. An overall or gown must be put on as soon as the sick-room is entered and removed before leaving. The fact that the air and dust of the room is charged with infection should be explained to the attendant. Damp-dusting and wet-mopping of floor surrounds are acceptable methods; the 'brush and pan' must be banished. When vacuum cleaners are used, the dust contained in the bag is heavily infected and must be emptied carefully.

The attendant must grasp the concept that the patient is the centre of a series of concentric circles of infection: this is most dense at the inner circle, and the constant endeavour must be to prevent spread outwards. The air and dust of the room form the important means whereby the outer circles become contaminated, so that all steps to reduce dust and the careless circulation of air which disturbs dust will tend to limit spread. These measures are not only of importance in preventing the infection of others; the patient himself, especially if nursed alongside others, may acquire secondary complications from the implantation (particularly in the respiratory tract) of organisms acquired from infected dust.

The use of a mask by the attendant is as a rule undesirable. If the attendant has a cold and the patient is under the age of a year, a mask is worth while, for at this period of life a very ill infant may have its chances of recovery greatly reduced by a secondary infection. An effective paper mask is now available which can be destroyed after use. It should be used only once and should not be touched by the hands when being worn. The wearing of a mask is often thought to infer a special efficiency in preventing infection, but it is worth emphasizing that among careless or untrained attendants the mask may constitute more of a danger than a safeguard.

The patient. All discharges emanating from the patient must be assumed to be infective.

Coughing and sneezing should be guarded against by the use of paper handkerchiefs. Sputum as well as nasal, aural or ocular discharges should be carefully collected in paper handkerchiefs and placed in paper bags to be burnt.

Vomitus should, if possible, be collected in a basin and immediately disposed of. The basin should be disinfected by wiping with weak lysol and washing in hot soapy water. If the linen is soiled, it should be steeped in disinfectant and then washed. Children who are ill often vomit unexpectedly, and the bed-linen may be saved by the use of towels, old sheets and pieces of plastic sheeting at the top of the bed or cot. Faeces and faeces-soiled bed-linen must be promptly removed and disinfected.

Strict asepsis is essential in attending to wounds. Steps should be taken to avoid soiling of pillows and bed-linen with discharge, for as this dries it may be shaken off to form infected dust. All fluids removed for testing (blood, cerebrospinal fluid) must be handled carefully and sent to the laboratory without delay.

Articles closely associated with the patient. The most important of these are the bedclothes, linen and towels. All of them become heavily contaminated and, if the bed is made vigorously, the air becomes heavily infected. The enclosing of the blankets in linen sheets diminishes this hazard and the attendant should be instructed to avoid vigorous movements of bedclothes and mattress. Feeding utensils should be kept separately for the patient. After each meal the dishes should be washed and scalded by pouring a kettleful of boiling water over them. Between meals the patient's dishes are kept in a bowl of hypochlorite solution. At the end of the illness books and papers should be burnt, but most toys can be adequately disinfected with soap and water.

Final domestic cleaning. A thorough domestic cleansing is all that is required for those infections which can be treated in the home. The process of laundering will effectively purify all bed-linen, clothing, etc. Bulky articles such as mattresses and carpets can be exposed to sunlight and fresh air, and the vacuum cleaner will be effective for cleaning. Sprays and gases have no place in the ritual except in the case of smallpox, when the responsibility will rest with the Medical Officer of Health.

ANTHRAX

Anthrax is an infection which is classed as an occupational risk, and in man is more or less confined to workers with animals or in wool, hair or hides. The importance of artificial fertilizers containing bone-meal must be borne in mind for this may explain the infection of individuals with no obvious occupational or other contact. The disease is seen principally in animal husbandmen and infection usually enters through minute wounds or abrasions on the exposed skin, giving rise after an incubation period of about 24 to 36 hours to a cutaneous lesion—the 'malignant pustule'.

Anthrax is not a notifiable disease, but information regarding cases occurring in factories and workshops must be forwarded to the Chief Inspector of Factories at the Home Office.

Preventive treatment. Although there is a considerable animal reservoir of infection in this country the disease is so well diagnosed by veterinarians that human anthrax from indigenous sources is very uncommon. By law, carcasses of infected animals must be either burned or deeply buried in lime and the area of ground fenced for some years. Thus, in the British Isles most cases arise from imported material—hides or bones being principally involved. As a result of legislation regarding the proper ventilation of factories, human cases of gastrointestinal or respiratory anthrax—invariably fatal in the past—are never seen in Britain. Factory legislation also ensures that protective clothing is worn and that workers are shown illustrations of the malignant pustule.

Great care must be taken in handling infected material. Workers with skin lesions should be excluded. Nurses or attendants must take all necessary precautions when handling infective discharges from the 'pustule' or the respiratory and intestinal tracts and the use of disposable polythene gloves is recommended. Contaminated dressings should be promptly burnt and discharges disinfected. Bedclothes, mattresses and bed linen must be subjected to steam disinfection.

A safe anthrax vaccine is now available. It is an alum-precipitated antigen prepared from the Weybridge strain of *B. anthracis* by the Lister Institute, Elstree. It is available free of charge through Public Health Authorities. The dose is 0·5 ml. intramuscularly, repeated after six weeks and again after 26 weeks, followed by annual booster doses. After the third dose up to 90 per cent. of those vaccinated possess antibody to anthrax. Local reactions are mild and transient; constitutional reactions are rare. Only those at risk need to be vaccinated. They are listed in the Ministry of Health Circular 1965, No. 19/65. Family doctors should warn their patients who are farm workers or gardeners (amateur and professional) that rubber gloves should be worn when handling bone-meal as it is occasionally infected with anthrax.

Curative treatment. Penicillin in large doses is highly effective; an initial injection of 2 mega units (1·2 g.) is followed by doses of 1 mega unit (0·6 g.) four-hourly. Anti-anthrax serum is obsolete and should not be used.

Many patients are apyrexial but the severity of the infection is indicated by the amount of local swelling and oedema. In infections of the face and neck, oedema has an additional significance as it may extend into the larynx and produce partial obstruction of the airway. Arrangements should be made to perform tracheostomy should the need for this arise. As clinical improvement becomes obvious the doses of penicillin may be reduced to 0·5 mega units (0·3 g.) but treatment should continue for 10 days. Secondary infection of the pustule may occur and the organisms may be penicillin-resistant. Additional specific therapy should then be given, based on the results of sensitivity tests.

Dressings are used because they reduce contamination of the bed-linen. Instructions should be given for burning the scab when it separates. In the most severe cases there may be considerable sloughing so that skin grafting may be required.

References
DARLOW, H. M. *et al.* (1956), *Lancet*, **2**, 476.
Report of the Committee of Inquiry on Anthrax, H.M.S.O., London 1959, paras 288 and 289.
Leading Article, *Lancet* (1965), **2**, 374.
Drug and Therapeutics Bulletin (1967), Vol. 5, No. 15.

CHICKENPOX
(VARICELLA)

Chickenpox is a viral disease of high infectivity. It is spread by droplet infection and perhaps by aerial currents. The incubation period is usually from 13 to 16 days. It is rarely less than 11 days or more than 20 days. The disease is probably infective for at least 24 hours before the appearance of the rash. The duration of infectivity is uncertain, but for practical purposes may be regarded as persisting until the last crust has separated from the skin.

Chickenpox is not a notifiable disease, but should smallpox be prevalent in a particular area, chickenpox cases may have to be reported to the local Public Health Authority.

Preventive treatment. There is no method of preventing chickenpox. Indeed attempts to avoid infection in childhood should not be made since, in the adult, chickenpox is almost always a more severe illness. The viruses of chickenpox and herpes zoster are identical and herpes zoster often produces chickenpox in susceptible contacts.

General management. The treatment of chickenpox is on general lines, no specific remedy being available. Even in mild attacks the patient should be confined to bed during the efflorescence of the eruption. When the rash is profuse it is wise to insist on rest in bed until the lesions have crusted. If there is a tendency to scratch the pocks, the hands

may be wrapped in lint or gauze, or the arms lightly splinted. If itching is intense, the application of either calamine lotion or 2·5 per cent. phenol in petroleum jelly or olive oil will give relief, or the skin may be dusted freely with a good sterilized talcum powder or with a powder consisting of zinc oxide (1 part) and starch (2 parts). Boric acid should be avoided.

Complications. In children, complications are rare. If severe secondary infection of the skin lesions occurs bacteriological examination should always be carried out and the appropriate antibiotic prescribed. In adults chickenpox is often a fairly severe and disabling infection; concomitant herpes zoster is seen occasionally, and encephalomyelitis and pneumonia are rare complications.

DIPHTHERIA

Diphtheria is now a rare infection in Britain. The disease has been practically abolished by prophylactic inoculation of children with toxoids. However, in recent years the tendency of parents to postpone immunization until their children are of school age has increased the likelihood of epidemics. Cases of diphtheria are re-appearing and some have been fatal.

Diphtheria is almost entirely a toxic disease. Although some slight tissue invasion takes place in severe infections, the organisms mostly remain localized to the site of inoculation from which the toxin diffuses by lymphatics and blood stream to all parts of the body. The ability of the host to neutralize toxin thus constitutes an almost complete defence; for, deprived of its toxic action, the diphtheria bacillus is a weak pathogen.

Patients and carriers constitute the main sources of infection. Usually the bacteria are carried in the throat or nose, the latter site being rather more common, so that in a search for a source of infection nasal cultures should never be omitted. Cutaneous diphtheria, often simulating a chronic sore, may be an unsuspected source of infection. Although in most instances infection is spread by droplet infection, contaminated milk, ice-cream and food have initiated local outbreaks.

The importance of early diagnosis of diphtheria cannot be too strongly emphasized. Careful examination of the fauces should be a routine procedure in every febrile patient. Apart from the presence of 'false membrane', marked faucial and palatal oedema, accompanied by an acute gross enlargement of the cervical glands, should, in a child, always be treated as diphtheria until proved otherwise.

Diphtheria is a notifiable disease. It has an incubation period of two to five days.

Prevention and epidemiological control. *The Schick Test* is used to determine susceptibility to diphtheria. The procedure is described in detail in manuals of infectious diseases, but it consists essentially in the intradermal injection of a measured quantity of diphtheria toxin. In the Schick-positive reactor—showing susceptibility to diphtheria—a patch of erythema develops at the site of injection of toxin.

Active immunization. Every child should be actively immunized against diphtheria during the first year of life. A preliminary Schick test is unnecessary.

Four vaccines[1] are available: purified toxoid aluminium phosphate (PTAP), alum-precipitated toxoid (APT), formol toxoid (FT) and toxoid antitoxin floccules (TAF). For children under 5 years two intramuscular injections, each of 0·5 ml., of one of the alum-toxoids with an interval of four weeks between injections will produce effective immunity. In older children or adults it is better to start with a small dose (0·2 ml.) and observe the degree of local reaction. If this is severe two further injections of 0·2 ml. with a four-week interval are advised. FT is not recommended since it is a weaker antigen and reactions are common in older children and adults. TAF is a good antigen and remarkably free from local reaction. It has the disadvantage that it contains horse-serum and may, therefore, have a sensitizing effect. Three injections of 1·0 ml. are required.

The first injection has no permanent immunizing effect. It is the subsequent doses which evoke a high level of antitoxin in the blood and confer immunity. The duration of this immunity is variable, but a child who has received the two immunizing doses may later have its immunity 'boosted' by a further single injection. Such a booster injection is essential before the child enters school at the age of 5 years.

Combined vaccines are now commonly used. For example, *diphtheria-tetanus adsorbed vaccine* is a good antigen and remarkably free from local

reactions in children. *Diphtheria, tetanus and pertussis vaccines* are best prepared without alum and in this form are good antigens, but should not be given before the age of 3 months in order to obtain a satisfactory response to the diphtheria and tetanus antigens. As it is so convenient to obtain this comprehensive immunizing effect with single injections, the method is recommended as a means of obtaining immunity during the first year of life.

General measures. For the control of an outbreak the first steps are the isolation of the patient. Contacts must be carefully examined for evidence of a sub-clinical infection. Particular attention should be paid to any person suffering from chronic nasal or aural discharge, or obviously unhealthy tonsils—or a suspicious cutaneous lesion—and the appropriate swabs taken for bacteriological examination.

The normal carrier rate in the general population is exceedingly low. Hence when a case of clinical diphtheria occurs it is important to try to identify the carrier by whom the infection was conveyed. After a preliminary warning to the bacteriologist when large numbers are involved, swabs should be taken from the nose *and* throat and from any suspicious lesion of all contacts. Since the typing of *C. diphtheriae* isolated from either the primary case or the contacts will take three to four days, this time may be usefully occupied in eliciting precise details regarding the immunization status of those involved. Contacts who have already received a full course in childhood can now be effectively boosted by a single injection of 0·2 ml. of an appropriate vaccine (PTAP). Persons who have never been immunized should be given active-passive immunization. To accomplish this 500 units of diphtheria antitoxin is injected into one arm at the same time as 0·5 ml. of PTAP is injected into the other arm. A note should be taken to ensure that these persons are given a further injection of 0·5 ml. of PTAP four weeks later to complete the active immunization course.

Any carriers disclosed by the bacteriological examination must be isolated in hospital and treated appropriately (p. 32). It is nowadays essential to ensure that the carrier state has been effectively eradicated before the individual is released from isolation.

Curative treatment. *A history of immunization must never lead the practitioner to ignore the possibility of diphtheria.* Indeed, it must be appreciated that mild diphtheria—usually due to *gravis*

---

[1] The term 'vaccine' was formerly confined to the description of materials which contained bacteria or viruses. It is now used to describe all antigenic substances designed to secure active immunity.

organisms—occasionally occurs in the inoculated and that such infections are usually atypical and may be more suggestive of tonsillitis. Further, although it is undoubtedly true that the disease in the immunized is often mild, failure to make an early diagnosis may result in the administration of serum too late to prevent nervous complications.

Antitoxin. An intramuscular injection of at least 8,000 units of diphtheria antitoxic serum should immediately be administered to any patient suspected to be suffering from the disease. The importance of *early* administration of antitoxin cannot be exaggerated. The doctor who 'wonders whether this might be diphtheria' is under an obligation to give serum at once. Swabs can then be taken. By the time full bacteriological investigations have been made, several days must elapse. These are the critical days: omission of antitoxin treatment at this stage may be fatal. There is considerable difference of opinion regarding the optimum dose of antitoxin in the treatment of diphtheria. Broadly speaking, mild attacks require 8,000 units intramuscularly; cases of moderate severity about 32,000 units intramuscularly; and severe or toxic attacks from 48,000 to 96,000 units divided between the intramuscular and intravenous routes. When the diphtheritic infection is limited to the larynx, 24,000 units of antitoxin are usually sufficient, and a similar dose is adequate in purely nasal diphtheria unless toxaemia is severe. Now that diphtheria antitoxin is a highly refined preparation, many physicians give the whole dose intravenously irrespective of the severity of the disease, but the method recommended above reduces the risk of anaphylactic shock (p. 59).

There is no satisfactory method of assessing the correct amount of antitoxin, so that it is better to err on the side of overdosage. There are good grounds for believing that a dose of 48,000 units is more than adequate for the most severe case of diphtheria and that it is never necessary to give more than 96,000 units.

The *route of administration* is very important. It is seldom appreciated that a considerable time elapses after intramuscular injection before 'peak' levels are attained in the blood stream. *All severe cases (i.e. where more than 32,000 units are to be given) must receive at least part of the dose intravenously.* In other words, the intramuscular route is the second-best and should only be used in mild or moderate cases. Intramuscular serum should be

given into the lateral aspect of the thigh. Before giving serum the doctor must be conversant with the possible dangers which may result, and the measures to be taken for their prevention and treatment are discussed on p. 59.

Other specific treatment. The bacteriological examination of the throat swab will include search for other pathogens—particularly *Str. pyogenes*—by suitable culture. Penicillin has a definite value in the treatment of diphtheria *after serum has been given.* In the first place it is of value in dealing with the superadded infection so often present; and secondly it hastens the disappearance of *C. diphtheriae* from the throat and reduces the risk of development of the carrier state. The dose must be large—2 mega units (1·2 g.) twice daily for five days—in order to ensure an adequate local concentration.

General measures. With the exception of the mildest attack, a case of diphtheria should not be treated at home unless adequate nursing attention is available day and night. From the moment that diphtheria is suspected, the patient must be confined to bed in a strictly recumbent position. Owing to the risk of toxic myocarditis, any attempt to sit up, reach over to a chair or bedside table, etc., must be prohibited. Indeed, in the most toxic forms the patient should not even feed himself. The period of recumbency varies from 14 days in mild attacks to eight weeks or longer in severe cases, according to the condition of the cardiovascular system and the occurrence of paralysis.

After the addition of a second and a third pillow at intervals of two clear days, the patient is permitted to sit up, and may leave his bed seven to ten days later. The rate of progress will vary according to the severity of the attack and the response of the cardiovascular system to increased exertion. This is assessed by a study of the pulse rate: a rising pulse rate means that convalescence is being unduly hurried. Care should be taken to curtail activity when the patient begins to walk.

Paresis of the extrinsic muscles of the eyes is common and reading should be restricted to avoid ocular strain.

Complications. The mitigation of serious toxic damage to the heart and vessels by the early application of the measures detailed above is the fundamental principle in the treatment of diphtheria. Once well-marked signs of cardiovascular weakness appear, the situation is grave and treatment other than skilful nursing is of little avail.

B*

The foot of the bed should be raised. Vomiting due to cardiac failure necessitates the replacement of oral feeding by the administration of intravenous infusions but overloading of the failing heart must be avoided. The mouth may be moistened with sips of water. Epigastric pain (caused by rapid enlargement of the liver), restlessness and anxiety are best relieved by repeated hypodermic injections of morphine: 2 mg. for a child of 2 years, 4 mg. at 5 years, and 5 mg. for a child of 10 years.

The poisoned myocardium is insusceptible to drug therapy on conventional lines. The various vasomotor or cardiac stimulants have no place in the treatment of circulatory failure in diphtheria. The administration of alcohol has nothing to commend it.

Apart from involvement of the pharyngeal and respiratory muscles, no anxiety need be felt regarding the outcome of post-diphtheritic palsies, since they gradually recover spontaneously within a few weeks though severe palsies may last for six months or longer. In palatal paresis the fluid part of the diet should be replaced by semi-solids. In pharyngeal paralysis the foot of the bed should be raised 18 in. and the patient nursed in the prone position. Saliva and mucus should be aspirated at frequent intervals from the pharynx and food administered by nasal tube. On the slightest indication of weakness of the intercostal muscles or diaphragm constant supervision is essential. The degree of respiratory dysfunction must be carefully assessed and the necessary preparations made for instituting mechanical assistance (p. 651).

Late generalized muscular weakness improves with graduated exercise, fresh air and a nutritious diet.

Convalescence. It is necessary to obtain three consecutive negative cultures from both throat and nose at an interval of one week before the patient is released from isolation. Even after a mild attack the patient should not resume school or work for at least a fortnight after isolation is stopped. The convalescent period may require to be prolonged to six months or even longer following severe toxic diphtheria. Strenuous exercise must be forbidden.

CARRIERS

The first essential in dealing with a persistent convalescent—or contact—carrier of morphological diphtheria bacilli is to make sure that the organisms are virulent. Carriers of non-virulent bacilli are not dangerous to the community and need not be segregated.

If the organism isolated is virulent, tests to disclose its antibiotic sensitivity should be requested. Erythromycin is usually particularly effective against *C. diphtheriae* and, while awaiting the laboratory results, its administration may be started. The daily dose of erythromycin is 30 mg. per kg. body weight and it is administered in capsules. This will ensure a high local concentration. Erythromycin should be continued for 10 days and during this time the carrier must be strictly isolated in order to prevent reinfection.

While treatment is proceeding the time can be used to make a detailed clinical and radiological examination of the mouth and upper respiratory tract since, in persistent carriers, it is common to find some local abnormality which serves to prolong the carrier state. At the end of the course of treatment it is advised that six negative cultures from the nose and throat should be obtained over a period of at least 14 days. This period should not be shortened for it is often found that negative swabs may give place to positive ones at the end of the series.

Should erythromycin fail, the question of further chemotherapy may be considered in light of the known sensitivity of the organism. However, when the examination of the nose and throat has disclosed some abnormality which should be corrected surgically it will usually be preferable to adopt this course for, in such circumstances, cure may prove exceedingly difficult with chemotherapy alone. The effective clearing of carriers is now all the more important because of the very low carrier rate in the community.

LARYNGEAL DIPHTHERIA

On the slightest suspicion that a child is suffering from a diphtheritic laryngitis, the practitioner should immediately inject 24,000 units of antitoxin and 1 mega unit of penicillin intramuscularly and arrange for the prompt removal of the patient to hospital. This is essential for bacteriological diagnosis and, when necessary, tracheostomy or intubation.

Laryngo-tracheo-bronchitis. The widespread practice of diphtheria immunization has resulted in the virtual disappearance of diphtheritic laryngitis; and yet 'croup' is still commonly encountered. The commonest form is that associated with a general inflammation of the respiratory tract. Although the condition is primarily a virus infection, secondary bacterial invaders are responsible for much of the subsequent damage. All ages may be affected, but because of the narrow laryngeal cleft in children, obstruction to respiration is usually confined to those under five years of age. In many cases *Staph. pyogenes* can be grown in pure culture from throat swabs. The organism has proved to be penicillin-resistant in such a high proportion of cases that penicillin should never be the antibiotic of first choice. Since other bacteria may be involved, treatment should be started with a tetracycline while the results of sensitivity tests are awaited; after more precise information is available, the suitable antibiotic can be chosen. Even after tracheostomy such cases often pursue a stormy course and require constant expert supervision. The use of a steam tent is often helpful.

BACILLARY DYSENTERY

Dysentery must now be regarded as an endemic infection in large cities. In all parts of Great Britain notifications of the disease have increased greatly in recent years, and in view of the mild nature of the symptoms it may be assumed that the notifications represent but a proportion of the actual incidence. It is no longer true to say that the maximal incidence is always in the summer months. Notifications have been high throughout the year, and in some years the peak has occurred in the first quarter. A large proportion of the patients are children under five years of age. In many cases a few loose stools may comprise the whole complaint and no precautions are taken to prevent the spread of the disease. Some convalescents may become carriers for long periods of time and act as a source of infection.

When a case of dysentery is diagnosed in a family it is usual to find some other members with the organism in their stools. Outbreaks in day nurseries and children's homes are common—and here again the diagnosis of one case will often lead to the discovery of a large number of carriers. Occasionally local epidemics have been traced to contaminated water supplies.

Unlike typhoid fever, the infection remains almost entirely localized to the bowel and agglutinins do not appear in the blood to any great degree. Apart from toxic absorption due to ulceration of the bowel, the main danger in severe infections arises from exhaustion of the patient by loss of fluid and electrolytes in frequent liquid stools. Such a degree of severity is fortunately unusual.

Rectal swabbing permits of prompt bacteriological diagnosis, but stool cultures give a higher rate of positivity.

Dysentery is a notifiable disease. In Britain the Sonne type is by far the commonest form of infection but Flexner dysentery accounts for a significant proportion of cases in certain urban communities. The incubation period is two to five days.

Prevention and epidemiological control. The control of ward and institutional outbreaks often presents a formidable task. All further admissions should be stopped and a close search made for carriers and missed cases, both among patients and staff. The bacteriologist should be brought into consultation at once, for the addition to his routine work will be considerable and he should therefore be forewarned. Plans should also be prepared for the separation of those found to give positive results and arrangements made for the sterilization of food utensils and bed-pans. Soiled napkins should be dropped direct into covered pails containing lysol. The nursing staff must be instructed regarding the method of transference of the infection and there must be perseverance in the campaign for repeated hand washing and a careful ritual of personal hygiene. The nurses should also be taught that the simplest case of diarrhoea may well be dysentery and that the occurrence of a loose or green stool should be reported at once.

The extent to which bacteriological freedom from infection prior to discharge is enforced must vary from case to case. When the patient is to return to a closed community—service personnel and children from nurseries—and when there is close association with food preparation it is desirable to obtain at least three negative bacteriological reports. When the patient is returning home, however, it is unnecessary to carry out protracted examinations, and the average case may be regarded as free from infection by the tenth day of illness.

Curative treatment. The majority of cases, due to Sonne and Flexner infections, run a mild course of three or four days and call for little medicinal treatment. The administration of specific serum to cases of Shiga infection is of undoubted value. The dose is up to 100 ml. and the injection should be given intravenously after suitable precautions (p. 59).

Specific chemotherapy is made difficult by the fact that organisms may develop resistance to substances which have previously been regarded as effective. Thus in many areas, the endemic strains of shigella are all sulphonamide-resistant and resistance to tetracyline and ampicillin is common. The practitioner is advised to maintain contact with the local bacteriologist, who will inform him of the prevailing pattern. Fortunately, most cases are mild in character and should not require specific therapy. For the obviously ill patient, strepto-mycin by mouth in a dosage of 500 mg. six-hourly for five days is recommended. If the organism is resistant to streptomycin, then neomycin by mouth in the same dosage will often be effective in eradi-cating the pathogen from the stools. The bac-teriologist's advice has particular importance when treating food-handlers or in attempts to eradicate persistent pathogenic organisms.

General management. The patient must be confined to bed but he may be allowed the use of a bedside commode. When the call to stool is incessant and the patient is exhausted the motions should be received into tow, which, when soiled, is collected and burnt. Such patients almost invariably need intravenous infusions to meet their water and electrolyte requirements.

Carriers. Persistent symptomless carriers are sometimes unmasked in the investigation of an outbreak. The strain isolated should be tested for sensitivity against a wide range of antibiotics effective against gram-negative organisms and an appropriate substance chosen.

THE ENTERIC FEVERS

(TYPHOID AND PARATYPHOID)

The annual occurrence in Britain of one or more outbreaks of enteric fever indicates that, in spite of sanitary precautions, the risk of contamination of water and food supplies with the enteric group of organisms still persists. *S. typhi* and *S. paratyphi B*, the organisms commonly met with in the British Isles, are excreted in the stools and urine during the course of the illness. The unsuspected ambulant patient, the missed case, the temporary carrier and the chronic carrier play a very important part in the spread of enteric fever; and as more and more people take holidays abroad the number of typhoid carriers is likely to increase. It is probable that even with efficient chemotherapy from 2 to 5 per cent. of all cases of typhoid fever become permanent carriers. The frequency of the chronic carrier state is higher in women than in men and this is unfortunate in the context of contamination of food in course of preparation. Faecal carriers are more common than urinary carriers but the latter are potentially more dangerous. The organisms are discharged intermittently in both stools and urine, so that repeated bacteriological examinations are essential before the carrier state can be excluded.

Although isolation of the pathogen from faecal and urinary specimens is the only exact method of identifying carriers, preliminary examination of the blood serum may serve as a useful screening test for carriers of *S. typhi* when large numbers of suspects have to be reviewed. Those with a high titre of Vi antigen should be singled out for full bacteriological examination.

Milk or milk products, prepared meats, uncooked vegetables, fruit and shellfish constitute the usual vehicles of infection. A nurse may contract the disease in the course of her duties; this usually indicates carelessness in the washing of hands. Nursing and ancillary staffs while on duty in enteric fever wards must be forbidden to eat any food there.

Typhoid and paratyphoid fevers are notifiable diseases. The incubation period of typhoid infec-tions is from 12 to 14 days, and of paratyphoid B from 10 to 12 days.

Prevention and epidemiological control. The control of typhoid fever is essentially a problem for the local Public Health Authority and embraces such factors as an efficient system of sewage disposal, a safe water and milk supply, the detection of carriers, the supervision of shellfish culture, the control of the house-fly and effective supervision of premises where food is sold or prepared.

Careful supervision of sewage and water is usual in the large towns, so that widespread epidemics of typhoid are now exceptional due to this cause. In country districts, however, defective cesspools, flooding or ineffective disposal of sewage are still commonly the source of localized outbreaks. Articles of food, especially cold meats and tinned ham and beef have now replaced water as the vehicle of infection, especially of paratyphoid fever, and here the towns are in as much danger as the country-side. Although day-to-day control by Public Health Departments forms an important part of the protection of the public, the early diagnosis of the infected case by the practitioner is of prime impor-tance both in stemming an incipient epidemic and in stopping it once it has started. The value of early blood culture in cases of continued fever must here be emphasized; and the golden rule is *to carry out a blood culture on any patient who has an unexplained pyrexia for more than three days.* A specimen of blood for agglutination tests should be submitted at the same time. The impression that it is only worth while to examine for agglutinins after the end of the first week of illness is quite erroneous. An early specimen may show their presence in low titre, and if a further examination in three or four days shows a rise in titre the diagnosis is almost certain. Of course, previous inoculation against typhoid or paratyphoid to a large extent invalidates the Widal test and no reliance can be placed on the results of a single examination in such persons.

The subdivision of many of the salmonella species by specific bacteriophages into a number of 'phage' types has been of great assistance in tracing the exact source of the epidemic. This has led to greater precision in attributing cases to a particular carrier. Typing may also be of value in indicating the place in the United Kingdom or abroad from which infection has come.

Where a number of cases occurs in a district, the practitioner will usually be informed by the local Medical Officer of Health, and co-operation with him in attempts to investigate the source of the epidemic will be of the greatest benefit. The practitioner is in a favourable situation for seeing *formes frustes* examples of infection and he should bear in mind the fact that many of the illnesses, especially of paratyphoid fever, are mild; diarrhoea may never occur and many cases masquerade as influenza, tonsillitis or bronchitis. In his daily practice, too, he should insist on the boiling of water and milk and in the avoidance of all foods eaten in a raw or partially cooked state. A campaign against flies should be instituted, and here the use of gammexane sprays and dicophane (DDT) play an important part.

Immunization. TAB vaccine (either phenolized or acetone-treated) usually contains in each ml. 1,000 millions of *S. typhi* and 500 millions each of *S. paratyphi A* and *B*. Cholera is often included in the vaccine (TABC) and this is a convenient way to immunize persons travelling to the East. The initial dose in adults is 0·5 ml. followed seven to ten days later by 1 ml.: 0·25 and 0·5 ml. may be administered to children between 3 and 10 years of age. A third injection of 1 ml. (adult) or 0·5 ml. (child) should be given one week later to persons who are going to live in an endemic area. The injection is given subcutaneously, and as systemic disturbance is liable to follow, any strenuous exertion should be avoided for 24 hours after each dose. Pulmonary tuberculosis, diabetes mellitus and chronic kidney or vascular disease are usually listed as contra-indications to inoculation, but when the person is to reside in an endemic area the risks of inoculation are less than the danger of acquiring the disease. The vaccine should not be administered during late pregnancy or during the course of an acute infection. The administration of a more potent vaccine intradermally (0·2 ml.) appears to be effective and to have fewer side-effects.

Protection is attained within two weeks of the final injection, and after lasting for some months gradually lessens over a variable period. When a person has to live permanently in an endemic area an occasional booster injection of 0·5 ml. should be given.

Curative treatment. *Chemotherapy.* Chloramphenicol may now be regarded as a specific form of therapy and should be given to every patient. For the best results early administration is desirable, although success may still be attained when the patient has already been ill for one to two weeks. The dose recommended is 1 to 2 g. daily for a period of 15 days—the long period being desirable to reduce the tendency to relapse. A high initial dose is unwise; it may precipitate a Herxheimer reaction in some severely ill patients. Treatment with chloramphenicol often produces remarkable improvement within 24 to 48 hours, especially when begun early, but it should be remembered when treatment is started late that, in spite of the patient's well-being, ulceration of the bowel and muscular degeneration resulting from toxaemia are still present. It is, therefore, essential to maintain complete rest in bed for a period of two to three weeks, until healing of the ulcerated bowel has occurred. Relapses are common, but fortunately they often respond to ampicillin which should be given by mouth in the high dose of 4 to 6 g. daily for not less than 14 days. When patients fail to respond to this treatment, it is worth while to treat symptomatic relapses or the asymptomatic carrier state with trimethoprim sulphamethoxazole compound. Here again treatment should be for a minimum of 14 days. This is still under trial.

General management. The patient should be isolated and must be barrier nursed. The maintenance of hygiene in the ward is described on

p. 24. Enteric fever, like diphtheria, is characterized by a toxaemia which may cause serious myocardial degeneration. Complete rest in bed and skilful nursing are therefore imperative.

The mouth and skin require regular and careful cleansing, and precautions have to be taken to prevent the development of pressure sores.

Retention of urine is liable to occur and should receive appropriate treatment. Inspection of the stools, abdomen, lung bases and heart should form part of the physician's daily routine examination.

Diet. Although treatment with chloramphenicol usually produces clinical improvement, if ulceration of the bowel has occurred, time for healing must be allowed. Thus, during the first week of treatment the patient should receive a low residue diet, and this precaution should not be relaxed until the signs of intestinal inflammation have subsided. During the early days of the illness a fluid diet should be administered. The use of a 'composite' food such as Complan (Glaxo)—even if only for a part of the diet—makes it easy to ensure that the intake is adequate. Towards the end of the first week, in addition to 2 pints of milk daily, such readily digestible articles as lightly boiled eggs, custard, ice-cream, junket, cream cheese, milk shakes, milk puddings, jellies, mashed potatoes with butter or gravy, prepared breakfast foods, stewed apples, plain chocolate, thin bread and butter, sponge cake, and minced chicken or beef may be included in the diet.

Complications. As soon as the infection has been effectively brought under chemotherapeutic control, the symptoms and signs which were formerly dreaded—persistent diarrhoea, meteorism and intense toxaemia—rapidly disappear or are prevented altogether. Nevertheless, ulceration may still be extensive and perforation or haemorrhage may occur. Again, despite clinical improvement, organisms may persist in the stool. Relapse, as has already been indicated, is a common occurrence and may occur even after the 15-day course of treatment.

Haemorrhage and perforation (pp. 232, 233). The practitioner must be on the lookout for these serious complications, especially during the third week of the illness. On the first appearance of blood in the stools or a sudden drop in temperature accompanied by a rising pulse rate, 15 mg. of morphine and 0·3 mg. of hyoscine should be injected without delay. Further treatment will depend on the severity or persistence of the haemorrhage but

preparations should be made for blood transfusion.

A surgical opinion must be sought immediately if perforation is suspected, but conservative management with continuing chloramphenicol therapy is nearly always preferable to operative treatment.

Phlebitis. Thrombosis in the veins of the lower limbs is a common complication during convalescence. The affected limb is immobilized in a light plaster of Paris splint for two weeks, after which passive movements may be started. Paracetamol (1·0 g.) may be given to relieve the early pain. The use of anticoagulants is contraindicated because of the danger of precipitating haemorrhage from the bowel.

Other complications. Many different tissues may be involved during the stage of septicaemia. Thus, there may be evidence of one or more of the following conditions: pneumonia, myocarditis, meningitis, cholecystitis; and the bones and joints may also be affected (arthritis, periostitis and osteomyelitis). Early diagnosis and adequate treatment with chloramphenicol has greatly reduced the frequency and severity of these complications.

Periostitis or osteomyelitis must be treated on surgical lines. Material from a bone abscess may contain typhoid bacilli, and soiled dressings should be handled with care.

Convalescence. The patient should be kept in bed for about 14 days after the temperature has returned to normal. By this time the danger of relapse is usually past. Six consecutive negative cultures for enteric organisms must be obtained at two- or three-day intervals from stools and urine prior to the release of the patient from isolation. Chloramphenicol is not bactericidal and persistent excretion of organisms is common during convalescence. If the patient's work is concerned with the preparation of food, specimens of faeces and urine should be examined six weeks after discharge from hospital and the Public Health Department should maintain an interest in the patient for a year.

Treatment of carriers. As was emphasized in the discussion of diphtheria carriers, the carrier state often superimposes itself upon some preexisting chronic condition and this makes the treatment of the established carrier far from satisfactory. Unfortunately many chronic carriers are unaware that they ever suffered from the disease. In the case of a urinary carrier, a full examination of the urinary tract is desirable, for it is occasionally possible to rectify a coexistent abnormality. The faecal carrier state is often associated with chronic cholecystitis and, perhaps for this reason, is commoner in women; modern methods of anaesthesia have so greatly reduced the hazards of surgical interference that cholecystectomy should be seriously considered in such cases. The operative procedure should be covered by ampicillin for five days before surgery and for at least 10 days thereafter. Ampicillin may be given by mouth pre-operatively and by intramuscular injection for three days post-operatively if the patient is vomiting.

There is still no method which can be guaranteed to eradicate organisms from the chronic carrier. Assessment of cure is made difficult by the fact that excretion of organisms is usually intermittent and, even without treatment, negative results may be obtained over a period of a few months. For this reason at least 12 months of freedom from excretion are essential before a carrier is regarded as cured. Promising results have been obtained by the oral administration of ampicillin, 1·0 g. six-hourly, along with probenecid, 1·0 g. twice a day. The treatment must be continuous and persistent over a period of three months. Short-term treatment is valueless. Erythematous rashes due to ampicillin therapy are a common occurrence. These may disappear without discontinuation of treatment. Occasionally, however, the rash may be severe enough to warrant withdrawal of the ampicillin. Alternative treatment would then be with trimethoprim sulphamethoxazole compound which should be given for up to three months in a dose of two tablets (trimethoprim 80 mg., sulphamethoxazole 400 mg. per tablet) twice daily by mouth. The only satisfactory test of cure is the examination of faecal specimens for pathogens and this should continue until negative results have been consistently obtained for one year.

It is impractical to expect the chronic carrier to remain in hospital during this long period of treatment and bacteriological follow-up. He (or more frequently she) may be allowed home under the supervision of the family doctor and the Medical Officer of Health who will be responsible for obtaining further faecal specimens for bacteriological examination. Before his dismissal from hospital, the members of the patient's household should be immunized with TAB vaccine.

Finally, it should be emphasized that in Britain, where endogenous enteric fever is now uncommon, the most rigorous steps should be taken to eliminate the carrier state after an acute attack. A device which has great value in monitoring individual households or the community as a whole is the 'sewer-swab'. These can be inserted into the domestic sewer pipe or main sewers and after remaining there for a period of days are submitted to special bacteriological examination. They often disclose unsuspected pathogens.

ENCEPHALITIS LETHARGICA
(EPIDEMIC ENCEPHALITIS)
(See p. 404)

ERYSIPELAS

Erysipelas is an acute infection of the skin by haemolytic streptococci. It is a notifiable disease which should, as a general rule, be treated at home.

Curative treatment. Penicillin is the drug of choice. The dose is 1 mega unit (0·6 g.) twice daily and complete cure can be effected within three days. Complications such as lymphadenitis, abscess formation and the effects of massive oedema do not occur when adequate doses of penicillin are given during the first few hours of the disease.

Patients who are sensitive to penicillin can be treated effectively with erythromycin estolate, 500 mg. twice daily for seven days, or clindamycin, 300 mg. six-hourly by mouth for seven days.

GLANDULAR FEVER
(INFECTIOUS MONONUCLEOSIS)

Epidemics of this acute infectious disease occur in schools and institutions, and sporadic cases are common among the general population. It is thought to be caused by a virus. Although susceptibility to the disease appears to be almost universal, the degree of infectivity is not high. For example, cases of glandular fever can be treated in a mixed ward with no ill results. Fever accompanied by acute enlargement of the lymph glands, particularly of the neck, is the form of the disease commonly met with in children. Febrile and anginose types occur in young adults. A mononuclear leucocytosis is characteristic of the disease. The Paul–Bunnell sheep-cell agglutination test has proved a valuable aid to diagnosis; agglutination in a titre of 1 : 160 or higher may be regarded as diagnostic. Unfortunately, the test is often negative in cases which otherwise seem typical. The bacteriologist should be informed if horse serum has been administered, since this causes false positive results.

Glandular fever is not a notifiable disease. The incubation period is usually between five and fifteen days.

Treatment. There is no method of prophylaxis against glandular fever nor is there any specific treatment.

Management of the disease is on symptomatic lines. The antibiotics have some value in the anginose forms of infection because of their effect upon the secondarily infecting organisms. A period of three to four days' treatment will usually suffice. If an antibiotic is given it should be benzylpenicillin, phenoxymethylpenicillin or erythromycin. On no account should ampicillin be administered for the reasons previously stated (p. 16).

The patient should be confined to bed until the temperature has been normal for one week and the glandular swelling markedly diminished. The febrile type with high and prolonged pyrexia lasting several weeks requires to be treated on the same lines as a case of enteric fever.

Meningitis, epistaxis, haematuria and conjunctivitis are rare complications.

Convalescence. Recrudescences are liable to occur. The illness may be prolonged because of myocardial damage or by hepatitis. Rupture of the spleen is a rare occurrence. Even after mild attacks, anaemia and slight debility often persist for several months and the patient should return gradually to normal activity. When convalescence is unduly prolonged, careful haematological examination is desirable, for some cases of reticulosis have an onset similar to infectious mononucleosis.

INFLUENZA AND VIRUS INFECTIONS OF THE RESPIRATORY TRACT

Although it is impossible to compute their total frequency, virus infections of the respiratory tract are certainly the commonest cause of illness in Britain. The rise in the notifications of pneumonia during winter, the new claims for sickness benefit under health insurance and the deaths in persons over the age of 65 years reflect the prevalence of such infections. The appearance of a more virulent virus such as *influenza A* swells the figures. It is

certain that in every winter a number of different viruses play a part in the seasonal epidemic and this complicates the problems associated with the preparation of vaccines for active immunisation (p. 57).

People in all age-groups are susceptible to infection, but for those at the extremes of life the illness is particularly hazardous. Respiratory virus infection is not only more common in children under the age of five years but, in the first year of life, the illness is more severe. Indeed, simple involvement of the upper respiratory tract without evidence of pneumonia—what would in the adult be merely a 'cold' —can produce in the infant a life-threatening illness. Again, in the elderly, degenerative processes, especially of the heart or lungs, make pneumonia a more frequent and serious complication, and the same can be said for patients at all ages suffering from chronic cardiac disease or chronic bronchitis.

It is probable that the majority of the common respiratory viruses reach the mucosa directly from the inspired air. This has two consequences. First, since cellular invasion is direct the presence of humoral antibody is relatively unimportant, at least so far as the initiation of infection is concerned. This may in part explain why immunity to these common infections seems so poor, and susceptibility to reinfection throughout life so common. Secondly, virus multiplication in mucosal cells deranges their metabolism and may ultimately destroy them. The alteration to cellular physiology, however, is non-specific. The response of the cell is limited and this means that the signs and symptoms and their localization in the respiratory tract can be the same for a number of viruses. In other words the same virus may produce a variety of illnesses and a number of viruses may produce the same type of illness. This makes a very confusing picture for the clinician, especially as the number of viruses known to produce respiratory infection is continually increasing. The table lists some of the more important of these viruses but it must be appreciated that each family contains a number of different sero-types. Precise determination of the responsible virus on the strength of clinical signs and symptoms is thus impossible. Detailed virological examination is required and such methods cannot be applied in every case.

Some viruses are more virulent than others and more likely to produce severe disease or death. This is illustrated by the constancy of the behaviour of the *variola virus* in the unprotected host compared

TABLE 2

Clinical Pattern	Influenza A, B and C	Para-influenza 1–4	Respiratory Syncytial Virus	Adeno-viruses	Picornaviruses (Enteroviruses and Rhinoviruses)
'Febrile Catarrh' and 'Influenza' .	++	+	+	++	+
Croup	+−	++	+−	+	+−
Bronchitis and Pneumonia in infants.	+−	+	++	+	+−
Bronchitis and Pneumonia in adults	+	+−	+−	+	+−
Cold	+−	+−	+−	+−	++

with the relatively mild disturbance usually produced by *herpes simplex*. The appearance of new antigenic variants of influenza A virus (as in 1918, 1957 and 1966) can be responsible for pandemics with a high mortality. An important aspect of virus virulence is the speed of multiplication which permits extensive cellular destruction and the overwhelming of the host's defences. Thus, in infection by influenza virus a particularly severe pneumonia may be produced by the virus itself. But in the majority of cases, the appearance of complications can usually be explained by a superimposed bacterial infection. The pathogens involved are those which are present in the nasopharynx. The pneumococcus is the organism most commonly isolated, but in children, *H. influenzae* and in adults *Staph. aureus* should be thought of, for these produce the most severe illnesses.

Antibiotics have no value in the treatment of the uncomplicated virus infections. Unless there is evidence of pneumonia or other indication of bacterial infection they should not be used. The importance of bacteriological examination in such cases is stressed, for the micro-organism may prove to be resistant to the normal antibiotic of first choice, namely, penicillin.

The incubation period of most of these infections is short—one to two days. Influenza is only notifiable when it is complicated by pneumonia.

Prevention and epidemiological control. There is no method whereby the spread of infection can be prevented. Free ventilation and avoidance of crowds are clearly advisable, but since many people suffering from minor degrees of illness continue with their daily work, the prevalent virus is constantly present in crowded trains and buses, so that the avoidance of contact is virtually impossible.

Killed virus vaccines have a limited place in active immunization against influenza. A major difficulty lies in the fact that the various strains of influenza virus behave differently as antigens. Thus vaccines to be effective must be prepared from strains which are producing the current infections. As the Asian strain of 1957 is still the prevalent virus there is some justification for immunizing selected groups in the population if they are at special risk (e.g. doctors, nurses and the staffs of certain public services) or because of their known susceptibility to severe infection (e.g. persons with chronic pulmonary or cardiac disease). For adults a single dose of 1·0 ml. subcutaneously in October or November is recommended since adults may be assumed to have had some past experience of the virus antigens and the injection has thus a booster effect.

Virus vaccines have been prepared from adenovirus strains but their use in the general population is not recommended.

Curative treatment. *General management.* Ideally any person with a febrile upper respiratory tract infection should be isolated from the community in bed until the temperature has returned to normal. Unfortunately, mankind is not so tractable and the ability to 'carry on' is regarded as a virtue. There is no specific serum or drug treatment of proven value, so that the mainstay is efficient nursing and treatment of symptoms (p. 24). The nursing procedures that require emphasis are the hygiene of the mouth, nose, eyes and skin. For the relief of discomfort, aspirin will usually suffice. Troublesome cough is best relieved by the administration of a sedative such as camphorated tincture of opium. Cyanosis is usually a sign of pneumonia and an indication for oxygen (p. 644).

Antibiotics. The response of post-influenzal pneumonia to chemotherapy is often unsatisfactory. At least part of the explanation for this is that in severe infections there is extensive damage to the mucosa of the upper respiratory tract and bacterial superinfection is correspondingly great. Two pathogens which have already been mentioned—*H. influenzae* and *Staph. aureus*—are particularly dangerous secondary invaders and their prompt detection warrants bacteriological examination of the sputum from patients with pneumonia during influenza virus epidemics. Tetracycline (2·0 g. during the first 12 hours) is advised as the antibiotic of first choice while bacteriological results are awaited. There is often scope for the use of either ampicillin (p. 15) or chloramphenicol (p. 11) in *H. influenzae* infections; the isolation of *Staph. aureus* will call for substantial doses of penicillin (p. 2) if the organism is non-penicillinase producing, or a cloxacillin (p. 6) if it is penicillinase-producing. Staphylococcal infections which fail to respond to these lines of treatment warrant the use of cephaloridine, cephalexin or clindamycin, the last two drugs having the advantage of being given by mouth (pp. 18 and 8).

In fulminating cases two dangers must be emphasized. In some the haemorrhagic pulmonary secretion is so profuse that the patient cannot rid himself of it quickly enough and is in danger of suffocation. In others the extensive ulceration of trachea and bronchi results in desiccation with extensive crusting. These patients can be successfully managed by tracheostomy, removal of secretions by suction, nursing in a highly humid atmosphere or even by the use of a mechanical respirator.

Other complications. Pyogenic complications may arise in the paranasal sinuses or middle ear. In this event there is less urgency in beginning treatment, and a bacteriological examination which includes sensitivity testing of any pathogens isolated should precede the onset of treatment. The antibiotic to be used may then be chosen with some precision. Toxic myocarditis must always be borne in mind, especially in the older patient.

Convalescence. The importance of an adequate period of convalescence after influenza must be impressed particularly upon the older patient. Owing to the toxic effect of influenza on the myocardium it is wise even in the mildest case to advise

rest in bed for at least three days after the temperature has settled. This applies particularly to those over the age of 35 years. In more severe attacks this period should be extended to one to two weeks. The response of the heart to increased exertion must be carefully watched, and a further rest enforced if this be unsatisfactory. Cough due to tracheitis is sometimes very persistent, but is usually relieved to some extent by the administration of a teaspoonful thrice daily of either elixir of methadone or camphorated tincture of opium. Infected nasal sinuses may be the exciting factor and should receive appropriate treatment.

MEASLES
(MORBILLI)

The measles virus is commonly spread by direct contact (droplet infection), particularly during the catarrhal stage of the illness, a stage at which measles is seldom diagnosed. Except for those who have previously suffered from the disease, susceptibility to measles appears to be practically universal. Although measles is always to be regarded seriously, it only constitutes a significant threat in the first 18 months of life when the complicating bronchopneumonia is a dangerous hazard.

In certain areas the first case of measles occurring in a household has to be notified to the Medical Officer of Health. Otherwise the disease is not notifiable. The incubation period is usually from nine to 11 days, but may vary from seven to 14 days.

Preventive treatment. *Passive immunization.* An attack of measles can be prevented or modified by the intramuscular injection of an appropriate dose of gamma globulin in the early stages of incubation. The dose of gamma globulin cannot be gauged with great accuracy because the content of antibody is variable and there are minor variations in its preparation. For the child between 1 and 3 years of age the dose should be from 250 to 750 mg. When given during the first few days of the incubation period such a dose will usually give complete protection, but when this is not attained, at least the subsequent attack is reduced in severity. The use of gamma globulin should be restricted to contacts under the age of 18 months or children who are seriously debilitated, for example, after recovery from whooping-cough or pneumonia.

Active immunization. Both a killed and a live attenuated virus vaccine are now available. The immunity obtained by using the killed vaccine is of relatively short duration and a proportion of those inoculated with it acquire the disease at a subsequent exposure; and there is the likelihood that an allergic state will develop. Killed vaccines are, therefore, not recommended. The live attenuated virus vaccine produces a satisfactory immunity which certainly lasts for some years. The vaccine is freeze-dried and reconstituted with 1·0 ml. of sterile distilled water before use. The injection is given subcutaneously. A proportion of the children inoculated (from 15 to 25 per cent.) develop moderately severe febrile reactions about a week after injection, while a few show evidence of a mild attack of measles.

At present vaccine is used mainly in those countries where the mortality from measles is high. In other communities where there are adequate standards of child health and where malnutrition is rare, measles is seldom a dangerous infection and prophylaxis by mass vaccination is hardly justifiable. Selective immunization, for example, of susceptible groups, such as young children in residential homes or of weakly infants, is a valuable measure.

General measures. Contacts who have not previously suffered from measles are usually excluded from school for three weeks from the date of onset of the last case in the house. No restrictions need be applied to children who have previously suffered from measles. When measles is prevalent, susceptible children should not attend parties, the cinema or other gatherings. The need to prevent exposure of children under 18 months of age should be stressed.

Curative treatment. *General management.* Isolation of the child at home is desirable although by the time the diagnosis is made the other children will usually have been infected. Since the main danger arises from secondary bacterial infection, isolation will reduce the chances of such infection from without. The nursing of the child calls for no special measures apart from attention to the eyes, nose and mouth. In the early stages photophobia is often troublesome and makes screening of strong light desirable. When there is much conjunctivitis and blepharitis, gentle cleansing with warm saline is useful and, after cleansing, the lids should be smeared with petroleum jelly to prevent sticking. The conjunctivitis usually clears in two to three days; if it persists, the possibility of corneal ulceration should be considered. So far as the nose and mouth

are concerned all that is required is frequent and gentle cleansing.

Tracheitis and laryngitis usually resolve quickly without treatment. In the young child or the adult they may give rise to more difficulty—in the former from partial obstruction of the airway and in the latter because of substernal pain from coughing. Inhalation of steam with Friar's balsam is usually effective in relieving the child although occasionally tracheostomy is required. In the adult camphorated tincture of opium or the elixir of methadone should be prescribed.

Prophylactic chemotherapy. Antibiotics have no therapeutic effect upon the virus stage of the infection. The patient is at risk only from secondary bacterial complications during the time that mucosal damage is being produced by virus. Once this period is past, convalescence is usually straightforward. Although the administration of antibiotics prophylactically as a routine during the early catarrhal stage might seem desirable it is not recommended. With the form of measles now prevalent complications occur in a small proportion of cases and should be treated as they arise. Benzylpenicillin by injection or phenoxymethylpenicillin by mouth are effective in most cases as the commonest pathogens are *Str. pyogenes* and pneumococcus.

Complications. *Bronchopneumonia.* Bronchopneumonia is the most serious complication. Benzylpenicillin, given intramuscularly, should be the antibiotic of first choice and, when this treatment proves effective, it is often possible to change to oral preparations (p. 5).

A mild degree of *laryngitis* is a common early symptom in measles. As a general rule during the catarrhal stage this is of virus origin and improves as the rash appears. When laryngitis arises *after* the appearance of the rash the possibility of diphtheritic infection should be kept in mind. If the child has not been immunized, a dose of 32,000 units of diphtheria antitoxin is desirable. Further treatment should be on the lines detailed on p. 193.

In the same way, *gastroenteritis* may be expected during the catarrhal or early rash stage as a natural part of the disease; its occurrence, thereafter, should raise the immediate suspicion of dysentery. The possibility of acute appendicitis should not be forgotten.

Infection of the middle ear cleft is perhaps the most important complication as its careless management may leave the child with a chronic suppurative otitis media. Thus inspection of the tympanic membranes is an important part of the final clinical examination. Bacteriological examination of any aural discharge is essential so that an appropriate antibiotic—given systemically—may be chosen.

Acute encephalitis can occur with this as with other virus infections. Although a severe infection is not common, recent studies have indicated that mild encephalitis occurs much more frequently than was previously suspected. Indeed the remote possibility of encephalitis is one of the reasons for caution in the use of live measles virus vaccine.

Convalescence. In an uncomplicated case the child may be allowed out of bed about the fifth to seventh day from the onset of the disease, and out of isolation on the tenth day.

MENINGOCOCCAL INFECTIONS[1]

Acute meningeal involvement must be regarded as only one form of meningococcal infection. Two other syndromes—acute fulminating septicaemia often with adrenal haemorrhage (Waterhouse-Friderichsen syndrome, p. 302) and chronic septicaemia usually unaccompanied by meningitis—are likely to be seen during epidemic periods. The practitioner should have them especially in mind during the first and last two months of the year when the annual prevalence is at its height. For the recognition of both, the first essential is to remember the possibility of their occurrence; the features are sufficiently definite to permit a clinical diagnosis with a fair degree of accuracy. Although uncommon, attention is drawn to their existence, for in one—chronic septicaemia—correct treatment achieves rapid cure and may, in some cases, prevent subsequent meningitis; while, in the other, only the most rapid diagnosis and immediate institution of proper measures hold out any possibility of recovery (p. 302). The whole course from onset to death of a case of acute septicaemia with suprarenal haemorrhage may take but a few hours. In many fulminant cases of meningitis, too, the extensive nature of the skin haemorrhages suggests the possibility of suprarenal damage; these cases should receive the appropriate treatment described below.

Such a concept of meningococcal infection is important because it draws attention to the mode of access of the meningococcus to the meninges. This route is—nasopharynx, blood stream, choroid plexus, meninges. Every case of meningococcal meningitis should be regarded as blood-borne. Treatment must thus be aimed not solely at the meninges but also at a systemic infection.

Meningococcal infections are notifiable. The incubation period is from three to seven days.

Prevention and epidemiological control. Carriers play an important part in the spread of the disease, and because of this it used to be regarded as valuable to search for carriers on the occurrence of a case. A simple routine examination of the nasopharynx on a single occasion may well fail to isolate the organism, although repeated examinations will often succeed. Indeed, in some carefully conducted studies it has been shown that practically all of the contacts were carrying the organism. This is especially the case in closed or semi-closed communities. Search for carriers has, therefore, been abandoned as a method of control. Fortunately, in the general population, case-to-case infection is not common and it is unusual to see more than one case in a household. In dormitories or army barracks the living quarters and the recreational accommodation should be reviewed. Measures for the control of dust such as wet-sweeping or oiling of floors are useful. The danger of overcrowded sleeping quarters and lecture halls is due to the periodic disturbance of dust by movement as well as to overcrowding. Good ventilation is thus of great importance. It is possible that minor upper respiratory tract infections assist in the spread of meningococci, and in army camps, after a case has occurred, patients suffering from such complaints should be closely examined—especially if there is fever or headache.

The giving of sulphonamides to contacts is now probably of limited value as studies have shown that many carriers of meningococci harbour sulphonamide-resistant organisms. A few penicillin-resistant strains are also found but this is not yet a problem in this country and the degree of penicillin resistance is relative. A course of phenoxymethylpenicillin in a dose of 500 mg. six-hourly for 10 days should eradicate the organisms. If the patient is sensitive to penicillin, erythromycin estolate, 500 mg. twice daily for 10 days, is a suitable alternative.

Where the disease is epidemic in a community, it is well to remember that the highest attack rate is upon the child population under five years. The practitioner should take every opportunity to reinforce the advice given at these times by the

[1] All manifestations of infection by the meningococcus in Great Britain are notifiable under the general title 'meningococcal infections'.

Medical Officer of Health through the press. Crowded places should be avoided; and the danger of sleeping in overcrowded and badly ventilated rooms must be emphasized.

MENINGOCOCCAL MENINGITIS
(CEREBROSPINAL FEVER; SPOTTED FEVER)

Curative treatment. The first essential, when meningitis is suspected, is to perform a lumbar puncture. The presence of acute bacterial infection will immediately be declared by the appearance of a turbid or frankly purulent fluid. The spun sediment of the CSF is then strained by Gram's method. The characteristics of any bacteria present will often indicate whether or not intrathecal therapy is necessary. For example, meningococci will show as Gram-negative diplococci. If they are present there are some authorities who believe that small doses of benzylpenicillin (not exceeding 20,000 units in 10 ml. of saline for the adult) given daily intrathecally for the first five days of the illness will influence the progress of the disease significantly. The immediate treatment is 1,000,000 units (0·6 g.) of benzylpenicillin given intramuscularly and a similar dose is administered at two- to four-hourly intervals, depending on the severity of the infection. The author considers that intensive therapy with benzylpenicillin alone is curative.

An alternative which is preferred by some clinicians is to give sulphadimidine by mouth in the doses recommended in the B.N.F. (initial dose 3 g.; subsequent doses up to 6 g. daily in divided doses). It is clearly possible to combine these methods of treatment, supplementing penicillin therapy with the oral administration of sulphadimidine. Sulphonamides must *never* be injected intrathecally. Alternatively, if a patient is known to react adversely to penicillins or to sulphonamides or both, cephaloridine is another form of therapy that may be used (p. 16).

Dehydration is often present and in the most severe infections may require energetic treatment by intravenous infusions. This is of special importance when full doses of sulphonamides have been given. Vomiting is often a marked feature of the early illness and, when sulphonamides were the standard method of treatment, the reduced renal flow resulting from dehydration could encourage tubular blockage. This risk does not arise with penicillin. It is important, however, to estimate the urea and electrolytes at the start of treatment and, in regard to fluid replacement, to be guided by the results obtained.

The assessment of progress is as a rule straightforward and in mild infections the obvious improvement of the patient makes special tests unnecessary. The severity of the illness is declared by the shocked state of the patient when first seen as well as by the initial features of the cerebrospinal fluid. In the most severe cases the fluid contains a large number of organisms, easily seen in a direct film, with most of them situated extracellularly. The sugar content may be less than 10 to 15 mg. per 100 ml. In such cases a lumbar puncture 24 hours later is prudent. When treatment has been effective, meningococci should be greatly reduced and should be mainly intracellular; in the most favourable cases indeed meningococci may not be seen and the sugar content of the CSF has often risen dramatically and may even approach normal levels. When this is the sequence of events further lumbar puncture is unnecessary and the progress of the infection can be gauged by the normal clinical evidence of improvement. When the fluid is still markedly turbid at this second lumbar puncture a further intrathecal injection of penicillin is indicated, and the results of bacteriological and chemical examinations obtained as quickly as possible. When the expected improvement has not occurred the systemic dose of penicillin should be given more frequently and the sensitivity of the meningococcus to different antibiotics should be assessed urgently. Daily lumbar puncture in such severe infections will be necessary until the results make it apparent that chemotherapy is being effective.

Complications. Involvement of cranial or peripheral nerves may be expected in from 5 to 10 per cent. of cases. An unduly gloomy view of such complications is unjustified; a considerable proportion clear up satisfactorily, though blindness, often cortical in type, is usually permanent. Acute arthritis—a result of the initial septicaemia—often occurs after treatment has stopped. It rapidly responds to a second course of therapy.

Convalescence. The patient may be allowed out of bed towards the beginning of the third week of illness. A lumbar puncture should be performed on or about the twenty-first day; the best criteria of recovery are a normal cell count and a normal content of sugar in the fluid, which should be clear. The patient may now resume normal activities and a four to six weeks holiday should be advised. Adult patients frequently notice a general weakness for some time after their recovery; their relatives often complain of the patient's excessive irritability. Such changes, however, gradually disappear.

Chronic Meningococcal Septicaemia

This condition is particularly to be expected during epidemics. Unfortunately, blood culture, which is the essential method of diagnosis, is not always positive. The bacteriologist should be advised regarding the type of case from which the culture has been taken. A course of phenoxymethyl-penicillin for 10 to 14 days should be given in a dose appropriate to the age of the patient. Alternative treatments would be erythromycin or cephalexin if the patient is sensitive to penicillin. Thereafter the patient should be observed for a few days for the recurrence of fever, headache, or skin rash.

Acute Meningococcal Septicaemia with Adrenal Haemorrhage

(See p. 302)

ACUTE MENINGITIS DUE TO OTHER BACTERIA

Meningitis due to pneumococcus, streptococcus, staphylococcus, E. coli and H. influenzae is almost always secondary to some other focus of infection. These conditions call for vigorous treatment with both sulphonamides and antibiotics. Close co-operation between physician, neurosurgeon and bacteriologist is essential. Pneumococcal meningitis carries the most serious prognosis. The following are the main principles of treatment:

Antibiotics. Penicillin is the antibiotic most generally useful and is given systemically in a dose of at least 500,000 units (0·3 g.) every four hours. Intrathecal administration is usually essential, the dose being 20,000 units (12 mg.) once daily. The testing of the bacterium originally isolated for sensitivity to a wide range of antibiotics is very important, especially in haemophilus and staphylococcus infections. Frequent bacteriological control of the cerebrospinal fluid during treatment is essential. Cephaloridine, 1 g. six-hourly or eight-hourly intramuscularly, is a suitable alternative to penicillin in the management of pneumococcal meningitis and it will also be useful if gram-negative rods are seen in a direct film of the cerebrospinal fluid. Intrathecally the dose of cephaloridine is 50 mg. once daily for adults; for children

the dose is reduced proportionately (see also pp. 16-17). When the infecting organism is H. influenzae and chloramphenicol is contraindicated (p. 11), ampicillin should be given by intramuscular injection in full dosage (pp. 15-16).

Repeated changes of treatment unsupported by precise bacteriological data are to be condemned. While antibiotic therapy is progressing, a sample of the patient's cerebrospinal fluid can be tested in vitro for its antibacterial activity. This procedure provides quantitative information on the effectiveness of the treatment. As a general rule antibiotic treatment should be continued for 10 days.

Relapse, blockage, encephalitis and brain abscess. These complications are much more liable to arise from the organisms mentioned above than after meningococcal meningitis and must be kept constantly in mind. There must be no hesitation in performing lumbar, cisternal or ventricular puncture; any indication of rising intracranial pressure, especially in streptococcal infections, should raise the suspicion of abscess formation. Electro-encephalography is most valuable in confirming the presence of an abscess and in helping to localize it. The co-operation of the neurosurgeon is essential. (See section on Nervous Diseases, pp. 402-403.)

Tuberculous Meningitis

(See p. 74.)

MUMPS
(EPIDEMIC PAROTITIS)

The infective agent in mumps is a virus which is present in the saliva during the acute stage of the illness. Infectivity probably persists from the onset of the first symptom until the swelling of the salivary glands has subsided. Although the parotid is the gland most frequently involved, it is well to remember that the submaxillary or sublingual salivary glands may be exclusively affected and that abortive attacks of mumps, owing to the lack of facial deformity, may readily be missed. Indeed, some cases present with meningitis, and parotid involvement either does not occur or develops as a secondary manifestation. The occurrence of a lymphocytosis in the blood is of some diagnostic value.

Mumps is not a notifiable disease. The incubation period varies from 12 to 26 days, but usually lies between 17 and 21 days.

Preventive treatment. *Specific prophylaxis.* Although the prevention of mumps by the use of gamma globulin prepared from the blood of convalescent patients—as in measles—is possible, it should rarely be practised. No attempt should ever be made to prevent mumps in a child under 12 years. Mumps is often a severe and distressing illness in adults; orchitis—the most serious complication—occurs only after puberty.

General measures. Strict isolation of the patient is unnecessary. By the time a diagnosis is made susceptible contacts will have become infected. This usually results in a crop of secondary cases, but it is thought that many people acquire immunity from sub-clinical infection. Contacts should be warned to expect symptoms after an incubation period of 14 to 21 days. If the disease develops, the patient should rest and seek medical advice. Exposure to infection should be avoided by women in the early months of pregnancy though it has not been proved that the virus of mumps produces foetal abnormalities.

Curative treatment. There is no specific treatment for mumps. The patient should rest until the swelling subsides. Difficulty in opening the mouth and pain on mastication are indications for the restriction of the diet to fluids and soft solids.

Hot dry cotton-wool or hot fomentations applied to the swollen glands will help to relieve pain and local discomfort. The mouth should be washed out with a solution of glycerin of thymol or other mild antiseptic preparation four times daily.

Treatment of complications. Orchitis usually develops when the parotid swelling is at its height and may be expected in approximately 20 per cent. of males above the age of puberty. The patient may have a very high fever, may look toxic and be extremely depressed. He will need constant reassurance that recovery is the rule. The scrotum should be swathed with cotton-wool and the inflamed parts supported either by a pillow placed between the thighs or by a suspensory bandage. The administration of corticosteroids for three to four days diminishes the testicular swelling. An initial dose of 40 mg. prednisolone per day should be gradually reduced as the oedema subsides. Analgesics may also be required such as 1 g. of aspirin or paracetamol, and in the early stages of the illness 100 mg. of pethidine may be needed to allow the patient to sleep.

Abdominal pain and vomiting are usually due to pancreatitis. A hot bag or hot fomentations applied to the site of the pain may give relief. If the pain is severe, 100 mg. of pethidine may be injected hypodermically.

Meningeal symptoms are not uncommon in some epidemics, and, if severe, can be relieved by repeated lumbar puncture. There is no effective treatment for acute labyrinthitis, which is fortunately very rare.

Convalescence. In children, convalescence is rapid. In the adult, mental depression often retards full recovery and this may be the result of encephalitis despite the absence of florid signs. In such cases the return to normal activity should not be hurried.

POLIOMYELITIS
(Infantile Paralysis)

Poliomyelitis in its classic form is a disease accompanied by paralysis and more or less severe constitutional upset. In the great majority of cases of infection, however, the disease is non-paralytic and the symptoms are merely those of a transient febrile disorder (*formes frustes*). Ample proof of the occurrence of clinically unrecognized infection is provided by the virologist who is able to show the presence of serum antibodies (a sound index of past infection) in a high proportion of the adult population—often in people who are unaware of having encountered the infection.

The virus enters the body by the mouth, multiplies in the cells of the intestinal mucosa, and is excreted in the faeces. The central nervous system is reached by way of the blood stream so that viraemia precedes the onset of clinical evidence of involvement of nerve cells. The infectivity varies greatly, but it would appear that the faecal excretion of virus is greatest in the most severe cases. Virus is present in the stool of all paralytic cases, the excretion slowly waning over a period of eight to ten weeks. In about half the patients, stool cultures become negative in three to four weeks.

Poliomyelitis is a notifiable disease. There are three serological types of poliomyelitis virus, of which Types 1 and 2 seem to be the more frequent epidemic producers. The incubation period probably varies widely although in most cases it lies between seven and ten days. Paralytic disease may also be produced by ECHO and Coxsackie viruses.

Prevention and Epidemiological Control
Specific prophylaxis. Two varieties of polio vaccine are available:
(1) The first (Salk-type) consists of formalin-killed viruses of the three antigenic types. This

material is injected intramuscularly or subcutaneously in doses of 1·0 ml. The first two injections are given with an interval of four weeks; a third dose after a period of six months is an essential part of the immunization programme and, indeed, it is desirable to give a fourth injection a year or two later. The vaccines which are now available have undergone careful safety tests; they contain an increased quantity of antigen, and are very effective in inducing a measurable humoral immunity. The widespread use of Salk-type vaccine has been responsible for a sharp decline in the incidence of poliomyelitis in the United States and Britain.

(2) The second (Sabin-type) vaccine consists of live attenuated polioviruses. It may be obtained in monotypic form (most commonly used in North America or in tri-typic form (mainly used in this country). This vaccine is easily administered: the dose is dropped on a lump of sugar or similar vehicle which is then taken by mouth. The live virus infects the cells of the gastro-intestinal tract so that it is excreted in the stool for a considerable time after administration. Subsequently antibodies can be demonstrated in the serum.

Both vaccines, in their present form, offer satisfactory immunity. With the killed virus vaccine this immunity is purely a humoral one so that, although poliovirus is prevented from reaching the central nervous system, intestinal infection can still occur. For example, a child who has been protected from paralytic polio in this way may nevertheless become infected with polio virus in his intestinal tract. Such a child, not suffering from overt disease, is a potential danger to susceptible members of the community, and all the more so because he is thought to be 'safe', having been immunized. Further, with the passage of time, immunity might be expected to wane in the older person, who would, however, be less inclined to present himself for booster injections. Finally, there is the slight inconvenience involved in its intramuscular injection.

The live attenuated virus vaccine is free from most of these disadvantages. The simplicity of its administration has meant that large townships have been immunized in a carefully organized, one-day programme. In the face of a rising incidence of the disease this could permit the application of the vaccine very rapidly—preferably using a monotypic vaccine of a type not causing the epidemic— and indeed this method would seem to have been successful in halting the progress of an epidemic. It may be that in such conditions an 'interference phenomenon' comes into play; the bowel cells become infected with the 'tamed' strain and prevent the 'wild' virus from successfully colonizing them.

The fear of 'antigenic shift'—the mutation of low virulence to higher virulence strains during intestinal passage—would not, in the event, seem to have been of practical significance. There is some evidence that minor antigenic change occurs but, having regard to the very large populations that have been successfully vaccinated, there has been no indication of harmful effects. Some cases of paralysis have occurred in vaccinated subjects, usually in adults, which could possibly be attributed to the administered virus. Such events, however, have been of the order of one in several millions vaccinated and absolute proof that the vaccine virus was responsible has often been lacking.

There probably exists a place for both vaccines. If the 'quadruple vaccine' (diphtheria, tetanus, pertussis and killed poliovirus combined) could be produced free from side-effects, there would be much to be said in its favour. It would, however, be unlikely to contribute to the eradication of the disease. There is ground for believing that a really intensive world-wide campaign, using the live attenuated vaccine, would be likely to interfere seriously with the natural history of the virulent poliovirus. The vaccine of choice, therefore, is that of the live attenuated form—preferably administered on a widespread scale during the non-polio season of the year. The virtual eradication of poliomyelitis by community immunization programmes has drawn attention to the possibility that some other enteroviruses—particularly *Coxsackie A7*— may produce a paralytic illness. This should be borne in mind when a person who has been well immunized develops an illness resembling poliomyelitis and arrangements should be made for full virus examination.

General measures. By the time a diagnosis of paralytic poliomyelitis is made it may be assumed that infection has been well distributed among the immediate contacts. This makes effective control very difficult. There is, however, agreement that the patient must be promptly and effectively isolated and this is best done by admission to an infectious diseases hospital. Children who have been in contact with the patient should be kept under strict medical surveillance for a period of three weeks from the date of last contact. Adult contacts may continue their occupation providing it does not entail mixing with children, as in the case of nurses and school-teachers. They should, however, abstain from all social activities for three weeks from the date of last contact; kissing or playing with young children must be strictly forbidden.

Any form of strenuous activity should be avoided. A contact who suffers from a febrile illness or who complains of any symptoms suggestive of an abortive attack of poliomyelitis should be strictly isolated until recovery ensues. Rest in bed should be insisted on for a period of at least one week. During epidemics the practitioner should advise mothers to ensure that children are not over-active and that they secure adequate rest. A short period of enforced rest immediately after the midday meal is a sensible measure.

It is now accepted that certain factors provoke and determine the nature of the predominant paralysis. For example, tonsillectomy may be followed by a severe form of bulbar infection. During periods of prevalence operations on the nose and throat should not be undertaken. Intramuscular injections may be followed by considerable local reaction and this has been associated with paralysis in the limb used for the injection. Alum-containing vaccines have been especially incriminated and for this reason immunization programmes are often temporarily suspended during periods of increased prevalence. This risk should be eliminated by ensuring that polio vaccination is carried out early in life and immunity maintained by 'booster' doses. Pregnancy renders women more vulnerable to infection by poliomyelitis, and therefore in the case of the expectant mother immunization with killed vaccine is desirable. Finally excessive muscular activity during the period when the person is infected with the virus may contribute to the development of severe paralysis. Hence, during periods of increased poliomyelitis prevalence additional caution is justified in the treatment of any unexplained febrile illnesses, for these may in fact be minor reactions to polio virus infection. After recovery from such illnesses energetic sports should be forbidden for a week or two.

Curative treatment. Neither convalescent serum nor gamma globulin has any effect upon the course of poliomyelitis, for by the time a diagnosis is made the virus is in the nerve cells and beyond the reach of antibody.

General Management

The minor illness. It is easy to seem overfearful of poliomyelitis, and there is no doubt that few infections rouse stronger emotional reactions in parents. Since the symptoms of the minor illness are vague and non-specific—fever, headache, vomiting or nausea, pain in the back, stiffness of the neck, drowsiness or irritability with, in the more severe forms, muscular pains or weakness—the condition will be recognized only when there is either a history of contact with a case of paralytic illness or when the disease is known to be present in the district. In such circumstances it is wise to deal cautiously with minor febrile illnesses and to counsel complete rest. The severity of subsequent paralysis may thus be diminished, if not completely prevented.

The major illness. This may be suspected when there is extreme irritability, muscle tenderness or pain or obvious paralysis. Spinal and neck stiffness is usual in these cases: hence the patient either cannot sit up, or when he does so cannot bend forward to make the chin touch the knees. Unnecessary examinations should be avoided; careful observation will permit accurate diagnosis and the full assessment of paralysis can await the disappearance of muscle pain and tenderness. This pain and tenderness can be most commanding but may be relieved by continuous hot flannel packs. The affected limbs should be placed in a position of rest by means of properly placed pillows and sandbags and by the use of a cage to take the weight of bedclothes. When the patient is being treated outside of hospital, the advice of an orthopaedic surgeon should be immediately obtained.

When the shoulder-girdle muscles are involved, the possibility of interference with respiratory function must always be kept in mind. Careful examination to exclude diaphragmatic paralysis must be made. The patient should be asked to count from one upwards to see how far he can get with a single breath. The test can be frequently repeated and forms a useful gauge of diminishing respiratory control. It is important to differentiate between respiratory insufficiency due to lack of muscle power in diaphragm and intercostals and that due to obstruction of the airways by mucoid secretions from loss of the power of swallowing. These latter cases—the true bulbar forms—often present as respiratory infections or pneumonia, and their early recognition is of great importance. Here the immediate need is the establishment of adequate drainage, which is best obtained in the prone position with the foot of the bed raised. Suction of the pharyngeal secretions must be frequently carried out and every care taken to ensure a clear airway. Contrary to the common belief, these purely bulbar cases, when properly managed, will usually recover; the patient who is in greatest danger is the one in whom there is a combination of spinal and bulbar involvement, when the most skilled medical and nursing care is essential. All preparations must be made to maintain respiration (p. 651).

When all muscle tenderness has disappeared, simple splints (e.g. Cramer wire) should be applied under the guidance of an orthopaedic surgeon, who should, in fact, be called upon to assist in the supervision of the patient from the onset of paralysis. The limb should never be encased in plaster but should lie in plaster shells or padded Cramer wire splints made to the individual's requirements so that daily gentle massage and passive movements of the affected limbs may be supplemented by the local application of hot packs. There is much to be said for the institution of fairly vigorous physiotherapy as soon as pain and tenderness have disappeared. After an isolation period of three weeks, arrangements should be made to secure continued orthopaedic supervision and treatment preferably by transfer of the patient to an orthopaedic hospital. It is important to see that those patients who have been regarded as 'non-paralytic' are brought back for review three to six months later. Minor degrees of paralysis—especially of spinal muscles—may easily be overlooked during the acute stage.

The early period of the major illness is often regarded as a time when there is 'nothing to be done'. This is not the case. As soon as tenderness is gone, movement should be begun—passive if the muscle group is powerless but with assistance against gravity where minimal contraction is present. Movement under water requires less muscle power and can be started early. The patient may be trained in simple muscle contractions which will enhance the chance of recovery. In other words, activity should be encouraged as soon as freedom from discomfort permits.

ORNITHOSIS
(PSITTACOSIS)

Human infection with the viruses of ornithosis usually arises through contact with diseased parrots, budgerigars or other members of the parrot family, but the disease may also be contracted from infected canaries, pigeons, finches or fulmar petrels. The infecting agent, which is either a large virus or a rickettsia, is excreted in the bird's droppings, and the portal of infection in man is probably the respiratory tract. Human case-to-case infection has been suspected but not proven.

An acute febrile illness with combined typhoidal and pneumonic symptoms occurring in a person who is closely associated with parrots, pigeons, etc., is probably ornithosis. The diagnosis can be confirmed most easily by the demonstration of a rising titre of antibodies in the blood.

Ornithosis is not a notifiable disease. The duration of the incubation period is uncertain, but may be seven days or longer.

Prevention and control. The control of the importation of birds of the parrot family has not eliminated the disease. Many indigenous birds are infected and, in recent years, pigeons have been the most important single source of human infection. The handling and petting of even apparently healthy domestic birds is the usual means of infection and the possession of such pets may be an important clue pointing to the clinical diagnosis.

Curative treatment. Tetracycline is rapidly effective against infection with the ornithosis group of viruses. The dose is 2 g. daily, give by mouth at six- to eight-hour intervals, reduced to 1 g. daily as the clinical condition improves.

Although isolation need not be enforced, it is probably wise to regard the patient as potentially infective. Sputum, urine and stools should be disinfected.

RUBELLA
(GERMAN MEASLES)

Rubella is a virus infection, spread by direct contact and possibly by fomites. There is no information available regarding the conveyance of infection by carriers. Infectivity appears to be limited to the prodromal and early eruptive stages of the illness.

Rubella is not a notifiable disease. The incubation period is usually from 14 to 18 days, but may vary from 12 to 21 days.

Preventive treatment. This may be of great importance. If a woman contracts the disease during the first few months of pregnancy her child may experience a phase of arrested growth and suffer from one or more congenital defects including cataracts, deafness and cardiac abnormalities. The excretion of virus by the infected infant may continue for some months and this constitutes a serious hazard to a contact who may not be aware at that time that she is pregnant. Again, there is some evidence that convalescents from natural infection may continue to harbour virus in the nasopharynx for some weeks. In these circumstances our whole outlook on this mild disease requires re-examination. Fortunately widespread epidemics are not frequent, but when they do occur every effort must be made to avoid exposure of women who are in the early stages of pregnancy. It is generally agreed that, when the opportunity arises, children—especially young girls—should be deliberately exposed to rubella. This procedure calls for expert supervision lest the infected children should introduce the disease into a household where a woman, unknown to herself, is in an early stage of pregnancy.

Gamma globulin—either from rubella convalescents or from ordinary adult serum—has a useful place in passive immunization. If ordinary adult gamma globulin is used the dose must be large— 750 mg. to 1·25 g. It is very important to obtain a specimen of the woman's serum *before* administering the gamma globulin. The presence in it of neutralizing antibody proves that she has previously had rubella and there is no need for further anxiety. Should there be no antibody, she is susceptible and careful assessment of the situation is desirable. The circumstances may warrant termination of pregnancy.

In recent years clinical trials of rubella vaccines have been undertaken. Pre-pubertal girls between the ages of $11\frac{1}{2}$ and $13\frac{1}{2}$ years have been vaccinated in London schools. This selection was made because in this group pregnancy is extremely rare. A further group of post-partum women were vaccinated one day after delivery as they were less likely to become pregnant in two months following parturition than at other times. In general there is no reason why any girl over the age of one year should not be vaccinated. It is more practical, however, to vaccinate children at school, and boys as well as girls could be vaccinated during their school years. The dose is standardized for all ages: 0·5 ml. of a reconstituted freeze dried vaccine containing not less than 1000 TCID.50 activity is administered by the subcutaneous route only.

Curative treatment. Treatment is purely symptomatic. The patient, especially if febrile, should rest for a few days. During this time the rash fades. The diet need not be restricted. The only complication of any importance is polyarthritis in adults. It is uncommon. This condition lasts two or three weeks and is temporarily disabling. Complete recovery invariably occurs.

SCARLET FEVER

Scarlet fever results from infection (usually of the throat) with *Str. pyogenes*. It occurs only if the streptococcus produces the specific toxin in the host and if the host is susceptible to that toxin. The typical rash (and perhaps some of the other signs) is produced by this toxin, which is, therefore, often referred to as the erythrogenic toxin. Since there may be wide differences both in the toxigenicity and in the host-susceptibility, there is great variation in the severity of the clinical syndrome. Many mild cases occur which are liable to be missed and spread the infection. People who have become immune to the toxin are not immune to streptococcal infection. When they are infected, a streptococcal tonsillitis may occur, and such persons, perhaps even more than carriers, play an important part in the spread of the disease and render control virtually impossible.

Although infection very commonly occurs through the medium of the 'missed case', the contamination of animate or inanimate materials by streptococcal discharges is also of importance. Infected milk is a common cause of epidemics. In hospital wards, the dust may contain streptococci, and measures to reduce dust form an important aspect of control. After recovery, cases of both scarlet fever and tonsillitis which have not been specifically treated may continue to carry streptococci in the throat or nose. Nurses (especially midwives), teachers and others who supervise the supply of milk to schoolchildren should be subjected to detailed bacteriological examination after recovery from the infection and before return to work.

Scarlet fever has a short incubation period—from two to five days—and is a notifiable disease.

Prevention and control. *The Dick test and immunization.* A skin test, analogous to the Schick test, can indicate the capacity of the individual to deal with the erythrogenic toxin. It now has no more than historic interest for, of course, it gives no indication of the individual's susceptibility to streptococcal infection. Control, by means of penicillin, of all forms of attack by *Str. pyogenes*, is so complete that it is undesirable to commend the further use of the test, or the need to invoke an antitoxic immunity, whether active (by the injection of increasing doses of toxin) or passive (by the use in therapy of a specific antitoxin).

Penicillin. Systemic penicillin will clear streptococci from the throat and, in ward outbreaks in hospital, the spread of the organism is limited by this treatment. In such conditions, with the patient under control, administration of oral phenoxymethylpenicillin for seven days usually suffices to break the chain of infection. Tetracycline-resistant strains of *Str. pyogenes* have been isolated but penicillin resistance has not occurred. The bacteriologist should, therefore, examine all strains to exclude bizarre examples of resistance.

General measures. The patient must be promptly and effectively isolated. Children who are contacts should be excluded from school for one week. When the patient is treated at home—as he should be—some local health authorities still insist on the remaining susceptible children of the household being kept away from school throughout the entire period of treatment—an action made completely unjustifiable by our knowledge of the spread of the disease and the rapid reduction of infectivity by penicillin treatment.

A quarantine period of at least one week must be strictly enforced in the case of adult contacts whose occupation entails the handling of milk or other foods or close contact with children. Such persons can be rendered free from infection by giving penicillin in full therapeutic doses. Cultures of throat and nose one week later are almost invariably found to be negative.

If an epidemic of streptococcal infection is to be stamped out in a residential school or institution, a knowledge of the type of *Str. pyogenes* responsible is valuable, so that cases of haemolytic streptococcal tonsillo-pharyngitis and carriers of the specific organisms may be isolated. Bacteriological assistance is obviously very important.

Curative treatment. *Chemotherapy.* Penicillin therapy rapidly eliminates *Str. pyogenes* from the throat and nose, and this has two important results: it renders the patient rapidly non-infective and it lessens the risk of complications—particularly rheumatic fever. Oral therapy with phenoxymethylpenicillin is effective but, if streptococcal infection of the tonsils is to be eliminated, must be continued for at least seven days. A single intramuscular injection of 300,000 to 900,000 units of benzathine penicillin—according to age—is an effective way of ensuring that the patient receives

adequate penicillin coverage over the whole period of his illness. Unfortunately the injection is rather painful. When the initial illness is severe, treatment should be started with four-hourly intramuscular injections of benzylpenicillin; as clinical improvement occurs, treatment can be terminated with a single injection of benzathine penicillin. The important point in the administration of penicillin is that it must continue for seven days if the infection is to be adequately suppressed. When it is stopped too soon, relapse is likely to occur. Indeed, a possible disadvantage of the use of penicillin is its interference with the development of immunity.

Serum treatment. The effectiveness of penicillin is such that the administration of antitoxin is now unnecessary.

Complications. Otitis media, nephritis and arthritis are the main complications, for the treatment of which the reader is referred to appropriate sections of this book. Nephritis is now recognized to be associated with infection by a few special types of *Str. pyogenes*—particularly type 12. The complication therefore tends to occur in certain epidemics only. Rheumatic fever, on the other hand, may occur after infection by any of the serological types. Penicillin therapy reduces to a minimum all of these complications which may, of course, occur after apparently mild infections. This is a strong argument for treating all cases with penicillin.

Convalescence. If the condition of the myocardium and the pulse rate are satisfactory, patients with uncomplicated scarlet fever may be allowed out of bed on the seventh day of the disease, and in suitable weather into the open air three days later. The treatment of the complicated case in no way differs from that advised elsewhere for the particular complication.

Carriers

The mere presence of *Str. pyogenes* in the fauces or nose cannot be regarded as a reliable index of infectivity. Nevertheless, a rich growth of this organism from either the throat or nose of certain persons, e.g. dairy workers, nurses, doctors, schoolteachers, may reasonably be regarded as an indication for continued isolation until the carrier condition has ceased. A course of systemic benzylpenicillin in doses of 0·5 mega units (0·3 g.) per day for seven days is usually effective, but bacteriological confirmation is, of course, essential. If this fails, surgical appraisal of the condition of the nasopharynx should be advised. Antiseptic applications to the fauces and pharynx are worthless.

SMALLPOX
(VARIOLA)

Two distinct varieties of smallpox are recognized—variola major and variola minor. The latter was at one time endemic in certain parts of the country; the former is always imported from abroad. Clinically the two types can be similar, but whereas the death rate of major smallpox is around 15 per cent., that of minor smallpox rarely exceeds 0·2 per cent. The minor form is due to a smallpox virus of low virulence and the disease breeds true. Vaccination is equally protective against both forms.

The virus of smallpox enters the body via the respiratory tract by droplet infection. A patient's bed-linen becomes heavily infected and the air of the room becomes charged with the virus. His clothing and personal belongings are necessarily contaminated as the virus appears capable of survival for long periods in the dry state. It follows that isolation of the patient must be complete and thorough disinfection of all clothing and other articles in the sickroom is essential.

Smallpox is a notifiable disease. The incubation period is usually 12 days, but may vary between 10 and 14 days.

PREVENTION

The control of smallpox is essentially a public health problem. Diagnosis of the initial case or cases rests, however, with the practitioner, and herein lies a grave responsibility; he must be constantly alert to the possibility that a patient has smallpox when that patient has recently returned from parts of the world where the disease is endemic. Early diagnosis, followed by prompt isolation of the primary case, the immediate vaccination and continued supervision of all contacts, and thorough disinfection of the patient's house and its contents are the essentials of successful smallpox control. *The practitioner should not hesitate, therefore, to confer with an experienced consultant regarding any patient who in his opinion might possibly be suffering from smallpox.* The misdiagnosis of the initial case or cases as chickenpox has been the starting-point of almost every recent smallpox epidemic in Britain.

There can be no doubt as to the wisdom of promptly removing every case of variola *major* to hospital. During an epidemic of variola *minor* hospital isolation is desirable so long as accommodation is available. In the event of continued spread of the minor form, circumstances may justify or necessitate home treatment. These matters of policy are for the local Medical Officer of Health to decide, but when a case of variola minor is treated at home, isolation of the patient should be strictly enforced and every member of the household vaccinated.

After the removal of the patient to hospital every known contact should be traced as quickly as possible and subjected to vaccination or revaccination. When possible close contacts such as members of the same household should be isolated either in their own home or in suitable isolation units so that they may be more closely observed. Adult contacts, once they have been vaccinated, may continue their occupations but should be kept under daily surveillance. Intimate contacts who have never been vaccinated are especially at risk. Such persons will, of course, be vaccinated at once but should, in addition, be given a subcutaneous injection of 1·5 to 2·0 g. of hyperimmune gamma globulin (prepared from persons recently vaccinated against smallpox).

Chemoprophylaxis

The most significant contribution to the control of smallpox epidemics has been the discovery that methisazone (N-methylisatin β-thiosemicarbazone) exerts a prophylactic effect against variola infections. The drug is given in a dose of 3 to 6 g. per day on each of three successive days. In the present state of knowledge the contacts, of course, should also be vaccinated. Although the drug has toxic effects (mainly nausea and vomiting) it seems possible that these are less in those who are contacts; certainly these side-effects were less frequent under field conditions abroad than they were in some British trials.

Vaccination

In this highly effective method of prophylaxis against smallpox, introduced by Jenner in 1798, vaccinia, or cowpox, is inoculated into the human subject. Vaccinia is now regarded as a disease attributable to variola virus modified as a result of its passage through animals.

The National Health Service Acts in Britain

have abolished compulsory vaccination in infancy. It is, however, recommended that vaccination should be part of the programme for child immunization and carried out *after* the age of 1 year. Contraindications to this general recommendation are: failure to thrive, the presence of septic skin conditions, chronic eczematous or other manifestations of an allergic nature, the suspicion of hypogammaglobulinaemia or *the fact that the individual is receiving corticosteroid preparations.*

Fresh glycerinated lymph, which is issued in sealed capillary tubes, should be used. The lymph should be stored in a refrigerator. The contents of a tube, once unsealed, must not be kept for use on a future occasion. The lymph must be expelled from the tube by a rubber teat—such as that used on an infant's feeding-bottle; *the mouth must not be applied directly to the tube.*

The usual site for vaccination is over the insertion of the left deltoid muscle, but for aesthetic and other reasons the inner and posterior aspect of the arm or the outer aspect of the thigh or leg may be chosen. The skin should be cleansed with soap and warm water, wiped with ether and *dried carefully.* The multiple-pressure method is recommended. To perform the operation a drop of lymph is first expelled on to the cleansed area. With the side of the tip of a sterile needle firm pressures are made through the drop of lymph on to the underlying skin; the pressure exerted should be sufficient to mark the skin, but not to draw blood. For a primary vaccination 10 to 12 pressures are adequate; for revaccination 20 to 30 should be made. Excess lymph may be blotted off immediately and no dressing is necessary. This method has the advantage that it produces a minimal amount of trauma and, therefore, of local reaction and subsequent scarring. It probably does not give such a long-lasting immunity as the older scratch method, but the protection it affords is sufficient for most people in countries where the disease is no longer endemic. In smallpox contacts, where the maximum degree of protection is required, the scratch technique is used, with two applications at least 3 cm. apart. The point of the needle is drawn over the skin with sufficient force to break the stratum corneum but not to cause bleeding. The length of the scratch mark should not exceed 1 cm.

The duration of immunity to smallpox after primary vaccination by the multiple pressure method is variable. Good 'takes' to revaccination may be obtained even after the lapse of only one year. A distinction must be drawn between the results of primary vaccination and revaccination. In the former the resulting lesion does not reach a maximum until about the eighth day; in the latter the maximum evolution is reached on the third to fifth day. This more rapid response to revaccination is one of the arguments for continuing the practice of primary vaccination in early childhood. If such a person is exposed, he will respond to revaccination in the early part of the incubation period and thus be more likely to escape the illness.

Both of these reactions indicate that the individual was susceptible to smallpox and has now been rendered immune. There is a dangerous tendency in revaccination to regard no reaction or slight local reactions which reach a maximum in 24 to 48 hours as proof of immunity. Such an interpretation is unacceptable, for there may be three other explanations. First, the vaccination may have been unsatisfactorily performed; second, the lymph may be inert; and third, the individual may be reacting merely to trauma or to the vaccine lymph. The last may be excluded fairly easily by carrying out a control vaccination with heated lymph. The others can only be excluded by performing the vaccination at least three times; at the last insertion an entirely different site should be chosen. Such persistence is unnecessary in children. It is essential if the person is travelling to a country where smallpox is likely to be encountered and when an International Certificate of Vaccination is required.

In the event of exposure to smallpox, vaccination should immediately be performed unless there is reliable evidence of successful primary vaccination within the previous three years or successful revaccination within the previous five years. The important words in the last sentence are 'reliable' and 'successful'. In case of doubt, revaccinate. Owing to the risk of vaccinial encephalitis, slight as it may be, primary vaccination should not be performed in adolescents unless they have been directly exposed to smallpox; exceptions to this general rule are nurses and medical students—for the possibility of unsuspected contact in such persons is always present.

Successful vaccination within the first four days of the incubation period may prevent an attack of smallpox.

Curative treatment. There is no specific treatment for smallpox. The constitutional disturbance of the prodromal stage is treated on the lines already laid down (p. 24). The diet at this stage is limited to fluids, and water must be administered freely.

Neither the thiosemicarbazones nor any other chemotherapeutic agent influences the maturation of the rash of smallpox from the maculo-papular to the vesicular stage, even when treatment is begun in the pre-eruptive phase. The administration of antibiotics in adequate dosage may, however, be helpful in diminishing the amount of pus formation. The classical secondary fever caused by absorption of bacterial toxins may thus be reduced and scarring diminished. On the other hand, the patient with severe confluent smallpox goes steadily downhill— despite intensive chemotherapy—and may show evidence of increasing toxaemia, presumably due more to the absorption of tissue breakdown products and widespread destruction of the epidermis than to any bacterial effects.

General management. During the papular and vesicular stages of the eruption the regular application of calamine lotion (B.P.) will help to allay the skin irritation. In variola minor such treatment will usually suffice, for in this form the rash often aborts, secondary fever is usually absent and the prognosis is uniformly good.

Iced compresses applied to the face and distal parts of the limbs, and frequently changed, will be found comforting in the confluent eruption of major smallpox. Prolonged warm baths, spraying with a 1 : 40 solution of phenol or smearing the skin with petroleum jelly with 3 per cent. phenol are alternative methods of treatment. In children the arms may require to be splinted or the hands bandaged to prevent scratching. Chloral hydrate given orally may give some relief and facilitate sleep; morphine aggravates skin irritation.

When the pocks begin to rupture, the patient, if not too ill, should be given a daily bath containing potassium permanganate. The application of starch or linseed poultices spread thinly on lint will hasten the separation of the scabs, and subsequent rawness of the skin can be alleviated by the application of sterile zinc oxide ointment.

Owing to the presence of the eruption on the mucous membranes, the eyes, mouth, throat, nose and larynx require careful treatment. Drops of 20 per cent. sulphacetamide solution should be instilled into the eyes four-hourly. Simple ointment applied to the margins prevents the lids from sticking together during sleep. The mouth and throat must be cleansed at regular intervals. Frequent inhalations of steam, impregnated with Friar's balsam or creosote, help to alleviate laryngeal and bronchial symptoms. Dysphagia may be lessened by sucking fragments of ice.

The fluid diet of the prodromal period requires to be supplemented by soft solids during the eruptive stage. Fresh fruit juice drinks sweetened with glucose must be administered freely throughout the illness.

Complications. Severe laryngitis sometimes necessitates tracheostomy. Bronchopneumonia is a common and frequently fatal complication. Keratitis and panophthalmitis are liable to occur in severe cases, particularly if the eyes have not been carefully treated from the beginning. Myocardial damage is often present and strict bed-rest must be enforced throughout. Haemorrhage, especially from the uterus, is fairly common in female patients with smallpox, and may necessitate transfusion with blood or plasma.

Convalescence. The patient should be kept in bed until the eruption has crusted and isolation must be continued until the last crust has separated from the skin. This period varies from three weeks in mild cases to three months or longer in severe attacks. Detachment of the crusts can be hastened by warm baths and the application of starch poultices, olive oil or simple ointment. The thick skin of the palms and soles may be softened by frequent soaking in hot water, and the buried crusts picked out with a sterile scalpel. A thorough soap-and-water bath and shampoo precedes the transfer of the patient to a non-infected room in which he puts on clean clothes.

In variola minor and in mild attacks of major smallpox, convalescence is usually rapid and the patient is fit for discharge from hospital or isolation as soon as he is free from infection. He may return to school or business in two to four weeks after release from isolation, but after severe attacks, several months may elapse before the patient is able to resume his normal activities.

TETANUS

The normal habitat of *Cl. tetani* is the intestinal tract of horses, cows and other herbivora. The bacilli are sometimes found in human faeces. Heavily manured soil is particularly liable to be contaminated with the highly resistant spores of this anaerobe. Introduced through a punctured wound commonly made by a splinter or nail, the bacilli or spores—particularly in the presence of pyogenic infection, laceration of tissues or a foreign body—tend to multiply and produce the powerful toxin which acts on the nervous system.

Although the potential risk of tetanus following deep wounds is well recognized, the very real danger of infection following superficial septic abrasions in children or mild septic skin lesions in farm workers is not sufficiently appreciated. Imperfectly sterilized catgut has been responsible for the development of post-operative tetanus.

Early diagnosis is very important. Stiffness of the jaw, pain in the neck or back increased by manipulation and associated with the characteristic facial expression should lead to immediate specific treatment.

Tetanus is not a notifiable disease. The length of the incubation period varies greatly and the duration from the onset of symptoms until the appearance of definite spasms has a very important bearing on prognosis. An incubation period of less than seven days indicates a severe case. When the prodromal period is less than twenty-four hours death is almost invariable.

Preventive Treatment

Passive immunization is an effective measure, but it must be understood that the method has its limitations. First, it must be carried out at the time of injury. Delay is dangerous. Secondly, passive immunization lasts for only two to three weeks, so that the patient could emerge from his temporary cover before the incubation period has elapsed, though by this time florid tetanus would be unlikely to develop. Thirdly, and most important, persons who have previously received horse serum in some form may develop serum sickness; such persons are liable to eliminate the antitoxin more rapidly, thus reducing the period of 'cover'. To these factors must be added the doctor's natural reluctance to administer antitoxin when a wound is apparently trivial—yet such wounds may be infected by tetanus.

On rare occasions, when treatment of the patient is possible within a few minutes of his being wounded, intensive penicillin therapy suffices; the clostridia are annihilated and toxaemia is prevented. In practice, however—for a variety of reasons—delay of an hour or more is not unusual. The patient's best interests are served by assuming that infection is established and that toxaemia has begun. He should therefore receive an intramuscular injection of penicillin (2 mega units), tetanus antitoxin (1,500 units) and tetanus toxoid (1·0 ml.). When it is known that the patient is sensitized to horse serum and seroprophylaxis is imperative, hyper-immune human gamma globulin should be injected. Supplies of this material are still limited and it should therefore be used judiciously. The medico-legal implications of tetanus prophylaxis should not be overlooked.

Such ideal alternatives do not allow for the fact that more than half of the cases of tetanus occur as a result of trivial wounds which never called for medical supervision. To some extent this might imply the success of passive immunization. The most important aspect of the argument, however, is that it underlines the need for active immunization. If this is given first in infancy in the form of triple vaccine, repeated at 18 months and again at school entry (when only diphtheria and tetanus toxoids need be given) the risk of tetanus is reduced to a minimum. In such persons the correct treatment, when wounding occurs years later, is the administration of a booster injection of 1·0 ml. of tetanus toxoid.

Finally, when a first injection of toxoid is given at the time of wounding (as part of the active–passive immunization) all necessary steps should be taken to ensure that the family doctor is informed so that he may complete the course with a second injection six weeks later.

Curative Treatment

The management of a case of tetanus calls for considerable medical and nursing skill, and even under ideal conditions the prognosis is poor. If tetanic spasms or convulsions have already begun they will be precipitated by physical disturbance including parenteral injections and venesection. It is, therefore, imperative to obtain the advice and practical help of an experienced anaesthetist. The patient may become manageable only after general anaesthesia has been induced. A substantial dose of chlorpromazine should then be injected (100 mg. intravenously). Although thiopentone may be required, it is unwise for the physician to give this drug unless he is prepared to cope with laryngeal spasm by performing intubation. During the immediate period of drug therapy and throughout the following few days the injections of chlorpromazine must be continued in doses of 50 to 100 mg. intramuscularly four to six-hourly; up to

2 g. of the drug may be needed daily. If the use of chlorpromazine proves to be unsatisfactory, it is necessary to use muscle relaxants, such as tubo-curarine or gallamine, treatment which in turn necessitates tracheostomy, the insertion of a cuffed endotracheal tube and starting mechanical respiration. The general management is that of the unconscious patient (p. 385). An intravenous drip of glucose-saline is set up. Fluid balance and serum electrolytes should be reviewed daily.

Tetanic spasms and convulsions are due to the action of tetanus toxin that has become fixed in the cells of the central nervous system. Such toxin is beyond the reach of antitoxin, and little benefit can be expected from injections of tetanus antitoxin. Nevertheless, it is usual to try to neutralize toxin that may still be in the blood and other tissues. The dose should not exceed 40,000 units injected intramuscularly. The intravenous route should not be used in order to reduce the risk of serum reaction. As supplies of hyper-immune human gamma globulin become readily available, this material will replace horse serum and the risk of serum reactions will be eliminated. Penicillin (1 mega unit) should also be given intramuscularly twice daily for five days in an attempt to eradicate persisting *Cl. tetani* from the wound.

In many cases the causative wound can be identi-fied. Often this will have closed or there may be evidence of deep ramifications into the tissues to produce conditions which encourage an anaerobic situation. Whenever possible, the wound should be excised and freely opened and the opportunity taken to ensure the removal of any necrotic tissue or foreign material. The wound should then be left open, although every attempt must be made to prevent any further bacterial infection.

There is no doubt that the institution of such specialized methods has greatly improved the prog-nosis even in the most severe cases. The progress to recovery of such cases makes it necessary to point out certain features of tetanus that were previously not observed. First, during the acute stage, periods of pyrexia—even hyperpyrexia—are sometimes seen. This should be managed by leaving the patient uncovered and by the use of fans. Secondly, it seems likely that late toxic effects on other organs of the body—notably the heart—may occur. Con-valescence should, therefore, not be hastened. Finally, it should be realized that the patient who has recovered from tetanus is not necessarily immune. Since his occupation may expose him

to further risk it is important, when the stage of complete recovery is reached, to proceed with a programme of active immunization with toxoid.

The patient should lie on a sponge-rubber mattress with the bedclothes supported by a cradle. Isolation is not essential. Trained day and night nurses are necessary. Noise must be excluded, the sickroom darkened and nursing duties performed quietly and preferably at time when the patient is deeply under the influence of sedatives (p. 461).

WHOOPING-COUGH
(PERTUSSIS)

Whooping-cough, due to *B. pertussis* and *B. para-pertussis*, is one of the serious infections of early childhood; it is particularly dangerous in infancy. The incubation period is 7 to 14 days. The disease is spread by droplet infection, and it is most infec-tive during the early catarrhal stage. Among adults whooping-cough is seen occasionally in its florid form; more commonly the illness is trivial, but the patient may unwittingly spread the infection in the community.

Early clinical diagnosis, in the catarrhal stage, is impossible; but a paroxysmal cough in a child is highly suggestive of the disease. Bacteriological diagnosis is made by examining pharyngeal swabs—preferably obtained by the nasal route. Swabbing must be completed before starting chemotherapy; tetracycline rapidly eliminates the organisms.

Preventive Treatment

Active immunization. Vaccination either prevents the disease or reduces its severity. The effectiveness of the vaccine as an antigen depends largely on the method of preparation. It must contain the three specific agglutinogens of *B. pertussis*. Vaccination should be completed during the first three months of life. This is not the ideal time for obtaining the best response, but the disadvantages of early vac-cination are less important than the hazards of whooping-cough in infancy. If vaccination is completed at about three months, a booster dose of vaccine should be given when a child is a year old. Convulsions and, rarely, neuropathies have been reported as complications of pertussis vac-cination. During epidemics of poliomyelitis vaccination against pertussis should be discon-tinued. If there is a previous history of convulsions vaccination should be withheld; and if a child has

C

a convulsion after the first dose of vaccine, no more should be given. Pertussis vaccine is often combined with other prophylactic inoculations (p. 58).

Chemoprophylaxis. The administration of ampicillin in therapeutic dosage is justifiable when infants have been in close contact with a case and are first seen in the early stages of the incubation period. Although the tetracyclines are effective in reducing the severity of the attack when treatment is begun early, there is some reluctance to use them in infants because they cause discoloration of the teeth and bones. As ampicillin has proved equally satisfactory, it is the drug of choice in the first year of life. Treatment should continue for 12 to 14 days. Chemotherapy produces little benefit once the infection is well established. When the diagnosis is made after the paroxysms of whooping have begun, chemotherapy is justified only for the treatment of complications.

General measures. The public, and indeed the medical profession, must be made to realize that pertussis is now the most serious infectious disease in infancy. When contact has been known to occur, the child should be excluded from such places as nursery schools during a quarantine period of three weeks. The rigorous application of this policy can be life-saving.

Curative Treatment

Specific treatment. Ampicillin is effective in reducing the severity of the attack only when it is started early, that is, in the first 14 days of the illness. A suitable preparation is ampicillin syrup (B.N.F.) containing 125 mg. in 5 ml. Children up to one year should have 2·5 to 5 ml. every six hours and children of one to five years, 5 to 7·5 ml. six-hourly. Treatment should be continued for 10 days. Recrudescence may occur if treatment is stopped prematurely. Once the whooping spasm is well established, antibiotics produce little or no benefit and should only be prescribed for the treatment of complications.

General management. Even when antibiotics are used, reliance must still be placed on measures designed to lessen the severity of the spasm and to prevent pulmonary complications. Isolation of the child reduces the risk of secondary infection. It is seldom justifiable to insist on strict rest in bed and it may be unwise. Movement promotes aeration of the lungs and it is undoubtedly true that the occurrence of atelectasis is as much to be feared as bronchopneumonia. For the same reasons the sickroom should be well ventilated, and indeed, if the weather permits, an hour or so in the open air daily is beneficial.

Paroxysms of coughing often cause physical and mental distress in a child and his nurse or attendant must always be near at hand to give help and reassurance. With young babies, the old-fashioned method of throwing the child across the shoulder and smartly patting his back often appears to be helpful: it assists the expiratory phase of the cough and encourages deep inspiration.

The feeding of the infant and young child presents a serious problem. A feed should be given immediately after a paroxysm; and the interval between normal feeds should be reduced to two hours. The fluid intake should be maintained by means of a variety of beverages containing added glucose. Ice cream, variously flavoured, is usually acceptable. In hospital the help of the dietitian should be enlisted. A fluid intake and output chart is often necessary. Parents should be warned that in most cases of whooping-cough some loss of weight is to be expected.

If the paroxysms become severe and frequent, sedatives provide the only method of relief. Drugs normally used as cough suppressants are often tried but are generally ineffective. The most important point in using sedatives is to ensure that the child sleeps through the night; the hypnotic recommended is the chloral elixir for infants (B.P.C.); the dose is 5 ml. for children aged one to five years. Tincture of belladonna is worthy of trial in severe cases, but to be useful the dose must be increased until dryness of the mouth and dilatation of the pupil herald undue toxicity. A preliminary dose of 0·1 ml. three times per day may need to be pushed to 0·5 to 0·6 ml. for a satisfactory response.

There is an undoubted nervous element in the paroxysm. Quietness in the sickroom is essential; any sudden disturbance of the child should be avoided.

Complications. Collapse of lung, bronchopneumonia, convulsions and gastroenteritis are serious complications and a frequent cause of death in young children. Epistaxis and other haemorrhages, whilst of comparatively common occurrence, are not of serious import. Well-marked cardiac dilatation may occur in severe cases. Otitis media is not uncommon. Residual infection and persistent coughing may lead to bronchiectasis.

For bronchopneumonia, a broad-spectrum antibiotic such as cephaloridine or cephalexin is to be preferred, for many of the so-called broncho-pneumonias are in reality atelectatic areas with secondary infection by a variety of organisms. Chemotherapy has not produced such clear-cut benefit in the bronchopneumonia of whooping-cough as compared for example with measles.

If a child suffering from pertussis has a convulsion, the parents should give him chloral elixir (B.P.C.). In hospital the best treatment is to inject 0·5 to 1 ml. of paraldehyde intramuscularly, repeating the dose in 30 minutes if necessary. Recurring and intractable convulsions are a grave prognostic sign.

Convalescence. Fresh air and plenty of wholesome food are the essential requirements in convalescence. Care must be taken to protect the child against other infectious diseases. If circumstances permit, a change of air to the seaside or to the country may prove very beneficial, particularly in patients with a persisting catarrhal condition of the lungs. Cod-liver oil is a valuable supplement to the diet if the child takes it willingly. If iron deficiency anaemia is present, iron should be prescribed. The tendency of whooping-cough to reactivate a latent tuberculous process should be borne in mind.

The paroxysmal cough may persist for months in some cases, but the duration of the cough is no measure of the infectivity. The child gradually becomes less infectious from the time of appearance of the whoop; and as a rule may be regarded as non-infective four weeks after the start of whooping, despite its continuation.

ACUTE SUPPURATIVE OTITIS MEDIA

Infection of the middle ear occurs almost invariably from the eustachian tube, the only exception being introduction of infection from the external ear through a pre-existing perforation. Infections involving the naso-pharynx are predisposing factors. These should always be considered when treatment is being planned. The common infecting organisms are *Streptococcus haemolyticus*, *Staphylococcus aureus* and *Streptococcus pneumoniae*. The most important part of the management of acute middle-ear infection is to give an adequate course of an effective antibiotic for seven to ten days. Benzylpenicillin remains the antibiotic of first choice and should be given by intramuscular injection, 500,000 units (0·3 g.) six-hourly for the first three days, followed by phenoxymethylpeni-

cillin, 250 mg. six-hourly by mouth for the rest of the course (p. 5). Smaller doses will be given to children. In early cases this regimen will usually abort the infection and thus prevent rupture of the ear-drum. If the drum has ruptured the choice of antibiotic will be decided after the purulent discharge has been cultured and antibiotic sensitivities have been determined.

When the drum is intact the use of ear-drops containing a local anaesthetic—with or without antibiotic—is not recommended; and if the drum has ruptured the use of such drops may lead to mixed infections with organisms causing difficulties with antibiotic treatment. Following rupture of the drum topical therapy may be clearly indicated from laboratory reports. In these circumstances antibiotic solutions can be instilled; and such preparations as bacitracin with neomycin can be used in this way, although they are too toxic for parenteral administration.

Pain can be relieved by analgesics (p. 440) and patients often obtain further relief from the application of warm cotton pads. Nasal decongestants produce shrinkage of the naso-pharyngeal mucosa and are helpful in hastening resolution. If, however, the ear-drum remains full and congested and there is persisting deafness after ten days, myringotomy will usually be required.

Therapeutic failure in middle-ear infections is often the result of inadequate antibacterial therapy. In general practice a careless patient may omit to take the full and adequate course of the antibiotic; on transfer to hospital the disease often responds to the same antibiotic regimen if it is under continuous supervision. Persistent reinfection from the naso-pharynx because of underlying chronic adenoidal, tonsillar or sinus infection should always be considered if middle-ear infections recur. These underlying infections call for radical surgical management. If there is radiographic evidence of chronic mastoiditis, radical surgery will usually be required in order to prevent further exacerbations of middle-ear infection.

SPECIFIC IMMUNIZATION AGAINST INFECTIOUS DISEASE

The prevention of a wide range of infectious diseases by means of specific vaccines has been one of the most important medical achievements of the present generation. It is, therefore, disappointing to record that in many areas of Britain there is a lack of concern both by the public and the medical profession to ensure that all children are protected in this way against the relevant diseases. Before reaching the age of 15 months, every child should have undergone specific immunization which will almost eliminate the possibility of acquiring five serious infections, namely, diphtheria, tetanus, pertussis, poliomyelitis and smallpox. Furthermore, a state of immunity will have been created which, following appropriate booster injections, may be expected to confer life-long protection from these infections.

The age at which immunization should be started is about the sixth month of life. This age is to be preferred for several reasons. Firstly, in the early months of life the immunological response to vaccines is probably less effective so that by delay we may expect a more lasting immunity. Secondly, reactions are less severe in the older infant. Thirdly, the antibody response may be blanketed by the continued presence during the first three months of life of maternal antibody. It is true that for one of these infections—pertussis—it is desirable to attempt immunization as early as possible since maternal antibody is not transferred and the most severe cases and some of the deaths are encountered in the first six months. None the less, it is preferable that the immune state against the other infections should be made as solid as possible in view of their continuing danger throughout childhood. For these reasons a starting time of six months is advised.

The interval between injections is also important. A successful immunization programme requires *three* injections (Table 3). Between the first and second of these the optimum interval lies between six and eight weeks and between the second and third there should be an interval of four to six months. This can be achieved by giving triple vaccine at 6, 8 and 12 months of age. Such a course of injections ensures a good state of immunity which should carry the child through to school age.

Entry to school starts a period when exposure to infection is enhanced so that it is appropriate that immunity should be boosted at this time. This may be done either by an injection of diphtheria-tetanus vaccine plus a course of oral polio vaccine

TABLE 3

IMMUNIZATION SCHEDULE

Age	Prophylactic	Interval	Remarks
During the first year of life.	Diphtheria/Tetanus/Pertussis and oral Polio vaccine. Diphtheria/Tetanus/Pertussis and oral Polio vaccine. Diphtheria/Tetanus/Pertussis and oral Polio vaccine.	Preferably after an interval of 6 to 8 weeks. Preferably after an interval of 6 months	The earliest age at which the first dose should be given is 3 months, but a better general immunological response can be expected if the first dose is delayed to 6 months of age.
*During the second year of life.	Smallpox vaccination.		Although the second year is recommended for routine vaccination, in individual cases and if special circumstances call for it vaccination may be carried out during the first year.
At 5 years of age or school entry.	Diphtheria/Tetanus and oral Polio vaccine; or Diphtheria/Tetanus/Polio vaccine. Smallpox revaccination.		With the exception of smallpox revaccination these may be given, if desired, at nursery school entry at age 3 years.
Before 13 years of age.	BCG vaccine.		For tuberculin negative children.
At 15 to 19 years of age or on leaving school.	Polio vaccine (oral or inactivated). Tetanus toxoid. Smallpox revaccination.		

*If measles vaccine is used this will be the preferred age.

or by a repeat injection of triple vaccine containing diphtheria, tetanus and inactivated polio vaccine. It is unnecessary and perhaps undesirable to include the pertussis component at this time. Unfortunately, many children who arrive at school have been given no previous injections whatsoever. For these children the full course of primary vaccination—three injections at the appropriate intervals along with oral polio vaccine—is essential.

Smallpox vaccination is now advised in the second year of life because the likelihood of serious reactions is thereby reduced. Although exposure to smallpox in early childhood is most unlikely in European countries, primary smallpox vaccination at this age should be regarded as part of a long-term experience in which revaccination at least twice—at school entry and at school leaving—is a continuing programme. Primary vaccination of the adult should always be undertaken with caution in view of the greater risk of serious reactions. Foreign travel is now often undertaken as a part of later school and undergraduate life. Visits of unvaccinated persons to foreign countries are to be deprecated.

In general, it is unsatisfactory to conduct too many immunization procedures at the one time. Thus there should be an interval of four weeks between the injection of a dead vaccine (such as triple vaccine) and a live vaccine (such as smallpox or polio). Furthermore, when two live vaccines are to be given their administration should be separated by a similar interval.

So far as other vaccines are concerned, BCG should be given before leaving school. The age of choice varies but there is much to be said for making the 10th year of life the age for a Mantoux test to be carried out and for negative reactors to receive the vaccine before the age of 12 years. Measles is the next infection which is likely to be brought within the immunization programme. Since most infants under the age of six months are immune (from the presence of maternal antibody) and since the immunity conferred by live vaccine is likely to be more durable if it is not administered too early, the best age for beginning vaccination with live measles vaccine is 12 months.

Finally, all vaccines which are to be injected must be given in individual doses by means of a sterile syringe and needle. Although the risk of serum jaundice is not high in this country, this is no argument for not using aseptic techniques. Merely changing the needle for each person, with a syringe containing several injections, is insufficient to eliminate the possibility of transference of infection. The only good practice is a disposable sterile syringe and sterile needle for each person.

SERUM REACTIONS

Refined serums have greatly reduced the risk of serum reactions. The fear of causing anaphylaxis, therefore, should not make the practitioner withhold serum when the need for it is clear. For example, 4,000 units of diphtheria antitoxin are contained in a bulk of approximately 1 ml.; with such preparations, given intramuscularly, the occurrence of late serum sickness is limited to not more than 5 per cent. of the patients to whom they are administered. Nevertheless, in sensitive people, serum reactions do occur even with refined serums, and when large quantities of these are given intravenously the danger of anaphylaxis is very real. The reactions which occur may be divided into two main groups: (1) due to acquired or inborn sensitivity of the patient to foreign protein; (2) due to causes other than allergy.

Reactions due to serum sensitivity. Two main types of *general* reaction may be encountered, namely, (*a*) anaphylactic shock, and (*b*) serum sickness. *Anaphylaxis* is an immediate reaction, is of rare occurrence, but may prove rapidly fatal. Dyspnoea, cyanosis, loss of consciousness and a thin, rapid pulse are the most common clinical manifestations. *Serum sickness*, characterized by pyrexia, urticarial rashes, joint pains and lymphadenopathy, usually occurs from 7 to 12 days after administration. In such patients there is, as a rule, no history of a previous injection of horse serum. *Accelerated serum sickness* occurs three to four days after administration and presents a similar clinical picture. These patients usually have a history of a previous injection of horse serum. As has already been explained, these reactions cause a more rapid elimination of antitoxin and this point must be remembered when a sustained antitoxin level is thought necessary.

An intense form of *local* reaction is occasionally seen (*local anaphylaxis* or the *Arthus phenomenon*). A history of previous administration of horse serum, often within a comparatively recent period, is usually obtained. There is intense local oedema and haemorrhage, and subsequently, there may be extensive sloughing of skin and even of muscular tissues.

Tests for sensitivity. There is no entirely satisfactory test for hypersensitivity to horse serum, for the intradermal, scratch and ophthalmic tests are difficult to interpret and the results are often equivocal. The greatest reliance must be placed upon the answers to two questions, which must be asked of patient or relative whenever a decision is taken to give serum. They are:

(i) Has the patient at any time in his life been given an injection of horse serum?

(ii) Is there any personal or family history of asthma, hay fever, infantile eczema or food allergy?

If the answer to either of these questions is 'Yes', the possibility of hypersensitivity should be assumed and appropriate precautions taken.

Methods of administration of serum. When a decision is taken to give serum, the required dose must next be estimated. The decision in regard to dosage is important for it will to a large extent indicate the route of its administration: for mild cases or for prophylaxis, the dose should be small and the intramuscular route suffices; for severe cases, the dose should be large and the intravenous route is desirable. The rules for the administration of serum may, therefore, be given under these two headings.

Intramuscular route. The answers given to the two questions already stated will divide the patients into three groups.

(*a*) Answers to both questions—No. The injection of the required dose of serum is then undertaken. The patient should, thereafter, be kept under observation for at least half an hour. If nothing untoward has occurred in this period, there is no cause for anxiety regarding serious symptoms. Serum sickness, may, however, occur in this group some seven to ten days later.

(*b*) Answer to question (i)—Yes. The patient should be given a trial dose of 0·2 ml. of serum subcutaneously and observed for half an hour. Should there be no evidence of any general reaction in this period, the main dose of serum may then be given intramuscularly. Should there be any evidence of general reaction, a course of injections of 0·2 ml. by the subcutaneous route should be continued at half-hourly intervals until the assessed total dose has been given.

(*c*) Answer to question (ii)—Yes. It is in this group that special caution is required. Adrenaline (1 : 1,000 solution) and hydrocortisone hemisuccinate should be available for immediate use if a reaction occurs. A trial dose of 0·2 ml. of serum diluted 1 : 10 in pyrogen-free distilled water should be given subcutaneously and the patient kept under observation for half an hour. If there is no general reaction, a second injection of 0·2 ml. undiluted serum should be administered subcutaneously. If, after a further period of half an hour, no reaction has been noted, the remainder of the estimated dose can be given by intramuscular injection. Should any reaction develop, the remainder of the serum should be given at half-hourly intervals in amounts of 0·2 ml. by subcutaneous injection. A quick-acting antihistamine (mepyramine maleate, 100 mg.) should be given by mouth at least half an hour before the injections are made.

There is no doubt that it is with patients who have an allergic history that the greatest risk arises. *For this reason, it is of particular importance to ensure that allergic subjects are actively immunized against the two main toxic diseases, diphtheria and tetanus, for which antitoxic serum is used.* When passive immunization must be undertaken in such persons the possibility of using a hyper-immune human gamma globulin should be considered. Limited supplies are available for use against tetanus and smallpox.

Intravenous route. Three points deserve acceptance as *absolute rules*. Firstly, no patient should receive an intravenous dose of serum as a preliminary step in treatment; an intravenous injection must *always* be preceded by an intramuscular injection which has been given at least half an hour, and preferably one hour, previously. Secondly, when an intravenous injection is to be given, the doctor must charge a syringe with 1 ml. of a 1 : 1,000 solution of adrenaline before beginning the injection of serum. Hydrocortisone hemisuccinate should also be available. Thirdly, an intravenous injection of serum should never be given to a patient who has a history of asthma or other allergic disorder, or who has shown a reaction to the trial doses described above.

Serum for intravenous injection should be gently warmed by standing the ampoules in hot water for a few minutes. It should be injected very slowly through a fine needle. The doctor must be prepared to stop the injection immediately if there is any evidence of distress such as a short unproductive cough or cyanosis. In such an event adrenaline must be administered intramuscularly at once.

The above regimen has been described somewhat dogmatically, because it is felt that it should constitute a regular habit. Confidence in the practice of so-called desensitization is unwarranted. There is no ground for the belief that a person can be effectively desensitized with two or three injections. The ritual merely creates a false sense of security. The system of trial injections suggested is an adequate safeguard against dangerous reactions; and the methods described are recommended as a standard practice.

Treatment of reactions. As already stated adrenaline (1 : 1,000), 0·5 ml. to 1 ml., and hydrocortisone hemisuccinate (100 mg.) are the standard remedies for anaphylactic reactions. The adrenaline should be given intramuscularly. *After* the adrenaline has been given 100 mg. of hydrocortisone hemisuccinate is injected intravenously. If the heart has stopped, cardio-pulmonary resuscitation must be started at once (pp. 97, 643). Serum sickness can be very upsetting to the patient, although not itself dangerous. Here again adrenaline is indicated; 0·25 to 0·5 ml. should be injected every few hours to abolish urticaria and relieve itching. The irritable rash may also be soothed by calamine lotion to which phenol (2·5 per cent.) may be added for its antipruritic effect. Aspirin, 300 mg. to 1 g., usually relieves the joint pains and general malaise. Antihistamine drugs are worthy of trial, but they act only by preventing *further* acute exacerbations. Corticosteroid therapy has an obvious place in the management of such reactions when they are severe, but this is no justification for using corticosteroids routinely.

Reactions not due to allergy. *Vasovagal attacks.* Very rarely the patient may collapse when the needle is introduced into the skin. The patient is suffering from a 'faint' or vasovagal attack, as recognized by the pallor of the face, bradycardia, weak pulse and low blood pressure. Treatment consists of lowering the patient's head to improve the circulation to the medulla. Occasionally it may be necessary to inject 5 mg. of metaraminol bitartrate intramuscularly. Measures described for the treatment of shock may also be indicated.

Thermal reactions. These reactions occur within 30 to 90 minutes of the injection of serum, and can be recognized by the presence of chill (rigor or shivering), rise in temperature, malaise and sometimes nausea and vomiting. The rigor is followed by sweating. Thermal reactions usually occur in those who have been given serum intravenously.

The chances of a thermal reaction are greatly reduced (1) if disposable apparatus (syringe, tubing or needles) is used for the injection of the serum; (2) if refined and concentrated serum is employed, for experience has shown it to be free from thermogenic substances; (3) if serum is administered very slowly.

During the stage of chill the patient should be kept warm with hot blankets and hot bottles. Hot fluids should be given along with 1 g. of aspirin repeated, if necessary, in one hour. If the temperature rises excessively, tepid sponging is often beneficial.

Further Reading

CHRISTIE, A. B. (1969). *Infectious Diseases: Epidemiology and Clinical Practice*. Edinburgh: Livingstone.
British Medical Bulletin (1969). Immunization against infections diseases. **25**, 2.

TABLE 4

DRUG THERAPY IN INFECTIOUS DISEASES

SUMMARY OF RECOMMENDED TREATMENT

Disease	Specific therapy (*drug of choice)	Symptomatic measures	Is prevention practicable? (general measures)	Passive immunization possible?	Active immunization possible?
(A) Bacillary Infections					
Anthrax (p. 28).	*Penicillin. Tetracyclines. Cephaloridine.	Local dressings.	Yes.	No.	Yes (see text).
Diphtheria (p. 29).	*Antitoxin. Penicillin. Erythromycin. Clindamycin.	Sedatives (barbiturates). Analgesics (morphine) (p. 440).	Yes.	Yes.	Yes.
Dysentery, bacillary (p. 33).	Streptomycin. Neomycin.	Opium. Belladonna, see text.	Yes (difficult in practice).	No.	No.
Enteric Fevers (p. 34).	*Chloramphenicol. Ampicillin. Trimethoprim/ sulpha.	See text (p. 36).	Yes (difficult in practice).	No.	Yes.
Erysipelas (p. 37).	*Penicillin. Erythromycin. Cephalexin. Clindamycin.	Analgesic/ Antipyretics (aspirin). Cold compress locally.	No.	No.	No.
Meningococcal Meningitis (p. 43).	Penicillin. Cephaloridine.	Analgesics. Hypnotics. Corticosteroids.	No.	No.	No.
Ornithosis (? rickettsial) (p 48).	*Tetracyclines. Chloramphenicol. Penicillin.	Analgesics. Sedatives.	Yes.	No.	No.
Scarlet Fever (p. 49).	*Penicillin. Erythromycin. Antitoxin (only if toxaemia severe). Cephalexin.	Analgesic/ Antipyretics. Cold cream is antipruritic.	Yes (Chemo-prophylaxis with penicillin).	Yes (never used).	No.
Tetanus (p. 53).	Antitoxin (limited value). Penicillin.	Chlorpromazine. Anticonvulsants. See text (p. 54).	Yes.	Yes.	Yes.
Whooping-cough (p. 55).	Tetracyclines (limited value)	Hyperimmune serum. Sedatives. Hypnotics. Cough depressants.	Yes (difficult in practice).	Yes.	Yes.

TABLE 4 (*continued*)

Disease	Specific therapy (*drug of choice)	Symptomatic measures	Is prevention practicable? (general measures)	Passive immunization possible?	Active immunization possible?
(B) Infections probably due to Viruses					
Chickenpox (p. 29).	None.	Antipruritics: Dusting powder. Antihistamines. Tetracyclines. Penicillin.	Yes, but undesirable in healthy children.	No.	No.
Glandular Fever (p. 37).	None.	See Convalescence (p. 38).	No.	No.	No.
Influenza. (p. 38).	None.	Antipyretic-analgesics. Antibiotics for Secondary Invaders (p. 40).	No.	No.	Yes (see text).
Measles (p. 40).	None.	Penicillin.	Yes, but undesirable in healthy children.	Yes, special circumstances (p. 40).	No.
Mumps (p. 44).	None.	See Complications (p. 45).	Yes, but undesirable in healthy children.	Yes (Convalescent Serum).	No.
Poliomyelitis (p. 45).	None.	See General Management (p. 47).	No.	No.	Yes.
Rubella (p. 48).	None.	None.	Yes, but undesirable in healthy children.	Yes, special circumstances (p. 49).	On trial.
Smallpox (p. 51).	None (Methisazone on trial).	Antipruritics. Antibiotics (p. 6). Hygiene of the skin (p. 25).	Yes.	No.	Yes.

3. Tuberculosis

J. W. CROFTON

INTRODUCTION

In countries which are economically advanced the prevalence of and mortality from tuberculosis have very greatly diminished since the introduction of chemotherapy. However, in the world as a whole the disease continues to be one of the main causes of death. The World Health Organization calculates that between 0·5 and 1 per cent. of the world's population are suffering from infectious pulmonary tuberculosis. Nevertheless, when proper treatment is given the outlook for the individual patient has changed immeasurably. Formerly his illness was all too often fatal, either by rapid progression or by a tragic staircase of alternating stabilization and relapse. At the present time, with few exceptions, the patient with tuberculosis can be assured confidently that the disease will be arrested by specific therapy. He should be able to return to a relatively normal life and his risk of relapse should be small.

In economically developing countries, misuse of chemotherapy has led to the emergence and spread of drug-resistant bacilli, now a diminishing problem in developed countries. Formerly half of those diagnosed as tuberculosis died from the disease, often after a series of improvements and relapses. The clinician must remember that the avoidance of death, relapse and drug resistance now depends on prescribing the right drug-combinations and making sure that the patient takes them for the necessary time.

PREVENTION

INFECTION AND HOST RESISTANCE

Tuberculosis is an infectious disease. Until recently in Britain most people were infected at some time in their lives, as shown by an almost universally positive tuberculin reaction in adults. It may be that this is no longer true, though the use of BCG now makes such an assessment difficult. At any rate, of those who do become infected only a relatively small proportion develop clinical disease. The outcome of any particular infection will depend on the relation between the host and the parasite. The size of the infecting dose will tend to be much greater for one who lives in an overcrowded dwelling in close contact with a patient who is coughing up large numbers of tubercle bacilli, especially if that patient does not know he has the disease and is taking no precautions against infecting others. Development of disease will also depend on the resistance of the host. The factors affecting host resistance are numerous. They cannot be discussed in detail here, but some of them must be mentioned because they concern prevention.

Though it is difficult to separate genetic resistance from environmental influences, it is probable that races which have been exposed to tuberculosis for many centuries have acquired an increased resistance through natural selection. Age is an important factor. Infants are much more likely to develop disease if infected and are particularly prone to the generalized miliary and meningitic forms. Children from the ages of 5 to 12 are less susceptible, but during puberty, adolescence and young adult life resistance is again lowered, progressive pulmonary tuberculosis being the main danger at these ages. After puberty there is a difference in the two sexes. Resistance in women is lowest in young adult life and rises sharply after the age of 40, but the susceptibility of males remains much the same throughout life. At the present time in Britain the majority of deaths among males are in old men and the prevalence of active pulmonary tuberculosis is highest in males over the age of 60.

Resistance is also affected by environmental factors. It is certainly lowered by malnutrition. Overcrowding, as already indicated, increases the liability to massive infection, but the stresses and strains of such an environment probably also lower resistance. The same is true of working conditions. Occupations involving exposure to silica lower the resistance to tuberculosis. Alcoholism has the same effect. There is evidence that heavy smoking is also an adverse factor. Chronic diseases may lower the resistance to tuberculosis, the most important of these being diabetes mellitus.

The significance of physical and mental strain is much more difficult to assess. Given sufficient sleep and an adequate diet, there is no evidence that physical strain is important. Many patients, on the other hand, seem to develop tuberculosis after a period of mental strain and worry. There is evidence that a loss of a near relation, a divorce or a broken engagement may be a precipitating factor.

Once an individual has overcome a primary tuberculous infection his resistance against further infection is enhanced. This is the principle underlying the induction of a harmless primary infection by vaccination with BCG (*Bacille Calmette-Guérin*).

METHODS OF PREVENTION

From what has been said it will be obvious that in the prevention of tuberculosis there are two main aims: the first is to prevent infection with the tubercle bacillus, for without this there can be no disease; the second is to increase the resistance of the community so that if a person in that community is infected he is more likely to overcome the invader without developing clinical tuberculosis. In the past there have been two chief sources of infection: cows' milk and the sputum of patients.

Infection from milk. Bovine tubercle bacilli derived from milk were formerly of importance in causing disease. This source of infection has now been controlled in Britain by rendering herds free from tuberculosis and ensuring, by regular tuberculin-testing, that this freedom is maintained. Pasteurization is an additional insurance. Older patients, previously infected with bovine organisms, are occasionally seen. Their recognition is important, as bovine tubercle bacilli are sometimes naturally resistant to PAS (para-aminosalicylic acid) and usually to pyrazinamide.

Infection from sputum. The prevention of infection from sputum is much more complex. Although tuberculous infection can theoretically be acquired from patients with discharging sinuses, etc., these sources are so much less important that they will not be considered here. Those who are coughing up infective sputum are much more numerous and are liable to be mixing with the community; worst of all, many do not know that they have tuberculosis. With the facilities now available in economically developed countries it should be possible to make all diagnosed cases of tuberculosis non-infectious, usually within a few months. Provided treatment is sufficiently prolonged, relapse is unlikely. This makes the discovery of cases doubly important, for if we could discover all cases in a community, we should be able to make them non-infectious. In this way tuberculosis could be eradicated, provided the community remained free from imported disease. For a number of years, of course, there would be breakdowns in those previously infected, as indeed is happening now in elderly men.

If the tuberculosis services are good, all patients known to be infectious can be adequately treated. It is, therefore, from the unknown pool of infection that the main danger arises. The most important preventive measures are those designed to reduce the size of this pool. The aim should be to diagnose all cases of pulmonary tuberculosis before they become infectious and to ensure by proper treatment that they never become infectious at all.

Miniature radiography. To put this programme into effect many difficulties have to be overcome. By major expenditure of time, energy and apparatus, it has been found possible to take miniature radiographs of 80 per cent. or more of the adult population of large cities within a few weeks. With the fall in prevalence of tuberculosis, the mass radiography of whole populations is now hardly economically justifiable, but selective radiography of special groups retains its importance in an eradication programme.

There are two main categories of people who require diligent study by miniature radiography. To some extent these two categories overlap. The first consists of groups ('*high incidence groups*') which are known to contain a particularly high proportion of active cases. These will give the highest yield for a given effort. The second includes groups ('*danger groups*') among which an unknown infectious case might do most damage by infecting others. These groups will consist of those in occupations which bring them into contact with large numbers of people.

In the first category ('*high incidence groups*') it has been found from experience that three groups yield a proportion of active cases well above the general average. The first consists of people showing any symptom that might be due to tuberculosis. In most areas in Britain facilities are now provided for general practitioners to refer patients direct to a static miniature radiography unit. The doctor should realize that the value of radiology is not confined to any particular age-group. It is particularly important to investigate middle-aged and elderly men, in whom there is a high incidence of both tuberculosis and carcinoma of the bronchus.

The incidence of tuberculosis in men inhabiting lodging houses is particularly high. It must be remembered that there is an appreciable 'observer error' in the reading of chest films. The practitioner should not hesitate to have a film repeated, even though reported as normal, if symptoms persist and are otherwise unexplained.

The second group which yields larger numbers of active cases consists of patients attending general hospitals, either as out-patients or in-patients, whatever their complaints. This group is not yet adequately covered in Britain.

The third group, which is at present fairly well covered, is that of household contacts of known cases of pulmonary tuberculosis. The primary responsibility for investigating contacts usually lies with the local chest clinic in association with the public health services, but the practitioner can do much to encourage their attendance. Another much smaller group in this category consists of diabetic patients, who should be examined radiologically at regular intervals. The number of active cases of tuberculosis shown by surveys of prisoners and mental patients is also well above the average. Immigrants from countries with a high prevalence of tuberculosis require particular attention.

For the protection of the public the second category ('*danger groups*') is particularly important, since a patient with unrecognized tuberculosis can disseminate the disease widely. In some parts of Britain teachers in schools and universities, who come into contact with a particularly susceptible population, have voluntarily agreed to regular examination. A similar scheme has been introduced for public transport workers in Edinburgh. Regular radiological examinations are equally important for many other persons dealing with children—nurses, school employees, etc. Other groups which should be included are those who in the course of their work come into contact with a large number of people in the day: food servers, shop assistants, hairdressers, barmen, cinema attendants, ticket collectors, dentists, doctors, and all hospital employees. The reader can readily extend the list. Little has been done about any of these groups in Britain, though some of them are effectively covered in other countries.

Mobile units may be used for 'cleaning up' operations. If there are repeated notifications among employees at a place of work, all employees should be examined radiographically in order to detect and treat the infectors. A similar survey is called for if there is a high incidence in any particular district of a town.

The optimum use of miniature radiography varies with the local situation. It is most important that the policy should be under constant review and should be revised when necessary to meet changing conditions. The rapid elimination of tuberculosis depends mainly on the intelligent use of this weapon together with efficient treatment.

Decreasing the chances of infection. The chances of infection may be decreased by the proper management of known cases of tuberculosis and by ensuring that the members of the community live, work, travel and play under conditions which will reduce to a minimum the danger to others of an undiagnosed case. Good ventilation and avoidance of overcrowding are important. Known cases of infectious tuberculosis should be promptly treated. In developing countries hospital isolation is impossible, but controlled studies of family contacts in Madras have shown that with careful management patients can be treated at home with little risk to their contacts, provided proper chemotherapy is given. If modern methods of treatment are properly applied, it should be possible to convert a positive sputum to negative in about 80 per cent. of cases within three months, in more than 95 per cent. within six, and in the remainder within 12 months.

Raising of host resistance. Methods of increasing the resistance of the community to tuberculosis are implicit in the above discussion of the factors underlying resistance. They are mainly matters of social action and of health education.

Immunization with BCG. BCG or *Bacille Calmette-Guérin* is a strain of bovine bacilli attenuated by prolonged growth in the laboratory. The aim of vaccination is to increase the patient's resistance by producing an artificial primary tuberculous infection with an organism which causes only a local lesion and some swelling of the adjacent regional lymph nodes. It follows that BCG is suitable only for those who have never been infected and are tuberculin-negative. In Britain the policy is to vaccinate those especially exposed to infection, such as the contacts of known cases of tuberculosis, nurses and medical students. This has been extended in most areas to children who are about to leave school. A large-scale controlled trial among urban school-leavers in England has conclusively shown the value of vaccinating this section of the population. The later incidence of tuberculosis was reduced by about 80 per cent. for at least five, and probably for 10 years after vaccination. A controlled trial in India showed a 60 per cent. reduction in the vaccinated group.

Vaccination is carried out by injecting intra-dermally in the deltoid region 0·1 ml. of the vaccine, now usually the freeze-dried type. After two to three weeks a small area of induration may be felt at the site of vaccination. It gradually increases to a little papule about 0·5 to 1·0 cm. in diameter. Between the fourth and the sixth week in most cases a small bleb appears on top of this papule and dries to a crust. The crust may become detached, leaving a little ulcer. Thereafter healing gradually takes place, although the papule may still be detectable up to 12 months. A small scar remains. A technique of multiple puncture vaccination is at present being explored but cannot yet be recom-mended.

There may be slight painless enlargements of the regional glands in the early stages. The only important complication of BCG is a glandular cold abscess which occurs in a very small proportion of cases. When an abscess develops it should be treated by aspiration; streptomycin and isoniazid should also be given in the usual doses (p. 68). Lupus-like reactions at the vaccination site have been described but are very rare. Erythema nodosum occasionally occurs, especially in infants. Among the many millions of people vaccinated with BCG there have been a few cases of fatal dissemination, mainly in children with hypo-gammaglobulinaemia. The risk of vaccination is therefore infinitesimal compared with the risk it is designed to avert. Nevertheless, those with hypo-gammaglobulinaemia or eczema should not be vaccinated.

After vaccination the tuberculin test will usually become positive in about six weeks if liquid vaccine has been used, in 10 to 12 weeks if the vaccine was freeze-dried. Until this has occurred, the individual is not protected and he should still be kept away from any known case of tuberculosis.

THE TREATMENT OF TUBERCULOSIS

GENERAL PRINCIPLES

Chemotherapy is now by far the most important factor in the treatment of tuberculosis. The aim is either to destroy the patient's population of tubercle bacilli or to reduce it to numbers easily handled by the patient's own defences.

Rest in bed and hospital treatment. Rest in bed is unnecessary in the treatment of pulmonary tuberculosis, provided that appropriate chemo-therapy is prescribed and the drugs taken. A carefully controlled trial has shown that patients with mild disease can be treated just as effectively at work as at rest in bed. A similar trial under bad social conditions in Madras has shown that patients treated at home, even when the home is a slum and the patient's diet very poor, do just as well as those on a good diet in hospital, provided that chemotherapy is adequately supervised. More-over, there is no more risk of infection of their family contacts. Home treatment, and indeed for many patients treatment at work, is therefore the proper course in most economically underdeveloped countries where the provision of adequate hospital beds is economically impossible and any available money is much better spent on drugs and on the adequate supervision of domiciliary chemotherapy.

In economically developed countries, although bed-rest is strictly speaking unnecessary, hospital treatment for the infectious patient ensures adequate supervised chemotherapy in the vital early months and also ensures that he is not infectious to the community. In present conditions in Britain it is reasonable to treat a patient who is almost symptom-free, whose sputum is negative on direct smear and in whom there is no appreciable cavitation on the X-ray film, without asking him to stop work, pro-vided that he is a reliable person who will take his chemotherapy conscientiously. A patient with more severe symptoms or extensive disease, whose sputum is positive on smear or concentration, or who is thought to be unreliable, is best admitted to hospital until three negative cultures have been obtained. If cultures are kept for two months before they are pronounced negative, most patients will stay in for a minimum of three months. If there are important social reasons and the patient is reliable, smear-negativity may be sufficient for discharge. The majority spend between three and six months in hospital but some severe cases, particularly unreliable individuals, may have to remain for a year.

In general, a patient who is febrile or toxic should be confined to bed, although only the very ill are not permitted to go to the lavatory. As soon as he is well enough he can increase his activities and as soon as he is non-infectious can return to work.

Even heavy physical work, provided his respiratory function is adequate, is no more than an indication for a somewhat longer period of chemotherapy after returning to work.

Smoking. Smoking encourages coughing, and coughing may help to keep cavities open. It should, therefore, be avoided. Nevertheless, it is better to allow the patient to smoke in moderation if forbidding him tobacco makes him miserable and uncooperative in carrying out the treatment prescribed.

Social aspects. To give a patient physical therapy without discovering, and as far as possible remedying, the social effects of his illness on his work, his finances and his family is to leave the job half-done. Rehabilitation, the fitting of the patient for return to ordinary life, should be considered soon after diagnosis. Nowadays this is much easier than formerly, for most patients can return to their former employment and the chronic patient with a positive sputum should no longer be a problem. Nevertheless, a few patients may need training for some other occupation, and it may be possible to start this in hospital. The advice of a medical-social worker should be fully utilized in this connection and all other social aspects of the patient's illness considered. If the patient has been living in overcrowded conditions, it may be desirable, both for his own sake and for that of his family, that he should be rehoused on discharge; most local authorities in Britain give priority for rehousing to those suffering from pulmonary tuberculosis.

CHEMOTHERAPY

Formerly, when a single drug was used, the tubercle bacilli of many patients became resistant to its action within a few weeks or months. Moreover, these resistant organisms could be passed on to others. Nowadays it is known that, by using proper combinations of two or more drugs, such resistance can almost invariably be avoided. When only a single drug is given, naturally resistant mutants may increase until they replace the population of sensitive organisms. The more severe the infection, the larger will be the number of bacilli and the more likely is it that resistant organisms will emerge. If a proper combination is used, each drug inhibits the mutants which have become resistant to the other. There are only a few combinations which are highly effective in preventing the emergence of resistant bacilli. Dosage is also important, especially in the case of para-amino-salicylic

acid (PAS). Errors on the part of either the patient or the doctor may, therefore, have very serious consequences, as once the organisms have acquired resistance it is usually permanent and the patient's whole future treatment may be jeopardized. On the other hand, combined drug therapy can be given indefinitely and remain effective. Unfortunately skill and experience are needed in the performance and interpretation of tests for drug resistance. In many centres the techniques used for testing drug resistance are unreliable. For further information on these problems special publications should be consulted.

Chemotherapy should be continued in the individual case until the physician is confident that the patient's population of tubercle bacilli is so reduced that his own defences will be able to handle the residue. This is not always easy to estimate. It is, therefore, wise to be on the safe side and give too much rather than too little treatment.

At the present time there are three standard drugs: streptomycin, isoniazid (isonicotinic acid hydrazide, sometimes known as INAH or INH), and para-aminosalicylic acid (PAS). Thioacetazone is a cheaper substitute for PAS in developing countries. Other drugs are used only when, owing to previous unsatisfactory chemotherapy or to primary infection with a resistant organism, the patient's bacilli are resistant to one or more of the standard drugs. It is possible that, with further experience, ethambutol and rifampicin (p. 72) may become standard drugs. Some of the characteristics of the individual drugs will be outlined in the following paragraphs. Combined drug therapy will then be discussed.

Streptomycin. The usual dose of streptomycin is 1 g. daily in a single intramuscular injection; sometimes 1 g. is given two or three times a week. For children the daily dose is 30 mg. per kg. body weight. The main toxic effects are disturbances of the vestibular apparatus and hypersensitive reactions. The vestibular damage from streptomycin gives rise to giddiness. The incidence of this is very low under the age of 40, but appreciable in older people. By giving intermittent or lower dosage, as indicated later, it can largely be avoided. A modification, dihydrostreptomycin, has been advocated as causing less vestibular damage, but is much more likely to produce deafness.

Hypersensitive reactions are not uncommon with streptomycin. They usually occur within four weeks of starting treatment, but sometimes later.

The most common symptom is fever, with or without a rash, though the latter occasionally occurs alone. Sometimes there is also enlargement of lymph glands. Any increase in fever occurring within four weeks of starting chemotherapy should be regarded as a sign of drug hypersensitivity until proved otherwise. The drug should be stopped immediately until the fever and, if present, the rash have disappeared. A test dose of streptomycin should then be administered; if the reaction has been mild, 500 mg. can be given; if severe, 100 mg., repeating with 250 mg. if there is no reaction to 100 mg. Within an hour or two there will be a reaction, usually slight pyrexia with or without a mild return of the rash. This is also allowed to subside and, after testing for hypersensitivity to the other drugs (see below), the patient should be desensitized. In the majority of cases an initial dose of 100 mg. is given, which is then increased every 12 hours by 100 mg. If the original reaction has been very severe it is well to start with a smaller dose. Sometimes there will be a mild reaction and the previous dose will have to be repeated or the patient be given a day's rest. It is usually possible to desensitize a patient within one to three weeks. Very rarely reactions are so severe that desensitization has to be carried out under cover of a corticosteroid drug.

Isoniazid. This synthetic compound is much the most effective of the antituberculosis drugs. It is given by mouth in the form of tablets or cachets in which it may be combined with PAS. The standard dose is 100 mg. twice a day, though a single dose of 200 mg. may be given; in combination with thioacetazone the dose must be 300 mg. For children the daily dose is 3 to 5 mg. per kg. body weight, administered once or twice daily. Higher doses given daily in combination with other standard drugs have certainly no more than a marginal advantage, except perhaps in tuberculous meningitis, for which up to 10 mg. per kg. is often given (p. 74). Nevertheless, it is now established that a large dose given twice weekly with streptomycin (p. 68) is effective. These large doses of isoniazid sometimes cause peripheral neuritis with burning feelings and paraesthesiae in the extremities, but in the usual doses the drug is almost nontoxic. Even hypersensitive reactions are very rare.

PAS (para-aminosalicylic acid). PAS is a synthetic drug. It is well absorbed from the intestinal tract and is, therefore, given orally. It is less effective against tubercle bacilli than either streptomycin or isoniazid and its main use is to prevent the emergence of resistance to these drugs. It is usually prescribed as the sodium salt. In Britain the dose is expressed in terms of this salt, although elsewhere it is expressed in terms of the acid. Potassium and calcium salts are also available. The individual dose should be not less than 5 g. of the sodium salt and this is given two or three times a day in combination with other drugs. For children the individual dose should be not less than 100 mg. per kg. body weight and the total daily dose not less than 300 mg. per kg.

The chief toxic effect of PAS is nausea. When severe, this may lead to vomiting. Loose stools are also common. The drug is available in various special preparations designed to avoid these effects, but not all such preparations are fully absorbed. The most reliable ways to give PAS are dissolved in tap water, in granules or enclosed in rice-paper cachets, containing 1 to 1·5 g., which are dipped in water and then swallowed with the aid of a draught of fluid. If nausea occurs, especially with higher doses, the dose may be reduced for a day or two and then again slowly increased. It often helps to take the drug towards the end of a meal. The doctor should avoid any suggestion that nausea may occur; with confident handling, patients experience little trouble. If loose stools cause serious inconvenience, small doses of tincture of opium (1 ml.) may be given for a few days and then gradually discontinued. An occasional patient is quite unable to tolerate PAS; ethambutol or rifampicin may be substituted.

Hypersensitive reactions are quite common with PAS. The usual manifestations are similar to those of streptomycin sensitivity and occur about the same time after starting treatment. If it is not realized that the fever is due to hypersensitivity and the drug is continued, hepatic damage with jaundice may occur and the rash may go on to exfoliative dermatitis. In severe cases symptoms of encephalitis may develop. Patients often become hypersensitive to both streptomycin and PAS. Only with very severe reactions may there also be hypersensitivity to isoniazid. When all three drugs have been used it is wise to test successively for hypersensitivity to isoniazid, streptomycin and PAS in that order. The normal test dose for PAS is 2 to 2·5 g., but if the reaction has been a severe one it may be wise to start with a dose as low as 100 mg. The drug is given by mouth and the reactions to be expected are the same as those with streptomycin. In a mild case it is sufficient to start desensitization with a dose of 500 mg., but in severe cases this will have to be reduced to 100 mg. or less. In some patients reactions even to low doses are so frequent that desensitization has to be 'covered' with a corticosteroid drug or a different drug substituted. Nevertheless, it is usually quite feasible to start with 500 mg. a day and to increase by 12-hourly increments—1, 1·5, 2, 2·5, 3, 4, 5 g., etc.—completing the process within one to three weeks.

Patients sometimes become hypersensitive to more than one drug. Test doses of all three standard drugs should therefore be given, whether or not there is a reaction to the first one tested. If there is hypersensitivity to only one drug, the other two can be given during desensitization. If there is hypersensitivity to two, it is dangerous to give the remaining drug covered by only a small desensitizing dose of a second drug; there is a risk of the patient's bacilli becoming drug-resistant during desensitization. Instead, one of the reserve drugs, preferably ethambutol (p. 72), should be given with the tolerated standard one, usually isoniazid, until desensitization to one or other of the standard drugs is completed.

PAS has an antithyroid effect. When given in high dosage for more than six months the patient may develop a goitre and sometimes even hypothyroidism. Both disappear if PAS is stopped. If it must be continued, the goitre will usually disappear with 0·1 mg. of thyroxine given daily. Larger doses may be necessary to combat hypothyroidism.

Laboratory tests for PAS resistance are technically difficult. If a patient's past experience of chemotherapy raises uncertainty about the sensitivity of his bacilli, it is wise to test at least three or four different cultures before pronouncing the strain sensitive.

In conclusion, it must again be emphasized that resistant bacilli commonly emerge if any of these drugs is given alone. Further, the bacilli may remain resistant indefinitely and may infect others. Resistance can readily be prevented by using correct drug combinations.

Standard Combination of Drugs

One of the greatest tragedies that can overtake a patient with tuberculosis is that his infecting organisms become resistant to the standard drugs. This can be avoided if his organisms are initially sensitive to the combination of drugs used, provided he adheres strictly to the therapeutic plan.

Initial lack of sensitivity may be due to the patient having received incorrect drug treatment previously. This problem is dealt with on p. 72. In a newly diagnosed patient it may be due to infection with bacilli which are already resistant, derived from some mistreated patient. This is widely known as 'primary' drug resistance. If a patient is treated with two drugs, and his organisms are already resistant to one of them, the bacilli are likely to become resistant to the second drug also. In order to avoid this, patients should be treated initially with all three of the standard drugs until the results of sensitivity tests are available. With the standard indirect sensitivity test this usually takes two to three months. By using three drugs, a proper combination will be available to the patient even if his organisms later prove to have been resistant to one of the three.

Before treatment is begun at least two specimens of sputum should be sent for culture in order that resistance tests may be carried out. If previous chemotherapy suggests the possibility of drug resistance, five or six specimens should be sent.

Satisfactory combinations of drugs can be summarized as follows:

Hospital patients under the age of 40. Streptomycin, 1 g. daily, *plus* sodium PAS, 5 g. three times daily, *plus* isoniazid, 100 mg. twice daily.

When it is known that the pre-treatment cultures were fully sensitive the PAS can be omitted while the patient is in hospital. Daily streptomycin and isoniazid is probably the most powerful combination.

Hospital patients over the age of 40. In older patients there is a risk of vestibular disturbance with the larger dose of streptomycin. In such patients the antibiotic can be given in a dose of 1 g. three times weekly with the dose of PAS and isoniazid as in younger patients. Theoretically there is a slight risk of drug resistance with this combination if the patient's organisms were primarily PAS- or isoniazid-resistant. Clinical experience suggests that this risk is very small. Nevertheless, it is now more common practice to reduce the daily dose to 500 or 750 mg. in older patients.

If streptomycin is being used intermittently, both PAS and isoniazid must be continued throughout the patient's stay in hospital.

In any patient in whom impairment of renal function is suspected, it is wise to control the streptomycin dosage by an estimation of serum levels. If the serum level of streptomycin 24 hours after a dose of 1 g. is higher than 1 mcg. per ml., streptomycin is not being normally excreted and the dose should be correspondingly reduced until the serum level does not exceed 1 mcg. 24 hours after a dose.

Mild cases treated as out-patients, and patients after discharge from hospital. It is convenient to treat such patients with drugs given by mouth. An appropriate dose is 5 g. sodium PAS together with 100 mg. isoniazid, given twice daily. Preparations containing both PAS and isoniazid are available in cachets, tablets or granules so that the patient cannot take one without the other. Nevertheless it is very important that he should take the full dose, for there is evidence that if the total dose is not attained the amount of PAS may be insufficient to prevent the emergence of isoniazid resistance in some patients. If newly diagnosed patients with mild disease are given this drug combination, there is a theoretical risk of the emergence of resistance to both drugs should his organisms be primarily resistant to one of them. This objection can be met by giving streptomycin daily, or three times a week, until the results of pretreatment resistance tests are available or until it is known that the sputum was culture-negative initially.

A useful alternative treatment after discharge from hospital is streptomycin 1 g. and isoniazid 14 mg. per kg., both drugs given in a single dose twice weekly. Pyridoxine, 10 mg., is also given to prevent toxicity from the high dose of isoniazid. The advantage of this combination is that the administration of both drugs can be readily supervised. The results are at least as good as those with daily isoniazid and PAS in conventional doses.

Failure to take drugs. A comparatively high proportion of patients treated at home may fail to take their drugs as instructed. This has been demonstrated by testing the urine for PAS. As the patient has to continue his chemotherapy for many months after he is feeling perfectly well, it is important that the physician should continually impress on him the vital necessity to take his drugs as directed if he is to avoid relapse. A patient with a newly diagnosed infection may be given the full daily dose of streptomycin, 1 g., isoniazid, 200 mg., and sodium PAS, 10 g., at a single administration under supervision, followed by twice-weekly high-dosage isoniazid, streptomycin and pyridoxine, as outlined above, after the sputum has become negative.

Corticosteroid drugs. Controlled clinical trials have shown that patients treated with corticosteroid drugs in addition to chemotherapy initially improve more rapidly, both clinically and radiologically, than patients treated with chemotherapy only. Nevertheless, there is ultimately little difference between the two groups. It is therefore justifiable to incur the risk of the undesirable side-effects of corticosteroids only if a patient is seriously ill. In such a patient the use of corticosteroids may ensure his immediate survival and give time for the antituberculosis drugs to take effect. A dose of 5 mg. of prednisolone may be given four times daily and continued for six weeks of more, after which the drug is gradually withdrawn. The use of corticosteroids in assisting the technique of desensitization has already been mentioned.

Other Antituberculosis Agents

The use of the newer antituberculosis agents is mainly for the patient known or suspected to harbour bacilli resistant to the standard drugs. This may occur because he has been infected with resistant bacilli, because he has been previously treated with an unsatisfactory combination of drugs such as intermittent streptomycin with daily isoniazid or daily PAS, or because he has failed to take his drugs as prescribed. If the patient has been treated with any form of unsatisfactory chemotherapy in the past it should always be assumed that his organisms may be drug-resistant until tests have proved the contrary. In many parts of the world a substantial number of patients harbour bacilli resistant to the standard drugs. They constitute a formidable therapeutic problem. Often in such circumstances no resistance tests are available. If the physician knows the exact combinations of drugs previously prescribed, whether the patient has taken them, the extent of the disease and the grade of infection as judged by the sputum, he can often anticipate the drugs to which the patient's organisms will prove resistant and plan his treatment accordingly. The weighing of the probabilities demands skill, experience and time; it is best left to the specialist.

The assessment of the therapeutic problem in patients with drug-resistant organisms and the selection of optimum combinations of the newer drugs call for close co-operation between physician and bacteriologist. In the following paragraphs brief notes will be given of some of the drugs available. This is followed by a review of possible drug combinations for particular types of case.

Ethambutol, a synthetic drug, is highly active against the tubercle bacillus. It is given orally in a single dose of 25 mg. per kg., this being reduced to 15 mg. after 60 days. Retrobulbar neuritis, reversible on stopping the drug, is a rare side-effect, but patients should have monthly tests of visual acuity.

Rifampicin. Rifampicin is a semi-synthetic derivative of an antibiotic, rifamycin-B. It is highly active against the tubercle bacillus and well-tolerated. It may, with ethambutol, eventually find a place in primary treatment. It is given daily in a single oral dose of 450 or 600 mg.; the latter has been the usual dose but the former may be adequate. Liver toxicity has occurred in patients with cirrhosis or other previous liver damage, and occasionally with no preceding liver disease. The colour of the drug may cause an overestimate of the serum bilirubin level. The drug produces a brown or red colour in the urine. Regular liver function tests should be carried out during treatment.

Pyrazinamide. Pyrazinamide is a substance chemically resembling nicotinamide. It is a powerful drug. Unfortunately it has potential toxic effects on the liver, and deaths have occurred from hepatic atrophy. It should, therefore, only be used initially in hospital, and hepatic function tests should be carried out at regular intervals. If any abnormality is detected, the drug should be stopped at least temporarily. Retention of uric acid may occasionally lead to joint pains resembling gout. The patient should avoid exposing his skin to sunshine, as photosensitivity may be enhanced. It is given orally in a dose of 40 mg. per kg. per day, divided into two equal doses with a maximum of 1·5 g. twice a day.

Ethionamide. This drug is a compound allied chemically to isoniazid, but there is no cross-resistance with it. It is given orally and is highly effective. Nausea and malaise are unfortunately common side-effects. These are less marked with the recently introduced modification, *prothionamide*, but hepatic toxicity sometimes occurs with both drugs. The optimum dose of either is 500 mg. twice daily. If this is not tolerated at least 500 mg. in a single dose should be given and may be taken last thing at night to minimize side-effects. Should there be marked intolerance, suppositories of 500

mg. may be tried, but the degree of absorption is uncertain.

Capreomycin, an antibiotic, will probably replace viomycin and kanamycin to which it is related, as it is less toxic and more effective. A dose of 1 g. daily is given intramuscularly. Its toxicity is similar to streptomycin with perhaps a higher risk of auditory damage. Electrolyte disturbances, possibly due to renal tubular dysfunction, may occur, usually after several months of treatment. Low serum levels of calcium, magnesium and potassium may result in depression, muscular weakness and tetany.

Cycloserine. Cycloserine has a definite but weak antituberculosis action. The main toxic effects have been psychotic disturbances, usually starting within a few days of beginning treatment, and convulsions. A number of unexpected suicides have occurred. It is given orally and to obtain maximum effect a dose of 500 mg. twice daily is desirable.

Thioacetazone. Thioacetazone is a form of thio-semicarbazone with a weak antituberculosis activity. It is given orally in a single dose of 150 mg. daily. Its main use is as a very cheap alternative to PAS in combination with isoniazid (p. 69). The chief hazards are hypersensitivity and hepatic toxicity. There is often cross-resistance with ethionamide.

With the possible exception of cycloserine, drug resistance emerges rapidly if any of these agents is given alone.

Suggested regimens for patients with organisms known or suspected to be resistant to the standard drugs are given in the following paragraphs.

The patient who has had previous chemotherapy. Relapse after previous chemotherapy may occur because treatment with a reliable drug combination has been too brief, in which case the bacilli should be sensitive to the drugs used. Alternatively, the previous drug combination may have been unreliable (for example, intermittent streptomycin with daily isoniazid or daily PAS and isoniazid in a severe case, both of which will result in an important percentage of failure). In this case the bacilli may be resistant to the drugs used. Treatment should be based on this assumption, though, pending the results of resistance tests, isoniazid at least should be added to the reserve drug combination (see below).

The patient with bacilli resistant to standard drugs. If the bacilli are resistant to only one of the three standard drugs, ethambutol or rifampicin may be substituted. If they are resistant to two standard drugs, ethambutol and rifampicin should be combined with the third. If resistant to all three standard drugs, rifampicin and ethambutol may be used with prothionamide, substituting pyrazinamide if prothionamide is poorly tolerated. Isoniazid may be added in case some bacilli are still sensitive to it.

Such patients will usually be left with one or more residual open cavities so that chemotherapy will have to be continued for two years. Should the disease be localized and should resection prove feasible, its timing requires careful judgment; the safest period is often about three months from the start of chemotherapy. A previously unused drug should be added over the operation period. Cultures should be taken from the resected lung and resistance tests carried out for all relevant drugs.

Preventive chemotherapy. Chemotherapy has been advocated as preventive treatment for tuberculin-negative individuals in close contact with an infectious patient and for young people with a strongly positive tuberculin test but no clinical or radiographic evidence of active tuberculosis. Treatment of the first group mainly arises in economically underdeveloped countries. It is not recommended because, if the patient who is the source of the infection is receiving adequate chemotherapy, he soon ceases to be dangerous. Moreover, when drugs are in short supply they are best reserved for patients with active disease. The treatment of those with strongly positive tuberculin tests as the only evidence of disease is more controversial. It is certainly justified in infants less than one year old and perhaps in children up to three years of age in whom the breakdown rate is high. Over that age it is low and routine treatment seems unjustified, though recent tuberculin conversion, a very strongly positive test or any evidence of ill-health might be regarded as indications in an individual case. If not treated, the child should be watched closely and treatment should be started if he develops any radiographic or other evidence of disease.

The treatment of patients with radiographically visible tuberculous lesions of doubtful activity creates difficult problems. Controlled trials have shown that the breakdown rate is reduced by chemotherapy. The decision must be based on a judgment as to the likelihood of activity in the lesion, the availability of drugs and the probability that the patient will take them regularly.

Although isoniazid alone has been advocated for any of these purposes it is wiser to give at least two drugs so as to ensure against the emergence of resistant bacilli. Either PAS with isoniazid or twice-weekly high dosage isoniazid with streptomycin may be given (p. 69). Either combination should be continued for at least a year.

PRIMARY TUBERCULOSIS

When a patient is first infected with the tubercle bacillus a lesion occurs both at the site of infection and in the regional lymph glands. This is known as the primary complex and it is usually in the lung and hilar lymph glands. Thanks to the increased safety of milk, primary lesions elsewhere are now uncommon.

Primary pulmonary tuberculosis. In primary pulmonary tuberculosis in children the hilar glandular component of the primary complex often predominates. The lymph glands may erode the wall of a bronchus resulting in atelectasis, exudation, caseous pneumonia or a combination of these, the lesion affecting a lobe or a segment. In the adolescent or young adult primary tuberculosis often appears similar to post-primary, with little radiological evidence of enlargement of hilar glands; it is treated in the same way as post-primary disease (p. 75). The following paragraphs therefore refer to the treatment of primary pulmonary tuberculosis in children.

Rest in bed. Children with primary tuberculosis are best treated at home provided that the social conditions are satisfactory. It is undesirable to separate a child from his home surroundings for long periods if it is avoidable. If the child is ill he should be kept at rest in bed in the first place. Radiographic changes may take many months to disappear. Hence there is little point in keeping the child in bed if he is clinically well and if he is having chemotherapy which will safeguard against progression. In fact, if he is running about, he is more likely to cough up the caseous material exuding from the lymph gland into his bronchus. This may also be encouraged by postural coughing.

Chemotherapy. Chemotherapy itself seems to have little effect on enlarged hilar or mediastinal glands or on lobar or segmental lesions which, for mechanical reasons, may actually develop under treatment. There is evidence that the latter regress more rapidly and leave less residua of bronchiectasis if a corticosteroid drug, such as prednisolone, is given. It should be continued for several months, otherwise relapse may occur. If the pulmonary component of the primary complex is large or progressive, it appears to be affected by chemotherapy in the same way as a post-primary lesion in the lung.

In spite of these limitations, chemotherapy should be given to all children with primary tuberculosis in order to control the tuberculous infection and to avoid the later development of tuberculosis elsewhere. In deciding the form of chemotherapy, careful account should be taken of the drug sensitivity of the bacilli from the individual by whom the child was probably infected if this is known. In simple primary tuberculosis the emergence of drug resistance is less probable than in post-primary pulmonary tuberculosis. In order to avoid injections, PAS and isoniazid may be given, the dose being adjusted to body weight (p. 69). In more severe disease it is wise to give all three drugs until the results of sensitivity tests are known or at any rate for the first three months. Chemotherapy should be continued for at least a year.

Bronchoscopy. In the presence of segmental or lobar collapse bronchoscopy has been undertaken to suck out the caseous material discharging from the gland into the bronchus. It usually has only a very temporary effect; the gland continues to discharge and the bronchus soon becomes blocked once more. The only definite indications for bronchoscopy are secondary infection beyond the block or, occasionally, massive atelectasis.

Erythema nodosum. Erythema nodosum is often associated with primary tuberculosis, but may also be due to other conditions. Chemotherapy should be given to such cases if there is clinical or radiographic evidence of primary tuberculosis. A strongly positive tuberculin test is also an indication, as such patients are more likely to develop overt disease later.

Sometimes a patient with erythema nodosum may continue to run a high temperature with recurrent crops of skin lesions and perhaps with swollen joints. This is especially common in middle-aged women. In such cases, if the erythema nodosum is associated with tuberculosis, the response of the temperature and other symptoms to chemotherapy is usually dramatic. Once started, chemotherapy should be continued for at least a year.

MILIARY TUBERCULOSIS

As soon as a diagnosis of miliary tuberculosis has been made, the treatment is relatively straightforward. Standard drug combinations should be given (p. 80). The patient should be admitted to hospital and nursed on lines appropriate to the degree of his illness. Patients very ill with tuberculosis, especially the miliary form and particularly in the older age-groups, may develop severe electrolyte disturbances, especially hypokalaemia. This may occur even days or weeks after starting treatment. The serum electrolytes should always be checked initially, and later if there is any deterioration. If there is hypokalaemia it is wise to give both potassium and sodium; the response is usually rapid.

The patient can be permitted to get out of bed for increasing periods as soon as his general condition permits. When he is clinically well, if home conditions are good and if it seems probable that he will take, or be given, his chemotherapy conscientiously, he can be allowed home.

The results of treatment for miliary tuberculosis are now very satisfactory, though a few patients, if they are admitted desperately ill, die in the first few days or weeks. Corticosteroid drugs, in addition to chemotherapy, may save some of these and should be given to all who are severely ill. An adult may be given prednisolone, 5 mg. four times daily; in children the dose should be appropriately reduced. In infants the disease is often diagnosed late and there is a higher mortality than in older children. Most patients who survive the first few weeks are likely to make a complete recovery. At least 15 months' chemotherapy should be given, and if there is any doubt about the rapidity of clearance of the lesions the treatment should be continued for longer.

TUBERCULOUS MENINGITIS

The treatment of tuberculous meningitis has been revolutionized by the introduction of chemotherapy. Formerly nearly all patients died. At present, with proper treatment, 80 per cent. or more recover. The chances of recovery depend largely on early diagnosis. If treatment is started while the patient is conscious the prognosis is good, but if the diagnosis is made only when the patient is unconscious it is very much worse.

A patient who is unconscious or suffering from severe cerebral irritability may constitute a difficult nursing problem. He has probably become wasted and both his skin and his mouth will require constant attention. Feeding is frequently difficult. With patience and persistence it is usually possible to feed with a spoon, but occasionally tube-feeding may be necessary.

Chemotherapy should be started immediately the diagnosis is made. It is uncertain whether intrathecal chemotherapy improves the results of treatment, but it is probably justifiable in the first week or two of therapy in a severely ill patient, in which case isoniazid is probably the best drug to use as it is the most powerful. Twenty-five mg. of pure sterile isoniazid in 2 to 3 ml. of sterile normal saline is injected slowly, being mixed with cerebrospinal fluid as it is injected. Oral PAS and intramuscular streptomycin in the usual dose (p. 68) are combined with isoniazid, 5 mg. per kg. twice daily. Pyridoxine, 10 mg. daily, is given to prevent peripheral neuritis. PAS and isoniazid should be continued for at least a year, though the dose of isoniazid can be lowered to 3 mg. per kg. as soon as the patient is clinically well. Pyridoxine can then be omitted. In mild, early cases the initial streptomycin can be omitted after a few weeks. Corticosteroid drugs are probably of value and should be used in all severe cases: prednisolone, 5 mg. four times daily (or double that dose initially in the desperately ill), may be given to an adult, cautiously withdrawing it after six weeks.

If the cerebrospinal fluid pressure is raised, lumbar puncture should be repeated daily or twice daily, with cautious removal of fluid, until the pressure becomes normal. Thereafter puncture is unnecessary unless progress is unsatisfactory. Provided the drugs are taken regularly and the tubercle bacilli were initially sensitive to them, the cerebrospinal fluid will return gradually to normal within 3 to 12 months. As soon as the patient is relatively well clinically, he may be allowed out of bed for increasing periods. If his home conditions are good it may be possible to discharge him after a few months' hospital treatment. The physician must, of course, be confident that treatment will be meticulously continued at home.

The majority of patients who recover from tuberculous meningitis do so completely. Occasionally there is residual mental impairment or some other neurological lesion, especially in patients admitted unconscious. After a year's treatment, or sometimes a little longer, the adult is usually able for work or the child for school; mild cases may be fit earlier. Where teaching is available in the children's ward, lessons can be started as soon as clinical symptoms disappear. Chemotherapy should be continued for at least 18 months.

PULMONARY TUBERCULOSIS

Duration of chemotherapy. The minimum duration of chemotherapy in a case of pulmonary tuberculosis should be 15 months. If the disease is more than minimal, treatment should be given for 18 months. Severe cases, and all those with residual open cavities, should receive chemotherapy for two years. On these regimens, if punctiliously carried out by the patient, relapse should be exceptional. Chemotherapy is most effective in acute exudative disease, but has a slower effect in other types. Seventy per cent. or more of cavities close as the result of prolonged chemotherapy. If cavities are going to close, they will usually do so within six months. In chronic fibrotic disease the radiological response to treatment is very much less impressive. Nevertheless, in all cases it is possible to make the sputum permanently negative, provided the bacilli are initially sensitive to the standard drugs.

The prognosis in pulmonary tuberculosis was formerly dominated by the presence of cavitation. Before the introduction of chemotherapy a patient with a residual cavity was almost certain to relapse, but since its use, relapse almost never occurs unless the patient harbours bacilli resistant to the standard drugs or fails to take his chemotherapy as prescribed. Large residual healed cavities may later become the site of secondary infection, not uncommonly fungal, and haemoptysis may occur without any evidence of tuberculous relapse.

Thoracic surgery. The era of extensive surgery for pulmonary tuberculosis has passed. Residual healed cavities occasionally need resection for one of the complications mentioned in the previous paragraph. Resection is sometimes desirable for localized disease in a patient with bacilli resistant to the standard drugs, especially if he has difficulty in tolerating the reserve drugs. A tuberculous empyema may occasionally require resection.

Further observation. Relapse in pulmonary tuberculosis can be detected early only by radiography of the chest or by sputum examination. Even though the relapse rate is now very greatly reduced, it is important for the patient to have regular follow-up examinations for a prolonged period. If he is still receiving chemotherapy he should be seen every 6 to 12 weeks and his urine should be tested for PAS to ensure that the drugs are being taken. The necessity for strict chemotherapy must be constantly impressed on him, for most relapses are due to the patient's failure to take his drugs as prescribed. After finishing chemotherapy he should be seen at least every 12 months until the disease has been quiescent for at least five years. Even after that it is wise for him to have a chest radiograph taken at least once a year.

Haemoptysis. Haemoptysis is a clinical feature which is alarming for both patient and doctor. Fatal haemoptyses do occasionally occur and usually kill the patient within a few seconds. Most haemoptyses for which there is time for treatment are unlikely to be serious. The first step is to reassure the patient, who is not unnaturally alarmed. He should be confidently told that the bleeding will cease in due course and will do him no harm. A sedative, such as phenobarbitone or even 10 mg. of morphine, can be given if necessary. If the patient is under effective chemotherapy, there should be no risk of spread of disease within the lung. Any increase in the shadows in the radiograph due to aspirated blood will disappear within a week or two.

TUBERCULOUS PLEURAL EFFUSION

Tuberculous pleural effusion, without obvious manifestations of intra-pulmonary tuberculosis, may occur at any age. Formerly between 15 and 30 per cent. of such patients later developed other post-primary forms of tuberculosis. Pleural effusions are absorbed more quickly as the result of adequate chemotherapy and the incidence of relapse with post-primary pulmonary tuberculosis should be negligible. If the diagnosis is certain the standard chemotherapy for pulmonary tuberculosis (p. 75) may be combined with prednisolone orally in a dose of 5 mg. four times a day for a few weeks, thereafter gradually lowering the dose. The pleura should be aspirated dry initially. Further aspirations will probably be unnecessary. Breathing exercises are instituted early to encourage the return of full movement of the diaphragm. Chemotherapy should be continued for a year, streptomycin being stopped when the patient leaves hospital.

It is usual to keep the patient in bed until he feels well. He can then slowly resume his activities over a few weeks and return to his normal work. It is wise to keep him under observation for at least five years. He should have a chest radiograph at least every three months while receiving chemotherapy and thereafter every 12 months until the end of the

fifth year. However, when full chemotherapy has been given relapse is unlikely.

OTHER FORMS OF TUBERCULOSIS

In general, the chemotherapy of the other forms of tuberculosis mentioned below is similar to that of pulmonary tuberculosis. In all forms it is advisable to continue drugs for at least a year, usually 18 months to two years, in order to prevent recurrence in the local site or elsewhere.

Tuberculous laryngitis. With the early use of chemotherapy this is now comparatively rare. It responds rapidly to drug treatment, the patient losing his symptoms usually within a few days. It may, however, take a month or two before the appearance of the larynx returns to normal.

Tuberculous bronchitis. Tuberculous bronchitis responds so well to chemotherapy that it is seldom necessary to define the degree of involvement bronchoscopically.

Tuberculous empyema. Tuberculous empyema occasionally complicates pulmonary disease or spontaneous pneumothorax in a patient with underlying tuberculosis. In the early stages it may be possible to deal with the fluid by repeated aspiration and the introduction of streptomycin in a dose of 3 g. in 10 to 15 ml. of distilled water every third day. Oral isoniazid and PAS are given at the same time. If there is a pyopneumothorax, both air and fluid should be aspirated, the aim being to obtain rapid re-expansion of the lung. When the empyema has been present for weeks or months, medical treatment may be ineffective owing to thickened pleura, in which case the empyema will have to be excised surgically under cover of chemotherapy.

Abdominal tuberculosis. Tuberculous peritonitis responds excellently to chemotherapy, though sometimes it is later complicated by intestinal obstruction due to adhesions. The patient may require a few weeks' rest in bed. Tuberculous enteritis and ileocaecal tuberculosis also respond well to a similar programme of treatment. However, in tuberculous enteritis there is usually severe pulmonary disease, the treatment of which will dominate the picture.

Superficial tuberculous lymphadenitis. The treatment of tuberculous lymphadenitis with drugs is not yet entirely satisfactory. Some cases appear to respond excellently, but in others the glands break down in spite of chemotherapy and later relapse is not unknown. If there is a large mass of glands it is best to advise rest in bed in hospital in the first place. If there is fluctuation, the pus should be aspirated from above. Standard chemotherapy should be given. The situation should be reassessed in six to eight weeks. In many instances the glands will by then be diminishing in size and the progress will be quite satisfactory, in which case the patient can be discharged from hospital to continue chemotherapy. If no progress has been made within six to eight weeks, it will probably save time to have the glands, or at least the larger ones, removed surgically. Sometimes it will be necessary to carry out surgical evacuation of pus deep to the fascia. The patient should be kept in hospital for two to three weeks after the operation, chemotherapy being continued. He can then be discharged to be treated with PAS and isoniazid, or with streptomycin and isoniazid in high dosage twice weekly.

In severe cases an attempt has been made to avoid the development of sinuses in the skin or the necessity for operation by combining prednisolone with antituberculous chemotherapy (p. 68). The initial results are often good, but the glands sometimes become fluctuant when the corticosteroid is stopped. The prednisolone should be continued for two to three months, chemotherapy being given along the lines already indicated.

Genito-urinary tuberculosis. Tuberculous epididymitis responds excellently to standard chemotherapy (p. 68) and surgery should never be necessary. Tuberculous cystitis also responds well. Decision on the right treatment of renal lesions is much more difficult. For patients with bacilluria without demonstrable alteration in the pyelogram prolonged chemotherapy is all that is required. On the other hand, if a patient's kidney is largely destroyed, nephrectomy should be advised. The patient's bacterial population should be considerably reduced by chemotherapy for three or four months before the operation is undertaken. Since the patient's condition is often greatly improved once the damaged kidney has been removed, there is little to be gained by further delay. In patients with moderate renal damage the present practice is to be conservative regarding surgery in view of the excellent results obtained from prolonged chemotherapy. The urine always becomes negative for tubercle bacilli and the relapse rate is negligible. The subsequent incidence of hypertension is low, though it does occasionally occur and may necessitate nephrectomy later. Surgery may sometimes

be necessary to dilate or repair a residual stenosis of the ureter. This may only become apparent as the lesion heals, so that regular pyelograms should be carried out at appropriate intervals during the first few months of treatment. There is some evidence that corticosteroids may reverse ureteric stenosis. If this is present, or if there is hydronephrosis, prednisolone should be given, as for severe pulmonary disease (p. 74). In all patients chemotherapy should be continued for at least 18 months, and in those in whom the renal damage is at all severe two years should be the minimum period of treatment.

Gynaecological tuberculosis. Tuberculous salpingitis usually reponds very well to chemotherapy. Even large masses may shrink in the most dramatic manner. Surgery should never be undertaken until chemotherapy has been given a thorough trial. Tuberculous endometritis also responds satisfactorily. Unfortunately fertility is restored in only a small proportion of patients, though ectopic pregnancy is not uncommon. As in other conditions, chemotherapy should be continued for one to two years.

Tuberculosis of bones and joints. Orthopaedic textbooks should be consulted for the surgical management of bone and joint tuberculosis. There must be close co-operation between physician and surgeon. Chemotherapy will greatly shorten the patient's stay in hospital, avoid some surgical procedures and allow other forms of surgery to be undertaken much earlier. It is usually possible to evacuate abscesses, remove sequestra and suture the wound without subsequent trouble. Tuberculosis confined to the synovia, particularly of the knee, responds excellently to chemotherapy, and operation should usually be avoided. Stabilizing operations may be needed for tuberculosis of the vertebrae and of the hip. Chemotherapy should be continued during the whole of the patient's stay in hospital and throughout the period of healing, usually for 18 months to two years. If this is done, relapse is exceptional.

Tuberculosis of the eye. A number of diseases of the eye, such as choroiditis or iritis, are thought sometimes to be due to a form of hypersensitivity to the tubercle bacillus. A diagnosis may have to be based on such indirect evidence as a marked skin sensitivity to tuberculin or an abnormality in a chest film. Such lesions appear to respond to prolonged chemotherapy, but it is difficult to say how far the improvement may not be the result of a natural remission. It is usually unnecessary to admit the patient to hospital, and PAS and isoniazid may be given at home. Local and systemic corticosteroid treatment should be given in addition to chemotherapy.

Tuberculosis of the skin. Tuberculosis of the skin is now uncommon. It responds well to chemotherapy. It is wise to continue treatment for a year after the lesions have become quiescent.

PREGNANCY

In general, it is best to postpone pregnancy until the disease has been quiescent for at least a year and chemotherapy completed. Breast-feeding may then be permitted and the infant given BCG at leisure. Nevertheless large numbers of entirely satisfactory pregnancies have been completed under chemotherapy without trouble to mother or child. But there have recently been suggestions that streptomycin might sometimes affect the hearing of the infant and that ethionamide might have a teratogenic effect. These risks must be very small, and if necessary must be accepted. Nevertheless, it seems wise, when possible, to avoid such chemotherapy during pregnancy.

Therapeutic abortion. With the success of chemotherapy, therapeutic abortion is seldom necessary. It will have to be considered if the patient's tubercle bacilli are drug-resistant and the physician is anxious not to add in any way to her burden. It may also be necessary in a patient whose respiratory function has been severely damaged by tuberculosis. The recent suggestions of a possible risk to the foetus from certain antituberculosis drugs may have to be taken into account. Therapeutic abortion after the end of the third month of pregnancy should be avoided as by that time the operation involves as much strain as parturition.

THE PREVENTION AND TREATMENT OF TUBERCULOSIS IN ECONOMICALLY UNDER-DEVELOPED COUNTRIES

Organization. In economically under-developed countries tuberculosis is usually the major public health problem and there is frequently inadequate finance and trained staff to deal with it. It is very important that the available money should be used to best advantage. Priority should be given to the provision of chemotherapy and to BCG vac-

cination. Hospitals or sanatoria are unnecessary and very expensive; only a few emergency beds should be provided, close to the out-patient clinics. Treatment should be domiciliary, which, when properly organized, has been shown in Madras to be just as satisfactory. Expensive radiological equipment should not be widely provided; diagnosis and therapeutic control should be based on smear examination of sputum, which is cheap and can be carried out by a technician. Initially culture and drug-resistance tests must be confined to a few laboratories with a primary responsibility to undertake sample surveys of the prevalence of resistance.

There is bound to be a shortage of doctors, but they can train intelligent technicians to undertake a large proportion of the routine tasks. Their work should be regularly checked by random sampling and by having them working in pairs. In principle, nothing should be done by a doctor which can be done by a technician trained *ad hoc* for tasks such as supervision of chemotherapy or examination of sputum. Much can be achieved by medical social workers trained to deal with the particular local problems. It is sound policy to provide a few teaching centres with good radiological and laboratory services, including facilities for drug-resistance tests. Such centres might take a special interest in patients with drug resistance and perhaps only these centres should have access to the expensive reserve drugs.

General methods. In general, the policy should be to control infectivity by good chemotherapy and initially not to extend case-finding beyond the capacity of the therapeutic services to cope with the patients found. To discover patients without giving them adequate treatment is to bring the whole service into disrepute. Initially case-finding should be by smear examination of the sputum, which detects the most infectious and dangerous cases; the aim should be to examine everyone who has a cough. If radiological equipment is not available a positive case should be confirmed by at least two further sputum examinations before starting treatment. Miniature radiography is not essential. It is expensive, difficult to maintain and often cannot reach much of the country. Initially, if available, it may be used as an aid to diagnosis by sputum examination. Later its use may be cautiously extended to case-finding, as the therapeutic services improve. BCG vaccination is a cheap preventive. Its value has not been so definitely demonstrated in underdeveloped as in developed countries but with certain provisos the evidence is sufficient to justify its widespread use.

Chemotherapy

In most underdeveloped countries there is at present a crisis in the treatment of tuberculosis because of the relatively high prevalence of drug resistance, primary and acquired. This has arisen because of bad treatment by doctors or laymen. Repeated short courses of chemotherapy keep patients alive and infectious. If bad combinations or single drug therapy are used, patients are kept alive but infectious and with resistant bacilli which they can pass on to others. Isoniazid alone has been used extensively because of the erroneous theory that isoniazid-resistant tubercle bacilli might lose their virulence for man. Even the knowledgeable and conscientious doctor may use indifferent therapeutic measures owing to inadequate supplies or economic stringency.

Chemotherapy is so vital that the provision, not only in theory but in practice, of the best chemotherapy which is economically possible must be the first charge on the money available. Certain compromises, which are less than ideal, may have to be accepted in the interests of economy. In these circumstances some failures are unavoidable. The aim is to minimize them. When trained doctors are available, no one else should have access to the relevant drugs. This is the only way to prevent the spread of drug resistance and to avoid wastage.

Initial chemotherapy. In view of the high prevalence of drug resistance, including primary resistance, it is desirable to initiate therapy with three drugs, especially in patients with smear-positive sputum. The three following alternatives are suggested. The first is known to be highly successful and is probably the best, but is relatively expensive. The second two are appreciably cheaper; they have not been proved in careful trials, but there are theoretical reasons for expecting a high degree of success.

1. Streptomycin, PAS and isoniazid daily, as suggested for economically developed countries (p. 68).

2. Streptomycin, 750 mg. daily or, with a little added risk, three times weekly, together with isoniazid, 300 mg., and thioacetazone, 150 mg., both in a single dose daily. This has been highly successful in East Africa and probably in India, but the sensitivity of tubercle bacilli and the side-effects of the drug seem to vary from country to country, so

that each country should carry out its own preliminary trial.

3. Streptomycin, 1 g., together with isoniazid, 14 mg. per kg., PAS 10 g., and pyridoxine, 6 mg., all given together, preferably under supervision, twice weekly.

One of these combinations should be given until the sputum becomes smear-negative. If they are all financially impossible one of the combinations given in the following section may be used as initial treatment, but the failure rate will be higher, especially in those with primarily resistant organisms.

Maintenance chemotherapy in severe cases or initial therapy in those with smear-negative sputum. In order of priority, as regards likelihood of success, one of the following may be given:

1. Streptomycin, 1 g., together with isoniazid, 14 mg. per kg., and pyridoxine, 6 mg., all given together, preferably under supervision, twice weekly.

2. PAS, 5 g., with isoniazid, 100 mg., both given twice daily.

3. Isoniazid, 300 mg., with thioacetazone, 150 mg., both given once daily in a single dose. This is almost as successful as PAS with isoniazid and has been extensively used in East Africa with relatively little toxicity, but its success and toxicity are less certain elsewhere (see above).

With a small budget isoniazid alone in a single dose of 200 mg. daily may be justifiable in the second year of treatment in those without residual cavitation or, if no X-ray is available, in those with less initial positivity.

Duration of chemotherapy. In smear-negative tuberculosis chemotherapy should continue for at least 12 months. Smear-positive cases should continue for 18 months. Although not proved, it seems likely that in the great majority of cases 18 months' treatment, properly taken, will ensure against relapse.

Control of chemotherapy. Except for emergencies, all treatment should be domiciliary. The necessity for conscientious drug-taking for many months after he feels well must be continuously impressed on the patient and his relatives, both by initial talks and by later propaganda through broadcasts to waiting patients, etc. Supervised chemotherapy at the clinic is ideal, with arrangements for pursuing non-attenders. Urine testing for PAS, in the clinic and the home, pill-counting, and checking that oral drugs have been collected, are other important measures.

Patients who have had previous chemotherapy. Such patients require careful assessment, taking into account the factors mentioned on p. 72. Having decided to which, if any, drugs his organisms are most likely to be resistant, the best available combination of other drugs should be used, employing the most intensive treatment which is practicable until the sputum becomes smear-negative. If isoniazid has been hazarded by previous unsatisfactory treatment it should not be relied on to prevent resistance to other drugs but may be added to the combination in the hope that at least some of the patient's organisms may still be sensitive to it, in which case it is the most powerful drug available. The added cost is small. The same reasoning applies to streptomycin, but it is much more expensive.

Return to Work

It is ideal to keep a patient off work until he ceases to be infectious, but this is impractical if his family will starve as a result. In many parts of the world the patient will have to start work as soon as he is physically able to do so. This should not delay his recovery or involve an important risk to others, provided he continues to receive the appropriate chemotherapy for the appropriate time.

BCG Vaccination

Vaccination offers a relatively cheap and probably effective method of preventing tuberculosis. In mass vaccination campaigns in developing countries there is now evidence that no harm comes from vaccinating the whole population without the time-consuming preliminary of tuberculin testing. The value of the vaccine given must be continually checked, both by laboratory tests and by ensuring on a sample basis that a high proportion of the tuberculin-negative individuals vaccinated subsequently become tuberculin-positive.

SUMMARY OF ANTITUBERCULOSIS CHEMOTHERAPY WITH STANDARD DRUGS

1. HOSPITAL PATIENTS
(a) *Under age 40*
   (i) Before results of resistance tests available:
   Streptomycin, 1 g., in single dose daily, intramuscularly,
   plus isoniazid, 100 mg. twice daily, orally,
   plus sodium PAS, 5 g. three times daily, orally.
   (ii) If organisms sensitive to all three drugs:
   Sodium PAS omitted during hospital stay.
(b) *Aged 40 or over*
   (i) Before results of resistance tests available:
   Either Streptomycin, 500 to 750 mg. daily, intramuscularly,
   or streptomycin, 1 g. three times weekly together with, in each case, PAS *plus* isoniazid as in 1(a)(i) above.
(c) *Children*
   (i) Before results of resistance tests available, if source of infection unknown and case relatively severe:
   Streptomycin 30 mg. per kg. in single dose daily intramuscularly,
   plus isoniazid 3 to 5 mg. per kg. daily, divided into not more than two doses,
   plus sodium PAS 300 mg. per kg. daily, divided into not more than three doses.
   (ii) If organisms sensitive to all three drugs, in mild cases, or after first three months of treatment with all three drugs:
   Sodium PAS *plus* isoniazid as in 1(c)(i).

2. PATIENTS OUT OF HOSPITAL
(a) *Newly diagnosed Adult Patients*
   Streptomycin 1 g. intramuscularly three times weekly,
   plus isoniazid 200 mg. orally given in one or two doses daily,
   plus sodium PAS 10 g. orally given in one or two doses daily.
   PAS and isoniazid to be given in the same cachets, tablets or granules.
(b) After sputum has become culture-negative or if initial cultures prove negative, or after discharge from hospital with culture-negative sputum:
   Either isoniazid *plus* sodium PAS as in 2(a)
   or streptomycin, 1 g. intramuscularly twice weekly, *plus* isoniazid, 14 mg. per kg. in a single oral dose twice weekly, *plus* pyridoxine, 10 mg. in a single oral dose twice weekly.
(c) *Children*
   (i) Newly diagnosed mild primary tuberculosis, if source of infection unknown or known to have bacilli sensitive to the standard drugs; or after preliminary treatment in hospital:
   Isoniazid *plus* sodium PAS as in 1(c)(i).
   (ii) Severe cases:
   Streptomycin *plus* isoniazid *plus* sodium PAS as in 1(c)(i).

References

CROFTON, J. & DOUGLAS, A. (1969). *Respiratory Diseases.* Oxford: Blackwell.
Fox, W. (1964). Realistic chemotherapeutic policies for tuberculosis in the developing countries. *Br. med. J.,* **1,** 135.
ROSS, J. D. & HORNE, N. W. (1969). *Modern Drug Treatment in Tuberculosis,* 4th Ed. London: Chest and Heart Association.

4 Diseases of the Heart and Circulation

Sir Ian Hill

The decision to institute treatment of a cardiac patient does not follow automatically on the diagnosis of heart disease. Not every victim of a valvular lesion or arrhythmia stands in need of drugs, though a majority require guidance and surveillance by the doctor. It is axiomatic in the management of cardiac patients, as in medicine generally, that accurate diagnosis must precede treatment, and in cardiology this implies more than a bald anatomical diagnosis of such-and-such a valvular deformity, vascular lesion or muscular impairment. In valvular disease, for example, it is not sufficient to conclude that a certain valve is affected, but it is necessary to determine the aetiology; to assess precisely the relative rôles and degree of incompetence and stenosis; and to take account of the size of the heart, both overall and of individual chambers, of arrhythmias, of secondary pulmonary vascular effects, and above all of the state of the heart muscle. Such a complete fourfold diagnosis (aetiological, anatomical, physiological, and assessment of cardiac grade), implies a full assessment of the individual patient, and its accuracy is reflected in rational treatment and prognosis.

For example, the management of aortic valvular disease due to syphilis differs fundamentally from that due to rheumatism; the management of a tight, pure mitral stenosis differs from that of a minor grade of narrowing, and from that of incompetence: the size of the heart is an index to prognosis, as are abnormal rhythms which may also demand treatment: and the exercise capacity of the individual has bearings on prognosis and on the need for treatment. This last, for example, is crucial in the management of the pregnant cardiac patient. Such a four-fold diagnosis is in no way cumbersome, and a simple dated entry on the patient's record card can summarize in a line what would require a page of conventional history and signs.

Complete, accurate diagnosis of the type advocated is of two-fold value. The natural history of the various forms of heart disease is well known, and from considerations of the nature and severity of the lesion, the size and rhythm of the heart, the degree of disability and the occurrence of such episodes as embolism or acute pulmonary congestion, it is possible to pin-point the stage the patient has reached, to estimate his prognosis and to guide him effectively in his affairs. Treatment based on such a complete appraisal is more rational and thus more effective than the simple prescription of symptomatic remedies, such as nitroglycerin for angina or digitalis for heart failure.

It must be emphasized that treatment of each patient poses an individual problem. There are general rules for guidance, but variations from one patient to the next in severity and stage of disease, in response to rest and reaction to drugs, are so wide that each case demands individual assessment.

It follows as a corollary that there is no 'blanket' prescription for any type of cardiac disease. Medication must be prescribed on specific indications for a specific purpose. Digitalis is not required by every patient with a murmur; nor does the diagnosis of a cardiac lesion carry an automatic prohibition on activity or on child-bearing. Failure on the part of the doctor to carry the diagnosis beyond the stage of valvular disease or arrhythmia too often leads to misguided treatment, and on occasion to unwarranted invalidism and much avoidable suffering.

CONGESTIVE HEART FAILURE

Congestive heart failure, by reason of its frequency of occurrence and the distress and suffering entailed, remains the main problem in cardiac therapeutics. Recent advances in our knowledge have brought better understanding of its genesis and of the causation of the oedema and dyspnoea which are two of its features. Its management, while still largely on traditional lines, has changed considerably in detail in recent years, particularly since the advent of new diuretic agents and the introduction of the refined digitalis glycosides. Yet it remains a condition difficult to treat effectively, and in which the results of treatment are extremely variable. Congestive cardiac failure, while commonly a terminal process, is not necessarily a precursor of early death. If relieved by treatment, it may resolve completely, and when a precipitating factor has been dealt with may not recur for many years, if ever; but from the nature of things the failure may be irreversible: e.g. a grossly scarred heart muscle following repeated infarctions or rheumatic inflammation may have insufficient healthy contractile tissue to meet the needs of the body even at rest. Again the valve lesion may be of such severity that no muscle can cope with the burden. Such may be the case in aortic stenosis; when failure eventually occurs in patients with this lesion it may prove intractable and progresses to death within a few months. The situation is quite different with mitral disease, in which repeated bouts of congestive failure may occur over a period of years, each possibly more severe and more resistant than the last, but with long intervening periods of reasonably good health. The general course is, however, downhill and leads eventually to a terminal state of intractable failure. At the other extreme, cardiac failure precipitated by a remediable cause such as thyrotoxicosis may be permanently abolished by efficient therapy. The importance of full and accurate diagnosis as stressed in the preamble is apparent.

The recognition of congestive heart failure presents no difficulty. The *assessment of its severity* may be less easy, but is of great importance, since it has a bearing on the urgency with which treatment is carried out. Congestive cardiac failure is seen in all grades, from a slight increase in the venous pressure in the neck with some enlargement and tenderness of the liver to the grossly water-logged patient, with sacral pad, hepatic enlargement, ascites, bilateral hydrothorax, and accompanying orthopnoea, insomnia and vomiting. It is important that the *type of cardiac failure* should be recognized, since not every patient with congestive failure has a low cardiac output. In patients with valvular disease, hypertension and ischaemic heart disease, failure with low output is the rule, but in other conditions, notably thyrotoxicosis and in some patients with heart failure secondary to respiratory disease or anaemia, the cardiac output is actually above normal despite the oedema and other features of heart failure. It is important to recognize this high-output type since its management differs from that of conventional low-output failure.

Further, in every patient presenting with cardiac failure it is important that a search be made for a precipitating cause. For example, a patient with a valvular lesion with which he has lived in reasonable equilibrium for many years, probably with some restriction of activity but with little serious disability, develops gross congestive failure, it may be in the course of a day or two or dramatically in a few hours. The doctor must always ask himself what circumstance has determined this sudden deterioration. Commonly an intercurrent respiratory infection is responsible, and this may well escape detection unless deliberately sought for, since the signs are obscured by those of failure. Pulmonary infarction is another common cause, as is a relapse of rheumatic infection in the younger age-group or the onset of an abnormal rhythm, particularly atrial fibrillation. In women of child-bearing age pregnancy is a recognized hazard to the cardiac patient. In older patients, particularly hypertensives, the sudden development of cardiac failure may have been determined by a myocardial infarction, often without pain and therefore easily overlooked, or by the occurrence of an abnormal rhythm, such as atrial fibrillation or paroxysmal tachycardia. Lastly, and especially in the older age-group, thyrotoxicosis as a cause of unexplained failure must be kept in mind. The diagnosis of such hyperthyroidism is not always obvious, since in elderly patients the conventional ocular signs and nervousness may be minimal. Recognition of the underlying cause of cardiac failure is obviously of great importance in relation to treatment and prognosis.

MANAGEMENT AND NURSING CARE

Increased physical activity imposes a demand which is met by increased cardiac output, and thus physical rest as a cardinal principle in the management of heart failure is well founded. In many cases rest in bed in a position of optimal comfort and the securing of sleep may result in the rapid onset of diuresis, loss of oedema and a general return of well-being. The position of the patient should be that which he finds most comfortable: patients with congestive failure are unable to lie flat. They should be propped up with a sufficiency of pillows or a backrest, day and night. Many, particularly the obese and those distended with ascites, are better to be nursed either sitting in an old-fashioned armchair with high back and sides, or in a cardiac bed, the head of which may be raised and the foot dropped, so that oedema tends to gravitate to the legs and buttocks, and relief of pulmonary congestion with corresponding increase in comfort results. In extreme cases, a bed table well padded with pillows can be placed in front of the patient, who can then lean forward with his folded arms resting on this support. The patient at complete rest must have meticulous nursing care: attention must be paid where ischaemia may lead to tissue necrosis and bed sores; the risk is increased when the skin of the back and heels is oedematous. To reduce energy expenditure to the minimum, skilled nursing is essential; these patients must be washed and fed and attended to in every way. While the use of a bed pan is usual, it should be remembered that the energy expended by a stout, elderly person in attempting to use it may be greater than that involved in lifting him gently over the bed on to a night commode. If it is proved that micturition has become impossible because of gross genital oedema, recourse must be made to an indwelling catheter despite the formidable attendant risks of infection.

The duration of rest in bed is variable and depends in large measure on the response to treatment. In patients in whom the signs of congestive failure resolve within a few days and particularly in those in whom a remediable cause has been found and treated, the period of rest in bed may be no more than 10 days. More commonly improvement occurs more slowly and a month in bed may be required before a gradual return to activity is permitted. When oedema is resistant to treatment, the period of rest in bed may be indefinitely prolonged. It should not be forgotten that patients confined to bed for prolonged periods—and particularly those in whom the circulation is slow as in congestive failure—are liable to develop venous thrombosis, commonly in the legs. This complication must be sought for by daily examination of the limbs and should be treated energetically with anticoagulants if detected (p. 185). Neglect of this precaution may lead to serious or fatal pulmonary embolism. It is important that a patient confined to bed for a considerable time should have appropriate physiotherapy to prevent excessive muscular wasting.

Restless nights with at best brief snatches of sleep are the common lot of the patient in cardiac failure. The securing of adequate sleep is of major importance. In general morphine is the most satisfactory drug for the purpose, at least in the early stages of the illness. With it a patient may be afforded untroubled sleep throughout the night with relief of

distress and general benefit. The usual dose is from 10 to 20 mg. hypodermically; in adults of heavy build, up to 30 mg. may be required. For most patients it is perfectly safe, but there are certain contraindications to its use. It is not a drug to be given thoughtlessly to those in whom a respiratory infection plays a major rôle in the production of failure, and above all it must not be given to a patient suffering from cor pulmonale or bronchial asthma, in whom morphine may be lethal. It is also dangerous and occasionally fatal in the patient with cardiac failure secondary to gross spinal kyphoscoliosis. For those who are sensitive to morphine (and they are more numerous than is generally supposed) another analgesic may be substituted, such as methadone or pethidine, or cyclizine can be given along with the morphine.

In many patients sleeplessness is due to dyspnoea, and therapy for its relief may lead to peaceful sleep without the use of hypnotics. For this purpose, aminophylline is the most satisfactory drug: in a dose of 500 mg. intravenously, given slowly and well diluted, it commonly gives dramatic relief. It is particularly valuable in the patient suffering from dyspnoeic failure in the later stages of hypertensive heart disease and it is specific in the treatment of Cheyne–Stokes respiration. Oral treatment with aminophylline (250 mg.) is less effective and is apt to be defeated by production of nausea; administration as a suppository containing 360 mg. is worthy of trial. When sleeplessness is due to pain, morphine or its analogues are, of course, indispensable.

While at the outset morphine is invaluable, it is not suitable for continuous therapy during the course of a long illness. Sleep may be promoted in the long-term case by milder hypnotics. Among these, choral hydrate has a deservedly high reputation, though it is greatly disliked by some patients on account of its unpleasant taste. The stabilized solid derivatives, dichloralphenazone in a dose of 1 to 2 g. and trichlorethyl phosphate, 1 g., are useful preparations. Alternatively one of the barbiturate drugs may be used such as amylobarbitone, 200 mg., quinalbarbitone sodium, 100 mg., or some equivalent preparation with the action of which the doctor is familiar. In critically ill patients in whom the use of morphine is for one reason or another inadvisable, an intramuscular injection of 8 to 10 ml. of paraldehyde is a safe hypnotic, 4 to 5 ml. being injected into non-oedematous tissues.

DIET AND SALT RESTRICTION

The patient with chronic venous congestion of stomach and gut and with an enlarged congested liver is intolerant of a rich or bulky diet. At the same time he requires a sufficiency of calories to meet his daily requirements, and as soon as his condition permits he must be given enough protein to meet his metabolic needs. In the early stages of treatment the diet must be light, small in bulk and mainly carbohydrate. Meals should be small and frequent rather than few and large; food should be taken dry and fluids given between meals. Since retention of salt is an essential cause of oedema, some restriction of sodium is usually necessary. Some of the popular proprietary glucose and fruit drinks contain a considerable quantity of sodium citrate, and are unsuitable for the patient in cardiac failure. There is no purpose in reducing the sodium intake in the food to the point of unpalatability and allowing the patient large quantities of the offending ion in a medicated fruit drink.

As recovery takes place a gradual return to a more liberal light diet may be permitted. A specimen diet, poor in salt content, will be found below.

The main ion retained by the body in cardiac failure is sodium; to some extent chloride is also retained, but passively. Restriction of the sodium content of the diet is useful, but to be effective must be strict. A truly salt-free diet is not only difficult to attain, but those containing as little as 200 mg. of sodium daily are unpalatable, badly tolerated by the patient, and may lead to deterioration in renal function. Generally speaking, a salt-poor diet will suffice—one in which sodium intake is restricted to approximately 1 g. daily. This can be achieved by avoiding salty foods, by using salt sparingly in cooking, by adding no salt to food at table and by taking no beverages rich in sodium such as are mentioned above. Until recent years the long-term prescription of salt-poor diets of this type was an important feature of the management of cardiac failure. With the advent of the newer diuretics, such drastic restriction of salt has become less imperative, though in some chronic resistant cases diets of this type are still useful.

SALT-POOR DIET
Approx. 1·25 g. Na. 1,700 Cal. NaCl 4 g.

Breakfast—
  1 egg or small piece of white fish.
  2 slices of bread.

Jelly marmalade if desired.
Butter from allowance.
Tea with sugar, and milk from allowance.

Mid-morning—
  Glass of fruit juice.

Dinner—
  Average helping of meat, fish, chicken, rabbit or tripe. Avoid ketchups and sauces.
  Small helping of vegetable. Small helping of potato.
  Fruit, stewed or fresh.
  Small helping of milk pudding made with milk from ration, or lemon sago or caramel custard, using milk and egg from allowance.

Tea—
  Small helping of meat or chicken or fish, or an egg.
  Tomato or other vegetable if desired.
  2 slices of bread. Butter from allowance.
  Jam or jelly if desired.
  Tea with sugar, and milk from allowance.

Supper—
  2 slices of bread or 2 tea biscuits.
  Tea with sugar, and milk from allowance.
  Helping of fruit, fresh or stewed.

Bedtime—
  Glass of fruit juice.

Allowance for Day—
  ¾ pint of milk.
  1 oz. of butter or margarine.

While restriction of sodium intake is desirable, the reverse is true of potassium. Depletion of body potassium is common in untreated cardiac failure and further reduction of the body stores is liable to occur under treatment with diuretics. Potassium deficiency potentiates the action of digitalis on the conducting system of the heart and on myocardial excitability and leads to dangerous toxic effects. Potassium supplements are most acceptably given as Sando-K. This preparation provides potassium in a form that is rapidly absorbed; it also contains enough chloride to correct the tendency to hypochloraemic alkalosis. Potassium Effervescent Tablets B.P.C. should not be used (p. 120). As an adjuvant, fresh fruit juice—a rich dietary source of potassium—is useful. Such natural juices, as opposed to the semi-synthetic proprietary beverages, have a low content of sodium and are well tolerated.

Salt substitutes are available for patients intolerant of the tasteless food implicit in a salt-poor diet. When one of these is chosen as a substitute, the physician should ensure that he is in fact prescribing a preparation containing potassium chloride and not a citrate or other salt of sodium which, of course, defeats the purpose of salt restriction.

Digitalis

Among the dwindling number of galenicals there stand preparations of the foxglove—drugs which have proved of supreme value in the treatment of cardiac failure. Yet it is true to say that few drugs are in practice more deserving of the epithet 'much abused'. It is unhappily true that the great potentialities of the drug are all too rarely realized as it is so often prescribed for the wrong indications, in inadequate or toxic doses, and with its actions insufficiently supervised. Various factors are responsible for this lack of precision in its use, including the complexity of its pharmacological actions, the multiplicity of preparations available, the difference in their equivalent doses and the variations in the response and sensitivity of patients to the drug. Admittedly, skill in its efficient administration can only be acquired through knowledge and experience, but effort in mastering its use is amply rewarded by the results obtained. The indications for its use are simple; its toxic effects are easily recognized; and by judicious administration of an appropriate preparation a desired effect is readily obtained. The variation in sensitivity from one patient to another can be met only by observation of the effects of a given dose in the individual concerned.

Indications for digitalis. The prime indication for the administration of digitalis is heart failure. This applies to both the congestive heart failure which is under discussion and the left heart failure with intense pulmonary congestion discussed on p. 95. Digitalis can also be used to control the ventricular rate in patients with atrial fibrillation (p. 124), when its action is so striking that for long it was considered that this was its principal indication. In heart failure with normal rhythm digitalis is also valuable, though the effect upon the heart rate is naturally less dramatic. It is also of use in the treatment of supraventricular paroxysmal tachycardia (p. 123). Digitalis is of no value in the control of simple sinus tachycardia, whether this be due to infection, to metabolic disorders such as hyperthyroidism, or to anxiety.

Cardiac catheterization has shown that in patients with congestive cardiac failure of low-output type digitalis simultaneously raises the cardiac output and lowers the venous pressure; which effect is primary has been the subject of debate, but there is evidence that some related preparations have a direct stimulant action on the heart muscle (e.g.

ouabain). In patients with atrial fibrillation the effect of digitalis in slowing the ventricular rate can be abolished by atropine, and yet the increased cardiac output due to the drug persists despite a marked rise in ventricular rate. Other actions of digitalis include relief of oedema and production of diuresis. The effect produced is independent of the preparation used, provided that equivalent doses are given.

Preparations of digitalis and its allies. A wide variety of preparations of digitalis is available and their multiplicity has led to confusion. It is wise for the practitioner to make himself thoroughly familiar with a few of these and to confine his prescribing to them. The preparation recommended is digoxin (B.P.). It is available as tablets (0·25 mg.) for oral administration and as an injection for intravenous use (1 mg. in solution in an ampoule). Other preparations, such as digitalis leaf, digitoxin (available as proprietary preparations) and ouabain (from *Strophanthus gratus* and used only by intravenous injection), though potent are used relatively infrequently. The pharmacological effects of 0·25 mg. digoxin are approximately produced by 100 mg. of digitalis leaf or 0·1 mg. of digitoxin. The effects of cumulation are seen with all preparations of digitalis, but in varying degree: they are most obvious when crude preparations are given orally, and are minimal when the pure glycosides, such as digoxin, are given orally or intravenously in appropriate doses.

The *equivalent* dosage of these various preparations is:

	Oral Route
Digoxin . . .	0·25 mg.
Digitalis tablet (B.P.) .	100 mg.
Digitoxin . . .	0·1 mg.

Intravenously, digoxin is given in doses of 0·5 to 1 mg.; the corresponding dosage of ouabain is 0·25 to 0·5 mg.

While the individual preparations of digitalis vary in rate of absorption, rate of destruction and persistence of effect, they all have similar pharmacological actions. In general they are slowly absorbed and the capacity of the body to destroy or excrete them is limited. This implies that if the daily dose is greater than the total destructive capacity of the body, cumulation will occur. The drugs are rapidly bound by the tissues and particularly by the myocardium. Persistence of action for a considerable period after stopping administration is therefore inevitable, and in the case of preparations of digitalis leaf and of digitoxin the effect may last for many days; the action of digoxin is less prolonged. Further, all exert their full activity only when a certain therapeutic level in the blood and tissues has been reached, and this unfortunately approximates to that at which toxic effects become prominent. It is a great disadvantage that therapeutic and toxic levels are so close together. In any discussion of the therapeutics of digitalis the great variation in individual response to these drugs must be taken into account. Some persons need only a half or a quarter of the average daily requirement to maintain an effective action, and at the opposite extreme there are others who may require three or four times the average dose. There is no way of foretelling which patient is sensitive and which resistant; this great individual variation in sensitivity renders both hazardous and suspect any scheme of calculating massive dosage on the basis of units of activity of the drug multiplied by the body weight of the individual.

The administration of digitalis to a patient involves two separate processes: (1) *digitalization*, i.e. administration over a short period in doses necessary to attain a therapeutic level in the blood and tissues, and (2) *maintenance* dosage, i.e. the long-term administration of an amount to balance that destroyed daily by the body and to maintain the therapeutic level attained by preliminary digitalization. The factor of individual variation in sensitivity referred to above operates in both phases.

Digitalization by mouth. Digitalization by mouth on the dosage schedules recommended below takes three or four days to accomplish. If the patient is in urgent need of digitalization, it is preferable to use an intravenous preparation rather than to adopt oral medication with massive doses as was once popular. In practice, cases demanding urgent digitalization are relatively infrequent and the majority of patients in failure respond well to gradual digitalization over a three-day period. Moreover, such cautious therapy avoids the risk of giving excessive amounts of the drug to an individual who may be highly sensitive to it. On an average the total dose required to digitalize a fully grown adult using digoxin is 4 tablets of 0·25 mg. followed by a single tablet of 0·25 mg. six-hourly until the full effect is obtained. It is essential that a patient on digitalis therapy should be kept under close observation for signs of toxicity

or overdosage, and that the administration be interrupted or the dosage reduced on their first appearance.

Digitalization by intravenous route. When an effect is required within half an hour, digitalization can be achieved by a single intravenous injection of digoxin. This is dispensed in ampoules containing 1 mg., the contents of which should be dissolved in 10 ml. of saline and injected slowly intravenously. More concentrated solutions tend to cause venous thrombosis. It is essential to ascertain whether the patient has already been digitalized and in fact whether he has had any digitalis for a period of one to two weeks previously. It is not sufficient to inquire of the doctor whether he has prescribed digitalis, since many cardiac patients have a stock of 'heart pills' among their possessions and, unknown to the doctor, the patient may have taken digitalis for several days before consulting him. The average dose for an adult is 1 mg. In some heavily built individuals this may be increased to 1·5 mg. without danger, whereas in others of smaller stature, 0·75 mg. would be sufficient. The effect is apparent within a quarter of an hour and is maximal within 30 to 40 minutes. If any doubt exists it is always safer to err on the side of low dosage, giving initially say 0·5 mg. only, and a further 0·25 mg. after one hour if necessary. In no circumstances should a total intravenous dosage of 1·5 mg. in six hours be exceeded.

Maintenance therapy. Efficient maintenance therapy implies recognition of two fundamental factors: first, that the daily dose of digitalis administered should balance that destroyed by the body; and secondly, that the therapeutic and the toxic doses of digitalis are uncomfortably close to one another. The average patient destroys or excretes between 0·5 and 0·75 mg. of digoxin daily and the maintenance dosage will lie as a rule within this range. The exact dose required for each individual patient must be found by trial and error, by close observation of the effects produced by a given dose and the adjustment of his dosage schedule in the light of this experience. There is a wide scatter in the daily requirements and some patients are kept in full therapeutic control with as little as 0·25 mg. digoxin a day five days a week; others require 1 mg. a day continuously over long periods. The position has been further complicated in recent years by the introduction of diuretics causing profound potassium loss, which in turn sensitizes the body to digitalis and potentiates its action. It is implicit

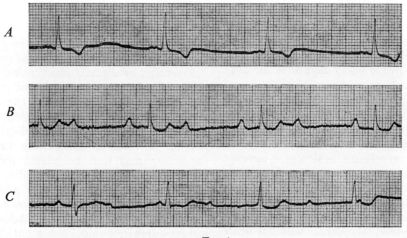

FIG. 1

E.C.G.s of three patients under treatment with digitalis, all showing a slow heart action. The rhythm is different in each. *A* shows sinus bradycardia, rate 42 per minute. *B* shows 2 : 1 heart block, ventricular rate 38 per minute. *C* shows complete heart block, ventricular rate 46 per minute. Note that the rate is actually fastest in the case of complete block.

Bradycardia of under 55 per minute is a signal to stop digitalis, and since clinical diagnosis of the nature of the rhythm may be difficult, an E.C.G. recording should be made.

that every patient receiving a maintenance dose of digitalis should be seen at frequent intervals, questioned regarding toxic symptoms and examined for signs of toxicity. The patient who takes a given dose of digitalis continuously seven days a week over long periods without toxic effects is probably having a daily ration which is less than the body's excretory capacity, so that his tissue level is steadily falling—to a level far below the effective one. It is because of this difficulty in keeping the tissue level at a therapeutic optimum just short of the toxic level that the writer prefers to administer digitalis for maintenance purposes on a five-day week schedule. The patient is instructed to take his daily ration each day from Monday to Friday inclusive, and to stop the drug on Saturdays and Sundays. The daily dose is adjusted in such a way that during a period of five days the patient is taking a total quantity of the drug which is just short of the amount known to produce toxic symptoms. He is warned that should he develop anorexia, headache or nausea toward the end of the week he should stop the drug and inform his doctor.

Toxic effects. Every doctor should be familiar with the toxic effects of digitalis and should be constantly on the lookout for their appearance. The commonest are gastro-intestinal on the one

hand, and cardiac arrhythmias on the other. The earliest side-effect is loss of appetite and squeamishness. If these symptoms are ignored and medication is continued, frank nausea, vomiting, headache and general malaise will supervene. Overdosage also produces striking effects on the heart rate and rhythm; there is excessive slowing of the ventricular rate to 50 per minute or less, arrhythmia due to extrasystoles and coupled beats (pulsus bigeminus)—a highly diagnostic arrhythmia which results when each normal beat is followed by an extrasystole. The extrasystoles may be too weak to reach the pulse at the wrist and may therefore escape detection unless the heart is auscultated. This is a most important sign and should be the signal for stopping the administration of the drug at once, since if it is continued the patient may develop ventricular paroxysmal tachycardia—a very serious condition. If this too is overlooked the patient is in peril from a fatal ventricular fibrillation. In other patients partial or complete heart block may occur, detected by the electrocardiogram or by the classical clinical features. It is important to remember that the ventricular rate in complete AV dissociation due to digitalis is commonly 40 to 50 per minute, much faster than in patients with organic disease of AV node and bundle, and hence

D

it may be overlooked. For the practitioner without an electrocardiograph it should be a golden rule that when a pulse falls below 55 or when an extra-systolic rhythm is found on auscultation, digitalis should be discontinued at once. These abnormal rhythms may persist for many days after the drug has been stopped.

There is another arrhythmia of importance, note-worthy for the difficulty attending its diagnosis. In a proportion of patients receiving digitalis the heart rate may increase as the full therapeutic level is reached and this may mislead the doctor to increase the dose. With increased dosage the rate remains unchanged or may increase further, and it is only when an electrocardiogram has been taken that the cause may be apparent—the development of supra-ventricular paroxysmal tachycardia with 2:1 heart block. In these circumstances an atrial rate of say 160 implies a regular ventricular rate of 80 per minute, neither so slow nor so fast as to arouse suspicion of digitalis toxicity. The recognition of this arrhythmia is important, since stopping digitalis therapy leads to the return of normal rhythm, while persistence with the drug may prove fatal. It is much commoner than was formerly suspected.

There are other toxic actions of digitalis, some common, some rare, and of less importance than those already discussed. Some patients, for example, develop neurological signs, particularly confusion or delirium; in others the initial diuresis may be succeeded by oliguria; disturbances of colour vision and bizarre complications such as gynaeco-mastia may occur.

Nausea and sickness may be so readily induced and of such intensity that an occasional patient cannot tolerate the drug. Digoxin, the glycoside of *Digitalis lanata* is less prone to provoke sickness than digitalis powder, but is not well tolerated by some patients. For the latter, the pure glycosides of *Digitalis purpurea* are the drugs of choice and Nativelle's Digitaline has for many years proved of value in these cases. It is supplied in pills of respectively 0·1 and 0·25 mg., and the average main-tenance dose is from 0·1 to 0·25 mg. per day. Similarly, other preparations of digitoxin may be used, supplied as pills of 0·1 mg., of which one or two pills daily will generally suffice to maintain digitalization. It is important that in all patients receiving digitoxin preparations a close watch should be kept on the cardiac rhythm, and if possible serial E.C.G.s should be taken. The usual symptoms indicating toxic levels with digitalis leaf

or digoxin may be absent and an abnormal rhythm or electrocardiographic changes may be the only indices that a safe dosage has been exceeded. In the writer's experience such preparations are required only in some 5 per cent. of patients.

Treatment of digitalis intoxication. Administra-tion of the drug must of course be stopped. Two measures are of real value: (*a*) The correction of proved potassium deficiency, using Sando-K (p. 120) by mouth: this alone is effective in a pro-portion of cases in suppressing toxic rhythms; the action may well be related to the lowered blood and tissue potassium in cardiac failure, parti-cularly in patients treated with potassium-losing diuretics; hypopotassaemia is known to potentiate the toxic effects of digitalis. (*b*) Administration of a beta-adrenergic blocking agent, for example, practolol. This relatively new drug is particularly effective in the control of arrhythmias induced by digitalis when given orally in a dosage of 50 to 100 mg. thrice daily. In emergencies it may be given cautiously intravenously say 5 mg. at a time, repeated if required to a total of 20 mg.

The frequency with which cases of heart block, pulsus bigeminus, paroxysmal tachycardia with block and other arrhythmias are now encountered in patients receiving digitalis, in comparison to their rarity in previous years, is impressive; the reason appears to be the increased use of those diuretics causing potassium loss.

Diuretics

The most important diuretics are those compounds which inhibit enzyme systems involved in sodium transport. Among these drugs the organic mer-curials (notably mersalyl) represented a major advance in the management of cardiac failure accompanied by fluid retention. However, the mercurials are now seldom used. They have been displaced first by a succession of benzothiodiazines (chlorothiazide, hydrochlorothiazide, bendroflua-zide and many others), and secondly (since 1966) by frusemide. This last drug, though not a benzo-thiadiazine, contains the same halogenated sulpha-moylbenzene group. It is a very powerful diuretic, producing—in full doses—an excretion of sodium twice as great as that resulting from the thiazides. Ethacrynic acid is another modern diuretic com-parable in potency with frusemide and acting on the kidney in the same way; but it is a derivative of aryloxyacetic acid and is chemically unrelated to the benzothiadiazines or to frusemide. When any of these potent diuretics fails to act satisfactorily on account of secondary hyperaldosteronism, spironolactone may be given simultaneously to antagonize the sodium-retaining action of aldosterone and thus to allow diuresis to occur. Acetazolamide, which owes its diuretic action to its power to inhibit carbonic anhydrase throughout the renal tubule, is not sufficiently potent, or dependable for routine therapeutic use. Similarly, triamterene, which promotes sodium excretion while conserving potassium, is of practical value only rarely as a supplement to mersalyl or the benzothiadiazines. Caffeine has a feeble diuretic action. Aminophylline given in full doses intravenously increases the renal blood flow; the action is fleeting but has been used to enhance the effects of other diuretics. Preparations of digitalis used in congestive heart failure characterized by oedema are classed as secondary diuretics because digitalis, in these circumstances, produces a sustained improvement in the renal blood flow.

The following paragraphs include a brief discussion of the nature of cardiac oedema and the merits of various drugs now in use as diuretics.

Oedema was at one time considered simply a consequence of increased hydrostatic pressure at the venous end of the capillaries. Such increased pressure tends to force fluid out of the capillaries or hinder its reabsorption from the interstitial tissues and was accepted as a cause of oedema, particularly affecting dependent parts as in cardiac failure. This increased intravascular pressure is to some extent augmented by lowered plasma osmotic pressure in many patients with cardiac failure, in whom a low total plasma protein concentration and particularly a low plasma albumin are common. It is now known that the cause of oedema is much more complex. The kidney plays a dominant role and retention of sodium, chloride and water plays an essential part. The low cardiac output in heart failure with impairment of renal blood supply, associated with a high pressure in the renal veins as part of the general increased venous pressure, seemed for a time the factor determining retention of water and electrolytes. It is now recognized that other aspects of renal physiology are involved. It is accepted that the filtration theory of renal function is correct and that a large volume of filtrate pours through the glomeruli into the renal tubules each minute. Of this, some 97 per cent. is reabsorbed in the tubules, together with a considerable quantity of sodium, potassium, chloride and other ions. Clearly, since the litre or litre and a half of urine normally secreted in a day represents only some 3 per cent. of the glomerular filtrate, any small change in the rate of reabsorption taking place in the tubules will have a dominant effect both on the volume of urine secreted and on the total quantity of fluid and electrolytes remaining in the body. It has become recognized that the primary defect in the genesis of oedema is increased reabsorption of sodium, of chloride and, as a secondary phenomenon, of water in the renal tubules.

Frusemide is a powerful diuretic with a prompt short-lived action. It appears to act on both the ascending limb of the loop of Henle and the distal convoluted tubule to inhibit sodium reabsorption. In addition it may antagonize the action of ADH on cell membranes. The diuretic activity is not affected by changes in acid-base balance. Given orally, it acts within an hour: given intravenously, in 30 minutes. The action is over in four to five hours but is intense, so that caution in administration must be observed particularly in elderly men, who may have prostatism. A diuresis of over six litres has followed administration of 200 mg., and such sudden loss of water and dissolved electrolytes may be hazardous. The oral dosage in severe heart failure should be of the order of 80 to 240 mg., the intravenous dose 20 to 60 mg. This latter is for patients in acute left heart failure, in whom the speedy action of the drug is of especial value. Frusemide does not cause disproportionate potassium loss, but with the massive diuresis hypokalaemia is a possible sequel to be foreseen and prevented by preliminary potassium loading if this is feasible. Frusemide has proved a most valuable new drug for the treatment of heart failure and is the diuretic of first choice.

The benzothiadiazine diuretics. The actions of all these drugs are similar and they differ primarily in their effective dosage, hydrochlorothiazide and hydroflumethiazide being some 10 times as potent on a weight to weight basis as chlorothiazide, while bendrofluazide is 200 times as potent. Their primary action is on sodium and chloride excretions, which are greatly increased. The effects on potassium and bicarbonate ions are less marked. The increased excretion of water is secondary to the salt loss. These drugs do not lose their effectiveness with continued administration as happens with carbonic anhydrase inhibitors, and their action is rapid. Their principal disadvantage is the production of potassium deficiency—an effect which results from their pharmacological action and hence is not truly toxic. Toxic effects, such as skin rashes and gastro-intestinal irritation, are uncommon. Another side-effect is their tendency to cause a rise in the blood uric acid. This may rarely be associated with a clinical attack of gout, and the drugs may precipitate an acute attack in individuals with no previous history of the disorder. The risk is increased in the subjects of gross poly-cythaemia, as, for example, in cyanotic congenital heart disease. This tendency may preclude their use in some patients. Their prolonged ingestion has also been shown to induce a diabetic state in up to 30 per cent. of patients after three years.

Equivalent doses of these drugs are: chloro-thiazide, 500 mg. twice daily, hydrochlorothiazide, hydroflumethiazide, 50 mg. twice daily, and bendro-fluazide, 5 mg. once daily, for three days in each week. It is wise to give at the same time potassium in a suitable form two or three times a day to balance potassium loss (p. 120). This may be very serious in a patient already depleted of that ele-ment and particularly in one who is fully digitalized.

There are many preparations on the market in-corporating one or other thiazide with a potassium salt. These are widely prescribed, but it should be realized that such fixed-proportion tablets allow no latitude for the individual patient's needs and further and more seriously, these enteric-coated tablets loaded with a salt may result in rapid absorption from a small area of mucosa with consequent localized venous thrombosis and have led to numerous instances of damage (haemorrhage or perforation) to the small intestine. These preparations should not be prescribed.

Organic mercurial diuretics. The most popular organic mercurial diuretic is mersalyl B.P., dis-pensed in ampoules of 2 ml. containing 10 per cent. of the sodium salt of mersalyl acid with 5 per cent. of theophylline in water. It should be administered by deep intramuscular injection; it is active when given intravenously, but by this route it can cause severe, even fatal, reactions; it should never be injected subcutaneously as it then causes intense irritation and may produce sloughing. A test dose of 0·5 ml. is given initially, followed next day by the full 2 ml. injection. The drug may be given on alternate days or every third day. The action can be enhanced by previous administra-tion of ammonium chloride 2 g. in tablets given orally two hours before the injection. Its action commences within an hour or two and persists for

8 to 12 hours. The drug should, therefore, be given in the morning, since if administered late in the day the patient's sleep may be disturbed. The effect of mersalyl on the water-logged patient may be dramatic: a diuresis of 2 or 3 litres is common, larger diureses up to 4 or 5 litres are sometimes observed, and on occasion a dramatic fluid loss of up to 8 to 10 litres has been recorded after a single injection. In a few patients the effect persists into the second day, but usually urinary output on the day following administration falls even below the oliguric level which obtained before the mersalyl was given.

Toxic effects occur infrequently. Dermatitis with erythema and urticaria are the commonest side-effects, but if cumulation occurs the signs of chronic mercury poisoning develop with hyper-salivation and evidence of renal damage. Any adverse effects arising from mersalyl should be treated immediately with dimercaprol (p. 563) which is a highly effective antidote.

RESISTANT CARDIAC FAILURE: SALT
DEPLETION SYNDROME

While in the majority of patients with congestive cardiac failure there is a prompt and adequate response to the usual measures of rest, digitalis and diuretics, there is a proportion in whom these remedies lose their effect, so that oedema persists or increases, and the response to individual doses of powerful diuretics becomes negligible; such patients pass into a state of resistant cardiac failure. In some there is biochemical evidence of a profound upset of the blood and tissue electrolytes, the so-called 'salt depletion syndrome' (p. 255).

It was once believed that this refractory state was induced by the treatment, and that depletion of sodium and chloride was responsible for it as well as for some of the untoward accompanying symp-toms. It is now clear that a complex mechanism is involved and that while depletion of sodium and chloride may occur this is rare and commonly sub-terminal. On the other hand, potassium depletion is recognized as a common and often dominant feature.

In a patient under treatment with a standard regimen of digitalis and diuretics, successive doses of diuretics tend to produce progressively smaller responses as the total accumulation of salt and water in the tissue spaces is reduced; the net water output falls and with it the daily output of sodium and chloride. As the patient approaches his dry weight—i.e. his weight free from oedema—the increase in water, sodium and chloride output after each injection of a mercurial or oral dose of a sulphamyl diuretic may become negligible. Thus depletion of body stores of sodium and chloride seldom occurs from the action of diuretics, unless drastic salt deprivation has been imposed, or until the terminal stages of the illness are reached. On the other hand, potassium excretion is increased as an integral part of the action of most diuretics, and despite the decreased excretion of water and sodium referred to above, potassium excretion in response to each dose may remain high. This leads eventually to a state of profound potassium depletion which may readily escape detection, since unhappily the serum potassium level does not reflect the tissue level. The potassium content of the cells becomes largely replaced by sodium, with serious effects on their metabolism and on the body as a whole. Short of employing a whole-body counter to measure the naturally-occurring radioactive ^{40}K such depletion of total body potassium can be established only by careful balance studies over a long period, during which the net daily intake and output of potassium are carefully measured. Such studies show that the body avidly absorbs and retains potassium without a corresponding rise in the blood level, indicating diffusion of the absorbed potassium into the depleted cells.

In some patients a low blood chloride and low blood sodium may be demonstrated—the so-called salt depletion syndrome. Such patients are commonly nauseated, weak, drowsy or confused and the condition is attended by a rising blood urea and evidence of azotaemia, progressing it may be to uraemic coma. This perilous state of affairs may be aggravated by any measure which drastically upsets the body equilibrium in respect of fluid and salt—for example, the withdrawal of a large quantity of fluid by abdominal or thoracic paracentesis. Even the use of Southey's tubes to drain subcutaneous oedema from the legs may result in a curious reaction on the part of the kidney, with active retention of ingested water leading to hydraemia, the consequent dilution lowering still further the blood sodium and chloride levels. This fall in the levels of sodium and chloride, formerly attributed to excessive urinary losses, is now realized to be due to a bizarre and active water retention by the body in the later stages of heart failure. The charts of a fatal case of hyponatraemia and hypochloraemia are shown in Fig. 2 (p. 92).

Management of 'resistant' failure. The successful management of a patient with resistant cardiac failure is a difficult therapeutic problem. Before concluding that a patient is actually in this resistant phase, however, every care should be taken to ensure that the diagnosis is accurate and that a false impression of resistance has not been produced. Each case should be carefully reviewed to ensure that a cause of continuing failure (active rheumatic carditis, respiratory infection, silent infarction, thyrotoxicosis) is not still operative, undetected and untreated.

Having excluded such factors, the next step is to review critically the treatment which the patient has had. Many patients, resistant under home conditions, respond rapidly to a hospital regimen, and it is clear that the complete rest enforced under ward discipline is commonly a major factor in the changed status. Particular attention should also be paid to the dose of digitalis which the patient has been having, and that he has actually taken the drug in the quantity prescribed and has not for one reason or another modified this dosage on his own initiative. Attention should also be paid to his intake of salt, since many patients reputedly on a salt-poor diet in fact take much more than is prescribed. Consumption of porridge made with salt, salt butter, certain proprietary fruit drinks and other articles of diet, may push the daily intake up to an undesirably high level. Lastly, in every resistant patient a check should be made of the blood levels of sodium, potassium and chloride to establish whether salt depletion is present, bearing in mind the warning that the level of blood potassium is not always an accurate guide to its concentration in the cells.

The first few days of treatment should be devoted to securing complete rest, to adequate digitalization and to the restriction of salt in the diet to a maximum of 500 mg. daily. After a few days during which the patient is stabilized on this regimen, and the response noted, diuretics should be given—mersalyl, thiazides, chlorthalidone, triamterene or frusemide in usual dosage (p. 88). If the resulting diuresis is unsatisfactory, adjuvant measures should be tried, e.g. the administration of ammonium chloride before the injection of mersalyl. Alternatively, the administration of aminophylline, 500 mg. intravenously an hour before 2 ml. of mersalyl is given intramuscularly, may cause a brisk diuresis.

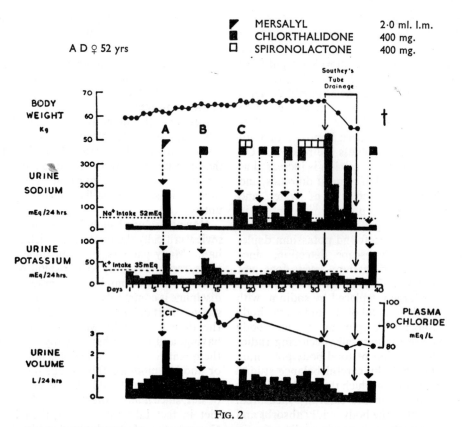

A D ♀ 52 yrs

◢ MERSALYL	2·0 ml. I.m.
■ CHLORTHALIDONE	400 mg.
□ SPIRONOLACTONE	400 mg.

FIG. 2

Graph of body weight, urinary electrolytes, plasma chloride and urine output over a six-week period in a patient with 'resistant' failure, illustrating effects of diuretics and spironolactone, development of hypochloraemia, and lethal effect of mechanical drainage of fluid.

This patient had gross heart failure which had failed to respond to digitalis and mersalyl at home. On a liberal intake of 1·5 g. salt (52 mEq./Na⁺) daily she showed oliguria and rising body weight in spite of digitalization and complete rest. Mersalyl at A produced a good diuresis with loss of fair amounts of Na⁺ *and* K⁺ in the urine. Chlorthalidone at B produced no effect on urine volume or Na⁺ excretion, but a brisk loss of K⁺. When this was repeated (C) along with a spironolactone a moderate diuresis and Na⁺ loss followed, lasting two days, while K⁺ loss was inhibited.

Further doses of diuretic with and without spironolactone produced moderate Na⁺ loss and slight sustained diuresis with no K⁺ loss.

During this time, despite a relatively high salt intake and only moderate Na⁺ loss, the plasma chloride was falling, while the body water was rising (increasing body weight).

Drainage by Southey's tubes led to gross loss of Na⁺ (300 mEq. in 5 days) and water (10 kg.=2 gallons). Hypochloraemia (80 mEq./l), and hyponatraemia led to death.

(By permission of Dr W. K. Stewart and the Editor, the *Lancet*)

It is in patients of this group that recourse may be had to the specific antagonist to aldosterone—a spironolactone. Aldosterone is an adrenal hormone, the secretion of which is not under the control of the pituitary but which is regulated by a complex feed-back system of volume sensors in the cardiovascular system. It actively promotes potassium excretion and conserves sodium—actions diametrically opposed to the needs of the oedematous

patient. Thus, the counteraction of its effect would be theoretically desirable and can be achieved in practice by the use of spironolactones. Aldactone-A, four times as potent as the original preparation, is given in 25 mg. doses together with a conventional diuretic. The drug is non-toxic and may induce a satisfactory diuresis in a patient otherwise resistant to mercurials or thiazides.

The crux of the matter in handling patients with

resistant cardiac failure is attention to detail—to strict rest, to digitalization, to salt restriction and to diuretic administration with such adjuvant therapy as outlined above. The truly resistant patient in whom cardiac failure defeats all attempts at treatment is generally in the terminal stage of his illness.

THE LONG-TERM MANAGEMENT OF THE PATIENT IN CARDIAC FAILURE

In the preceding pages attention has been devoted to the management of cardiac failure in its extreme forms as met with in hospital practice. Such management generally involves several weeks of intensive therapy, after which the patient is discharged to his home. There, over a period of months or years, he will require skilled supervision by his family doctor. Many patients who have been in gross failure and who have been rescued by treatment can be maintained in a state of relative well-being, fit for a fair amount of activity and possibly even able to continue their normal occupations provided their treatment is closely supervised. It is with this highly important aspect of treatment that the following paragraphs are concerned.

As a first step after convalescence, the patient should take stock of his whole environment and activities with a view to reducing expenditure of energy to within his cardiac capacity. Attention by the doctor to matters of detail is of inestimable value: for example, the avoidance of fatigue and exposure to inclement weather on the way to and from work may be more important to the individual than the nature of his occupation, since many patients with sedentary work can carry on without ill effects provided they are not exhausted by the effort of getting to it. So also in the home, by attention to such apparently trivial details as the location of bedroom and lavatory the patient may be spared fatigue. In the case of a patient whose home is in an upstairs flat a certificate by the doctor recommending a ground-floor house may result in appropriate action by the local housing authority. The patient who continues at work, perhaps with some difficulty, should be encouraged to spend at least eight hours in bed each night and should be advised to take things quietly at weekends. A day's rest in bed each week—be it Saturday or Sunday—is of great value and can readily be achieved. The only exception is the housewife, whose work goes on seven days a week, and these circumstances call for special arrangements. It may be possible to arrange for her to spend a part of each day resting, say in the afternoon from 2 to 4, once the midday dinner is over and before the children come home from school. It may be possible to arrange through the Social Services for home help of one sort or another—a woman may come in, at public expense or partially subsidized by the state, to do the heavy housework; cooked meals may be provided by one of the voluntary services; young children may be cared for in a crèche. The doctor who is familiar with the patient and family and with the particular environmental conditions may be of great help in giving advice about these matters.

On the major question of occupation the doctor's guidance may be of great value. Manifestly many will be unable to continue their previous occupation once they have suffered from congestive failure. Arduous manual labour is out of the question, and to re-engage in such employment is to court disaster. It is often possible for the doctor to suggest a suitable occupation for young people. In the case of the middle-aged or elderly individual, particularly the wage-earning man, it may be difficult to secure a niche in industry into which the handicapped person can be fitted. There are, however, facilities in rehabilitation centres for the training of patients in new skills, and up and down the country factories have been established in which sheltered employment can be given to those unfitted by physical handicap for the rough and tumble of ordinary industrial conditions. Some occupation even for the gravely handicapped is of the greatest therapeutic value and conversely prolonged unemployment through sickness is demoralizing. The conscientious family doctor will endeavour to secure employment appropriate to his patient's capabilities, and will encourage him in every way to continue wage-earning so long as circumstances permit.

COR PULMONALE

Heart failure secondary to respiratory disease deserves special consideration, since it differs from ordinary heart failure not only in the underlying physiological derangements but in its treatment. In this country cor pulmonale is generally secondary to chronic bronchitis and emphysema (pp. 194, 197). The prevalence of chronic bronchitis in this country has led to its being called 'the English disease'—displacing rickets from this nickname in the continental literature. In a small proportion of cases cor pulmonale develops as a sequel to other diseases such as pulmonary fibrosis and pneumoconiosis, and lesions with infiltration or destruction of the lungs, for example by lymph-spread carcinomatosis, sarcoidosis or infiltration by Hodgkin tissue. In countries where schistosomiasis is endemic, a form of cor pulmonale due to infection of the lungs is prevalent.

While chronic bronchitis and emphysema lead over the years to progressive limitation of effort, congestive heart failure is a late event in their course, occurring after many years of winter cough as an episode precipitated by respiratory infection. Contrary to traditional teaching, the progressive destruction of the pulmonary vascular bed in emphysema produces little effect on the right heart, and no rise in the pulmonary arterial pressure occurs in the uncomplicated case. This is related to the enormous capacity of the normal pulmonary vascular bed and the great reserve area of respiratory epithelium in health. Nevertheless, when such an individual develops an acute capillary bronchitis or bronchopneumonia with patchy atelectasis, the resultant anoxia leads to a steep rise in the pulmonary arterial pressure which in turn places a considerable load on the right ventricle. Bronchospasm and 'air-trapping' add to the anoxia. Cardiac failure tends to develop rapidly, and such patients are soon in desperate straits, with oedema, venous engorgement in the neck and hepatic enlargement. Owing to anoxia they are cyanosed, and this may be intensified by the polycythaemia which accompanies emphysema. The clinical picture differs from that of heart failure in valvular or ischaemic heart disease in that warm flushed hands and extremities are characteristic, the pulse is bounding and of full volume and sinus rhythm is usual, atrial fibrillation being uncommon. This clinical picture of a hyperkinetic circulation is related to the high cardiac output in such patients which may in fact be two or three times the normal, so that the condition falls into the group of 'high-output failure' (p. 82). In some patients far advanced in their course, the cardiac output falls and the peripheral coldness and small pulse of conventional cardiac failure develop with the low-output state. Superimposed on the cardiovascular symptoms are those of hypercapnia affecting the central nervous system.

In patients with 'high-output failure' digitalis is in general disappointing, and lacks much of its effect in conventional cardiac failure. Its use was once considered contraindicated, since a high venous pressure is necessary for the maintenance of the high output in turn necessitated by anoxia. Digitalis, however, still has a place in the treatment of failure in cor pulmonale, though its use must be tempered with caution.

Since the failure is precipitated by anoxia, infection and bronchospasm, the prime need is treatment of those factors. The administration of suitable antibiotics is the first step and such treatment should be vigorous (p. 2).

The oxygen saturation of the arterial blood in such patients can fall as low as 65 or 70 per cent., i.e., to that of the mixed venous blood of a normal person, and clearly relief of anoxia is of paramount importance. Administration of oxygen, however, must be cautious, since precipitate exposure of the patient to high oxygen concentrations may have serious consequences. Every doctor and every nurse should be aware of this therapeutic paradox, whereby a blue, conscious, dyspnoeic patient placed in an oxygen tent may rapidly become pink and comatose. If oxygen administration is continued the patient will die. The explanation is that such patients are not only anoxic but hypercapnic, the partial pressure of carbon dioxide in the blood rising to a high level. At such levels of pCO_2 the respiratory centre becomes insensitive to its normal stimulus, and the patient's respiration is controlled by oxygen-lack. When this is relieved by giving oxygen the breathing becomes shallow, hypercapnia increases and the blood carbon dioxide mounts to a level which produces unconsciousness and unchecked leads to coma and death. The danger attendant on the administration of oxygen to such patients has led many to avoid giving it to them. This is clearly against their best interests, since they require oxygen desperately, and it is the duty of the doctor to administer it in such a manner that distress and anoxia are relieved without the hazards of hypercapnia. This can be done by giving oxygen at a relatively low concentration (2 or 3 litres per minute) so that anoxia is to some extent mitigated but the risk attendant on its complete relief avoided. The patient must be kept under close observation so that with the development of drowsiness or even natural sleep oxygen may be discontinued and the patient allowed to become anoxic and awake. One type of mask utilizes the Venturi principle to supply oxygen in a safe and effective range of concentration. The practice is all too widespread today of denying oxygen to such desperately anoxic patients on the basis of the dangers attendant on its use (p. 644).

Many patients respond rapidly to the control of infection and of anoxia. The relief of bronchospasm and clearing of airways are highly important (p. 215). Digitalization, if adopted, should be done gradually, the effect on the individual patient being closely watched. Diuretics are also of value and it is in this condition that acetazolamide can on occasion play a useful rôle, since in hypercapnia the substrate for the carbonic anhydrase inhibitor is abundantly present.

The after-care of patients who have recovered from cardiac failure secondary to respiratory infection should be directed to the prevention of recurrences (p. 195). It is unhappily true that heart failure of this type is commonly a sub-terminal event; few patients so affected survive more than two years after their first attack.

LEFT HEART FAILURE

The clinical picture of left heart failure is distinctive and should not be readily confused with any other condition—with one exception. Cardiac asthma is well named, since the urgent, commonly nocturnal, dyspnoea of left ventricular failure is associated with bronchospasm in a considerable proportion of cases. This may lead to confusion with bronchial asthma—a serious error which may cost the patient his life as the treatment of the two conditions is quite different. It is particularly important before administering morphine to a suspected case of left ventricular failure to ensure that the diagnosis is correct since the giving of morphine to a patient with bronchial asthma may prove fatal.

Treatment of left heart failure is a matter of great urgency. The patient may recover spontaneously from his attack or may die in the course of half an hour. Efficient remedies are available and prompt intervention may save life.

The time-honoured remedy for cardiac asthma is morphine, and provided the diagnosis is certain, its administration is safe and effective. The dose depends on the weight of the patient and the route of administration. An average subcutaneous dose is 15 mg., but this may be increased to 20 or even 30 mg. in heavily built adults. The action of the drug is apparent in 15 to 30 minutes. A much speedier action is obtained by intravenous injection, and for this purpose a correspondingly smaller dose is desirable, say 5 to 10 mg. given slowly. The effect appears within two or three minutes and the doctor may at his discretion repeat the same or a smaller

dose in say 15 minutes if this is desirable. Since attacks of cardiac asthma commonly occur early in the morning and the practitioner is called from his bed to attend the desperately ill patient, it is probably wise to resort to the intravenous route and for the doctor to sit by the bedside of the patient till the full effect has been achieved.

Aminophylline is also a valuable drug in this condition: although it stimulates the respiratory centre it causes relaxation of the bronchioles and thus gives relief from dyspnoea. When there is any shadow of doubt as to the nature of the attack, aminophylline is the drug of choice. It is given by slow intravenous injection, well diluted in 10 ml. of saline, in a dose of 500 mg. The action is prompt and usually dramatic.

The rapidly acting diuretic, frusemide, given intravenously in a dose of 20 to 40 mg., is of great value and has supplanted mersalyl and other diuretics for this condition. Its intense though brief action occurs within minutes of its injection.

If facilities are at hand, the administration of oxygen by a disposable plastic mask is highly effective (p. 649). The rate of administration should be from 4 to 6 litres per minute.

In an emergency when no drugs are available venesection may be life saving. The amount withdrawn should be from 10 to 20 oz. (300 to 600 ml.), but the essence of the procedure is the *rapid* withdrawal. A wide-bore French's needle is thrust into the ante-cubital vein, and the procedure is cleaner if a length of rubber tubing is attached so that the blood may drain into a container. In an emergency the ante-cubital vein may be snipped with scissors or nicked with a scalpel. Arrest of bleeding is readily achieved by pressure with a pad and bandage. The effectiveness of venesection depends on the sudden reduction in the venous return to the right heart; this reduces right ventricular output and diminishes pulmonary congestion, thus enabling the overloaded left heart to cope with the influx from the lesser circulation. 'Bloodless venesection' achieved by reducing the venous return through cuffs applied to the four limbs may achieve a similar result without the hazard of inducing anaemia should the procedure require to be repeated. For this purpose two ordinary sphygmomanometer cuffs are applied to the arms and two broad cuffs to the thighs. These are pumped up to a pressure somewhat above the venous pressure to obstruct the venous return. It is important that when the patient has recovered from the acute

D*

attack the cuffs should not all be released simultaneously, since sudden flooding of the right heart with the trapped blood may cause recurrence of pulmonary congestion. It is wiser to release the cuffs one by one, keeping the patient under close observation.

In pulmonary oedema there is exudation of fluid into the lungs and constant cough with profuse watery pink-stained expectoration. In such cases much benefit can be achieved by suction through a catheter passed into the pharynx or (in the unconscious patient) into the trachea. In hospital the catheter can be connected to a suction apparatus, commonly an electric motor and pump, but alternative improvised methods may have to be used.

The treatment of the acute attack by no means completes the treatment of left heart failure: the patient who has suffered such an attack is in as much need of intensive treatment with rest, digitalis and diuretics as any other patient with cardiac failure. Many patients, particularly in the middle-aged hypertensive group, are intolerant of restriction and feel so well next day that they wish to return to work. They must be firmly dissuaded from doing so and should be treated by rest in bed for some three to four weeks. Digitalization may be achieved rapidly with 1 mg. digoxin intravenously; the administration of diuretics will be necessary and they should be given as already described for congestive heart failure (p. 86). Further, in all patients who have suffered an attack of left heart failure the underlying cause (hypertension, myocardial infarction, mitral stenosis) must be identified and treated. In this as in every other cardiac condition precise and complete diagnosis is of prime importance. To label a patient 'cardiac asthma' without identifying and dealing with the underlying cause is clearly inadequate.

CORONARY ARTERY DISEASE

Patients who suffer from disease of the coronary arteries present with a wide variety of symptoms of every grade of severity. On the one hand the clinical history may be dominated by an episode of myocardial infarction with prolonged pain, shock and a serious protracted illness; such episodes may recur time and again in a particular patient. At the other extreme there are those who suffer transient restriction of effort due to pain, varying from trivial discomfort to extreme distress. Some patients combine both syndromes and suffer for years from angina of effort with superimposed attacks of myocardial infarction. There is every justification for considering these patients collectively, whatever be their dominant symptoms, and their general management over the years does not differ from one group to the next. In so far as treatment of the acute episode is concerned, the management of myocardial infarction is conveniently considered separately from that of angina of effort. It will be noted that the term myocardial infarction is used rather than coronary thrombosis, for there is good evidence that while clotting in a coronary artery is a common cause of myocardial infarction it is by no means invariable and infarction of the heart muscle without coronary thrombosis is common.

MYOCARDIAL INFARCTION

Introduction. The treatment of patients suffering from myocardial infarction has not altered materially during the past few years, but important changes have taken place in the general management of the patient as a casualty. It is widely recognized that these patients are most liable to sudden death from cardiac arrest or ventricular fibrillation during the first few hours of the illness. At this time, therefore, continuous supervision by experienced physicians and nursing staff is highly desirable. It can be achieved in two ways. First, the flying-squad ambulance can bring to the patient most, if not all, of the apparatus and drugs which may be needed to save his life should he develop a cardiac dysrhythmia while he is at home—or elsewhere—and also while he is being transported to the nearest suitable hospital. Secondly, during his first few days in hospital the patient should be accommodated in a Coronary Care Unit where his cardiac rhythm can be monitored and where a trained team of physicians and nurses is constantly available to give appropriate treatment should an emergency arise. These procedures should always be adopted if the facilities described are available. Unfortunately the methods are not always practicable for geographical reasons, and in any case their organization is always costly. Not surprisingly, therefore, only a small minority of patients enjoy these advantages; and the family doctor is obliged to do the best he can in the circumstances that confront him.

Immediate treatment may be considered under four headings: the relief of pain; the management of shock; monitoring in an 'intensive care' unit; and the resuscitation of the apparently dead.

Relief of pain and removal to hospital. The immediate treatment consists in securing absolute rest in bed and the relief of pain by administration of morphine in full doses. Should the attack occur when the patient is at work or away from home, he should immediately be given hypodermically 15 to 20 mg. of morphine and should be sent to hospital by ambulance. He must be assisted to undress, and should from the outset be spared all avoidable exertion. The severely shocked patient should not be undressed or bathed. Since the greatest risk to life is in the first 24 to 48 hours, early hospitalization is advisable. It is unwise to allow a woman to undertake single-handed the nursing of a relative or other patient with this disorder. The day and night nursing and the lifting involved impose too great a strain, and the patient is naturally disposed to ease the burden by doing things for himself.

The amount of morphine required is variable. The initial dose of 15 to 20 mg. should be repeated without hesitation in an hour should pain be unrelieved, and further doses may be required. In severely shocked patients caution must be exercised since lack of effect from repeated subcutaneous injections may be due to non-absorption of the drug. For the later doses, oral administration of 15-mg. tablets by an attendant under medical direction is satisfactory. The drug exerts no deleterious effect on the heart. Morphine is invaluable because it relieves pain and abolishes anxiety: adequate doses are conducive to sleep, and complete rest is of prime importance. Nausea and vomiting are common symptoms in heart failure—including the acute failure seen in myocardial infarction—and they can be relieved by giving morphine. Nevertheless, these symptoms also commonly occur as side-effects of morphine—especially in women, so it is wise to give an anti-emetic, e.g. cyclizine, along with it. It is important to assess accurately the significance of nausea and vomiting and to be more cautious in the doses given to old people. Many physicians prefer diamorphine (5 to 10 mg.); it is less likely to cause vomiting because the analgesic action is achieved with doses about half those of morphine. In recent years, pentazocine (p. 443) has been used as an alternative to morphine and diamorphine. In doses of 30 to 60 mg. subcutaneously it produces adequate analgesia without the unwelcome side-effects of morphine, but its action may last only one or two hours.

Treatment of shock. Shock in cases of coronary occlusion varies markedly in degree. Profound shock develops in a minority of patients with massive infarcts, and in general is associated with a grave prognosis. Some desperately ill patients, however, do respond to treatment and may go on to a smooth convalescence, so that every effort should be made in every case. It is in these severely shocked patients that oxygen administration is of conspicuous value. To be effective, it should be given in high concentration (say 6 to 7 litres per minute) continuously for many hours by means of a polythene mask (p. 649).

Large intravenous infusions carry a serious hazard by overloading the damaged myocardium, and adrenaline and ephedrine are contraindicated on account of their cardiac actions. Noradrenaline has a marked vasoconstrictor action without the cardiac accelerator and augmentor actions of adrenaline. It raises the blood pressure by peripheral action. It is given intravenously by drip in a concentration of 8 mg. per litre. The rate of infusion is regulated according to the blood pressure response and is generally of the order of 10 mcg. per minute. There is now available a number of synthetic pressor agents (e.g. metaraminol) administered in the same way by intravenous drip, and these have been extensively investigated. Unfortunately the initial expectations have not been justified by results and the mortality among patients with severe shock, despite such treatment, varies in the reported series from 60 to nearly 100 per cent. The writer's personal experience has been correspondingly disappointing, and he places more faith in the administration of oxygen than in the use of pressor drugs.

Soon after the occurrence of myocardial infarction the clinical picture may be dominated by the onset of cardiac asthma (left ventricular failure) or paroxysmal tachycardia with a high ventricular rate. Appropriate measures should be taken to deal with these complications (pp. 95, 123).

Intensive care units and cardiac resuscitation. Every patient who has suffered a major myocardial infarction is, particularly during the first few crucial days, at risk of sudden death from cardiac arrest or ventricular fibrillation. Modern electronic devices and the techniques of external cardiac massage and mouth-to-mouth artificial respiration have led to many apparently hopeless cases being rescued. Time is of the essence for successful resuscitation, since after cardiac arrest lasting only some four minutes irreversible damage to the brain ensues. It is essential, therefore, that the onset of an attack is signalled at once, and that all staff (junior doctors, nurses) should be familiar with the life-saving measures employed while skilled help and modern apparatus are summoned. (See *ventricular fibrillation*, p. 125 and *cardiac arrest*, p. 126.)

The practicability of saving such patients has led to the institution in larger hospitals of Intensive Care Units, to which patients at risk can be admitted, and where monitoring and resuscitation equipment are available. It is possible for an alarm signal (light or buzzer) in the nurses' station to be triggered by the patient's heart rate falling below or rising above predetermined figures, and for electrical pace-making to cut in automatically in cases of ventricular standstill. If ventricular fibrillation is demonstrated on the oscilloscope, defibrillation is attempted by external electrodes or by their direct application to the exposed heart. The gross metabolic acidosis which develops rapidly in such patients must be promptly corrected by intravenous bicarbonate or lactate, otherwise attempts to restore cardiac action are fruitless. The staff of such units must all be trained in resuscitation procedures. Short of such units, suitable equipment can be mounted on a trolley, which is brought to the scene of the emergency in response to an alarm call to the hospital telephone exchange, the operator simultaneously summoning medical help (cardiologist, anaesthetist). Inevitably, the initial decision to attempt resuscitation has often to be taken by junior nursing or medical staff. It follows that they must be formally instructed in the principles and practice of cardiac resuscitation; and there is no satisfactory alternative to demonstration-lectures when all equipment can be examined and tested.

The proportion of patients saved is not high but an overall mortality of 33 per cent. in ordinary wards can be reduced to about 13 per cent. in such units. The barriers to their widespread introduction are capital expenditure and scarcity of skilled staff. The few successes amply compensate for the labour and expense involved. Ethical problems naturally arise—e.g. how far one is justified in attempting resuscitation in old, ill subjects far advanced in serious cardiac or other disease. Nevertheless, many 'coronary deaths' occur in young men, and in such the full resources of modern therapy must be deployed.

Treatment of myocardial infarction during the first month. The best guide to the practitioner in handling a patient with myocardial infarction is a

knowledge of the natural history of the disease so that, aware of the hazards besetting the patient, he may be ready to forestall disaster or treat complications. By far the largest number of deaths

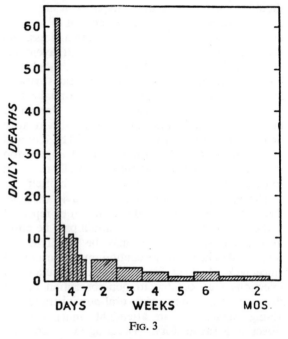

Fig. 3

Deaths in myocardial infarction in relation to stage of illness. (After G. E. Honey and S. C. Truelove, 1957. *Lancet* **1**, 1155. By permission of the authors and the Editor, the *Lancet*.)

occur within the first 24 hours after onset and a high percentage of the remainder within the first week. Thereafter they are relatively infrequent and scattered more evenly over the first six weeks. Figure 3 shows graphically this striking predominance of deaths in the early hours and days. On analysis the major causes of death are recurrence of infarction, abnormal rhythms, left heart failure and persistence of intractable shock. These, therefore, are the conditions which it must be our aim to treat. The later deaths result from congestive cardiac failure or left ventricular failure, from systemic or pulmonary embolism, and from cardiac rupture, while recurrent infarction accounts for a smaller number. Accordingly, during the later weeks therapy should be directed towards prevention or treatment of these various complications.

Prevention of recurrent infarction. In patients in whom the infarction is caused by coronary thrombosis, it would be logical to prevent spread or recurrence of clotting by giving anticoagulants. The pros and cons of anticoagulant treatment are discussed below. Such treatment cannot of itself have any direct effect on the death rate from such complications as shock, arrhythmias or left heart failure.

Dysrhythmias. Any arrhythmia may occur after myocardial infarction: not all are dangerous and not all demand treatment. The commonest is the occasional *ventricular extrasystole*. Sometimes these may be frequent and may in the course of a few hours lead on to *ventricular paroxysmal tachycardia*. In cases with numerous ventricular extrasystoles it is therefore wise to give lignocaine hydrochloride by intravenous drip at the rate of 1 to 2 mg. per minute as a prophylactic measure (p. 125). The treatment of paroxysmal tachycardia is dealt with on p. 125. A second common and serious arrhythmia is *atrial fibrillation*. When this occurs with a high uncontrolled ventricular rate it commonly precipitates congestive failure and may place the patient in peril. In such cases it is justifiable to digitalize the patient along the lines detailed on pp. 85-88. *Heart-block* is a not uncommon accompaniment of myocardial infarction. Recently corticosteroids have been widely used with equivocal results. Generally the rhythm returns to normal in the course of a few days without specific treatment. Otherwise management should be along the lines detailed on p. 126.

Later complications. These complications are treated along standard lines (pp. 81, 95).

Of the *later complications* of myocardial infarction *cardiac rupture* can neither be foreseen nor prevented, but its occurrence is less frequent in patients nursed strictly in bed while scar tissue is being formed.

Embolism either in the lungs or in the systemic vascular bed is a frequent complication, and is responsible for a considerable proportion of the fatalities occurring after the first few days. Pulmonary embolism arises as a rule from peripheral venous thrombosis, though on occasion a clot from the right ventricular cavity may be swept into the lungs. Systemic embolism occurs from an intracardiac clot forming over a roughened endocardium. The incidence of both types is markedly reduced by anticoagulant therapy (see below).

Anticoagulant Therapy

Anticoagulants have been used for over 25 years in the acute phase of myocardial infarction but there is still much controversy as to their value. The author believes that anticoagulants have a definite but limited value. They are not effective in reducing the mortality from shock, arrhythmias or cardiac failure, and cases of recurrent infarction occur in patients under anticoagulant treatment in whom tests for prothrombin time indicate adequate therapeutic action. Their main effect is the reduction in thrombo-embolism and there is general agreement that they thus effect a significant reduction in mortality.

Assessment of their value has proved difficult, since many factors interfere with a straightforward evaluation. For example, in patients admitted to hospital on the second or a later day after infarction, the overall mortality is lower than in those admitted on the first day of illness, since those treated are the survivors of the first supremely dangerous 24 hours. Variations due to the age and sex of the patient, to the severity and extent of the infarction, and to the condition of the heart muscle before infarction occurred introduce major complicating factors. Only by comparison of large series of treated and untreated (control) cases, carefully matched in respect of all these factors (age, sex, severity, degree of shock, duration of illness, etc.) can a reliable impression be obtained as to the value of anticoagulants. Many such series have been published, some comprising large numbers of cases, and widely divergent assessments of their value have been reached. Generally the most striking benefits are in men around the age of 50 without serious previous myocardial lesions. By contrast in patients over 65 of either sex, and in those who have suffered a series of previous infarctions with consequent scarring of the muscle, the results are unimpressive.

Some physicians divide cases of myocardial infarction into 'good risk' and 'bad risk' classes. The bad risk patients are those with persistent pain, severe shock, arrhythmias or failure, who have had previous myocardial infarctions, or with a systemic disorder such as diabetes. The good risk group are those without such ominous features. It is claimed that among good risk patients the mortality without anticoagulant treatment is so low that the risks attendant on its use are unjustifiable, and this treatment should be reserved for patients of the bad risk group. The writer believes that this is an unjustifiable simplification, since we deal with individuals and not with groups. A patient when first seen may be little shocked with all the criteria of a small infarction, and yet in the course of 24 or 48 hours may develop an extension of his lesion and rapidly pass into the bad risk category. Nor is it possible to predict in which individual this deterioration may occur. For this reason patients with myocardial infarction in the younger age-group (up to 50 years) should be given anticoagulant treatment when the condition is first diagnosed, irrespective of the severity of the original attack. When there are other visceral lesions anticoagulants are contraindicated. Fatal haemorrhage has occurred in a patient who has had no dyspeptic symptoms for over a decade, but with an old peptic ulcer history; and similar disasters have occurred from cerebrovascular embolic accidents complicating the coronary attack before admission to hospital.

All patients receiving anticoagulants must be kept under close observation for signs of overdosage (purpura, lowered capillary resistance, microscopic haematuria) and estimations of blood coagulation time and/or prothrombin index must be done (p. 189). The known antidotes should be at hand. It is helpful and safe for a single initial intravenous dose of heparin (15,000 units) to be given by the family doctor as soon as he has established the diagnosis of coronary occlusion. Continuation of the treatment and its laboratory control can be achieved in hospital.

It is usual to administer heparin for 48 hours after admission to hospital, meantime giving phenindione or warfarin orally. Thereafter their action is sufficient for the heparin to be discontinued. Treatment with phenindione or warfarin should be continued for two to four weeks depending on initial assessment of severity and duration of rest in bed, and then the dose is gradually tapered off. While the writer's main experience has been with phenindione and he still uses it in practice, it should be noted that there is a growing body of opinion that warfarin is preferable as an oral anticoagulant. The daily dose of phenindione varies from 25 to 150 mg. and of warfarin from 3 to 10 mg. according to the blood prothrombin level.

Other treatment. Vasodilators are useless in myocardial infarction, and should not be given, particularly as shock is commonly severe and the blood pressure already low.

The type of diet recommended for cases of severe congestive failure (p. 84) will prove generally suitable; it is easily taken and readily assimilated.

Purgation should be avoided. The instillation of two ounces of olive oil into the rectum, followed by a saline enema in the morning, is a safe and effective method of opening the bowels.

Duration of rest in bed. The duration of confinement to bed varies with the severity of the case. Where intense and prolonged pain, profound shock and the electrocardiographic pattern of transmural infarction indicate an extensive lesion involving the whole thickness of the ventricular wall, the patient should be kept in bed for six weeks. There are real risks to life throughout the first few weeks in such a case (recurrence, embolism, rupture of the softened area of muscle, failure), and these are increased by exertion. After six weeks or so these risks are greatly reduced, and a gradual return to activity can be permitted. On the other hand, a single attack of pain lasting half an hour, not associated with shock, and with an electrocardiogram indicating a limited area of superficial damage only, would warrant a cautious return to activity in one to two weeks. The return to activity must be gradual; the patient is first allowed to sit up in bed, to feed himself and to wash and to shave, to sit dangling his legs over the bed for short periods, and finally to get up and about before leaving hospital. The question of his future activities must then be considered.

Difficulty will often be experienced in persuading a patient to stay in bed for the prescribed period, since frequently he feels perfectly well within a few days. The difficulty is naturally greatest in mild cases, or in patients who have had no pain. Explanation that the heart has been damaged, and that it takes some weeks to heal properly, will usually render the patient amenable to discipline. But one must be careful not to induce a state of undue apprehension of the hazards, for much anxiety may result and more harm than good be done. The attitude of the doctor towards his patient is important. The patient is generally aware of the seriousness of his condition. An attitude of unrelieved gloom on the part of the attending physician is both inhuman and unjustifiable. The risks to be run during convalescence must be kept in mind but must not be used as a bogey to frighten a patient into submission. Not the least of the patient's risks is that of developing a cardiac neurosis which may be more crippling than his organic lesion.

Patients who have suffered an attack of myocardial infarction, whether or not residual angina of effort persists, should in their after-care be treated on the same lines as the subjects of effort angina.

ANGINA OF EFFORT

Treatment of attacks. It is unusual for a patient to be seen by his doctor while actually in the throes of effort angina. The attacks are of short duration and occur while the patient is about his daily business, and the pain is likely to have abated spontaneously before a doctor reaches the patient. When pain has lasted without intermission for half an hour or more the case should be regarded as one of myocardial infarction and treated as such. The same applies to patients previously free from angina or suffering from attacks of only moderate severity who suddenly develop attacks of great frequency on slight exertion. Such patients are commonly labelled cases of 'acute coronary insufficiency'. Some at least suffer occlusion of coronary arterial twigs, leading to patchy infarction and later to small scars in the myocardium.

The patient who is habitually seized with praecordial pain while walking soon realizes that continued effort aggravates his discomfort, and learns to stand still when pain comes on. In many cases this suffices to relieve the pain promptly, and no medication is required. In more severe or resistant cases one or other of the quickly acting nitrites usually affords relief, and the subjects of effort angina frequently carry such preparations for emergency use. The preparation of choice is the official tablet of glyceryl trinitrate containing 0·5 mg. While relief may follow as little as 0·25 mg., 0·5 mg. is usually required and sometimes 1 mg. or exceptionally 2 mg. may be necessary. The patient should be instructed to chew and suck the tablets, as absorption is most rapid from the buccal mucous membrane.

The action of glyceryl trinitrate lasts only a few minutes, but this is usually adequate. Nevertheless, compounds having a prolonged action have been introduced. It is appropriate here to remind the reader that however potent a vasodilator may be for the coronary vessels of healthy animals, its action on the rigid, sclerosed or calcified coronary arteries of anginal subjects is to say the least problematical. The relief from pain afforded by many vasodilators (not excluding nitroglycerin) may be due rather to peripheral action and decreased cardiac load than to direct action on the coronary vessels. Examples of long-acting coronary vasodilators include pentaerythritol tetranitrate, prescribed in doses of 20 to 60 mg. twice or thrice daily, of which the vasodilator action is certainly longer than that of nitroglycerin,

yet carefully controlled clinical trials of its action in angina have shown it to be less effective. One of the most promising of the long-acting preparations is nitroglycerin dispensed in tablets prepared to release the drug in small quantities over a prolonged period. These tablets contain much larger doses than the therapeutic single dose of 0·5 mg.—up to 2 mg. or even 30 mg. The gradual solution of the matrix in the gut over a number of hours produces a prolonged effect. These slow-release tablets are not recommended for quick relief of an acute attack of angina, but are designed to afford protection from attacks over several hours.

Various mono-amine oxidase inhibitors (iproniazid, isocarboxazid, nialamide) have been claimed to be effective long-acting coronary vasodilators, but such action as they possess is outweighed by their potential toxicity.

Beta-adrenergic blocking agents are of value in some cases. Propranolol is effective but has a tendency to produce bronchospasm in some individuals. It has been superseded by practolol which is more specific in its cardiac action and devoid of effect on the bronchi, etc. These drugs slow the pulse and lower the blood pressure and they have an action also in oxygen sparing. Their action is not primarily due to vaso-dilatation. The oral dose of propranolol is 20 to 30 mg. thrice daily (occasionally larger doses are required); and of practolol 50 mg. twice daily initially, rising to a maximum daily intake of approximately 600 mg.

After subsidence of an episode of pain many patients are able to resume walking or other activity where they left off, but should be warned to adopt a slower pace than that which provoked the pain.

General management of patients with coronary disease. The treatment of actual attacks of pain should be looked upon as a minor part of the management of coronary disease. Reduction in the number of attacks is of greater importance, and much can be done to achieve this end. More will be accomplished by regulation of life at work and play, of habits regarding meals and the use of alcohol and tobacco, and by advice on other mundane matters than by the administration of drugs. Attempts have been made to modify the progress of the atherosclerotic process by measures to lower the blood cholesterol level and to prevent recurrent infarction with long-term anticoagulant therapy. It is a travesty of our therapeutic knowledge to make a diagnosis of effort angina and to send the patient away merely with a supply of nitroglycerin and instructions to chew a tablet when pain is felt.

Many patients are overweight and in them reduction in weight is probably the most potent therapeutic measure. A reduction of body weight by 10 to 20 per cent. greatly eases the burden on the heart, and frequently results in a striking improvement in the exercise tolerance without the use of drugs. The sufferer from angina should be encouraged to attain a weight slightly under the average for height, age and sex. This can be achieved by simple dietetic restrictions, provided the co-operation of the patient is secured (p. 340). Attacks commonly occur when exercise is taken soon after a meal: heavy meals are to be avoided, and a rest or short sleep after lunch or dinner may reduce the frequency of attacks.

The family physician, from his knowledge of the patient's habits and mode of life, is best qualified to instruct him as to what to do and what to avoid in his daily routine. Many of these patients are active business men around 50 years of age, and careful consideration of their habits and circumstances will reveal the steps to be taken to reduce the demands on the circulation. *In all subjects of angina, and probably in all men over 50, sudden strenuous unaccustomed exertion is dangerous.* The writer has repeatedly seen cases in which such activity (e.g. cranking a car, shovelling snow, hurrying with a suitcase for a train) has immediately preceded the onset of myocardial infarction. The avoidance of business worries, delegation of as much work as possible to juniors, the giving up of committee work involving strain, etc., all require consideration. Physical effort can be reduced considerably by taking thought—securing office or bedroom on the ground floor, if there is no lift; going late to the office and leaving early, thereby avoiding the rush hours of commuting; cutting down the weekend golf from two strenuous days to an easygoing round, and so on. In men employed in heavy manual labour, or in vocations demanding physical effort (postmen, rent collectors, shopkeepers, etc.), it may be difficult to reduce exertion at work without jeopardizing their livelihood. In certain cases it may be necessary to advise a change of occupation or to recommend retiral. Each patient demands individual assessment, and sound judgment in weighing the risk involved by continued work against the financial worry and hardship that follow invalidism. Certain occupations should never be permitted to the subjects of angina,

because of the risk not only to themselves but to others—e.g. drivers of locomotives, buses, etc.; and the fitness of any patient to drive his car must be determined, and periodically reviewed.

Whatever other measures are taken to spare the heart, it is always possible to arrange that the patient can have at least eight hours' sleep each night; and he can spend Saturday afternoon and Sunday in bed if required. At the outset of treatment in severe cases considerable improvement follows an initial period of two to three weeks' rest in bed. The relief may persist after return to activity, and the increased cardiac reserve is shown by improved exercise tolerance. Periodic spells of rest in bed are of value to many patients.

The use of nitroglycerin to relieve angina of effort has been dealt with above. This drug can also be effectively used *in anticipation* of exertion which would ordinarily cause pain: a few minutes before the extra effort is called for the patient may chew one or two tablets of the B.P. preparation. Attacks produced regularly by climbing a flight of stairs may thus be prevented, or the strain of an important business meeting undertaken without discomfort. Many tablets can be taken daily over long periods without untoward results. For example, in patients with *angina decubitus* attacked by pain on turning in bed, sitting up for a meal, or straining at stool, anything from 10 to 20 tablets may be necessary to keep the patient free from pain throughout the day. This is important and is insufficiently appreciated, since it is common to find patients on a doctor's advice attempting to cut their daily consumption of nitroglycerin to a minimum. The ambulant patient, using vasodilators to prevent attacks, must be warned that they are intended to allow him to pursue his essential daily business at a slower pace and are not to be taken with the object of allowing him to return to a more strenuous mode of life.

The use and value of long-acting vasodilators have been discussed on p. 101. A combination of theophylline and ethylene diamine (aminophylline, B.P.) is efficient as a coronary vasodilator when injected intravenously, but has little place in the treatment of angina of effort. Oral medication is of limited value because adequate doses result in nausea and vomiting. The combination of 200 mg. of aminophylline with 250 mg. of aluminium hydroxide gel permits higher dosage with less gastric upset.

The place of surgery in the treatment of angina is discussed on p. 133.

Reduction of blood cholesterol. During the last 30 years increasing attention has been paid to the correlation between the incidence of coronary artery disease and high blood cholesterol levels. The average blood cholesterol levels in individuals of different races show a parallelism to the incidence of coronary disease, both being at their highest in the Western world and at their lowest among the Bantu of South Africa. Further, diseases associated with a high blood cholesterol level such as diabetes mellitus and myxoedema, have a high incidence of myocardial infarction. The blood lipo-protein pattern has some bearing on susceptibility to coronary disease, and the sex differences in the alpha and beta lipo-protein proportions are paralleled by the relative susceptibility of the sexes to myocardial infarction. Understandably efforts have been made to lower the blood cholesterol in order to diminish the incidence of myocardial infarction. Whether such attempts are misguided or justified is a matter which the writer believes is not yet fully determined. It is well, however, to review the methods in use so that the physician is familiar with them.

DIET. Reduction of the cholesterol intake is of only transient value in depressing the blood cholesterol level. On a *cholesterol-free diet* the level falls initially over a period of weeks but soon starts to climb and reaches its pre-treatment height despite continued consumption of the strict diet; endogenous cholesterol synthesis is responsible. On the other hand, diets rich in *unsaturated fatty acids* produce a significant and sustained fall in blood cholesterol level and this despite the continued ingestion of substantial quantities of saturated fats. Such unsaturated fatty acids are generally of vegetable origin and occur in quantity in maize (corn) oil, safflower and sunflower seed oil and many other products; they occur also in sardine and pilchard oil as well as in the familiar olive oil. The more active unsaturated fatty acids contain two or more double bonds, for example linoleic acid, linolenic acid and arachidonic acid. By taking about 50 g. of such an oil daily the blood cholesterol level may be reduced. Commercial preparations are widely available, incorporating such oils in margarines, cheese preparations, and salad and cooking oils, so that the requisite quantity may be incorporated in the diet without drastic alteration in its palatability or nature.

NICOTINIC ACID. Nicotinic acid is a vasodilator producing flushing of the skin after ingestion of moderate doses. Large doses (300 mg. thrice daily) may produce a sustained fall in the blood cholesterol level. Such doses initially cause side-effects of flushing and palpitation which subside with continued administration. It is noteworthy that nicotinamide is devoid of this cholesterol-lowering action.

HORMONES. The sex difference in the lipoprotein pattern suggests that female sex hormones might affect the α/β ratio and protect males from coronary disease. The feminizing effects of the female sex hormones and the metabolic actions of analogues of thyroxine outweigh their usefulness.

CLOFIBRATE (ethyl-α-p-chlorophenoxy-isobutyrate) is a most promising drug which has a cholesterol lowering action without serious side-effects. It does, however, potentiate anticoagulant drugs.

CHOLESTEROL SYNTHESIS INHIBITORS. These drugs have been abandoned on account of their side-effects.

IN SUMMARY, the author is of the opinion that the evidence is insufficient that the rate of progress of coronary disease can be stayed by drastic intervention in the dietetic habits of individuals or by the ingestion of drugs to lower the blood cholesterol level. Obesity and over-eating are on general grounds detrimental to the subjects of coronary disease, and such dietetic measures as are required to achieve weight-reduction are eminently justifiable. It is probably sound practice to attempt to reduce the cholesterol concentration in those patients having very high blood levels, and the author uses clofibrate for this purpose. Tobacco smoking is known to increase susceptibility to coronary disease. Abstinence from smoking is mandatory in patients with ischaemic heart disease, and advisable for everyone.

Long-term anticoagulant therapy. Attempts have been made to reduce the incidence of recurrence of myocardial infarction among those who have survived an attack by prolonged administration of anticoagulant drugs and several large and carefully controlled series have been reported. Such is the variability of the course of the disease in different individuals that evaluation of such treatment is as difficult as of the value of the drugs in acute infarction, but there is some evidence that among men of the younger age-group, under 50 years old, a fair reduction in relapse rate and mortality over the first year at least is achieved. In older men and in women the benefits are problematical. It is the author's practice to offer such protection as long-term anticoagulant treatment affords to men with a history of infarction in the age-group under 50 and to some patients who have suffered a recurrence of infarction within a few months of the original attack.

The preparations available for long-term anti-coagulant therapy are listed elsewhere (Table 6, p. 189) with recommendations regarding dosage, laboratory control, antagonists and contraindications.

ACUTE CIRCULATORY FAILURE

The treatment of acute circulatory failure occurring in the course of infections is discussed on pp. 31 and 111. Collapse due to haemorrhage and to surgical shock is discussed on pp. 146 and 232 respectively. The treatment of collapse due to syncope is dealt with below.

SYNCOPE

Sudden loss of consciousness, brief or prolonged, from circulatory causes occurs under a wide variety of conditions, some of cardiac origin and others unconnected with the heart itself. It varies in importance from a trivial incident to one of the utmost gravity.

Vaso-vagal attacks. Recurrent fainting attacks, while most frequent in asthenic girls, occur in either sex at any age and are not associated with cardiac disease. Generally the patient has some warning of the impending attack and is able to sit or lie down before becoming unconscious. Provided she is laid flat, the clothes around the neck loosened and the tongue prevented from falling back to block the airway, recovery is usually rapid. Attempts on the part of sympathetic well-wishers to force brandy or other stimulants between the lips of the unconscious patient should be discouraged, since an aspiration pneumonia is a possible sequel. Smelling salts are no longer included among the contents of a lady's handbag, and their lack seems to have little effect on the rate of recovery. The most important aspect of the management is probably the establishment of the diagnosis. Fainting attacks can occur following haemorrhage which, if it is into the gut, may not be immediately apparent. Again sudden loss of consciousness may occur as the result of a subarachnoid haemorrhage, cerebral embolism, and a host of other non-cardiac conditions.

Cough syncope. In a number of people fainting is regularly precipitated by a heavy bout of coughing—the post-tussive or cough syncope. Prevention by cough sedatives or the avoidance of known irritants (e.g. tobacco smoke) is the only treatment.

Carotid sinus syndrome. Recurrent syncopal attacks in patients in the older age-group may be due to a hypersensitive carotid sinus reflex. In such persons light cutaneous stimulation of the neck over the bifurcation of the carotid artery may lead to syncope. This may occur as a result of turning the head to one side, thereby compressing the carotid sinus, particularly if the subject is wearing a tight collar. Vagal inhibition of the heart and vasodilatory vascular effects predominate in different cases, while in others cerebral features are predominant. If the diagnosis is established, treatment is surgical denervation of the affected sinus which generally effects a cure.

Syncope due to low cardiac output. In patients with severe stenotic lesions of the aortic or pulmonary valves, it may be impossible for the cardiac output to rise with exercise, and syncope is likely to occur during strenuous activity. A similar mechanism is responsible for syncope occurring during physical activity in patients with established complete heart block; in these individuals the heart rate is fixed at about 30 per minute and acceleration with exercise is impossible. This again leads to deficient cardiac output under stress, impaired cerebral blood supply and syncope.

Cases of valvular stenosis with such symptoms should be considered as candidates for surgical relief. The patient with established complete block must be cautioned to live within his cardiac reserve or provided with a pacemaker (p. 122).

Postural syncope. Postural hypotension, a fall in blood pressure with the assumption of the erect posture, may be sufficiently severe to cause fainting. Severe postural hypotension of this type is uncommon: it is now most often due to treatment with hypotensive drugs, and should be regarded as an indication for reviewing the dosage of such preparations (p. 114). It may also follow operations for hypertension, e.g. extensive bilateral sympathectomy.

In such patients some improvement may be effected by simple mechanical means—the application of a tight abdominal binder when the patient is lying flat in bed and before he rises. This prevents to some extent pooling of the blood in the splanchnic bed, which is largely responsible for the profound drop in pressure in the erect posture. The action of vasoconstrictive drugs such as noradrenaline is too short to be of value in this condition, but 15 to 30 mg. of ephedrine given orally half an hour before rising may be helpful.

Syncope due to primary cardiac causes. While in infancy marked tachycardia can be tolerated without upset of cerebral function, attacks of paroxysmal tachycardia in the adult, and particularly in the elderly, are generally associated with loss of consciousness if the heart rate is over 200 per minute. The incoordinate ventricular activity of ventricular fibrillation is comparable with cardiac arrest in its effects. At the other end of the scale very slow heart action, as may occur in long-standing complete heart block, may also be associated with loss of consciousness. Cardiac stand-still, occurring in the course of an Adams–Stokes attack or at the onset of a coronary infarction, leads to unconsciousness of greater or longer duration and may be fatal (p. 126).

Adams-Stokes Attacks

The management of Adams-Stokes attacks is described on p. 126.

Cardiac Resuscitation. Reference has been made in the section on the cardiac arrhythmias (p. 126) to cardiac resuscitation. Such measures have a valuable rôle to play in other conditions, e.g. in electrocuted individuals or in those who suffer cardiac arrest or ventricular fibrillation during a surgical operation. Such apparatus is now widely distributed and readily available in hospitals, and medical and nursing staff should be familiar with its use. Time is the over-riding factor in successful resuscitation, for after more than three or four minutes of cardiac arrest permanent anoxic cerebral damage is inevitable. Artificial respiration is as important as maintaining the circulation, and in default of electrical apparatus, bold and timely recourse must be had either to external cardiac massage or to thoracotomy (p. 127). The importance of the immediate correction of metabolic acidosis cannot be overemphasized.

The procedures for dealing with cardiac arrest are described on pp. 126-127.

PULMONARY EMBOLISM

When a major embolus becomes impacted in a large branch of the pulmonary artery, the patient is struck down without warning and may expire in a few minutes. When the embolus is smaller survival is possible, but despite skilled treatment the patient's life is commonly in danger for some days.

For the largest emboli no treatment is available short of the heroic operation of embolectomy, for which surgical facilities are rarely at hand at the moment of catastrophe. If the material is available, a streptokinase intravenous infusion is worthy of consideration, but the treatment must be started without delay. The essence of treatment lies in prevention, and too much stress cannot be laid on prophylaxis.

The patient who survives a major embolic accident is shocked, dyspnoeic, apprehensive and in pain. The most effective immediate remedies are 15 to 30 mg. of morphine subcutaneously and the liberal administration of oxygen. In severely shocked patients the giving of analeptic drugs, such as nikethamide, 5 ml. intravenously, may be of some value. Relief for the labouring right heart may be afforded by a rapid venesection, the indication being the degree of distension of the veins in the neck. Anticoagulants should be instituted at once, starting with 10,000 to 15,000 units of heparin intravenously; continued treatment with anticoagulants is maintained along the lines detailed on p. 189. Pleural effusion develops in some patients surviving a major pulmonary infarction and this may require repeated aspiration.

Prophylaxis. The essential causal factor in pulmonary embolism is migration of a clot from either the venous system or the right atrium, through the right ventricle to the pulmonary artery. Formation of clots in the right auricle is favoured by atrial fibrillation of rheumatic or other origin, while venous thrombosis occurs in a wide variety of conditions associated with immobilization in bed, with or without previous surgical operation. Much can be done to prevent their development by prophylactic anticoagulants. The incidence of pulmonary infarction after gynaecological and orthopaedic operations, particularly in elderly people with a fractured neck of femur, can be dramatically reduced by such treatment. Phlebothrombosis in leg veins commonly occurs in patients in medical wards and attention to mobilization of the patient and daily examination of the legs for evidence of venous thrombosis or tenderness may forestall serious embolic accidents, though even with the greatest care these may occur. The administration of anticoagulants to such individuals as a routine is advisable. Patients with atrial fibrillation, who are all liable to pulmonary and systemic embolism, should be afforded protection by long-term anticoagulant therapy, which reduces the incidence of such embolic incidents to ten per cent. of that in the unprotected.

THE INFECTIONS

Rheumatic Carditis and Rheumatic Fever

The incidence of acute rheumatic fever has fallen dramatically in this country over the last 30 years— a fortunate circumstance, since treatment remains unsatisfactory. Sulphonamides, penicillin and corticosteroids have all in turn been found in greater or less degree disappointing. Rest in bed and the administration of salicylate or corticosteroids remain the mainstays of treatment.

Penicillin. Penicillin does not affect the course of rheumatic fever or carditis but is used in treatment to eliminate persistent (tonsillar) streptococcal infection and to prevent reinfection. A week's intensive course of benzyl penicillin is given at the outset followed throughout the patient's stay in hospital and after discharge with phenoxymethyl-penicillin by mouth. Such treatment is given along with salicylates or other anti-rheumatic drug.

Corticosteroids. In some patients with severe pancarditis in whom the administration of salicylates pushed to toxic limits has failed, corticosteroids may produce striking improvement, leading to disappearance of fever and arthritis and to rapid resolution of the cardiac affection. In others, however, the hormones fail to influence the condition, and there is no means of predicting which patients will respond. Prednisolone is preferable to cortisone, since its salt-retaining action is less marked. The other recognized side-effects have not proved troublesome in the relatively short courses required in acute carditis. It is well to reserve its use for acute cases under institutional care.

Rest. The child who develops acute or subacute rheumatism should be confined to bed in hospital till all the signs of rheumatic activity have subsided. Good nursing is essential, and during an active carditis the patient should not be allowed to do anything for himself. The achievement of complete physical rest in young children without acute symptoms always presents difficulty, but confinement to bed should be maintained even although the child is moving about in bed; to allow such a child up greatly increases the demands made on the heart and circulation. During the period of fever, with accompanying profuse perspiration, careful toilet of the skin is necessary and will lessen the risk of sweat rashes. The diet should be fluid and light, as for any other febrile condition. The duration of rest in bed is discussed below.

Salicylates. Salicylate has generally been regarded as being without action on the progress of the carditis, though exerting a striking and specific effect on the fever and arthritis. Recent work suggests that it may produce similar effects to cortisone and corticotrophin through the pituitary–adrenal system. When the blood salicylate level is maintained between 30 and 40 mg. per 100 ml., not only are fever and arthritis abolished but the E.S.R. returns more quickly to normal and the duration of the disease is shortened.

If the condition has to be treated without biochemical control, the drug must be given in doses sufficient to produce the symptoms of mild salicylate intoxication. So-called drug resistance is in many cases due to under-dosage. The daily dose varies with age and weight. The guide to the dose in any individual case is clinical: the abolition of joint pains and of pyrexia, or the development of mild symptoms of salicylism (deafness, tinnitus, etc.). In children overbreathing is often the first sign of excessive dosage. For adults, doses of 1·5 to 2 g. two- or three-hourly will be required, a total of 12 g. per day being commonly sufficient. In children the effective daily dose varies from 4 to 8 g. per day, according to age. The old practice of giving sodium salicylate with bicarbonate simply enhances excretion, and necessitates giving twice the amount of salicylate to produce a given effect. Such doses may produce gastric irritation which may be the limiting factor in dosage. When sodium salicylate is badly tolerated, soluble aspirin may be prescribed as tablets to be dissolved in cold water immediately before use. Dosage again has to be pushed so far as the tolerance of the patient permits. The intravenous administration of salicylate has no appreciable advantage over oral administration and the risk of toxic reactions is much increased (p. 547).

Once fever and pain have subsided—generally within a few days, or when symptoms of salicylism have appeared, the dosage of salicylate should be reduced. The drug should not be entirely discontinued, but should be administered in smaller doses so long as the rheumatic process remains active. The maintenance dose is that which will just suffice to keep pain and fever in abeyance, and for an adult is generally from 6 to 7 g. per day. Recurrence of acute symptoms is common when the maintenance dose is reduced to as low as 4 g.

per day. Should such recurrence occur, the dose must be temporarily increased.

Local treatment for the affected joints should be simple. Wrapping in cotton-wool and bandaging to secure rest suffice during the few days of acute pain. The application of liniments is valueless. Care is essential in patients in whom pain lasts more than a few days, since, contrary to general teaching, permanent joint affection may occasionally result from rheumatic fever. Continuous immobilization of joints carries the risk of later limitation of movement. Passive movement through the maximum range, short of causing pain, should be performed daily as soon as the most acute symptoms subside, and immobilization during the rest of the day should be in the best orthopaedic position.

Focal sepsis. In rheumatic fever a focus of streptococcal infection in tonsils or upper respiratory tract may remain active throughout the course of the disease. Penicillin, used as suggested above, has rendered it rare nowadays for the physician to be faced with the serious decision of advising tonsillectomy at the risk of provoking a severe and possibly fatal exacerbation. The risk is such that every effort should be made to eradicate streptococci by antibiotics rather than hazard tonsillectomy. Cover by antibiotics should be given before operations on teeth or tonsils in apparently quiescent rheumatic cases.

Routine tonsillectomy of healthy children does not protect them against subsequent attacks of rheumatic fever, nor after a first attack does it appreciably lessen the risk of recurrence of rheumatism. It is wise to advise tonsillectomy only when the local condition is such as would demand operation in a non-rheumatic case, to choose the time for operation with great care and to provide antibiotic cover.

Duration of rest. The question of how long a patient with rheumatic carditis is to be kept in bed is not easily answered and no hard-and-fast rule can be laid down. Certainly in all cases with clinical evidence of *active* carditis, rest in bed should be prolonged so long as the signs of activity persist, and this may extend over a period of months. It is wrong, however, to prolong rest after signs of activity have disappeared. Not only is an established, static valvular lesion not benefited by such treatment, but there is evidence that moderate exercise is beneficial for the subjects of early valvular disease.

The criteria for determining quiescence of carditis are important. A valvulitis of sufficient intensity to produce eventual gross fibrosis may persist with very little clinical upset. Pulse rate and temperature may be normal and cardiac enlargement absent even though active infection persists in the valves. Sinus arrhythmia is not a safe indication that the heart has escaped damage, and the duration or degree of joint involvement bears no relation to the extent of the cardiac lesions. Subcutaneous nodules when present indicate persistent rheumatic activity, but their absence does not exclude active carditis. Certain electrocardiographic changes when present are indicative of active myocarditis. The return of the blood sedimentation rate (E.S.R.) to normal is generally a guide to recovery; but it is not infallible, as in congestive failure it may return to normal. Such cases, however, are easily recognized, and the question of allowing the patient up does not arise. Now and then a normal E.S.R. persists in a patient showing no signs of failure while other evidence of carditis is obvious. Conversely, a raised E.S.R. does not necessarily indicate carditis, for many conditions increase it. Other criteria of cessation of activity are gain in weight in children if not due to oedema, stabilization of the position of the apex beat and of physical signs in the heart, and a stable pulse rate, particularly during sleep.

Children who have suffered from repeated attacks of carditis may develop a severe and occasionally fatal acute pancarditis. The handling of such a case can be as sad a task as any that a doctor has to face; ordinary measures fail to arrest or retard the disease, and treatment is symptomatic. In such fulminating cases corticosteroids have on occasion proved valuable, but in a proportion these drugs, too, fail to stay the course of the disease.

Convalescence. When the period of complete rest in bed is over, the return to activity should be gradual and carefully supervised. Any recrudescence of the rheumatic process should be met by a prompt return to complete rest.

The child who has weathered rheumatic carditis is frequently sent for a short period to a convalescent home, and then returns to school and to full routine. This is unsatisfactory, and is probably responsible for much later disability. Convalescence should be protracted in healthy surroundings with facilities for schooling.

After-care. On discharge from such an institution, or after convalescence at home, the child should return gradually to activity, the limitation of effort being determined by the extent of the cardiac damage. In cases with mild but quiescent valvular lesions full activity is allowable with a prohibition only on such strenuous exertions as competitive sports. A patient with gross myocardial damage and hypertrophy must, however, lead a quiet, sedentary life. Careful follow-up with periodic assessment of general health and cardiac condition is essential, and any sign of renewed rheumatic activity demands prompt measures—rest in bed, etc. It is understandable that such solicitous after-care may well engender a cardiac neurosis—a point always to be borne in mind.

The prevention of recurrent streptococcal infection is important, by the long-continued administration of penicillin either by the monthly injection of a long-acting preparation (0·9 g. benzathine penicillin, B.P.) or the oral administration of 250 mg. of phenoxymethyl penicillin twice daily.

The choice of a future occupation should always be made under the guidance of the doctor. Instances of young adults with advanced cardiac lesions engaged in strenuous occupations are all too familiar, and would not occur if after-care were efficient. It is vital that the education of a child should not be neglected during long periods of semi-invalidism. Many rheumatic children leave school at sixteen years with much less than average schooling and are driven on to the unskilled labour market. Better education means greater ability to secure a sedentary occupation which will not lead so soon to a cardiac breakdown. There is ample scope for the doctor, in village or city, to make himself acquainted with local industries, and by direct approach to employers to secure the right niche for the individual patient. Light, skilled crafts (wood- and leather-work; radio mechanics; precision instrument making, watchmaking, etc.) are remunerative, make little call on physical strength and maintain the patient's interest and independence. Often the journey to and from work or school, and the exposure to inclement weather involved, impose greater strain and risk of relapse than the actual physical strain of employment.

It is implicit that diagnosis must be accurate. When such important matters are involved as the whole future of a young patient, his choice of vocation or her fitness for marriage and child-bearing, it is surely incumbent on the doctor to exercise the greatest care. As diagnosis is admittedly often difficult, the doctor should seek specialist and radiological help before pronouncing an opinion. A thoughtless remark after a superficial examination may have disastrous consequences.

Subacute Bacterial Endocarditis

Prior to the discovery of penicillin, subacute bacterial endocarditis was almost invariably fatal; today, with efficient antibiotic treatment the picture is entirely different and the majority of those affected may be saved. The mortality, and of almost equal importance the degree of residual disability, depend on two factors—the stage at which treatment is begun and its thoroughness. If diagnosis is delayed for weeks, or months, irreparable damage to a valve may occur, so that even if recovery results the heart may be so handicapped that progressive cardiac failure is inevitable. Further, the disease once firmly established becomes more difficult to eradicate. As regards thoroughness of treatment, short courses of penicillin for two or three weeks, while yielding a high initial recovery rate, are associated with a considerable relapse rate and a bad overall prognosis.

Early treatment presupposes early diagnosis, and this in turn depends on the diagnostic acumen of the individual doctor. Cases of subacute bacterial endocarditis, like those of every other disease, come first under the observation of the general practitioner, and it is he who should consider this possibility in every case of obscure or unexplained fever occurring in a patient known to suffer from rheumatic or congenital heart disease. The disease may even occur with no history or signs of a valvular lesion, especially when the infection is implanted on a congenital bicuspid aortic valve. A further group of cases is now being diagnosed with increasing frequency, namely in adults over the age of 50, in whom unhappily the diagnosis is commonly not suspected until the disease is far advanced.

The diagnosis of subacute bacterial endocarditis may be missed in cases of congenital heart disease with a left-to-right shunt (ventricular septal defect, patent ductus arteriosus) since in these emboli are carried not to the systemic circulation but to the lungs, and the characteristic peripheral embolic phenomena so common in the rheumatic case are lacking. Such patients may suffer repeated episodes of respiratory illness, a curious recurrent pneumonic condition, the significance of which may be overlooked. Diagnosis may be further complicated by the injudicious use of penicillin or other antibiotics. These, given in short courses for apparently minor infections, may for a time control fever and inflammation, so that the possibility of subacute bacterial endocarditis may not be considered, and even if it is the diagnosis may be discarded because blood cultures taken after antibiotics have been given are likely to be negative.

When a doctor suspects subacute bacterial endocarditis on clinical grounds every attempt should be made to isolate the organism. Repeated blood cultures should be undertaken, and a higher percentage of positive results will be obtained if these are done in series of three on any one day. A spike of temperature should suggest the withdrawal of blood for culture on three occasions at hourly or two-hourly intervals, and this process should be repeated on successive days till four or five batches have been sent for examination. No antibiotics should be administered until such tests have been carried out, but treatment should be started without delay as soon as the cultures have been taken.

The isolation of the organism and the determination of its sensitivity to penicillin and other antibiotics decide both the choice and the dose of antibiotic to be given. Not all cases are due to the *Streptococcus viridans*, a proportion being due to other organisms varying widely in resistance to penicillin. This is particularly true of *S. faecalis*, a commonly highly resistant organism which may gain access to the blood stream from the urinary tract. In a proportion of patients no organism is isolated from the blood and a significant number of abacterial cases occur even when investigations are carefully carried out. The incidence is reduced if blood cultures are made sufficiently frequently and with appropriate techniques. As soon as a number of blood cultures have been made these abacterial cases should not be denied vigorous treatment.

Antibiotics. For the average case from which a fully sensitive *S. viridans* has been isolated the standard course of treatment consists of the intramuscular injection of 3 g. benzylpenicillin daily in divided doses, continued over a period of 56 days. It may seem cruel to inflict four or five painful injections daily over a period of eight weeks, particularly to a child, but the author has still to be convinced that procaine penicillin or oral preparations of penicillin are equally effective; the disease is of such gravity that it is imperative to pursue treatment in the most effective fashion. When the organism recovered is more resistant than usual this dosage may have to be increased even up to 12 g. daily, and an adjuvant antibiotic added, for which purpose streptomycin, 1 g. daily by intramuscular injection, is usually the drug of choice. The broad-spectrum oral antibiotics of the tetracycline group are not of great value in treatment of subacute bacterial endocarditis, though on occasion an organism may be recovered which is sensitive to one member of the group and resistant to penicillin or streptomycin (e.g. *Coxiella burneti*, Q Fever). When a very high blood level of penicillin is desired the renal tubular-blocking action of probenecid (p. 3) may be employed. The desired result is achieved without greatly increasing the dose of antibiotic.

General treatment. The general treatment of a patient with subacute bacterial endocarditis is that for any febrile infective illness, modified by the severity of the cardiac lesions present. In the patient whose valves are so grossly damaged and whose heart muscle is so poisoned by toxaemia that he is in cardiac failure, complete rest and treatment along standard lines for congestive heart failure will be required for weeks or months. Anaemia and malnutrition must be treated appropriately. Those patients in whom the infection has been diagnosed and treated at an early stage, and in whom cardiac enlargement and valve damage are minimal and failure absent, need only be kept in bed for two to three weeks, after which a progressive increase in activity may be allowed.

Embolism. Major embolic accidents, affecting the cerebral circulation or other important systemic arteries, are frequent and account for a considerable proportion of fatalities. Such accidents are unfortunately not reduced by anticoagulants which have no place in the treatment of this disease. Death from embolism is most likely to occur in patients with large crumbling vegetations—that is in patients who have suffered from the disease for a considerable period before a correct diagnosis has been made and treatment commenced. The overall mortality from these embolic accidents is of the order of 10 per cent.

Septic foci. Every patient with known rheumatic or congenital heart disease should be subjected to regular dental survey so that early sepsis can be detected and dealt with. No such patient should be allowed to retain a dead crowned tooth, as apical infection in such a case is probable and may escape notice since it may be painless. Dental extractions should always be carried out under protection with benzyl penicillin administered by injection an hour or two before and for two or three days after the dental operation. Similarly, infections of the urinary tract in such individuals should be efficiently treated, since it is known that *S. faecalis* may gain entry to the blood stream from such a focus. Patients under treatment for subacute bacterial endocarditis should also be carefully investigated for septic foci and if these are found they should be dealt with while the patient is under the protection of an antibiotic. Failure to eliminate a septic focus may lead to repeated reinfection and relapse of the endocarditis.

Prognosis. Even with efficient treatment the prognosis varies considerably with the stage at which treatment is begun. The overall recovery rate today is of the order of 75 per cent. Patients diagnosed and treated at a late stage and who may already be in cardiac failure, have a much worse prognosis, the recovery rate being 50 per cent. or less, and the survivors tend to lapse at an early date into cardiac failure. When patients are treated at an early stage the recovery rate is about 90 per cent. and residual disability may be slight.

Pericarditis

A patient suffering from acute pericarditis, whatever the aetiology, should be nursed at complete rest in bed. For those with acute rheumatic carditis, the general lines of treatment are as described under that heading. In tuberculous cases the therapeutic measures are those appropriate to tuberculosis (p. 68). Cases which occur in association with pyogenic infections (haemolytic streptococci, staphylococci, pneumococci, etc.) are treated with the appropriate antibiotic (pp. 3–23), the possibility of the development of a purulent effusion being kept in mind. The so called benign non-specific variety (due to, for example, Coxsackie virus) generally clears up rapidly without specific treatment and without residual disability. Pericarditis occurring in the course of disseminated lupus erythematosus responds, like the other manifestations of this protean disorder, to treatment with corticosteroids.

The relief of pain may call for treatment, though many patients suffer surprisingly little discomfort even when pericardial friction is audible. Mild analgesics such as aspirin or paracetamol may suffice, but severe pain may necessitate the administration of 15 mg. of morphine with the customary proviso regarding its potential dangers in young children.

A large effusion may embarrass the cardiac action or interfere with respiration by causing partial collapse of the left lung. These symptoms may be severe enough to warrant aspiration of the pericardial effusion. Tapping must be carried out promptly with the appearance of the signs of tamponade—rising venous pressure and pulse rate, onset of cyanosis, increasing dyspnoea and general distress. Aspiration is also a routine diagnostic procedure when bacteriological examination of the fluid is necessary, or when the presence of pus has to be excluded. For diagnosis the aspiration of a few millimetres of fluid will suffice, but to relieve tamponade the aspiration of several hundred millilitres may be necessary. The technique of paracentesis is described on p. 638. In malignant involvement of the pericardium, rapid re-accumulation of effusion after paracentesis is common; for this, local radiotherapy may be given by instilling into the sac a radioactive isotope of gold. This is done under the guidance of a radiotherapist, familiar with the details of procedure, dosage requirements and isotope hazards to personnel. The treatment is only palliative.

Pus in the pericardial sac is an indication for surgery. Drainage may be established by open operation, with resection of ribs, or by a closed method, by insertion of a tube through the soft tissue of an interspace and the maintenance of suction. Both methods yield good results, and the choice must lie with the surgeon. Specific antibiotics should be used systemically and locally.

In non-purulent cases recovery with absorption of the effusion is the rule, except in the terminal acute pericarditis which occurs in the last stages of uraemia and other cachectic conditions. Convalescence may be slow, and there is no efficient method of hastening absorption of the fluid. Repeated assessment of the size of the effusion and of the patient's general state will guide the physician in his decision as to when to allow the patient to move about in bed, when to allow him up, etc. Patients on recovery from the acute attack may be allowed a fair amount of exercise, but should be re-examined from time to time during the ensuing years to detect the development of other lesions or of chronic constrictive pericarditis. When pericarditis occurs as part of a polyserositis, joint supervision by physician and thoracic surgeon is desirable, for operation may be indicated at a stage before hard scar tissue or calcified deposits have formed. Chronic constrictive pericarditis is a surgical problem (p. 133).

Circulatory Failure in Acute Infections

In the circulatory failure which occurs in acute infections such as lobar pneumonia or septic abortion, two factors are at work: central, due to failure of the poisoned heart muscle, and peripheral, due to dilatation of the poisoned small vessels. Exhaustion or apoplexy (p. 302) of the adrenals plays an important role in the syndrome of bacteraemic shock. This peripheral failure is generally more important than central (cardiac) failure. Even in diphtheria, many of the deaths are due to peripheral failure, though in some cases the specific action of the toxin on the heart causes sudden (cardiac) death, often many days after the subsidence of the acute infection.

Once circulatory failure has developed, the prospects of successful treatment are poor. It is then too late for efficient specific therapy, and efforts to stimulate the heart or the peripheral vessels are disappointing. The treatment of toxaemic circulatory failure lies in its prevention by early and adequate treatment of the causal infection. In diphtheria, for example, timely administration of antitoxin greatly reduces the incidence of dangerous circulatory failure. Similarly in pneumonia, early and specific treatment with antibiotics obviates later intractable toxaemic effects. In diseases for which no specific treatment exists general measures to reduce toxaemia are employed to the best of our ability.

In view of the adrenal factor there are logical grounds for using corticosteroids as replacement therapy despite the known disadvantage of their depressing immunological responses. In practice their use has been justified by the results, and hydrocortisone is a potent weapon in combating toxaemic shock. Intramuscular hydrocortisone, 100 to 200 mg. daily should be given for its depot action, while for its speedy effect the water-soluble hydrocortisone hemisuccinate should be given intravenously. The dosage should be 10 mg. per hour, best given as say 30 mg. added to a pint of dextran infusion fluid, given by drip. An appropriate antibiotic should be administered simultaneously in high dosage. While some apparently desperate cases of toxaemic shock in acute infections may be rescued by hydrocortisone, the results of treatment of peripheral failure late in the course of an infection are unsatisfactory. In fact, once such failure has developed, death is likely in spite of all therapy, unless the natural defence mechanisms succeed in overcoming the infection, as in the crisis phenomenon of lobar pneumonia. Of drugs acting on the heart, digitalis is the most widely employed; its use in pneumonia was once traditional, though its value is now discredited. The old controversy as to its value is hardly relevant in these days of efficient antibiotics.

Many other drugs once enjoyed a reputation as cardiac stimulants, and were widely used in conditions of toxaemic circulatory failure—strychnine and diffusible stimulants. It is now recognized that they have no direct cardiac action and that we do not possess any drug which can whip an exhausted or poisoned heart to renewed activity.

Focal Sepsis in relation to Heart Disease

The rôle of focal septic infection in the aetiology of heart disease is uncertain apart from the production of subacute bacterial endocarditis which has been discussed (p. 109). It is possible that septic foci may be of aetiological importance in some cases with heart block of milder grades or with obstinate extrasystolic irregularities. In such cases, removal of the foci is desirable and is generally without risk if suitable prophylactic measures are taken by pre- and post-operative treatment with penicillin (p. 4).

It is held by some physicians that a few patients with cardiac pain and congestive failure may owe their condition to toxaemia from an infected gallbladder. Others contend that chance association determines the simultaneous occurrence of the two conditions. Those who suffer from cholecystitis are of the habitus and age in which arterial degeneration and its sequelae of angina and myocardial failure are common. The evidence in favour of the so-called gall-bladder heart is not convincing, and operations for removal of the gall-bladder should be undertaken only when there are clear indications, apart from the cardiac condition, to justify the step. The high mortality attending this operation in patients with hypertension, obesity and impaired myocardial efficiency should be kept in mind.

SYSTEMIC HYPERTENSION
(HIGH BLOOD PRESSURE)

INDICATIONS FOR TREATMENT

Hypertension is a physical sign and not a disease. Although about 20 per cent. of the adult population have a systolic blood pressure above 160 mm. Hg., only about 10 per cent. have a raised diastolic blood pressure. A raised systolic blood pressure alone is not dangerous and needs no treatment. The mean blood pressure is nearer the diastolic than the systolic level, so a raised diastolic blood pressure is much more important; throughout the rest of this section when the word 'hypertension' is used it refers to *diastolic* hypertension.

Sustained hypertension can lead to *hypertensive heart disease* with eventual left ventricular hypertrophy and even failure; it can also produce *hypertensive vascular disease* which can seriously damage many organs, notably the kidneys, the brain, the retinae and the myocardium. Hypertension predisposes to atheroma and in pregnant women increases the risk of perinatal mortality.

Not all patients with diastolic hypertension need to have their blood pressure reduced. The prognosis of moderate hypertension in elderly women is very good, so drastic treatment is unnecessary. Mild sustained diastolic hypertension may never produce serious hypertensive cardiac or vascular disease. Some patients with hypertensive vascular disease already have ischaemic damage to the heart or brain. A considerable reduction of their blood pressures might lead to further failure of perfusion of an already ischaemic organ, or even to actual infarction.

It is often hard to decide which patients should be energetically treated. As a general rule the blood pressure should be lowered substantially in patients who already have evidence of hypertensive heart disease or hypertensive vascular disease, or if the sustained level of the diastolic pressure at rest is so high that the development of these conditions can reasonably be forecast.

Before treatment, patients should be carefully investigated with a view to establishing three things: (1) the cause of the hypertension, in case it is curable, (2) the severity of the hypertension, so that appropriate management can be devised for each patient, (3) any contraindications to the drastic lowering of blood pressure, e.g. cardiac or cerebral ischaemia.

By careful investigation a small but increasing number of patients can be identified in whom the hypertension is caused by a potentially curable condition. These conditions must constantly be borne in mind, for it is tragic if a patient with curable hypertension either dies with his underlying disease undiagnosed, or is made to endure, unnecessarily, the rigours of a prolonged regimen of hypotensive drugs.

These causes, which can usually be cured surgically, are aortic coarctation, unilateral renal disease, phaeochromocytoma, Cushing's syndrome and primary hyperaldosteronism. For details of their diagnosis the reader is referred to standard textbooks.

THE MEDICAL TREATMENT OF HYPERTENSION

Although these causes of hypertension are extremely important because of the chance of a radical cure, they are rare; and unfortunately the great majority of patients either have hypertension secondary to bilateral renal disease, or what is called 'essential' hypertension. If it is decided that treatment is necessary, there is no alternative to the use of drugs that lower the blood pressure.

The object of treatment with hypotensive drugs must be to reduce the patient's blood pressure to normal levels, or as near normal levels as he can tolerate, and to keep it there for as long as possible throughout each 24 hours for the rest of his life. This is a difficult undertaking, made no easier by the wide choice of drugs now available. When powerful drugs are used, the management is exacting and time-consuming for doctor and patient alike. It is best started in hospital, and later continued in special out-patient clinics, for careful attention to detail is needed to avoid the risks of uncontrolled hypertension, on the one hand, and those of dangerous hypotension on the other.

Ideally, a hypotensive drug should have a dependable and consistent clinical effect; it should be fully absorbed after oral administration in a predictable time; the patient should not become resistant to its effect, and undesirable side-effects should be minimal. No such drug is yet available, but those available range from relatively mild hypotensive agents that have few unpleasant or dangerous side-effects, to those with extremely powerful hypotensive effects that themselves may be dangerous, and, in addition, with unpleasant or potentially dangerous side-effects.

The selection of a drug must always be a matter of personal choice, based on the ideal criteria described, but also, and most importantly, on personal familiarity based on experience. A practitioner should make himself thoroughly acquainted with the use of the one or two drugs in each of the groups to be described, and confine his prescribing to those with which he is familiar.

It is now clearly established that the expectation

of life of moderately and severely hypertensive patients is substantially greater when their blood pressures are controlled. It is likely that the same may be true of young patients with milder, but sustained, hypertension.

Blood-pressure reducing drugs can be divided roughly into two groups: those with a relatively mild action—mainly the diuretics—and those with a powerful action, e.g. adrenergic-blocking drugs.

To gauge the maximal hypotensive effect of a drug the blood pressure should always be recorded with the patient standing. When starting the treatment of a severely hypertensive patient who is confined to bed, the head end of the bed should be raised on 12-inch blocks to obtain the full effect.

Orthostatic hypotension in treated patients is much commoner than is generally appreciated, and can be dangerous in patients who already have

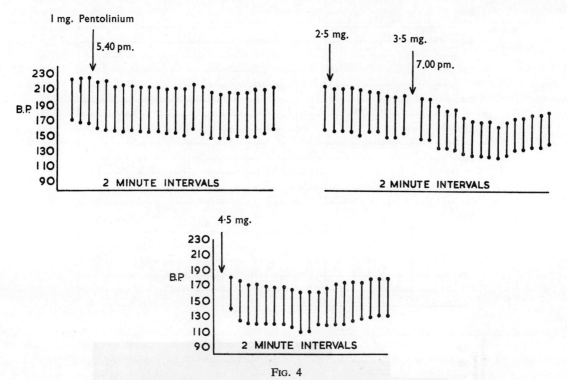

FIG. 4

Frequent blood-pressure records, over a period of about 2 hours, to show adjustment of dosage when using a hypotensive drug with a rapid but short action (subcutaneous pentolinium).

Powerful Hypotensive Drugs

These drugs have many different pharmacological effects, but their chief action is through blockade or damping of adrenergic neural transmission.

When a normal person stands up from the lying position his blood pressure is maintained by vaso-constriction of the arterioles and veins of his legs, brought about reflexly by adrenergic stimulation. If these reflexes are interrupted by adrenergic-blocking drugs, blood pools under the influence of gravity, and the central blood pressure falls. Two important practical points emerge from these facts.

impaired coronary or cerebral perfusion. It is aggravated by peripheral vasodilatation, standing suddenly or for long, a diminished blood volume and, in the case of some drugs of the guanethidine group, by exercise—especially in the morning. Patients should be warned against lying too long in hot baths or in the sun, and the dose of their drug may have to be reduced if they go to a warmer climate. They should be taught to get out of bed slowly, sitting on the edge of the bed for a few minutes before standing upright. If they feel dizzy they should sit down. The physician should be aware that the acute administration of diuretics may reduce the blood volume, and hence the blood pressure. An elderly man should be particularly careful when he gets out of bed during the night to empty his bladder. The combination of cutaneous vasodilation from the warm bed, sudden standing,

strokes; and patients with frank uraemia, unless there are facilities for dialysis at hand. Dialysis alone may, of course, control the hypertension of renal failure.

Dosage. It is impossible to forecast what dose

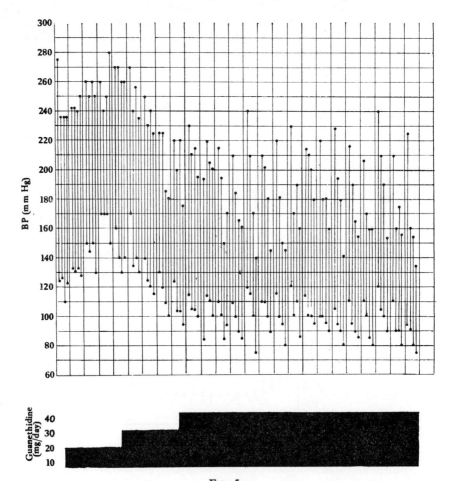

FIG. 5

Daily blood-pressure records to show response to a slow-acting hypotensive drug (guanethidine). The four readings shown for each day are respectively the blood pressures measured with the patient lying, sitting, standing, and standing after exercise. They are all recorded in the morning. Note the effect of exercise.

and the emptying of a full bladder may cause hypotensive syncope.

The use of powerful hypotensive drugs is usually contraindicated in three groups of patients: those with cardiac ischaemia, although one may have to take a calculated risk in patients who have malignant hypertension and coronary artery disease; patients with cerebral ischaemia, for example, elderly people with a history of blackouts or

of any particular drug will eventually be needed to control the blood pressure of any individual patient. Thus, every time the physician starts treatment with a powerful hypotensive drug he is embarking on an acute therapeutic experiment. The dose of the drug must be determined by carefully observing the patient's response to it. Success depends on a knowledge of the duration of action of the drug given by any particular route. Trial and error—

starting with a small dose, and gradually increasing it—will establish the dose of the drug needed to reduce the blood pressure to the required level, and also how often the drug needs to be administered. This necessarily involves frequent measurement of the blood pressure with the patient lying or sitting, standing, and also standing immediately after exercise, if the patient is fit enough. (Figs. 4 and 5.)

Once the correct dose of the drug has been established, accurate control of the blood pressure can be maintained only by regular recording of the blood pressure. Even when the blood pressure is apparently stabilized by a constant dose, some patients, quite unpredictably, become resistant to the effects of a particular drug, and this tolerance can only be detected by frequent follow-up measurements of the blood pressure.

Undesirable effects of hypotensive drugs. These are of two kinds: (1) too much of the action desired, causing hypotension as described above, and (2) true side-effects, for example nasal congestion or 'stuffiness'. When ganglion-blocking drugs were used, paralytic ileus was a side-effect that could be fatal. Nowadays most side-effects are a nuisance only, and many can be countered by using other drugs, or in other ways.

Mild Hypotensive Drugs

These drugs may be used alone for patients who have no evidence of hypertensive vascular or cardiac disease, but whose blood pressure is regarded as putting them at risk. They may also be used as adjuvants to more powerful drugs. By combining, say, an adrenergic-blocking drug with a diuretic, a satisfactory control of the blood pressure may be achieved with fewer undesirable side-effects from the powerful drug. Diuretics and reserpine are the most valuable drugs in this group.

THE MANAGEMENT OF MILD HYPERTENSION

There is increasing evidence that even mild hypertension is ultimately associated with morbidity. Many patients with mild hypertension merely need to be kept under review, but drug treatment should be carefully considered for those in whom other factors predisposing to vascular disease are present. These include heavy cigarette-smoking, lack of physical activity, excessive weight, abnormal glucose tolerance and raised serum cholesterol levels. Since these factors, together with hypertension, predispose to vascular disease they should be corrected as effectively as possible.

Diuretics. As well as potentiating the action of more powerful hypotensive drugs, the long-term administration of diuretics such as the benzothiadiazines reduces the blood pressure, possibly by depleting the body of sodium. It takes some weeks for the blood pressure to fall maximally on this regimen, so the use of a long-acting diuretic is logical, for example chlorthalidone, 50 mg. daily. Patients who have long-term diuretic therapy must, of course, be carefully supervised for the detection of hypokalaemia, hyperuricaemia, overt gout, or thiazide-induced diabetes. Many physicians routinely give potassium supplements. This simple treatment often suffices to control the blood pressure of mildly hypertensive patients, and they are not usually troubled with postural hypotension or side-effects.

Reserpine. If treatment with long-term diuretics alone is not effective, reserpine may be added to the regimen. It depletes the post-ganglionic nerve endings of noradrenaline, and, given by mouth, gradually reduces the blood pressure over a few weeks. It may produce nasal congestion, but the most serious side-effect of long-term treatment is depression with a possible risk of suicide. Depression, however, very rarely occurs with the recommended dose of 0·1 mg., given three times a day.

THE MANAGEMENT OF MODERATE HYPERTENSION

For patients in this group drugs which block adrenergic transmission are usually required.

Methyldopa. Like many drugs that interfere with the autonomic nervous system, methyldopa has several pharmacological effects, but clinically it acts mainly by damping down adrenergic transmission. After a single dose the blood pressure starts to fall in two to five hours; the peak effect is often within about four hours, and some effect may sometimes last for 24 hours. Methyldopa Tablets B.P. (500 mg., 250 mg. and 125 mg.) are used. Treatment can be started with 250 mg. twice daily, and the dose increased in amount and frequency, one tablet at a time, at intervals of not less than three days, to a maximum of about 3 g. daily. Higher doses can sometimes be given.

With high doses there is some postural hypotension, increased by exercise, but some authors have found that the lying blood pressure is more satisfactorily controlled than with other drugs of this group. Side-effects are usually mild: drowsiness for a few days after the treatment begins, or after the dose has been raised, nasal congestion, skin rashes and, occasionally, drug fever. About 20 per cent. of patients taking methyldopa have a positive Coombs' test but the incidence of haemolytic anaemia is low. Antinuclear factor is found in some patients. Tolerance to methyldopa develops fairly commonly. If this cannot be countered by the addition of a diuretic, one of the drugs in the next group may have to be used.

THE MANAGEMENT OF SEVERE HYPERTENSION

ISMELIN

Guanethidine. Given by mouth, guanethidine is slowly and incompletely absorbed, slowly metabolized and slowly excreted. The patient therefore needs to take only a single dose daily, but it may be three or four days before the effect on the blood pressure becomes apparent. It is not possible to forecast whether a particular patient will need 20 mg. or 120 mg. a day; adjusting the dose may take several weeks (Fig. 5). Guanethidine Tablets B.P. contain 10 or 25 mg. As usual, the fall of blood pressure is greater on standing than while lying, and is very much greater during exercise, especially in the morning, when hypertensive patients have a lower plasma volume than at any other time of day. This exertional hypotension is a major hazard in the use of guanethidine. Patients hurrying to work in the morning can become faint. One such patient, complaining of morning weakness, was found while standing to have a blood pressure of 220/130 mg. Hg.; immediately after walking up two flights of stairs the blood pressure had fallen to 90/40 mm. Hg.

Diarrhoea is perhaps the commonest and most troublesome side-effect, but it can frequently be controlled by Codeine Phosphate Tablets B.P. Bradycardia is common, as is nasal obstruction; some patients complain of pain in the parotids, especially after eating. Although men are not made impotent, as they were with ganglion-blocking drugs, they frequently experience failure of ejaculation. Some patients complain of weakness and depression, and many patients gain weight because of fluid retention. A few actually become oedematous and need a diuretic.

This list of side-effects should not hide the fact that guanethidine is still the most dependable of the adrenergic blocking drugs. Control of the blood

pressure is reasonably smooth, the oral dose need only be taken once a day and, most important of all, resistance to the drug rarely develops.

When establishing a patient on guanethidine, or other drugs in this group, it is extremely important that the blood pressure should be taken *with the patient standing, immediately after exercise, in the morning*. This is the only way in which the maximum effect of any dose can be assessed. Sometimes exertional hypotension in the morning may demand a dose of guanethidine that is inadequate to control the blood pressure in the afternoon and evening. This effect can sometimes be lessened by using a smaller dose of guanethidine and a diuretic as an adjuvant, but a single small dose of another short-acting hypotensive drug may have to be given in the afternoon.

DECLINAX

Debrisoquine. Given by mouth debrisoquine is well absorbed from the gut, and after an effective single dose the blood pressure begins to fall in two to four hours. The hypotensive effect lasts from 8 to 24 hours, but usually less than 12 hours. The starting dose is usually 10 mg. twice daily and increments may be made every second or third day. Average daily requirements have ranged from 10 to 300 mg. Postural and exertional hypotension are often a problem. Failure of ejaculation, diarrhoea, nasal congestion and tiredness are common side-effects. Tolerance develops much more frequently than to guanethidine.

ESBATAL

Bethanidine. Given by mouth as Bethanidine Tablets B.N.F. this drug is well absorbed and fairly rapidly excreted. The blood pressure begins to fall one or two hours after a single dose, reaches its lowest level within four hours to five hours and has usually returned to the original level within 12 hours. It is therefore necessary to give a dose two or three times daily. Postural and exertional hypotension are often severe, and it is therefore prudent to use 5 mg. (half a tablet) as a starting dose. Increments can be made every second or third day. Diarrhoea is less frequent with bethanidine than with any other drugs in this group, but all the other side-effects of the group are present. Tolerance is common and is a serious drawback. The great advantage of bethanidine is its speed of action.

THE MANAGEMENT OF HYPERTENSIVE EMERGENCIES

Occasionally it is essential to reduce the blood pressure quickly. The need is commonest in accelerated ('malignant') hypertension. In patients whose hypertension is in the accelerated phase the vascular disease includes fibrinoid necrosis, and the retinae show haemorrhages and exudates. They are at risk from failure of vision due to retinal damage or from extensive damage to other organs. Oral bethanidine will usually reduce the blood pressure within a few hours, but if immediate action is indicated pentolinium is regarded as the drug of choice. Pentolinium Injection B.P. 1·0 mg. is given subcutaneously and blood pressure readings are made every five minutes. When the pressure begins to rise (usually within half an hour) further doses, increased if necessary, are injected to keep the blood pressure under control (Fig. 4). The head of the bed should be raised. For a very rapid effect pentolinium can be given by intravenous drip. The starting dose should be 0·5 mg. or less; if there is no response within about five minutes the dose can be doubled and then increased until the desired effect is obtained. If the drug is used in this way for more than one to two days resistance develops quickly. Pentolinium is a powerful ganglion blocker and its effects in acute arterial hypertension are of therapeutic value. Like many other drugs of this kind, however, it is not sufficiently selective for long-term use; it blocks both cholinergic and adrenergic activity and thus tends to produce side-effects— especially in the alimentary tract—which are entirely unacceptable. Even during a short course of treatment the patient must be carefully observed for signs of bladder dysfunction (retention of urine) and paralytic ileus.

Pulmonary oedema from hypertensive heart disease should be treated as for left ventricular failure due to any other cause (p. 95). It is true that it responds well to acute reduction of the blood pressure, but the physician must be cautious, because pulmonary oedema from any cause can raise the diastolic pressure to high levels for some hours, and before deciding to reduce the blood pressure with drugs the physician would have to be certain, from other evidence, that the pulmonary oedema was the result of hypertension, rather than vice versa.

Severe hypertension is sometimes associated with focal cerebral symptoms and signs. The differential diagnosis of cerebral haemorrhage, thrombosis and hypertensive encephalopathy can be extremely difficult. A hypertensive patient who develops a stroke should not have his blood pressure reduced until about a week has elapsed unless the case is one of malignant hypertension. Even then, initial treatment should aim at a moderate reduction only.

LONG-TERM MANAGEMENT

Hypertensive patients treated by drugs must be regularly reviewed for the critical control of the blood pressure, the avoidance of undue side-effects, and the detection of tolerance. It is an unfortunate fact that many patients feel less well with their hypertension controlled by treatment than they do with quite dangerous blood pressures and no drugs. They must learn to accept this fact as the price they must pay for a better life-expectancy.

HEART DISEASE AND PREGNANCY

Pregnancy is a natural hazard to the young female cardiac patient, and the frequency of the problems to which the association of the two conditions gives rise may be gauged from the fact that between 1·5 and 3 per cent. of all women attending antenatal clinics are found to have cardiac lesions. The great majority (90 per cent.) are cases of rheumatic valvular disease; a much smaller proportion have congenital malformations; ischaemic heart disease in the pregnant woman is rare. The association of hypertension and pregnancy is considered on p. 119.

Pregnancy imposes a severe strain on the cardiovascular system of handicapped patients and in a considerable proportion the heart cannot withstand the additional burden so that cardiac failure in one form or another ensues. The increased load on the circulation is in part imposed by the metabolic demands of the pregnant state, but there are also haemodynamic factors of considerable importance. The placental circulation acts as an arterio-venous shunt, imposing a considerable burden on the heart. Further, during pregnancy the blood volume increases progressively in the early months to reach a peak at or about the 32nd week and thereafter falls towards normal. The load imposed by this increased volume is then at its maximum, which explains why disability is usually maximal at that time and may later regress.

The diagnosis of heart disease in a woman seen for the first time during pregnancy can be difficult. Every cardiologist can recall patients in whom murmurs heard during pregnancy suggest a valvular lesion and yet on re-examination after delivery no murmurs are heard and there is no clinical evidence of heart disease. Probably the increased cardiac output associated with the high blood volume during pregnancy is responsible for these transient murmurs.

The best guide as to how a woman with a cardiac lesion will withstand pregnancy is afforded by her previous history. The first question is to determine how far she was handicapped before the pregnancy began. The woman who previously had little or no disability is unlikely to come to serious harm during its course, and conversely the woman who before pregnancy was already seriously handicapped or in failure will certainly be in danger so long as the pregnancy continues, and in fact well into the puerperium. Other factors to be considered are first the age of the patient, as the risks increase steeply with advancing age; secondly, the parity, since successive labours are likely to be shorter and to impose less burden on the heart; thirdly, the previous obstetric history in so far as the cardiac complications of pregnancy were concerned; fourthly, her circumstances, such as wage-earning and domestic duties which may or may not permit her to rest adequately; fifthly, the co-existence of other complicating disorders such as anaemia and renal disease; and sixthly, obstetric factors (disproportion, etc.).

One class of case constitutes a striking exception to these general rules—the patient with a tight mitral stenosis, probably with a small heart and normal cardiac rhythm, who develops episodes of acute paroxysmal dyspnoea due to pulmonary congestion secondary to left atrial failure. Although such patients may have in the intervals little breathlessness or other handicap, they are in peril, and it is in this group that there is a relatively high proportion of fatal cases. In such patients mitral valvotomy during pregnancy may save life (p. 131).

Probably the most important single factor in the safe management of the pregnant cardiac patient is regular careful antenatal supervision. In most hospitals there is a close liaison between the obstetric unit and the cardiologist. Thus the early signs of incapacity or failure can be detected and dealt with, decisions as to interruption of pregnancy can be taken jointly, and during the final obstetric management of the case the advice of the physician will be available to deal with heart failure or any other emergency which may arise either at term or in the puerperium. With such care the maternal mortality can be reduced to a very low figure in comparison

with the high mortality among women who continue their pregnancy unsupervised and who seek medical advice only when driven to do so because of serious incapacity. Although patients seek help at all stages of pregnancy it is convenient to consider the management of those seen for the first time during each of the three trimesters. Some broad guiding principles, however, may first be considered.

The general rules as to obstetric management are relatively simple. In the first place, interruption of the pregnancy, if this is deemed necessary, should not be carried out later than the third month; thereafter the risks of interference are greater than the risks of allowing the pregnancy to proceed, so that a patient seen for the first time in the fourth month or later even if she is in failure should on no account be subjected to therapeutic abortion. Again, when as the result of good management, a patient has successfully reached the last few weeks of pregnancy, a decision has sometimes to be taken regarding the manner of delivery, whether per vaginam or by Caesarean section. The consensus today is against Caesarean section, which formerly was carried out about the 37th week as an operation of election to spare the mother the strain of labour. The risks involved, however, are greater than if the woman is allowed to go to term, and the infant mortality is considerably higher. Provided there are no obstetrical complications, a forceps delivery can usually be achieved without difficulty, and fortunately many of the infants born to these women are small. It should be emphasized that the more serious the patient's cardiac condition appears to be on admission to the obstetric unit, the more important it is not to interfere with the pregnancy until the cardiac failure has been controlled; only then should obstetrical interference be considered. This rule applies at all stages of pregnancy. As stated above, interruption of pregnancy after the third month is unwise. A decision to perform sterilization should not be used as an argument in favour of Caesarean section; this can be carried out at a later date when the hazards of pregnancy have been surmounted. It should be remembered that the risks are not over when the woman has been delivered of her child; cardiac failure may supervene in the puerperium and may prove fatal.

First trimester. During the first trimester important decisions must be taken regarding the management of the individual patient. In these the practitioner is guided by the factors enumerated above, forecasting the likelihood of a stormy or peaceful pregnancy from the previous history. Where there has been no previous disability a patient seen in this period should be reassured and supervised at regular intervals; as the pregnancy advances she should be encouraged to rest more than the average pregnant woman, particularly in the later months. When there has been some previous handicap or the history of some cardiac complication in a previous pregnancy, the risks of continuing the pregnancy should be explained to the patient and her husband and the advisability of therapeutic abortion considered. When the patient has been seriously incapacitated or has developed cardiac failure, or when serious failure has complicated previous confinements, termination of pregnancy should be strongly advised. If the patient is already in failure when seen, as emphasized above, no interference with the pregnancy should be permitted until the failure has been relieved. Thereafter its termination is advisable.

Second trimester. From the fourth month onwards interference with the course of the pregnancy is contraindicated, and the management of the patient consists of the assessment of the degree of handicap and of the treatment of cardiac failure if this is present. Even in patients with little disability it is wise to insist on additional rest in the afternoons and at weekends and in those more seriously affected complete rest in bed may have to be imposed even at this early date. Appropriate treatment with diuretics, salt restriction and digitalis will assist the patient through the remaining months of her pregnancy.

Third trimester. Patients who pass through the first six months of pregnancy without ill effect and who develop signs of failure in the third trimester will require admission to hospital and treatment, but in general they are likely to improve in the last weeks of the pregnancy and may be less upset by labour than might be expected. It must be reiterated that no matter how severe the failure or how desperate the handicap surgical obstetrical interference at this stage is contraindicated.

Puerperium. Cardiac failure after delivery is a very serious matter: the spontaneous amelioration which occurs with reduction of blood volume in the later weeks of pregnancy cannot be expected, since the blood volume has already returned to normal. The death rate among patients in failure at this stage is high and the failure is often refractory to treatment. When for one reason or another breastfeeding is undesirable, it should be remembered

E

that oestrogens given to suppress lactation favour water and sodium retention.

Advice on child-bearing. Young married women and their husbands frequently ask advice on this matter, and the doctor must be prepared to guide them to the best of his ability. It is a great mistake to defer pregnancy in a young patient who is married and desires a child. If she is fit to have a child she should be encouraged to have one, since with each year that passes she will become less tolerant of the strains involved. Pregnancy carries no undue risk for the woman who is little handicapped by her lesion, though for the woman whose capacity for effort is already restricted pregnancy is a grave hazard. A thoughtless ban imposed by a doctor playing for safety may be productive of much distress and unhappiness, and it is unfortunate that such prohibitions are widely enforced without due consideration. When the patient's handicap is definite though not gross, and when the practitioner anticipates that—at least in the later weeks of pregnancy—the patient is likely to be in failure and confined to bed, the position should be explained to the prospective mother. Many women are more than willing to accept a risk in their desire to have a child, but in such patients repeated pregnancies should be discouraged. One baby may be safely achieved; a second child after a year or two may be feasible, and on family grounds is highly desirable to avoid the disadvantage of the only child.

It is commonly forgotten that the burden imposed by child-bearing does not cease with delivery. Caring for the child during infancy and early childhood may impose on the mother a greater strain than the pregnancy. Where there are two or three children in the family under the age of 5 the physical load on the mother with cardiac disease may be formidable.

Hypertension in Pregnancy

High blood pressure during pregnancy occurs under two different circumstances: a woman with established hypertension may become pregnant; or a patient with a normal blood pressure may in the course of pregnancy develop a toxaemia of which hypertension is a sign.

If a patient known to have hypertension becomes pregnant she must be kept under close observation throughout its course. Apart from the dangers of hypertension itself, the risk of a superimposed toxaemia of pregnancy is greatly increased in hypertensive patients, nearly half of whom develop toxaemia. With close antenatal supervision any tendency for the pressure to rise as the pregnancy progresses can be detected, and appropriate measures instituted. In the milder cases enforcement of rest, restriction of sodium in the diet and the use of reserpine usually suffice to maintain the pressure at a safe level. The persistence of a high pressure, above, say 150/100 for several weeks at a time, leads to deterioration in the health of the mother and commonly results in the death of the foetus, so the hypertension should be vigorously treated. The ganglion-blocking agents are contraindicated in this condition, as they tend to increase foetal mortality, but treatment with reserpine and chlorothiazide (pp. 88, 115) should be continued for the remainder of the pregnancy. The termination of pregnancy should be considered, particularly if the foetus is viable, when persisting hypertension is associated with albuminuria and a progressive gain in weight due to fluid retention.

Hypertension may persist into the puerperium and occasionally dangerous acute hypertensive episodes occur during that stage. These demand treatment along similar lines.

THE CARDIAC ARRHYTHMIAS

A cardiac arrhythmia calls for treatment only when the abnormal rhythm threatens to interfere with cardiac efficiency. Occasional extrasystoles, or even short bouts of paroxysmal tachycardia, may occur in healthy hearts with no effect on cardiac efficiency. Minor degrees of heartblock and atrial fibrillation with a slow ventricular rate may be indications of cardiac damage, but do not in themselves limit the capacity for effort. In the management of all arrhythmias attention should be directed primarily to the maintenance of ventricular efficiency, and in some atrial disorders, for example fibrillation, this can be done without fundamental change in the abnormal rhythm.

An adequate analysis of disorders of the cardiac rhythm is possible only be means of the electrocardiograph. It is particularly important that patients with paroxysmal arrhythmias should have an electrocardiogram recorded during a paroxysm. This is the only way of establishing the diagnosis and formulating the correct treatment.

The treatment of arrhythmias includes physiological manœuvres such as carotid sinus pressure, physical methods including electrical shock and pacing, and drugs.

(A) DRUGS AND ARRHYTHMIAS

Digitalis

Although the chief action of digitalis is to abolish or relieve cardiac failure, it is the drug of choice for the treatment of some cardiac arrhythmias (p. 124). It also requires to be considered as a common cause of potentially dangerous changes in cardiac rhythm. These occur more readily in patients depleted of potassium, and modern diuretics easily produce hypokalaemia. The use of digitalis in combinations with potent diuretics, cation-exchange resins or steroids, is particularly liable to lead to digitalis intoxication. If it is suspected that an arrhythmia may have been caused by digitalis the drug must be stopped at once. Any other potassium-lowering drugs should also be stopped. Any potassium losses must quickly be made good. Potassium should be given by mouth in a form that is rapidly and well absorbed and does not cause dyspepsia or cause intestinal ulceration. Many of these patients have lost both potassium and chloride, and there are therefore sound physiological reasons for giving both potassium and chloride; only in this way will a hypochloraemic alkalosis be corrected. Potassium Effervescent Tablets B.P.C. contain no chloride and should not be used. 'Sando-K' contains suitable amounts of both ions and is rapidly effective.

Digitalis-induced fast arrhythmias should be treated at once, with either propranolol or practolol (see below), or with phenytoin sodium. Electrical cardioversion is absolutely contraindicated. Phenytoin Injection B.N.F. contains 250 mg. in a vial, and this dose, suitably diluted, should be infused intravenously over 3 to 5 minutes, the electrocardiogram being monitored simultaneously to detect bradycardia or heart block. Nausea, vomiting and a feeling of nervousness are symptoms of toxicity.

Beta-adrenergic-blocking Drugs

Propranolol acts on the heart not only by blockade of beta-adrenergic receptors, increasing the refractory period of a–v conduction, but also directly, by actions similar to those of quinidine. It slows the sinus rate and increases the refractory period of the a–v node. Like quinidine it depresses the power of cardiac contraction. It is often valuable in the treatment of supraventricular arrhythmias, particularly those induced by digitalis overdosage. Propranolol Tablets B.P. (10 or 40 mg.) may be given by mouth three or four times a day; the total dose in 24 hours may vary between 60 and 160 mg. If the situation is so urgent that Propranolol Injection B.P. has to be given intravenously, the initial dose should not be more than 0·5 mg. (0·5 ml.). At least 30 seconds should elapse, to allow the drug to reach the heart, before further small increments are given. Propranolol may induce intense bronchospasm in asthmatics.

Practolol is a new drug in this group and is said to have important advantages over propranolol: it is cardioselective and does not cause bronchospasm; side-effects are uncommon (rashes and mild gastro-intestinal upsets have been recorded); and its use is not contraindicated in the presence of signs of cardiac failure—but preliminary treatment for cardiac failure should be given. The usual dose by mouth is 100 mg. twice daily, but higher doses may be required; by intravenous injection the dose is 5 mg. and this may be repeated if necessary. Overdosage may cause bradycardia or hypotension: this calls for atropine sulphate 1 mg. intravenously followed by orciprenaline 0·5 mg. intravenously.

Lignocaine hydrochloride

Many of the drugs used to treat dysrhythmias have a local anaesthetic action, and this well-known local anaesthetic has a powerful, antiarrhythmic effect, by diminishing ventricular excitability. In high doses it decreases the power of cardiac contraction. *Lignocaine* has become the drug of choice for ventricular arrhythmias associated with acute cardiac infarction. Lingocaine Hydrochloride Injection B.P. should be given intravenously in a dose of about 1 to 2 mg. per kg. body weight, for an almost immediate effect. It is rapidly metabolized by the liver, so its action stops within 10 to 20 minutes, unless there is liver damage. Frequent injections, or a continuous intravenous drip at a rate of 1 to 2 mg. per min. may therefore be needed for prolonged control. Two hundred milligrams given intramuscularly produces a blood lignocaine level similar to that of 50 mg. intravenously, but only after a delay of about 15 minutes. Hypotension, visual disturbance and depression or irritability of the central nervous system are toxic side-effects; but if the dosage and rate of administration are carefully supervised, side-effects are rarely seen.

Procainamide, like quinidine, depresses both the myocardium and conducting tissue. It is absorbed rapidly and completely. After an oral dose the peak plasma concentration is reached in one or two hours and a significant amount is still present after six hours. When oral doses are given three to four times a day a steady plasma level is reached after about 48 hours. Undesirable effects include confusion, anorexia, nausea, vomiting, sweating, diarrhoea, drug fever and hypotension. Agranulocytosis and a syndrome resembling SLE have been reported, but only in patients having the drug regularly for over six weeks; patients should therefore be warned to report a sore throat or gums or other symptoms. Ventricular dysrhythmias and disturbances of conduction can also occur. Nevertheless, the drug is safer than quinidine, since there is not the same fear of sudden ventricular fibrillation. Long-term treatment should be avoided.

Procainamide hydrochloride tablets, B.P. contain 250 mg. Procainamide injection, B.P., is available in 10-ml. ampoules containing 100 mg. in 1·0 ml. It is best given by mouth in a dose determined by trial in each patient. Intravenous administration should be reserved for emergencies such as ventricular tachycardia. Procainamide is more effective in controlling ventricular than supraventricular arrhythmias.

B. PHYSIOLOGICAL MANŒUVRES

These aim at stimulating the vagus nerve, to slow the heart.

Carotid sinus pressure. This is an important manœuvre because it can be used both in the clinical diagnosis, and for the treatment, of some of the dysrhythmias. With the patient propped up, one carotid artery is gently palpated at the level of the upper border of the thyroid cartilage (Fig. 6). The physician should listen to the patient's heart, using his stethoscope, throughout the manœuvre. With his thumb he presses the carotid artery firmly for several seconds; massaging gently gives a stronger stimulus. The moment the cardiac rhythm alters, the pressure must stop. If the rhythm does not change, the other carotid sinus should be stimulated, but both carotid sinuses should never be pressed together. If possible the manœuvre should be monitored by an electrocardiograph. It should be avoided during the early stages of a cardiac infarction and where there is evidence of a previous cerebral vascular accident.

It is difficult for a patient to stimulate his own carotid sinus, though some learn to do so. *Other vagus-stimulating manoeuvres include:* holding the breath and bending forward; tickling the pharynx until retching occurs; swallowing something very cold, like ice-cream; Valsalva's manœuvre (forced

period of cardiac standstill caused by the shock, normal sinus rhythm often returns.

This technique can be used electively, by operators with some special experience, to convert, say, atrial fibrillation to sinus rhythm (electrical 'cardioversion'). For this a D.C. shock is best,

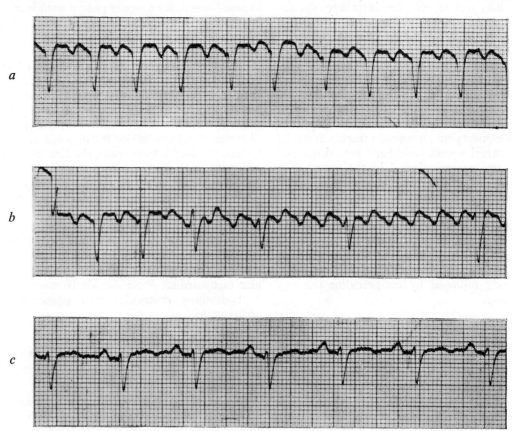

FIG. 6

Effect of carotid sinus stimulation in a patient with atrial flutter (E.C.G. Lead II).

(*a*) atrial flutter with 2 : 1 *a–v* block (ventricular rate 150/min.).
(*b*) carotid sinus pressure increases *a–v* block progressively.
(*c*) return to sinus rhythm shortly after (*b*).

expiration against closed nose and mouth); Müller's manœuvre (forced inspiration against closed glottis). Patients can easily perform these 'tricks'.

C. PHYSICAL METHODS

1. **Electrical defibrillation.** A high-energy electrical shock (50 to 400 watt-seconds or joules) applied across the thorax from a suitable apparatus often produces complete depolarization of the heart and may end any tachyrhythmia. After the short

electronically synchronized so that it avoids the vulnerable (T-wave) period of the cardiac cycle. To stop ventricular fibrillation timing is not important. Elective cardioversion of long-standing tachyrhythmias should not be performed on patients who have had digitalis within 48 hours, and they should preferably first have been stabilized on an anticoagulant to reduce the risk of embolism after the resumption of sinus rhythm.

2. **Electrical pacing.** For the short-term treat-

ment of ventricular asystole, *external pacing* can sometimes produce a heart beat. Electrodes are applied to the chest wall and stimulating impulses of 50 to 150 volts at about 60 per minute are applied through the thorax by a suitable apparatus. If this is ineffective, or for long-term pacing in patients with complete heart block, *endocardial pacing* is needed. This involves cardiac catheterization and the direct stimulation of the endocardium by impulses of about 1 to 10 volts. It is a specialist cardiological procedure. For intermittent ventricular asystole, 'on-demand' internal pacemakers are available, whose impulse formation is inhibited by the patient's heart beat, and which therefore only come into action when needed.

THE SUPRAVENTRICULAR ARRHYTHMIAS

1. Sinus arrhythmia. Sinus arrhythmia is physiological, causes no symptoms and needs no treatment.

2. Sinus tachycardia and bradycardia. The significance of variations in sinus rate and hence their treatment, depends on their underlying causes rather than the speeds themselves. Sinus tachycardia must be distinguished clinically from atrial flutter or supraventricular tachycardia. Carotid sinus pressure gradually slows the rate, which then gradually increases again. Sinus bradycardia may be confused clinically with heart block, but an electrocardiogram will distinguish the two conditions. Sinus bradycardia complicating cardiac infarction may contribute to a low cardiac output, and is therefore serious. It should then be treated with atropine sulphate 0·4 mg. to 0·6 mg. by subcutaneous injection every 4 to 6 hours, or, in coronary care units, by pacing. In acute vasovagal episodes the same dose may be given intravenously. Atropine is contraindicated in glaucoma and prostatism.

3. Supraventricular ectopic beats. Unless ectopic beats are causing symptoms they should be ignored. If palpitation is distressing, smoking, alcohol and caffeine should be forbidden, and the patient should be encouraged to take gentle exercise in the open air. If a sedative is required, 30 mg. doses of phenobarbitone can be given at 2 p.m. and 6 p.m.

4. Supraventricular tachycardia. (a) *Paroxysmal supraventricular tachycardia.* Supraventricular tachycardia is usually paroxysmal, often occurring in normal hearts and in young people. Carotid sinus pressure either has no effect, or stops the paroxysm dramatically.

The best chance of ending a paroxysm of supraventricular tachycardia occurs very early in the attack. The patient should be taught to try the various physiological 'tricks' described above as soon as the palpitation starts. If these do not stop the paroxysm, carotid sinus pressure should be tried: it sometimes restores sinus rhythm. If it fails, the eyeballs can be pressed hard, but this is unpleasant.

These 'first aid' measures may not stop the tachycardia. The patient must nevertheless be reassured. At this stage many physicians give an injection of morphine, and this alone may stop the paroxysm. If not, digitalis is probably the most useful drug. So long as no digitalis has been given for some weeks it should be administered by intravenous injection—0·5 mg. digoxin, followed by 0·25 mg. by mouth six-hourly. The alternative is to give 1·0 mg. digoxin by mouth, followed by 0·25 mg. six-hourly until the patient is digitalized.

Paroxysms of supraventricular tachycardia may be rare events, but they may be distressingly frequent. When this is so, a tranquillizer (p. 423) should be prescribed in the first instance. If this does not prevent attacks maintenance digoxin should be used (p. 86). This often reduces the number of paroxysms and shortens their duration.

(b) *Paroxysmal atrial tachycardia with* a–v *block (PATB).* This dysrhythmia is important because, although it can arise spontaneously, it is more often provoked by digitalis poisoning.

Clinically, it may be impossible to distinguish PATB from atrial flutter, or even, when the degree of *a–v* block is very variable, from atrial fibrillation. Sometimes it can be hard to distinguish PATB and atrial flutter, even with an E.C.G. Carotid sinus pressure increases the *a–v* block in both.

When atrial tachycardia with *a–v* block is thought to be caused by digitalis the drug should be stopped, and propranolol or practolol and potassium should be given as outlined above.

5. Atrial flutter. Atrial flutter often supervenes in the diseased heart. It is a rather capricious rhythm, easily giving way to sinus rhythm on one hand or to atrial fibrillation on the other. It can be paroxysmal; rarely, it becomes established. Occasionally it results from digitalis poisoning. Carotid sinus pressure increases *a–v* block while the pressure lasts, so the ventricular rate may slow abruptly to, say, half the rate, and may then increase in a stepwise manner (Fig. 6).

When atrial flutter is diagnosed in a patient who

has not had digitalis the flutter should preferably be treated by cardioversion. A D.C. electric shock with an energy content as low as 50 watt-seconds will often convert flutter to sinus rhythm. If the apparatus is not available atrial flutter should be treated by digitalis, given in full doses to the limits of tolerance. In some cases the flutter will give way to atrial fibrillation; if this happens the digitalis should be continued for a few days and then suddenly stopped. In some patients the rhythm will then change to sinus rhythm; others will continue to have atrial fibrillation, and digitalis may again be needed to control the ventricular rate and prevent cardiac failure. In some patients digitalis merely increases the degree of *a–v* block, thus slowing the ventricular rate; atrial flutter with a high degree of block may then become established as the permanent rhythm. Usually ventricular rate and cardiac performance can be permanently controlled by digitalis.

6. **Atrial fibrillation.** Atrial fibrillation may cause no symptoms, or only palpitation, unless the ventricular rate is very fast and the heart damaged, when a low cardiac output or reduced ventricular filling may cause ischaemic pain or even heart failure. Sometimes, when the ventricular rate is slower than usual, it may be hard to distinguish atrial fibrillation from frequent ectopic beats or from atrial flutter with changing block. The diagnosis should always be confirmed by an E.C.G.

Atrial fibrillation can occur in paroxysms or become established as a permanent rhythm.

(a) *Paroxysmal atrial fibrillation.* This can be divided into 'lone' and 'symptomatic'.

Lone paroxysmal atrial fibrillation occurs in healthy people; it is a source of inconvenience but the patient must be reassured. Paroxysms may be precipitated by alcoholic or other excesses; here the treatment is obvious. If the paroxysms are short and infrequent, no specific treatment may be needed. If they are frequent and prolonged, or cause disagreeable palpitation, the patient should be treated with maintenance digoxin (p. 86).

Occasionally a single transient episode of atrial fibrillation may complicate pneumonia or a head injury, but usually *symptomatic paroxysmal atrial fibrillation* is associated with heart disease or thyrotoxicosis. Sooner or later, atrial fibrillation becomes established as the permanent rhythm. The treatment must be directed primarily to the cause, for example thyrotoxicosis, but if the heart is enlarged or paroxysms are troublesome

the ventricular rate should be controlled by digitalis. Stopping the paroxysms by cardioversion does not prevent their recurring. If paroxysms recur frequently the patient should receive digitalis permanently.

(b) *Established atrial fibrillation.* Here again, lone and secondary forms exist. In either case long-continued atrial fibrillation, whatever the aetiology, predisposes to systemic thromboembolism and most physicians think such patients should have long-term anticoagulant therapy.

(i) Lone established atrial fibrillation is relatively rare. The ventricular rate is typically under 100 a minute in the untreated patient, and the prognosis is usually good. No attempt need be made to restore sinus rhythm by drug therapy; only when exercise causes frequent disagreeable palpitation need digitalis be used, to reduce the ventricular rate and to prevent the onset of heart failure. Cardioversion is usually ineffective.

(ii) Secondary established atrial fibrillation is common. The arrhythmia has become established as a complication of heart disease or thyrotoxicosis. When the ventricular rate is excessive it should be reduced by digitalis therapy. The aim of the treatment is to improve ventricular filling and so increase the cardiac output as much as possible. Once a patient with established atrial fibrillation needs digitalis he should continue to have it indefinitely.

(c) *Conversion of established atrial fibrillation to sinus rhythm.* It is often possible to convert established atrial fibrillation to sinus rhythm by electrical cardioversion (see above), but unless the underlying cause can be removed, fibrillation will usually recur sooner or later. There are two situations in which there is a good chance of sinus rhythm being permanently re-established: after the otherwise successful treatment of thyrotoxicosis, and, with less certainty, when atrial fibrillation persists in patients with mitral stenosis after a successful valvotomy.

Before the development of elective D.C. cardioversion, atrial fibrillation was sometimes converted to sinus rhythm with quinidine. In the absence of facilities for cardioversion, it would still be possible to use this method. Nevertheless, cardiologists are sharply divided in their attitudes to this question because of the dangers of quinidine therapy. Anyone who considers using quinidine for this purpose, should first read the review of the subject by Goldman (1960).

The restoration of normal rhythm often raises the cardiac output a little. However, most patients with atrial fibrillation manage well if their ventricular rates are adequately controlled by digitalis.

The Ventricular Arrhythmias

1. Ventricular ectopic beats. These cannot be distinguished clinically from supraventricular extrasystoles and are often provoked by similar factors, but they can be suspected where there is pulsus bigeminus. This disorder is characteristic of digitalis overdose. If ventricular premature beats cause troublesome palpitation, and do not stop on adopting a more moderate way of life, they can usually be suppressed over a short period by procainamide, 250 mg. four times daily or by practolol, 100 mg., by mouth twice daily.

Ventricular ectopic beats are potentially dangerous in patients who have suffered a recent cardiac infarction. If an ectopic beat occurs in the vulnerable period of the cardiac cycle occupied by the top of the T-wave ('R on T') it can trigger ventricular tachycardia or fibrillation. Ventricular ectopic beats coming as often as 5 to 6 per minute in patients with a recent cardiac infarction, particularly if they are multifocal in origin, or coming in salvos, should be suppressed by an injection of lignocaine, 100 mg. intravenously, and controlled thereafter by a lignocaine infusion, as described above.

2. Paroxysmal ventricular tachycardia. Ventricular tachycardia is a relatively rare arrhythmia, but often a grave one, because it usually arises in a heart already seriously damaged by chronic disease or a recent infarct; digitalis poisoning can also cause it.

The ventricular rate is high, usually over 180 to 200 beats a minute. Carotid sinus pressure has no effect whatever. If the paroxysm continues long, heart failure follows, or ventricular fibrillation leads to sudden death.

Digitalis is usually contraindicated in ventricular tachycardia, for it may change the rhythm to fatal ventricular fibrillation. It is best treated by electrical cardioversion. If this is impracticable, the drugs of choice are lignocaine or procainamide; and as ventricular tachycardia in a patient with heart disease is a real medical emergency, therapy must be given intravenously by carefully controlled infusion. This treatment should be given in hospital and continuously monitored by an electro-cardiograph. Rest and sedation must be ensured The blood pressure is checked frequently. If the blood pressure falls excessively the infusion is stopped and a pressor solution is infused instead (Metaraminol Injection B.P.).

If the tachycardia cannot be controlled and congestive failure threatens life, digitalis may have to be given as a last resort, notwithstanding the risk of causing ventricular fibrillation. An electrical defibrillator should be at hand.

3. Ventricular fibrillation. The only reliable treatment of ventricular fibrillation is *electrical defibrillation*, followed by cardiac massage and assisted ventilation if necessary. Unless the arrhythmia develops where a defibrillator is immediately available, the circulation will have to be sustained by external cardiac massage and artificial ventilation until a defibrillator is reached. (See 'Cardiac Arrest' below.) If the patient cannot be brought to a defibrillator lignocaine, 100 mg., can be given intravenously and cardiac massage continued. If this does not help, a direct intracardiac injection of procainamide, 100 mg., can be tried.

Heart-block

Partial Heart-Block

The treatment of minor grades of heart-block is directed towards elimination of the cause. Drugs cannot increase conductivity of damaged *a-v* conducting tissue, although atropine may occasionally reduce the grade of block. In many cases a long PR interval or Wenckebach periods are caused by digitalis poisoning (see above). Others occur in active carditis, and for these patients the treatment is that of their acute rheumatism. After acute cardiac infarction Wenckebach periods are usually associated with inferior cardiac ischaemia and are transient. Dropped beats, by contrast, are usually associated with massive anterior necrosis and carry such a grave risk of complete heart block that the patient should be carefully monitored for the necessity of cardiac pacing.

Digitalis is contraindicated in partial heart-block because it may further depress *a-v* conduction and increase the grade of block.

High-grade Heart-Block

2:1, 3:1 or even higher grades of fixed-ratio *a-v* block, are often permanent. The prognosis is poor; many patients develop complete heart-block, sometimes with Stokes-Adams attacks.

Stokes-Adams Attacks

These are transient attacks of cerebral ischaemia due to inadequate cardiac output caused by a change of cardiac rhythm. Loss of consciousness is a feature of a typical attack, but minor failures of cerebral perfusion may cause only transient dizziness. The cardinal signs that differentiate Stokes-Adams attacks from other causes of convulsions or syncope (p. 104) are the absent pulse and the characteristic flush that appears when consciousness returns.

Both fast and slow arrhythmias have commonly been recorded in Stokes-Adams attacks. During a single attack there may be more than one rhythm, with fast and slow rhythms succeeding each other, or two fast rhythms alternating, e.g. ventricular fibrillation and tachycardia. Between attacks the E.C.G. may show normal sinus rhythm or high-grade heart-block. If during an attack the heart cannot sustain the cerebral circulation for more than about three minutes complete recovery is rare.

Complete Heart-block

Complete heart-block may suddenly complicate cardiac infarction, but if the patient survives, the heart-block is often transient. Established complete heart-block is usually due to irreparable lesions of the conducting tissue, and is therefore not, itself, amenable to treatment by drugs.

When the ventricles beat independently of the atria, with an idioventricular rate of 30 to 50 per minute, hardly increased by exercise, the patient must learn to live within his exercise tolerance and be warned against strenuous exertion which can lead to syncope.

Management of High-grade Heart-block and Stokes-Adams Attacks

If the patient is symptomless, and the idioventricular rate is fast, as in cases of congenital origin, no treatment is needed. If there is cardiac failure, or a history of Adams-Stokes attacks, an attempt should be made to increase the ventricular rate. This can be done either by drugs or electrically.

Adrenergic amines increase the ventricular rate, and the most useful is isoprenaline. One 20-mg. Isoprenaline Tablet B.P. should be allowed to dissolve under the tongue while the rhythm is monitored by E.C.G. If ventricular ectopic beats appear isoprenaline is contraindicated, and electrical pacing should be used instead. If there are no

extrasystoles a delayed-release preparation of isoprenaline hydrochloride ('Saventrine') should be tried. Each tablet contains 30 mg. and should be swallowed whole. Treatment should start with two tablets (60 mg.) six-hourly and the dose should be increased in amount and frequency until either the heart rate is satisfactory, the dose reaches a maximum of 720 mg. daily, or ventricular ectopic beats appear. If a patient with complete heart-block develops congestive heart failure digitalis need not be withheld. It should, however, be given cautiously, and stopped if it provokes Stokes-Adams attacks.

The best treatment of an actual Stokes-Adams attack is a thump on the sternum, followed by the treatment for cardiac arrest (see below). Drug treatment is difficult for various reasons. The rhythm is unknown, the circulation has stopped, and the only rational way of giving drugs for that particular attack would be by direct intracardiac injection.

When Stokes-Adams attacks occur often, maintenance isoprenaline can be very valuable. It has the great advantage that it can be given when ventricular arrest alternates with ventricular tachycardia or fibrillation in the same patient.

If long-acting isoprenaline fails to control Stokes-Adams attacks or heart failure in a patient with high-grade heart-block electrical pacing (see above), of the 'on-demand' type, is the best treatment.

Cardiac Arrest

When the heart fails to maintain the cerebral circulation for about 3 minutes the brain may become so damaged that the patient, even if he survives, may remain in a decerebrate state. When circulatory arrest occurs in a patient whose heart 'does not deserve to die' emergency treatment must be started at once, by whoever recognizes the arrest. The crucial signs are coma, absent pulse and respiration, and dilated pupils. There are just 3 minutes in which to start and maintain an effective circulation. Waiting for a second opinion, recording the blood pressure, giving intravenous injections, or oxygen, are a dangerous waste of time.

The patient must at once be laid on his back on a hard surface, e.g. the floor, and his legs raised for a moment. Someone must thump the precordium hard once or twice: this alone will sometimes start the heart beating.

The patient's airway should be cleared, his neck

should be flexed, his jaw should be tilted forward and his head back. Artificial respiration must then be started, if necessary by the mouth-to-mouth method, the lungs being inflated by blowing hard through the patient's mouth. As soon as possible intubation and more efficient assisted respiration should be substituted.

External cardiac massage should also be started immediately. With one hand placed on top of the fist, the sternum is firmly pressed not faster than about 60 times a minute, so that each depression of 3 to 5 cm. squeezes the heart between the sternum and spine. Ribs may crack, but this is a minor complication.

The efficient management of cardiac arrest needs several people, but until help arrives the single-handed attendant must do his best. The lungs should be inflated by mouth-to-mouth respiration two or three times between each group of six to eight sternal depressions.

The cause of arrest in most cases is ventricular fibrillation. As soon as possible, therefore, electrical defibrillation should be attempted, without waiting for identification of the rhythm by E.C.G. If a defibrillator is not immediately available, or if defibrillation is ineffective, closed-chest massage and artificial respiration must be continued until the rhythm is accurately diagnosed and the appropriate treatment given.

If the E.C.G shows asystole, and facilities for electrical pacing are not available, an intracardiac injection of 5 ml. of 10 per cent. calcium chloride may occasionally restore sinus rhythm. If asystole persists, cardiac massage should be continued and 5 ml. of a 1 : 10,000 solution of adrenaline (Adrenaline Injection, B.P., diluted 1 : 10) should be injected into the heart.

Whatever the cause of arrest, metabolic acidosis must be combated by frequent intravenous injections of 8·4 per cent. sodium bicarbonate. This solution contains 1 mEq. in 1 ml. The patient's bicarbonate requirement (mEq./1.) can be estimated approximately by the formula $0.3 \times$ Body weight (kg.) $\times$ Base Deficit (mEq./1.). About half of this amount should be supplied by intravenous infusion.

The reappearance of a normal E.C.G. pattern should not encourage any relaxation of effort. Closed-chest cardiac massage and assisted respiration must be continued until the arterial pulse and blood pressure show that the heart is mechanically supporting an adequate circulation.

E *

SURGERY IN THE TREATMENT OF CARDIAC DISEASE

For certain cardiac conditions relief may be obtained by extra-cardiac operations, as for instance by sympathetic nerve section in cases of angina pectoris or hypertension or by thyroidectomy in cases of heart disease caused by thyrotoxicosis. Improvements in the techniques of surgery and anaesthesia have, however, made operations on the heart itself a commonplace of modern treatment.

SURGERY IN RELATION TO CONGENITAL HEART DISEASE

It is usually the family doctor or the school medical officer who first makes the diagnosis of a congenital cardiac abnormality. A full examination is then made in hospital to define its nature and to assess its suitability for surgical operation. The application of surgery to the relief of congenital heart disease has produced remarkable advances. New methods are constantly being explored and the combined resources of the biochemist, the physician and the surgeon are now employed as a routine.

In general the risks associated with operative surgery are directly proportional to the extent of the structural defect, and inversely proportional to the judgment, experience and skill of those responsible for the patient. Thus simple ligation of a patent ductus arteriosus by a surgeon technically competent in this field, carries a mortality no higher than that of appendicectomy. On the other hand, where the structural defects are multiple and complex the risk is correspondingly increased, with a high mortality even in the hands of an experienced team in a well-equipped unit. Nevertheless, operation may be justifiable because, without such treatment, the prognosis of a particular lesion may be grave.

Operations on the heart may be classified into three groups. First and simplest are those which necessitate thoracotomy without actual interference with the heart. Into this category come ligation of the patent ductus, resection of coarctation of the aorta and those cases of Fallot's Tetralogy in which anastomosis is made between a subclavian artery and a branch of the pulmonary artery. The hazard in these is slight, provided always that the surgeon is experienced, that he has the assistance of a competent anaesthetist and a well-trained nursing team, and that the pre-operative diagnosis is accurate.

In the second group where repair of a septal defect or division of a stenosed pulmonary valve under direct vision is in question, the problems are more formidable. For a time hypothermia was the method of choice, whereby the patient was chilled to a predetermined temperature around 30° C. and after occlusion of the great veins, pulmonary artery and aorta, the heart was arrested by injection of potassium or neostigmine. This allowed the surgeon to open the right atrium and explore and deal with a septal defect. Cardiac arrest for several minutes under these hypothermic conditions is harmless because the vital cerebral functions are protected by the low body temperature.

The increasing safety of cardio-pulmonary by-pass techniques, using a heart-lung pump, has led to wide adoption of this method even for closure of simple atrial septal defects. It is essential in cases involving ventricular septal defects and in all complex malformations. It demands not only costly and complicated apparatus but a highly trained team, not of surgeons only but of technicians, biochemists and blood coagulation specialists. The early high overall mortality (up to 20 per cent.) has fallen dramatically to a quarter of that figure in the last few years and to a very low level in the simpler procedures (e.g. closure of atrial septal defects).

The justification for such operations is the poor prognosis in patients left untreated. It should be borne in mind that complete well-being and lack of disablement in a child, the subject of congenital heart disease, are no guides to his future progress. From what is known of the natural history of the different lesions one may predict with some accuracy the probable outcome in individual cases. For example, children with a patent ductus arteriosus are continually subject to the hazard of superimposed subacute bacterial endarteritis—a condition difficult to diagnose and fatal if untreated. Moreover, those who escape such infection are liable to develop irreversible cardiac failure in early middle life, by which time operation becomes hazardous. Again, the subjects of atrial septal defect are rarely handicapped in childhood or early adult life, but a large proportion develop cardiac failure in their twenties or thirties and operation at this stage is much more serious than in the young subject as yet free from pulmonary hypertension. Similar considerations apply to patients with coarctation of the aorta, a condition compatible with full activity for many years but which in time leads to the inexorable consequences of sustained gross hypertension with the risk of aortic rupture, cerebral haemorrhage, and left ventricular failure. Hence operation is advisable in the young subject.

In some congenital lesions operation has to be undertaken for the relief of symptoms. In Fallot's Tetralogy the handicap may be such that the child is confined to the house, unable to undertake ordinary activities or to attend school: operation may restore a considerable measure of activity. In cases of severe pulmonary stenosis, in which the right ventricular pressure is extremely high and the muscle grossly hypertrophied, many patients suffer syncopal attacks and there is a constant risk of sudden death on exertion: in these patients also operation has to be undertaken at an early stage. Finally, while operations on very young children are not as yet widely practised, there are certain conditions which lead to progressive cardiac failure at an early age, even in infancy. Outstanding among these are cases of transposition of the great vessels. Such patients commonly die in the first few months after birth. It has recently become possible to relieve the condition and prolong life by a balloon-catheter technique—rupturing the atrial septum to allow mixing of oxygenated with venous blood. Others are occasional cases of coarctation of the aorta of great severity and some cases of patent ductus arteriosus with a large shunt and a raised pulmonary blood pressure. Operations for both these conditions have been carried out successfully in infants a few weeks old.

All infants with congenital cardiac lesions should be referred to a paediatric cardiologist as soon as possible, in view of the very high mortality among them in the first few months of life. Not every child, the subject of congenital heart disease, is suitable for surgical treatment. A considerable proportion of those deeply cyanosed in early infancy have highly complex malformations irremediable by present methods. For example, correction of transposition of the great vessels is hazardous and commonly unsatisfactory and there are a number of other conditions (tricuspid atresia, common truncus, etc.) for which treatment at present is impracticable, even with the most skilled surgeon and the most complex equipment. It is appropriate, therefore, to consider some of the common lesions and the indications and risks of their surgical correction.

Patent ductus arteriosus. In patients with uncomplicated patent ductus—usually recognized in early childhood or when the child is examined on first going to school—operation carries a low mortality. It is advisable, preferably between the ages of four and six in view of the risk of subacute bacterial endarteritis and of intractable cardiac failure developing in later life. As noted above, occasional cases accompanied by cardiac failure in infancy may have to be operated on at a very early age.

Coarctation of the aorta. This lesion notoriously shortens life. Operations for its relief are safest when carried out in childhood or before puberty. When performed after the age of 20 they are more hazardous and particularly so after the age of 30. The rising mortality is associated with the progressive arterial degeneration of increasing age. The operative mortality in skilled hands is low and the results are good. Untreated, these patients are in peril during strenuous activity, and in women during labour, from the risk of aortic rupture, cerebral haemorrhage and left ventricular failure. On the other hand, if a patient over the age of 30 is found by chance to have coarctation of the aorta and is symptom-free he is best left untreated.

Atrial septal defect. Defects in the atrial septum are common and vary in position and size. The common defect high in the septum (ostium secundum) may be large and may lead to an enormous increase in the pulmonary blood flow, which in turn puts a strain on the right heart and leads to pulmonary vascular changes. Such patients commonly experience symptoms in their twenties and soon develop failure. Operation in skilled hands carries a low mortality, but calls for either the induction of hypothermia and a short cardiac arrest or for cardio-pulmonary by-pass. Before operation is undertaken in patients with an atrial septal defect it is most important that a precise diagnosis be reached, including an estimation of the magnitude of the shunt, the state of the pulmonary vessels, and in particular the site of the defect. Defects low in the septum (ostium primum) are commonly associated with defects of mitral and tricuspid leaflets and with free communications between the two atria and between the two ventricles. Correction of this defect is hazardous and demands assisted circulation from a cardio-pulmonary by-pass pump. A serious operative hazard is permanent complete heart block from an ill-placed stitch.

Pulmonary stenosis. There is wide variation in the severity of this lesion. Many children with pulmonary stenosis have a loud murmur, little disability and little upset in cardiac haemodynamics. In others the stenosis is extreme, the right ventricular pressure very high and the right ventricular muscle grossly hypertrophied. Operation is not indicated in every case and many people with slight degrees of pulmonary valvular stenosis may live to an old age with little handicap. On the other hand those with severe stenosis are generally short-lived. The decision to operate should be reached only after careful assessment of the individual case, utilizing ancillary methods of investigation, including cardiac catheterization.

The original blind transventricular section of the valve has been superseded by division under direct vision through the opened pulmonary artery under hypothermia or with the heart-lung pump. The operative risk is not great and the results excellent.

Aortic stenosis. Similar considerations apply to this lesion as to pulmonary stenosis. All grades of severity occur from slight to severe and operation is indicated only in a proportion of cases. The original operations were performed by a blind transventricular valvotomy, but today it is preferable to operate under direct vision through the opened aorta. Such operations on the left heart demand a cardio-pulmonary by-pass.

Ventricular septal defect. In this lesion all grades of severity occur from the classical Maladie de Roger with a tiny orifice high in the septum to patients with a gross defect several centimetres in diameter. Contrary to general medical belief ventricular septal defect is not a benign lesion, and only the smallest defects are compatible with a long unhampered life. Larger defects lead to gross pulmonary plethora, to a rising pulmonary blood pressure and to early failure and death. Repair of lesions of any but minimal size is, therefore, justifiable in view of the bad prognosis which they carry. Palliative operations may be done on very young children with gross lesions (for example, 'banding' of the pulmonary artery. Such operations demand the full resources of cardio-pulmonary by-pass techniques and a skilled and experienced team. Detailed pre-operative investigation by cardiac catheterization, etc., is essential.

Fallot's tetralogy. This syndrome is of great importance on two counts: first, its frequency, and secondly, the severity of the handicap it imposes. It constitutes a high proportion of all cases of cyanotic congenital heart disease surviving into later childhood and early adult life, and in fact some two-thirds of such children have this particular combination of lesions. A much smaller proportion of very young cardiac patients have Fallot's Tetralogy, since many cyanosed infants have lesions of other types which in the majority are incompatible with prolonged survival, e.g. transposition of great vessels. The frequency of this tetralogy in later childhood and adolescence is so great, and its susceptibility to treatment so striking, that every cyanosed child with congenital heart disease should be reviewed with this diagnosis in mind. This entails detailed investigation in a specialized clinic.

Various operations have been practised for relief of the condition. The original operation devised by Blalock—anastomosis of one subclavian artery to the corresponding branch of the pulmonary artery— gave relief from cyanosis and remarkable increase in effort tolerance to a large number of handicapped children. A similar procedure is Pott's operation, in which a small fenestration is made between the aorta and the pulmonary artery in the form of an artificial ductus. The mortality from these operations is not high and the relief afforded is considerable. The objection to both operations is that they are only palliative: they give relief by increasing the blood flow to the lungs but do not correct the other deformities of the tetralogy—the pulmonary stenosis, the ventricular septal defect and overriding aorta. Other operations have been devised to cure the whole syndrome—division of the stenosed pulmonary valve, and closure of the ventricular septal defect. These demand the by-pass technique described above for cases of ventricular septal defect, while the stenosed pulmonary valve may be divided as described on p. 129. These procedures carry a considerably higher mortality than the simple operations first practised, but when successful are believed to be more satisfactory. Whether the improved results are sufficient to counterbalance the increased risk is a matter of some debate.

Other congenital cardiac lesions. Of the other congenital lesions many are extremely complicated and few are at present amenable to surgical correction. For example, transposition of the great vessels, in which the aorta rises from the right ventricle and the pulmonary artery from the left, has been tackled by attempts to transplant the two venae cavae and the four pulmonary veins to the respective venous and arterial atria. These operations are in general disappointing and the mortality prohibitive. Similarly operations for tricuspid

atresia, common truncus, and comparable malformations are at present beyond the scope of surgery.

General Management of Patients with Congenital Heart Disease

Diagnosis. With readily available surgical facilities and rapidly advancing techniques it is essential that every patient, the subject of a congenital cardiac lesion, should have the benefit of skilled assessment by a cardiologist and surgeon at an early stage. It is no longer sufficient for the doctor to label a patient 'congenital heart disease' or even to diagnose a specific lesion clinically. The patient must be assessed in detail so that not only the precise anatomical diagnosis is established but the severity of the lesion, the extent of pulmonary vascular changes and other secondary effects gauged, and the necessity for and feasibility of operation determined.

Infection. The subjects of congenital heart disease are notoriously liable to superimposed subacute bacterial endocarditis, with the exception of those with an atrial septal defect who display a curious relative immunity to this disease. It should be remembered that operation on the malformation does not necessarily prevent the later development of such an infection—for example, in Fallot's Tetralogy where a Blalock operation has been performed, or in pulmonary stenosis where the valve has been divided, there are many instances on record of subsequent subacute bacterial infection. On the other hand, the surgical correction of a patent ductus arteriosus or coarctation generally precludes the later development of this infection.

All patients with such lesions should have regular dental supervision and should be treated with penicillin as a prophylactic a few hours before and for a few days after dental extraction.

Cerebral thrombosis. Children with severe cyanotic congenital heart disease commonly have a gross polycythaemia with haemoglobin levels of 125 per cent. or more. In such cases when haemoconcentration occurs due to dehydration secondary to vomiting or diarrhoea, intravascular clotting is liable to occur, commonly in the cerebral circulation. The risk is greatest in infancy, when such dehydration is readily induced by infections. In patients who survive, the resultant hemiplegia adds an additional burden to the handicapped child and may be a deciding factor against later cardiac surgery.

The doctor must, therefore, be careful to prevent or to treat promptly such dehydration, particularly in infants. When early signs of cerebral thrombosis are detected, it is justifiable in an infant to do a small venesection (20 ml.) and give a very small dose of 250 to 500 units of heparin.

Activity. Patients with congenital heart disease and loud murmurs are commonly more severely restricted in their activities through over-solicitous advice from parents or doctor rather than by physical incapacity. It should be emphasized that the loudness of a murmur is no guide to the severity of the lesion. Some children with conspicuous murmurs have trivial defects which do not hamper growth, development or physical activity, while others with faint murmurs may be grossly handicapped. In general, it is wise to allow the child to exercise to the limit of his tolerance. Clearly far-reaching decisions regarding choice of a career, fitness for marriage and parenthood and indulgence in athletics should not be taken by the doctor unless the most careful attention has been given to detail of diagnosis in the individual case; this generally implies investigation in a specialized clinic.

Surgery in relation to Rheumatic Valvular Disease

By far the greatest number of operations on hearts affected by rheumatic valvular disease are carried out for the relief of mitral stenosis. Operations for aortic stenosis are relatively infrequent, and surgical treatment for incompetence of either mitral or aortic valves today taxes the resources of surgeons all over the world.

Mitral stenosis. Operations for mitral stenosis, originally introduced and abandoned many years ago, have now won a dominant place in the management of rheumatic valvular disease. The lesion is so common and so disabling that every practitioner should review all his patients with mitral disease with the possibility of operation in mind, and should refer all likely cases to a cardiac unit for assessment and decision. In the past we were too conservative and operation was often unduly delayed; many patients had been severely disabled for some 7 years, operation having been deferred on the grounds that though there were gross physical signs of disease, the handicap was moderate rather than extreme. The ill effects of such procrastination are now apparent and today operation is done at an earlier stage. When he operates earlier the surgeon deals with a younger

patient whose tissues are relatively healthy; myocardial degeneration may be slight and the mitral valve is not likely to be irretrievably damaged. Heavily calcified valves present formidable difficulties and the greater incidence of calcification in male subjects may be one of the reasons why the operation in men is generally less successful than in women. Inefficient division of calcified commissures is a common cause of a poor result, and while re-stenosis of a fully divided valve can occur, the cause of recurrent symptoms is much more frequently a suboptimal 'split' at operation.

The mortality from mitral valvotomy in skilled hands is about 4 per cent., including patients with considerable calcification or significant incompetence; in pure stenosis with pliable cusps the mortality should not exceed 2 per cent. Preoperative assessment of the anatomical lesion and of other factors (age, rheumatic activity, heart size, rhythm, myocardial function and degree of disability) is essential if optimal results are to be obtained with a low mortality.

The selection of patients for operation is of great importance. The ideal patient is the handicapped person in whom mitral stenosis is an isolated lesion, the heart is not grossly enlarged, failure is absent or controlled, and active rheumatic carditis absent. Atrial fibrillation *per se* is no contraindication, but generally occurs in older patients and indicates a damaged heart muscle and a less favourable prognosis. Associated mitral incompetence, unless trivial, contraindicates simple valvotomy, as do more than minor grades of aortic incompetence. Aortic stenosis associated with mitral stenosis may be dealt with simultaneously at the same thoracotomy. As regards age, operations under the age of 20 are inadvisable (though sometimes imperative) on account of the risk of rheumatic relapse. At the other extreme, patients over 50 are probably past the optimum age for safety and maximum relief. The average age of patients coming to operation in most series and in the writer's experience has been between 35 and 45, but there is a general consensus that patients should increasingly be selected for operation at a younger age. In India and elsewhere in the tropics the course of rheumatic heart disease is greatly accelerated, and operations under the age of 20 are common, and in children under 10 not infrequent.

OPERATION AND CHILD-BEARING. Young women with significant mitral stenosis as an isolated lesion should be considered for valvotomy before marriage and pregnancy, and women who have had failure or disability during a pregnancy should be advised to have operative treatment three or four months after delivery. Operations during a pregnancy can generally be avoided by careful antenatal care, but if necessary valvotomy can be carried out up to the sixth or seventh month with little added risk to the mother and no ill-effect on the foetus.

Results. The immediate post-operative results are usually good, with prompt relief of symptoms and increase in exercise capacity; many patients on discharge from hospital indulge in activities which for years had been impossible. Such is the power of faith that some improvement is noted for a time even in many found at operation to have irremediable lesions, but in these early deterioration is apt to occur.

When the late results, say five years after operation, are reviewed some two-thirds of those treated surgically are found to be in satisfactory health with significant relief of symptoms. Some patients show remarkable improvement, working a full day in industry or in the home, and withstanding repeated pregnancies without upset. Others are less well, particularly those in whom grossly calcified or incompetent shrunken cusps were found at operation, or in whom adequate division of both commissures for one reason or another was not achieved. With the passage of time more patients notice deterioration in their capacity for effort; 10 or 12 years after valvotomy many are sadly handicapped. Re-stenosis of the valve may demand further operation which in turn may yield a good result. About one-sixth of those surviving the post-operative period succumb to failure or embolism within five years. Both the death rate and the proportion of poor results are significantly higher in men.

Aortic stenosis. Aortic valvular stenosis with gross physical signs may be tolerated for many years with minimal disability: the orifice must be reduced to about 25 per cent. of the normal area before symptoms become urgent. When they do occur, the prognosis becomes grave: angina of effort, syncope and cardiac asthma are ominous and frank congestive failure sub-terminal. Since long unhampered survival with gross signs is common, it is difficult to determine when surgical relief should be called for, especially since operation carries a fairly high mortality.

The original operation of blind transventricular valvotomy has been replaced by open operation under hypothermia and/or by-pass with insertion of a graft or prosthesis as required.

Valve replacement surgery. For two decades isolated pure stenosis of the mitral valve was the only lesion capable of surgical relief with a low mortality and good results. Incompetence of either the aortic or mitral valve was surgically intractable, and aortic stenosis is a dubious proposition. The development of by-pass techniques, of plastic repair and of grafts and prostheses have made it possible to consider a surgical approach to all valve defects. Potential candidates for such operations are familiar to every doctor, general practitioner and specialist alike, and outnumber those with pure mitral stenosis.

Where a valvular lesion is causing regurgitation it is often feasible for the surgeon, under the unhurried conditions of the by-pass technique, to effect a plastic repair of the valve by appropriate stitching. In others, and in aortic cases, a prosthesis (Starr valve) can be inserted at a cost of £70 to £90 for the valve alone, excluding costs of hospital care, surgeons' skill and ancilllary services. Weighed against the operative mortality and possible benefit such financial implications are trivial. In some centres, excision of a diseased aortic valve is followed by grafting a healthy valve from a cadaver, e.g. a fatal accident subject; or the patient's own pulmonary valve can be transplanted to the aortic ring, and a prosthesis inserted in the pulmonary orifice. Nevertheless a successful operation is not the end of the story: platelet thrombi may form on the new valve, and lead to systemic embolism, with disastrous consequences; or a fungal subacute endocarditis may supervene in patients drenched prophylactically with broad spectrum antibiotics. However promising the initial results, the long-term value of such operations is as yet uncertain.

The assessment of individual patients for such radical surgery should be a function of special cardiac units with an experienced staff.

Heart transplants. Only a very small minority of doctors are called upon to take decisions regarding referring a patient for a heart transplant, and still fewer to decide regarding the acceptance of such an individual for the operation. On the other hand any doctor is liable to be involved in discussion or even lively argument over this controversial subject with some of his patients or with members of the lay public, and every doctor should be informed as to the present status of this operation. The writer is not concerned here with the ethics of the matter, but simply with its practicability.

The number of heart transplants done all over the world is testimony that any skilled surgical team is capable of carrying out the actual operation. It is also clear from the published results that the problem of rejection of the transplanted organ by the recipient has not been solved. In many cases rejection is immediate and complete; in others it is delayed but nevertheless relentless. In suppressing the body's immune responses, one inevitably incurs the penalty that the defences are down against infections of all kinds. Thus if the patient tolerates the transplanted heart he may also fail to react normally to an invading pathogenic micro-organism and be destroyed by it.

While rheumatic valvular heart disease remains prevalent and is a considerable problem, progress in valvular surgery and replacement is such that transplantation of a fresh heart is not called for in such cases. The great field in which 'a new heart for old' is desperately needed is in ischaemic heart disease, where the muscle may be so badly scarred by repeated myocardial infarctions and where the coronary arteries are so stenosed that nothing short of a new heart will ensure the patient's survival. Ischaemic heart disease is rife. In a town of say 200,000 population several hundred men die each year of this disease. If only a fraction, say 10 per cent., of these men are judged on other grounds to be suitable to receive a new heart then we must plan for a load of about 50 patients per year for cardiac transplantation in this small city alone. This would entail a cardiac team doing one operation per week, with an incredible strain on the scarce resources of skilled nurses, immunologists and all the other supporting staff in such a unit. Further, this demands that each week a young healthy heart must be found for transplantation immunologically compatible with the recipient, a heart coming from some young person killed in a motor accident or otherwise dying within easy reach of the cardiac centre, since delay in transporting the heart to theatre militates against the chance of its survival. Overall, the writer believes that cardiac transplantation on this scale is not a practical proposition in the immediate future.

Pericardial disease. Surgery may be required in purulent pericarditis; the indications for free drainage by open or closed methods are more or less as in cases of pleural empyemas.

In cases of chronic constrictive pericarditis where the layers of pericardium are matted together and possibly extensively calcified, operation is difficult and may be hazardous, but when successful is rewarding. The type of operation varies from case to case, but an extensive decortication of the heart may be necessary, stripping the mass of scar tissue and calcium salts which impede its contraction. Technical difficulties may be great, and the surgeon must often be content with partial operations. Early operation, before the formation of dense scar tissue and plaques of calcium, is advisable.

Such operations offer such good prospects of relief with a moderate mortality that all patients in whom constrictive pericardial disease has been diagnosed should be referred to a medico-surgical cardiac unit.

Operations for the Relief of Cardiac Pain

The indication for surgical treatment in angina is pain, persistent over two or three months, of such severity and frequency as to cause great suffering. The time factor in this definition is important, since patients initially bedridden through severe angina may recover spontaneously in a month or two and operation should not be considered till it is clear that spontaneous remission is unlikely. Such crippled patients constitute a very small proportion of cases of angina, but their state is pitiable: it has been aptly summarized as 'too sick to live and not ill enough to die'. As a corollary radical treatment has been defined as 'that which the doctor would hesitate to recommend for himself'.

Operative measures fall into three groups: (*a*) attempts at revascularization of ischaemic muscle by omental grafts or implantation of an internal mammary artery; (*b*) thyroidectomy; and (*c*) section of nerves carrying pain. *Revascularization* alone holds promise of cure as opposed to palliation, but operations of this type are generally disappointing and are little practised. *Thyroidectomy*, achieving relief of pain through lowering the B.M.R. with lessened demands on the circulation, has been replaced by ablation of the gland with radioactive iodine (^{131}I). With this there is no operative mortality, the mental and physical stress of operation are avoided and good results are claimed. The very simplicity of the treatment, however, encourages its use on inadequate grounds. It should be remembered that the resulting myxoedema is notoriously a cause of coronary disease. *Interruption of the pain pathways* may be secured by resection of the stellate and upper dorsal ganglia, or by injection of the ganglia with a sclerosing fluid (alcohol). Preference for one or other method varies with individual surgeons; in skilled hands either yields good results. The injection—a minor procedure performed under local anaesthesia, is effective when skilfully performed, though fatal syncope has occurred during an injection. In some cases an obstinate intercostal neuritis results from implication of posterior roots in the resulting scars. Sympathectomy demands open operation and, as a rule, general anaesthesia. The operative mortality is low, and many of the possible pitfalls of blind injections are avoided. A troublesome neuritis may follow the operation; it is most liable to occur where traction on the brachial plexus has occurred through difficulty in exposure of the ganglion, which is deep-seated and rather inaccessible. Horner's syndrome on the operated side is an inevitable sequel. After such operations many severe cases of angina decubitus are restored to a fair degree of activity and may be able to take up light work. Absolute relief from pain cannot be promised in any individual case, but is usually achieved. The tenure of life in coronary disease is notoriously uncertain, and an occasional unforeseen death in such patients should not too readily be attributed to the operation. Mackenzie's objection that operation by relieving pain abolished the red light that signalled danger in over-exertion, has been exaggerated. Some patients, freed from pain by operation, are still conscious of a sense of oppression on exertion, which indicates that the limit has been reached.

It must be emphasized that such measures are reserved for the exceptional case of angina. They have no place in therapy until it has been established that the patient is not suffering from the acute type with spontaneous remission after a few weeks of rest and medical treatment. The administration of radioiodine is temptingly easy, but it must not be forgotten that success with the isotope spells permanent myxoedema. The very gross manifestations of hypothyroidism can be mitigated by giving small doses of thyroxine. On balance the patient may, therefore, feel that this is not an excessive price to pay for release from chronic intractable pain. Nevertheless, the physician's approach should be cautious rather than heroic in what may be a self-limiting disorder.

Surgical Treatment of Hypertension

The demonstration in the experimental animal that ischaemia of one kidney could lead to severe and progressive hypertension, and that removal of the diseased organ led to its regression, opened a new line of approach to hypertension in man. In some patients in whom unilateral kidney disease is accompanied by high blood pressure, removal of the functionless and ischaemic kidney is followed by striking and lasting clinical improvement. They constitute only a small percentage of hypertensives, but in the investigation of all younger patients with high blood pressure, say under the age of 45 years, and in all of those with symptoms suggestive of renal (non-nephritic) disorder, an intravenous pyelogram should be made with later retrograde pyelography if necessary. This is commonly supplemented by a detailed study of the response of the two kidneys to a water and salt load, so-called split-function studies, which may reveal impairment of function at an earlier stage than is shown by excretion pyelograms. Renography using a radio-active isotope is a valuable new technique if facilities for it are available. Should the indications warrant the risk involved, aortography may be done: a fine catheter is introduced into a femoral artery and passed back into the upper abdominal aorta; radio-opaque medium is injected and its progress through the aorta and its branches recorded on films. Deficient blood supply to one kidney may be demonstrated, and the relatively rare cases of hypertension due to unilateral kidney disease (hydronephrosis, calculus, pyelonephritis) or to unilateral renal ischaemia from thrombosis or stenosis of a renal artery may be detected and the patient referred for surgery (endarterectomy, arterial graft or nephrectomy).

Severe hypertension in a young subject should always lead the examiner to feel the femoral pulse at the groin to exclude coarctation of the aorta—a condition unlikely to be overlooked if this simple routine is followed (p. 129).

A small proportion of cases of hypertension are due to a functioning tumour of the adrenal medulla (phaeochromocytoma) which is more typically associated with paroxysmal hypertension and such a cause should be sought. Operations for removal of a phaeochromocytoma are rendered reasonably safe only by our possession of powerful specific drugs, and by meticulous attention to detail in their use. Phentolamine cuts short the paroxysms of extreme hypertension and is given intravenously before and during the operation (e.g. when the surgeon handles the tumour). Alternatively, the sudden profound fall in pressure—it may be to catastrophically low levels—which follows excision of the noradrenaline-secreting adenoma is counteracted by intravenous infusion of noradrenaline acid tartrate B.P. (p. 97) and by restoration of blood volume by transfusion. These infusions may require to be kept up for 24 to 48 hours after operation, the blood-pressure being constantly observed.

Subtotal Thyroidectomy in Cases of Thyrotoxicosis
The subject is discussed on p. 293.

CARDIAC NEUROSES

Patients with imagined heart disease or who fear its development are relatively uncommon in the wards of hospitals, since in general they are dealt with in out-patient departments. They constitute, however, a considerable proportion of those seen by physicians in consulting practice, and are common on the lists of the family doctor. They may be as seriously crippled by their imaginary heart disease as those with organic lesions and are deserving of our sympathy and skill.

In the popular imagination the heart occupies a pre-eminent position among the organs of the body —the seat of the emotions, the fountain of life, the very core of one's being. This attitude to the heart is embodied in phrases and figures of speech in everyday use—a person is 'warm-hearted', or his 'heart leaps for joy'; he gives himself 'heart and soul' to a project; in a moment of suspense his 'heart stands still'. It is understandable that while a man may regard with comparative equanimity a statement that his liver or his kidneys are diseased, the slightest doubt cast upon the integrity of his heart causes serious alarm. In many patients such a doubt has first been raised by a doctor. Among patients with effort syndrome, all young soldiers without organic cardiac lesions, the author found that a high percentage had been told by at least one doctor, and in some by several, that they had heart disease. Reference has been made in the section on rheumatic carditis (p. 108) to the ease with which suspicion regarding the soundness of the heart can be engendered in a patient, and the doctor must constantly be on his guard lest by word or deed he conveys such an impression to a sick person. In other cases the genesis of the cardiac neurosis lies in over-solicitude on the part of parents toward an ailing child; over-protection of a child on the supposed grounds of 'a weak heart' is a potent source of mischief in later life. Frequently the possession of 'a weak heart' is subconsciously used by patients to avoid unpleasant tasks or duties, as for instance the young man who is thereby rendered unfit for military service, the young woman unfit for childbearing or housework, or the work-shy male who finds in his heart disease an excuse which justifies his idleness. The patient with imagined heart disease, unconscious of his real motive, may use it to wring sympathy and even a measure of protection from his family. Understandably a patient whose life has been orientated round a conviction of having heart disease, or who has escaped military service on such grounds, is likely to resist strongly any suggestion that the heart is in fact sound; commonly he rejects the verdict and seeks a doctor who will confirm the diagnosis and preserve the prop of his comfort or self-respect.

In a proportion of patients with so-called functional cardiac symptoms there is underlying organic heart disease. A young woman with mitral stenosis of minimal degree, whose disability from this lesion is at most slight, may have a superimposed cardiac neurosis which can be crippling. Men who have weathered the storm of a myocardial infarction may later develop functional pains in the chest, regarded by them as anginal and crippling in their results. It is most important in the management of patients that any such underlying organic lesion should be detected, assessed at its true value, and admitted in assessing the patient's final condition.

Diagnosis. A detailed discussion of the diagnosis of functional heart disease is beyond the scope of a textbook of treatment, but the practitioner should be aware of the symptoms of which these patients complain. Commonest possibly is left inframammary pain, differing in site, nature, duration and relationship to effort from true ischaemic pain (angina); other frequent symptoms are breathlessness, disproportionate to the exercise taken and on analysis commonly found to be sighing respiration quite unlike cardiac dyspnoea, weakness and easy fatigue, vertigo, 'black-outs' and palpitation.

Treatment. It is essential to take the history carefully and to make a thorough clinical examination. This should be reinforced by such ancillary methods of investigation—X-ray, electrocardiogram, etc.—as the physician believes necessary for the proper assessment of the case. On occasion, when a murmur is present which the physician believes is significant of a minor grade of pulmonary stenosis or mitral disease, it may be wise even to subject the patient to intensive investigation by cardiac catheterization. Armed with such information the doctor is in a strong position to reassure the patient categorically regarding the nature of his disability. If treatment is to be successful it is essential to gain the confidence of the patient, a confidence based on a realization that the doctor has taken every care to assess the importance of the symptoms, to detect any clinical or other abnormality present, and that he is competent to give a valid opinion on the findings. It is most important, in order to retain the trust of an apprehensive patient, that the doctor should acknowledge freely the presence of a murmur if such is heard. Others may have in the past drawn attention to it and if the physician denies its existence his opinion will be dismissed as worthless. If he admits that the murmur is present but goes to considerable trouble to assess its significance by modern methods, the patient is more likely to accept his evaluation and his reassurance.

So too in the case of a patient who complains of pain in the chest, full investigation is followed by a detailed explanation of why his particular symptoms arise from innocent causes. If the physician accepts that pain is present, admits all its unpleasant sequelae as claimed by the patient, and draws a clear distinction between such pain and the true pain of myocardial ischaemia, the patient will generally accept the distinction. This acceptance is in the last analysis based on trust in the doctor's honesty and professional competence.

It is not always easy, however, to convey reassurance in this way. It has been well said that the patient with true angina comes to the doctor making light of his symptoms, and hoping against hope for the reassurance which inwardly he knows will be denied him. The cardiac neurotic on the other hand comes to the doctor exaggerating his symptoms, over-dramatizing his case and hoping to be told there is an organic basis for his complaints. It is difficult to break down a barrier backed by such resistance on the part of the patient and by subconscious desires for the retention of the symptom.

Rehabilitation. In attempting to get a patient fit to resume work and take his place in ordinary life, the doctor faces considerable difficulties which are all the greater the longer the cardiac neurosis has lasted. When a life-long belief in the presence of cardiac disease has led a patient into a particularly sheltered existence it may be impossible to dispel

his fears and to rehabilitate him. Similarly, when a man has been excused military service because of a wrong diagnosis of cardiac disease, it may be impossible to get him to accept in later life that in fact his heart is sound, since to admit this to himself would destroy his self-respect. It is clear that in treating a patient suffering from imaginary heart disease, one is dealing with complex problems of motivation which a sympathetic and shrewd doctor may evaluate but which the unaided patient may be unable to resolve; on occasion the skilled assistance of a psychiatrist is essential.

One may divide patients with imaginary heart disease into two broad groups: there are those who, impatient of the restrictions imposed on their activities, are anxious to have the diagnosis refuted and to be allowed to lead a normal life; and there are those who from use and wont, or from deep-seated unconscious motives of which they are unaware, are prepared to accept the invalid status conferred on them by their cardiac condition. In general the first group respond quickly to reassurance while the second are notoriously refractory. In the latter the acceptance by the patient that heart disease does not exist may be followed shortly by substitution of imaginary disease in some other organ.

Among young men called up for military service the condition of effort syndrome is common and from the nature of the environment it is sometimes possible to arrange for considerable numbers of such people to be treated in batches. A thorough medical examination as described above is followed by drafting to a physical training unit, where graduated exercises are performed over a period of several weeks, and where it is generally arranged that increasing proficiency is rewarded by increasing privileges as an incentive. In such circumstances a considerable proportion of the affected men make a remarkable recovery, but in others the treatment fails. During the last war (1939-45) such failures usually drifted into a neuropsychiatric unit, the cardiac neurosis being simply one expression of a deep-seated inadequacy of personality.

From time to time a patient is encountered who has been bedridden for years on account of imaginary heart disease, and his rehabilitation presents a difficult problem. It is essential to remove him from the over sympathetic home environment, admitting him to hospital for initial investigation and subsequent encouragement in activity. The process is tedious and time-consuming, and demands a high degree of co-operation from nursing and medical staff. One such patient under the writer's care, a girl who had been confined to bed for 11 years following an attack of rheumatic fever and in whom there was no clinical or radio-logical evidence of cardiac disease, eventually returned to full activity after three months in hospital. During this time she had endless encouragement from physiotherapists and medical staff, but it was fully two months before her trust was gained and she realized that undertaking unaccustomed activity brought no aftermath of distress. Not the least of the obstacles to her rehabilitation was the attitude of her mother, who eventually had a nervous breakdown when she found the girl, on whom as a cardiac cripple she had lavished affection and care for over a decade, was no longer dependent on her.

Such a person may become the focus of sympathy and interest for the whole family, around whom the household may, as it were, revolve. Returning home after successful rehabilitation, the patient finds that from being the centre of attention in the family he is relegated to a minor rôle. It is not surprising that faced with the alternatives of existence as an ordinary person in a humdrum job or returning to semi-invalidism and to being the focal point for family benevolence, he relapses promptly into his former invalid state.

The problem of iatrogenic heart disease deserves consideration. Over the years doctors have been guilty of serious shortcomings: one should recall that until the days of Mackenzie many a boy was kept in bed for months on account of a sinus arrhythmia, while other children were similarly restricted on account of innocent cardiac murmurs. Today, possibly the brunt of iatrogenic illness falls on the middle-aged sufferers from hypertension and from coronary disease. Implicit in the modern control of high blood pressure is the need for continued accurate observation of the patient, and the frequent visits to the doctor's consulting room or hospital out-patient department may not only prove disturbing to a sensitive patient but may encourage

him to believe that slight variations in his blood pressure are of major importance. Similarly, hypochondriasis may be encouraged among patients receiving long-term anticoagulant therapy who have to come repeatedly to hospital for prothrombin checks. So too the publicity given in the lay press to the frequency and gravity of coronary disease, and to the alleged importance of cholesterol levels in its genesis and prevention, leads to considerable anxiety. The trust imposed by many patients in instrumental aids (electrocardiography, ballistocardiography) as guides to their progress and capabilities is evidence of how misleading is much modern medical practice.

References

Dynamics of Heart Failure
McMichael, J. (1952). *Br. med. J.*, **2**, 525, 578.

Cardiac Arrhythmias
Resnekov, L. (1964). *Post-grad. med. J.*, **40**, 381.

Cardiac Arrest
Portal, R. W. (1964). *Ibid.* **40**, 370.

Myocardial Infarction
Killip, T. & Lambrew, C. T. (1966). *A. Rev. Med.*, **17**, 447.
Lieberman, J. S. & Wright, I. S. (1960-61). *Prog. cardiovasc. Dis.*, **3**, 43.
Turner, R. W. D. (1964). *Post-grad. med. J.*, **40**, 369.

Quinidine
Goldman, M. J. (1960). *Prog. cardiovasc. Dis.*, **2**, 465.

Digitalis
Hoffman, B. F. & Donald, H. S. (1965). *Prog. cardiovasc. Dis.*, **7**, 226.

Diuretics
Laragh, J. H. (1967). *Ann. intern. Med.*, **67**, 606.

Hypertension
Lee, R. E. (1965). *Prog. cardiovasc. Dis.*, **8**, 101.

Propranolol
Besterman, E. M. M. & Friedlander, D. H. (1965). *Post-grad. med. J.*, **41**, 526.
Hamer, J., Grandjean, T., Melendez, L. & Sowton, G. E. (1966). *Br. Heart J.*, **28**, 414.

Practolol
Gent, G., Davis, T. C. & McDonald, A. (1970). *Br. med. J.*, **1**, 533-535.

5. Diseases of the Blood Vessels of the Limbs and the Effects of Cold

D. M. DOUGLAS

NORMAL BLOOD FLOW IN LIMBS

The blood flow through a limb varies with the cardiac output; it also depends on the calibre of the vessels, which in turn is controlled by the tonus of the smooth muscle in their walls. In the case of the vessels supplying the skin, tonus is controlled by vasoconstrictor fibres from the sympathetic nervous system, whereas vessels to muscle are controlled by chemical substances produced by muscle activity. Circulating adrenaline causes constriction in skin vessels and dilatation in those to muscle. For normal work and repair of minor injuries rapid adjustment of the amount of blood flowing to skin and muscle is necessary and this is possible only if both the vessels and controlling mechanisms are normal.

PATHOLOGICAL PROCESSES WHICH REDUCE BLOOD FLOW

Flow through arteries may be reduced by occlusive disease or by spasm.

Occlusive Vascular Disease

Sudden vascular occlusion is usually due to an embolus originating in the heart (atrial fibrillation, myocardial infarction) or less commonly in an atheromatous ulcer. Gradual occlusion is almost always due to atherosclerosis in which the wall of the vessel is thickened and the lumen narrowed by fibro-lipid deposits. In young people thrombo-angiitis obliterans may be responsible. Rarely it is due to arteritis (juvenile, temporal, polyarteritis nodosa, collagen diseases), polycythaemia vera or long-standing vasospastic disorders. The cause of vasospastic disease is unknown but the patients are hypersensitive to cold. It is also often seen in workers who use vibrating tools such as pneumatic drills and power saws.

Acute arterial occlusion. ARTERIAL EMBOL- ISM. The features of arterial embolism are sudden pain and numbness in the limb. Loss of power, pallor and mottling of the skin then occurs. The digital pads become shrunken and the veins are empty. The limb becomes cold and anaesthesia spreads towards the trunk. The muscles swell and contract; in the leg the heel is pulled up. The degree of the ischaemia depends upon the collateral circulation. When vessels are affected by atheroma the outlook is bad and of course the higher the occlusion the worse the prognosis. In a young patient with healthy vessels brachial emboli rarely cause gangrene of the hand.

TREATMENT. *Embolectomy.* With the advent of the Fogarty catheter, the treatment has radically changed. This long fine catheter with a balloon attachment can be introduced into an artery under local anaesthesia and the embolus removed. Unless there are strong contraindications such as late diagnosis with established gangrene, this technique should normally be used in limb emboli of any magnitude, though in the case of small emboli it is unnecessary.

Following embolectomy general measures such as reflex heating of the trunk with an electric blanket, anticoagulants such as heparin warfarin (p. 189) and analgesics should be used. Whisky is useful because it has the treble effect of allaying anxiety, relieving pain and causing vasodilatation.

Local care of the limb. The ischaemic limb should be covered with a light blanket and exposed to room temperature. It should never be heated. Points of pressure should be padded and a limb cage applied to prevent pressure on the toes. The head of the bed may be raised on nine-inch blocks to aid arterial flow. The limb must be kept clean and dry by washing, drying and the application of dusting powder.

Chronic arterial occlusion. The symptoms of chronic arterial occlusion in limbs are pain in the muscles during exercise (intermittent claudication), coldness and numbness of the digits, and, in advanced cases, rest pain which is most troublesome when in bed at night. The skin may show loss of hair, flushing on dependency and pallor on elevation. Irregular growth of nails and slow healing of epithelial injuries are common.

Intermittent claudication, the commonest symptom of chronic arterial occlusion is usually felt in the calf, less commonly in the sole of the foot or gluteal muscles. It is a curious fact that it is rarely felt in the extensor muscles.

GENERAL TREATMENT. Since atherosclerosis is a generalized disease, coronary and cerebrovascular disease should be sought and treated. Diabetes, if present, should be controlled. Cigarette smoking should be forbidden especially in young people. The value of postural exercises is doubtful but the advice to walk slowly and use a stick usually allows an increase in walking distance.

DIET. There is increasing evidence that, apart from heredity, diet is the most important contributing factor in the cause of atherosclerosis. However, there is no evidence that diet has any effect on the established disease. It is a matter of commonsense however to reduce weight when claudication is present.

PREVENTION OF INJURY TO THE ISCHAEMIC LIMB. Excessive heat or cold may injure the skin of an ischaemic limb. The aim should be to avoid extremes of temperature by wearing warm woollen clothing in winter and by forbidding the patient to warm his feet at a fire. Hot bottles should not be applied to the feet at night. In general, it is wise for patients with ischaemic limbs to remain indoors in cold weather.

FOOTWEAR. The best form of footwear is the soft leather boot with a fleece lining which protects against cold but does not press excessively on prominences. Within it, the patient should wear woollen socks. Patients should be warned against any form of tight-fitting footwear, though this is seldom acceptable advice for women.

CARE OF SKIN AND NAILS. The feet should be kept scrupulously clean and a dusting powder used. If there is any evidence of epidermophytosis, a fungicide (p. 582) should be incorporated in the dusting powder. Great care should be taken with the trimming of nails which should be cut long to avoid damage to the nail bed. Chiropodists and relatives dealing with such patients should be warned of the danger of corn-cutting and of keratolytic plasters. If ulceration, infection or hard cracked skin is present, the affected part should be soaked in warm (37° C.) water containing a mild disinfectant such as chlorhexidine (0·5 per cent.). When slough is present, a moist dressing of Eusol held in position by tube gauze is sometimes beneficial.

MANAGEMENT OF GANGRENE. When gangrene affects only part of a digit or digits, conservative measures are occasionally successful. These are to wait until the area separates spontaneously, keeping the part dry in the meantime.

However, much more commonly, the gangrene spreads giving rise to severe night pain for which powerful analgesics are required. The use of vasodilator drugs is generally ineffective, though phenoxybenzamine, isoxsuprine, inositol nicotinate, tolazoline and many others have been tried.

A decision must then be made as to whether a major amputation (usually at or above the knee) should be advised or whether an attempt should be made surgically to improve the circulation. This may be achieved by lumbar sympathectomy or arterial grafting or both. Usually amputation is advised in patients over seventy, vascular surgery being reserved for patients in their fifties and sixties. The results of the latter are unpredictable but occasionally gratifying salvage of a limb is achieved. If a major amputation is carried out, it is essential that early consultation with the regional limb-fitting centre should be arranged so that the patient may be transferred there as soon as possible after operation. With modern light walking pylons, it is to be expected that most patients will be walking within a month of operation even in the older age-groups.

ANTICOAGULANT THERAPY. There is little evidence that long-term anticoagulant therapy is of any value in occlusive vascular disease. The situation is comparable to their use in occlusive coronary or cerebrovascular disease. Until there is better evidence of benefit, it is hardly justifiable to submit these patients to the inconvenience of regular attendance at anticoagulant clinics.

SOCIAL SERVICES. Most patients with intermittent claudication who are manual workers have to seek sedentary or indoor employment. Retraining and re-settlement clinics play an integral part in the management of the condition. It is important to adopt an optimistic approach, emphasizing that while claudication is a nuisance it is not of itself a serious symptom. Most patients live for many years after its onset. The important objective is to learn to live with the disability. The state of other important arteries, especially the coronaries, should be assessed as a matter of routine; if they are affected the prognosis should be guarded.

Vasospastic disease. RAYNAUD'S PHENO-

MENON. This is commoner in young women than men. It consists of the appearance of pallor and numbness in one or more of the fingers. The condition is thought to be due to excessive spasm of the digital vessels in relation to cold but there is recent evidence that increased blood viscosity and cryoglobulins may also be concerned. The condition is usually precipitated by cold but it occasionally occurs during emotional disturbances. It also occurs in scleroderma and obliterative arterial disease of the arms. Its course is variable; it may improve, remain static, or deteriorate and give rise to digital gangrene.

The disorder is said to be less common in North America where the houses are well heated. In this country the symptoms are much worse in winter when the majority of the people start work in a chilled condition. The wearing of adequate warm clothing and the avoidance of chilling during dressing and the taking of a good breakfast usually results in improvement. Vasodilator drugs (p. 101) may be tried but they are not usually helpful.

If the condition is severely disabling or results in ulceration of the digits, sympathectomy may be carried out. In the case of the legs, the results are good and long lasting, but in the case of the arms the results, though initially satisfactory, are disappointing in the long run. However, the attacks are not usually as severe as before. Sympathectomy does not help in scleroderma.

ERYTHROCYANOSIS. A complaint of cold blue legs is not uncommon in young women in cold climates. There is often an increased deposit of fat in the region of the ankles where patches of ischaemic fat necrosis may develop leading to indolent ulcers.

General treatment is the same as for Raynaud's disease but lumbar sympathectomy in severe cases is usually well worth while.

Effects of cold. CHILBLAINS are localized swellings which occur on the dorsum of fingers and toes in children and young people and are believed to be due to localized vasodilatation which results from cold injury. General treatment is the same for Raynaud's phenomenon and erythrocyanosis; and many patients with erythrocyanosis suffer from chilblains. Care should be taken to avoid directly heating the affected parts in front of fires. Temporary relief of discomfort can be obtained by the application of an ointment containing 1 per cent menthol in soft paraffin. When ulceration has occurred the treatment is that for any ulcerated

skin lesion but 5 per cent. compound tincture of benzoin is a comforting dressing.

FROSTBITE. Frostbite has become more common in this country following the development of ski-ing, winter hill climbing and also the commercial use of deep freezing of food. It may affect the hands, ears or tip of the nose. The area becomes white and numb and the danger is that the patient may be unaware of it.

Frostbite is more easily prevented than cured; suitable wind- and chill-proof clothing with a Parka hood to protect the face should be worn. During exposure to cold, inactivity is dangerous. Once frostbite has occurred, the patient should return to a warm environment whenever possible. Failing this the frostbitten area should be completely covered. During recovery there is intense vasodilatation and severe pain which may require morphine for its relief. Blistering and oedema are common and local death of tissue may occur. This should always be treated conservatively by exposure to room temperature (20° C.). The eventual tissue loss may be gratifyingly small. Amputation is seldom required. Blisters should be treated by aspiration under sterile conditions and antibiotics only used if infection occurs.

IMMERSION FOOT. This condition occurs after shipwreck or in trench warfare when the feet are immersed for long periods in water below 15° C. The feet become swollen and numb and later may blister and show patches of gangrene.

Treatment is the same as for frostbite with the addition of elevation of the limbs if swelling is severe. Final loss of tissue is often surprisingly small.

Venous thrombosis. This often occurs in the saccular parts of superficial *varicose veins* and is a method of natural cure. The affected area is red and tender. There is little risk of pulmonary embolism unless the thrombus extends into the deep veins. Treatment consists of the application of a firm pad of sorbo rubber over the segment, held in place by a crepe bandage from the toes to well above the thrombosed segment. The patient is encouraged to walk. Resolution may take several weeks. Anticogaulants are not advised, but phenylbutazone 100 mg. thrice daily for five days relieves pain and hastens resolution. Surgical treatment of the varicosities may be undertaken after resolution.

MIGRATORY PHLEBITIS. This rare condition usually occurs on the dorsum of the foot or in the line of a normal saphenous vein. It may be an early sign of thromboangiitis obliterans or of an unsuspected cancer of the pancreas, lung, nasopharynx, stomach or thyroid. Local treatment is hardly necessary but if thromboangiitis is suspected, long-term anticoagulants may be employed. Epidermophytosis must be treated if present.

Deep venous thrombosis. This is a serious complication of operation, childbirth, or debilitating illness. It carries a risk of fatal pulmonary embolism and every effort must be made to prevent its occurrence.

Preventive measures include early ambulation after operation (48 hours), physiotherapy and leg exercises during confinement to bed and the use of prophylactic anticoagulants in high-risk patients.

Treatment of established deep venous thrombosis depends upon the time when first diagnosed. Within 48 hours of the first appearance of the hot, swollen and cyanosed limb thrombectomy using a Fogarty catheter may be employed with good effect. It is essential to use operative venography to establish that the thrombectomy is complete.

When seen later in the illnesses, the treatment is conservative, by elevation of the foot of the bed on 9-in. blocks, by the use of heparin and warfarin as anticoagulants (p. 186), and by the administration of analgesics (p. 440). The use of low molecular weight dextran as an intravenous infusion has not received general acceptance.

When pain and swelling have subsided, a firm elastic bandage should be applied from toes to groin and the patient encouraged to walk. This is usually possible in three weeks.

As a long-term policy these patients should sleep with the end of the bed elevated and an elastic stocking should be worn until the tendency to swelling has disappeared—and this may take many years. The risk of gravitational ulcer is very real unless great care is taken to prevent chronic venous stasis by exercise and elastic support. The patients should be carefully instructed in the use of elastic stockings: women should have at least three suspenders per stocking and men should wear a woman's suspender belt to which the stockings are attached. It is essential that wrinkling of the stocking at any level should be avoided. At rest, the patients should keep the leg raised above the level of the heart by lying on a sofa. Sitting in a chair with the leg dependent is the position which, more than any other, will aggravate swelling and venous engorgement.

6. Disorders of the Blood

R. H. GIRDWOOD

INTRODUCTION

The doctor who is attempting to decide whether or not a patient is anaemic cannot rely on the presence or absence of pallor, since the colour of the skin depends in part on the state of contraction of the capillaries, and the facial appearance may be misleading. It is wasteful and unfair to the patient to indulge in empirical therapy without first confirming the diagnosis, noting the type of anaemia, and discovering its cause.

CLASSIFICATION

Treatment can be placed on a more rational basis if the practitioner has some simple but clear conception of the classification of disorders of the blood.

The Anaemias

ANAEMIAS DUE TO DEFICIENCY OF FACTORS ESSENTIAL FOR NORMAL BLOOD FORMATION
(a) Iron deficiency
1. Chronic nutritional hypochromic anaemia, including the Plummer Vinson syndrome.
2. The hypochromic anaemia of pregnancy.
3. Hypochromic anaemia of infancy and childhood.
4. Post-haemorrhagic anaemia, acute and chronic.
(b) Deficiency of vitamin B_{12} or folic acid.
1. Addisonian pernicious anaemia.
2. Megaloblastic anaemia of pregnancy.
3. Megaloblastic anaemias of infancy.
4. Megaloblastic anaemia in malabsorptive disorders (gluten enteropathies and idiopathic steatorrhoea, tropical sprue).
5. Megaloblastic anaemia associated with disease of the small intestine (e.g. regional ileitis, reticuloses).
6. Megaloblastic anaemia associated with operations on the gastro-intestinal tract or with blind loops or fistulae.
7. Megaloblastic anaemia due to fish tapeworm infestation.
8. Nutritional megaloblastic anaemia.
9. Megaloblastic anaemia of liver disease.
10. Megaloblastic anaemia due to drugs, including certain anticonvulsants, folic acid antagonists and pyrimethamine.
11. Megaloblastic anaemia in generalized malignancy, leukaemia, di Guglielmo's disease and myelofibrosis.
(c) Ascorbic acid (vitamin C deficiency).
The anaemia of scurvy (p. 358).
(d) Thyroxine deficiency.
The anaemia of myxoedema (p. 154).
(e) Pyridoxine (vitamin B_6) deficiency—one form of sideroblastic anaemia.

ANAEMIAS DUE TO EXCESSIVE BLOOD DESTRUCTION (HAEMOLYTIC ANAEMIAS)
(a) Due to intrinsic red cell defects.
(b) Due to extrinsic mechanisms.

ANAEMIAS DUE TO APLASIA OR HYPOPLASIA OF THE BONE MARROW (USUALLY PANCYTOPENIA)
Aplastic and hypoplastic anaemia.
1. Idiopathic.
2. Secondary.

ANAEMIAS OF UNCERTAIN ORIGIN
Due to chronic infection, uraemia, rheumatoid arthritis, liver disease or widespread malignant disease.

Miscellaneous Disorders of the Blood

THE SYNDROME OF PORTAL HYPERTENSION (Splenic anaemia, Banti's disease).

HAEMOCHROMATOSIS

HAEMORRHAGIC DISEASES
(a) Due to defects in the clotting or fibrinolytic mechanisms, e.g. haemophilia, Christmas disease, hypoprothrombinaemia, fibrinogenopenia.
(b) The purpuras:
(i) Due to abnormality of the capillaries.
(ii) Due to defective production or excessive destruction of platelets (thrombocytopenic purpura).
(iii) Due to excessive production of platelets (thrombocythaemia).

AGRANULOCYTOSIS

INFECTIOUS MONONUCLEOSIS (p. 37).

DISEASES OF THE RETICULO-ENDOTHELIAL SYSTEM
(a) The Myelo-proliferative Diseases:

Cell Series	Resulting Disorders
Erythrocyte	Erythraemic myelosis
	Polycythaemia vera
Platelet	Primary thrombocythaemia
Lymphocyte	Acute lymphoblastic leukaemia
	Chronic lymphatic leukaemia
Granulocyte	Acute myeloblastic leukaemia
	Chronic myelogenous leukaemia
Monocyte	Monocytic leukaemia
Plasma Cell	Multiple myeloma
Fibroblast	Myelofibrosis
Osteoblast	Myelosclerosis

(b) The Reticuloses:
(i) Lymphadenoma (Hodgkin's disease), lymphosarcoma (including follicular lymphoblastoma) reticulum cell sarcoma, etc.
(ii) Diseases of lipoid storage: Gaucher's disease and Niemann–Pick disease.
(iii) Eosinophilic granuloma: Hand-Schüller-Christian disease and Letterer-Siwe syndrome.
(iv) Macroglobulinaemia.

THE ANAEMIAS DUE TO IRON DEFICIENCY

Iron-deficiency anaemia is much more common than other types in all parts of the world. It develops after haemorrhage, acute or chronic, and it is common in pregnancy, in women of reproductive age and in infancy.

Chronic Nutritional Hypochromic Anaemia

(*Hypochromic anaemia, chronic microcytic anaemia, simple achlorhydric anaemia*). Chronic nutritional hypochromic anaemia is an iron-deficiency anaemia occurring especially in women of child-bearing age, particularly those of the low-income group. The most important factor in its causation is the ingestion of a diet of low iron content, insufficient to meet the demands imposed by menstruation and pregnancy. Foods rich in iron such as liver, meat, eggs, oatmeal and green vegetables should be taken in adequate quantity.

Treatment is considered under the following headings: (1) general measures; (2) drug treatment (iron, ascorbic acid); (3) symptomatic treatment.

General measures. The haemoglobin level usually falls gradually over several years. Accordingly, the patients become, to a considerable extent, acclimatized to a low level of haemoglobin and can often undertake moderate exertion with little disability despite a severe degree of anaemia; this is in contrast to the state of shock which occurs in patients with acute haemorrhage even when the haemoglobin is only moderately reduced to 7 or 8 g. per 100 ml. Nevertheless, until iron therapy has improved the anaemia, the amount of activity undertaken should be reduced to such a level that dyspnoea, palpitation, giddiness and tiredness are avoided.

Drug treatment. IRON. It is now generally agreed (1) that iron is absorbed in the ferrous state mainly from the duodenum and upper jejunum; (2) that the ferrous salts are more efficacious than similar doses of the ferric salts; (3) that the use of preparations of iron in combination with folic acid is seldom justified except in pregnancy; and (4) that parenteral iron therapy is not often required.

Provided that complicating factors such as haemorrhage or infection are absent, a rise in the haemoglobin level of at least 1 g. per 100 ml. per week should result from efficient oral iron therapy. The following preparations are those most frequently used:

Preparation	Usual Dose, thrice daily	Iron Content, (mg. per day)
Ferrous sulphate	200 mg.	180
Ferrous fumarate	200 mg.	180
Ferrous gluconate	300 mg.	108
Ferrous succinate	150 mg.	105

All the above preparations are available as tablets. Five tablets daily of ferrous gluconate or ferrous succinate are needed to give the same amount of iron as three tablets daily of ferrous sulphate. A useful liquid preparation is Fersamal Syrup which contains 140 mg. of ferrous fumarate (equivalent to 45 mg. of iron) in 5 ml.

Tablets are more convenient than fluid preparations because they are easily carried and do not blacken the teeth and tongue. If dysphagia is present, a fluid mixture is obviously preferable. With regard to cost, ferrous sulphate is much cheaper than the other forms of iron available in tablet form. Intolerance to iron preparations is probably largely psychological, and ferrous sulphate is recommended as the preparation of choice.

The great majority of patients will experience no significant side-effects from taking one 200 mg. ferrous sulphate tablet thrice daily, provided that the tablet is always taken after meals. However, some may complain of nausea, constipation or diarrhoea. It is important to emphasize to the patient that any upset which occurs is often transient and it may be advisable to start treatment with one tablet daily for two or three days, then two tablets daily for a further few days before giving the optimal dose of one tablet thrice daily

If ferrous sulphate causes upset despite the precautions mentioned above, it is justifiable to change to ferrous fumarate or gluconate and, if these fail to a proprietary controlled release preparation such as Ferro-Gradumet (Abbott). This is a ferrous sulphate tablet in which it is claimed that little of the mineral is released in the stomach. One tablet contains 105 mg. of elemental iron, and although there is controversy about the value of such preparations, it may be that in certain instances one tablet daily will be effective and satisfactory.

The period likely to elapse before the haemoglobin level returns to normal will usually vary from one to three months, depending mainly on the initial level. Treatment should be continued for one month thereafter to provide adequate stores of iron. In women past the menopause, maintenance treatment is seldom required because of the decreased demands for iron. In women of reproductive age iron therapy should always be recommended if pregnancy occurs. Apart from this, further treatment is unlikely to be necessary unless menorrhagia is present, but a haemoglobin estimation should be made once or twice a year.

The oral administration of iron produces such satisfactory results that parenteral therapy is rarely indicated. There is no doubt that it is used far too often, and without clear indications, and it should be noted that the rate of haemoglobin rise is not necessarily more rapid when iron is given by injection. It may be required for the patient who has a true intolerance to iron given orally, but this is uncommon provided the precautions discussed above are taken. It is indicated in patients with hypochromic anaemia who fail to respond satisfactorily to adequate oral therapy because of malabsorption, but such cases are rare. Its use is justified when severe hypochromic anaemia is discovered late in pregnancy because it fills the body stores and may perhaps produce more rapid regeneration of haemoglobin than oral iron. However, if the anaemia is not diagnosed until very late in pregnancy, so that it would be impossible by the use of parenteral iron alone to bring the haemoglobin to a satisfactory level before the onset of labour, one should not hesitate to transfuse blood in addition. Parenteral iron has also been recommended for the treatment of the hypochromic anaemia associated with rheumatoid arthritis which is notably resistant to oral iron. Lastly, its use is justified when it is likely that the patient, despite assurance and explanation, is neglecting to take the prescribed doses of oral iron. Such cases are common and it is important to realize that comparisons of the efficacy of parenteral and oral iron therapy may lead to erroneous conclusions in out-patient practice. Frequently patients who have been regarded as refractory to iron by mouth respond very satisfactorily to the same dose of the same preparation in hospital where its regular administration can be supervised.

The following preparations of iron for parenteral use are available:

A preparation developed for intramuscular use is iron dextran injection B.P. (Imferon). It is available in ampoules of 2 ml., 5 ml., or 20 ml., and these contain 50 mg. of iron per ml. The dose required depends upon the haemoglobin level and body weight, and it is advisable to give 2 ml. in the first instance. If no untoward reaction occurs, continue with 5 ml. daily or every second day. A total adult dosage of 20 to 40 ml. may be needed, depending on the severity of the anaemia.

Pain and tenderness frequently occur at the site of injection. A brownish discoloration of the overlying skin is common and for this reason injections, especially in women, should be given deeply into the upper and outer quadrant of the buttock.

General reactions occur rarely and are usually mild, consisting of headache, dizziness or vomiting. Bizarre effects have been reported, e.g. conjunctivitis and swelling of the eyelids. Reactions may be delayed for several hours after injection, so that, in the case of out-patients, the first manifestation may not appear until the patient is at home. Adrenaline (0·5 ml. of a 1 in 1000 solution subcutaneously) or an antihistamine drug such as chlorpheniramine maleate 10 to 20 mg. intravenously or intramuscularly is of value in both the early and delayed mild reactions.

Unfortunately experimental work in animals (rats and mice) has shown that sarcomata may be produced by the injection of large amounts over a long period. The relationship of these findings to human medicine is obscure. The doses used in animals were, weight for weight, many times greater than the therapeutic doses in humans, but if the effect is mainly due to the local concentration of the compound at the injection site, the objection to its use in man is still valid. Moreover, the development of sarcomata in animals did not appear until some time had elapsed after the injections, and it is impossible to be dogmatic that similar lesions will not occur in humans, having regard to the different life-span of the species. For these reasons and because there is an alternative and safer preparation we feel that iron dextran should not be given intramuscularly. It has also been advocated as an intravenous infusion, the whole iron requirement being given slowly in a single dose diluted in sodium chloride injection (B.P.), starting with ten drops per minute for ten minutes under medical surveillance.

With any iron preparation given by injection there can be more severe reactions than those referred to above, and this is particularly so when administration is by the intravenous route. There may be severe bronchospasm, pain in the back, and circulatory collapse. Iron dextran should not be given by the intravenous route to children, and in the adult, hydrocortisone sodium succinate 100 mg. should be at hand for intravenous injection if a reaction occurs. Iron dextran should not be given intravenously to asthmatics.

A more satisfactory preparation for *intramuscular* use is the iron sorbitol injection (Jectofer). It also contains 50 mg. of iron per ml. and each ampoule contains 2 ml. The recommended single dose is 1·5 mg. of iron per kg. of body weight by deep intramuscular injection. The trial dose is calculated on the basis of the patient's initial haemoglobin concentration, assuming that about 250 mg. of iron will cause a haemoglobin increase of 1 g. per 100 ml. of blood. Headache, dizziness, nausea and vomiting have occurred particularly when it has been given together with iron by mouth. The explanation for this may be that iron sorbitol is absorbed very rapidly into the blood stream, where it becomes bound with transferrin. If previous oral iron has reduced the iron-binding capacity by combining with most of the available transferrin, iron sorbitol may pass into the plasma unchanged and produce this toxic effect. This can usually be avoided if the injections are not started until oral iron therapy has been discontinued for a few days. However, such reactions may also occur in pregnant women suffering from folic acid deficiency. It seems, too, that this preparation of iron may exacerbate pyelonephritis; hence it should not be used in those with a history of urinary infection. The patient receiving injections of iron sorbitol may be disconcerted by the urine turning black on standing, probably because the excreted iron is converted into iron sulphide. So far there are no reports of sarcomata following the injection of iron sorbitol in animals although some instances of a fibroma-like tumour have been reported. Iron sorbitol must *not* be given intravenously.

An iron carbohydrate preparation (Astrafer) is available for intravenous use

ASCORBIC ACID. Vitamin C is recognized to be one of the factors essential for normal haemopoiesis. In some cases of iron-deficiency anaemia without frank manifestations of scurvy, a supplement of ascorbic acid may augment the effects of iron. This is likely to occur only when the diet has been deficient in ascorbic acid as well as in iron.

Symptomatic treatment. When satisfactory iron therapy is undertaken, the haemoglobin level rises and, as it does so, all the manifestations of chronic nutritional hypochromic anaemia rapidly disappear in the great majority of cases.

DYSPHAGIA. Mild degrees of dysphagia disappear as the anaemia diminishes. Severe and persistent dysphagia (Plummer–Vinson syndrome, Paterson–Brown Kelly syndrome) may be associated with web formation in the pharynx, and its relief may necessitate using bougies or cutting the obstructing membrane. The possibility of carcinoma developing in the pharynx should be kept in mind if dysphagia recurs.

MENORRHAGIA. If menorrhagia is present, the problem is really one of chronic post-haemorrhagic anaemia rather than of chronic nutritional hypochromic anaemia. However, since it is usually impossible to assess accurately the severity of menstrual blood loss from the history, it is convenient to discuss this symptom here. Minor degrees of menorrhagia may disappear when the anaemia is corrected. If a satisfactory rate of haemoglobin regeneration fails to occur despite adequate iron therapy, it is probable that the loss of blood is considerable, and the patient should have a gynaecological examination to rule out organic disease. If menorrhagia continues so that the anaemia cannot be fully relieved by iron therapy, the induction of an artificial menopause may have to be undertaken but such haemorrhagic disorders as thrombocytopenic purpura must first be excluded.

When a patient has iron deficiency anaemia and the cause is not obvious, investigations must be thorough. Failure to respond may be due to the patient not taking her treatment, to malignancy, infection, uraemia, thalassaemia or a haemoglobinopathy, or to sideroblastic anaemia (p. 154).

Hypochromic Anaemia of Pregnancy

The development of some degree of iron-deficiency anaemia during pregnancy is so common that the routine administration of iron to all pregnant women is justified as a prophylactic measure. The haemoglobin should be estimated at the first antenatal visit, and if it is less than 12·4 g. per 100 ml. (85 per cent.) iron should be given by mouth (p. 143) for the rest of the pregnancy and one month afterwards. In women whose initial haemoglobin is above this level, the start of iron therapy may be postponed, but it should always be given from the 24th week to term and for a month afterwards. The value of this procedure has now been clearly demonstrated. It should prevent the discovery of severe anaemia for the first time late in pregnancy, when blood transfusion might be necessary to bring the haemoglobin to a safe level rapidly before the onset of labour and possible post-partum haemorrhage. The prevention of folate depletion in pregnancy is discussed on p. 152.

Nutritional Hypochromic Anaemia of Infancy and Childhood

Since an adequate store of iron in the foetal liver is of importance in maintaining a satisfactory blood level in infancy, iron should always be given to the mother during pregnancy (p. 145). This is desirable not only from the point of view of prevention of anaemia in the infant but probably also as a means of improving its general nutrition.

A rapid fall in the haemoglobin level occurs during the first two months of extra-uterine life. No method of treatment can prevent this fall, which is physiological. Recovery normally occurs during the next 18 months, but there are various factors which may prevent or retard this improvement. The first of these is low birth weight occurring as a consequence of prematurity or otherwise. All children of low birth weight should receive iron therapy from the second month. The second indication for prophylactic iron therapy in infancy is the presence of an infection. Even a mild infection in infants may cause anaemia and retard blood regeneration—hence the administration of iron for some weeks following infection is a sound general rule. Mild degrees of anaemia may occur in infants between 6 and 18 months as a result of parental ignorance or poverty. For instance there may be undue delay in the change to a mixed diet, or the latter may be of poor quality. Accordingly the practitioner should institute iron therapy in all infants who appear to be pale, easily fatigued and not thriving.

Iron. A palatable, efficient and non-irritating preparation of iron in liquid form which can be added to the infant's feed is the ideal. In the British National Formulary there are two such preparations, viz. ferric ammonium citrate mixture paediatric (B.P.C.) and ferrous sulphate mixture paediatric (B.P.C.). Each is flavoured, and the curative dose is 5 ml. thrice daily up to the age of 1 year and 10 ml. thrice daily up to 5 years Only half these amounts are necessary for prophylaxis. A proprietary preparation such as ferrous fumarate syrup (Fersamal Syrup) costs little more but is more palatable.

Parenteral iron therapy may be indicated in infants with a true intolerance for oral iron or when it is clear that the mother is not carrying out the treatment recommended. Sorbitol citrate (Jectofer is usually satisfactory and is given intramuscularly.

Iron-deficiency Anaemia in Men

In most cases chronic blood loss is the cause, and investigation and treatment should follow the lines laid down on p. 148, particular attention being directed to the possibility of malignant disease of the alimentary tract. If blood loss can be excluded, the possibility of gluten enteropathy should be kept in mind (p. 237). Occasionally, however, hypochromic anaemia which cannot be attributed to either of these causes is seen in the male during late adolescence or early adult life. Probably it is produced by a combination of deficient iron intake due to faulty diet, and increased requirements for iron due to rapid growth in childhood and adolescence. Treatment is on the same lines as for chronic nutritional hypochromic anaemia of women (p. 143), but since the demands for iron in adult men are very low in the absence of external blood loss, treatment seldom has to be continued after the diet has been corrected and the anaemia has been cured.

Post-haemorrhagic Anaemia

Extravascular blood loss may be acute or chronic and it is necessary to describe the treatment of these two conditions separately.

ACUTE POST-HAEMORRHAGIC ANAEMIA

Acute post-haemorrhagic anaemia is due to the sudden loss of a large amount of blood or to repeated smaller haemorrhages occurring in rapid succession.

Arrest of haemorrhage. In some cases haemostasis may be secured by ligature of or pressure on the bleeding point—for example, if there is a severed artery, extra-uterine gestation with bleeding or rupture of a superficial varicose vein. In other cases, as in haemorrhage from a peptic ulcer, operation may be indicated. Lastly, the haemorrhage may be part of a general blood disease such as thrombocytopenic purpura, haemophilia or acute leukaemia, and mechanical arrest of the haemorrhage may be impossible.

Treatment of shock. The degree of shock which follows a sudden loss of blood depends on several factors. The principal ones are the amount and rate of blood loss, the age and previous health of the patient and, in accidents and major operations, the concomitant effects of tissue trauma and previous exposure to cold. The decision to give intravenous fluids depends on a proper appreciation of these factors.

The sudden loss of 500 ml. of blood will not produce symptoms of shock in a healthy adult, as is clearly indicated from everyday experience with blood donors. When symptoms arise, they are usually psychological in origin rather than the result of lowered blood volume. Definite symptoms of shock appear when 1 l. of blood is lost rapidly and death may occur if the figure approaches 2 l. If the loss is spread over 24 hours, the symptoms are less severe and the prognosis correspondingly better. Infants and old people stand acute haemorrhage relatively badly, and this is particularly true if there is a history of previous debility or ill-health.

A patient suffering from acute post-haemorrhagic anaemia and shock should immediately be placed in bed. He should have blankets over him, but at this initial stage of treatment he should not be warmed by hot bottles, an electric blanket or other means, since peripheral vasoconstriction is the natural response to shock and is beneficial. When the blood volume has been restored by blood transfusion, the patient should be warmed since continuing vasoconstriction may be harmful. A suitable dose of morphine should be injected intramuscularly and repeated in two hours if necessary. The dose required is the minimum necessary to allay apprehension and restlessness, and to control pain if present. For an adult, 15 mg. and for a child of 6 to 12 years, 5 to 10 mg. is sufficient for the initial dose. Morphine is of less value if given subcutaneously rather than intramuscularly because of delay in absorption and the possibility that repeated doses may be absorbed together, resulting in features of overdosage. With it may be given an intramuscular injection of 50 mg. of cyclizine hydrochloride to prevent vomiting.

The foot of the bed should be raised on blocks, the patient being kept flat on his back except for a low pillow under his head. In severely exsanguinated patients awaiting blood transfusion, the limbs should be bandaged with crêpe bandages from below upwards.

Since the essential cause of shock in acute haemorrhage is the resulting low blood volume, the restoration of this is undoubtedly the most important therapeutic procedure. When haemorrhage is only slight, all that may be required is an adequate amount of water by mouth. The giving of 600 ml. of fluid per hour for three or four hours may make good the fluid deficiency. If, however, there is evidence of shock, fluid must be given intravenously (p. 626). For this purpose saline, dextran 110 (B.P.), plasma (liquid or dried) and whole blood are available. Of those, blood must take first preference, since it is of the correct viscosity and osmotic pressure and effectively increases the oxygen-carrying capacity. Second in order of merit is plasma. If neither is available, dextran 110 (6 per cent. in normal saline) should be used. This is a polymer of glucose produced by the fermentation of sucrose by the action of *Leuconostoc mesenteroides*, and has a molecular weight of 110,000. (Lower molecular weight dextran is unsuitable as it is so rapidly excreted). However, it causes increased rouleaux formation and may make blood grouping difficult. With increasing weight, dextrans may progressively interfere with blood coagulation and hence dextran 110 should not be used if there is thrombocytopenia or a coagulation defect. It should also be avoided if there is established renal failure with anuria.

Saline and glucose saline pass out of the blood and into the tissue spaces within a few minutes of their injection and hence cannot be recommended for the restoration of blood volume, although they are of the greatest value in correcting dehydration and chloride depletion from such causes as excessive vomiting and diarrhoea. If 600 ml. of blood is given it will, on the average, raise the haemoglobin level by about 1 g. per 100 ml. with a concomitant increase of blood volume and blood pressure. The amount of blood required depends upon the severity of the shock, the degree of anaemia present and whether bleeding is continuing, but usually at least 1 litre will be needed. Similar quantities of plasma or dextran are indicated if blood is not available, but if dextran is used, quantities greater than 2 litres should not be given unless absolutely necessary because disturbances in blood clotting may occur. In addition, blood for grouping and compatibility tests should be withdrawn before the dextran infusion begins.

Indications for blood transfusion. It is unwise to rely solely or mainly on a blood count, since for some hours after acute haemorrhage the haemoglobin level and packed cell volume may be little altered. Moreover, a falling haemoglobin level does not necessarily prove that haemorrhage is continuing; it may be due to haemo-dilution. In some centres it is possible to estimate the circulating red cell volume using radioactive chromium, but if there are signs of shock in the supine position this indicates a loss of about a third of the blood volume. The signs of deterioration are a rising pulse rate ($\frac{1}{2}$ hourly chart) and a progressive fall in blood pressure, sighing respiration, uneasiness and restlessness, coldness and clamminess of the skin, pallor, general weakness and impairment of mental faculties. When the pulse rate is over 100 per minute and the systolic blood pressure below 100 mm. Hg., haemorrhage has usually been severe. If the systolic pressure falls below 80 mm. Hg., the prognosis is very grave unless immediate blood transfusion is given.

Blood transfusion should preferably be given by the continuous drip method. By this means 2 to 3 litres of blood can be introduced over 24 hours, usually with complete restoration of the blood volume and with the lowest possible risk of producing acute heart failure and pulmonary oedema, or causing aggravation or recurrence of the haemorrhage due to a sudden increase in the blood pressure. In a healthy person suffering from haemorrhagic shock as the result of an accident or wound, the first 600 ml. may be given in 15 minutes and, if bleeding is continuing, it may be necessary to administer further blood at this rate.

When the bleeding point has been effectively secured and the state of shock adequately treated, recovery will occur without further intravenous therapy. On the other hand, when the bleeding point cannot be secured easily, it is usually desirable to make immediate arrangements to have suitably cross-matched blood available even if the initial degree of shock is not marked, since recurrence or increase in the severity of the haemorrhage may suddenly precipitate the patient into a dangerous state of collapse. Moreover, it is wise, especially in cases of haemorrhage from the alimentary tract, to consult a surgeon before the state of severe collapse has developed. In this way operation may be carried out with less delay if recurrent haemorrhage should make it necessary.

The great upset in the dynamics of the circulation which follows severe haemorrhage necessitates the continuation of complete rest in the recumbent position, warmth and good nursing for at least a week after restoration of the blood volume. Thereafter, treatment comprises removal of the causal condition where possible. A preparation of iron (p. 143) should be given by mouth at an early stage in treatment and continued until the haemoglobin level has returned to normal and for four weeks afterwards.

CHRONIC POST-HAEMORRHAGIC ANAEMIA

The treatment of chronic blood loss is considered under two headings: (a) removal of the cause and (b) treatment of the anaemia.

Removal of the cause. The most frequent cause of this form of anaemia, especially in males, and the one most likely to be missed, is occult bleeding from the gastro-intestinal tract. Patients with haemoglobin levels even below 5 g. per 100 ml. are often unaware that they are losing blood by this route. The occult bleeding may come from varicose veins in the oesophagus and stomach, ulcers of stomach or duodenum, hiatus herniae, malignant tumours or polypi of the gastro-intestinal tract or from haemorrhoids. The taking of aspirin may be a factor. The orthotolidine reaction for the recognition of occult blood in the stools is a very valuable test. In many countries the comonest cause is infestation of the small intestine with the parasites *Ancylostoma duodenale* or *Necator americanus*. Other causes of chronic blood loss are excessive haemorrhage from the uterus resulting from the presence of tumours, polypi or endocrine dysfunction, repeated nose-bleedings, and chronic blood diseases such as thrombocytopenia or haemophilia. In the great majority of cases of obscure hypochromic anaemia the gastro-intestinal and urogenital tracts should first be investigated as possible sources of haemorrhage. When the cause of the haemorrhage has been discovered, treatment directed to its removal must be instituted. It should be noted that the diet frequently prescribed for diseases of the gastro-intestinal tract is low in iron and vitamin C and may accentuate the anaemia if these deficiencies are not corrected.

Treatment of the anaemia. This consists of the administration of full doses of iron, together with the general measures outlined under chronic nutritional hypochromic anaemia (p. 143). If the source of bleeding has been removed, the chances of relapse after the blood count has been brought to normal are insignificant and, therefore, in general, maintenance treatment with iron is not required.

PERNICIOUS ANAEMIA AND OTHER MEGALOBLASTIC ANAEMIAS

When the term 'macrocytic anaemia' is used it indicates that the red cells in the peripheral blood are abnormally large. In many cases the underlying cause is a macronormoblastic bone marrow (e.g. in haemolytic anaemia, acute leukaemia, etc.). In others the marrow is megaloblastic and the term 'megaloblastic anaemia' is then used.

Classification and Pathogenesis of the Megaloblastic Anaemias

A clinical classification of the megaloblastic anaemias is given on p. 142. The factors that can convert a megaloblastic marrow to the normoblastic state are the cobalamins (vitamin B_{12} group of substances), folic acid (pteroylglutamic acid) and folinic acid (the citrovorum factor).

The cobalamins (*vitamin B_{12} group of substances*). In discussions of metabolic processes the general term used is vitamin B_{12} though the metabolically active substance in the liver is probably a coenzyme form. Two substances are available for therapeutic use. These are cyanocobalamin, which contains cobalt and a cyano group, and hydroxocobalamin in which the latter group is replaced by a hydroxyl one. Neither form has any chemical relationship to folic or folinic acid. Hydroxocobalamin is retained in the body better than the cyano form and maintains the serum B_{12} at a higher level without extra cost. Accordingly it is the drug of choice.

Folic acid. This substance is present in the green leaves of plants and also in animal tissue such as liver and kidney. Folic acid is a member of the vitamin B complex and is an essential factor for the growth of certain bacteria such as the *Lactobacillus casei* and for the normal growth and development of a variety of animals. The name folic acid is frequently used to include a group of analogues with similar activity in various biological systems, but in clinical work it is restricted to the chemical substance, pteroylglutamic acid, which is available in 5 mg. tablets or in solution for injection. There is usually no object in using the parenteral route, as oral administration is simpler and as effective, except in malabsorptive disorders when an intramuscular injection of folic acid should be given for two or three days at the start of treatment.

Folinic Acid is chemically related to folic acid and has the same effects as folic acid but is not available commercially.

THERAPEUTIC INDICATIONS

Vitamin B_{12}, folic acid and folinic acid all play a complex rôle in various metabolic processes including nucleic acid metabolism, and although anaemia is usually an obvious sign of deficiency, it should be realized that this is only one facet of a generalized depletion. Although the inter-relationship between these factors has not yet been completely determined, the indications for their use in treatment are already clearly established.

Vitamin B_{12}. Injections of hydroxocobalamin should be given in Addisonian pernicious anaemia, because here the development of megaloblastic blood formation is a direct consequence of defective absorption of vitamin B_{12}. This results from a failure of production by the stomach of intrinsic factor which is necessary for its passage through the wall of the lower ileum. Total gastrectomy will have a similar effect, and in a proportion of patients who have undergone partial gastrectomy the remaining intrinsic factor-bearing area may be destroyed by gastritis. This rarely occurs after gastroenterostomy. Juvenile pernicious anaemia is due to lack of intrinsic factor with or without achlorhydria, and this leads to deficiency of vitamin B_{12}. A genetically determined abnormality of vitamin B_{12} transport has also been described. When there are strictures or fistulae of the small intestine, blind or stagnant loops may be colonized by bacteria and these have the ability to utilize vitamin B_{12}, resulting in a deficiency in the host. A similar cause may be responsible for megaloblastic anaemia in patients with jejunal diverticula. The fish tapeworm (*Diphyllobothrium latum*) commonly found in people living in the region of the Baltic, also deviates vitamin B_{12} from those who harbour the worm in the alimentary tract. Since absorption of vitamin B_{12} occurs in the lower ileum, resection or disease of this area will lead to its deficiency. In all these cases treatment or prevention of the anaemia must be with hydroxocobalamin, but, if it is possible, the cause of the trouble should be eliminated (e.g. removal of a blind loop; elimination of the fish tapeworms).

Folic acid. Megaloblastic anaemia of pregnancy is usually due to folic acid depletion, but in countries where malnutrition is rife there may be vitamin B_{12} deficiency in addition. Megaloblastic anaemia of infancy has usually been due to lack of folic acid in goats' milk or dried milk preparations, but occasionally is due to gluten enteropathy. The administration of certain anticonvulsant drugs may lead to deficiency of folic acid.

Dual deficiency. In patients with malabsorptive disorders of the sprue type and in nutritional megaloblastic anaemia the deficiency may be of folic acid, vitamin B_{12} or both, and a response to treatment with folic acid does not necessarily mean that a concomitant deficiency of vitamin B_{12} does not exist. It should be realized, however, that there are geographical variations in the predominant deficiency because of differences in dietetic habits. For example, the Vegans, a very strict vegetarian group which has many members in Europe, develop nutritional megaloblastic anaemia from deficiency of vitamin B_{12} rather than of folic acid. Nutritional deficiency of cobalamins has been reported in Hindu women living in Great Britain. In our experience about 85 per cent. of patients with idiopathic steatorrhoea have malabsorption of folic acid, while about 60 per cent. of such patients fail to absorb vitamin B_{12} satisfactorily. In organic disease of the small intestine such as reticuloses or regional enteritis, it is also common to have malabsorption of both folic acid and vitamin B_{12}.

If a patient suffering from vitamin B_{12} deficiency is treated with folic acid alone, there will be a haematological response, but this treatment *must not* be employed because neither folic acid nor folinic acid will prevent the development of subacute combined degeneration of the cord, and the haematological response may not be maintained.

In the megaloblastic anaemias a superadded deficiency of iron may be a feature. In these circumstances it will be necessary to supplement treatment by giving iron (p. 143). This is commonly desirable even in Addisonian pernicious anaemia.

Addisonian Pernicious Anaemia

When the patient is critically ill, with a blood count of approximately 1 million red cells and a haemoglobin content of 3 to 4 g. per 100 ml., the question of immediate blood transfusion arises. The clinical condition of the patient, as judged by the degree of circulatory failure rather than by the blood level, must be the deciding factor. If it is concluded that the delay of four or five days which must elapse before improvement can occur as a result of treatment entails a risk to life which should not be taken, a blood transfusion should be given at once.

Undoubtedly blood transfusion in such severely anaemic patients should not be undertaken without a full realization of the risks involved, the most important of which is the possible occurrence of acute pulmonary oedema and death. This catas-

trophe is due to a failure of the weakened myocardium to withstand the effects of the increase in blood volume which accompanies transfusion. Accordingly, packed red cells should be given rather than whole blood. The cells should be transfused very slowly, 500 ml. (i.e. the red cells derived from approximately 1 litre of blood) being given in not less than six hours, and the transfusion should be preceded by an intravenous injection of frusemide. Exchange transfusion is thought by some to be safer than simple transfusion in very anaemic adults. The volume removed should exceed the volume given by about 200 ml. Thus, 1,200 to 1,700 ml. of blood might be removed from the femoral vein or one in the arm and 1,000 to 1,500 ml. of packed cells given into a vein in the opposite arm. In less urgent cases, in which some doubts exist regarding the need for immediate transfusion, the patient's blood group should be determined so that a transfusion can be given without delay should the necessity arise.

When the diagnosis of pernicious anemia has been established, an intramuscular injection of 1,000 mcg. of hydroxocobalamin should be given and repeated three days later. Thereafter a weekly injection of 250 mcg. of hydroxocobalamin should be given until the red-cell count is normal.

Within two or three days the reticulocyte increase will have started and a marked subjective improvement will be noted. Very occasionally at the commencement of treatment a patient requires to have folic acid in a dosage of 5 or 10 mg. daily for a week in addition to hydroxocobalamin, perhaps because there are insufficient stores of folic acid remaining for normal erythropoiesis to be resumed. Folic acid must not be used alone for the treatment of Addisonian pernicious anaemia, for it does not prevent the onset of subacute combined degeneration of the cord and may even accelerate its production.

A preparation of iron (p. 143) should be given twice a day after meals and continued for two months in all patients receiving their initial treatment, since an iron shortage is apt to arise owing to the exceedingly rapid production of erythrocytes. Iron may increase the anorexia and dyspepsia so frequently present in the severe relapse stage of pernicious anaemia; accordingly, the administration should be delayed until after the occurrence of the reticulocyte crisis, by which time the marked clinical improvement of the patient will enable it to be well tolerated.

Should a relative of a patient with pernicious anaemia become weak and listless or develop other symptoms of anaemia, neurological features or mental disturbance, this may be because he or she is suffering from the same disease. Patients with pernicious anaemia and their relatives may have auto-antibodies not only to gastric cells but also to thyroid tissue, and the incidence of both thyrotoxicosis and myxoedema is greater in pernicious anaemia than in the general population. Other not uncommon complicating diseases are gastric carcinoma and diabetes mellitus.

Pre-operative measures. Should an emergency arise during the relapse stage of pernicious anaemia requiring an operation which cannot be delayed, intensive parenteral treatment should be undertaken immediately (1,000 mcg. of hydroxocobalamin intramuscularly) and preparations for blood transfusion made so that it can be given immediately if required. Patients in the remission stage of pernicious anaemia should receive hydroxocobalamin before undergoing any major operation.

Maintenance treatment. Since neither cyanocobalamin nor hydroxocobalamin produces a cure but is a form of substitution therapy, maintenance treatment must be continued for life. This point should be carefully explained to patients.

The amount of hydroxocobalamin required to maintain a normal blood level varies in different individuals, often for no apparent reason. A suitable dose of hydroxocobalamin is 1,000 mcg. at intervals of four to eight weeks. Theoretically, the time between injections could be greater than this, provided the hydroxo form is used, but there is no virtue in attempting to use the minimal effective dose. Iron is not required if it has already been prescribed during the first two months of treatment. An ordinary well-balanced mixed diet is all that is necessary. Maintenance treatment with parenteral liver extracts, oral liver preparations, hog's stomach or oral cyanocobalamin with or without intrinsic factor is not recommended, and the value of depot preparations of cyanocobalamin for intramuscular use (cyanocobalamin zinc tannate or cyanocobalamin zinc tannate aluminium monostearate) has not been established.

Subacute Combined Degeneration of the Spinal Cord

Prophylaxis. Lesions of the cord rarely if ever develop in pernicious anaemia if the blood count is maintained within normal limits. It must be

F

emphasized, however, that symptoms cannot be relied upon as an indication of the blood level. Many patients receiving inadequate maintenance therapy have no symptoms although the blood count may be subnormal, e.g. Hb. 11·5 g. per 100 ml., R.B.C. 3·5 to 4 million. It is in such cases that the incidence of subacute combined degeneration of the cord is highest. It is of great importance, therefore, that blood counts should be done at regular intervals (preferably every six months) during maintenance treatment. If the red-cell count falls below 4·5 million in the case of women or 5 million in men, maintenance treatment is inadequate and should, therefore, be increased. In many blood clinics routine red-cell counts are not carried out in the supervision of patients with pernicious anaemia, reliance being placed on determination of the haemoglobin level and examination of a stained blood film. Since only the expert may be able to detect macrocytosis in a stained film, the red-cell count should always be estimated if there is a fall in the haemoglobin level. The danger of spinal cord lesions developing when folic acid is employed as the sole therapeutic agent for initial and maintenance treatment is referred to on p. 150.

It should be remembered that subacute combined degeneration may rarely occur in any of the conditions which give rise to a deficiency of vitamin B_{12}, e.g. deficient dietary intake, following gastric operations, small intestinal fistulae and anastomoses, jejunal diverticulosis and resection of the terminal ileum.

Treatment. The management of the disabilities due to subacute combined degeneration is described on p. 372. All that need be said here is that patients with pernicious anaemia showing signs of neurological involvement are usually given more frequent injections of hydroxocobalamin than those with a comparable blood picture but without neurological changes. This intensive treatment should possibly be continued for at least six months after the blood count has reached normal, the maintenance dose of 1,000 mcg. being given weekly instead of every six weeks. At the same time remedial exercises should be employed. By these means many patients who are bedridden may be able to lead a useful life, while those with less severe involvement of the spinal cord may return to full employment.

Optic atrophy. Occasionally, optic neuritis has been reported in pernicious anaemia, and the serum vitamin B_{12} level has been found to be low in tobacco amblyopia. It has been suggested that tobacco smoke may lead to chronic cyanide intoxication. Further information is required, but it is safe to say that in tobacco amblyopia or Leber's optic atrophy, *hydroxocobalamin* must be given. *Cyanocobalamin* may cause blindness to develop rapidly.

MEGALOBLASTIC ANAEMIAS OTHER THAN ADDISONIAN ANAEMIA

Megaloblastic Anaemia of Pregnancy and the Puerperium

This is usually due to folate deficiency, because the body stores of folate, unlike those of vitamin B_{12}, may be insufficient for the demands of pregnancy. Recurrent abortion may sometimes be due to folate depletion.

The treatment of megaloblastic anaemia of pregnancy or of the puerperium is to give 10 mg. of folic acid daily by mouth. If the degree of anaemia is so severe as to endanger life, one or more transfusions of blood should be given while awaiting the effect of folic acid, and ideally the serum vitamin B_{12} level should be estimated. If it is normal this excludes Addisonian pernicious anaemia complicated by pregnancy, but if it is slightly lowered this may be due merely to haemodilution. However, it is safer to give hydroxocobalamin injections in addition to folic acid if the serum vitamin B_{12} level is low, and further investigations can be carried out when the pregnancy is over.

A deficiency of iron is also usually present in this condition and accordingly iron should be prescribed simultaneously with folic acid. Treatment can be discontinued after the puerperium and the restoration of a normal blood level.

Biochemical tests suggest that some 20 per cent. of pregnant women in certain regions of the United Kingdom have a degree of folate depletion. Although there is a very slight danger that one might be giving folic acid alone to a patient with unsuspected Addisonian pernicious anaemia, it is, nevertheless, reasonable to give a prophylactic dose of folic acid daily in pregnancy, in addition to iron by mouth. More than a dozen proprietary preparations are available for this purpose; one providing 300 to 500 mcg. of folic acid and about 80 mg. of ferrous iron per day should be chosen.

In underdeveloped countries where malnutrition is a serious problem there is a particular need for folic acid, but a dual deficiency of this and vitamin B_{12} may exist in pregnancy.

Megaloblastic Anaemia of Infancy

This occurs in infants whose diets are markedly deficient in protein, folate and ascorbic acid, and who in addition may be suffering from infections and diarrhoea. Although the disease is very rare in the United Kingdom and Eire it is being recognized with increasing frequency in underdeveloped countries as a complication of kwashiorkor (p. 350). The anaemia responds to treatment with folic acid, but maintenance treatment is not required if the dietetic errors are corrected. In coeliac disease anaemia is usually due to iron deficiency, but the occasional case with a megaloblastic anaemia will respond to folic acid therapy. Very rarely in infancy and childhood there are patients with pernicious anaemia and they may have hydrochloric acid in the gastric juice although the intrinsic factor is absent. These patients should be treated with hydroxocobalamin by injection.

Megaloblastic Anaemias due to the Disorders of the Gastro-intestinal Tract

Radioactive techniques for the determination of vitamin B_{12} absorption, and microbiological methods for the assessment of folate absorption and serum vitamin B_{12} and folate levels, have contributed greatly to an understanding of the megaloblastic anaemias due to disorders of the gastro-intestinal tract and have led to a more rational therapeutic approach. In every case the cause of the underlying disease of the small intestine must be investigated and appropriate treatment prescribed.

Megaloblastic anaemia in malabsorptive disorders (*gluten enteropathies, including coeliac disease and most cases of idiopathic steatorrhoea; tropical sprue*). Here malabsorption of folate is more common than malabsorption of vitamin B_{12}, but in the adult there may be impaired absorption of both. Nevertheless, folic acid, in a dose of 10 to 20 mg. daily by mouth, usually causes reversal of the megaloblastic marrow to normoblastic erythropoiesis and a rapid improvement in the blood picture. In cases with severe anaemia, initial parenteral treatment for two or three days with folic acid, 15 mg. daily, is recommended. In coeliac disease of children the complete withdrawal of gluten from the diet (p. 486) will cure the anaemia and the other clinical abnormalities, and maintenance treatment with folic acid is not required. It is not certain that the disorder formerly known as idiopathic steatorrhoea is, in the adult, always associated with gluten sensitivity, and certainly some adults do not respond to a gluten-free diet even if it is continued strictly for six months. In these patients maintenance therapy with folic acid will be necessary. The dosage needed for this purpose is variable, but is probably around 5 to 10 mg. daily. Since about two-thirds of the adult patients have malabsorption of vitamin B_{12}, it is advisable to administer a monthly injection of 1,000 mcg. of hydroxocobalamin as a prophylactic against neurological complications.

Tropical sprue may occur sporadically or in an epidemic form, and it is sometimes difficult to distinguish it from nutritional megaloblastic anaemia. In any event benefit will ensue from the administration of folic acid, although vitamin B_{12} may be needed in addition. It should be remembered that gluten enteropathy is occasionally seen in tropical countries.

Megaloblastic anaemia associated with organic disease of the small intestine. In conditions such as tuberculous enteritis, regional enteritis, reticuloses and Whipple's disease, the disease of the intestinal wall or lymphatic drainage system may cause malabsorption of folate and vitamin B_{12}. In addition to treatment of the primary condition, if this is possible, anaemia should be treated with iron and, if it is megaloblastic, with folic acid and hydroxocobalamin. In the reticuloses there is, however, the possibility that folic acid will aggravate the primary disease, and in regional ileitis malabsorption of vitamin B_{12} is the likely deficiency.

Megaloblastic anaemia in association with operations on the gastro-intestinal tract or with blind loops or fistulae. In this group the deficiency is of vitamin B_{12} and there are several possible mechanisms.

Lack of intrinsic factor. Total gastrectomy invariably produces a megaloblastic anaemia provided the patient lives long enough. The liver usually contains enough vitamin B_{12} to last for three or four years. Megaloblastic anaemia may also follow partial gastrectomy or, more rarely, gastroenterostomy; in these cases secretion of intrinsic factor fails as a result of damage to the gastric mucosa from a spreading gastritis originating at the site of the anastomosis.

Absence or disease of the absorbing area. Vitamin B_{12} is normally absorbed from the terminal ileum, and extensive disease or resection of this area may result in megaloblastic anaemia. Apart from the treatment of the cause, if this is possible, therapy is the same as for pernicious anaemia (p. 150).

The presence of an abnormal bacterial flora. This arises as the result of destruction or utilization of vitamin B_{12} by a quantitatively abnormal bacterial flora in blind or stagnant loops of small intestine. These anomalies may result from short-circuiting operations, fistulae or strictures involving the small intestine; jejunal diverticulosis can produce similar effects, the diverticula constituting small stagnant pockets. Steatorrhoea occurs in a considerable proportion of cases with such abnormalities. As might be expected from the bacterial aetiology, the oral administration of a broad spectrum antibiotic such as oxytetracycline in a dosage of 250 mg. four times daily may produce a haematological response but the duration of this response is extremely variable, and this is not suitable treatment for the anaemia. Megaloblastic anaemia due to a blind or stagnant loop should be treated by the parenteral administration of hydroxocobalamin in the same manner as for Addisonian pernicious anaemia (p. 150). Occasionally folic acid is required in addition, but since the primary deficiency is of vitamin B_{12}, it must never be given alone because of the danger of precipitating subacute combined degeneration of the cord. Where possible, surgical correction of the intestinal abnormality should be undertaken, since it may result in permanent cure of the anaemia and of any existing diarrhoea and steatorrhoea.

Megaloblastic Anaemia due to Fish Tapeworm Infection

A megaloblastic anaemia develops in a small proportion of individuals harbouring the fish tapeworm (*Diphyllobothrium latum*). The worm utilizes the dietary vitamin B_{12} at the expense of the host. Expulsion of the worm will usually relieve the anaemia, but treatment should be supplemented with hydroxocobalamin. If re-infection does not occur, maintenance treatment will not usually be required, but it is important to be sure that the patient does not have Addisonian pernicious anaemia.

Nutritional Megaloblastic Anaemia

In many parts of the world, particularly the tropics, where malnutrition is rife, a megaloblastic form of anaemia occurs both in males and in females. Not unnaturally it is particularly common during pregnancy when the foetus depletes the malnourished mother of her stores of folate and vitamin B_{12}.

The exact nature of the deficiency has varied in different geographical areas, and complicating factors have been malaria, ankylostomiasis and tropical sprue. There have been numerous reports of failure of response to vitamin B_{12} therapy with a subsequent remission when folic acid was given, and it is undoubtedly true that folate deficiency has been the main problem in many instances. Nevertheless, modern methods of investigation have confirmed the belief that a dual deficiency of vitamin B_{12} and folate is common in nutritional megaloblastic anaemia, and hence it is reasonable to supplement folic acid in a dosage of 10 to 20 mg. daily by injections of hydroxocobalamin in a dose of 250 mcg. weekly.

Anaemia due to iron deficiency is very much more common than nutritional megaloblastic anaemia, and it will respond only to iron and not to folic acid or hydroxocobalamin. Sternal marrow examination may, therefore, be necessary to differentiate the conditions in the tropics because iron deficiency may be so marked that a combined deficiency of iron and folic acid or vitamin B_{12} is not easily recognizable in the peripheral blood.

A group of very strict vegetarians, the Vegans, many of whose members are Europeans, have such strong views about an acceptable diet that some will not eat honey because it is produced by bees. These sincere but misguided people may develop subacute combined degeneration and megaloblastic anaemia from vitamin B_{12} deficiency.

There have been reports from various parts of the United Kingdom of the occurrence of nutritional megaloblastic anaemia from folate deficiency in elderly people taking inadequate diets. In some areas this has been found to be more common in the aged than Addisonian pernicious anaemia. Many of these patients do not have scurvy, but a coincidental deficiency of ascorbic acid might be expected.

Megaloblastic Anaemia of Hepatic Disease

Megaloblastic blood formation is very rarely seen in patients with cirrhosis of the liver and may be due to deficiency of folate or vitamin B_{12} consequent on the ingestion of a very poor diet in which the calories are largely derived from alcohol. More commonly the macrocytic blood picture is associated with a macro-normoblastic bone marrow. It is not surprising, therefore, that treatment with a cobalamin or folic acid is usually ineffective. Moreover, the prognosis depends not so much on the severity and type of anaemia but on the degree and progress of liver damage.

Megaloblastic Anaemia due to Drugs

Megaloblastic anaemia occasionally occurs when epileptics have been undergoing treatment with certain anticonvulsant drugs, e.g. phenytoin and primidone, possibly because these drugs have a certain structural similarity to pteroylglutamic acid and compete with it in various metabolic cycles. Treatment consists of the administration of folic acid for as long as the anticonvulsant drug is required.

Megaloblastic anaemia may also follow the administration of folic acid antagonists, including the antimalarial drug, pyrimethamine.

Anaemia in Myxoedema

The anaemia of myxoedema is usually moderate in degree and normocytic or macrocytic in type. Associated iron deficiency is not uncommon. The clinical picture may strongly suggest pernicious anaemia, but treatment with hydroxocobalamin is usually ineffective, except in the very rare cases where a megaloblastic bone marrow is present or the serum vitamin B_{12} level is low. Administration of thyroxine produces a slow improvement in the blood count. Associated iron deficiency must be corrected.

PYRIDOXINE RESPONSIVE ANAEMIA
(*A form of sideroblastic anaemia*)

Patients suffering from this rare type of anaemia usually have the characteristic peripheral blood picture of chronic iron-deficiency anaemia, but fail to respond to iron therapy; in contrast to the classical case of iron-deficiency anaemia they have a high serum iron level and an increased deposition of stainable iron in the bone marrow and other tissues. If haemolytic anaemia, uraemia, thalassaemia and other more common causes of refractory anaemia can be excluded, the possibility that the anaemia is due to pyridoxine deficiency should be considered, but it should be noted that this is likely to be a genetically determined abnormality rather than a form of nutritional deficiency. It is believed that pyridoxine plays an essential rôle in the early stages of haem synthesis. During the last few years cases of anaemia have been reported in which a partial or complete response has followed its administration. The vitamin is usually given subcutaneously in a dose of 50 to 100 mg. daily for four to seven days, followed by oral maintenance treatment of 25 mg. daily. In some instances the bone marrow has been megaloblastic and this abnormality has responded to pyridoxine. In others it has been necessary to give folic acid in addition. If there is no response to pyridoxine therapy within two weeks it is unlikely to be of value. There are many other blood disorders in which sideroblasts may be found in the marrow.

HAEMOLYTIC ANAEMIAS

The haemolytic anaemias comprise a group of widely differing causation in which there is evidence of excessive blood destruction as demonstrated typically by the finding of bilirubinaemia, urobilino-genuria and an excess of reticulocytes.

Haemolytic anaemias may be classified as follows:

Haemolytic Anaemia due to Intrinsic Red Cell Defect

1. Hereditary spherocytosis (congenital haemolytic anaemia, familial acholuric jaundice).
2. Hereditary non-spherocytic haemolytic anaemia.
3. Hereditary elliptocytosis (ovalocytosis).
4. Paroxysmal nocturnal haemoglobinuria.
5. Racial haemolytic anaemias (haemoglobinopathies):
    (a) Thalassaemia.
    (b) Sickle cell disease.
    (c) Other hereditary haemoglobinopathies.

Haemolytic Anaemia due to Extrinsic Mechanisms

1. Idiopathic auto-immune haemolytic anaemia.
2. Symptomatic haemolytic anaemia.
3. Paroxysmal cold haemoglobinuria.
4. Haemolytic disease of the newborn (p. 478).
5. Transfusion with incompatible blood (p. 634).
6. Haemolytic anaemia due to infections and infestations.
7. Haemolytic disorders due to drugs, chemicals or plants.
8. March haemoglobinuria.
9. Porphyria.

Haemolytic Anaemia due to Intrinsic Red Cell Defect

Hereditary spherocytosis (*congenital haemolytic anaemia, familial acholuric jaundice*). The problem of treatment resolves itself into a simple one, namely, whether splenectomy should be undertaken and, if so, when. Opinion varies on this matter, particularly in mild forms of the disease, when the patient is more jaundiced than ill. Many authorities believe that splenectomy should be advised in every case when the diagnosis is made, because of the occurrence of serious complications in a high percentage of cases at some later period in the disease. The principal complications which may

endanger life and greatly enhance the risk of operation are cholelithiasis and cholecystitis, and severe haemolytic or aplastic crises. On the other hand, since the familial form of the disease has been recorded in successive generations in people who were able to carry on their occupations with little or no ill-health, other authorities do not consider that splenectomy is indicated in the milder cases of this group. We believe that, since it is impossible to foretell with certainty the future of even the mildest case of acholuric jaundice, it is wiser to advise operation while the patient is in good health than to risk the serious complications already mentioned. There should be no hesitation in offering this advice if the anaemia is in any way affecting the patient's physical and mental health and causing a loss of efficiency. Additional reasons for advocating splenectomy are a past history of haemolytic or aplastic crises or a history of the disease occurring in a severe form in relatives, since it has been shown that the course of the disease runs fairly true to type in different members of the same family. In a female patient there is the additional hazard of superadded iron deficiency from menstrual loss. Moreover, the anaemia is sometimes aggravated by pregnancy, when occasionally megaloblastic change may be found in the marrow because of superadded folate depletion. There is, therefore, even more justification for advising splenectomy in the female patient with hereditary spherocytosis. Splenectomy should also be considered if a patient is going to reside in an area where surgical treatment is not readily available. When the haemolytic anaemia commences in infancy or early childhood, the dangers of biliary complications are remote, and provided health is not impaired by anaemia, splenectomy may be safely postponed until the child is 10 or 12 years of age, when the procedure is attended by less risk.

Should acute inflammation of the gall-bladder, necessitating laparotomy, occur in a patient with acholuric jaundice, it is generally advisable to limit the operative procedure to the gall-bladder and to undertake splenectomy later. The interval between the operations should not, however, exceed a few months, since the excessive haemolysis will continue until splenectomy is performed and calculi may form in the bile ducts. If a chronically diseased gall-bladder with or without stones is found during an operation for splenectomy, the opportunity should then be taken to correct the biliary disease. Severe haemolytic or aplastic crises require treatment by blood transfusion. Blood must be matched very carefully and administered by slow drip. Treatment with corticosteroids is ineffective in this type of haemolytic anaemia, but splenectomy almost always cures the anaemia and abolishes the increased haemolysis, even although the intrinsic red cell defect remains.

Hereditary non-spherocytic haemolytic anaemia. Clinically this condition resembles hereditary spherocytosis, but the red cells are not spherocytic or abnormally fragile in saline. The response to splenectomy is often unsatisfactory.

Hereditary elliptocytosis (*ovalocytosis*). In this condition the red-cell abnormality is inherited as a Mendelian dominant. Most patients are not anaemic and have no symptoms, but in a proportion there is evidence of haemolysis. If a patient with elliptocytosis is anaemic it is essential to eliminate other causes such as iron deficiency; if haemolysis is a predominant feature, splenectomy may be beneficial. Fortunately most patients require no treatment.

Paroxysmal nocturnal haemoglobinuria. In this rare disorder there develops an abnormality of the erythrocytes which results in haemoglobinuria during the night or on awakening in the morning. The age of onset is usually in the third or fourth decades and there may be chronic haemolytic anaemia and splenomegaly. In mild cases no treatment is necessary, but if the condition is severe it will be necessary to give transfusions of packed red cells. The giving of plasma may cause haemolysis of the patient's cells. Splenectomy is rarely beneficial.

Racial haemolytic anaemias. This group of conditions is more commonly referred to as the hereditary haemoglobinopathies and it includes a wide range of haematological disorders in which, as a result of genetic mutations, there is a disorder of haemoglobin synthesis affecting the globin moiety. This is a complex subject since further abnormal haemoglobins are constantly being discovered and the terminology is difficult, but the abnormality in each instance is in the sequence of amino acids in the polypeptide chains of the globin portion of the haemoglobin molecule. In some of the haemoglobinopathies excessive haemolysis is a feature, in others there is iron deficiency anaemia that does not respond to iron therapy, while in many of the conditions there is no clinical abnormality.

THALASSAEMIA. In the homozygous form (thalassaemia major) there is severe anaemia and death may occur in infancy. Although excessive haemolysis is a feature, the anaemia is hypochromic and microcytic. The red cells contain large amounts of foetal haemoglobin (haemoglobin F), the remainder being normal adult haemoglobin (haemoglobin A or A_2). The heterozygous form (thalassaemia minor) is usually much less serious and the blood picture is that of a mild microcytic and sometimes hypochromic anaemia with but little evidence of haemolysis. The name was given to the condition because it was so frequently found in races inhabiting countries around the Mediterranean sea, but it is a widespread disorder and 'refractory iron deficiency' in Great Britain may be due to thalassaemia minor.

The only method of treatment is by blood transfusion because there is no cure for thalassaemia, no response to iron therapy, and splenectomy should be avoided unless there is a marked haemolytic element.

SICKLE-CELL DISEASE. In this condition, which is common in Negroes but very rare in other races, the presence of the abnormal haemoglobin S causes changes in the shape of the red cells. In the heterozygous state (sickle-cell trait) there is usually no anaemia, but in the homozygous form haemolytic anaemia and sometimes multiple thromboses and infarcts of various organs may occur.

Blood transfusions are indicated if haemolysis is severe, but it is likely to prove impossible to maintain a normal haemoglobin level in a patient with sickle-cell disease. Splenectomy is seldom of value, as it usually does not alter the course of the disease. In sickle-cell anaemia, surgical operations should be avoided if they are not essential, infections should be treated at the earliest possible moment and, if an affected female patient survives to adult life, the hazards of pregnancy must be borne in mind. There may be similar dangers in patients who have genes for haemoglobin S combined with other abnormal haemoglobins, such as C. Those with haemoglobin S and thalassaemia, or S and C are said to be liable to develop sickling, splenic infarcts and haemolytic crises because of lowering of the oxygen tension if flying above 4,000 feet.

Folate deficiency is common in association with sickle-cell disease, and a prophylactic dose of 5 mg. of folic acid should be given daily. In a sickle-cell crisis, folic acid therapy is particularly important. In areas where malaria is endemic, children with sickle-cell anaemia should have constant antimalarial prophylaxis.

Other haemoglobinopathies. In most there are no clinical features and treatment is not required.

Haemolytic Anaemias due to Extrinsic Mechanisms

Idiopathic acquired haemolytic anaemia. The so-called idiopathic form of haemolytic anaemia in which a familial trait cannot be discovered occurs mainly in adult life. The disease may occur in acute, subacute or chronic forms. Most cases are due to circulating auto-antibodies to which the patient's erythrocytes are susceptible. This is in contrast to hereditary spherocytosis and the racial haemolytic anaemias in which the cause of the haemolytic process is the production of abnormal erythrocytes or abnormal haemoglobins respectively. The direct antiglobulin test (Coombs' test) indicates that the patient's red cells are coated with the antibody.

There is a warm-antibody type of haemolytic anaemia in which the auto-antibody is active at 37° C. and a cold-antibody type where it is active at a lower temperature. The former is strongly adsorbed on to the red cells, but the latter is present in large amounts in the plasma. In the cold-antibody type there may be features of the Raynaud phenomenon. One form which occurs after infections, particularly virus pneumonia, clears up without specific treatment.

BLOOD TRANSFUSION. In the subacute and chronic case in which the anaemia is mild or moderate in degree, blood transfusion will usually not be required. In the acute case the haemolytic process may be so severe that within a few hours the patient may become severely anaemic and shocked. A transfusion of 1 litre of blood should be given immediately and should be repeated several times if necessary. The dramatic clinical improvement that often follows blood transfusion probably depends as much on the dilution of the lysin in the patient's plasma by the normal transfused plasma as on the addition of the donor's red blood corpuscles to the patient's blood. Blood transfusion during a haemolytic crisis, however, is a potentially dangerous procedure, since it sometimes precipitates an increase in the haemolytic process. This danger is greatly reduced if the donor blood is closely matched to that of the recipient and given very slowly. The transfusion should be carried out under cover of steroids. The anuria following blood transfusion is not due to precipitation in the renal tubules of haemoglobin released by haemolysis of the trans-fused cells but is a manifestation of acute tubular necrosis.

Except in a small proportion of cases, the results of blood transfusion are transitory. In such patients a decision must, therefore, be reached as to whether to start steroid treatment or to proceed at once to splenectomy.

CORTICOSTEROID THERAPY. Since remissions of varying degree occur in 50 to 75 per cent. of patients with idiopathic acquired haemolytic anaemia when given corticosteroids, this form of treatment should be tried before splenectomy is contemplated. A dose of 60 mg. of prednisolone should be given daily for at least three weeks before such therapy is abandoned. In a small proportion of cases a dramatic improvement occurs with complete suppression of the haemolytic process and this continues after stopping steroid treatment. In such cases splenectomy should be postponed, but the patient must be kept under careful observation for signs of a relapse. In most cases, unfortunately, when the drug is stopped or reduced below a certain level the haemolytic process becomes active again. For patients who fail to respond initially to corticosteroid therapy or have only a partial response, splenectomy is advised, and this should not be delayed since a prolonged course of corticosteroids with inadequate response will only add to the problems of the surgeon and the patient.

SPLENECTOMY. The question of splenectomy for acquired haemolytic anaemia is a difficult one. As many different types of haemolytic disorders are embraced by this designation, it is essential, before coming to a decision to operate, that the physician makes certain that he is dealing with the auto-immune form and not haemolytic anaemia secondary to conditions such as lymphadenoma or leukaemia. The rationale of splenectomy in idiopathic acquired haemolytic anaemia is based on the belief that the spleen may be the organ mainly responsible for the elaboration of auto-antibodies. Since splenectomy produces substantial improvement in only approximately 50 per cent. of cases of idiopathic acquired haemolytic anaemia, it seems likely that other important sources of antibody production and red cell destruction are present in those patients who fail to respond to the operation. Attempts may be made with radio-active chromate-tagged red cells to assess prior to operation the extent to which increased destruction of erythrocytes is occurring in the spleen, but it is not always possible to predict the success or failure of splenectomy in this way. If the patient has received corticosteroids within the previous two years the operation should be covered by adequate corticosteroid therapy. In patients responding satisfactorily to splenectomy a rapid rise in the red-blood count occurs, since the bone marrow is extremely hyperplastic, and a gain of half to one million cells per week may be confidently expected. The rapid rate of regeneration begins to slow down as the count approaches 3·5 to 4 million, and at this stage iron may have to be given. The general measures regarding rest, nursing, etc., in a case of haemolytic anaemia are identical with those required in any case of anaemia of similar severity, and are described on p. 143.

For those patients who fail to respond adequately to splenectomy, an attempt should be made to bring the haemolytic process under control by further steroid therapy. Should this fail, the prognosis is poor, but an attempt may be made to reduce the amount of auto-antibody formed by inhibiting the activity of the lympho-reticular tissue, and some success follows the use of mercaptopurine or the related drug azathioprine.

Symptomatic haemolytic anaemia. This may be found accompanying such conditions as Hodgkin's disease, chronic lymphatic leukaemia, disseminated lupus erythematosus, reticulum-cell sarcoma, carcinomatosis, etc. The treatment is that of the primary condition, supplemented by blood transfusion. Should the haemolytic element be so great that transfusions have to be repeated frequently and at shortening intervals, steroid therapy should be given a trial. Splenectomy is seldom indicated, but may be considered if the disease is very chronic and haemolysis a prominent feature.

Paroxysmal cold haemoglobinuria. In this disorder rapid haemolysis leading to haemoglobinaemia and haemoglobinuria occurs when the patient enters a warm atmosphere after having been exposed to cold. The cause is usually unknown, but occasionally syphilis is responsible. It should be remembered, however, that a false positive Wassermann reaction may be found in various types of haemolytic anaemia. The condition can be recognized by the Donath–Landsteiner test.

Prophylaxis, which should include avoidance of all forms of chilling, e.g. washing the hands in cold water or drinking cold fluids, is an important part of the treatment.

When syphilis is the cause, thorough and pro-longed antisyphilitic treatment should be instituted, and it is claimed by some authorities that this is usually successful and may cause disappearance of the autohaemolysin from the blood.

During an attack the body should be kept warm and plenty of fluids should be given by mouth. Should anuria develop, the treatment described on p. 275 should be instituted. If anaemia results, iron therapy (p. 143) should be given. These measures are equally applicable to all types of haemoglobinuria.

Haemolytic anaemia due to infections and infestations. An acute form of haemolytic anaemia may result from septicaemia, but this is rare and the anaemia present is more likely to be due to toxic inhibition of the bone marrow or to interference with iron metabolism.

Haemolytic anaemia occurs in malaria (p. 513) and, in Peru, from infection with *Bartonella bacilliformis*, the latter disease being known as Oroya fever. Reference has already been made to haemolytic anaemia in virus pneumonia.

The treatment is that of the causative disease, but blood transfusion may be required.

Haemolytic anaemia due to drugs, chemicals or plants. A number of drugs and chemicals, including certain gases and insecticides, can give rise to haemolytic anaemia, but they differ in the way in which they do this. Thus phenylhydrazine and the war gas, arsine, will cause haemolysis in any individual by destruction of red cells. Haemolysis is also commonly caused by lead and by certain snake venoms. Some drugs such as acetanilide, dapsone, dimercaprol, nitrofurantoin, para-aminosalicylic acid, phenacetin, probenicid and sulphonamides very rarely cause haemolytic anaemia. It is now known that in some instances, such as haemolytic anaemia following the administration of primaquine, a not uncommon complication in Negroes, the red cells of the affected person are deficient in glucose-6-phosphate dehydrogenase. This enzyme is involved in a step necessary for the reduction of oxidized glutathione. Without sufficient reduced glutathione the erythrocytes are susceptible to damage by potential oxidants such as primaquine, and related 8-aminoquinolines. It is possible that naphthalene may cause haemolysis in a similar manner, and that sensitivity to some drugs including sulphonamides is brought about in this way. Other drugs, particularly methyldopa, may become adsorbed on the surface of red cells and induce antibody formation resulting in haemolysis.

Favism is a haemolytic disorder, often associated with haemoglobinuria, that is found particularly in Sardinia, Sicily and Calabria, but has been reported in individuals of Italian or Greek origin living elsewhere, and occasionally in other races. The acute attack of haemolysis is brought on by contact with the pollen or ingestion of beans of the plant *Vicia fava*. These patients have a similar red cell defect to those who are sensitive to primaquine.

The treatment of these conditions involves the immediate cessation of the administration or ingestion of the offending agent. Blood transfusion may be necessary and in certain conditions such as lead poisoning (p. 559) it will be necessary to eliminate the substance from the body. The Inspector of Factories must be notified if there is believed to be an industrial hazard.

March haemoglobinuria. In this condition haemoglobinuria occurs after exercise and lasts for a few hours. It occurs only if the exercise is undertaken in the erect posture, but there is frequently evidence of a renal tubular defect. There is recent evidence that trauma to the heels and soles of the feet in prolonged walking or running may be the precipitating factor, and sponge rubber pads within the boots or shoes may be useful in prophylaxis.

Porphyria. The porphyrias are a group of metabolic abnormalities characterized by the excretion in abnormal quantities of substances that are either precursors or by-products in the metabolic pathways leading to the formation of haem. It is convenient to divide the porphyrias into five types:

(a) ACUTE INTERMITTENT. This is inherited as a Mendelian dominant, and is probably due to an enzyme defect in the liver. During attacks there may be colicky abdominal pain, vomiting and constipation. Frequently there is peripheral neuropathy, and sometimes mental abnormalities occur. Skin sensitivity is not a feature. Chlorpromazine is of value in relieving symptoms, and in an acute attack benefit may be obtained from the administration of corticosteroids. Physiotherapy is likely to be required. If respiratory paralysis occurs, tracheostomy and intermittent positive pressure artificial respiration may be needed. The patient should be informed about the condition, and since attacks are often precipitated by barbiturates, sulphonamides, alcohol, griseofulvin or contraceptive pills, these *must* be avoided. Anaesthesia with thiopentone may be lethal. The condition should

F*

be looked for in relatives, who may also have to avoid these drugs

(b) CUTANEOUS HEPATIC. This may be inherited as a Mendelian dominant, but can be acquired. Excessive amounts of uroporphyrins are formed by the liver and these are photosensitizing. Hence there is light sensitivity and skin lesions occur. The condition is found rarely in alcoholics but is common in the Bantu. A severe epidemic occurred in Turkey because of contamination of wheat with the pesticide hexachlorobenzene. Treatment consists in protecting the skin and avoiding agents that cause liver damage.

(c) MIXED. In this form there are features both of photosensitivity and of acute intermittent porphyria. It is common in South Africa amongst white people of Dutch extraction. The treatment and precautions are as for (a), and the skin has to be protected.

(d) CONGENITAL (ERYTHROPOIETIC) PORPHYRIA. This is inherited as a Mendelian recessive and is very rare. There is light sensitivity, but also haemolytic anaemia, splenomegaly and fluorescence of the teeth. There is no treatment other than skin protection and blood transfusion.

(e) ERYTHROPOIETIC PROTOPORPHYRIA. This is inherited as a Mendelian dominant and is more common than (d). Skin protection is necessary because of photosensitivity.

PANCYTOPENIA, APLASTIC AND HYPOPLASTIC ANAEMIA

Pancytopenia results from a loss, complete or partial, of the cells in the bone marrow that form erythrocytes, leucocytes and platelets. If the erythroblasts are the cells particularly affected the term aplastic anaemia is used, but if the condition is less severe it is called hypoplastic anaemia.

The conditions may be idiopathic or secondary to a recognizable cause, particularly the drugs chloramphenicol and phenylbutazone, and it should be realized that a single short course of chloramphenicol in normal dosage can be responsible.

CAUSES OF PANCYTOPENIA, APLASTIC OR HYPOPLASTIC ANAEMIA

Physical Agents

    (a) The heavy metals: gold, mercury, silver, bismuth, arsenic, lead.

    (b) The benzol compounds: benzol, trinitrotoluol, dinitrophenol, paraphenylene-diamine, gamma-benzene-hexachloride (Gammexane).

(c) Drugs used for their effect on blood cell formation: methotrexate, nitrogen mustards, chlorambucil, mercaptopurine.

(d) Other drugs: carbutamide, chloramphenicol, chlordiazepoxide, chlorpheniramine, chlorpropamide, colchicine, indomethacin, mepacrine, meprobamate, methoin, neoarsphenamine, oxyphenbutazone, phenylbutazone, potassium perchlorate, streptomycin, sulphamethoxypyridazine, tolbutamide, troxidone. Many others have been reported as occasionally causing pancytopenia or aplastic anaemia.

(e) Poisonous gases: carbon monoxide, methane, mustard gas, nitrous oxide.

(f) Radio-active materials and X-rays, radium, radon gas, thorium.

In certain occupations there is a hazard because of exposure to physical agents that may cause aplasia of the marrow:

(a) Benzol: rubber workers, dry-cleaners, tanners, varnish and paint workers, gilders, feather workers, milliners, printers and tinners are engaged in occupations in which benzol is used for its solvent properties.

(b) Lead: painters, plumbers, etc.

(c) Trinitrotoluol: munition workers.

(d) Gases: soldiers, sewer workers, mine workers.

(e) Radio-active substances: luminous-paint workers, workers with X-rays, radium and radio-active isotopes.

Infections and Intoxications

Although aplasia is rare, hypoplasia of the bone marrow sometimes results from infections. Occasionally, particularly in children, inhibition of the bone marrow may rapidly take place if the infective process is extremely severe, e.g. in typhoid fever and miliary tuberculosis. Hypoplasia can also occur in long continued chronic infections, but the introduction of antibiotics has greatly reduced the importance of infections as a cause of bone marrow depression.

Terminal Stages of Certain Diseases

Bone marrow inhibition may be a feature of the terminal stages of renal failure.

Replacement of the Bone Marrow by Neoplastic Cells or by Fibrous Tissue

This may occur in leukaemia, carcinomatosis and myelofibrosis.

Other Associations

Rarely a familial form of aplastic anaemia occurs, possibly due to an inborn error of metabolism. More rarely still, adults develop hypoplasia of the marrow in association with a tumour of the thymus gland and myasthenia gravis (p. 411). Occasionally a patient, believed to be suffering from aplastic anaemia, is subsequently found to have leukaemia.

Whenever pancytopenia, hypoplastic or aplastic anaemia is thought to have resulted from the taking of a drug, the fact or the suspicion should be notified to The Committee on Safety of Drugs, Queen Anne's Mansions, Queen Anne's Gate, London, S.W.1.

TREATMENT

In all cases of aplastic and hypoplastic anaemia the general measures suitable for the degree of anaemia as outlined on p. 143 should be instituted.

When anaemia is so severe that life is endangered (p. 146), blood transfusion should be undertaken at once. If all marrow elements are depleted, fresh whole blood may be used at least at the commencement of treatment, but it is likely that repeated transfusion will be needed, possibly at short intervals. Packed cells should then be given and may have to be continued at intervals for many months or even years. It may prove possible to maintain the haemoglobin level only at about 8 to 10 g. per 100 ml. If bleeding is troublesome, platelet transfusions may be of great value. In this way symptomatic relief may be given and time is secured to enable the physician to search for and if possible remove the causal factor. Occasionally spontaneous improvement occurs. If a diagnosis of aplasia of the marrow is irrefutable, no form of treatment is likely to stimulate marrow regeneration; but because the precise diagnosis is often doubtful, most physicians try the effect of haematinics (iron, hydroxocobalamin, folic acid). It is most important to remember that in Addisonian pernicious anaemia there is leucopenia and thrombocytopenia, sometimes leading to skin haemorrhages. Occasionally, when there has been difficulty in obtaining marrow, an incorrect diagnosis of aplastic anaemia has been made.

Oxymetholone, a synthetic derivative of testosterone, has given a good response in some children and adults. It is administered by mouth in a dosage of 4 mg. per kg. of body weight daily. The drug may be continued for several months, but the dosage should be halved when there is evidence of a remission. The drug is not so hepatotoxic as testosterone, but liver function tests should be done. There may be some increase of weight during its administration.

Alternatively, prednisolone, 60 mg. daily, may be tried. It may reduce transfusion requirements, prevent transfusion reactions and, by its action on capillaries, reduce bleeding.

A consideration of the classification of the aetiological factors as outlined above will indicate the investigations and treatment required in individual cases.

Injections of dimercaprol should be tried (p. 561) if aplastic anaemia is due to gold or arsenicals. Thymectomy has occasionally relieved the anaemia when a tumour of the thymus gland was present.

The patient should be kept alive with blood transfusions and the other remedies mentioned should be continued, if necessary, for months or even years, in the hope that bone marrow regeneration will occur. This may lead to haemosiderosis from iron overload after many transfusions have been given. The intramuscular injection of 500 mg. of the iron chelating agent desferrioxamine twice daily will remove at least 10 mg. of iron daily, but there is the practical difficulty that the patient may tolerate injections badly.

ANAEMIAS OF UNCERTAIN ORIGIN

Refractory normochromic or hypochromic anaemia without hypoplasia of the marrow may be found in chronic infection, uraemia, rheumatoid arthritis, liver disease and widespread malignant disease, and treatment consists mainly of attempts to control the primary condition.

THE SYNDROME OF PORTAL HYPERTENSION

(*Splenic Anaemia, Banti's Disease*). This is more a syndrome than a disease and in its commonest form it may be described as a chronic condition characterized by splenomegaly and hypochromic anaemia with leucopenia and thrombocytopenia, no enlargement of lymphatic glands and a tendency to haemorrhage from the alimentary tract.

Before the diagnosis is accepted, the following conditions, in which anaemia and splenomegaly may occur, must be eliminated: (1) the reticuloses, e.g. lymphadenoma (p. 182); (2) the leukaemias (p. 176); (3) myelofibrosis (p. 181); (4) the haemolytic anaemias (p. 155); (5) acute and chronic infectious diseases with splenomegaly, e.g. infective endocarditis, malaria, schistosomiasis and kala-azar; (6) chronic nutritional hypochromic anaemia (p. 143). Portal hypertension may be secondary to hepatic cirrhosis or to thrombosis, congenital anomalies or other lesions in the portal or splenic veins. The leucopenia and thrombocytopenia are believed to be due to hypersplenism, but the anaemia is mainly due to bleeding from oesophageal varices.

TREATMENT

Treatment may be considered under the headings operative measures and symptomatic treatment.

Operative measures. The beneficial effects claimed for splenectomy and other operations rest mainly on anatomical and mechanical foundations.

In patients with portal hypertension the advisability of surgical treatment must be based on an assessment of the degree, type and site of obstruction to the portal circulation. The obstruction may be intrahepatic or extrahepatic in site, but cirrhosis of the liver is the principal cause of portal hypertension. Surgical treatment offers the only hope of reducing the portal hypertension and decreasing the liability to bleeding from varices. The clinical history and physical examination, together with the assessment of liver function by special tests and by biopsy, play an essential part in deciding on the advisability of operation and the most suitable surgical procedure. If advanced liver cirrhosis is present and the patient's clinical state is poor, surgical intervention is contraindicated. If the pathological changes in the liver are only moderate, slight or absent, while the dangers of haemorrhage from oesophageal or other varices are great, operation should be undertaken. An assessment of the case may be made pre-operatively on the basis of the results of a trans-splenic portal venogram, or on the findings at laparotomy. If the portal hypertension is due to intrahepatic block or to extrahepatic block in the portal vein, splenectomy alone will fail to relieve the portal hypertension. It was because of this knowledge that operations were devised to shunt the portal blood into the systemic circulation. This can be accomplished by anastomosing the splenic vein to the left renal vein or the portal vein to the inferior vena cava, and the results are more satisfactory than those obtained from resection of the lower end of the oesophagus and upper part of the stomach to remove the area carrying the varices. When the block is extrahepatic and in the splenic vein, splenectomy alone may cure the syndrome and remove the danger of haemorrhage. Splenic vein obstruction is much less common than obstruction of the portal vein.

Although splenectomy alone may not influence materially the mechanical factors which lead to bleeding in intrahepatic block and extrahepatic block in the portal vein, it may be of value in reducing the tendency to bleed if the platelets are markedly reduced, as is not uncommonly the case. The presence of severe neutropenia due to hypersplenism may be an additional reason for splenectomy in the syndrome of portal hypertension.

Symptomatic treatment. The general treatment of the anaemia in this syndrome is on the lines indicated on p. 143. The use of a Sengstaken tube to exert pressure on the varices has been largely discontinued, as it may lead to ulceration and is ineffective when the haemorrhage arises from varices in the gastric fundus. Vasopressin (20 units intravenously over ten minutes) may reduce the portal pressure by constricting splanchnic arterioles, but is risky treatment and contraindicated if there is myocardial ischaemia.

DIET. Food liable to injure mechanically the gastric and oesophageal varices should be excluded from the diet or irritating components removed. The following articles should be excluded—highly seasoned and indigestible foods, condiments and pickles, the skins and pips of fruits, nuts, etc.—and coarse vegetables and fruits should be passed through a sieve and served as purées or fools. When cirrhosis of the liver is present, the dietetic instructions given on p. 248 should be followed.

IRON. The response to iron preparations given by mouth is frequently good.

BLOOD TRANSFUSION is of great value in the treatment of shock following the severe haemorrhages which occur in portal hypertension. By this means patients may be tided over emergencies and life may be prolonged for years. Iron therapy should be started immediately after the transfusion. Blood transfusions should be discontinued only when there is clear evidence that an advanced stage of liver failure has been reached or when haemorrhages are recurring at short intervals and operative procedures to relieve the portal hypertension cannot be undertaken. At this stage of the disease the mental misery entailed by the constant fear of another haematemesis is of such a degree that it makes it inadvisable to attempt to prolong life. Palliative treatment is then directed to promoting mental tranquillity and sleep.

For the treatment of cirrhosis of the liver, ascites and haematemesis, see pp. 248–249.

HAEMOCHROMATOSIS

It may be difficult to distinguish between haemochromatosis and portal cirrhosis with siderosis. The factors involved in the latter are increased absorption of iron due to excessive intake of alcohol, together with a shortened red-cell life-span and reduced utilization of iron because of nutritional deficiencies of folic acid and pyridoxine. Skin pigmentation, gonadal atrophy (p. 304), diabetes (p. 316) and an increased saturation of the serum total iron-binding capacity can occur in both disorders. Usually the deposition of iron in the liver as revealed by liver biopsy is greater in haemo-

chromatosis than in cirrhosis with secondary siderosis, but no clear dividing-line can be drawn. It is probable that primary haemochromatosis is due to an inherited defect of iron metabolism leading to increased absorption of iron from a normal diet, but various modes of inheritance may occur. The relatives of patients with primary haemochromatosis should be carefully observed and when a significant increase of iron stores occurs, as judged by liver biopsy, repeated venesection may minimize or prevent serious hepatic and pancreatic damage.

Treatment of established haemochromatosis consists essentially of treatment of diabetes when it is present (p. 316) and a reduction of iron stores by repeated venesection. Usually 500 ml. of blood is withdrawn every day or every second day until there is mild anaemia and the serum iron is below normal. Thereafter venesections are repeated with sufficient frequency to maintain this state of affairs, usually weekly. The chelating agent desferrioxamine is less effective: 200 to 500 mg. intramuscularly or intravenously twice daily can produce a negative iron balance of 10 to 50 mg. daily whereas 500 ml. of blood contains approximately 200 mg. of iron.

METHAEMOGLOBINAEMIA AND SULPHAEMOGLOBINAEMIA

Methaemoglobinaemia is usually caused by the taking of drugs which preferentially oxidize haemoglobin, and in sufficient quantity they may overcome the normal reducing mechanisms of the red cells. For example, nitrates may be converted to nitrites by intestinal bacteria and may then produce methaemoglobinaemia after absorption. Aniline dyes may cause it by penetration of the skin, and even dyed blankets may be responsible. Other offending drugs are acetanilide, phenacetin, sulphonal, potassium chlorate and certain sulphonamides such as sulphathiazole and sulphapyridine, but not sulphadiazine or sulphadimidine. There are also a number of hereditary forms of methaemoglobinaemia.

It is not usually necessary to treat patients for hereditary methaemoglobinaemia, and in drug induced forms it is usually sufficient to stop the administration of the offending agent. If, however, there is evidence of anoxaemia, the best treatment is to give methylene blue intravenously, a dose of 1 to 2 mg. per kg. being given over a five-minute period in a 1 per cent. solution. This can be repeated in an hour, but the total amount administered should not exceed 7 mg. per kg. Another, less effective, form of treatment is to give ascorbic acid by mouth in a dosage of 300 to 500 mg. daily. This may be useful for cosmetic reasons in certain congenital forms of the disease, but is of no value in a group of such patients who suffer from a haemoglobinopathy due to the presence of haemoglobin M.

Sulphaemoglobinaemia is due to the presence of a haemoglobin derivative not normally found in red cells, and once it is formed it remains until the erythrocytes are destroyed. Sulphaemoglobin is almost always produced by drugs, particularly phenacetin and acetanilide. Congenital sulphaemoglobinaemia is extremely rare. No form of drug treatment will remove the sulphaemoglobin. The drug should be stopped and, if from some other cause there is respiratory distress, blood transfusion or exchange transfusion may be necessary.

THE HAEMORRHAGIC DISEASES

Introduction. The diseases included in this section are characterized by an increased tendency to bleed.

Although there is no rigid separation, it is useful to consider the haemorrhagic states in two categories, viz. the 'purpuras' and the 'coagulation defects'. The purpuras are characterized by bleeding into the skin (petechiae), or from mucous membranes with resulting epistaxis, gastro-intestinal bleeding or menorrhagia. Small superficial haematomata are common. However, deep-seated and large haematomata are the characteristic feature of clotting disorders, e.g.—haemophilia. A small incision, such as is made by a needle in the skin, may give prolonged bleeding in thrombocytopenic purpura but is not likely to cause a problem in haemophilia. The deeper wound of dental extraction in thrombocytopenic purpura may create little difficulty but is always a problem in haemophilia. The latter disease occurs in two distinct grades: it is regarded as mild where the patient has a problem only following a severe haemostatic challenge such as tooth extraction, tonsillectomy or major trauma. In other respects these patients lead a normal life. On the other hand, the severely affected haemophiliac has no protection against physiological haemostatic stress and therefore has spontaneous bleeding into areas such as the knee joints. This is probably because normal people seem to sustain small haemorrhages

into such joints, with no untoward consequences because their haemostatic system is normal.

The following classification of bleeding disorders is proposed as a useful working basis for the practitioner, but it must be understood that in some of the purpuras (that is in conditions listed under B and C below), capillary damage and thrombocytopenia may coexist. Furthermore, in von Willebrand's disease there is not only a coagulation defect but also an abnormality in platelet function, and the patients characteristically have the mucous membrane type of bleeding.

A. DEFECTS IN THE COAGULATION MECHANISM

1. Haemophilia (deficiency of anti-haemophilic globulin, i.e. factor VIII)—sex-linked recessive genetic abnormality.

2. Christmas disease (deficiency of Christmas factor, i.e. factor IX)—sex-linked recessive genetic abnormality.

3. von Willebrand's syndrome—unlike 1 and 2 which only affect males, this condition is genetically determined but affects males and females and is characterized by a prolonged bleeding time which is not a feature of haemophilia or Christmas disease, by mucous membrane bleeding, a deficiency of factor VIII and a demonstrable abnormality of platelets *in vitro*.

4. 'Hypoprothrombinaemia' (deficiency of prothrombin i.e. factor II usually with associated deficiencies of factors VII, IX and X).
    (a) in haemorrhagic disease of the newborn.
    (b) in biliary obstruction and intestinal disorders such as malabsorption and ulcerative colitis.
    (c) in severe hepatic disease.
    (d) from anticoagulant drugs of the coumarin/indanedione type.

5. Fibrinogenopenia (deficiency of fibrinogen i.e. factor I). This condition is usually acquired and is often due to intravascular coagulation, but is occasionally from excessive fibrinolysis and sometimes from a combination of both mechanisms. Genetically determined deficiency of fibrinogen occurs, but is excessively rare.

B. DEFECTS IN, OR DAMAGE TO THE CAPILLARIES (NON-THROMBOCYTOPENIC OR VASCULAR PURPURA)

1. Infections (usually severe in degree and particularly if a septicaemia is present) with *Streptococcus haemolyticus* and *viridans*, meningococcus, *B. typhosus*, *B. diphtheriae* *M. tuberculosis* (especially in miliary forms), the rickettsiae or typhus fever and the viruses of measles, smallpox etc.

2. Idiosyncrasy to drugs, e.g. sulphonamides, barbiturates or carbromal.

3. Occasionally in the terminal stages of cardiovascular failure. Here purpura of the lower limbs in particular may appear.

4. Avitaminosis—scurvy.

5. Allergic states, including Schönlein's and Henoch's purpura.

6. Hereditary telangiectasia.

7. Senile purpura.

C. Defective Production or Excessive Destruction of Platelets (Thrombocytopenic Purpura)

1. Primary: idiopathic thrombocytopenic purpura.

2. Secondary: due to (a) exposure to X-rays or radio-active substances, (b) other blood diseases, e.g. pancytopenia, leukaemia or hypersplenism, and sometimes in reticuloses or the syndrome of portal hypertension, (c) myelomatosis, myelofibrosis and other myeloproliferative syndromes, also secondary malignant disease of the bones and the bone marrow, (d) other systemic disease, e.g. disseminated lupus erythematosus, thrombotic thrombocytopenic purpura, (e) drug sensitivity: drugs can produce thrombocytopenic purpura by severe marrow damage, frequently in association with depression of other formed elements of the blood. This occurs with phenylbutazone or chlorambucil. Occasionally it may be due to a sensitivity phenomenon causing excessive peripheral destruction of platelets as with quinidine, (f) severe infections.

D. Excessive Production of Platelets—Thrombocythaemia

It is surprising to find that an excessive number of platelets may paradoxically sometimes cause thrombosis and on other occasions a haemorrhagic defect.

In a haemorrhagic state it is clearly important to establish the diagnosis both by clinical and laboratory means. The overall clinical context may well establish the diagnosis. Thus a careful history and examination will readily indicate that a patient has scurvy, and details of the family history may well establish that the condition is haemophilia or Christmas disease. Examination of the purpuric lesions of the skin will often indicate whether it is vascular or thrombocytopenic purpura because vascular purpura usually has an accompanying inflammatory component.

In a majority of patients, however, some confirmatory laboratory investigation will be required but it is important to select the most applicable test to confirm the diagnosis. Common screening procedures include the clotting time, the one-stage prothrombin time, the platelet count, the bleeding time and some form of capillary resistance test. In the clotting of blood, prothrombin is converted to thrombin by the thromboplastin system; this latter is either extrinsic (having tissue components as well as plasma factors) or intrinsic (components from entirely within the blood) Thrombin clots fibrinogen to form fibrin. The investigation known as the kaolin cephalin clotting time is a test of the intrinsic thromboplastin system and if an abnormal result is obtained then specific factor assays may well be needed to define the defect, particularly estimations of factors VIII and IX.

Haemophilia

Haemophilia is an hereditary disease due to a deficiency of antihaemophilic globulin (factor VIII). As indicated above it may occur as a severe condition with chronic disabling involvement of the joints from haemarthroses or as a very mild condition in which the patient has a problem only after a major haemostatic challenge. The patients are often at greater risk from bleeding into tissues than from external blood loss. Any internal bleeding therefore must be treated as vigorously as external bleeding. For example, a haematoma in the neck or at the base of the tongue may cause respiratory obstruction. Males only are affected but the condition is transmitted by the female. The daughters of an affected man will all be transmitters and can be so identified. Amongst the family of a transmitter female, 50 per cent. of the daughters will be transmitters and 50 per cent. will be non-transmitters. The problem is to identify between the transmitter and the non-transmitter female in such a context.

The physician will not infrequently find himself consulted for genetic counselling in respect of this disease. The daughters of a haemophilic man should be told that they are transmitters and that the risks of passing the disease on to subsequent generations are as indicated above. With the daughters of a transmitter or the sisters of an affected male the definition may be difficult or impossible. Some of these women have low levels of factor VIII and can be identified as transmitters but the finding of a normal level of factor VIII in such a female does not exclude the woman being a transmitter. The decision ultimately of course is with the patient and there may be a case for giving contraceptive advice and suggesting adoption of children. The genetic counselling may also have to be tailored to the grade of the defect, and this remains constant in a family. Where the disease is of high grade then the family should be strongly discouraged from producing more affected members. When it is very mild then the advice may be altered accordingly.

The severely affected haemophiliac necessarily has many absences from school and work, and appropriate social and other supportive measures have to be adopted. It is clearly important that the haemophilic child should have the best possible education, and home tuition may be needed. Thereafter, the patient frequently has difficulty in maintaining employment, and social help is essential. While the severely affected patient should have his physical activities limited, the mildly affected patient should not be over restricted. The dangers of operative procedures such as tonsillectomy or tooth extraction must be clearly understood by all grades of haemophilic patients. In the interval between major episodes, the most important other single medical issue is to ensure that adequate conservative dental care is provided. In this way the necessity for extraction of teeth at a later date is much reduced.

Haemophilia centres. There have been established organized centres throughout Britain at which the diagnosis and usually the treatment of bleeding episodes can be undertaken. At these centres advice is also given to the parents of the patients and a haemophilia identity card is issued with information about the diagnosis, blood group and other points of detail.

The centres listed in the haemophilia scheme are given on pp. 171–172.

Treatment during an attack of bleeding. Recent work has established several important principles. The abnormal haemostasis can be corrected by infusing a sufficient quantity of the missing plasma factor. If the factor VIII can be extracted from 3 to 5 litres of blood and given once daily to a haemophilic patient then the factor VIII level of that patient can be sustained at a normal level; if this occurs, healing of the bleeding area will occur at the normal rate. The problem is that the half-life, *in vivo*, of administered factor VIII is approximately nine hours; the patient therefore has to receive a sustaining infusion daily in order to keep the level of factor VIII raised. The factor VIII level in the blood can be measured in the laboratory. It should be appreciated in the diagnosis and treatment of haemophilia that a normal clotting time does not mean that the factor VIII level of the blood is normal. As little as 1 per cent. of factor VIII in the blood may render the whole blood clotting time normal, and more specific factor assays are required to follow therapy.

The materials available to treat haemophilia are as follows:

1. ROUTINE BANK BLOOD. This will be required to supply red cells appropriate to that lost but should not be relied upon as significantly raising the factor VIII level. Fresh whole blood will obviously provide a small amount of factor VIII as well as red cells, but again cannot be viewed as producing a really sustained level of factor VIII.

2. FRESH PLASMA OR FRESH FROZEN PLASMA. Fresh plasma can be collected from freshly donated blood by centrifugation, but its use is restricted by the administrative inconvenience of the procedure and by the fact that enormous amounts of plasma have to be infused to produce satisfactory levels; as indicated above the amount of plasma is of the order of 3 to 5 litres. It is administratively more convenient to supply fresh frozen plasma; it is separated from the red cells, immediately frozen and maintained at −20° C. until used. There is some loss of potency but this provides a useful form of therapy for lesser incidents in haemophilia.

3. CONCENTRATES OF FACTOR VIII. Two of these are available. In the first place there is Lyophil. This is dried fraction of plasma which is prepared by blood-processing units at great cost and often with significant loss of potency in the factor VIII level. Nevertheless, these preparations have made a very valuable contribution to therapy. The most widely used concentrate of factor VIII is cryoprecipitate: in the preparation of this, blood is collected in a two plastic bag system involving centrifugation, transfer of plasma to the secondary pack, and rapid freezing followed by thawing at 4° C. overnight. The secondary pack contains the cryoprecipitate; most of the supernatant plasma on top of the cryoprecipitate can be transferred back on to the top of the red cells and used for routine transfusion purposes. The availability of cryoprecipitate has been a major advance in the therapeutics of the disorder.

A small number of patients treated with human sources of factor VIII develop an inhibitor to factor VIII, rendering therapy thereafter extremely difficult.

4. ANIMAL PREPARATIONS OF FACTOR VIII —PORCINE AND BOVINE. These are very powerful materials but after a period of a week to ten days it must be assumed that the patient is now sensitized to the particular animal protein and fatal anaphylaxis is a possibility. Local treatment has very considerable limitations in the management of haemophilia. Excessive pressure, for example on the site of bleeding, may create a greater problem than the original injury. If the blood is forced back into the tissues instead of being allowed to escape externally it may cause pressure on vital structures. Local treatment of a wound should

mean so far as is possible leaving the wound undisturbed until healing is complete. If replacement therapy has been given, healing may occur at the normal rate. If, for any reason, replacement therapy has not been given, then a much longer time than normal will have to be allowed for the wound to heal.

A problem of recurring frequency in the management of these patients is haemarthrosis. The correct treatment for this is far from clear; if sufficient supplies of factor VIII are available, adequate replacement therapy is indicated and when this is attained aspiration of the joint may be attempted. It will often be found, however, that the volume of blood which can be aspirated is disappointingly small because it has already clotted within the joint. Aspiration should certainly not be attempted unless adequate replacement therapy has been established.

Protection of a local site is not however without merit, provided the pressure employed is not excessive. For example, dental extraction should be accompanied by the skilful construction of an acrylic resin dental splint which is placed in position when the tooth has been extracted. This protects from the tongue or food any soft friable clot that is filling the socket. Procedures involving excessive pressure or cauterization which merely increase the area to heal must be avoided. Local haemostatics are disappointing and tend to be swept away by blood issuing from a wound. For this to be successful the haemostatic material must arrive in the wound as replacement therapy through the circulation—i.e. by the giving of factor VIII.

In respect of dental extraction it may be possible to do single tooth extraction with minimal replacement therapy and with appropriately constructed dental splints. If it is intended to remove a large number of teeth in a single operative procedure then very adequate therapy must be given. Anaesthesia should not be by nerve block as this may result in a dangerous tissue haematoma. However, infiltration of the local tissues around the tooth will produce adequate anaesthesia without this hazard. Skilled dental extraction is of the utmost importance. Surgical dressings soaked in Russell's viper venom or thrombin are put in the socket but the operator must not place too much reliance on such local haemostatic applications. Stitching of the sockets should usually be avoided as this merely provides an increased area of trauma from which haemorrhage can occur. In the management of

epistaxis excessive packing should not be relied upon and if nasal packing is used, it should be with absorbable material.

Christmas Disease

The principles of management here are similar to those in haemophilia, except that the appropriate therapeutic materials for replacement therapy are less widely available. In most centres, fresh frozen plasma is the mainstay of therapy. Christmas factor is well preserved in fresh frozen plasma but again there are the problems of giving adequate amounts to produce satisfactory levels. The survival *in vitro* of factor IX is better than that of factor VIII and so also is the survival *in vivo*. Nevertheless, daily infusions with replacement therapy are required to sustain levels of the missing clotting factor in just the same way as with haemophilia.

In a few very specialized centres, factor IX concentrate preparations are available, but the majority of transfusion services throughout the United Kingdom do not produce it. Such concentrates also contain large amounts of factors II, VII and X.

von Willebrand's Syndrome

As indicated above this is categorized by deficiency of factor VIII and possibly of another plasma factor called the von Willebrand's factor. Moreover, there is a demonstrable disturbance of the patient's platelets. This disease affects males and females and is characterized by bleeding from the mucous membranes manifested particularly by epistaxis, gastro-intestinal bleeding and menorrhagia. Cryoprecipitate is extremely effective therapy for this condition and the rise in factor VIII which occurs is similar to that in haemophilia, but is better sustained, suggesting that the cryoprecipitate also contains some precursor material of factor VIII which the von Willebrand's patient can utilize for the synthesis of effective factor VIII. Pregnancy in these patients is a major challenge to the haemostatic mechanism and cryoprecipitate should be administered as soon as labour begins.

'Hypoprothrombinaemia'

Prothrombin or factor II is seldom deficient alone and any such defect is usually accompanied by deficiencies of factor VII, IX and X. The term 'hypoprothrombinaemia' however is still in common usage to cover this multifactorial defect which may arise as the consequence of vitamin K deficiency or administration of coumarin or indandione drugs or salicylates. Vitamin K deficiency is seen in obstructive jaundice and malabsorption. It is also seen in other severe and prolonged diarrhoeas such as ulcerative colitis. In severe parenchymal disease of the liver (cirrhosis), all these factors may well be deficient and additionally there may be a diminished concentration of other coagulation factors, e.g. fibrinogen. In haemorrhagic disease of the newborn there is a deficiency of prothrombin and other coagulation factors. Healthy newborn infants have lower concentration of them than have adults, but in the state of haemorrhagic disease in the newborn the level of the factors is extremely low and this produces haemorrhage.

In the management of hypoprothrombinaemia, whatever its cause (either vitamin K deficiency or drug induced) the practising physician should become familiar with the use of phytomenadione (vitamin K_1) and not the other vitamin K preparations. The reason for this is that many of the other synthetic and particularly the water-soluble vitamin K preparations are not effective in antagonizing the coumarin/indandione drug defect. Where the patient is an adult and there is evidence of deficiency, then a dose of 25 mg. of phytomenadione intravenously or by mouth depending on the degree of urgency, will correct the abnormality. As the preparation is not entirely absorbed from the intestine, it is probably preferable to administer the material intravenously. In the reversal of the coagulation defect produced by the coumarin/indandione drugs the dosage of vitamin K_1 should be adjusted to the particular situation in which the patient is found. If he has a major haemorrhage and a decision is taken that anticoagulant therapy has to be abandoned, then 50 mg. of phytomenadione can be given intravenously. In doing this, however, the physician should appreciate that this action will render the patient resistant to the effects of the anticoagulant drug if these are reintroduced. Where the patient is bleeding and it is intended to recommence anticoagulant therapy, a dosage of phytomenadione of the order of 15 mg. should be given. Where the results of suitable tests cause the physician concern but the patient is not bleeding, a dosage of the order of 5 mg. will restore the results of the test to those desired in normal therapy. In the management of haemorrhagic disease of the newborn, 1 to 2 mg. of phytomenadione intramuscularly will correct the abnormality.

Phytomenadione does not carry the hazard of some of the water-soluble vitamin K preparations which may cause or aggravate haemolysis.

Fibrinogen Deficiency

Fibrinogen deficiency arises for a number of reasons. It can arise because fibrinogen is used up in an intravascular site from continuing intravascular coagulation. It may be that occasionally excessive fibrinolysis is the mechanism causing disappearance of the fibrinogen; this happens, for example, during a streptokinase infusion. It is probable that there are some situations in which both intravascular coagulation and excessive fibrinolysis are giving rise to the problem.

In the vast majority of clinical situations involving fibrinogen depletion the basic mechanism is likely to be intravascular blood coagulation. This may happen with metastatic tumour formation. Possibly, some such tumours destroy vascular endothelium and blood is then directly in contact with tumour tissue. It is likely that in acute obstetrical disasters the fibrinogen depletion is due to intravascular coagulation. Such acute situations should be managed by replacement with fresh blood and fibrinogen supplements. Most of these are short-lived clinical storms, and when the obstetrical problem has been resolved, for example by delivery of the child, then the haemorrhagic state ceases and fibrinogen returns to normal concentrations.

Particularly with widespread metastatic tumours there may be more complex defibrination problems in which heparin therapy can restore the fibrinogen to normal and stop bleeding. The number of occasions when this is applicable is limited because usually the metastatic disease is so widespread that there is no real therapeutic issue. If, however, such a patient is having troublesome bleeding, heparin may be used to give relief. Sometimes laparotomy may be considered if it is believed that the tumour tissue is not widely disseminated. In such patients the fibrinogen level should be corrected by intravenous heparin administration and when the fibrinogen level has been raised heparin should be stopped and operation carried out forthwith.

In a small number of patients as indicated, the problem of excessive fibrinolysis with haemorrhage can occur during streptokinase therapy. In these circumstances the treatment is to administer epsilon amino caproic acid, 5 gm., by intravenous infusion over 30 minutes and a gram per hour thereafter for

5 hours. If epsilon amino caproic acid (EACA) is given, then fibrin laid down while it is in circulation will be unlysable because of the incorporation of the EACA. For this reason the use of this therapy is theoretically hazardous where the patient's problem is primarily one of defibrination with continuing intravascular coagulation. In a fibrinolytic state the survival of fibrinogen degradation products may for some hours interfere with normal fibrin polymerization and cause continuing haemostatic failure despite the reversal of the fibrinolytic effect.

Purpura

Vascular purpuras. The vascular purpuras can be recognized by a physician with some experience because of the characteristics of the lesions. The lesion has an inflammatory component as well as evidence of haemorrhage into the skin. Vascular purpuras are often categorized along with thrombocytopenic purpuras but in a sense represent an entirely different problem. They do not indicate exsanguination but are merely indicators of an underlying disease process which it may or may not be possible to delineate further. A whole range of conditions are now known to be associated with small vessel disease and cause the accompanying skin lesions. Henoch-Schönlein syndrome is one well-known example of a broad spectrum of conditions.

Senile purpura on the backs of the hands and forearms is common and of no clinical relevance except that it requires recognition.

Thrombocytopenic purpura. As indicated already the bleeding in this condition is usually into the skin or below it as small bruises. Bleeding deep into the muscles and tissue planes is unusual. Bleeding may also occur from mucous membranes giving epistaxis, gastro-intestinal bleeding and menorrhagia. Intracranial bleeding does undoubtedly occur but is probably much rarer than many of the accounts of this disease would indicate. Retinal haemorrhages are common in many thrombocytopenic conditions but are surprisingly uncommon in idiopathic thrombocytopenic purpura. They are more commonly found in the thrombocytopenia of severe pernicious anaemia, leukaemia, pancytopenia or marrow replacement by tumour.

The most important diagnostic issue in thrombocytopenic purpura is to be confident of the platelet count. There is, however, no simple relationship between the number of platelets and the severity of the bleeding; it is unusual to have a major problem unless the platelet count is less than 50,000 c.mm. and usually in frank haemorrhage from thrombocytopenia it is much lower. In idiopathic pancytopenia a low platelet count is a common feature and in the recovery phase the rise in platelets may lag significantly behind the improvement in the red and white cells. Indeed, the patient may be left with a normal haemoglobin level and white cell count, but still be markedly thrombocytopenic.

MARROW DYSFUNCTION. In purpura after the administration of drugs a distinction needs to be made between agents which can be expected to induce marrow hypoplasia and others which do so because of some sensitivity phenomenon affecting the individual. A regular and predictable effect can be found after administration of busulphan, chlorambucil, cyclophosphamide, folic acid antagonists, mercaptopurine or nitrogen mustard, to quote only a limited number of these agents now used in treatment. As an occasional effect in susceptible individuals the following drugs may be mentioned though again this list is not exhaustive: acetazolamide, chloramphenicol, chlordiazepoxide, frusemide, indomethacin, meprobamate, oxyphenbutazone, phenylbutazone, pyrimethamine, streptomycin, sulphamethoxypyridazine and troxidone. No particular form of therapy can be counted on to restore marrow function and the chief principles of treatment should be to avoid further exposure to possible toxic substances and to keep the patient in reasonable health by transfusion of fresh platelet rich blood or plasma platelet concentrates. There should be avoidance of intramuscular injections as these may produce troublesome haematomata. Steroid therapy probably deserves a limited trial and some control of bleeding may occur even although the platelet count is unaffected. If, however, no improvement has occurred in four weeks the likelihood is that the risks of continuous steroid therapy will be greater than any possible benefit. It is doubtful whether a small maintenance dose of steroid has any non-specific advantageous effect on the vascular component of capillary haemostasis. Such treatment is probably not indicated except when there is a definite relationship between the administration of steroids and the maintenance of the platelet count. Other hormone preparations such as oxymetholone (p. 160) may be tried. The question of splenectomy may arise in these patients but is unlikely to be beneficial and is not advised.

In neoplastic disease of the bone marrow the therapeutic issue is obviously that of the underlying problem and need not be dealt with further in this section.

It is important to remember that the dominant presenting feature of megaloblastic anaemia may be thrombocytopenia with purpura. Once the diagnosis is made and treatment commenced the marrow will respond with a very brisk outpouring of platelets at the same time as the reticulocyte count starts to rise.

Thrombocytopenia probably due to excessive destruction of platelets in the peripheral circulation.
DRUG SENSITIVITY. It is important to appreciate that there are two main mechanisms whereby drugs can cause thrombocytopenia. In the one already described the thrombocytopenia is due to marrow damage from the drugs. In the variety now to be considered the drug action is on the peripheral platelet, where it is thought that the drug acts as a hapten to the thrombocyte and the resulting antigen causes an antigen/antibody reaction. The sequence of events is that the patient is recognized to become rapidly thrombocytopenic on ingestion of the drug, but as soon as the therapy is stopped the platelet count returns to normal. When such a patient has recovered from the effects of the drug and the platelet count is again normal, then the thrombocytes in a specimen of blood removed at that time and studied *in vitro* can be shown to aggregate in response to addition of the drug. This mode of action has been shown with certainty with the following drugs: antazoline (an antihistamine), apronal, quinidine, quinine and sulphamethazine. It is probable that other drugs including the barbiturates, thiazide diuretics and some antidiabetic compounds, in particular chlorpropamide, produce thrombocytopenia in the same way but the evidence so far produced is not entirely complete. No treatment is usually required other than withdrawal of the drug.

ACUTE INFECTIONS. These may be associated with thrombocytopenia. This is seen at the most acute phase of certain infectious diseases, for example smallpox, typhoid fever, and infectious mononucleosis. Much more common than thrombocytopenia at the height of an acute infection is thrombocytopenia after almost any of the commoner infective illnesses of childhood, such as measles, rubella, chickenpox or mumps. The purpura or other manifestations of thrombocytopenia is usually seen 10 to 21 days after the onset of the preceding illness suggesting a hypersensitivity to the action of the causative agents. Some of these patients are wrongly thought to have idiopathic thrombocytopenic purpura and it may well be that in others given this diagnostic label the acute infecting agent has not been recognized.

Idiopathic thrombocytopenic purpura (ITP). The acute form of this disease is most often seen in childhood but no age is exempt. The onset commonly follows an infective illness. Apart from the purpura, physical examination is usually negative. It is unusual for the spleen to be palpable and a very definite splenic enlargement is against the diagnosis of idiopathic thrombocytopenic purpura. This condition usually runs a self-limited course ending in a spontaneous and permanent remission after a period of 10 days to a few months. After a three-month period it must generally be accepted that the patient is no longer suffering from acute idiopathic thrombocytopenic purpura but that the disorder is of the chronic variety. Chronic idiopathic thrombocytopenic purpura usually starts insidiously and is predominantly a disease of young adults, affecting women three times more often than men. Usually a history is obtained of easy bruising for some months, with crops of petechiae or with menorrhagia. In the peripheral blood film such platelets as are seen may be giant and irregular in size. In all cases of idiopathic thrombocytopenic purpura, but particularly in patients with persistent leukopenia, laboratory and clinical evidence should be sought for diffuse lupus erythematosus.

When untreated, idiopathic thrombocytopenic purpura may run a fluctuating course sometimes with long periods of freedom from symptoms although the platelet count may never return to normal. There is not infrequently a poor correlation between the platelet count and the clinical manifestations. These patients may have serious haemorrhage from the nose, the alimentary tract or the uterus, but the bleeding is seldom acute and profuse in this disease except at the onset. A fatal cerebral haemorrhage is relatively rare after the first few weeks of the disease.

In the treatment of this disorder, blood transfusion will be required if significant blood loss has occurred. If there is evidence of continuous bleeding then the transfused blood should be freshly collected. In discussing the management of this condition one can only lay down certain general guide lines and the appropriate treatment of each case must be decided on its own merits. It is usual to give 60 mg. of prednisolone daily when the patient is first seen but obviously such doses cannot be maintained for long periods because of side-effects. It is obviously unwise to treat a young patient suffering from idiopathic thombocytopenia with steroids over a long period when there will be resulting dwarfism. The dangers of long-term corticosteroid therapy in adults are described elsewhere (p. 452). If the platelet count rises to normal the dosage of steroids should be gradually reduced and withdrawn completely. In some patients the platelet count will rise, perhaps spontaneously, while the patient is being treated with corticosteroids and after withdrawal of the therapy there is no longer a problem because the platelet count is maintained. In a further group of patients the platelet count falls when the steroid therapy is withdrawn and it may be justifiable to have a second short trial of 60 mg. of prednisolone. If the dosage is reduced after two weeks and the platelet count again falls, splenectomy should be carried out under adequate corticosteroid cover. In a further group of patients there will be no rise in the platelet count at all and splenectomy should be done. In the chronic case without evidence of dangerous bleeding it may be justifiable to wait for three months in the hope of spontaneous remission. If, for any reason, splenectomy cannot be carried out or if thrombocytopenia persists after splenectomy then the physician has to take a decision whether the continuing thrombocytopenia or the continuing administration of corticosteroid drugs is the greater of the two risks. On the whole the latter is the more dangerous. Many patients live for years with reduced number of platelets and experience nothing more alarming than a recurrent series of subcutaneous haematomata or skin petechiae. It cannot be denied that intracranial haemorrhage has been known to occur, but this is very unusual in long-standing idiopathic thrombocytopenic purpura.

Before proceeding to splenectomy the chances of success or failure should be clearly explained to the patient or the relative. There have been varying results in different published series, but an optimistic view is that approximately half the patients in the situations indicated above with a low platelet count subjected to splenectomy have an immediate rise in the platelet count and this is maintained. In about a quarter of the patients there is no rise in the platelet count but sometimes there is less evidence of the bleeding tendency after splenectomy. In the remaining quarter of the patients the platelet count rises after splenectomy but the rise is not sustained and a fluctuating course of the platelet count and of the clinical condition may follow.

Surgery must be carried out under full corticosteroid cover, intravenous corticosteroid administration being used at the time of the operation. The platelet count is followed in the immediate post-operative phase and if a satisfactory response is occurring a very significant increase is usually found in the platelet count within 24 hours of operation. Thereafter, in those responding well, the platelet count may rise significantly before settling down at about the normal level. When this is found to occur the corticosteroid therapy can be tapered off, starting two to three days after the operation unless there is some new complicating feature. When a satisfactory platelet response has not been obtained then the problem is more difficult, but corticosteroids should certainly be continued until the wound has healed. Thereafter, even if the platelet count has not risen, it is our practice to reduce and discontinue corticosteroid therapy, believing that the risk of this treatment in the long-term is greater than the risk of bleeding. Best results can be forecast in these patients where the platelet count rises well above normal by the third or fourth day after operation. Unfortunately there is no way of predicting pre-operatively which patients will respond to splenectomy. In many previous accounts of this topic the issue has been raised of an accessory spleen causing the failure of response to splenectomy. This possibility can be explored by a chromium labelled red cell technique and evidence to suggest splenic tissue would justify re-exploration of the abdomen.

In the follow-up of patients with apparent idiopathic thrombocytopenic purpura it will be found that a small proportion develop unequivocal evidence of disseminated lupus erythematosus. For this and other reasons all patients should be placed on long-term out-patient follow-up.

Idiopathic thrombocytopenic purpura during pregnancy can create a difficult problem. If clinical manifestations are severe, corticosteroids may have to be given as previously indicated, although there is slight evidence to suggest that cleft palate may occur in the infant. If thrombocytopenic purpura persists, splenectomy may be performed in late pregnancy possibly combined with caesarian section. In coming to a decision as to the policy in any individual it should be recalled that many patients with thrombocytopenia have been delivered without special risk of bleeding.

Infants born to mothers with idiopathic thrombocytopenic purpura are more likely than not to be thrombocytopenic at the time of birth even though the mother's thrombocytopenia may have gone into remission as a consequence of splenectomy. The probability is that this form of neonatal thrombocytopenia is due to the transfer of a platelet antibody across the placenta from the mother's circulation to that of the infant. Although death has been known to occur in this condition the majority of the infants recover, the disease process burning itself out over a period of ten days to three weeks. The most dangerous time for the infant is during delivery of the mother and in the first few days of life. Platelet transfusions may be indicated.

Haemorrhagic thrombocythaemia. Paradoxically not only does thrombocytopenia cause haemorrhage but thrombocythaemia also may do so. Sometimes thrombocythaemia is associated with thrombosis. Thrombocythaemia may be idiopathic and may occur as one feature of the myeloproliferative syndrome, even with normal red and white cell counts. It may be a feature of chronic myeloid leukaemia or polycythaemia vera. The commonest manifestations are gastro-intestinal bleeding, epistaxis, and bleeding from the gums and mouth. External ecchymoses may be seen. The spleen is often enlarged. On the other hand the condition of hyposplenism due to splenic atrophy may be found and thrombocythaemia may be a consequence of splenectomy. The marrow usually shows marked hyperplasia of the megakaryocytes. The treatment of choice is the use of radioactive phosphorus in a dosage of three to four millicuries. This dosage may be larger in patients where there is accompanying polycythaemia. Splenectomy is not indicated as this will aggravate the problem.

Hereditary haemorrhagic telangiectasia. The lesions in mucous membranes, particularly in the nose, bleed periodically and often profusely, leading to severe anaemia. Cauterization of the nasal lesions is often necessary, and although this may stop the bleeding for a time, recurrences are the rule. There is now reasonable evidence that treatment with oestrogens is often effective in reducing haemorrhage from mucous membranes,

including epistaxis. Small doses (0·25 to 1 mg. daily by mouth) of ethinyl oestradiol are recommended. The post-haemorrhagic anaemia should be treated with iron.

Thrombotic thrombocytopenic purpura. In this condition vast numbers of platelet thrombi occur in small vessels probably secondary to a lesion of the endothelium with intravascular coagulation. Haemolytic anaemia and transitory focal neurological lesions accompany the haemorrhagic manifestation and point the way to the diagnosis. At a theoretical level there may be a place for heparin but the value of this is unproven. Equally corticosteroids may be worth a trial but in most of the patients that have been recorded, death has occurred.

ABERDEEN: Professor A. S. Douglas or Dr A. A. Dawson, Department of Medicine, Foresterhill, Aberdeen. (Aberdeen 23423)

BELFAST: Dr M. G. Nelson, Department of Clinical Pathology, Royal Victoria Hospital, Belfast. (Belfast 30503)

BIRMINGHAM:
Dr M. J. Meynell, Haematology Department, Queen Elizabeth Hospital, Edgbaston, Birmingham. (021-472-1311)
Dr J. Stuart, Department of Haematology, The Children's Hospital, Ladywood Middleway, Birmingham, 16. (021-454-4851)

BRADFORD: Dr R. Turner, Royal Infirmary, Bradford. (Bradford 42200)

BRISTOL: Dr A. B. Raper, Department of Medicine, The Royal Infirmary, Bristol. (Bristol 2-2041)

CAMBRIDGE: Professor F. G. J. Hayhoe, Haematology Clinic, Department of Medicine, University of Cambridge, Hills Road, Cambridge CB2 1QT. (Cambridge 45171)
(At night and at weekends please telephone Addenbrookes Hospital—Cambridge 55671—and ask for Professor Hayhoe's Senior House Officer.)

CARDIFF: Dr A. L. Bloom, Department of Haematology, Royal Infirmary, Cardiff. (Cardiff 33101)

CARLISLE: Dr A. Inglis, Department of Pathology, Cumberland Infirmary, Carlisle. (Carlisle 23444)

DERBY: Dr C. R. R. Wylie, Royal Infirmary, Derby. (Derby 47141)

DUNDEE: Dr G. R. Tudhope, Therapeutics Unit, Maryfield Hospital, Dundee. (Dundee 40011)

EDINBURGH:
Professor R. H. Girdwood, University Department of Therapeutics, The Royal Infirmary, Edinburgh, EH3 9YW. (031-229-2477, Ext. 2523)
Dr S. H. Davies, Department of Haematology, The Royal Infirmary, Edinburgh, EH3 9YW. (031-229-2477, Ext. 2099)

EXETER: Dr J. O. P. Edgcumbe, Department of Pathology, Royal Devon & Exeter Hospital, Exeter. (Exeter 72261, 59261)

GLASGOW: Dr G. P. McNicol, Department of Medicine, Royal Infirmary, Glasgow, C.4. (041-552-3535)
(If not available ask for the Receiving Physician.)

HULL: Dr L. S. Sacker, Department of Pathology, Kingston General Hospital, Beverley Road, Hull. (0482-28631)

INVERNESS: Dr I. A. Cook, Royal Northern Infirmary, Inverness. (Inverness 34411)

LEEDS: Dr W. Goldie, St. James's Hospital, Leeds, 9. (Leeds 3-3144)

LIVERPOOL: Dr T. Black, Liverpool Royal Infirmary, Pembroke Place, Liverpool L35 PU. (051-709-5511)

LONDON:

Professor P. L. Mollison, Haematology Department, St Mary's Hospital, Praed Street, Paddington, London, W.2. (01-262-1280)

Professor R. M. Hardisty, Haematology Department, The Hospital for Sick Children, Great Ormond Street, London, W.C.1. (01-405-9200, Ext. 331)
(At night and at weekends please ask hospital telephone operator for the Resident Assistant Physician.)

Dr P. Barkhan, Department of Haematology, Guy's Hospital, London, S.E.1. (01-407-7600)

Professor J. V. Dacie, Postgraduate Medical School, Hammersmith Hospital, Ducane Road, Shepherds Bush, London, W.12. (01-743-2030, Ext. 28) (Blood Transfusion Laboratory)

Dr H. B. May, Haematology Department, The London Hospital, Whitechapel Road, London, E.1. (01-247-5454)

Professor W. M. Davidson, Haematology Department, King's College Hospital, Denmark Hill, London, S.E.5. (01-274-6222)

Dr C. A. Holman, Haematology Department, Lewisham Hospital, High Street, Lewisham, London, S.E.13. (01-690-4311)

Professor J. W. Stewart, Bland Sutton Institute of Pathology, The Middlesex Hospital, Mortimer Street, London, W.1. (01-363-8333)

Dr Katherine M. Dormandy, The Haemophilia Centre, The Royal Free Hospital, (N.W. Branch), Lawn Road, London, N.W.3. (01-794-4561)

Professor T. A. J. Prankerd, Haematology Department, University College Hospital, Gower Street, London, W.C.1. (01-367-5050)

Dr G. I. C. Ingram, Department of Haematology, St Thomas' Hospital, London, S.E.1. (01-WAT-9292, Ext. 2268)
(At night and at weekends, please ask hospital telephone operator for the Doctor on Duty for Haemophilia.)

Dr J. G. Humble, Haematology Department, Westminster Hospital, St John's Gardens, London, S.W.1. (01-828-9811)

Professor J. L. Stafford, Haematology Department, St George's Hospital, Tooting Grove, London, S.W.17. (01-672-1255)

MANCHESTER: Professor M. C. G. Israels, Department of Clinical Haematology, The Royal Infirmary, Manchester, M13 9WL. (061-273-3300)

MARGATE: Dr H. Sterndale, Isle of Thanet District Hospital, (Margate Wing), St Peter's Road, Margate, Kent. (Thanet 20222)

NEWCASTLE: Dr T. H. Boon, Royal Victoria Infirmary, Newcastle-upon-Tyne, 1. (Newcastle 25131)

OXFORD: Dr Rosemary Biggs, Dr C. Rizza, Oxford Haemophilia Centre, Churchill Hospital, Oxford OX3 7BP. (Oxford 64841, Ext. 575)
(After 5 p.m. and at weekends, please ask for the doctor on call for the Haemophilia Centre.)

PORTSMOUTH: Dr J. P. O'Brien, Central Laboratory, St Mary's General Hospital (East Wing), Milton Road, Portsmouth. (Portsmouth 22331)

SHEFFIELD: Dr E. K. Blackburn, The United Sheffield

Hospitals, Department of Haematology, The Royal Infirmary, Sheffield S6 3DA. (Sheffield 20977)
(At night and at weekends please ask for the doctor on call for the Haemophilia centre.)

AGRANULOCYTOSIS

(AGRANULOCYTIC ANGINA; GRANULO-CYTOPENIA; MALIGNANT OR PRIMARY NEUTROPENIA)

Agranulocytosis is a disorder usually characterized by acute onset, pyrexia, necrotic lesions mainly in the buccal cavity and marked leucopenia with extreme lowering or complete absence of neutrophil polymorph cells. Rarely the course of the disease is chronic with periodic exacerbations. The condition is due to arrest of granular white cell formation in the bone marrow.

Severe leucopenias may also occur in septicaemia, acute infectious fevers, acute leukaemias and aplastic anaemia, and as a terminal event in long-continued debilitating diseases. Leucopenia is occasionally a pronounced feature of Addisonian pernicious anaemia or other forms of megaloblastic anaemia.

We are concerned here, however, with the prevention and treatment of a condition which may be idiopathic or due to certain drugs or chemicals. The latter have become the main cause for concern, with the development of powerful new therapeutic agents and insecticides. Apart from drugs which may cause granulocytopenia as a component of pancytopenia (p. 159), it is accepted that leucopenia or agranulocytosis may occur as an idiosyncrasy or hypersensitivity to amidopyrine, arsphenamine, chloramphenicol, chlordiazepoxide, chlorothiazide, chlorpheniramine, chlorpromazine, chlorpropamide, frusemide, imipramine, mepacrine, meprobamate, oxyphenbutazone, perphenazine, phenidione, phenylbutazone, prochlorperazine, promazine, promethazine, pyrimethamine, streptomycin, sulphadiazine, sulphafurazole, sulphamethoxypyridazine, sulphapyridine, thiouracils, tolbutamide, and troxidone. This list is not exhaustive, and to it must be added insecticides such as chlordane and gamma benzene hydrochloride, also certain hair dyes and rinses. It will be noted, too, that certain drugs may cause granulocytopenia in some individuals, but thrombocytopenia, pancytopenia or even haemolytic anaemia in others.

The development of agranulocytosis may bear no relationship to the amount of the drug taken, and when a patient has recovered, a minute dose may cause an immediate fall in the granulocyte count. There is no way of predicting that an individual may be one who will react to a drug or chemical in this way and so the occurrence of sore throat, unexplained pyrexia or pneumonia should immediately raise the suspicion of granulo-cytopenia. A white cell count should be done and, if the results warrant it, the drug must be stopped at once.

General measures. The general nursing and care of a patient with agranulocytosis are the same as for any acute febrile illness. The diet in the acute phase should be fluid or semi-solid in consistence because of the dysphagia which is frequently a troublesome symptom. Nursing in isolation is advisable.

A simple mouth-wash, such as diluted compound of glycerin of thymol (B.P.C.) or 50 per cent. hydrogen peroxide in water, should be used every two or three hours. The local application of peni-cillin by spray, by insufflation or by pastilles is not recommended. The application of an ice bag to the neck may relieve the pain in the throat, but severe pain calls for the use of morphine subcutaneously.

Curative treatment. In every case of agranu-locytosis exhaustive inquiries should be made regarding drugs taken by the patient as drug treat-ment is much the most common causative factor, and any preparations with leucotoxic properties should be withdrawn at once. Since the cause of death in agranulocytosis is directly attributable to bacterial invasion of the tissues and blood stream, the most important measure is the prevention and cure of infection. Penicillin, which seldom causes blood dyscrasias, is the drug of choice provided the patient is not sensitive to it, and the leucopenia has not followed the administration of this antibiotic. It should be given by mouth as phenoxymethyl-penicillin, but throat swabs should be taken to establish the sensitivity to antibiotics of any infecting organisms. If the infection is not ade-quately controlled, blood cultures should be taken, and pending the results of the laboratory tests it may be thought advisable to employ another oral antibiotic such as ampicillin or tetracycline. Daily leucocyte counts should be undertaken and treat-ment can safely be discontinued a day or two after the neutrophil polymorphs have returned to nor-mal; in most cases, this satisfactory state is reached in seven to ten days after the onset.

In the great majority of cases due to drugs, the treatment described above is all that is necessary.

In some idiopathic cases, however, the neutropenia may persist and treatment with prednisolone may then be tried. Reference has already been made to the leucopenia of megaloblastic anaemia, and it is important to be sure that the patient does not suffer from deficiency of vitamin B_{12} or folic acid.

Blood transfusions are sometimes helpful in patients with severe infection, anaemia and marked debility. The patient's leucocyte count, however, cannot be raised substantially or for long by this means.

Prevention of relapses. All patients with agranu-locytosis due to drugs should be warned against taking the offending preparation in any form in the future. In the United Kingdom The Committee on Safety on Drugs should be informed by comple-tion of a yellow reporting card.

Cyclical Agranulocytosis

This rare condition is characterized by periods of complete or almost complete absence of neutrophil polymorphs, recurring every three to four weeks and lasting usually for four or five days. Penicillin given parenterally is the treatment of choice for each relapse. A wide variety of other remedies has proved valueless, but steroid therapy may be effective in reducing the degree of the neutropenia. Splenectomy is well worthy of a trial if, as is usual, the condition persists.

Chronic Neutropenia

This condition may be primary or it may complicate many diseases characterized by splenic enlargement such as Hodgkin's disease, lymphosarcoma and splenic anaemia. It is generally regarded as a manifestation of 'hypersplenism', and chronic thrombocytopenia may accompany the neutropenia. Recurrent infections are liable to occur if the neutro-penia is severe. Good results follow splenectomy in many of the primary cases, and in this group steroid therapy sometimes produces a dramatic improvement. In the secondary group splenectomy may be justified if other procedures, radiotherapy and chemotherapy are not followed by a satisfac-tory response (p. 169).

DISEASES OF THE RETICULO-ENDOTHELIAL SYSTEM

There is no general agreement about the classi-fication of these diseases, and, indeed, histologists and pathologists do not agree amongst themselves as to which cells should be included in the reticulo-endothelial system. However, it is convenient to divide the diseases into two groups: (a) the myelo-proliferative diseases; and (b) the reticuloses. (Some authorities recognize three groups: myelo-proliferative disorders, lymphoproliferative disorders and reticuloses, but this classification will not be used here.)

Reticulo-endothelial tissue is widespread throughout the body in spleen, liver, marrow, lymph nodes and other situations. One view is that from the stem cell, the reticulum cell, are derived not only the macrophages of the tissues, but also endothelial cells, all the blood cell precursors and the fibroblasts. In the group of diseases under consideration there is an uncontrolled ('malignant') proliferation either of the parent cell, the reticulum cell (reticulum cell sarcoma) or of one of the series of cells derived from it (the leukaemias, polycythaemia vera, etc.).

In the myelo-proliferative diseases the cell series affected is one which is normally present in the marrow and the mature cells derived from it appear normally in the blood stream. This is true except in the case of myelofibrosis where proliferation in the marrow affects mainly fibroblasts, but this condition is closely related to myeloid leukaemia and thrombocythaemia so that its inclusion in this group is justified.

In the reticuloses (for example, reticulum cell sarcoma, Hodgkin's disease, lymphosarcoma) the proliferating cells do not normally appear in the blood stream and, as a rule, the proliferation occurs first in an extra-medullary situation, for example, one or more groups of lymph nodes. Accordingly it is convenient to consider this group separately. It should be realized, however, that in reticulum cell sarcoma, lymphosarcoma and certain uncommon diseases related to them, the proliferating cells may gain access to the blood stream in the advanced stages of the disease, giving rise to a blood picture very similar to that of leukaemia. Leuko-sarcoma is the term sometimes applied in these circumstances.

THE MYELOPROLIFERATIVE DISEASES

Most of the diseases in this group are closely related, and a transition from one type to another is not infrequent. For example, primary polycy-thaemia very seldom occurs in a pure form with excessive production of red cells alone; there is usually an accompanying increase of the myeloid series of cells in the blood stream and of platelets (thrombocythaemia), and sometimes the condition terminates as frank chronic or acute myeloid leukaemia. Similarly, in myelofibrosis and thrombocythaemia an increase of myeloid cells is common and, again, transition to chronic myeloid leukaemia may occur. Acute leukaemias do not become chronic (although their progression may be considerably slowed by appropriate therapy), but chronic leukaemias often show the clinical and haematological features of acute leukaemia in the terminal stages.

Erythraemic Myelosis

Acute erythraemic myelosis (acute erythraemia, di Guglielmo's disease) is a rare condition of acute onset and rapid course with death in a few weeks. It is best regarded as an uncontrolled proliferation of erythroblasts in the marrow with a failure of most of them to form erythrocytes. Accordingly there is severe anaemia, and, although many erythroblasts appear in the peripheral blood, the reticulocyte count is low. Leucopenia and thrombocytopenia are present as a result of the erythroblastic proliferation, and hepatosplenomegaly and pyrexia are usually found. Blood transfusions are of temporary benefit and prednisolone may be tried. Mercaptopurine is also worth giving although there is little likelihood of success.

Subacute and chronic forms of the disease with survival for as long as a few years are now recognized. Again blood transfusions are the mainstay of treatment. The intense erythroblastic hyperplasia may result in depletion of folic acid so that megaloblasts may appear in the marrow, but neither folic acid nor hydroxocobalamin slows the progression of the disease. The cautious use of mercaptopurine or busulphan merits trial.

Polycythaemia Vera

(*Erythraemia; Vaquez's disease; Osler's disease*). In this condition there is considerable erythroblastic hyperplasia, but, in contrast to erythraemic mye-losis, the production of erythrocytes is much increased. This results in an increase in the volume and viscosity of the blood.

Before treating the patient for polycythaemia vera one must exclude the following causes of a high red-cell count: (*a*) local congestion, e.g. Raynaud's disease, or incorrect use of a venous tourniquet in taking blood; (*b*) diminution of plasma volume (relative polycythaemia), e.g. after severe sweating, vomiting or diarrhoea; (*c*) erythrocytosis secondary to factors causing incomplete oxygenation of the blood, e.g. chronic cardiac and pulmonary disease, living at high altitudes; (*d*) a haemoglobin level as high as 17·5 g. per 100 ml. and a red-cell count as high as 6·0 million per cu. mm. may be normal in men; (*e*) polycythaemia may be present in Cushing's syndrome and may occur in association with tumours, especially of the kidney.

Treatment. Five methods of treatment are available: (1) venesection; (2) radioactive phosphorus; (3) irradiation with X-rays; (4) busulphan or (5) pyrimethamine.

VENESECTION. Because of the high blood volume, a large quantity of blood must be withdrawn if significant benefit is to follow; little relief is likely unless at least 1 litre is withdrawn at each venesection. Owing to the greatly increased blood viscosity, the following modifications of the usual technique should be made: (1) a wide-bore needle should be used, and the rubber tubing attached to this and leading to the receptacle for collection of the blood should be short and thoroughly washed with sodium citrate solution or heparin before use; (2) the needle should be inserted into the vein in the direction opposite to that of the blood stream; (3) a negative pressure should be maintained in the receptacle to hasten the rate of flow through the tubing.

There is no doubt that venesection gives more rapid relief of symptoms than any other form of treatment. When symptoms are severe it should always be used, and repeated if necessary.

It is, however, unsatisfactory as the sole method of treatment. Its effect is transitory and, even if repeated at frequent intervals, the red-cell count and blood viscosity may continue to be increased even when the haemoglobin level is normal. Moreover, venesection does not lessen the thrombocythaemia which is one of the factors leading to increased susceptibility to thrombosis in this disorder.

RADIOACTIVE PHOSPHORUS, ^{32}P. This has a short half-life of 14 days and emits only beta particles. It is deposited in bone and so the isotope exerts its effect on the actively proliferating cells of the bone marrow. It is simple to administer orally, or, better still, intravenously as a solution of sodium acid phosphate. The usual dose for a man is five, and for a woman four millicuries. The general upset which sometimes follows radiotherapy does not occur.

Usually the platelet count falls first and the degree and rapidity of this fall help to predict the subsequent reduction of the red-cell count. The patient often experiences subjective improvement after a month and the red-cell count falls during the succeeding two months. If the response is inadequate another smaller dose of radioactive phosphorus should be given. A satisfactory remission usually lasts for one to three years, and, when relapse occurs, the treatment is repeated.

Irradiation with X-rays. This was the treatment of choice before radioactive phosphorus became available. Wide-field or 'bath' radiotherapy was usually employed.

The incidence of acute and chronic myeloid leukaemia may be increased in patients who have been treated with ^{32}P or radiotherapy but this effect, if it occurs, does not become manifest for a considerable number of years, and the risk is offset by the satisfactory remissions produced.

BUSULPHAN. It has been claimed that busulphan in the same initial dosage as for chronic myeloid leukaemia (p. 179) is a satisfactory alternative method of treatment that is unlikely to cause leukaemia. The maintenance dose is 2 mg. once or twice daily.

PYRIMETHAMINE. This folic acid antagonist has given satisfactory results in many instances. The initial dose of 25 mg. daily usually needs to be given for four to six weeks. The dose is then reduced to half and when the haematocrit reading is 50 per cent., treatment should be stopped. It is resumed when a steady increase in the packed cell volume occurs.

SYMPTOMATIC TREATMENT. Most of the symptoms disappear when a satisfactory remission follows treatment with radioactive phosphorus. If thrombotic episodes continue, long-term anticoagulant therapy (p. 187) should be instituted. Dyspepsia should be treated by a light easily digested diet together with alkalis, and the frequent occurrence of peptic ulceration in patients with polycythaemia vera should be borne in mind. Haemorrhage, e.g. epistaxis, helps to relieve the plethora, and measures to stop it should not be undertaken unless large amounts of blood are being lost.

Primary Thrombocythaemia

A marked increase in the number of circulating blood platelets is quite commonly seen in polycythaemia vera, in the early stages of chronic myeloid leukaemia, and in myelofibrosis (secondary thrombocythaemia). The primary form is rare and occurs when the proliferative process affects the megakaryocytes exclusively or almost so. In the later stages, the characteristic features of chronic myeloid leukaemia may develop. The platelet count is very high, often over 1 million per cu. mm. (normal range 200,000 to 400,000). The patients, who are almost always over middle age, are prone to develop recurrent venous thromboses, and, paradoxically, haemorrhages in the skin, from mucous membranes or in any organ. The haemorrhagic tendency may arise because of functional inadequacy of the platelets.

Treatment. Most authorities recommend radioactive phosphorus (p. 175) as the treatment of first choice. Alternatively, busulphan in the same dosage as for chronic myeloid leukaemia (p. 179) may be tried. Busulphan is sometimes successful in inducing a temporary remission when radioactive phosphorus has failed.

THE LEUKAEMIAS

The treatment of the various forms of leukaemia is being actively investigated throughout the world, and a large number of chemotherapeutic agents has been developed. Some have proved to be of value in prolonging life, while others have soon been discarded either as a result of ineffectiveness or because of side-effects. Any form of treatment that makes life even more distressing for the unfortunate victim of leukaemia or for his relatives is not justifiable.

The main drugs that merit consideration in the treatment of the leukaemias or reticuloses are listed in Table 5.

Acute Lymphoblastic Leukaemia

This type of leukaemia is common in children and rare in adults. There is currently much interest in establishing whether or not life can be prolonged without undue misery by a combination of drugs instead of a single therapeutic agent. The likelihood of improvement is greater in children than in adults.

Drugs that merit consideration are prednisolone, mercaptopurine, methotrexate, cytosine arabinoside, vincristine sulphate, cyclophosphamide and daunorubicin. The initial treatment must be in hospital and some believe that it should be in an area of strict isolation. This in itself, while logical if an attempt is being made to destroy the majority of leukaemic cells, inevitably with destructive effects on other cells in the bone marrow, is hardly justifiable because of the distress that is lilely to be caused.

Corticosteroids. Prednisolone or prednisone may be used in doses of 60 mg. daily for adults and 30 to 40 mg. daily for children. Much larger doses have been given, but the results of such heroic therapy do not justify its continuation. Maintenance is usually with a reduced dosage once remission has been induced. Corticosteroids usually bring about a remission more rapidly than any other therapeutic agent given alone, but this form of treatment by itself is not the optimal way to deal with the problem. *Corticosteroids are better combined with other drugs in an attempt to induce a remission* (p. 177), but they may be used alone when other drugs are ineffective. In lymphoblastic leukaemia, about 60 to 70 per cent. of children have a good remission with prednisolone alone, while in the adult the figure is nearer to 40 per cent.

Mercaptopurine. This hypoxanthine analogue has for some time been used by itself or in combination with prednisolone as the treatment of choice in acute lymphoblastic leukaemia, but it is now more commonly employed for maintenance (p. 177). The dose for initial treatment or for the early stages of maintenance in children or adults is 2·5 mg. per kg. of body weight daily by mouth. When mercaptopurine is used alone, no beneficial effects are likely until a few weeks have elapsed, when, in favourable cases, the white-cell count falls with an accompanying rise in the haemoglobin and platelets. At this stage the dosage should be reduced (usually to about 50 mg. daily in the adult), but it is advisable to do bone marrow examinations every eight weeks because the reappearance of blast cells may precede changes in the peripheral blood and necessitate a change of therapy. Mercaptopurine may cause nausea, vomiting and diarrhoea. Rarely there has been liver damage.

Methotrexate. This folic acid antagonist has been used more in children than in adults. Its serious disadvantage is that it may cause oral and gastro-intestinal ulceration, and it sometimes leads to alopecia or hepatic necrosis. It used to be given in a dosage of 2·5 to 5 mg. daily by mouth, and this amount frequently had to be reduced because of oral ulceration or other alimentary disturbance rather than marrow depression. More recently the dose has been related to body surface, the patient receiving 20 mg./m.² twice weekly orally or intramuscularly. According to the formula of Du Bois and Du Bois (1916), $S = W^{0 \cdot 425} \times H^{0 \cdot 725} \times 71 \cdot 84$ where S = body surface in sq. cm., W = weight in kg. and H = height in cm. Nomograms are available to expedite the calculations. Alternatively $\log S = \log W \times 0 \cdot 425 + \log H \times 0 \cdot 725 + 1 \cdot 8564$. As always, the length of the course depends upon the response and side-effects. The drug is used more for maintenance than for initial treatment.

The meninges may be involved in acute lymphoblastic leukaemia, and this leads to nausea, headaches, convulsions, papilloedema or cranial nerve palsies. This involvement can be treated with intrathecal methotrexate in a dosage of 0·2 mg. per kg. of body weight on alternate days for four days. The course can be repeated a week later if necessary.

Cytosine arabinoside. This is a pyrimidine antagonist which inhibits the synthesis of DNA. It has been given intravenously in a dose of 3 mg. per kg. of body weight daily for 5 to 10 days in the initial treatment of acute lymphoblastic or acute myeloblastic leukaemia. It is perhaps more useful in the latter condition, but side-effects may be troublesome, and the value of the substance is not yet certain.

Vincristine sulphate. This is an alkaloid derived from the periwinkle plant (*Vinca rosea*) and it may be used intravenously for initial therapy of acute lymphoblastic leukaemia, usually in combination with other drugs (*v. infra*). It cannot be given intramuscularly. The recommended dosage is 2 mg./m.² of body surface once weekly, but not exceeding 3·5 mg. Vincristine should rarely be given for more than three doses. The drug is toxic to the autonomic and central nervous systems and causes muscle weakness in the limbs, larynx and ocular muscles, together with constipation, paraesthesia and unexplained pain in the pre-auricular and submandibular regions. Alopecia, insomnia, headache and depression may occur.

Cyclophosphamide. This alkylating agent has a certain amount of effectiveness in a number of malignant disorders. It is usually given orally, but the intravenous route is available for patients who are troubled by vomiting. One possible use is in acute lymphoblastic leukaemia, particularly in maintaining a remission. The drug may cause severe bone marrow depression if the dose is not carefully controlled. A suitable initial dosage by the oral route is 3 mg. per kg. of body weight daily. If it is given intravenously the dose should be 15 mg. per kg. weekly, but results are less satisfactory. If the fluid intake is not adequate there may be bladder irritation, and alopecia is another possible side-effect.

Daunorubicin. This antibiotic is produced by two strains of *Streptomyces coeruloerudibus*. It is known in the United States as Daunomycin and in the United Kingdom the name Rubidomycin is commonly used. It is effective against gram-positive organisms, but has such a serious effect on the bone marrow that it can only be used to induce a remission in acute leukaemia and possibly neuroblastoma. It is usually employed in combination with other drugs, or when the disease is resistant to agents such as prednisolone and vincristine. Daunorubicin is given intravenously, 1 mg. per kg. being administered daily for 1 to 5 days, but diluted to a concentration of 1 mg. in 20 ml. of normal saline. It may cause heart failure if several courses are given, and the total dose should never exceed 14 mg. per kg. of body weight. Side-effects include thrombosis of veins, buccal ulceration, nausea and vomiting and alopecia. The drug must not be allowed to leak out into the tissues, and blood counts must be carried out daily.

Combined therapy. The aim of combined therapy as currently practised is to use a group of powerful drugs to initiate a rapid remission in acute lymphoblastic leukaemia, attempting to eradicate the entire leukaemic cell population in the process. Unfortunately, this will not be successful, and maintenance therapy with other drugs is needed to reduce still further the persisting population of leukaemic cells. This has been tried in children and in adults, but is still largely experimental. In a trial carried out by Mathé and his colleagues in Paris, the patients were isolated in pathogen-free rooms, and the initial treatment was with a combination of prednisolone, vincristine and daunorubicin. Maintenance was with successive courses of methotrexate, mercaptopurine and cyclophosphamide. On the whole, the results of such trials are not sufficiently encouraging to justify the upset engendered in a family when a patient has to be nursed in an isolation unit and it is known that the illness will be fatal in any case. However, in the routine *initial* management of acute lymphoblastic leukaemia a combination of prednisolone and vincristine sulphate has given encouraging results. For *maintenance*, mercaptopurine, cyclophosphamide or methotrexate may then be used, and each time relapse occurs the combination of prednisolone and vincristine sulphate can be tried again. Another drug is then used for maintenance.

Other methods of treatment. Active immunotherapy with B.C.G. alone or together with irradiated leukaemic cells has been used by the Paris group in the treatment of acute lymphoblastic leukaemia after chemotherapy has been stopped. B.C.G. was given every fourth day during the first month and then once a week. This appeared to prolong remissions. Trials by other workers using Bordetella pertussis vaccine have been less successful and all that can be said is that this is a new method of approach.

SUPPORTIVE MEASURES. Blood or platelet transfusions will be required for marrow depression, and oral antibiotics may be necessary because of increased susceptibility to infection. An adequate fluid intake may be needed to minimize irritation of the bladder by drug metabolites. Hyperuricaemia may occur and require treatment with allopurinol (p. 460).

Chronic Lymphatic Leukaemia

This type is most common in elderly patients, usually over the age of 65. The disease may be only slowly progressive, and treatment need not be undertaken as soon as the diagnosis is established, but should be postponed until one or more of the following indications have arisen: (*a*) the lymph nodes or spleen have become so much enlarged that they cause discomfort or pain, or produce other undesirable features, e.g. evidence of hypersplenism or pressure effects; (*b*) significant anaemia has appeared (haemoglobin less than 70 per cent.); (*c*) haemorrhagic manifestations have occurred; (*d*) the white-cell count has risen to about 100,000 per cu. mm. or higher; (*e*) acute lymphoblastic leukaemia has supervened.

Chlorambucil. This nitrogen mustard derivative is given by mouth, initially in a daily dose of 8 mg., which should be reduced to a maintenance one of about 2 mg. daily when a satisfactory response has been obtained. The dosage must be carefully controlled by frequent blood counts to avoid the occurrence of aplastic anaemia. Some patients need courses at infrequent intervals, and others require a small dose daily. Survival may be for many years. There is, fortunately, freedom from side-effects when chlorambucil is used.

Splenic irradiation. This form of treatment may be tried in the common type of case with moderate anaemia, a white-cell count of 100,000 per cu. mm. or more, and moderate enlargement of the spleen, liver and lymph nodes. It is given in small daily doses and the white-cell count often falls by 10,000 to 15,000 per day. Treatment should be stopped when the white-cell count is about 10,000 per cu. mm., but if the rate of fall is precipitous, it should be stopped earlier. In favourable cases the haemoglobin level rises, and the size of lymph nodes and liver diminishes. The white-cell count slowly rises over the ensuing months, but a year or more may elapse before further treatment is required.

Radiotherapy may be given to groups of glands large enough to cause embarrassment if visible in the neck, or discomfort in the axillae or groins. Enlarged mediastinal glands may be treated in the the same way before they give rise to pressure effects. Usually it is possible to deal with only one group of glands in this way, because the treatment causes a rapid fall in the white-cell count. This fall usually lasts for a shorter time than that which follows splenic irradiation, and accordingly the remission induced is less satisfactory.

Gross splenomegaly alone, causing discomfort or pain, may be treated by radiotherapy even in the absence of the other indications mentioned above. The daily dose should be related to the initial white-cell count, but, even in aleukaemic cases, it may be possible to reduce the size of the spleen without a dangerous fall in the white-cell count by giving daily doses of about a quarter of those usually used. Irradiation sickness is treated with trifluoperazine, 1 mg. three times daily, and an intramuscular injection of pyridoxine, 50 mg. daily.

Corticosteroids. A severe degree of haemolysis often occurs in the course of chronic lymphatic leukaemia. Prednisolone in sufficient dosage to control the haemolytic process should then be given. Initially 60 mg. daily may be required, but in many cases this can be gradually reduced to about 30 mg. daily or less without recurrence of notable haemolysis. Another possible indication for prednisolone is severe anaemia or a platelet count below 75,000 per cu. mm. The lymphocyte count may continue to rise in the early weeks of corticosteroid therapy, but thereafter fall, with a coincidental rise in erythrocytes and platelets. When the disease is under control, treatment should be with chlorambucil.

Splenectomy. If radio-chromium studies have indicated that haemolysis is occurring exclusively, or almost so, in the spleen, splenectomy may rarely be justified. After the operation, reticulo-endothelial tissue elsewhere may become the site of haemolysis. Treatment with corticosteroids will then have to be instituted and continued indefinitely.

Antibiotics. Patients with chronic lymphatic leukaemia are very prone to infections. This is due in part to the small number of polymorph leucocytes in the circulation, and in part to the hypogammaglobulinaemia which is very common in the late stages of the disease. Oral penicillin should be given as a prophylactic measure, and the appropriate antibiotic when any infection occurs. Gamma globulin can be given by injection for disorders in which it is deficient, but it is in very short supply, and its use for long periods in a disease which is inevitably fatal, is not justified.

In the late stages of the disease, the clinical and haematological features of acute lymphoblastic leukaemia may appear. The treatment described on p. 178 should then be instituted.

Acute Myeloblastic Leukaemia

This type of leukaemia occurs both in childhood and adult life. When it occurs in adults, it may be preceded by months of increasing ill-health, lassitude, dyspnoea and anorexia. This represents the phase of 'pre-leukaemia' in which the marrow is in an aplastic or hypoplastic state and there is 'refractory' anaemia. When the disease is established and the typical blood picture of acute leukaemia appears, the progression is just as rapid in adults as in children, death occurring after a few weeks or months.

TREATMENT. The treatment of acute myeloblastic leukaemia in adults or children is even less satisfactory than that of acute lymphoblastic leukaemia. Daunorubicin and cytosine arabinoside may be used to initiate remission (p. 177), or a combination of vincristine and prednisolone can be tried. Maintenance can be with prednisolone or mercaptopurine (p. 176).

Supportive measures. Blood or platelet transfusions may be required and may strain the resources of transfusion services. Oral antibiotics may be necessary to prevent or treat infection.

Chronic Myelogenous (Myeloid) Leukaemia

This type of leukaemia is common in patients of middle-age or over. The initial symptoms are those of moderate anaemia or are due to massive enlargement of the spleen.

TREATMENT. The methods of treatment available at present can be expected to prolong life beyond the average survival only to a slight extent, which is about three years from the onset of symptoms when no treatment is used. This is not to say, however, that treatment is unimportant, because, by its use, the patient's well-being and efficiency are much improved and he may be able to lead a near-normal life until a few months before death.

Busulphan. This is a sulphonic acid ester resembling nitrogen mustard (p. 182) and having a similar cytotoxic effect, except that its action is limited almost entirely to the myeloid cells; it has little effect on lymphoid tissue. The usual dosage initially is 4 mg. daily. In favourable cases the effects are the same as with splenic irradiation, viz. reduction of splenomegaly and leucocytosis with an increase in the haemoglobin and red-cell count. Dosage should be reduced to a maintenance level of 1 to 2 mg. daily before the white-cell count has reached the normal range and this dosage should be continued until relapse occurs despite continued treatment. Some patients have been maintained in good health for two to three years by this treatment. Allopurinal (p. 460) may be given to prevent secondary gout.

Busulphan is a simple form of treatment and the patient need not be admitted to hospital although he will have to attend at frequent intervals for the blood counts which are essential if dosage is to be adequately controlled. Patients who are resistant to busulphan will not benefit from treatment with other alkylating agents.

Irradiation with X-rays. This is less satisfactory than treating with busulphan. However, when radiotherapy is used the grossly enlarged spleen usually shrinks and may indeed become impalpable; the very high white-cell count gradually falls and, because splenic irradiation usually produces a reduction of myeloid proliferation throughout the body, this is usually accompanied by an increase of the haemoglobin level and red-cell count. The dosage necessary to produce a satisfactory remission varies from case to case and it should always be controlled by blood counts, including platelet counts, two or three times a week during treatment. The rate at which the white-cell count falls is the best guide. Treatment should always be stopped before this reaches the normal range, and the more rapid the fall the earlier should treatment be discontinued. When relapse occurs, as it usually does after about a year, further irradiation to the spleen should be given.

Irradiation sickness, with malaise and vomiting, may occur in the course of treatment if megavoltage radiotherapy is not used. Many drugs have been tried both in the prevention and treatment of this side-effect, but none has proved entirely successful. Chlorpromazine, in a dosage of 25 mg. thrice daily, is often effective. In some patients pyridoxine, 50 mg. intramuscularly daily, or pyridoxine hydrochloride, 10 mg. four times a day by mouth, may result in relief of symptoms.

Blood transfusion. If a satisfactory haemoglobin level is not produced by busulphan or splenic irradiation, blood transfusion should be given to raise it to at least 11 g. per 100 ml.

In the late stages of the disease, the condition frequently shows the clinical and haematological features of acute myeloblastic leukaemia and the methods of treatment described for this condition (p. 178) should then be used.

Monocytic Leukaemia

This type of leukaemia occurs in both childhood and adult life. It has an acute or, at least, a subacute course, with death in a few months; chronic forms rarely occur. This applies to the Naegeli type in which the marrow shows proliferation of cells both of the monocytic and myeloid series, and the Schilling type where monocytic cells alone proliferate. In addition to the usual features of acute leukaemia, hypertrophy and ulceration of the gums and enlargement of the liver out of proportion to the size of the spleen, are common findings.

Monocytic leukaemia is even more refractory to treatment than acute myeloblastic leukaemia, but initial therapy with mercaptopurine and prednisolone together should be tried. If this fails, vinblastine sulphate (p. 177) may be given in a dosage of 0·1 to 0·15 mg. per kg. of body weight intravenously weekly. Results have been rather poor.

Multiple Myeloma

This disease, which mainly affects people over the age of 50, is usually characterized by multiple tumours of plasma cells in the bone marrow, with progressive anaemia which may be of the leuco-erythroblastic type, or hypoplastic with leucopenia and thrombocytopenia. The tumours invade the cortex of bones causing pain, swelling or pathological fractures which are particularly common in the lumbar vertebrae. Sometimes it presents as a solitary tumour. Usually the plasma cells are confined to the bone marrow, so that sternal puncture is necessary to establish the diagnosis, but occasionally they gain access to the blood stream giving a leukaemic picture (plasma cell leukaemia). The disease is a rapidly progressive one, usually causing death within two or three years of the onset of symptoms.

TREATMENT. The rare case of solitary myeloma is best treated by local excision if it is in an accessible situation.

Radiotherapy. In patients with localized areas of bone destruction and pain, irradiation of the involved areas is the treatment of choice. The tumours may be destroyed and recalcification of bone may follow.

When the disease is generalized with diffuse pain, anaemia, pyrexia and loss of weight and strength, treatment is much more difficult, but the following drugs sometimes prove beneficial.

Melphalan. This alkylating agent is phenylalanine nitrogen mustard. It is usually given orally in a dose of 0·15 mg. per kg. of body weight for seven to ten days, but repeated blood counts are essential. The white-cell and platelet counts may continue to fall for three weeks or more after a course of treatment. After about seven weeks a further course may be given, and others thereafter. Improvement may continue for many months. Nausea, vomiting, diarrhoea and alopecia are possible side-effects. If there is impaired renal function, special care is needed (see below).

Cyclophosphamide. This is an alternative method of treatment in an initial dosage of 150 to 200 mg. daily by mouth for a week. When evidence of bone marrow depression has ceased, a maintenance dose of 100 mg. daily can be given. Frequent blood counts are necessary, and alopecia may occur.

Prednisolone. This form of treatment is indicated where there is thrombocytopenia. If there is hypercalcaemia or evidence of renal failure, it is perhaps best to give prednisolone in a dose of 60 mg. daily together with 4 mg. of melphalan daily. The dose of the former should be reduced as improvement occurs, and the latter should be stopped after two weeks. It can be recommended after about three weeks in a dose of 2 mg. every second day, depending on the blood counts.

Myelofibrosis

This disease of the older age-groups is insidious in onset and runs a chronic course, sometimes passing into the stage of chronic myeloid leukaemia after an interval of some years. The spleen is always greatly enlarged due to myeloid metaplasia (extra-medullary haemopoiesis), and the liver is often enlarged from the same cause. Most cases show

daily and this is reduced gradually to the lowest dose which will control the haemolysis.

Splenectomy. This may prove fatal and is justifiable only (a) if the size of the spleen is such as to cause very marked discomfort or if there are repeated splenic infarcts, and (b) when there is considerable haemolysis which cannot be controlled by moderate doses of corticosteroids or azathio-prine and when it can be shown, by radio-chromium studies, that haemolysis is occurring exclusively, or almost so, in the spleen.

TABLE 5

Drugs used in Treating the Leukaemias or Reticuloses

Type of Drug	Drug Employed	Usual Route of Administration	Believed Mode of Action
Corticosteroid	Prednisolone	Oral	Uncertain, but is
	Prednisone	Oral	lymphocytolic
Alkylating agents	Busulphan	Oral	Cytotoxic, possibly by
	Chlorambucil	Oral	alkylation of guanine
	Cyclophosphamide	Oral or i.v.	in DNA
	Melphalan	Oral or i.v.	
	Mustine hydrochloride	i.v.	
Antimetabolites	Methotrexate	Oral, i.v., i.m. or intrathecal	Folic acid antagonist
	Mercaptopurine	Oral	Purine antagonist
	Azathioprine	Oral	Purine antagonist
	Cytosine arabinoside	i.v. or i.m.	Pyrimidine antagonist
Plant alkaloids	Vinblastine sulphate	i.v.	Produce metaphase arrest
	Vincristine sulphate	i.v.	
Antibiotics	Daunorubicin	i.v.	Uncertain
	Actinomycin C	i.v.	Actinomycins seem to
	Actinomycin D	i.v.	associate with DNA and inhibit its function
Enzyme	1-asparaginase	i.v.	Destroys asparagine
Methylhydrazine derivative	Procarbazine hydro-chloride	Oral or i.v.	Suppresses mitosis by prolonging interphase

moderate anaemia which is often of the leuco-erythroblastic type. Thrombocythaemia may occur. The marrow is increasingly replaced by fibrous tissue or bone and trephine of the iliac crest is likely to be required to provide a specimen. Some degree of haemolysis is common.

TREATMENT. If there is no haemolysis or splenic discomfort, blood transfusions at intervals to keep the haemoglobin at a reasonable level (10 g. per 100 ml.) may be the only treatment necessary for several years. Overloading with iron may necessitate treatment with desferrioxamine (p. 162). Folate deficiency may occur and require treatment.

Corticosteroids. Prednisolone should be given if haemolysis occurs. The initial dose is 60 mg.

THE RETICULOSES

The reticuloses are characterized by uncontrolled proliferation of reticulum cells, some of which show differentiation along certain lines. It is customary to include under this title Hodgkin's disease, reticulum cell sarcoma, lymphosarcoma and certain less well-defined conditions such as follicular lymphoma and essential macroglobulinaemia. In Hodgkin's disease (lymphadenoma) there is pro-liferation of reticulum cells, some of bizarre type (Reed–Sternberg cells), but some differentia-tion has also occurred and varying numbers of fibroblasts and myeloid cells, including eosinophil leucocytes, are present. The acuteness of the disease process is inversely proportional to the degree of differentiation. Thus in reticulum cell sarcoma (Hodgkin's sarcoma), which is a rapidly progressive disease, reticulum cell proliferation occurs, with little or no differentiation into more mature cell types. At the other end of the scale are cases of local paragranuloma in which proliferation of reticulum cells is slight and the lesions consist mainly of fibrous tissue and myeloid cells. Here the course is very chronic extending over many years.

Hodgkin's Disease (*Lymphadenoma*)

From what has been said above it will be apparent that the rate of progression of Hodgkin's disease varies considerably. In the 'average' case, there is first enlargement of a group of superficial lymph nodes, often in the neck, with little or no disturbance of general health. Later the disease becomes more generalized with involvement of more lymph nodes and of the liver, spleen and marrow. At this stage systemic upset is prominent and the patient shows anaemia, pyrexia, loss of weight and jaundice which may be of the obstructive type or due to haemolysis. The diagnosis should always be confirmed by biopsy of one or more enlarged superficial lymph nodes, or, if these are not involved, by liver biopsy, which establishes the diagnosis in a high proportion of cases when general symptoms are present.

TREATMENT. In cases of local paragranuloma, excision of the involved nodes, if they are in an easily accessible situation, is indicated. Following operation it may be many years (10 or more) before there is recurrence in another situation.

Local radiotherapy. This is the best form of initial treatment for most cases of Hodgkin's disease, where, in the early stages of the illness, only one group of lymph nodes is involved. Recurrence in the treated region is unlikely when treatment has been adequate. In the more chronic cases, some years may elapse before further irradiation is required because of recurrence of the disease in another site.

In some cases involvement of several groups of glands is present when the patient is first seen, e.g. enlargement of nodes in both sides of the neck and in the mediastinum. Here wide field radiotherapy is preferable to chemotherapy unless there are systemic disorders (loss of weight and pyrexia) or involvement of liver and spleen.

Irradiation sickness is more likely when wide field therapy has to be used. Its treatment is mentioned on p. 178.

Chemotherapy is indicated when the disease has become generalized with widespread involvement of lymph nodes, enlargement of liver and spleen, pyrexia and loss of weight.

Chlorambucil. This can be given intermittently or as a prolonged course. In the latter event, the usual dose is 6 to 8 mg. daily by mouth depending on body weight. Its main advantages are that it seldom leads to systemic upset, and marrow depression develops slowly so that it is usually possible to discontinue treatment before the stage of irreparable damage.

Improvement, when it occurs, is slow. Often patients begin to feel better about three or four weeks after the start of treatment, and objective evidence of amelioration, such as diminution in size of lymph nodes, liver and spleen and lessening or absence of pyrexia may appear within six weeks. If no improvement at all is apparent in six weeks the drug should be discontinued. In favourable cases full doses are continued for four to six months provided that blood examinations, which should be done at frequent intervals, do not show evidence of serious marrow depression. When the white-cell count falls below 3,000 per cu. mm. or the platelet count below 100,000 per cu. mm., treatment should be stopped.

Complete or near-complete remissions lasting for six months or longer may be achieved. When relapse occurs a second course of treatment should be given, but improvement is likely to be less and of shorter duration.

Nitrogen mustards. These nitrogen analogues of mustard gas are powerful cytotoxic agents. The *bis* compound, methyl-bis (β-chlorethyl) amine hydrochloride, is available commercially as a dry hygroscopic powder in ampoules containing 10 mg. (mustine hydrochloride). Immediately before use the powder is dissolved in 10 ml. of sterile normal saline. Administration is by the intravenous route, and it is best to inject the solution into the rubber tubing of a freely flowing saline infusion, because it is a powerful irritant and it is essential to ensure that none of it escapes into the tissues.

It is probably best to give injections at intervals of three days so that toxic effects can be assessed after each injection. Each dose should be 0·1 to 0·15 mg. per kg. of body weight and should not exceed 10 mg. Four or five injections may be given followed by an injection once a week if the response is favourable.

Side-effects are common. Nausea and vomiting

should be treated in the same way as irradiation sickness (p. 178). Blood counts should be undertaken daily and treatment should be stopped if evidence of serious marrow depression appears.

This form of treatment is used mainly when a rapid effect is essential because of the patient's poor general condition. If the results are favourable, treatment with chlorambucil should be started later.

Cyclophosphamide (p. 177). This may be tried in those patients who derive no benefit from chlorambucil. It is usually given by mouth in an initial dose of three 50 mg. tablets daily. The main danger is agranulocytosis which may occur very rapidly. Alopecia may also result. Accordingly, frequent blood counts are necessary throughout the course of treatment. When amelioration is produced dosage should be reduced to one 50 mg. tablet daily.

Vinblastine sulphate. This is an alkaloid derived from the periwinkle (*Vinca rosea*) which is sometimes useful in generalized Hodgkin's disease. It should not be confused with vincristine sulphate (p. 177). It probably acts as an antimetabolic agent and accordingly may cause marrow depression. For this reason it should not be used if the leucocyte count is less than 4,000 per cu. mm. It is given intravenously in weekly doses starting with 0·1 mg. per kg. body weight and increasing to 10 to 15 mg. total dose weekly for at least six weeks, depending on the leucocyte and platelet counts. It may be possible thereafter to maintain improvement with a smaller dose every two weeks. Neuromuscular disorders may occur as well as mental depression.

Procarbazine hydrochloride. This cytotoxic agent is a methylhydrazine derivative which has the advantage of being effective when given by mouth, usually in a daily dose of 150 to 200 mg. It is certainly worth trying when the disease process is refractory to other treatment. The drug tends to cause nausea and vomiting.

Corticosteroids. When systemic symptoms such as pyrexia and weight loss are not controlled by the therapeutic measures described above, and when haemolysis or haemorrhagic manifestations are present, prednisolone should be given. The usual initial dose is 60 mg. daily and when a favourable response is achieved, this is reduced to a maintenance one of 20 to 30 mg. daily. In a few cases the response is dramatic and the improvement may last for several months.

Blood transfusions. If anaemia is prominent and

G

does not improve as a result of the measures outlined above, transfusions of whole blood or packed cells should be given at intervals to maintain the haemoglobin at a reasonable level (10 g. per 100 ml.).

Lymphosarcoma (*including follicular lymphoma*)

In the early stage the marrow and blood picture are normal. As the disease advances the proliferation of lymphosarcoma cells becomes more widespread and the marrow becomes infiltrated. Hence, differentiation from aleukaemic lymphatic leukaemia becomes difficult, but the distinction is largely academic. In some cases the lymphosarcoma cells appear in the blood stream and the picture is very similar to that of chronic lymphatic leukaemia.

TREATMENT. This should be on the same lines as for Hodgkin's disease (p. 182), viz. radiotherapy to the site of involvement in the early stages when the disease is localized, and chemotherapy, with chlorambucil as the drug of first choice, when the disease is too widespread to be controlled by irradiation. The indications for corticosteroids and blood transfusions are the same as in Hodgkin's disease. When other agents fail, vinblastine sulphate, mercaptopurine, or azathioprine may be tried.

Reticulum Cell Sarcoma (*Hodgkin's Sarcoma*)

In this condition proliferation of reticulum cells, with little or no differentiation into more mature cells, occurs first in one situation, e.g. a group of lymph nodes and, as the disease progresses, involvement becomes more widespread (liver, spleen and bone marrow). The course is usually more acute than in Hodgkin's disease but remission, sometimes of long duration, may be induced by treatment.

TREATMENT. Radiotherapy, when the disease is confined to a group of lymph nodes, is often followed by a long remission. Later, when the disease is more widespread, chlorambucil (p. 182) should be tried but it is usually less effective than in Hodgkin's disease and lymphosarcoma. Corticosteroids should be used when a haemorrhagic state or haemolysis is present, and blood transfusions should be given to counteract severe anaemia.

Macroglobulinaemia

In this condition it seems that macroglobulins are produced by abnormal cells which may be plasma cells, lymphocytes or intermediate forms and these may be found in the bone marrow in large numbers. There may be difficulty in deciding whether the patient suffers from myeloma, lymphosarcoma, aleukaemic lymphatic leukaemia or a variant. The usual treatment of this last is with chlorambucil. However, the writer has had remarkable results in one patient who was given initial treatment with a corticosteroid for several years. When a severe relapse then occurred there was a dramatic response to azathioprine, in an initial dosage of 50 mg. thrice daily together with prednisolone 40 mg. daily.

Diseases of Lipoid Metabolism (*Gaucher's disease; Niemann–Pick disease*)

There is no specific treatment for these conditions. The presence of hypochromic anaemia is an indication for the administration of iron (p. 143). In Gaucher's disease splenectomy is seldom justified because the operation may cause hepatic enlargement to occur more rapidly. It is occasionally indicated, however, because of hypersplenism or if the spleen causes severe symptoms because of its size. Splenectomy is of no value in Niemann–Pick disease, and radiotherapy is not helpful in either condition.

Eosinophilic Granuloma (*Hand–Schüller–Christian disease; Letterer–Siwe syndrome*)

In the past Hand–Schüller–Christian disease was included in the group of diseases of lipoid metabolism, but it is now known to be a form of eosinophilic granuloma. Radiotherapy may cause disappearance of the tumours and of the osteolytic areas in bones. The Letterer–Siwe syndrome is the acute form of the condition and it is usually seen in infants and children. There may be benefit from corticosteroid therapy.

7. Anticoagulant Therapy

A. S. DOUGLAS

INTRODUCTION

The object of conventional anticoagulant therapy in thrombo-embolic occlusive vascular disease is to limit the extension of intravascular fibrin deposition; fibrinolytic or thrombolytic enzymes have been used to remove unwanted fibrin deposited in the vascular tree.

Arterial thrombus has an organized structure which consists of a head of aggregated platelets and a fibrin tail; the platelet head may be of such size that quite apart from the fibrin tail it is capable of producing arterial occlusion. The histological structure of thrombi differs from that of blood clot which is formed when blood is allowed to clot in a glass tube; *in vitro* the platelets are distributed evenly throughout the clot. Venous and arterial thrombi have a similar histological structure, but in venous thrombi the platelet component is diminished and the structure approximates more closely to that of a clot formed *in vitro*.

Though anticoagulant drugs do undoubtedly interfere with fibrin formation, they can have only a limited and prophylactic rôle in therapy by preventing extension of intravascular thrombus formation; they do not significantly affect platelet aggregation in the critical early stage in thrombus formation. It is probable that much platelet aggregation can occur without significant fibrin formation; however, the larger aggregates of platelets in the head of the thrombus are held together by fibrin. It can be shown that fibrinolytic (or more correctly thrombolytic) therapy not only dissolves the fibrin tail of a thrombus but also splits the head into numerous small fragments which, on histological examination, have the structure of platelet aggregates; presumably these fragments are held together by fibrin.

Conventional anticoagulant drugs which interfere with fibrin formation may, therefore, interfere in a limited way with the formation of the platelet head of the thrombus and, relatively more effectively, with the fibrin tail. There is evidence also that prolonged administration of these drugs increases the rate of recanalization of blood vessels, presumably by shifting the balance of normal haemostatic equilibrium towards fibrin removal as compared with fibrin deposition. The functional benefit of the recanalization remains in some doubt.

Mechanism of Interference with Fibrin Formation by Anticoagulant Drugs

In clinical practice the only drugs which require to be considered are heparin and the oral anticoagulant drugs of the coumarin and indanedione type.

Fibrinogen is converted to fibrin by the proteolytic enzyme thrombin. When certain stimuli arise, a sequence of events is set in motion to convert prothrombin, a proenzyme, to thrombin. This occurs under the influence of the thromboplastin system. This can be derived entirely from within the blood (intrinsic or blood thromboplastin), or it may include a tissue as an essential component reacting with certain coagulation factors from the blood (the extrinsic or tissue thromboplastin system).

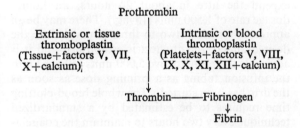

Prothrombin		
Extrinsic or tissue thromboplastin (Tissue+factors V, VII, X+calcium)		Intrinsic or blood thromboplastin (Platelets+factors V, VIII, IX, X, XI, XII+calcium)
	Thrombin——Fibrinogen	
	Fibrin	

Heparin is immediately effective as an anticoagulant when administered intravenously, interfering with the formation of intrinsic or blood thromboplastin and so with prothrombin conversion. Any small amounts of thrombin which may form are antagonized by heparin, which also inhibits the thrombin-fibrinogen reaction.

The coumarin or indanedione drugs produce their anticoagulant effect after an interval of 36 to 48 hours, by inhibiting the synthesis and hence reducing the concentration in the circulation of prothrombin and the factors needed in prothrombin conversion (factors VII and X in the extrinsic system and factors IX and X in the intrinsic system). The delay phase before the anticoagulant effect is observed is likely to be due to the survival time in the circulation of factors which have already been synthesized.

There is some recent evidence that the fall in the concentration of these coagulation factors has two explanations: it is probable that these drugs cause a block in the production of the relevant coagulation factors, and at the same time cause the production of proteins similar to, but not chemically identical with factors II, VII, IX and X. These similar but defective proteins may interfere with the relevant intermediate coagulation reactions in such a way that they have an inhibitory or anticoagulant action.

HEPARIN

The methods of administration are: (1) continuous intravenous infusion; (2) intermittent intravenous injection; (3) subcutaneous or intramuscular injection.

Continuous intravenous method. In this technique 35,000 units (350 mg.) of heparin should be added to a litre of 5 per cent. glucose or normal saline. The infusion should be started at a rate of 20 to 25 drops per minute—this is the rate which would expend the litre in about 24 hours, an hourly dosage rate of 1,500 units (15 mg.). There may be an appreciable period (two to three hours) before the desired anticoagulant effect is established and it is advisable therefore to give 5,000 units (50 mg.) into the infusion tubing as a priming dose as soon as the drip has been started. The whole blood-clotting time requires to be estimated by a standardized technique every two hours to maintain the coagulation time at two to three times the control value. Since the performance of these tests may take a half-hour or longer once the anticoagulant effect has been established, it becomes clear that this is almost a full-time occupation for one doctor or technician. The careful, prolonged supervision of the heparin administered in this way, coupled with the necessary blood examination, renders it too cumbersome for other than occasional use. The large volume of fluid, which may be contraindicated by the patient's condition, is a further disadvantage of the method, but this can be overcome by the use of a mechanical syringe driver, which delivers very small volumes of fluid over a long period. A continuous infusion of heparin by any of these methods may, despite the anticoagulant action of the heparin, give rise to superficial thrombophlebitis.

If there was good evidence that the continuous route gave better therapeutic results than the intermittent intravenous route, then more physicians would make the effort required to use this technique. There has, however, to the author's knowledge, been no controlled clinical trial of one method compared with the other. The author uses heparin in this way in patients with pulmonary embolism during the induction phase until the coumarin effect has been established and also following vascular clearing by thrombolytic therapy.

Intermittent intravenous method. The effect of a single intravenous injection of heparin is almost instantaneous. With doses of 10,000 to 15,000 units (100 to 150 mg.) the blood drawn immediately afterwards is incoagulable; some anticoagulant effect will last four to six hours. In a proportion of patients, by six hours the coagulation time will have returned to near normal but increasing the dose of heparin produces only a very small prolongation of the duration of effect. Using this method, heparin should be given in a dosage of 5,000 to 7,500 units (50 to 75 mg.) every four hours, or 10,000 units (100 mg.) every six hours, or 15,000 units (150 mg.) every eight hours. When it is thought preferable to leave the patient undisturbed during the night, then the following schedule can be used:

7 a.m.	12 noon	5 p.m.	11 p.m.
10,000 units	10,000 units	10,000 units	15,000 units
(100 mg.)	(100 mg.)	(100 mg.)	(150 mg.)

A variety of indwelling intravenous devices can be used to avoid the problem of repeated injections.

Intramuscular heparin. This method of administration is not recommended as there are serious disadvantages; these include the variability of effect, the risk of accumulation of effect and the painful haematomata at the injection site.

SIDE-EFFECTS OTHER THAN HAEMORRHAGE. Hypersensitivity reactions are very infrequent; but they may be alarming, and deaths have been reported but very rarely. The reactions include sneezing, rhinitis, conjunctivitis, urticaria, difficulty in expiration and praecordial tightness. In any patient with a previous history of allergic disease it is advisable to give a test dose of 1,000 units before proceeding to the full initial dose.

Fever has been ascribed occasionally to heparin, but this also is rare.

Transient alopecia developing three to four months after the heparin administration has been reported, but is infrequent.

Antagonist to heparin. When it becomes necessary to neutralize heparin urgently, protamine sulphate must be given intravenously. The potency of batches both of heparin and of protamine sulphate vary, but the usually accepted dose of protamine sulphate is 1·0 to 1·5 mg. for 1 mg. (100 units) of heparin. When heparin is given intravenously the quantity of protamine required for neutralization falls rapidly with the lapse of time following the administration of heparin. Hexadimethrine bromide should no longer be used as a heparin antagonist because of reported toxicity to the kidney. The need for a heparin antagonist usually arises as a consequence of haemorrhage of sufficient severity to warrant reversal of the anticoagulant effect.

Heparin neutralization may also be necessary before a surgical operation or other procedures, e.g. a chemical sympathectomy in a patient heparinized for acute arterial obstruction.

Clinical Uses of Heparin

(1) For the induction of anticoagulant therapy for 48 hours prior to the coumarin effect becoming established (pp. 100, 101, 141, 396); (2) in acute arterial occlusion; (3) in haemodialysis and in cardiac surgery involving extracorporeal circulation; (4) in the treatment of some patients with haemostatic failure due to intravascular coagulation.

COUMARIN AND INDANEDIONE DRUGS

These are derived from 4-hydroxycoumarin and from indane-1 : 3-dione.

COUMARIN DERIVATIVES	INDANEDIONE DERIVATIVES
Phenprocoumon	Phenindione
Warfarin sodium	Diphenadione
Nicoumalone	Anisindione
Cyclocoumarol	Chlorphenylindanedione
Dicoumarol	
Ethyl biscoumacetate	

Sensitivity reactions. It is now established that serious and sometimes fatal sensitivity reactions to the indanedione derivatives can occur whereas the coumarin drugs appear to be free, or almost free, from this hazard. Sensitivity reactions have been widely reported from phenindione; they may develop at any time from within a few days to as late as six weeks—the majority occurring at three to four weeks.

The following serious sensitivity phenomena have been reported when using phenindione: (1) skin rashes—the rash is usually erythematous and macular but may progress to exfoliative dermatitis and in such circumstances has been fatal; (2) pyrexia; (3) diarrhoea—this may be a bloody diarrhoea or steatorrhoea and fatal 'ulcerative colitis' has been reported; (4) neutropenia, agranulocytosis and thrombocytopenia—these may occur singly or in combination, and deaths have occurred; (5) hepatitis and nephropathy—these may occur singly or together and deaths have been reported.

Phenindione gained popularity in Britain as an oral anticoagulant with an intermediate duration of activity. It has been said that the safest anticoagulant drug is the one with which the clinician has the most experience, and for this reason some physicians will probably continue to use this drug. Setting aside this argument, there is now, however, a strong case for using warfarin sodium in preference to phenindione. Warfarin sodium has a similar duration of action and the dosage is approximately one-tenth that of phenindione and a change of drug is not difficult; but if a patient has already been stabilized for many months on longterm therapy with phenindione it is probably unjustifiable to change, as the period of danger from sensitivity has passed.

Haemorrhagic side-effects of coumarin and indanedione drugs. The incidence of haemorrhage reported depends on how closely the patients are studied for evidence of bleeding. Minor haemorrhage, such as microscopic haematuria, epistaxis, rectal bleeding, small bruises, subconjunctival haemorrhage, bleeding from shaving cuts, oozing from the gums, are two or three times as common as major incidents, which include macroscopic haematuria, haemoptysis, haematemesis or melaena or intracranial bleeding.

Provided the physician in charge of the patient is experienced in the use of the drug of his choice, it is improbable that the risk of haemorrhage is affected by the choice of drug in this group. It can be claimed that once haemorrhage has started there is some advantage in having a short-acting rather than a long-acting drug, but the ready availability of vitamin K_1 vitiates this argument.

Factors producing an increased risk of haemorrhage. There is an increasing risk with advancing years and the incidence of bleeding is probably twice as great in the decade 70 to 80 years as it is in the 30 to 40 age group. The general condition of the patient may predispose to bleeding; the more ill the patient, the greater the risk. Inexperience and divided responsibility in the control of therapy also increases the frequency of haemorrhage. Neglect of established contraindications and the concomitant administration of certain other drugs will increase the risk. Salicylates, in addition to the production of haemorrhage by gastric erosion, produce the same disturbance of blood coagulation as that produced by coumarin or indanedione drugs, and there may therefore, be a summation of effect.

Specific haemorrhagic complications. *Renal.* Microscopic haematuria is probably the commonest form of haemorrhage in patients on coumarin therapy. Haematuria in itself has generally not been fatal, but death has occurred in patients in whom one manifestation of defective haemostasis was renal haemorrhage.

Gastro-intestinal bleeding. About one-quarter of all deaths occurring as a direct consequence of this treatment have been due to massive gastro-intestinal bleeding from previously unsuspected peptic ulcer. Intestinal obstruction is a well-documented complication, due to bleeding into the wall of the bowel. Retroperitoneal haemorrhage may also occur. Rectal bleeding is usually from haemorrhoids and is seldom serious. If bleeding occurs in the alimentary tract when the effect of the drug is not excessive, then a pathological lesion should be sought.

Cardiovascular. The development of congestive failure makes the patient more sensitive to coumarin drugs and dosage may require adjustment.

Pulmonary. Pulmonary interstitial haemorrhage occurs as a complication of therapy and the clinical and radiological features may resemble pulmonary embolism.

Neurological. Subdural haematoma is a well-known complication and should always be considered in patients on treatment who develop headache and mental or neurological abnormalities. Patients who sustain even trivial head injuries while on anticoagulants should be followed with this possibility in mind.

Ophthalmic. Subconjunctival haemorrhages are common but usually harmless complications of therapy.

Skin. Minimal skin purpura and small spontaneous bruises are not uncommon. The platelet count should be performed to check that the purpura is not thrombocytopenic, especially if the drug used is phenindione when thrombocytopenia may occur as a toxic reaction. Haemorrhagic cutaneous necrosis is a complication of anti-coagulant therapy with coumarin or indanedione drugs, usually affecting the breast; in this there is extensive haemorrhage into the skin with ensuing necrosis and the skin may slough, leaving an ulcerated area; and this may necessitate skin grafting.

Muscle. Haemorrhage into muscle is unusual but of all the possible sites bleeding into the rectus sheath is the most common. Such patients may present to the surgeon as abdominal emergencies.

Pregnancy, puerperium and menstruation. There can be no doubt that coumarin therapy given to the pregnant patient carries a significant haemorrhagic risk to the foetus. This is not surprising since even the normal infant has a moderate deficiency of those factors which are diminished in amount by the anticoagulants that are given by mouth. There have been several reports of intra-uterine death due to haemorrhage in the foetus. If there is an urgent requirement for anticoagulant therapy during pregnancy, then heparin is the only drug which may be used. Oral anticoagulant drugs do not cause a haemostatic problem in the puerperium or in relation to menstruation. If given in the puerperium, the child should not be breast-fed because the drug is excreted in the milk.

Antagonist to coumarin and indanedione drugs. When it is necessary to counteract the effect of coumarin and indanedione drugs, vitamin K_1 should be used. The dosage given orally or intra-venously will depend on the clinical situation. When there is haemorrhage and a firm decision is taken that anticoagulants will not be reintroduced, a dose of 25 to 50 mg. should be given. Dosage of this order will render the patient resistant to further treatment for about two weeks. When there is haemorrhage, but the intention is to continue therapy, 15 mg. should be given to reduce the effect of the drug without cancelling it. When the routine test shows an excessive effect but the patient is not bleeding, 5 mg. should be given.

Laboratory control. The effect of oral anticoagulant therapy should be checked 48 hours after the start of treatment and thereafter daily or every second day until stabilization is attained. When the patient is on long-term therapy it may be sufficient to check the laboratory result every three to six weeks.

Enormous differences in drug dosage may result from different methods of laboratory control. This difficulty arises because many laboratories introduced different types of thromboplastin into the one-stage prothombin time as described by Quick in 1935. For example, acetone-extracted brain in a one-stage prothrombin time with a clotting time of twice the control value represents a much more intensive drug effect than twice the control value using a saline extract of brain. The need for a national and international standard thromboplastin is now widely accepted. This will be conducive to uniform practice in treatment. Further, there has been confusion in the expression of results, depending on whether the laboratory used the prothrombin index or the percentage as read off a saline dilution curve or made from adsorbed plasma. Methods of laboratory control such as 'thrombotest' and '2-7-10 reagent' are in no sense extraordinary but they have certain small advantages in that they make it possible to compare procedures in different centres.

The following levels of drug effect are suggested—

Using one-stage prothrombin time (with saline extract of brain)	'Thrombotest' '2-7-10 Reagent'
2 to 2½ times the control value	8 to 15 per cent.

Dosage. In Table 6 recommendations are given regarding initial doses of the more commonly used oral anticoagulant drugs and average maintenance doses. The latter must, of course, be determined for each individual patient.

Contraindications to long-term out-patient and short-term in-patient therapy. Some of the contra-indications to long-term therapy do not exclude a patient from short-term management.

General. (1) Any patient who is judged to lack sufficient intelligence to carry out the treatment or whose attendance at the clinic is irregular on account of occupation or other personal difficulties (long-term); (2) any patient who is a chronic alcoholic (long-term); (3) pregnancy (long-term and short-term); (4) any patient who may need intensive salicylate therapy (long-term).

Gastro-intestinal (long-term and short-term). (1) peptic ulcer; (2) hiatus hernia; (3) hepatic disease; (4) steatorrhoea (from any cause).

Cardiovascular (long-term and short-term). (1) Malignant hypertension; (2) any retinopathy; (3) subacute bacterial endocarditis.

TABLE 6

	Loading Dose during first 36 to 48 Hours (mg.)	Maintenance Dose	
		Range (mg.)	Average (mg.)
Phenprocoumon	27–39	0·75 to 6	3 to 4·5
Warfarin sodium	25–30	3 to 21	7·5 to 9
Nicoumalone	36–52	2 to 12	5
Cyclocoumarol	125–200	12·5 to 50	25
Dicoumarol	400–500	25 to 150	75
Ethyl biscoumacetate	1800–2400	150 to 900	450
Phenindione	200–300	25 to 200	100

Renal. (1) Blood urea over 60 mg. per 100 ml. (long-term); (2) known surgical disorder of the kidneys (long-term and short-term).

Neurological (long-term and short-term). (1) Previous cerebrovascular accident—unless embolic; (2) recent surgery or trauma to the central nervous system.

Haematological (long-term and short-term). Any patient known to have pre-existing haemostatic defect.

Therapeutic use of coumarin and indanedione drugs. SHORT-TERM THERAPY. (1) Venous thrombosis and pulmonary embolism (pp. 103-104).

(2) Superficial thrombophlebitis (p. 140). The vast majority of these patients should not be treated by anticoagulants because the condition is usually a manifestation of varicose veins. They should remain ambulant, but if for any reason such a patient has to be confined to bed, anticoagulant therapy should be given to prevent extension to the deep venous system

(3) Acute myocardial infarction (p. 99).

(4) Cerebrovascular disease—(*a*) cerebral venous

thrombosis (p. 398); (*b*) stroke in evolution (p. 396); (*c*) completed stroke (p. 397). In (*b*) and (*c*) anticoagulant therapy is *not* recommended (see text).

LONG-TERM THERAPY. (1) Rheumatic heart disease with emboli (pp. 105, 124).

(2) Long-term therapy after myocardial infarction (p. 103).

(3) Angina pectoris—the precise rôle of anticoagulant therapy in patients with angina has not been finally assessed, though there is at least one well-designed trial showing considerable reduction in death rate, and patients with acute or subacute coronary insufficiency or so-called 'ingravescent angina' should be given anticoagulant therapy.

(4) Cerebrovascular disease—(*a*) transient is-chaemic attacks—most of the available evidence indicates that anticoagulants have a rôle in this condition; (*b*) completed strokes—most of the available evidence suggests that no significant benefit is to be gained from anticoagulant therapy.

Malayan pit-viper venom: Arvin: Ancrod. Patients bitten by the Malayan pit-viper have defibrination due to a form of intravascular coagulation. The fibrin which is formed is abnormal and unstable and is thought to be removed by the reticuloendothelial system. A fraction has been prepared and used in patients and administered in such a way that controlled defibrination can be maintained for days or weeks. The possible rôle of this phenomenon in human therapeutics is under investigation.

8. Diseases of the Respiratory System

I. GORDON and I. W. B. GRANT

THE PREVENTION OF UPPER RESPIRATORY INFECTIONS

Virus infections. Many viruses are now known to cause diseases of the respiratory tract, ranging from minor upper respiratory infections, such as acute coryza and acute pharyngitis, to more serious infections, such as acute bronchitis and pneumonia. These respiratory viruses include influenza, parainfluenza and respiratory syncytial viruses, adenoviruses, rhinoviruses and many others. Although certain viruses are usually associated with a particular clinical syndrome (e.g. sore throat, pharyngoconjunctival fever), many of them are capable of infecting any part of the respiratory tract, causing clinical patterns varying from acute coryza to pneumonia.

Respiratory virus infection is often a minor illness causing only mild disability in healthy adults; but secondary bacterial infection may lead to serious complications, such as bronchitis and pneumonia, in elderly and debilitated persons, patients with heart disease and, in particular, those with chronic bronchitis, asthma and bronchiectasis. These people should avoid contact with persons in the early stage of these infections, and also should not use public transport or enter crowded places of public entertainment. Patients who are seriously incapacitated by chronic cardiac or pulmonary disease should try to remain indoors throughout the winter, and should always do so during cold and foggy weather.

Ideally, patients with acute respiratory infections should isolate themselves in their homes during the first 24 to 48 hours of the illness; failing this, they should avoid contact with others. Doctors, dentists and nurses have a special responsibility in this respect and should take particular care to avoid infecting their patients.

Vaccines. The claims made for bacterial vaccines in the prophylaxis of the common cold cannot be substantiated, and their use is, therefore, not recommended. Immunization against some types of influenza viruses and adenoviruses is effective.

Influenza virus vaccine is in an inactivated form and is prepared from virus grown in the allantoic cavity of the chick embryo. The vaccine usually contains recently isolated strains of A and B viruses likely to be prevalent in the approaching season. After a single dose of the vaccine, it is claimed that a maximum level of antibodies appear in about two weeks, and that significant protection will be afforded for 6 to 12 months. The vaccine is administered subcutaneously and local reactions are rare. It should not be given to those who have shown hypersensitivity to eggs. It has been recommended that for fuller protection, a second dose of vaccine should be given one to two months after the first. Immunization should, therefore, be given annually to all persons with chronic debilitating disease particularly those suffering from cardiac or chronic respiratory disease. Key personnel, such as doctors, nurses, policemen, etc., should also be offered vaccination.

Adenovirus vaccine (types 4 and 7) has been remarkably effective in preventing infection in military centres. Since only a small percentage of acute respiratory infections in the general population is caused by adenoviruses, vaccination, except in closed communities, is not indicated.

Streptococcal infections. The common lesions caused by *Str. pyogenes* are acute tonsillitis and pharyngitis to which older children are particularly susceptible. Infection usually occurs from direct contact with an infected person or carrier, and isolation and treatment of the individual in the early stages of infection may help to prevent the spread of the disease. Streptococcal infections can be rapidly aborted by penicillin. Thus, the prophylactic administration of this antibiotic may limit an outbreak of streptococcal infection in closed communities, e.g. schools. Penicillin is also of great value in the prevention of streptococcal infection in those children who have had rheumatic fever or rheumatic carditis (p. 106).

TREATMENT OF UPPER RESPIRATORY INFECTIONS

Acute Coryza

This is the first manifestation of many virus infections. It is seldom confined to the nose and is particularly liable to extend to other parts of the

G*

respiratory tract where secondary bacterial infection frequently develops.

Symptomatic treatment. Nasal obstruction can be temporarily relieved by the local application of vasoconstrictor drugs to the congested mucous membrane. The preparation of choice is ephedrine nasal drops B.P.C. which may be used three or four times daily. This may provide temporary symptomatic relief and may promote drainage of infected nasal sinuses. There is no evidence that other vasoconstrictor agents contained in the many proprietary preparations are superior to ephedrine and some of them may be harmful if used to excess. Antihistamine drugs are valueless in this condition and should not be prescribed.

Treatment of the established condition. Ideally all sufferers from acute virus infections should stay at home for 24 to 48 hours in a well-ventilated but warm room kept at an even temperature, in the hope that extension of bacterial infection to the nasal sinuses, larynx and bronchi will be prevented.

Aspirin may relieve fever and headache and a dose of 600 mg. may be taken three or four times a day. The tablets should be crushed and taken in milk or soluble aspirin tablets should be dissolved in milk or water. If dry cough is troublesome at night 4 to 8 ml. of linctus pholcodine may be prescribed with a hot drink. Antibiotics, whether given systemically or applied locally to the nose, are not indicated in the treatment of uncomplicated coryza, but tetracycline or ampicillin may be useful in preventing secondary bacterial infection of the bronchi and lungs in patients with chronic bronchitis and emphysema (pp. 194, 197).

One of the most useful forms of local treatment at this stage of the illness is the inhalation of steam medicated with Friar's balsam, menthol or eucalyptus. If an inhaler designed for the purpose is not available, a jug which will hold approximately 2 pints should be half-filled with water from a kettle that has been 'off the boil' for a few minutes, thus reducing the risk of scalding the patient's face or cracking the jug. One teaspoonful of Friar's balsam is added to the hot water for its sedative effect, while the addition of 2 drops of oil of eucalyptus will stimulate a freer flow of secretion. The jug is surrounded by a towel the ends of which are gathered together to form a funnel through which the patient inhales the vapour. It is advisable to keep the eyes outside the funnel in order to avoid irritation from the medicated steam. Drainage of infected sinuses may be facilitated by the application of ephedrine nasal drops B.P.C., 10 to 15 minutes before the inhalation of steam.

Acute Sinusitis

Acute sinusitis may occur in viral infections of the upper respiratory tract. Pain over the maxillary or frontal sinuses indicates blockage of the ostia of the sinuses by oedematous mucous membranes, and efforts should be made to relieve the obstruction and thus to promote drainage of the sinuses by prescribing inhalations of compound tincture of benzoin combined with the instillation of ephedrine nasal drops (B.P.C.). When purulent nasal discharge occurs, indicating secondary bacterial infection, a short course of a wide spectrum antibiotic may be useful.

Chronic Sinusitis

In all patients with chronic lung disease, e.g. chronic bronchitis or bronchiectasis, it is important to treat chronic sinusitis if this is present. Its severity may be assessed by radiological examination of the sinuses, and if gross changes are demonstrated, the patient should be referred to an Ear, Nose and Throat Surgeon for further investigation and treatment which will probably include proof puncture and lavage.

Acute Tonsillitis and Pharyngitis

Primary bacterial infection, usually caused by *Str. pyogenes*, may give rise to a severe illness characterized by fever, pharyngeal and tonsillar exudate and cervical adenitis. Milder forms of streptococcal infection may be difficult to distinguish from pharyngitis caused by virus infection. The rare occurrence of diphtheria should not be forgotten.

Streptococcal infections. It is important that infection with *Str. pyogenes* should be recognized, since penicillin therapy is rapidly effective. If the physician is uncertain whether a sore throat is due to a streptococcal or to a virus infection, penicillin should be administered at once, but swabs should first be taken from the tonsils or posterior pharynx and sent for bacteriological examination. Penicillin is effective against all strains of haemolytic streptococci and is the antibiotic of choice. In the average case phenoxymethylpenicillin should be administered by mouth in a dose of 250 mg. four times a day for seven days. If the patient is severely ill with high fever, benzylpenicillin should be given in a dose of 600 mg. twice daily by intramuscular injection, and when the temperature reaches normal oral penicillin may be substituted. In patients adequately treated with penicillin, fever and constitutional symptoms usually subside within 48 hours, though sore throat and tender cervical lymph node enlargement commonly persist for a few days longer. A course of penicillin for seven days is necessary to prevent the development of a carrier state. If symptoms of hypersensitivity to penicillin have occurred previously, tetracycline or erythromycin may be given in a dose of 250 mg. four times a day for seven days. Sulphonamides are not advised. When fever is present, rest in bed is essential and the usual measures recommended for the febrile state should be instituted. Swallowing may be painful, but an adequate intake of fluids must be encouraged.

Local treatment is not required in mild cases of streptococcal sore throat. Gargles are of little value, but when the throat is painful, lozenges containing local anaesthetics, e.g. benzocaine compound lozenges B.P.C., usually give temporary relief; after sucking a lozenge the patient may be able to swallow fluids or liquid nourishment without much discomfort. Inhalations of medicated steam (p. 192) are soothing and often allow the patient to swallow fluids more easily.

When the cervical lymph nodes are markedly enlarged and tender, the local application of heat may bring some relief. This complication almost invariably responds to penicillin: abscess formation is rare. Peritonsillar abscess has also become a rarity since the introduction of penicillin. A very small percentage of acute cases of streptococcal tonsillitis and pharyngitis develop sequelae— rheumatic fever and acute nephritis—one to three weeks after the local symptoms have subsided.

Virus infections. Local symptomatic measures such as those advised for streptococcal tonsillitis and pharyngitis are also of value for the relief of sore throat caused by virus infection. Aspirin in a dose of 600 mg. three or four times a day is usually an effective analgesic for those patients who may complain of headache in addition to sore throat.

Acute Laryngitis

When acute laryngitis occurs it is usually associated with infection of other parts of the upper respiratory tract. In severe cases, the patient should stay in bed and be given inhalations of medicated steam (p. 192). To expedite recovery, it is essential to rest the larynx by abstaining from speaking and smoking. When pain in the neck is troublesome, the application of heat by means of a rubber hot-water bottle or electric pad will bring relief. Compound benzocaine lozenges may be sucked half an hour before food if there is pain on swallowing. Painful and unproductive cough should be treated by pholcodine linctus in a dose of 4 to 8 ml. The treatment of croup and acute laryngotracheo-bronchitis in children is dealt with on p. 32.

Chronic Laryngitis

Hoarseness is the predominant symptom. The diagnosis of chronic laryngitis should never be made until malignant disease has been excluded by laryngoscopic examination.

Obvious aetiological factors such as excessive smoking and drinking must be firmly dealt with, and a change of occupation may have to be considered if the patient works in a dusty atmosphere.

The application of drugs is of little value in the treatment of chronic laryngitis though the inhalation of medicated steam (p. 192) may give some symptomatic relief. Excessive use of the voice should be discouraged; indeed complete rest of the voice for short periods may be advisable.

ACUTE BRONCHITIS

This is an acute inflammation of the mucous membrane of the trachea and bronchi caused by virus or bacterial infection. An initial virus infection is often followed by bacterial infection. The further the inflammation spreads down the bronchial tree, the more serious will be the systemic manifestations, but no sharp dividing-line exists between tracheitis, bronchitis, bronchiolitis and bronchopneumonia.

In mild cases of *tracheitis* in healthy persons, the general measures outlined below may be sufficient to control the infection. Patients with *acute bronchitis* may be seriously ill, especially if elderly and debilitated or suffering from chronic bronchitis, asthma or cardiovascular disease. In these patients, there is always the danger of extension of the infection to the lungs, and those with severe systemic disturbance should be treated as outlined in the section on pneumonia (p. 201). The treatment of acute bronchitis occurring as a complication of chronic bronchitis presents special problems and is described on p. 196; the treatment of laryngotracheobronchitis and capillary bronchitis in infants is dealt with on p. 32.

General measures. The patient should be confined to bed in a warm room in an attempt to prevent paroxysms of coughing. Hot drinks help to promote expectoration and may be given in the form of tea, coffee, cocoa, etc. The patient and his visitors should be forbidden to smoke.

Specific therapy. Chemotherapy is not indicated in cases of mild tracheitis with little systemic upset.

In acute bronchitis of *moderate severity*, an antibiotic should be administered even if fever is absent. Penicillin is usually adequate for these cases and may be given orally in the form of phenoxymethyl-penicillin in a dose of 500 mg. four times a day. Penicillin is less effective in persons with acute infective exacerbations of chronic bronchitis than in acute bronchitis occurring *de novo*. Tetracycline or ampicillin is, therefore, recommended for acute bronchitis in patients with chronic respiratory disease.

In *severe attacks* of acute bronchitis, most patients will respond to tetracycline or ampicillin given in a dose of 500 mg. four times a day.

Antibiotic therapy need not be continued for more than seven days. By this time marked clinical improvement will almost certainly have occurred, cough should not be troublesome and the pus should have cleared from the sputum. In rare cases, fever and the expectoration of purulent sputum persist in spite of chemotherapy. In these circumstances, the physician must (a) review the diagnosis and arrange forthwith for radiological examination of the chest and (b) consider whether the bronchitis is due to an organism insensitive to the antibiotic being administered. Examination of a specimen of sputum by a bacteriologist, together with sensitivity tests, will sometimes help in the selection of the appropriate antibiotic although, in general, these examinations are not of much practical value in this type of case. In hospital practice, however, cross-infection with *Staphylococcus pyogenes* must always be considered.

Symptomatic treatment. In the early stages of acute bronchitis the patient has an irritating, dry cough, often with some degree of breathlessness and wheeze, and occasionally pain or discomfort behind the sternum. These symptoms will usually subside rapidly after treatment with an antibiotic is started.

Cough. A sedative cough mixture or linctus should be prescribed when a painful non-productive cough is exhausting the patient and preventing rest and sleep. The two most suitable preparations are 4 to 8 ml. of either linctus methadone or linctus pholcodine (B.P.C.). When cough becomes pro-

ductive, drugs which suppress it should be avoided because of the danger of retention of secretions in the respiratory tract leading to aspiration pneumonia. A dry, painful cough is often associated with tenacious sputum which is difficult to expectorate, but can often be loosened by hot drinks or by the inhalation of steam. An effective prescription which has stood the test of time is sodium chloride compound mixture (B.P.C.) in doses of a tablespoonful in a tumblerful of hot water three or four times a day. Steam may be inhaled as described in the treatment of acute coryza (p. 191). A better method, which is particularly valuable in children, is the use of a steam tent in which steam from a kettle is led into a canopy erected over the head of the bed.

Expectorant cough mixtures were formerly prescribed on a large scale in the belief that they liquefied bronchial secretions and facilitated their expulsion, but they have not been shown to have a therapeutic action. Very few physicians now advocate expectorant cough mixtures and we do not recommend their use. Persistent cough after apparently adequate treatment may be due to chronic sinus infection or to broncho-pulmonary disease, such as bronchiectasis, tumour or tuberculosis. Here, further investigation is clearly essential.

Breathlessness and wheeze. Some patients with acute bronchitis may develop a clinical picture resembling that seen in bronchial asthma. When these symptoms are mild they usually respond to bronchodilator drugs. If these prove ineffective, treatment with corticosteroids should be started at once (p. 218) in combination with chemotherapy.

Retrosternal Discomfort. For retrosternal soreness, the local application of heat to the chest is of value. It is best to use a rubber hot-water bottle, filled to a third of its capacity to keep it lax and suitably covered with blanket cloth. An electrically warmed pad, when available, is a useful alternative.

CHRONIC BRONCHITIS

This is the name given to the clinical syndrome in which cough and sputum, and in some cases wheeze, have persisted or recurred frequently for a period of a year or longer. It is believed that the earliest feature of chronic bronchitis is excessive secretory activity of the mucous glands and goblet cells in response to the inhalation, for a prolonged period, of irritant substances contained in dust, smoke or fumes. These irritants may be encountered as specific occupational hazards, e.g. in mining and heavy industry, or may be discharged into the atmosphere of cities and large towns by factory and domestic chimneys. The fact that chronic bronchitis is more prevalent in Britain than in any other country in the world is mainly the result of failure to control atmospheric pollution. Britain's generally damp and cold climate may, however, be an aggravating factor. The high humidity of the atmosphere not only reduces the rate of smoke dispersal but, by dissolving some of the irritant gases such as sulphur dioxide and sulphur trioxide and converting them into acids, potentiates their action on the bronchial mucosa. Tobacco smoking, particularly of cigarettes, is an even more important cause of bronchial irritation. In some cases the onset of chronic bronchitis may date from a severe respiratory infection. An inherited constitutional predisposition is usually postulated to explain why a relatively small proportion of the many people exposed to these aetiological factors develop chronic bronchitis.

In its initial stages, chronic bronchitis may be nothing more than an excessive response to bronchial irritation and, as such, it is potentially reversible. In most cases, however, infection with *Str. pneumoniae* and/or *H. influenzae* supervenes at a relatively early stage. The infection involves not only the bronchi but also the bronchioles and their related bronchopulmonary lobules, many of which are destroyed by suppuration at each episode of infection. The development of recurrent infection leads to progressive destruction of lung tissue and eventually to respiratory insufficiency and cor pulmonale.

Wheeze is a variable feature in the clinical picture. In many cases it is due merely to inspissated mucus clinging to the bronchial walls and narrowing the airway. Wheeze of this type occurs mainly or solely in the mornings and clears after sputum is expectorated. In some patients, however, treatment is required along the lines recommended for chronic asthma (p. 216).

PREVENTION

From what has been said regarding the aetiology of chronic bronchitis, the following would appear to be the most important preventive measures: (1) the discouragement of the habit of cigarette smoking by intensive propaganda directed particularly at young people; (2) the reduction and, if possible, the elimin-

ation of general atmospheric pollution from industrial and domestic sources; (3) the improvement of working conditions, particularly in heavy industry, so as to reduce to a minimum the concentration of dust, smoke and irritant gases in factory buildings; (4) the prevention of respiratory infection and the prompt and effective treatment of all types of acute respiratory infection, especially acute bronchitis and pneumonia.

TREATMENT

Before a diagnosis of chronic bronchitis is accepted and treatment started, the chest should always be examined radiologically to exclude diseases such as bronchial carcinoma and pulmonary tuberculosis.

It is seldom possible to reverse the bronchial and pulmonary changes which have already occurred in an established case of chronic bronchitis, and treatment is essentially palliative. Nevertheless, a great deal can be done by conscientious medical care to reduce the severity of symptoms and possibly even to limit the rate of progression of the disease. Treatment is based on four main principles: (1) the prevention of further bronchial irritation; (2) the treatment of respiratory infection; (3) the control of symptoms; (4) the treatment of complications.

The prevention of further bronchial irritation. There is convincing statistical evidence that tobacco smoking is a factor of major importance in maintaining and aggravating bronchitis, the inhalation of cigarette smoke being particularly harmful. Patients are usually loath to give up tobacco, but we have seen so much benefit arising in those who have stopped smoking that we strongly advise all bronchitics to do so. Patients with chronic bronchitis often assert that the first cigarette in the morning helps them to bring up sputum and that they could not do without it. In many cases, however, the abandonment of smoking results in a marked reduction of morning cough and sputum, and renders the 'therapeutic' cigarette unnecessary.

Since atmospheric pollution is an undisputed cause of chronic bronchitis and some of its acute exacerbations, it would be logical to advise patients with this condition to move permanently to a region where pollution is absent or negligible and the climate is warm and dry. Unfortunately, such a favourable environment does not exist in any part of the United Kingdom and patients seeking it must go to the Mediterranean, South Africa, New Zealand or the West Indies. Such advice is very seldom economically or socially acceptable, but occasionally a move from a heavily polluted city to a country district may be practicable and, to a limited extent, beneficial.

A careful inquiry should always be made into the atmospheric conditions at the patient's work. Occasionally it may be possible to reduce exposure to dust by the use of a respirator or by improving ventilation in the factory or workshop, but in many cases nothing will be really effective short of a complete change of occupation. This will often be impracticable and will almost inevitably involve the patient in a serious reduction in income. Such advice should, therefore, not be given lightly.

The aggravation of bronchitic symptoms in foggy weather is well recognized, and all patients who can do so should remain at home with the doors and windows closed during periods of fog. There is indeed much to be said for advising severe chronic bronchitics who are retired or unemployed to remain indoors throughout the winter. Those who can afford to spend the winter abroad in a warm dry climate may derive great benefit from doing so.

The treatment of respiratory infection. Patients with chronic bronchitis are extremely prone to develop acute bacterial respiratory infection which may take the form of acute bronchitis or pneumonia. Bacterial infection in these circumstances is often preceded by a virus infection of the upper respiratory tract which may predispose to bacterial invasion. The most reliable indication of bacterial infection is the expectoration of purulent or muco-purulent sputum. Acute infection not only aggravates symptoms but may be expected to increase whatever permanent pulmonary damage has already been sustained; it must always be treated promptly and energetically. The most common pathogenic organisms found in the purulent sputum of chronic bronchitics are *Str. pneumoniae* and *H. influenzae*, occurring singly or together. Penicillin, being effective against *Str. pneumoniae* but not against *H. influenzae*, is thus of limited value, controlling the infection in only 50 to 60 per cent. of cases. Much better results can be obtained from the use of (1) a combination of benzylpenicillin, 300 to 600 mg. twice daily, and streptomycin sulphate, 500 mg. to 1 g. twice daily, by intramuscular injection, (2) tetracycline, 250 to 500 mg. four times daily by mouth, (3) ampicillin, 250 to 500 mg. four times daily by mouth, or (4) a combination of trimethoprim (80 mg.) and sulphamethoxazole (400 mg.) (Bactrim or Septrin),

2 tablets twice daily by mouth. The last should be used only if the others have proved ineffective as information on the frequency and severity of their side-effects is still incomplete. Very large doses of ampicillin have a bactericidal effect on *H. influenzae* and a seven-day course of 1 g. four times daily may control infection of this type for several weeks. Although expensive, it should be used in intractable cases. Streptomycin should not be given if there is renal insufficiency.

Treatment with penicillin and streptomycin, which involves twice daily injections, is unsuitable for domiciliary practice, but because it is effective and inexpensive it is still being used in hospital, particularly when the illness is acute and the patient is febrile. Tetracycline, ampicillin and trimethoprim/sulphamethoxazole combinations have the advantage of oral administration and are effective in the vast majority of cases. Chloramphenicol should not be used now that equally effective and less toxic drugs are available.

A seven-day course of an antibacterial agent usually brings an infective exacerbation of chronic bronchitis under control, but many patients will require two or three such courses every winter. It is particularly important that treatment be started immediately pus appears in the sputum; the sooner treatment is begun, the more rapid will be the response and the better chance will there be of preventing further bronchopulmonary damage. An intelligent patient may be issued with a small stock of tetracycline or ampicillin and instructed to start treatment whenever he notices the sputum becoming purulent.

In a few cases infection is so severe and persistent or so frequently recurrent that intermittent courses of antibacterial therapy are insufficient to keep it under control. In such cases continuous suppressive treatment with an antibiotic is worth a trial. Tetracycline and ampicillin are the most suitable drugs for this purpose, but neither is ideal because in some cases side-effects cause the treatment to be abandoned, while in others it fails to control the infection. Failure may be due, especially in hospital patients, to replacement of the usual pathogens by drug-resistant staphylococci or gram-negative bacilli. Bacteriological examination of the sputum should, therefore, be undertaken whenever a patient receiving continuous suppressive treatment with tetracycline or ampicillin is not making satisfactory progress.

After treatment is started, it is essential to review

critically the response to tetracycline or ampicillin at an early stage in order to make certain that the infection is being adequately controlled. A dose of 250 mg. four times a day should be prescribed, and a morning specimen of sputum should be inspected twice weekly for a fortnight. If the last two specimens are not free of pus, it is unlikely that a useful effect will be obtained, and the treatment should be stopped. If the sputum is cleared of pus, treatment should be continued at least throughout the winter.

It must be emphasized that continuous antibiotic therapy in chronic bronchitis is of value only when infection is present. It has no place in the treatment of chronic bronchitis with consistently mucoid sputum.

It is undesirable to treat pregnant women and infants with tetracycline for long periods as this may produce a brownish-yellow discoloration of the deciduous teeth.

The control of symptoms. *Cough and sputum.* There are few chronic bronchitics who do not wake up in the morning with an ineffective cough, a feeling of tightness in the chest and a slight wheeze. Such patients may derive considerable benefit from a hot drink or an alkaline mixture (sodium chloride compound mixture, B.P.C.) in hot water taken, if necessary, with a bronchodilator drug such as ephedrine or salbutamol. This should be followed by a purposeful bout of coughing and expectoration. If this simple ritual is practised every morning, the patient may be spared many paroxysms of tiresome unproductive coughing later in the day.

If the patient is expectorating larger quantities of sputum, postural coughing should be given a trial (p. 210). Our views on the traditional expectorant cough mixtures have already been stated (p. 194). Nocturnal cough should be suppressed by a sedative cough linctus only if it is unproductive of sputum.

When the sputum is mucoid, these are the only measures from which the patient is likely to benefit. There is, for example, no good evidence that the inhalation of detergent solutions or of mucolytic drugs, including bromhexine (Bisolvon), in the preparations at present available is an advance on earlier methods of liquefying tenacious sputum. The inhalation of fine droplets of plain water from an efficient nebulizer operated by air or oxygen under pressure is just as effective.

Wheeze and breathlessness. Breathlessness accompanied by wheeze, when due to reversible airways obstruction, can generally be relieved by a bronchodilator drug such as adrenaline, salbutamol, aminophylline or ephedrine (pp. 216-219). Where asthmatic features are particularly severe, however, it may be necessary to give a short course of treatment with a corticosteroid preparation (p. 216) or even, in exceptional cases, prolonged treatment of this kind (p. 217). In general, the bronchodilator drugs and the corticosteroids are less effective in this type of case than in true bronchial asthma. Infection, which often aggravates wheeze and breathlessness, must always be promptly treated (p. 196).

Treatment of complications. The treatment of the two chief complications of chronic bronchitis, viz. respiratory failure and pulmonary heart disease, is dealt with on pp. 198 and 93 respectively.

Other Measures

Obesity, which aggravates exertional dyspnoea, must be corrected by dieting. Regular exercise in the fresh air should be encouraged except during damp and foggy weather. Remedial exercises under expert supervision may help to correct faults of breathing and posture which are so common in patients with chronic bronchitis. Physiotherapy of this type is of particular value in the prevention of chest deformity in children and adolescents.

EMPHYSEMA

This term, in the clinical as distinct from the pathological sense, is commonly used to denote the state of ventilatory insufficiency which ultimately develops in many cases of chronic bronchitis and, less frequently, in other chronic respiratory diseases such as bronchial asthma. Rarely, emphysema may occur without obvious cause. The pathological features in so-called chronic bronchitis and emphysema show considerable variation from case to case. Disorganization and destruction of normal pulmonary structure are common to all; the variations chiefly involve the extent and degree of lobular suppuration, pulmonary fibrosis and alveolar distension and disruption. There is progressive impairment of ventilatory function leading to ventilatory insufficiency and finally to respiratory failure in which, even at rest, the oxygen pressure of arterial blood is reduced (normal=80–100 mm. Hg.) and the carbon dixoide pressure increased (normal=36–44 mm. Hg.). The onset of respiratory failure commonly follows a period of alveolar hypoventilation resulting from partial obstruction of the bronchi during an exacerbation of bronchitis or an attack of asthma. Pulmonary hypertension is liable to develop whenever there is a prolonged period of hypoxia and the increased load on the right ventricle often causes congestive heart failure, especially when the hypoxia and pulmonary hypertension are suddenly aggravated by a respiratory infection.

TREATMENT

As the pulmonary changes in emphysema are irreversible, any treatment can have only three limited objectives: (1) the prevention of further bronchopulmonary damage; (2) the prevention and treatment of respiratory failure and of right-sided heart failure; (3) the alleviation of dyspnoea.

The prevention of further bronchopulmonary damage depends upon the efficient management of chronic bronchitis and bronchial asthma (p. 194). The most important measures in the prevention and management of respiratory and cardiac failure are the control of respiratory infection by antibacterial agents, the maintenance of a clear airway and the correction of alveolar hypoventilation. The detailed management of respiratory failure is described below.

Symptomatic measures which have been recommended for the alleviation of dyspnoea include breathing exercises, oxygen therapy and the treatment of obesity.

There is no doubt that in emphysema pulmonary ventilation is mechanically inefficient; too little use is made of the diaphragm, and the cervical muscles are pressed into service, even though these so-called accessory muscles of respiration function by the cumbersome method of lifting the entire thoracic cage. Breathing exercises designed to correct these faulty methods are, however, of limited value. Large emphysematous bullae may compress lung tissue capable of functioning effectively, and surgical ablation of such bullae may, in carefully selected cases, be followed by a considerable improvement in respiratory function.

Patients with a severe degree of ventilatory insufficiency often obtain substantial symptomatic benefit from the inhalation of oxygen. Given for a few minutes after washing, bed making, defaecation or similar exertion, the relief it brings to a patient in severe respiratory distress may be considerable. The National Health Service has now made pro-vision for oxygen to be supplied to such patients in their homes. A portable apparatus for the administration of oxygen can be provided on loan by the hospital service (p. 650). This may enable patients otherwise rendered bed-fast by respiratory distress to walk about the house in relative comfort and even to go out occasionally.

Obese patients will always derive some symptomatic benefit from a reduction in weight. As many obese emphysematous patients are incapable of much physical activity, weight reduction may be difficult to achieve and a diet of 800 Cal. or even less may have to be prescribed. In advanced cases with severe hypoxia, however, marked loss of weight may occur spontaneously.

Drugs are of little or no value in the treatment of emphysema itself, but must, of course, be used for the control of respiratory infection and bronchospasm. Patients with intolerably distressing dyspnoea may benefit from chlorpromazine in a dose of 25 to 50 mg. thrice daily, which presumably acts by making them less conscious of their respiratory difficulty. Consideration must always be given to the nature of the patient's occupation and to his conditions of work. If his job is too heavy or if his place of work is particularly damp or dusty, an attempt should be made, with the help of resettlement agencies, to find him more suitable employment.

RESPIRATORY FAILURE

Respiratory failure can be defined as a state in which respiratory function is so seriously impaired that the partial pressures of oxygen and carbon dioxide in the arterial blood cannot be kept within the normal range. Dyspnoea at rest and central cyanosis, the two cardinal clinical features of respiratory failure, are often accompanied by neurological manifestations of hypoxia and hypercapnia (muscle twitching, mental confusion and coma) and also in many cases by congestive cardiac failure. The diagnosis can readily be confirmed by estimation of the partial pressures of oxygen and carbon dioxide and of the pH of a sample of arterial blood. In most patients with respiratory failure the arterial oxygen pressure at rest is below 50 mm. Hg. and if the failure is of ventilatory origin the carbon dioxide pressure is usually above 60 mm. Hg.

Ventilatory failure is likely to supervene in patients with chronic bronchitis and emphysema when they develop acute respiratory infections. In this type of respiratory failure, hypoxia is accompanied by retention of carbon dioxide (hypercapnia) which is probably the chief cause of the headache and drowsiness of which these patients may complain, particularly when oxygen is administered. The congestive cardiac failure which frequently accompanies respiratory failure is the result of pulmonary hypertension caused by hypoxia. Respiratory failure due to alveolar hypoventilation may also occur in a variety of other conditions such as bronchial asthma, kyphoscoliosis, gross obesity and paralytic poliomyelitis.

Respiratory failure of a different type occurs when the normal balance of ventilation and perfusion within the lung is disturbed, as in less advanced cases of chronic bronchitis and emphysema, and in all forms of interstitial lung disease. This type of respiratory failure differs from that due to generalized alveolar hypoventilation in that reduction of arterial oxygen partial pressure is not accompanied by retention of carbon dioxide.

TREATMENT

Acute ventilatory failure is a serious medical emergency, but is often amenable to energetic treatment. The patient is generally a middle-aged or elderly man with chronic bronchitis and emphysema who has recently developed an acute respiratory infection and has relapsed in the last day or two into a state of respiratory distress, accompanied by mental confusion or even coma. The patient's increasing difficulty in expectoration and deepening cyanosis may have been noticed by observant relatives.

The therapeutic problem in these cases is fourfold: (1) to clear the air passages of secretion; (2) to increase alveolar ventilation; (3) to increase the oxygen content of the inspired air; and (4) to treat the complication which precipitated respiratory failure, usually infection, but less commonly bronchospasm.

Even the most energetic treatment of respiratory infection is unlikely to have much effect on respiratory function for 24 to 48 hours, and control of bronchospasm also takes time. The correct policy, therefore, is to give urgent attention to the first three items mentioned above. The action required under each of these headings will depend on the degree of ventilatory failure which should, wherever possible, be accurately assessed by measurement of the partial pressures of oxygen and carbon dioxide in arterial blood, and of the pH (pp. 644-646).

Incipient Ventilatory Failure

At this stage the patient is fully conscious and co-operative; he has only a moderate degree of central cyanosis, is capable of coughing fairly effectively and has an arterial carbon dioxide pressure of less than 60 mm. Hg. In such a case the following measures are usually sufficient to increase and maintain alveolar ventilation until the process which precipitated respiratory failure has been controlled.

Supervised coughing. The patient is visited by a nurse or physiotherapist at hourly or half-hourly intervals and encouraged to make strenuous efforts to cough up sputum.

Oxygen. Controlled oxygen therapy (p. 648) must be given continuously by Ventimask, Edinburgh mask or nasal cannula (p. 649), starting with an estimated concentration of oxygen in the inspired air of about 28 per cent. If this causes drowsiness or an increase in the arterial carbon dioxide pressure, the concentration should be reduced to 24 per cent. Such patients would then be regarded as having moderately severe respiratory failure and should be treated accordingly.

No drug (opiate or barbiturate) with a depressant action on the respiratory centre should on any account be prescribed. Indeed, large doses of any hypnotic must be avoided, since expectoration should be encouraged whenever the patient is awake. Restless patients or those unable to sleep should be given either 1 g. of triclofos by mouth or 5 to 10 mg. of diazepam intramuscularly.

Moderately Severe Ventilatory Failure

At this stage the patient is confused and drowsy but can be roused; breathing is shallow and cyanosis fairly marked; cough is ineffective and secretions can be heard rattling in the larynx and trachea; the arterial carbon dioxide pressure is usually above 60 mm. Hg. If the condition of a patient with incipient ventilatory failure fails to respond to treatment or if he presents *de novo* with moderately severe ventilatory failure the following regimen should be adopted:

The bronchi should be cleared of secretion by aspiration through a bronchoscope or, if that is not possible, by suction applied to a polythene tube passed into the trachea and bronchi by means of a laryngoscope. The improvement in ventilation and oxygenation obtained in this way is often sufficient to restore the patient's ability to cough effectively so that he can then resume regular supervised coughing.

Oxygen. In all cases controlled oxygen therapy (p. 648) must be given, starting with an inspired oxygen concentration of 24 per cent.

Respiratory stimulants. Nikethamide, 2-4 ml., combined with aminophylline, 500 mg., should be injected intravenously every one to two hours or more frequently according to the patient's level of consciousness and depth of respiration. These drugs can be injected as a bolus into the tubing of an intravenous drip in order to spare the patient frequent venepunctures.

Dichlorphenamide, a carbonic anhydrase inhibitor, stimulates respiration by producing a severe metabolic acidosis. It is occasionally of value in severe chronic ventilatory failure when hypoxia and hypercapnia cannot be controlled by other measures, but the drug is potentially dangerous and should not be used unless facilities are available for monitoring the arterial blood gas pressures and pH.

Severe Respiratory Failure

At this stage the patient is semiconscious or comatose, deeply cyanosed, incapable of coughing and in danger of drowning in his secretions. If there is time or opportunity to measure the arterial carbon dioxide pressure, it will probably be about 80 mm. Hg., or even higher if oxygen has been given. Only immediate action by a well-equipped and practised team is likely to save the patient's life. The following regimen is now standard practice in such cases:

(1) A bronchoscope is passed at once (an anaesthetic is usually not required) and the trachea and bronchi are cleared of secretions. Toilet of the pharynx and larynx is performed at the same time.

(2) As soon as the bronchoscope is withdrawn, 5 to 10 ml. of nikethamide is injected intravenously. In most cases consciousness is quickly but temporarily restored. When this occurs, the patient must immediately be encouraged to cough up sputum.

(3) Controlled oxygen therapy (24 per cent. inspired air concentration) must be given to correct cerebral hypoxia which is the chief danger to life in this condition.

(4) If these measures are not effective, a cuffed tube should be passed through the mouth into the trachea and connected to an intermittent positive-pressure apparatus (p. 652). Aspiration of bronchial secretions with a 'whistle-tip' rubber catheter should be carried out every half to one hour at first and at longer intervals as the amount diminishes.

The patient should be turned from side to side at regular intervals to ensure that secretion is removed from both main bronchi. It may be possible to discontinue artificial ventilation after 24 to 48 hours, and to maintain the improvement in the patient's condition by controlled oxygen therapy, supervised coughing and respiratory stimulants. In some cases, however, a longer period of artificial ventilation may be required and tracheostomy must then be undertaken.

(5) Congestive cardiac failure, when present, should be treated with diuretics (p. 88). Digoxin is seldom of any immediate value, but it may be given later, together with a diuretic in regular dosage and a low salt diet, if signs of congestive cardiac failure persist.

It should always be borne in mind that resuscitative measures of this kind involve patients in a good deal of physical discomfort and mental anguish. They should, therefore, be undertaken only when there is a reasonable prospect of success. The criterion of success should not be mere survival, but survival in a reasonably comfortable state. Patients who have been respiratory cripples for months before the illness which precipitated failure are quite unsuitable for this form of treatment. Those with fairly good respiratory function who have been rapidly plunged into respiratory failure by a severe infection often make a remarkable recovery and may survive in relatively good health for several years.

The treatment of respiratory failure in interstitial lung disease is described on p. 222.

THE PNEUMONIAS

Since the discovery of effective bacteriostatic and bactericidal drugs for the treatment of pneumonia, it is usual to classify the pneumonias, as far as is possible, on an aetiological basis. Not all of them can be classified bacteriologically, since in the individual patient several other factors may also be concerned. It is convenient, however, to divide them into two main groups—specific pneumonias and aspiration pneumonias.

THE SPECIFIC BACTERIAL PNEUMONIAS. These may be caused by (a) *Streptococcus pneumoniae* (pneumococcus), (b) *Staphylococcus pyogenes*, (c) gram-negative bacilli, such as *Klebsiella pneumoniae* (Friedländer's bacillus) and (d) *Mycobacterium tuberculosis*.

In this group, the pathogenic organisms can be

isolated from the sputum during life or from the lung at autopsy in pure or almost pure culture. By far the most common organism in these cases is *Str. pneumoniae*, the cause of pneumococcal pneumonia, which was previously referred to as lobar pneumonia. During an influenza epidemic, though *Str. pneumoniae* will probably remain the most common causative agent in cases of pneumonia, staphylococcal infection may cause a fulminant illness ('*influenzal-staphylococcal*' pneumonia).

THE SPECIFIC PNEUMONIAS CAUSED BY VIRUSES, BEDSONIAE, MYCOPLASMATA AND RICKETTSIAE. Several viruses are known to cause pneumonia, and certain organisms resembling viruses—bedsoniae, mycoplasmata and rickettsiae—can produce a similar type of illness. The viruses include those of influenza, measles and chickenpox, respiratory syncytial virus and adenovirus, but in some cases the development of pneumonia may be due not to the virus itself but to secondary bacterial infection. Bedsoniae of the ornithosis (psitticosis) group, *Mycoplasma pneumoniae* and *Rickettsia (Coxiella) burneti* (Q-fever) may all cause specific pneumonias resembling those produced by viruses.

THE ASPIRATION PNEUMONIAS. The organisms causing this group of pneumonias consist of bacteria derived from the upper respiratory tract and the mouth, e.g. pneumococci, staphylococci, streptococci, *H. influenzae* and rarely anaerobes such as Vincent's spirochaetes and fusiform bacilli. Aspiration pneumonias may arise in a variety of ways.

Diffuse aspiration bronchopneumonia. This type of pneumonia results from an extension of infection from the widespread aspiration of infected secretions into the alveoli from the smaller bronchi. In elderly, bedridden patients, too weak to cough effectively, a similar type of aspiration pneumonia may develop, when secretions, infected by organisms of low virulence derived from the upper respiratory passages, gravitate to the lung bases (*hypostatic pneumonia*).

Localized aspiration pneumonia. The least serious type of pneumonia in this group is *benign aspiration pneumonia*. A cold in the head accompanied by purulent sinusitis is followed by the aspiration of pus into the lower respiratory tract. The pneumonia may be of such a mild degree as to be recognizable only by radiological examination of the lungs.

Occasionally *acute suppurative pneumonia* de-velops, and when the suppuration is localized and intense, a lung abscess develops. During operations on sinuses, teeth and tonsils, the aspiration of septic material may lead first to atelectasis and then to aspiration pneumonia.

Similarly, during and after operations on the thorax and abdomen, tenacious secretion may be aspirated from the upper respiratory passages leading to bronchial obstruction and pulmonary collapse, which is readily followed by infection—the so-called *post-operative aspiration pneumonia*.

Pneumonia may also result from the aspiration of pus from a pre-existing suppurative lesion of the lung, e.g. bronchiectasis or lung abscess, into a healthy portion of lung.

The most important single factor in the production of aspiration pneumonia is inadequate drainage of the respiratory passages. Thus, aspiration pneumonia will be facilitated by suppression of the cough mechanism by drugs or anaesthesia, by severe pain in the chest or abdomen or by physical weakness. Patients with pre-existing bronchial or pulmonary disease are particularly susceptible.

TREATMENT

The treatment of the pneumonias will be dealt with as follows (1) general measures, (2) symptomatic treatment, (3) specific therapy, (4) the treatment of complications.

General Measures

Before the discovery of sulphonamide drugs and antibiotics, the treatment of pneumonia consisted essentially of good nursing and symptomatic treatment. Specific chemotherapy has shortened the duration of the illness dramatically. Nevertheless, the physician will have to care for many cases of pneumonia in which chemotherapy is less effective and the illness more severe and protracted. Examples of such cases are bronchopneumonia in the elderly and in chronic bronchitics, and staphylococcal pneumonia complicating influenza. Here good nursing is essential, and in the case of influenzal-staphylococcal pneumonia, there are special problems which can only be dealt with adequately in hospital. Many patients with pneumonia may be treated in their own homes, but if the conditions there are unsatisfactory admission to hospital should be recommended. If it is decided to treat the patient at home, he should be nursed in a warm room with plenty of fresh air. Skilled nursing is essential for the elderly.

The patient should be permitted to assume the position in bed which he finds most comfortable. In general, this is in the inclined position, the back being supported by pillows or a back rest. In old and debilitated persons the nurse should alter the patient's position in bed from time to time in order to prevent the pooling of secretions in dependent parts of the lungs. Encouragement to cough up sputum at regular intervals is also of great importance. Ample amounts of fluid must always be given.

The danger of thrombosis in the deep veins of the calf muscles must always be remembered and measures taken to prevent it (p. 141). The legs should be inspected daily in patients liable to this complication. Active and passive movements of the lower limbs and deep-breathing exercises should be regularly carried out as soon as the patient's condition permits. Other nursing measures are described in the section on the general management of the febrile state (p. 24).

Symptomatic Treatment

Pain in the chest. With modern chemotherapy, the duration of pain is generally so short that simple measures, e.g. a hot-water bottle and a mild analgesic, are adequate to control it. If not, methadone, 5 to 10 mg. by mouth, or pethidine, 50 to 100 mg. by intramuscular injection, may be given, but as such drugs are apt to depress cough and respiration, they should be used with caution, particularly in patients with impaired respiratory function and much bronchial secretion. Morphine, which has a similar but even more powerful effect, is best avoided altogether. Strapping of the chest for the relief of pleuritic pain is undesirable, since by restricting movement of the chest wall it may cause bronchial secretions to be retained and result in interference with resolution or even in pulmonary collapse.

Cough. In the early stages of the illness, when cough is painful and unproductive, methadone linctus (B.P.C.), 4 to 8 ml., may be prescribed. When sputum is present, the patient should be encouraged to cough at regular intervals and thus clear his respiratory passages. There is no evidence that the so-called expectorant cough mixtures are any more effective in pneumonia than in acute bronchitis.

Insomnia. Relief of pain in the chest and of distressing dry cough will often help the patient to sleep. Routine nursing attention must not be neglected. Sponging with tepid water, rearranging the bedclothes, placing the patient in a comfortable position, getting him to pass urine and giving him a hot drink, are simple measures which are often effective. Adequate sleep is important in the elderly patient and hypnotics will often be required. Barbiturates are best avoided in the elderly, since they so often produce mental confusion and restlessness. Triclofos (1 to 2 g) and nitrazepam (5 to 10 mg) are useful alternatives: When these fail, diazepam, 10 mg by intramuscular injection, is usually effective. Alcohol, particularly in those accustomed to taking it regularly, often promotes rest and sleep.

Hypoxia. Hypoxia (p. 644) is common in pneumonia. The presence of even slight central cyanosis in a patient with pneumonia must be regarded as a serious development to be treated immediately by the administration of oxygen in high concentration (p. 647). Patients in whom the pneumonia has supervened on chronic respiratory disease may require controlled oxygen therapy.

Delirium. Any patient with a temperature of 39° C. or higher may become delirious, but when the temperature is reduced by tepid sponging the mental confusion usually subsides rapidly. When delirium is associated with central cyanosis it is probably the result of cerebral hypoxia, and the continuous administration of oxygen is essential. Unfortunately, patients who are mentally confused, restless and apprehensive are often violently intolerant of oxygen masks and some form of sedation is required to permit the administration of oxygen. The dilemma with which the doctor is faced in these circumstances is that in order to quieten the patient he may be forced to administer a drug which is liable to depress respiration and thus aggravate hypoxia. There is no satisfactory solution to this problem, but for rapid control of delirium chlorpromazine and paraldehyde are more effective than barbiturates and safer than opiates. The recommended dosage for chlorpromazine is 50 to 100 mg. intramuscularly or intravenously and for paraldehyde 4 to 8 ml. intramuscularly. Whenever either of these drugs is given, the patient must be closely watched for signs of respiratory failure.

Specific Therapy

Specific therapy must be started on the basis of the clinical diagnosis before the physician has knowledge of the infecting organism and its sensitivity to antibiotics. Since the majority of cases of pneumonia are caused by *Str. pneumoniae*, penicillin should be started by intramuscular injection without delay. In all seriously ill patients and in those with chronic bronchitis, emphysema or asthma, both penicillin and streptomycin are required. The addition of streptomycin may be of considerable advantage in combating infection with *H. influenzae* an organism commonly found in the sputum in chronic bronchitis. As an alternative, ampicillin, which is effective against both *Str. pneumoniae* and *H. influenzae*, may be given by mouth in a dose of 500 mg. four times a day. If staphylococcal pneumonia is suspected on clinical grounds, it should be assumed that the organism may be resistant to penicillin, streptomycin, the tetracyclines and ampicillin. Accordingly, in these cases cloxacillin or sodium fusidate, combined with erythromycin, should be used from the start, since staphylococci in this country have not so far shown much resistance to these antibiotics.

Immediately before treatment is started, a specimen of sputum should be sent to a bacteriological laboratory for culture and for tests of sensitivity of the predominant organism to penicillin and other antibiotics. While this is the usual practice in hospital, it is certainly not indispensable. When the bacteriological reports become available, the physician should also assess the clinical response to the antibiotic used, bearing in mind that there are sometimes disparities between the results of the sensitivity tests carried out on culture media and the effectiveness of an antibiotic in a particular patient. It has been shown that in almost one-third of cases of pneumonia no pathogenic organism is isolated from the sputum. Why this should be so has not yet been determined, but the response to treatment has usually been the same as in those cases in which a pneumococcus has been isolated from the sputum.

Pneumococcal pneumonia. Penicillin is the drug of choice in the treatment of pneumococcal pneumonia, but patients who have previously exhibited hypersensitivity to it should be given tetracycline or erythromycin.

Penicillin (benzylpenicillin B.P.) should be administered intramuscularly in an initial dose of 600 mg. which may be repeated at 12-hourly intervals for three or four doses. Thereafter, if the clinical response has been satisfactory and the temperature has fallen to normal, penicillin may be continued by mouth in the form of phenoxymethylpenicillin, 250 mg. four times a day. To prevent recurrence of infection, treatment should be main-

tained until the temperature has been normal for at least four days. In most cases of pneumonia, penicillin thus given produces dramatic clinical improvement and a rapid fall in temperature.

If there has been no response to penicillin within 48 hours, the physician should (*a*) review the diagnosis of pneumonia and consider the possibilities of pulmonary infarction, infection distal to bronchial carcinoma, pulmonary abscess, empyema or tuberculous pleural effusion and (*b*) consider the possibility that the pneumonia is caused by organisms insensitive to penicillin. If a specimen of sputum has been sent to a bacteriological laboratory for culture and sensitivity tests before the start of treatment, a report should now be available which may be of great value in determining the correct form of specific therapy. If no such information is available and staphylococcal pneumonia is not suspected, an antibacterial agent with a wide therapeutic range (tetracycline, ampicillin or a trimethoprim-sulphamethoxazole combination) should be substituted.

Tetracycline, ampicillin, erythromycin or trimethoprim-sulphamethoxazole. The usual dosage of the first three drugs is 500 mg. four times a day until the temperature has returned to normal; thereafter it can be reduced to 250 mg. four times a day. Trimethoprim-sulphamethoxazole combinations (p. 2) are prescribed in a dose of 2 tablets twice daily.

Chloramphenicol. Now that other equally effective antibiotics are available this potentially dangerous drug should not be used.

Staphylococcal pneumonia. Staphylococcal pneumonia is an important complication of influenza although there is evidence that the virus by itself may occasionally cause death from haemorrhagic tracheobronchitis and bronchopneumonia without demonstrable staphylococci or other pathogenic organisms in the lungs at necropsy. Nevertheless, combined infection with these two organisms is notoriously liable to produce a type of pneumonia which is always serious and often rapidly fatal. Staphylococcal pneumonia may also occur *de novo* or secondary to a focus of staphylococcal infection elsewhere in the body.

All patients suffering from staphylococcal pneumonia present special features often requiring measures which are not available at home. Accordingly such patients should be transferred to hospital at the earliest opportunity. The administration of an antibiotic to which the staphylococci are sensitive is obviously of vital importance. In recent years, staphylococci resistant to benzyl penicillin and tetracycline have become increasingly prevalent and selection of the correct antibiotic is often difficult. If penicillin has been administered initially, and the patient is making satisfactory progress, it should be continued until the results of sputum culture and tests of sensitivity become available. If, however, there has been no clinical improvement, if it is suspected that the patient is harbouring resistant staphylococci, or if the illness is of a fulminant character, he should immediately receive an antibiotic or preferably a combination of antibiotics to which the staphylococci are unlikely to be resistant.

Initially, 500 mg. of cloxacillin and 500 mg. of erythromycin should be given four times a day by mouth, but if the patient is gravely ill they should both be given intravenously in half the oral dose for the first 24 hours. When the results of sensitivity tests are available appropriate modifications in treatment can be made. Other antibiotics which may prove effective against staphylococci include cephaloridine, lincomycin and sodium fusidate. The disadvantage of the last drug is that it is available only for oral administration. Although there are very few reports of *in vitro* resistance to either cloxacillin or sodium fusidate this is unfortunately not an absolute guarantee against a fatal outcome in fulminating staphylococcal pneumonia. The prognosis is, however, much more favourable if treatment with the correct antibiotic is begun at the earliest possible stage and continued for two to three weeks.

When hypoxia is present, oxygen should always be administered continuously in a high concentration. A restless patient is often better nursed in an oxygen tent (p. 648). The treatment of peripheral circulatory failure (bacteraemic shock) which is a frequent and serious complication of staphylococcal pneumonia is discussed on p. 111.

In so-called *influenzal-staphylococcal* pneumonia, the trachea and bronchi occasionally become obstructed by a haemorrhagic, necrotic, purulent exudate. It is of the utmost importance to recognize the clinical picture of partial respiratory obstruction, since death from asphyxia may be averted by timely aspiration of the tracheal and bronchial exudate by bronchoscopy or tracheostomy (p. 199).

Staphylococcal respiratory infection followed by pneumonia may be a serious hazard in hospital wards and the hospital staphylococcus is almost invariably resistant to penicillin and tetracycline. Furthermore, patients treated with these antibiotics, particularly chronic bronchitics, are susceptible to secondary infection by this organism. Ideally, when resistant staphylococci are prevalent in a hospital ward, all patients suffering from chronic bronchitis or other chronic respiratory infections should be confined to single side-rooms. This is seldom feasible and the best that can usually be done to prevent cross-infection is to isolate all patients who are known to be disseminating staphylococci.

Pneumonia due to Gram-negative organisms. Pneumonia caused by Gram-negative bacilli is an uncommon but serious illness and usually occurs in elderly patients suffering from chronic bronchitis, diabetes mellitus and other debilitating diseases. The organisms—*Klebsiella pneumoniae, Escherichia coli, Pseudomonas aeruginosa, Haemophilus influenzae* and various strains of *Proteus vulgaris*—may be grown in pure culture from the sputum. Antibiotics such as tetracycline, ampicillin, kanamycin and colomycin should be given initially, but guidance in the choice of an antibiotic will be indicated by the results of the sensitivity tests of organisms cultured from the sputum or blood. Gram-negative organisms may be isolated from the sputum of patients who have had antibiotic therapy in high dosage for a week or longer, but in these cases the organisms are not usually pathogenic and they disappear when the antibiotic is stopped. All patients from whom Gram-negative organisms are cultured should be kept under close observation since there is always a possibility that they may develop septicaemia with peripheral circulatory failure (bacteraemic shock) (p. 111).

Pneumonia due to *Klebsiella pneumoniae* causes massive lobar consolidation with cavitation, especially affecting the upper lobes, and permanent damage to the lungs may result. Streptomycin together with chloramphenicol is the treatment of choice and should be given until the sensitivities become known. Streptomycin is given in a dose of 1 g. intramuscularly twice daily with 250 to 500 mg. of chloramphenicol by mouth six-hourly. As soon as the temperature falls to normal, the dose of streptomycin should be reduced to 500 mg. twice daily and given for three or four days longer, while chloramphenicol is continued for a further week if the organism is sensitive to it. In elderly persons, streptomycin may cause vestibular dysfunction and deafness, but provided renal failure is not present these toxic effects seldom appear if the total dose of the drug given is less than 10 g.

Tuberculous pneumonia. See p. 75.

Pneumonia due to bedsoniae. This infection (ornithosis or psittacosis) is rare in Great Britain. The recommended treatment is tetracycline in a dose of 500 mg. four times daily for a week.

Pneumonia due to mycoplasma pneumoniae (*Eaton agent*). This may cause pneumonia, particularly in young adults. The illness, which is usually mild, normally responds to treatment with tetracycline in a dose of 500 mg. four times daily.

Virus and rickettsial pneumonia. No specific therapy is available against the viruses of influenza and measles. The secondary bacterial infection should be treated on the lines already described.

Occasional outbreaks of pneumonia caused by adenoviruses and other respiratory viruses have been reported in schools and Service establishments. The illness is a benign one and antibiotics are scarcely necessary, nor is there much evidence that they are effective.

Pneumonia occurs in Q fever. The treatment recommended is tetracycline given orally in a dose of 500 mg. four times a day. When the patient is afebrile, the dose may be reduced to 250 mg. four times daily.

The Aspiration Pneumonias

The main principle in the prevention of aspiration pneumonia is the effective drainage by both posture and coughing of secretions in the lungs and bronchi in all cases of respiratory infection. Maintenance of the cough mechanism is important. The inhalation of infected material from sinuses, tonsils and teeth during sleep and following operations in these regions should be remembered as a cause of aspiration pneumonia and precautions taken to eliminate this risk. In patients with bronchiectasis or lung abscess, postural coughing at regular intervals prevents this type of pneumonia which arises from the aspiration of infected material from a diseased to a healthy part of the lung.

DIFFUSE ASPIRATION BRONCHOPNEUMONIA. This type of pneumonia is commonly seen in elderly persons with chronic bronchitis of long standing and is often a more serious illness than pneumococcal pneumonia. The antibiotic regimen of choice is benzylpenicillin, 300 to 600 mg. together with streptomycin, 500 mg. to 1 g., administered intramuscularly twice daily for approximately seven days. Alternatively, tetracycline or ampicillin may be given for the same period in a dose of 500 mg. four times daily. Vigorous measures to promote expectoration by coughing and by posture must be instituted. Many of these patients will be too ill or too breathless to tolerate postural drainage, but much can be achieved merely by encouragement to cough, which should be given frequently by a nurse or physiotherapist. Ventilatory failure is a common complication when patients with advanced chronic bronchitis and emphysema develop diffuse aspiration pneumonia. The treatment of this complication is described on p. 197.

LOCALIZED ASPIRATION PNEUMONIA. The most common form is benign aspiration pneumonia caused by inhalation of bacteria from the nose or nasal sinuses. The diagnosis is made from the finding of segmental consolidation on the chest radiograph. The condition is best treated with tetracycline or ampicillin, 250 mg. four times a day for seven days. Drainage of infected secretions should be encouraged by postural coughing.

POST-OPERATIVE ASPIRATION PNEUMONIA. This type of pneumonia is sometimes of the diffuse variety but more often of the localized aspiration type. The onset is usually sudden and occurs during the first 24 to 48 hours after the operation. Initially, there is atelectasis secondary to bronchial obstruction caused by retention of inspissated mucus or purulent secretion. Numerous factors predispose to sputum retention, but if steps are taken to correct these beforehand, the liability to post-operative pulmonary complications will be greatly reduced.

Prophylaxis before operation. Non-urgent operations should always be postponed in patients with acute bronchitis or even a cold in the head. This should also be advised in patients with chronic bronchitis who are producing purulent sputum. Such patients should be treated with an appropriate antibiotic (p. 5) combined with postural drainage and breathing exercises. Smoking, which is an important factor in producing chest complications, should be forbidden for at least two weeks prior to operation. Obesity should be corrected by dieting if time permits.

Prophylaxis after operation. After all major operations the position of the patient should be changed at least every four hours. The nurse should remove the pillows, place the patient on each side in turn, and instruct him to cough. After abdominal and thoracic operations, coughing is painful but must be encouraged. It will be easier for the patient to cough if a nurse supports the wound firmly with her hand. Constricting bandages around the lower part of the chest and abdomen interfere with expansion of the lower lobes and should never be allowed. The suppression of cough, for example by pain in the wound, is a potent factor in the production of atelectasis, and a small dose of morphine, not more than 10 mg., may relieve the pain sufficiently to enable the patient to cough without discomfort. Larger doses of morphine are contraindicated, since they depress the cough reflex, and not even a small dose should be given to patients with emphysema. Atropine should not be used after operation as it increases the viscosity of bronchial mucus.

Treatment. The main aim of treatment is to help the patient to dislodge and cough up the inspissated secretions which are obstructing the bronchi. In most cases this can be done by simple measures, the most effective being encouragement to cough. If the patient is not too distressed, coughing should be carried out in the prone position with the foot of the bed raised and the pillows removed, so that the bases of the lungs are uppermost. This position is usually the correct one, since the bronchi to the lower lobes are those most commonly obstructed. Additional measures include hot drinks at frequent intervals and the inhalation of salbutamol if wheezing is present. To prevent or combat infection a combination of penicillin and streptomycin or alternatively tetracycline or ampicillin, should be administered in every case. Cyanosis and dyspnoea call for the continuous administration of oxygen.

If the above measures fail and atelectasis still persists at the end of 24 hours, bronchoscopy should be carried out to remove obstructing secretions.

Complications of pneumonia

A mortality rate of about 5 per cent. is still recorded in pneumonia, and this can be attributed to a number of causes. It is still a dangerous illness in old people; sometimes there is delay in treatment or the bacterial infection is overwhelming, and often patients with chronic disease of the lungs or co-existing heart disease fare badly when they contract pneumonia. With modern treatment the incidence of complications is low, but some of them may be fatal if they are not recognized at an early stage and adequately treated.

Circulatory failure. Circulatory failure in pneumonia may present in the form of either cardiac failure or peripheral circulatory failure which not uncommonly co-exist.

Cardiac failure. Where circulatory failure is primarily central, its most common causes are atrial fibrillation and pulmonary heart disease (cor pulmonale).

Atrial fibrillation, supraventricular and other dysrhythmias may develop in the course of pneumonia, especially in elderly patients, and if these persist for more than two or three days with a rapid ventricular rate, congestive cardiac failure is likely to supervene. The patient should be rapidly and fully digitalized (p. 86), and if frank congestive heart failure with peripheral and pulmonary oedema is present, other measures will be required, e.g. a low salt diet and diuretics. Digitalization often leads to the restoration of sinus rhythm, but when the dysrhythmia persists, a maintenance dose of digoxin may have to be continued indefinitely.

If pneumonia occurs in a patient with advanced chronic bronchitis and emphysema, pulmonary hypertension may be produced or aggravated. This frequently leads to right ventricular failure, which must be treated along the usual lines (p. 93). The main cause of the pulmonary hypertension is hypoxia which must be relieved by controlled oxygen therapy (p. 648). It is also imperative to treat the pneumonic infection as speedily as possible.

Peripheral circulatory failure. This remains one of the commonest causes of death in pneumonia. It tends to occur in the elderly and in fulminant and inadequately treated cases. It is probably due to a combination of septicaemia or bacteraemia, hypoxia and hypovolaemia. Patients with pneumonia due to Gram-negative organisms may suffer sudden and profound circulatory failure (bacteraemic shock). Prompt administration of the correct antibiotic is of vital importance in these cases.

Hypovolaemia must be corrected by infusion of glucose or dextran, with monitoring of the central venous pressure to avoid circulatory overload.

The administration of corticosteroids when peripheral circulatory failure has developed is a matter on which there is some controversy. The results of corticosteroid therapy have in general been discouraging though some spectacular recoveries attributed to this therapy have been recorded. If it is decided to use corticosteroids, hydrocortisone sodium succinate, should be given intravenously in a single massive dose of 1 to 3 g. as soon as signs of peripheral failure become apparent and the dose may be repeated in an hour or given by intravenous drip.

The results of the administration of vasopressor drugs to combat hypotension in circulatory failure have been disappointing and when this complication supervenes in pneumonia their use is probably contraindicated.

Pleural effusion. Serous fluid in the pleural cavity occasionally complicates pneumonia, particularly of the pneumococcal type. Before the advent of specific therapy such pleural effusions rapidly became purulent, but treatment of the pneumonia with antibiotics usually prevents the development of empyema. Whenever an effusion is suspected, aspiration of the fluid should be carried out (p. 637). A specimen of the fluid should be sent for culture. Further aspiration should be undertaken if the effusion recurs. In most cases, no pathogenic organisms will be cultured from the fluid.

Delayed resolution. The physician's responsibility for the patient with pneumonia does not end until complete resolution has occurred. This may be delayed because of senility or structural disease of the lung (advanced chronic bronchitis, fibrosis, bronchiectasis, neoplasm). Often no cause can be found. Investigations to eliminate bronchiectasis and bronchial carcinoma may have to be undertaken and appropriate treatment instituted. Bronchoscopy should always be considered in middle-aged and elderly patients with unresolved pneumonia since partial bronchial obstruction due to carcinoma may be responsible for the delay in resolution. In other cases of delayed resolution, postural coughing followed by breathing exercises should be undertaken several times a day and a prolonged convalescence advised.

Convalescence

The patient should be allowed out of bed as soon as possible after the temperature has reached normal. In patients with chronic bronchitis early discharge from hospital should be encouraged to avoid further respiratory infection, which is so prevalent in hospital during the winter months. If home conditions are not suitable, a holiday at a convalescent home should be recommended.

LUNG ABSCESS

A pulmonary abscess may develop without apparent cause, or it may complicate the suppurative type of aspiration pneumonia, bronchial carcinoma, or bronchiectasis. It is a common sequel to the inhalation of a foreign body. Similarly, it may follow operations on the mouth and nasopharynx when there has been aspiration of infected tissue and blood clot into the bronchi.

The prevention and treatment of post-operative chest complications are of importance in the prophylaxis of pulmonary abscess (p. 205). If circumstances permit, every patient who is about to undergo a major surgical operation under general anaesthesia should first receive local treatment for any sepsis in the mouth and throat.

Before treatment is started, an attempt should be made to discover the cause of the pulmonary abscess. In all cases the sputum must be examined bacteriologically to discover, if possible, the causal organism. Bronchoscopy or bronchography will often be necessary to determine whether the abscess is secondary to bronchial neoplasm or to bronchiectasis, though such investigations may have to be delayed until after the acute phase of the illness.

The introduction of antibiotics has had a dramatic impact on the treatment of pulmonary abscess. External drainage of the abscess, formerly a common procedure, is now very seldom required and, provided there is no complicating factor such as tumour or empyema, conservative treatment is almost invariably successful.

Conservative Treatment

The objects of conservative treatment are (1) to improve the patient's general condition and relieve symptoms; (2) to control the infection by antibiotics; and (3) to keep the abscess cavity or cavities drained by postural coughing.

General measures. These differ in no essential detail from those recommended for pneumonia (p. 201). Although complete healing of an abscess takes much longer than the resolution of a pneumococcal pneumonia, the acute phase of the illness is seldom protracted now that antibiotics are available. Once the pyrexia subsides, there is no need to keep the patient in bed merely because a radiographic abnormality persists. Indeed, it is usually advantageous to have the patient up and about at this stage. A close watch should be kept for complications such as empyema and cerebral abscess, which are now fortunately rare.

Antibiotics. Benzylpenicillin by intramuscular injection should be given initially, as many of the organisms responsible for the production of pulmonary abscess are sensitive to this antibiotic. When the results of bacteriological examination of the sputum are available, a change in antibiotic may have to be made, but this decision should take into account not only the *in vitro* sensitivity of the organism but also the patient's clinical progress.

The duration of chemotherapy in lung abscess is important. Treatment should be continued for a period of at least four weeks.

Postural drainage. This should be performed at least thrice daily for half an hour until the cavity cannot be seen radiographically and the sputum has become mucoid. When the abscess is situated in an upper lobe, postural coughing is carried out, first in the upright position and then in the lateral position, with the affected lung uppermost. If the abscess is in the right middle lobe, the patient lies on his back with a pillow under the right side and the foot of the bed slightly raised. If the lesion is in a lower lobe, the foot of the bed is raised about 12 inches and the patient lies supine, in the lateral position or prone, depending on which segment the abscess occupies.

Bronchoscopy, although useful as a diagnostic measure, has no part to play in the routine treatment of lung abscess. Unless the patient is very weak, the pus can be expectorated just as efficiently as it can be aspirated through a bronchoscope.

Surgical Treatment

In the very rare instances where conservative treatment fails, the patient may require some form of surgery. At an early stage, if there is no response to chemotherapy, the patient may develop grave toxaemia from an undrained or inadequately drained abscess. In these circumstances external drainage may be required. Alternatively, the patient may recover fairly well from the acute phase of the illness, but in spite of chemotherapy the abscess cavity may persist or irreversible bronchiectasis may supervene. Such sequelae are best treated by resection of the affected lobe or segment, the results of which are generally satisfactory.

EMPYEMA

Acute Empyema

Acute empyema may complicate any type of pneumonia. Before the introduction of antibiotics most cases were secondary to pneumococcal pneumonia but this type of empyema has now become much less common. A more important cause of empyema is aspiration pneumonia derived from infection in the upper respiratory tract, or occurring as a complication of bronchiectasis or of bronchial obstruction by a carcinoma. Staphylococcal pneumonia is another fairly common cause of empyema, especially in children. Rarely, an empyema occurs as a complication of a pulmonary infarction or subphrenic abscess.

The diagnosis of empyema is established by the aspiration of pus from the pleural space. In contrast with serous fluid, pus is not spontaneously absorbed from the pleural space even if it has become sterile following treatment with an antibiotic. On the contrary, with the passage of time the pus tends to become thicker and the walls of the empyema cavity more rigid.

It is thus clear that the primary objective in the treatment of acute empyema must be the evacuation of all the pus at the earliest possible stage and the prevention of its reaccumulation. This can best be achieved by continuous drainage of the empyema at its most dependent point by means of a tube inserted either through an intercostal space or following rib resection.

Many of the bacteria responsible for acute empyema are sensitive to penicillin and, pending bacteriological confirmation, benzyl penicillin should be given intramuscularly in a dose of 600 mg. twice daily on the assumption that the organisms are sensitive to it. Provided that tuberculosis can be excluded, this assumption is also justifiable if pus obtained from a patient already treated with penicillin is found to be sterile.

If a penicillin-resistant organism is isolated from the pus, an antibiotic to which it is sensitive should be substituted.

Surgical treatment. The help of a thoracic surgeon should be sought when the empyema is first diagnosed. If the patient is febrile and toxic, the pus is thin and the empyema has not become localized by adhesions, closed drainage is established by means of a self-retaining intercostal catheter connected to a water seal drainage system (p. 637). When the patient's general condition is satisfactory, when the pus is thick and the empyema is localized by adhesions, rib resection and open drainage through a wide-bore tube into a dressing is preferable as this procedure allows infected fibrin clot to be removed from the pleural space.

Chronic Empyema

The two chief causes of this are: (a) delayed or inefficient treatment of an acute empyema, resulting in the formation of a rigid cortex of organizing fibrin on the surface of the lung, which is thus prevented from re-expanding; (b) disease in the underlying lung, such as bronchial carcinoma, bronchiectasis or tuberculosis, which not only initiates the pleural infection but also prevents its healing by rendering the lung incapable of full re-expansion.

In both groups the presence of a broncho-pleural fistula may be an important factor in producing and maintaining a chronic empyema.

The first group of cases should be treated by decortication of the lung or by resection of the whole of the empyema sac.

In the second group treatment depends on the nature of the underlying disease. When a bronchial carcinoma or bronchiectasis is present, the infected pleural sac is resected along with the primary lesion if practicable; otherwise drainage is instituted. When a chronic empyema is due to tuberculous infection of the pleura secondary to pulmonary disease, the infection must first be controlled by repeated aspiration of the pus and by antituberculous chemotherapy (p. 68). Often it will be possible to secure obliteration of the pleural space in this way. In many patients, however, some form of surgery is ultimately required. This generally consists of resection of the pleural sac along with the diseased lung, lobe or segment. Operation should not, however, be undertaken until tubercle bacilli can no longer be cultured from the sputum or from any pus remaining in the pleural space.

BRONCHIECTASIS

There are wide variations in the clinical picture of bronchiectasis. Occasionally the condition is discovered on routine radiological examination and is symptomless. Other patients may complain only of recurrent respiratory infection or of repeated haemoptysis. The classical picture of bronchiectasis viz. toxaemia, foetid sputum and gross clubbing of the fingers, is now seldom seen in Britain. There is, however, a large intermediate group in which health is not impaired for many years despite the expectoration of large amounts of sputum. The type, stage and localization of the disease as well as the age, social circumstances and general health of the patient are factors which must be taken into consideration in determining the most suitable method of treatment.

PROPHYLAXIS

A history of one or more attacks of pneumonia, usually in childhood, is of such frequent occurrence in bronchiectasis as to suggest that failure to secure complete resolution of the inflammatory process is a factor of great aetiological importance. Accordingly, the family doctor should realize the essential need for thorough and prompt treatment of all forms of pneumonia in children and adolescents. He should also ensure that radiographs of the chest are taken to confirm that complete resolution of the pneumonia has taken place. If resolution is incomplete, intensive physiotherapy, including postural drainage and inspiratory breathing exercises, must be given, and antibiotic therapy must be resumed if there is anything to suggest that the infection has not been completely controlled. If pulmonary collapse is present, the possibility of bronchial obstruction by a tuberculous lymph node, a tumour, a foreign body or a collection of tenacious secretion should be investigated by bronchoscopy and, whenever possible, the obstructing agent should be removed.

As persistent infection of the nasal sinuses and teeth is one of the most important factors in initiating and maintaining infection in the bronchial tree, such conditions should receive attention.

TREATMENT

Since the introduction of antibiotics the prognosis and treatment of bronchiectasis have been substantially modified, mainly because it is now possible in most cases to control the acute exacerbations of infection which have been responsible for most of the mortality and for much of the morbidity from the disease. Many patients with advanced bronchiectasis can be kept alive and in reasonably good health for many years; those with relatively mild or intermittent symptoms are no longer in the same danger of progressing to the advanced stage.

For these reasons all patients with bronchiectasis, with the exception of those in whom repeated haemoptysis is the chief symptom, should in the first instance be treated conservatively. Subsequent management will depend partly on the initial clinical and radiological assessment and partly on the response to conservative treatment.

As far as treatment is concerned, it is possible to

place any case of bronchiectasis in one of three categories. The *first* includes all those patients whose symptoms are adequately controlled by conservative measures, whatever the extent of the disease. Surgical treatment is not indicated, but these patients should always be kept under observation so that if intractable symptoms develop resection can be reconsidered.

The *second* category comprises those unfortunate patients in whom conservative measures fail and who cannot be offered surgical treatment either because the disease is too widespread or because co-existing chronic bronchitis, bronchial asthma or emphysema would gravely increase the hazards of the operation and diminish the prospects of its achieving a satisfactory functional result.

In the *third* category, intermediate between the first two, are those patients whose symptoms are not adequately controlled by conservative measures but in whom the disease is sufficiently limited in extent to permit its complete surgical extirpation without seriously impairing respiratory function.

The greatest care must be taken in selecting patients for surgical treatment. It is, for example, particularly important to be certain that the symptoms are in fact due to bronchiectasis and not to generalized chronic bronchitis, with which it is frequently associated.

The surgical treatment of bronchiectasis achieves its greatest success in young subjects, particularly children, in whom the disease is confined to a single lobe, as demonstrated by bronchography and in whom there is little or no clinical evidence of bronchitis or asthma. Cases of more extensive bronchiectasis, up to the equivalent of one lung, can be successfully dealt with surgically, but it must be remembered that the more extensive the resection the more vital it is to be sure that the remaining lung tissue is capable of sustaining respiratory function. Even a mild degree of chronic bronchitis and emphysema should be regarded as a contraindication to extensive resection for bronchiectasis. Nothing is gained by relieving a patient of cough and sputum if thereafter he becomes a respiratory cripple. This danger is especially serious in older patients, as respiratory function normally declines with age. Bronchiectasis should seldom be treated surgically after the age of 40 until conservative treatment has been given a prolonged trial and the patient's respiratory function has been assessed.

Repeated severe haemoptysis constitutes a special indication for surgical treatment. Difficulties may arise when the bronchiectasis is too extensive for total resection and the source of the bleeding cannot be established with sufficient certainty for a local resection to be performed; here, treatment must be expectant until the site of the bleeding has been determined.

The practical aspects of the two types of treatment, conservative and surgical, will now be considered.

Conservative Treatment

The aims of conservative treatment are twofold: (1) to control respiratory infection by antibiotics, and (2) to prevent pus from accumulating in the dilated bronchi by postural drainage.

Antibiotics. The problems presented by infection in bronchiectasis are similar to those in chronic bronchitis (p. 194). Thus, antibiotic therapy has a vital part to play in the control of acute exacerbations of infection. Infection is often perpetuated by the tendency for pus to accumulate in the dilated bronchi but if this can be prevented by postural drainage, the control of symptoms seldom presents insuperable difficulties.

If the sputum is purulent or foetid, tetracycline or ampicillin, 250 to 500 mg. four times daily, should be given by mouth, and intensive postural drainage should be started at the same time. Antibiotic therapy should be continued until the sputum is mucoid. Thereafter, postural drainage should normally suffice to keep the infection in check. An antibiotic should be used to control every further exacerbation of infection.

Chronic sinusitis, which is a frequent accompaniment of bronchiectasis, must be dealt with as thoroughly as possible, because it may be an important factor in maintaining infection in the dilated bronchi (p. 192).

Postural drainage. The importance of this measure has already been emphasized. Its chief value is in those cases in which one or both lower lobes are involved. The upper lobes drain naturally by gravity when the patient is in the erect position. For drainage of the lower lobes the patient is instructed to lean over the edge of the bed with the head well below the level of the body, which is supported by placing the hands on the floor, so that the bases of the lungs are uppermost. A basin is placed on the floor to catch the expectoration. This posture should be adopted twice daily, on rising in the morning and before retiring at night, for a period of 10 to 20 minutes. For elderly or weak patients unable to tolerate this method, raising the foot of the bed as high as the patient will tolerate may be almost as satisfactory. To loosen sputum prior to postural drainage a hot drink will be found useful, as will the inhalation of steam medicated with compound tincture of benzoin (a teaspoonful to a pint of hot water.)

Aspiration of the pus through a bronchoscope seldom has any advantage over postural drainage. It should not be employed unless there is any clinical or radiological evidence to suggest that the pus is obstructing a large bronchus.

Surgical Treatment

The indications for surgical treatment have already been discussed. The type of operation performed must depend on the location and extent of the disease. With modern operative and anaesthetic techniques the mortality is very small and the results are good. Bad results are almost invariably due to faulty selection of cases or to inadequate pre-operative care. The most common mistake is to attempt to treat surgically patients whose bronchiectasis is too extensive or whose repiratory reserve is inadequate. It is essential that a full assessment of the patient's respiratory function be made before surgery is contemplated. If pre-operative preparation is unsatisfactory, the patient will be liable to post-operative collapse or pneumonia through the aspiration of pus into healthy portions of lung. No patient should be submitted to operation until, by the conservative measures already described, his sputum has been reduced to a minimum. Anaemia must always be corrected before operation is undertaken. Patients who have had severe haemoptyses may require preliminary blood transfusion.

RESPIRATORY DISEASES CAUSED BY FUNGI

Most fungi encountered by man are harmless saprophytes, but some species may in certain circumstances infect lung tissue or promote damaging allergic reactions. The term *mycosis* is applicable to diseases caused by fungal infection. Systemic factors which predispose to this type of infection include metabolic disorders and toxic states, such as diabetes mellitus, uraemia and chronic alcoholism, diseases such as leukaemia and myelomatosis, in which immunological responses are disturbed, and certain therapeutic agents such as corticosteroids, immunosuppressive drugs and deep X-rays, which impair the body's defences against infection. Local factors, such as tissue damage by suppuration or necrosis and the elimination of the competititve influence of a normal bacterial flora by antibiotics, may also facilitate fungal infection.

The commonest respiratory mycosis is *aspergillosis*. In this condition inhaled air-borne spores of *Aspergillus fumigatus* lodge and germinate in pulmonary cysts or bullae, 'healed' tuberculous cavities (p. 75), dilated bronchi, lung abscess or pulmonary infarcts. In most cases the fungal infection remains localized to the site of the original lesion, but occasionally, when resistance is low, it may extend into adjacent normal lung tissue, or via the bronchi into the opposite lung, with the production of extensive pulmonary necrosis and grave systemic disturbance.

When a pre-existing pulmonary cavity is infected by *A. fumigatus*, a large spherical mass of fungal mycelium may form within the cavity, producing on X-ray examination a tumour-like lesion to which the term *mycetoma* or *aspergilloma* is applied. This type of lesion usually produces no specific symptoms, but is occasionally responsible for recurrent haemoptysis.

Candida albicans is a normal commensal of the skin and alimentary tract, but multiplication of the organisms may, when the bacterial flora is suppressed by antibiotics, produce superficial mycotic lesions. Buccal candidosis or 'thrush' is a common condition in these circumstances. Occasionally, in debilitated subjects, the lesions extend downwards into the respiratory tract, with the production of *bronchial* or *pulmonary candidosis*.

Other mycoses which may involve the lungs, all of which are rare, include nocardiosis (*Nocardia asteroides*), cryptococcosis (*Cryptococcus neoformans*), mucormycosis (*Mucorales spp.*), blastomycosis (*Blastomyces dermatitidis*), and sporotrichosis (*Sporotrichum schenekii*). Only the first three of these conditions have been encountered in Britain. In a somewhat different category are histoplasmosis (*Histoplasma capsulatum*), and coccidioidomycosis (*Coccidioides immitis*), which are endemic in certain areas of North America and Africa, and produce local or systemic granulomatous lesions resembling tuberculosis.

TREATMENT OF THE PULMONARY MYCOSES

This is difficult and unsatisfactory. Conditions such as diabetes mellitus, uraemia and alcoholism, which may have predisposed to fungal infection, must be vigorously treated, and the administration of immunosuppressive drugs and corticosteroids should be stopped, whenever this can be done without risking a relapse of the primary disease. Antibacterial agents, particularly wide-spectrum antibiotics, should be withdrawn whenever a diagnosis of respiratory mycosis is made.

Antibiotics active *in vitro* against many species of fungi are available, but they all have serious disadvantages in clinical practice. Nystatin and natamycin, for example, are not absorbed from the gut, and are too toxic for intravenous administration. They are thus of no value in the treatment of severe systemic mycoses, but are fairly effective *topical* fungistatic agents. Nystatin mixture (N.F.), used as a mouthwash, is the treatment of choice for oral thrush, but natamycin, given by inhalation, is preferable for fungal infections of the trachea and bronchi, such as aspergillosis and candidosis. In these conditions natamycin is administered as a 2·5 per cent. suspension in an aqueous aerosol in a dose of 2·5 to 5 mg. three or four times daily, until the fungus is eliminated from the sputum and the mucosal lesions have resolved. Natamycin by inhalation is of no value in the treatment of aspergilloma, as the lesion is invariably situated in an underventilated portion of lung, and little of the inhaled aerosol can reach it. Any which does is unlikely to have any effect on a bulky mass of fungal mycelium. Provided an aspergilloma is not causing symptoms, it is usually left untreated, but if haemoptysis occurs, and pulmonary function is not seriously impaired, surgical treatment may be indicated. Formal resection of the lobe or segment containing the aspergilloma carries a high morbidity, but a satisfactory result can sometimes be obtained by evacuating the fungal mass through an incision on the surface of the lung, and irrigating the cavity with natamycin solution through a small intercostal drainage tube for 6 to 8 weeks.

Amphotericin B, a powerful antifungal agent, is also poorly absorbed when given by mouth, and is liable to produce severe toxic damage to the kidneys and bone marrow, in addition to fever and nausea, when administered intravenously. In patients with severe systemic mycoses, however, no effective alternative treatment is available, and the risks associated with these serious side-effects have to be accepted. The initial dose of amphotericin in such cases should be in the region of 0·25 mg. per kg. body weight, injected intravenously on alternate days. The dose should be gradually increased, side-effects permitting, over the course of 1 to 2 weeks to a maximum of 1 mg. per kg. body weight, and continued at this level until a total of 3 g. has been given.

Actinomycosis, which was formerly included amongst the fungal diseases, is now regarded as a bacterial infection. It is caused by *Actinomyces israeli*, a septate anaerobic organism, which exists as a commensal in the human mouth. It presumably gains access to the lungs by aspiration, and may produce a widespread suppurative lobular pneumonia. Empyema, often bilateral, and associated with persistent chest wall sinuses, may develop at a later stage, or occasionally *de novo*. The infection usually responds to benzylpenicillin, given by intramuscular injection in a dose of 1·2 g. 6-hourly for six weeks. *A. israeli* is occasionally resistant to penicillin, and in such cases an appropriate antibiotic should be selected on the basis of information obtained from sensitivity tests.

Fungal allergic reactions may cause bronchial asthma (*A. fumigatus* and *Cladosporium herbarum*), pulmonary eosinophilia (*A. fumigatus*) or allergic alveolitis (*Micropolyspora faeni*, *Thermoactinomyces vulgaris*, *Coniosporium corticale*, and *Aspergillus clavatus*). The treatment of these conditions is described in the section on allergic disorders of the respiratory system (p. 213).

ALLERGIC DISORDERS OF THE UPPER RESPIRATORY SYSTEM

Allergic Rhinitis

This is a disorder in which there are episodes of nasal congestion, watery nasal discharge and sneezing. It may be *seasonal* or *perennial*. The seasonal form is due to a Type I antigen-antibody reaction in the nasal mucosa. The antigens concerned are pollens from grasses, flowers, weeds or trees. Grass pollen is responsible for hay fever, the most common type of seasonal allergic rhinitis in Britain, and this disorder is at its peak between May and July. Perennial allergic rhinitis may be a specific reaction to antigens derived from house dust, fungal spores or animal dander, but similar symptoms can be caused by physical or chemical irritants, such as pungent odours or fumes, including strong perfumes, cold air and dry atmospheres. In this context the term 'allergic' is a misnomer.

Prevention. In the seasonal type an attempt should be made to avoid exposure to pollen, or at least to reduce it to a minimum, for example by avoiding country districts and keeping indoors as much as possible, with the windows closed, during the pollen season. An antihistamine drug taken daily throughout the pollen season will often prevent attacks of hay fever. If this form of treatment is ineffective, or if it causes intolerable drowsiness, hyposensitization with a grass pollen extract is always worth a trial, although claims for improvement in 70 to 90 per cent. of cases are difficult to evaluate since the term 'improvement' is seldom clearly defined. Alum-precipitated pyridine extracts, such as Alavac P (Bencard) or Allpyral G (Dome) should usually be prescribed, as these extracts appear to be as safe and as effective as aqueous extract, and involve a much smaller number of injections (8 or 9). Emulsions of pollen extract in mineral oil should be avoided, as they have been reported to produce subcutaneous oil granulomata.

The prevention of perennial rhinitis consists of avoiding, as far as possible, exposure to the various aetiological factors mentioned above. Specific hyposensitization is of no value.

Treatment. The following symptomatic measures are applicable to both seasonal and perennial allergic rhinitis:

1. Antihistamine drugs, such as chlorpheniramine maleate (Piriton), 4 to 8 mg. thrice daily, or meclozine hydrochloride, 25 to 50 mg. in the morning, often provide considerable or even complete relief of symptoms.
2. Local measures which may be of some value are (*a*) decongestant nasal sprays, using a 1 per cent. solution of ephedrine hydrochloride in saline and (*b*) eye drops of 1 per cent. ephedrine in saline to relieve conjunctival irritation, which often accompanies the nasal symptoms.
3. Patients failing to respond to these measures may obtain symptomatic relief from the use of a hydrocortisone or betamethasone nasal spray four times daily.

Intramuscular injections of a 'slow-release' corticosteroid preparation given at intervals of 10 to 14 days during the pollen season have been advocated for the treatment of very severe hay fever. Although often very effective, this is an undesirable form of treatment, but circumstances may arise in which it can be justified, for example in a school teacher or university lecturer who finds incessant sneezing an intolerable handicap and embarrassment. A suitable preparation contains methylprednisolone acetate (Depo-medrone), which is given in a dose of 80 mg. by intramuscular injection at appropriate intervals.

In some cases of perennial allergic rhinitis, when all other forms of treatment have failed, the symptoms may be relieved temporarily by cauterization of the inferior turbinates. Many patients with this condition develop nasal polyps, and these may have to be removed surgically if they cause nasal obstruction.

BRONCHIAL ASTHMA

Bronchial asthma is a clinical syndrome of which the characteristic features are paroxysmal wheeze and dyspnoea caused by increased resistance to the flow of air through narrowed bronchi. The changes in the bronchial wall which reduce the size of the lumen are not precisely understood and may not be the same in every case. It is, however, clear from clinical observation of patients with asthma that the bronchial obstruction varies in degree and is potentially reversible. Probably the two processes chiefly concerned are (1) abnormally sustained contraction of the bronchial musculature (bronchospasm) and (2) oedematous swelling of the bronchial mucosa. The presence of tenacious mucus in the smaller bronchi is another possible cause of reversible airway obstruction. It may operate in conjunction with the other two processes but it is probably not capable of producing asthma independently. There is at present no method of determining the relative importance of bronchospasm and bronchial mucosal oedema in an individual patient. Furthermore, so far as human bronchial asthma is concerned, we have little knowledge of the factors which disturb the normal function of the bronchial musculature and mucosa, and the ways in which they operate.

Despite this lack of information on the pathogenesis of bronchial asthma, many conflicting views on its aetiology are strongly held and vigorously expounded. There is much circumstantial evidence to suggest that hypersensitivity to foreign proteins or other substances is capable of producing bronchial asthma, especially in children. The removal of such substances from the patient's environment or the neutralization of their effects by the injection of gradually increasing doses of the allergen or allergens concerned (hyposensitization) may give satisfactory results, but only in a minority of cases.

It is widely recognized that emotional instability is a prominent feature in many asthmatic patients, and attacks may be precipitated by psychological trauma or stress, often of a relatively minor nature. Only rarely, however, can these factors be clearly identified as the *primary* cause of bronchial asthma. Furthermore, even when asthma seems to have a predominantly emotional basis, psychiatric treatment seldom meets with success.

Respiratory infection may also be an important aetiological factor in bronchial asthma. In some cases bacterial infection can precipitate an asthmatic attack, which subsides when the infection is controlled by an antibiotic. In other cases, however, it seems that asthmatic bronchial obstruction predisposes to the development of bacterial infection, and this may explain why the effect of antibiotic treatment is often disappointing. Virus infections of the respiratory tract may also play some part in the production of asthmatic attacks but specific treatment is not yet available for these cases.

If these observations are valid it is clear that in the production of asthmatic attacks three factors may operate—an allergic factor, psychological trauma and respiratory infection. It would, however, be idle to pretend that these factors can be identified or successfully treated except in a small number of cases. Nevertheless, in every patient suffering from asthma, especially children, these causes should be considered during detailed history taking. In suitable cases, skin testing should be performed. In most cases, however, the physician will have to rely on purely empirical therapeutic measures. These, when judiciously applied, are capable of maintaining most patients with bronchial asthma in a reasonably satisfactory clinical state.

Clinically, asthma may be episodic or chronic. In *episodic* asthma, more common in children, adolescents and young adults, brief phases of dyspnoea and wheeze occur with virtually no interval symptoms, and bacterial infection is a relatively infrequent complication. In *chronic* asthma, which is more common in middle-aged and elderly subjects, there is more or less continuous wheeze and exertional dyspnoea, fluctuating in severity; it is usually accompanied by symptoms of bronchitis and often complicated by respiratory infection. The management of episodic asthma differs in many important respects from that of chronic asthma and

these two subjects will be discussed separately. *Status asthmaticus*, in which dyspnoea and wheeze become unremitting and very severe, may supervene at any time in either type of asthma.

THE MANAGEMENT OF EPISODIC ASTHMA

In the vast majority of cases, episodic asthma is a relatively benign condition which can be easily controlled by simple therapeutic measures, but some less fortunate patients may have frequent episodes of moderate severity or even status asthmaticus.

Although there is good evidence that bronchial asthma is often due to antigen-antibody reactions provoked, for example, by pollens, mites and fungal spores, the practical problem of preventing or controlling such reactions still remains. The avoidance of exposure to these ubiquitous allergens is seldom practicable, and hyposensitization, except perhaps in the case of grass pollen asthma, is not an effective form of treatment. Efforts to reduce the environmental concentration of some allergens may, however, meet with limited success. When the clinical history and the results of skin tests suggest that sensitivity to house dust is an important aetiological factor, it is rational to vacuum the patient's mattress at regular intervals, or if necessary to seal it with polythene sheeting, in order to prevent the escape of dust containing large numbers of mites (which are chiefly responsible for the antigenicity of house dust), and to remove dust-harbouring soft furnishings from the bedroom. Asthma caused by contact with domestic animals, or by the ingestion of certain foods, or of drugs such as aspirin, can usually be prevented by avoiding the offending allergen, but isolated allergies of this type are uncommon.

In some patients a history of respiratory infection preceding each episode of asthma suggests an infective aetiology, and they often benefit from antibiotic treatment. If started soon after the onset of infection, antibiotic therapy may prevent the development of asthma. If given later its effect is less apparent, but a gradual improvement in asthmatic symptoms is often observed after infection has been controlled.

Occasionally, the onset of individual episodes of asthma may be related to emotional tension or to incidents of psychological trauma. If these situations can be resolved by social adjustments or by superficial psychotherapy, the asthma may improve considerably or even subside completely.

It is more often the case, however, that primary aetiological factors either defy recognition or cannot be effectively treated even when known to exist. In these circumstances reliance must be placed on empirical measures for the control and, if possible, prevention of episodes by the administration of bronchodilator drugs or corticosteroids.

TREATMENT OF AN ASTHMATIC ATTACK

The patient should be allowed to take up the position which he finds most comfortable, either propped up in bed or sitting in a chair. Ephedrine, 30 to 60 mg. by mouth, may be sufficient to abort a mild attack, but modern β-adrenergic receptor stimulant drugs, such as salbutamol (4 mg.) or orciprenaline (20 mg.), are more effective bronchodilators. These two drugs, particularly salbutamol, are also less liable to produce palpitation and tachycardia, and are gradually replacing ephedrine for the oral treatment of asthmatic attacks. The same two drugs can, perhaps even more effectively, be given by inhalation from pressurized dispensers. A Ventolin inhaler provides a metered dose of 100 μg. of salbutamol, and an Alupent inhaler 750 μg. of orciprenaline. For maximum bronchodilatation two doses ('puffs') should be inhaled at a time, the second five minutes after the first. The relief obtained usually lasts for 2 to 3 hours. It is possibly unsafe to repeat the inhalation within this period. Isoprenaline, which is also available for inhalation from a pressurized dispenser, has a more pronounced action on cardiac β-receptors than the other two drugs, and is potentially more dangerous in the presence of hypoxia. It should therefore not be used in the treatment of asthma.

Adrenaline injection (B.P.), 0·2 to 0·5 ml. subcutaneously, occasionally relieves an attack which has failed to respond to inhalations of salbutamol or orciprenaline, but it may be no less dangerous than isoprenaline in hypoxic subjects. In these circumstances aminophylline, 250 to 500 mg. injected slowly intravenously, is safer and often more effective; it is available as Aminophylline injection, B.P. and 10 ml. contains 250 mg.

The oral administration of aminophylline and of derivatives such as choline theophyllinate seldom controls attacks of asthma. The same is true of many widely advertised proprietary combinations of ephedrine, aminophylline or one of its derivatives and a barbiturate. In some of these preparations

the individual components are present in inordinately small doses.

PREVENTION OF ASTHMATIC ATTACKS

Drugs. The efficacy of ephedrine and aminophylline, and of the countless derivatives and combinations of these and other drugs which are now available, in preventing attacks of asthma is extremely limited despite the large sums of money spent by the National Health Service each year on these preparations. It may be possible, however, to prevent nocturnal episodes of asthma by prescribing a sedative combined with a small dose of ephedrine if the latter does not cause insomnia. One of the safest and most effective sedatives is promethazine hydrochloride, the antihistaminic effect of which is probably irrelevant to its use in this context. It is given in a dose of 25 to 50 mg. at bedtime. Patients with asthma should always have a salbutamol (Ventolin) or orciprenaline (Alupent) inhaler at the bedside so that it is available for immediate use should an attack develop during the night.

Hyposensitization. There is little evidence that this form of treatment is effective in bronchial asthma unless the patient has a clear-cut allergy to grass pollens, confirmed by skin sensitivity tests. Details of the diagnostic preparations are provided by manufacturers. Claims for the efficacy of a mite-fortified house-dust extract have not yet been substantiated, but patients who are sensitive to animal dander occasionally benefit from specific hyposensitization.

Disodium cromoglycate. It has been shown that this drug interferes with the release of spasmogens derived from antigen-antibody reactions in the bronchial wall, and it is regarded by many as a major advance in the control of bronchial asthma, particularly in patients with demonstrable sensitivity to external allergens. It has, however, still to stand the test of time in clinical practice. It is usually prescribed as Intal Compound, which is a combination of disodium cromoglycate and isoprenaline, but is also available as the pure substance (Intal). Both preparations are administered by inhalation with a special device (Spinhaler) 3 to 5 times per day. Each dose of 20 mg. is supplied in a sealed capsule (Spincap).

Breathing and postural exercises. It is extremely doubtful if breathing exercises can help to prevent attacks of asthma or to limit the pigeon chest deformity which is liable to develop when the

H

condition starts in childhood. Exercises designed to correct the faulty posture common in asthmatic subjects may, however, be of some value.

THE MANAGEMENT OF CHRONIC ASTHMA

Although bronchodilator drugs may provide substantial relief of symptoms for short periods, some form of maintenance treatment must be given if a patient with chronic asthma is to be kept tolerably free from wheeze and exertional dyspnoea. An additional therapeutic problem is the susceptibility of these patients to respiratory infection. If the sputum becomes purulent or if any other symptoms or signs of infection develop, an antibiotic should always be prescribed, with the dual purpose of eliminating a factor which may aggravate the asthma and preventing the bronchopulmonary damage which this type of infection is liable to produce (p. 195). Allergic and emotional factors are probably of less importance in chronic than in episodic asthma and it is seldom that hyposensitization or psychological treatment is of any value. Not infrequently, however, the asthma itself causes severe mental stress and sedation with a barbiturate or with a phenothiazine derivative may help to ease the patient's discomfiture, although it seldom has a direct effect on the respiratory symptoms.

Bronchodilator drugs are less effective in chronic than in episodic asthma. In many cases, however, a fair measure of temporary relief can be obtained from regular inhalations of bronchodilator aerosols, such as salbutamol or orciprenaline, but patients must be warned that these drugs may be dangerous if used to excess. The standard dose of two 'puffs', the second five minutes after the first, should not be taken more frequently than once in every 2 to 3 hours. Regular oral administration of the same two drugs is effective in some cases, the recommended doses being 4 mg. of salbutamol or 20 mg. of orciprenaline every 4 hours. Combinations of ephedrine, a theophylline derivative and a barbiturate (such as Franol, Tedral and Amesec) have achieved wide popularity but are of doubtful efficacy. Aminophylline suppositories have a useful place in the control of asthma during the night but here again there are obvious limitations to the frequency of administration. Aminophylline and its derivatives given by mouth have little effect in chronic asthma, as an adequate dose is often not tolerated because of the side-effects of nausea and vomiting. Choline theophyllinate is less liable to cause gastric disturbance than the parent substance. The dose should be increased gradually from 100 mg. four times daily to the limit of tolerance, which is usually reached at a dose of 200 mg. four times daily, but even at this level the results are frequently disappointing.

Corticosteroids

In many cases of chronic asthma treatment with bronchodilator drugs fails to keep the symptoms in check and until recent years such patients were forced to lead lives of frustrating and often intolerable respiratory distress. All these patients are now potential candidates for prolonged corticosteroid therapy. This form of treatment, although not without danger, can offer in properly selected cases a very substantial measure of symptomatic relief. In children it can also bring about the correction of a severe 'pigeon chest' deformity. The mode of action of corticosteroids is not fully understood but is believed to be related to their anti-inflammatory effect. This effect is suppressive, not curative, and a recurrence of symptoms of chronic asthma can be expected, sooner or later, if treatment is withdrawn.

Two conditions must be satisfied before a patient is considered suitable for prolonged corticosteroid therapy: (1) the chronic asthma must be causing a severe degree of disability which cannot be influenced by other measures; (2) a specific effect on ventilatory function tests must be demonstrated by observing the patient's response to a short preliminary course of treatment with a corticosteroid.

It is usually possible to arrive at a correct decision on the first point by careful history taking, but the second requires the help of a physician experienced in the management of chronic asthma and facilities for the performance of simple tests of ventilatory function. For that reason it is desirable that all patients likely to require prolonged corticosteroid therapy should be referred to a hospital where their suitability for this form of treatment can be accurately assessed. If that is not done, there is a danger that patients who do not show a genuine response to corticosteroids will be needlessly exposed to the risks of a potentially dangerous form of treatment. These risks will be all the greater if the doctor supervising it lacks experience in the use of corticosteroid drugs. It is not even safe to sanction, say, a month's uncontrolled trial of corticosteroid therapy as many patients who fail to show a specific response to treatment seem to become dependent on these drugs, and it may then become difficult or even impossible to discontinue their use.

When a patient is admitted to hospital for an assessment of his response to corticosteroids, treatment is withheld (or inert control tablets resembling the drug to be used may be given) until daily tests of ventilatory function (forced expiratory volume or peak expiratory flow rate) provide a stable base-line from which the effect of treatment can be evaluated. The patient is then given a fairly large dose of corticosteroid, e.g. prednisolone, 5 mg., four times daily, for seven days. Daily function tests are continued and if a sharp rise in forced expiratory volume or peak expiratory flow rate is observed, starting 24 to 72 hours after the first dose of prednisolone, it can be accepted that the patient's chronic asthma is responsive to corticosteroid therapy. In such cases it can be confidently predicted that a similar response will be obtained whenever corticosteroids are given in future and that prolonged treatment, if it is required, will maintain complete or almost complete freedom from asthma. Not infrequently, however, patients given a seven-day course of corticosteroid therapy have a remission of symptoms lasting for several weeks or even for a few months. It is possible to keep many of these patients well by occasional courses of corticosteroid, given whenever asthmatic symptoms cannot be kept at a tolerable level by bronchodilator drugs. In other cases, however, the remissions which follow courses of corticosteroid are so short that some form of maintenance treatment has to be given, either in a small daily dose or in a larger dose given intermittently, e.g. on three consecutive days per week.

Although many of the synthetic corticosteroids can safely be used for a single course of treatment, certain preparations are less satisfactory than others for prolonged treatment. Cortisone and dexamethasone are liable to cause sodium and water retention, and triamcinolone and betamethasone to produce muscular weakness. Methylprednisolone is inordinately expensive and has no special merit. Most of the experience with this form of treatment has been obtained with prednisolone, and on present evidence it remains the drug of choice.

All corticosteroids, when given for long periods, are capable of producing serious side-effects and this problem is a constant challenge to those engaged in the study of prolonged corticosteroid therapy. As the incidence of side-effects is directly proportional to the dosage employed, every effort should be made to keep the dose at the lowest level which will prevent the asthma from interfering with the patient's activities. In many cases this can be achieved by a daily dose of 10 mg. or less of prednisolone but occasionally a dose of 15 mg. or even 20 mg. may be required. Another method of reducing the total dosage of corticosteroid is by giving a larger dose (e.g. 20 mg. per day of prednisolone) on three consecutive days in every seven or on two consecutive days in every four, leaving the patient without treatment on the other days. With intermittent treatment of this type the incidence of serious side-effects is very low and most patients find that these short bursts of treatment are sufficient to prevent recurrence of symptoms during the periods when corticosteroids are withheld. Some patients, particularly children, are, however, unsuitable for intermittent treatment and have to be given a maintenance dose of corticosteroid every day.

The dose required to keep chronic asthma controlled is not constant even in the individual patient, and status asthmaticus of varying degrees of severity may supervene from time to time, even when the maintenance dose of corticosteroid may previously have seemed adequate. On such occasions it is seldom sufficient to advise a slight increase in the maintenance dose. It is much safer to raise the dose immediately to the equivalent of 20 to 60 mg. daily of prednisolone and, as soon as the symptoms subside, to reduce it within the course of a few days to the usual maintenance level.

In patients who require daily treatment with a dose equivalent to 10 mg. or more per day of prednisolone side-effects are frequently encountered. Although the management of serious side-effects is broadly similar to that adopted in patients with rheumatoid arthritis (p. 453), it must be appreciated that attempts to withdraw corticosteroid therapy from patients with severe chronic asthma may be immediately followed by the development of severe status asthmaticus. Provided the need for corticosteroid therapy has been clearly established, it is safer to continue treatment and take steps to correct the side-effects or limit their consequences. A corticosteroid-induced peptic ulcer may heal if prednisolone is given in the form of enteric coated tablets, e.g. Deltacortril (enteric), or as prednisolone disodium phosphate. Osteoporosis may be prevented, or perhaps even corrected, by a high calcium intake and the administration of an anabolic steroid.

Once corticosteroid therapy has been established for chronic asthma it usually has to be maintained for several years, possibly even for the rest of the patient's life. The need for continued treatment is probably dictated more often by persistence of the asthmatic state than by the development of so-called 'corticosteroid dependence'. In children, adolescents and young adults, in whom chronic asthma is often a self-limiting disorder, it may be possible to reduce the dose of corticosteroid progressively and in some cases to withdraw the treatment completely after two to three years. In older subjects a very gradual reduction in dose can often be effected, but present experience suggests that complete withdrawal of treatment can seldom be achieved.

Corticotrophin. Although corticotrophin has the advantage over the corticosteroids of not causing suppression of pituitary-adrenal function it has other drawbacks and is not recommended for the treatment of chronic asthma in adults. There is, however, some evidence to suggest that it is less liable than corticosteroids to retard growth in children.

If a child whose growth is retarded requires a daily maintenance dose of more than 5 mg. of prednisolone, the substitution of corticotrophin should be considered.

The change-over from prednisolone to corticotrophin should be carefully monitored by plasma cortisol estimations, and admission to hospital is usually necessary. Prednisolone should not be withdrawn until it has been shown that the dose of corticotrophin gel normally used in the conversion procedure (40 units in adults and 20 units in children) increases the plasma cortisol concentration after a period of four hours to at least 20 μg. per 100 ml. Once this stage has been reached, prednisolone can safely be withdrawn, and the dose of corticotrophin should then be adjusted to the patient's requirements. A dose of 20 to 30 units once daily is a common maintenance dose in adults, but this can usually be reduced as the functional capacity of the adrenals improves. Twice-weekly injections may be adequate in some cases if slow-release tetracosactrin zinc phosphate complex (Synacthen Depot) is used. The effective dose, as in the case of corticotrophin gel, depends on the responsiveness of the adrenals, and may vary from 0·25 to 2 mg. This preparation has the advantage over corticotrophin gel of being less liable to produce general reactions, but twice-weekly injections are not always effective, and some patients still have

to be treated by daily injections of corticotrophin gel. These should be given *twice daily* if a patient on a maintenance dose of either corticotrophin gel or slow-release tetracosactrin develops a recurrence of asthma. Provided the adrenals are functioning normally, the hypothalamo-pituitary-adrenal response to stress is not impaired by prolonged corticotrophin therapy, but if a patient has recently been receiving regular treatment with corticosteroids, pituitary-adrenal function may still be impaired, and exposure to stress then demands the temporary addition of a corticosteroid preparation, such as hydrocortisone sodium succinate intravenously or cortisone acetate intramuscularly.

Treatment of status asthmaticus. Status asthmaticus, the term used to describe a very severe and prolonged episode of asthma, may occur as a complication of either episodic or chronic asthma. It is more common, and usually more dangerous, in chronic asthma, and carries a significant mortality unless the patient can be promptly admitted to a hospital with adequate facilities for dealing with this type of emergency.

By definition, status asthmaticus is resistant to bronchodilator drugs, but corticosteroids are almost invariably effective if started in time. In a case of average severity prednisolone should be given by mouth in a dose of 20 mg. 6-hourly on the first day, 10 mg. 6-hourly on the second, and 5 mg. 6-hourly thereafter. Patients who are gravely ill should receive 100 mg. of prednisolone by mouth in the first 12 hours, along with hydrocortisone sodium succinate intravenously in a dose of 100 to 200 mg. 4-hourly during the same period. Oxygen should be administered in a concentration of 60 per cent. (6 *l.* per minute by M.C. mask), with suitable precautions to detect hypercapnia (p. 648), which is, however, usually a late development in status asthmaticus. Dehydration, which increases the viscosity of the sputum, must be corrected, if necessary by intravenous fluids. If in spite of this treatment the patient's condition continues to deteriorate, and particularly if the partial pressure of carbon dioxide in the arterial blood rises above 50 mm. Hg., oro-tracheal intubation with intermittent positive-pressure ventilation should be carried out (p. 647). Very few patients require tracheostomy. Except during artificial ventilation, hypnotics should be used with great caution, and opiates must never be given. Diazepam, 5 to 10 mg. intramuscularly, is relatively safe, and may promote relaxation and sleep. As status asthmaticus is often complicated by respiratory infection, which may not always be readily recognizable in the early stages, a suitable antibiotic (Table 1) should be administered in every case.

There is considerable controversy in regard to the use of bronchodilators in status asthmaticus. Sympathomimetic drugs, such as adrenaline and isoprenaline, have often been blamed for sudden deaths from cardiac arrest in patients with this condition, and there is some evidence that these drugs are particularly dangerous when given to hypoxic subjects. It may therefore be safer to give aminophylline in a dose of 250 to 500 mg. in 10 to 20 ml. sterile water by slow intravenous injection. When the patient is being adequately oxygenated, however, subcutaneous Adrenaline Injection B.P. in a dose of 0·2 to 0·5 ml. is relatively safe and often effective. Isoprenaline should not be used in status asthmaticus, but salbutamol by inhalation in a dose of 200 μg. (2 'puffs' from a pressurized dispenser) may provide temporary relief in less severe cases, with little danger of producing cardiac side-effects. This drug can also be administered by intermittent positive-pressure ventilation, using a Bird or Bennett apparatus driven by 40 per cent. oxygen and connected to a tightly fitting face mask. This treatment should not be given for more than three minutes, but can be repeated at hourly intervals if necessary. It appears to be safe, and may be dramatically effective.

Reports of the finding of large amounts of tenacious mucus obstructing the smaller bronchi in fatal cases have led some physicians to advocate bronchoscopy and bronchial lavage to permit the removal of such secretions by aspiration. In most cases the mucus responsible for the bronchial obstruction is far beyond the range of the bronchoscope, but bronchial plugs situated more peripherally can sometimes be dislodged by squirting normal saline solution, warmed to body temperature, into the segmental orifices. This procedure is, however, apt to cause an increase in the degree of hypoxia, which may be dangerous. It should therefore be employed only as a last resort.

In the vast majority of cases, treatment with corticosteroids moderates the distress of status asthmaticus within 8 to 24 hours. Although symptoms may persist for a few days afterwards, the initial improvement, once it has occurred, is usually maintained, and the danger of death rapidly recedes. The usual procedure when the patient begins to recover is to continue treatment with prednisolone in diminishing dosage for 10 to 14 days. Corticosteroids have, however, only a temporary suppressive effect, and asthma frequently recurs a few weeks, or even a few days, after treatment is stopped.

When a general practitioner is called to a patient with status asthmaticus, one of the most important and difficult decisions he will have to make is whether or not to send the patient to hospital. There can be no hard and fast rules, but transfer to hospital is strongly advisable in the following circumstances: (1) if there is a previous history of severe status asthmaticus, (2) if there has been no response to bronchodilator drugs, and (3) if there is central cyanosis, tachycardia of over 120 per minute, or arterial pulsus paradoxus. If there is likely to be a delay in the patient's admission to hospital, corticosteroid therapy, if it is not already being given, should be started at once with an initial dose of 20 mg. of prednisolone, and oxygen should be administered if facilities are available. The chief advantage of having patients with status asthmaticus in hospital is that they can be kept under constant skilled observation, and can be transferred to an intensive care area if the need arises.

PULMONARY EOSINOPHILIA

This term is used to describe a heterogeneous group of conditions in which transient pulmonary shadows on the chest radiograph are associated with an eosinophil count in the peripheral blood of more than 400 per cu. mm.

In *simple pulmonary eosinophilia* (Loeffler's syndrome) these features are accompanied in some cases by a slight cough and a mild febrile illness, but in others by no symptoms at all. The condition is usually a manifestation of hypersensitivity to a drug such as PAS, nitrofurantoin or a sulphonamide, or to an intestinal parasite such as *Ascaris lumbricoides*. Treatment should be directed to eliminating all potential causes of the allergic reaction. Any drug to which hypersensitivity may have developed should be withdrawn, and treatment with anthelmintic drugs should be given for intestinal parasitic infestations.

Asthmatic pulmonary eosinophilia is due in most cases to allergic reactions in the bronchi and lungs to *Aspergillus fumigatus*. The lesions are of two types: (1) segmental or sub-segmental (occasionally lobar) collapse caused by occlusion of the related bronchus by a mucinous cast coated with eosino-phils, which often contain fungal hyphae, and (2) areas of pulmonary infiltration in which the alveolar spaces and alveolar walls contain numer-ous eosinophils and varying numbers of lympho-cytes and plasma cells. The first type of lesion is more common than the second. The radiographic appearances reflect the pathological changes—collapse of a segment (or of a larger or smaller bronchopulmonary unit) in the first type, and an ill-defined pulmonary opacity in the second. These lesions may recur at intervals for many years any-where in the lungs, but more often in the upper lobes. Bronchiectasis frequently develops in collapsed bronchopulmonary segments.

Treatment. This can be very difficult. Efforts to eliminate the fungus from the respiratory tract by regular inhalations of natamycin (p. 20) seldom succeed. Antihistamines are of no value, but corticosteroids (p. 216) may relieve the asthma, and at the same time prevent recurrent pulmonary infiltrations and the formation of new bronchial casts. If these cannot be dislodged by postural drainage they should be extracted through a bronchoscope. Failure to deal effectively with bronchial casts is an important factor in the pro-duction of bronchiectasis; and this is usually too widespread for surgical treatment to be undertaken.

Tropical pulmonary eosinophilia, which occurs mainly in India, is thought to be an allergic reaction to microfilariae in the lungs. The illness usually responds to treatment with the antifilarial drug, diethylcarbamazine (p. 534).

Pulmonary eosinophilia persisting or recurring for weeks or months in the absence of asthma may be an early manifestation of *polyarteritis nodosa*, the treatment of which is described on p. 458.

Extrinsic Allergic Alveolitis

This term is used to describe a group of conditions in which the inhalation of certain types of organic dust produces a diffuse allergic reaction in the walls of alveoli and bronchioles. There is a cellular exu-date consisting of polymorphs, lymphocytes and plasma cells, and small epitheloid granulomata may also be seen. These changes cause decreased pul-monary compliance and ventilation-perfusion in-equalities. They are presumably also responsible for the widespread coarse crepitations heard on auscultation, and for the diffuse micro-nodular shadowing seen on the chest radiograph. The diag-nosis is confirmed by the detection in the serum of precipitating antibodies against the relevant antigen. The causes of extrinsc allergic alveolitis include thermophilic actinomycetes (farmer's lung, mush-room worker's lung and bagassosis), *Aspergillus clavatus* (malt worker's lung) and avian protein in pigeon and budgerigar droppings (bird-fancier's lung). The symptoms usually subside when expos-ure to the dust ceases. In severe cases, however, a corticosteroid preparation should be given for 2 to 3 weeks, starting with 40 to 60 mg. of prednisolone per day. Severely hypoxic patients may require oxygen in high concentration (60 per cent.).

INTRATHORACIC NEW GROWTHS
Malignant Tumours

The prevalence of bronchial carcinoma has risen steeply during the past 30 years. In men it now far exceeds pulmonary tuberculosis as a cause of death in Britain, and has become the most common type of malignant tumour. Hopes for its prevention are at present based on the evidence that it is caused by the smoking of tobacco, especially cigarettes, and to a lesser degree by pollution of the atmosphere by industrial and domestic smoke in cities and towns. The disease is thus in theory preventable, and it is now imperative to dissuade all young persons from ever starting to smoke cigarettes.

Surgery. Radical surgery affords the only prospect of cure. Provided the operation can be undertaken before the tumour has extended beyond the lung, the number of successful results is by no means negligible, 25 to 30 per cent. of cases sur-viving for more than five years. The number of patients in whom operative treatment is practicable is, however, extremely small, probably between one-tenth and one-fifth of all cases. Generally this is because the tumour has reached too advanced a stage before it is detected, but operative treatment may also be prevented by old age, poor general condition or respiratory insufficiency.

As soon as the diagnosis is made, whether con-clusively by bronchial biopsy or presumptively from the radiological appearances, a decision must be taken for or against surgical treatment. The in-vestigations required for this purpose include a com-plete clinical examination, bronchoscopy, radio-logical examination of the lungs, mediastinum, diaphragm and oesophagus, and tests of respiratory function. Surgical treatment is contraindicated by:

(1) serious cardiovascular or renal disease; (2) distant metastases, the commonest sites being the supraclavicular lymph nodes, the liver, the skin, the brain and the skeleton; (3) severe impairment of respiratory function, which is usually due to chronic bronchitis and emphysema; (4) invasion of the mediastinum, as shown by paralysis of either hemidiaphragm or of the left vocal cord. Horner's syndrome, a brachial plexus lesion, localized displacement of the oesophagus, or obstruction of the superior vena cava or trachea; (5) direct or metastatic involvement of the pleura, which in doubtful cases should be confirmed by pleural biopsy; (6) proximity of the tumour to the main carina, making its resection technically impossible.

If none of these contraindications is present, the patient should be referred to a surgeon for thoracotomy. Pneumonectomy is generally the operation of choice, but if the lesion is localized to a single lobe, lobectomy is preferable, particularly if the patient is over 65 years of age or if his respiratory function is impaired. In expert hands the risks of the operation itself are slight, but even after a technically successful pneumonectomy or lobectomy the tumour recurs in about 70 per cent. of cases within five years.

Radiotherapy. If surgical treatment is contraindicated, radiotherapy may be given. If the tumour is small, radical irradiation with a linear accelerator, which allows much higher doses to be applied without damage to the skin or superficial tissues, may produce results comparable with those of surgery. Even when the tumour is too extensive for radical treatment, palliative doses may provide useful symptomatic relief in patients with superior vena caval obstruction, tracheal compression, pain due to invasion of the chest wall or skeletal metastases. Occasionally, too, radiotherapy may relieve repeated haemoptysis or bronchial obstruction with its sequelae of pulmonary collapse and suppuration.

Cytotoxic drugs. These agents have at present only a very small place in the treatment of bronchial carcinoma. They are never curative, are less effective than radiotherapy and produce more severe and less predictable side-effects. Probably their most useful application is in the treatment of malignant pleural effusion. Reaccumulation of fluid can often be prevented by the intrapleural injection of 20 mg. of mustine hydrochloride, followed 48 hours later by evacuation of the fluid by aspiration or intercostal drainage.

Mustine or cyclophosphamide can be given intravenously to relieve pain caused by chest wall invasion or skeletal metastases. This form of treatment may keep patients almost pain-free for a few weeks, but if repeated when the pain recurs it is usually less effective and is liable to damage the blood-forming tissues. A maintenance dose of cyclophosphamide by mouth is sometimes advised after intravenous treatment, but in the authors' experience this is of little value and is not without danger. The intravenous administration of a rapidly acting cytotoxic drug, such as mustine, is of particular value in the treatment of patients suffering from tumours compressing the trachea or main bronchi, in whom the application of deep X-rays, which initially causes tumour swelling, may increase the degree of obstruction, even to the point of asphyxia. In these circumstances, a single dose of mustine hydrochloride (0·4 mg. per kg. body weight), which produces tumour shrinkage, apparently without initial swelling, should always precede treatment with deep X-rays.

Cytotoxic drugs in bronchial carcinoma are, in practice, valuable only for the relief of specific complications such as those mentioned above. Any benefit obtained is invariably of short duration, but it can be very useful because it may allow opiates to be withheld until a later stage in the illness. This is particularly important when a patient seems likely to survive for some months and there is a danger, if opiates are started too soon, that they will have become ineffective when he has still some weeks to live.

Symptomatic treatment. Sooner or later symptomatic treatment will be required for the relief of pain, cough and breathlessness. Drugs such as codeine compound tablets, methadone and pethidine should be used initially, but later most patients will require opiates which also relieve anxiety. A mixture containing morphine, 15 mg., and cocaine, 10 mg., flavoured with sugar and alcohol is often remarkably effective in relieving pain and raising morale. This mixture may at first be required only at night, but later increasing doses may have to be given every few hours. Ultimately, increasing doses of morphine or diamorphine by subcutaneous injection are necessary. Chlorpromazine in a dose of 50 to 100 mg. thrice daily is of value in the relief of pain and mental distress and may be prescribed in combination with opiates; it may also be valuable in suppressing the nausea and vomiting caused by opiates.

NON-MALIGNANT TUMOURS

Bronchial adenoma. This tumour generally consists of a small intrabronchial lesion with a large encapsulated extra-bronchial extension. The portion of the tumour situated within the bronchial lumen can be removed through the bronchoscope but, as the extra-bronchial extension remains, recurrence is almost invariable. It is, therefore, necessary to resect the pulmonary lobe or segment containing the tumour along with the bronchus from which it arises.

Benign mediastinal tumours and cysts. These should generally be removed surgically as soon as they are discovered because most of them produce symptoms sooner or later. Some do so by their size alone, others become infected and a few undergo malignant change. The operative mortality is very small.

PULMONARY FIBROSIS

Pulmonary fibrosis has a variety of causes. It occurs, for example, after infections in which there has been damage to pulmonary structure, such as tuberculosis and suppurative pneumonia. In these conditions the fibrous tissue merely repairs the parenchymal damage and is not responsible for any specific symptoms. Prompt and efficient treatment of the primary disease will limit the extent of the fibrosis, but there is no treatment for the fibrosis itself.

In another group of conditions the fibrosis represents a reaction to different types of pulmonary lesion. In *silicosis* and other forms of pneumoconiosis (p. 571) fibrous tissue forms round particles of silica lodged in the pulmonary lymphatics (focal fibrosis). The type of fibrosis which follows *radiotherapy* involves the alveolar walls (interstitial fibrosis) and is the sequel to monocytic cellular exudation. If the whole thorax has been irradiated, the effect of interstitial exudation and fibrosis may be to make the lungs rigid and to impair the transfer of oxygen from the alveoli into the blood. Such patients may become intensely dyspnoeic and seriously hypoxic. Similar changes may occur in *sarcoidosis* (p. 223), in some of the *connective tissue disorders* (p. 458), and in another condition of unknown aetiology, namely, *cryptogenic fibrosing alveolitis*.

Treatment. Diseases in which the lesions are 'interstitial', that is, in the alveolar walls, may respond to corticosteroid therapy. In irradiation damage and sarcoidosis the remission produced by corticosteroids may be permanent, but in order to reduce the likelihood of relapse, treatment should be maintained for three or four months in cases of irradiation damage and for at least six months in cases of sarcoidosis. The response to treatment in cryptogenic fibrosing alveolitis is unpredictable, often only partial and seldom permanent. It is more often favourable in women under the age of 40 than in other subjects. Treatment should be maintained for at least two years and may have to be continued for the rest of the patient's life. Where the pulmonary lesions are a manifestation of one of the connective tissue disorders, the prognosis is determined chiefly by the lesions in the other organs, particularly the kidneys.

In our experience, prednisolone is still the most suitable drug for all types of interstitial lung disease. Initially, 15 to 20 mg. should be given daily in three or four divided doses. This should be continued until no further improvement in dyspnoea and pulmonary function tests can be observed, and serial radiographs suggest that no further clearing of the pulmonary shadowing can be expected. Thereafter a very gradual reduction to a maintenance dose of 10 to 12·5 mg. per day should be made. If the dose is reduced too rapidly or if the treatment is abruptly withdrawn, there may be a sudden and serious relapse which is apparently caused by a recurrence of the exudative phase of the condition. In that event the dose must be immediately increased to twice the initial level and subsequent reduction made with even greater caution than before.

Respiratory failure in interstitial lung disease differs from that due to alveolar hypoventilation in that retention of carbon dioxide and respiratory acidosis do not occur. Oxygen can, therefore, be given freely in these conditions without the risk of inducing carbon dioxide narcosis. Unfortunately, by the time this stage is reached the pulmonary changes responsible for the respiratory failure are generally irreversible and no treatment is of any avail.

PNEUMOCONIOSIS

Although in the past the term pneumoconiosis was used to include all diseases of the lungs due to the inhalation of various kinds of dust, it is now normally reserved for diseases due to silica, asbestos and coal dust. The prevention and social repercussions of pneumoconiosis are fully discussed on p. 571.

The symptomatic treatment of pneumoconiosis differs in no essential respect from that of chronic bronchitis (p. 194) and emphysema (p. 197). The treatment of pulmonary tuberculosis complicating the pneumoconiosis of coal-workers is described on p. 75.

SARCOIDOSIS

Sarcoidosis is a systemic granulomatous disease of undetermined aetiology and pathogenesis. Mediastinal and superficial lymph nodes, lungs, liver, spleen, skin, eyes, parotid glands and phalangeal bones are the organs most frequently involved. The diagnosis can usually be confirmed by histological examination of a cervical lymph node or by a Kveim test.

Sarcoidosis may present in a subacute or a chronic form. Subacute sarcoidosis is usually a benign and self-limiting disorder. One of its most common manifestations is bilateral enlargement of the hilar lymph nodes which is often accompanied at the onset by erythema nodosum, pyrexia and polyarthralgia. Only symptomatic treatment is required in such cases except when the clinical features are persistent and severe, when it may occasionally be necessary to give a short course of corticosteroid therapy. If prednisolone is used, treatment should be started with a dose of 20 mg. per day and this is gradually reduced after about a fortnight until the treatment is withdrawn in four to six weeks.

As subacute sarcoidosis occasionally fails to remit spontaneously and may then pass on to the chronic form of the disease, all patients in whom the diagnosis is made should be kept under observation for a minimum period of five years.

Chronic sarcoidosis is a more serious condition than the subacute form. Involvement of vital organs such as the lungs, heart and kidneys may cause irreversible structural damage, progressive impairment of function and death. Ocular sarcoidosis may lead to blindness and lesions of the skin and subcutaneous tissues (e.g. lupus pernio) may produce serious disfigurement. The manifestations of this form of sarcoidosis can often be suppressed by corticosteroid therapy but, except in a few cases which undergo spontaneous remission while corticosteroids are being given, they are liable to recur whenever treatment is stopped. Although many patients require to be treated for long periods,

H*

this does not detract from the value of corticosteroids, as in many instances the potential danger from side-effects is much less than that of allowing chronic sarcoidosis to progress unchecked. In many patients with pulmonary disease, for example, the development of secondary interstitial fibrosis and all its grave consequences can be postponed indefinitely by quite a small daily dose of prednisolone.

Indications for corticosteroid therapy. Corticosteroids should be reserved for those patients, most of them with chronic sarcoidosis, in whom the disorder is liable to have a fatal outcome or to cause permanent disability or serious disfigurement. On that basis corticosteroid therapy is recommended when the following indications are present:

1. Active ocular sarcoidosis (local corticosteroid therapy is inadequate in this condition).
2. Pulmonary sarcoidosis.

    Corticosteroids should be given if during a two-month period of observation there is evidence of clinical or radiological deterioration or of progressive impairment of pulmonary function. Treatment should also be advised if radiological changes fail to clear spontaneously after a four-month period of observation.
3. Persistent hypercalcaemia or hypercalciuria, which may lead to the development of renal calcinosis.
4. Involvement of the central nervous system.
5. Myocardial sarcoidosis.
6. Disfiguring cutaneous lesions.
7. Persisting hepatomegaly or splenomegaly.

Dosage and duration of corticosteroid therapy. The correct maintenance dose of corticosteroid in sarcoidosis is the smallest amount of the drug which will suppress clinical and radiological evidence of activity. This is seldom more than 10 mg. per day of prednisolone or the equivalent dose of one of the other synthetic corticosteroid preparations, and may be as little as 5 mg. per day in some cases. It is advisable at the start of treatment to prescribe a higher dose, e.g. 15 to 20 mg. per day, to bring the more florid features of the disease under control, but this can usually be reduced to maintenance level within a few weeks.

Corticosteroid therapy should be given in the first instance for a period of six months except on rare occasions when corticosteroids are being used to control transient manifestations of subacute sarcoidosis (p. 223). An attempt should then be made to withdraw treatment by reducing the dose gradually over a period of four to six weeks. In the event of a relapse, corticosteroid therapy must be resumed for a further period. Life-long treatment may be required in some particularly chronic cases.

Opinions are divided on the need for coincident antituberculosis chemotherapy, but most physicians believe it is unnecessary. This view, however, is opposed by those who still consider sarcoidosis to be, in many instances, an atypical form of tuberculosis.

PULMONARY EMBOLISM AND INFARCTION

The treatment of *massive pulmonary embolism* is described on p. 105.

PULMONARY INFARCTION

This condition is caused by an embolus derived in most instances from thrombi in the superficial or deep veins of the legs or in the femoral or iliac veins.

Treatment. Unless there are contraindications, all cases of pulmonary infarction must be treated with one of the anticoagulant drugs. These agents have no action on an established venous thrombus in the legs or elsewhere but by restricting the production of fibrin, prevent the formation of new thrombus, which may become detached and give rise to further pulmonary embolism. Retrograde extension of the thrombus in the pulmonary arterial system may also be prevented by anticoagulants. Treatment is thus directed to the prevention of further pulmonary embolism. Established pulmonary infarcts usually resolve without other treatment; analgesics are given if pleuritic pain is present.

It is rational to keep the patient at rest in bed until the thrombus has had time to become less friable and more firmly adherent to the wall of the vein. A period of 10 days is usually sufficient for these changes to occur; thereafter the patient can be permitted to resume normal activity fairly rapidly. Before being allowed up, however, he should practise active movements of the lower limbs, the most common site of venous thrombosis, in order to prevent the development of dependent oedema. If a lower limb becomes swollen before or during treatment, the foot of the bed should be elevated and when the patient is up an elastic stocking should be worn.

The management of anticoagulant therapy is described in detail on p. 186. In most cases of pulmonary infarction a course of treatment for three to four weeks is sufficient to prevent further venous thrombosis and pulmonary embolism. Occasionally, however, thrombosis or embolism recurs before or after treatment is stopped; in such cases anticoagulant therapy will have to be maintained for several months. Prolonged anticoagulant therapy is also indicated in the rare condition of multiple pulmonary emboli occurring over a period of months or years, often without clinical evidence of infarction, and leading eventually to pulmonary hypertension and cor pulmonale.

Provided the diagnosis is correct and adequate facilities are available for estimating the prothrombin concentration, there are few contraindications to anticoagulant therapy in pulmonary infarction. Anticoagulant drugs are contraindicated by active peptic ulceration, recent haematemesis and melaena, hepatic disease, malignant hypertension or by a haemorrhagic diathesis. Persistent haemoptysis or a slightly blood-stained pleural effusion should not be regarded as a contraindication, nor should it cause treatment to be interrupted. If a patient develops hypersensitivity to an anticoagulant drug, treatment may be continued by substituting another preparation or, if necessary, by reverting to the use of heparin (p. 186).

In patients with venous thrombosis of the legs who have further pulmonary emboli in spite of well-controlled anticoagulant therapy, surgical treatment will have to be considered. This may have to be more frequently recommended in cases where anticoagulants are contraindicated.

Before the operation, the site of the venous thrombosis should be localized by means of ^{125}I-labelled fibrinogen technique or by phlebography. When thrombosis is demonstrated in the femoral veins or distally, both superficial femoral veins are usually ligated below the termination of the profunda. In the case of thrombus in the iliofemoral veins, thrombectomy is performed, preferably as early as possible, since delay reduces the chances of complete removal of the thrombus. In rare cases, in which well-controlled anticoagulant therapy and surgical procedures have failed to prevent recurrent pulmonary emboli, caval thrombectomy or the operation of plication of the inferior vena cava may have to be considered. These procedures, which carry a high mortality, will very seldom be necessary.

Pulmonary infarcts may become infected by various organisms, but this is uncommon except with large infarcts. In such cases the development of a lung abscess or an empyema is always a serious event but prophylactic antibiotic therapy in pulmonary infarction is not recommended because of the danger of cross-infection by drug resistant staphylococci and gram-negative bacilli. The best method of prevention is the prompt isolation of patients with large pulmonary infarcts. If a lung abscess or empyema develops, it should be treated as described on pp. 207 and 208. Anticoagulant therapy should be given at the same time if it is believed that there is a risk of further venous thrombosis in the legs.

Prevention. The prevention of venous thrombosis and pulmonary embolism is discussed on p. 141.

SPONTANEOUS PNEUMOTHORAX

Spontaneous pneumothorax results most commonly from the rupture of an emphysematous bulla or the tearing of a pleural adhesion at its pulmonary attachment. Occasionally, it may be due to the rupture through the visceral pleura of a superficial tuberculous focus or a pulmonary abscess.

If there is a large broncho-pleural fistula, e.g. following the rupture of a tuberculous cavity or pulmonary abscess, pleural infection almost invariably supervenes, with the production of a pyopneumothorax. The treatment of tuberculous pyopneumothorax is described on p. 76 and that of non-tuberculous cases on p. 197.

In most instances, however, the pneumothorax is of the so-called benign variety due to the rupture of a subpleural emphysematous bulla. The fistula is small and usually closes almost immediately, the air is gradually absorbed, the collapsed lung re-expands and the pleural space does not become infected. Occasionally the fistula persists as a small valvular opening, in which case the intra-pleural pressure rises above atmospheric level, the lung collapses completely and ventilation of the opposite lung is impaired by mediastinal displacement. The state of 'tension' pneumothorax which results may, if untreated, prove fatal.

Treatment. The first decision to be made after the diagnosis is reached is whether or not emergency treatment is required for the relief of intrapleural tension. Urgent dyspnoea, especially if accompanied by cyanosis, suggests that a tension pneumothorax is present and calls for the immediate insertion of an intercostal drainage tube into the pleural space (p. 638). The tube should be connected either to a water-seal drainage system or to a one-way valve, which allows air to escape from, but not to re-enter, the pleural space. In a dire emergency, if facilities for this procedure are not available, the pleural space can be decompressed by inserting a wide-bore needle connected to an improvised water-seal drainage system.

Complete re-expansion of the lung is usually obtained within 24 hours of the insertion of an intercostal tube. Although the fistula generally closes as soon as the visceral and parietal pleural surfaces come into contact, it is advisable to keep the tube in place for five or seven days to ensure that the fistula seals off completely and to encourage the formation of pleural adhesions, which may prevent further episodes. If the pneumothorax is accompanied by a pleural effusion, the fluid can either be drained through the catheter by suitable posturing or aspirated with a syringe and needle at another site.

All other cases of spontaneous pneumothorax fall roughly into two categories: (1) the pneumothorax is small and the degree of dyspnoea is slight; (2) the pneumothorax is large and dyspnoea is moderately severe.

Patients in the first category require no treatment apart from rest, but the chest should be examined radiologically at weekly intervals until re-expansion of the lung is complete. The second category includes all cases in which the lung is more than one-third collapsed. Absorption of the air in these cases may take several weeks, and the period of disability can and should be reduced by the insertion of an intercostal tube, as described for the treatment of 'tension' pneumothorax.

The same general principles apply to the treatment of patients with an active tuberculous lesion in the underlying lung, with one important exception. If a pleural effusion develops, particularly if tubercle bacilli are found in the fluid, re-expansion of the lung must be secured with all possible speed in order to prevent the formation of an empyema. Regardless of the size of the pneumothorax, an intercostal tube should be inserted in all such cases.

Every case of spontaneous pneumothorax should be investigated in an effort to discover its cause. Radiologically, the appearance of the underlying lung in the presence of a pneumothorax (especially if it is large) may be misleading, as intrapulmonary disease, particularly tuberculosis, may be obscured by collapse. The examination must, therefore, be repeated after the lung has re-expanded. If there is any sputum it should be examined repeatedly for tubercle bacilli. Thoracoscopy seldom helps in diagnosis or treatment, and in most instances can safely be omitted.

If an active tuberculous lesion is found, specific chemotherapy (p. 75) should be started at once. In most cases, however, no such abnormality is found and a non-tuberculous cause can be assumed. Rarely, a tuberculous lesion appears in the lung long after the patient has recovered from a pneumothorax. It is, therefore, a wise precaution to continue observation for six months.

Recurrent spontaneous pneumothorax. When this occurs on the same or opposite side, it should be treated by the induction of an artificial pleurisy to stimulate the formation of adhesions between the visceral and parietal pleural surfaces. This can often be achieved by injecting an irritant substance into the pleural space such as 2 ml. of a 25 per cent. suspension of kaolin. Parietal pleurectomy will be necessary if these methods of treatment prove ineffective.

Chronic spontaneous pneumothorax. When a valvular fistula persists for months or even years it can seldom be successfully treated in the same way as the acute type of tension pneumothorax. Owing to thickening of the visceral pleura, the lung cannot re-expand and decortication has to be performed.

SPONTANEOUS HAEMOPNEUMOTHORAX

Haemorrhage may occur into the pleural space following spontaneous pneumothorax as a result of the rupture of a pleural adhesion. This condition can often be treated successfully by the aspiration of blood and air, but it may be necessary in some cases to insert two intercostal tubes, one at the base to evacuate the blood and the other below the clavicle to remove the air. If bleeding continues or the pleural space becomes filled with blood clot, thoracotomy will be required.

9. Diseases of the Alimentary System

W. P. SMALL and D. J. C. SHEARMAN

INTRODUCTION

Great changes have taken place in the management of gastro-intestinal disease in recent years and many traditional methods of treatment have been called into question and re-appraised with the help of new methods of study. Thus the investigation and management of gastro-intestinal disorders has become increasingly specialized. The specialist skills required to carry out management have made obvious the need for a combined approach by physician and surgeon in order to solve difficult and complicated problems. In many hospitals, this concept of a unification of medical and surgical procedures has been taken a step further with the formation of teams or units which include radiologists, pathologists, psychiatrists and biochemists. The facilities thus established for the intensive investigation and scientific control of the management of alimentary disease have advantages both to the patient and the doctor. There are opportunities for the perfecting of special techniques, for the postgraduate training of nursing and medical staff, and for the concentration of specialized equipment.

If treatment is to be effective, not only must it be controlled during its administration, but its long-term effects must also be known. An important part of management is therefore the follow-up of patients. Because many disorders of the alimentary tract occur in young people and tend to run a chronic course, long-term follow-up is essential not only to allow adjustment of the patient's treatment but also to assess the results. Even when operation has been carried out, the doctor is not absolved from the after-care of the patient who has undergone, for example, bowel resection or an operation for duodenal ulcer.

Many of the functional disorders of the alimentary tract, such as the dyspepsias or the irritable bowel syndrome, present chronic or recurrent problems calling for careful and long-continued support from the physician.

DISEASES OF THE MOUTH

The mouth and tongue may be affected in a variety of systemic disorders, or by vitamin or mineral deficiencies, and are sometimes involved in reactions to drugs. Most of the lesions respond adequately to treatment of the underlying disorder, to the administration of vitamin or mineral supplements or to withdrawal of the offending drug.

Ulcer of the Tongue

Although this may be secondary to irritation from a sharp or damaged tooth it is wise to regard all ulcers, present for longer than a few weeks, as possibly malignant. A biopsy should be carried out and if the tissue is malignant, radiotherapy and/or surgery instituted. Patients with leucoplakia (firm whitish areas on the tongue or in the mouth), should be kept under close review, as this may be a pre-malignant lesion.

Aphthous Stomatitis

In this condition periodic outbreaks of small painful ulcers occur on the buccal mucosa and tongue. Pellets containing 2·5 mg. of hydrocortisone may be helpful and in very severe cases it has been suggested that very low doses of steroids (5 mg. of prednisolone daily) given over many weeks may reduce the severity of the disorder. In other cases, pain can be alleviated by sucking tablets which contain local anaesthetic.

Thrush

This fungal infection tends to occur in debilitated patients and in those who have received broad-spectrum antibiotics for a prolonged period. For local oral lesions, 0·5 per cent. gentian violet may be used as a paint. For more severe cases, oral nystatin 500,000 units, three to four times per day is indicated.

Vincent's Stomatitis

In this infective condition, the treatment of choice is parenteral penicillin (p. 3).

DISEASES OF THE OESOPHAGUS

Difficulty in swallowing, with or without pain or regurgitation, is the dominant symptom of oesophageal disease. The ability to swallow is so fundamental to survival that dysphagia inevitably causes anxiety to the patient. A failure to appreciate this aspect of oesophageal disease risks the erroneous assumption that symptoms due to a genuine and perhaps serious organic cause are of psychiatric origin.

The Paterson-Kelly syndrome (Plummer Vinson syndrome). This is characterized by dysphagia and atrophy of epithelial cells in the mouth, oesophagus and stomach. There may be iron-deficiency anaemia. Barium swallow and oesophagoscopy may reveal the presence of a mucosal web, but more commonly there is no abnormality. The oesophagoscopy often relieves the dysphagia although the web remains. If there is anaemia, treatment by oral and sometimes parenteral iron is effective (p. 143), but surveillance for life with a yearly oesophagoscopy is advisable to prevent relapse and to ensure immediate treatment if malignant disease should supervene. This condition is suspected of being pre-cancerous.

Pharyngeal pouch. As a result of incoordination of the inferior constrictor of the pharynx, abnormally high pressures may develop in the pharynx and lead to herniation of mucosa posteriorly in the gap between the constituent parts of the sphincter. Difficulty in swallowing thus precedes the development of a pouch. As this increases in size it causes distortion of the oesophageal orifice and compression of the upper oesophagus with exacerbation of the dysphagia.

For a time, the patient can gain a measure of relief by compressing the pouch and thus emptying its contents. The treatment is surgical resection, after careful pre-operative cleansing of the sac, and under antibiotic cover to prevent mediastinal infection. If the pouch remains untreated there are dangers of chronic ulceration and carcinoma from stagnation of food, and acute or chronic chest infection from the inhalation of collected food and secretions.

Achalasia of the cardia. This is a motility disorder of the whole oesophagus. Failure of the lower end to relax is associated with progressive atony and flaccid dilatation of the rest of the organ. It is a slowness or a difficulty in swallowing that characterizes this disease and the patient may take hours over a simple meal. The true diagnosis may not be suspected until pneumonia or mass radiography leads to chest X-ray. The large quantities of food residue contained in the capacious oeso-

phagus are readily inhaled, and there is a special risk if a general anaesthetic be given to the unprepared patient.

Treatment is surgical after adequate cleansing of the oesophagus. This pre-operative preparation may require repeated oesophageal lavage with one or more oesophagoscopic removals of solid particles of food. Forcible dilatation of the cardio-oesophageal junction, sufficient to cause muscle rupture, can be effective and can be achieved either by the passage of a hydrostatic dilator through an oesophagoscope, or laparotomy. The endoscopic method is difficult and not without danger of perforation. Undoubtedly the most satisfactory method of treatment is Heller's operation (cardiomyotomy) whereby the muscle at the cardio-oesophageal junction, and for some distance above and below, is slit leaving the mucosa intact. One possible complication of the operation may be oesophagitis. This is caused by reflux through the now incompetent oesophagogastric junction, so that the precautionary addition of vagotomy and drainage at the time of myotomy is advisable.

Other motility disorders. Abnormal oesophageal motility or spasm leading to pain and dysphagia may occur in the elderly or secondary to emotional stress. After exclusion of organic disease, anticholinergic drugs may be prescribed, and the patient's life so ordered that precipitating factors such as dietetic indiscretions, exhaustion and mental stress are avoided as far as possible.

Carcinoma of the oesophagus. The outlook in this disease has been radically changed by the introduction of improved methods of radiotherapy. In some centres the chance of cure has been increased with the use of the linear accelerator. In less favourable cases, it produces worthwhile palliation. Radiotherapy is suitable for squamous growths in the upper and middle thirds of the oesophagus. Adeno-carcinoma, which is often situated at the lower end and arises from the stomach, is relatively unresponsive to radiotherapy and is treated by resection. The operation is formidable and particularly in the elderly it carries a high risk. Prior to radiotherapy or operation, anaemia and dehydration should be corrected (fluids intravenously and blood transfusion), and parenteral feeding may be required.

Palliative measures in extensive and recurrent oesophageal disease raise ethical problems. The complete dysphagia that prevents the swallowing of saliva can be alleviated by the insertion of a tube through the oesophagoscope or at laparotomy, but to make a gastrostomy or a jejunostomy merely as palliation is not considered proper; nor is it worth while, for the cause of death is usually inhalation pneumonia rather than starvation.

Oesophagitis. Peptic oesophagitis is the usual form and is due to the reflux of gastric secretions through an oesophago-gastric junction rendered incompetent by hiatus hernia. Acute oesophagitis causes heartburn and intermittent dysphagia, whereas in chronic oesophagitis a stricture has usually developed, with consequent dysphagia, but the heartburn is often less severe. Oesophagitis may also be due to other agents such as bile and intestinal juice.

Peptic oesophagitis. At the stage of reflux and heartburn, treatment depends on the severity of the symptoms and the presence or absence of predisposing causes. The heartburn of pregnancy associated with increased intra-abdominal pressure is treated symptomatically with alkalis, and the avoidance of a sloppy diet. When hiatus hernia is a complication of obesity, weight reduction will often relieve symptoms entirely. Where there is free reflux, it may be necessary to begin medical treatment by a period of bed rest, two-hourly alkalis, elevation of the head of the bed on wooden blocks, and the provision of pillows enough to ensure that the patient sleeps propped up. This raising of the head of the bed must be adopted as a permanent arrangement. Work must be arranged to avoid stooping and some aspects of daily life, such as scrubbing floors and weeding the garden, become virtually impossible. Women must be encouraged to avoid the wearing of all tight and restrictive abdominal clothing. While rigid adherence to a medical regimen secures relief, the hardship is considerable, and most patients whose symptoms persist after weight reduction are best treated by operation. This entails repair of the hernia through the chest or abdomen and the treatment of any concomitant duodenal ulcer usually by vagotomy and drainage.

When stricture formation complicates peptic oesophagitis, stretching of the stricture temporarily improves the dysphagia, but it creates a risk of recurrence of the heartburn and an exacerbation of the oesophagitis. In many of these patients the oesophageal fibrosis has resulted in shortening of the oesophagus so that replacement of the oesophago-gastric junction below the diaphragm becomes impossible. However, a satisfactory symptomatic response can be obtained by concentrating on the nature of the reflux rather than on its occurrence. Partial gastrectomy or vagotomy and drainage will reduce gastric secretion and by so doing will relieve symptoms and secure healing of the stricture. This operation must be a last resort because there is some possibility that a biliary oesophagitis will occur. If dysphagia persists after vagotomy and drainage or partial gastrectomy it is then safe to stretch the stricture with bougies, either swallowed by the patient or introduced through an oesophagoscope. Daily self-bouginage with a Hurst's mercury bougie is often a satisfactory method of restoring the patient's confidence in the ability to swallow, and at the same time it allows gradual stretching of the stricture. It is seldom necessary to continue bouginage for more than a few weeks, for in the absence of persistent gastric hypersecretion, the stricture, once stretched is unlikely to recur.

Biliary oesophagitis. This occurs particularly after high or total gastrectomy but it can take place after any gastric operation. Severe ulceration of the lower oesophagus can occur as a result of reflux of bile and pancreatic secretions. For treatment, alkalis are of no value and attention must be paid to small dry meals and to posture. If it remains a severe problem this may be due to failure to repair a hiatus hernia, a badly functioning anastomosis between stomach and jejunum or duodenum, or adhesions causing an afferent loop syndrome. Laparotomy should be undertaken for repair of hernia and perhaps the construction of an entero-anastomosis of the Roux-en-Y type.

DISEASES OF THE STOMACH
Peptic Ulcer

This is a common disorder and a large proportion of the population will probably suffer from it at some time in their lives. It follows that the great majority of ulcers will heal spontaneously. Other ulcers will not heal but symptomatic treatment over the years will provide control acceptable to the patient. Occasionally, intensive medical therapy or surgery may be required. A peptic ulcer can occur in the oesophagus, stomach, duodenum, or in the jejunum after operations on the stomach, and the aetiology of the ulcer may differ for each of these sites. Thus it might be expected that there will be differing responses to any one treatment depending on the site of the ulcer.

MEDICAL TREATMENT OF UNCOMPLICATED GASTRIC AND DUODENAL ULCER

Rest in bed. During a severe exacerbation of ulcer symptoms, rest in bed nearly always brings relief. In hospital, this commonly takes only three to four days, though at home such treatment may fail because rest is incomplete, or more significantly because many of the surrounding irritations and stresses of life are not removed. Thus a severe episode which does not respond to bed rest at home plus the measures listed below should be treated in hospital.

Diet. 'Gastric diets' of milk, fish, etc., are not necessary. Some physicians advise them because they emphasize to the patient that there is some need to avoid dietary excesses, but in general the patient should receive a well-balanced nutritious diet. Meals should be regular, small and frequent, and gastric stimulants such as tea, coffee and alcohol should be avoided. Patients with long-standing symptoms may be malnourished and should be encouraged to take a normal diet with vitamin supplements.

Smoking. The patient should be strongly advised to stop smoking. This is particularly important if operation is being considered. Cessation of smoking allows a more rapid healing of gastric ulcers.

Harmful drugs. Many drugs have been shown to produce gastric ulceration by acting on gastric mucus or on gastric epithelial cells. Such effects are produced by aspirin, corticosteroids, indomethacin and phenylbutazone. If a gastric ulcer develops in a patient who is receiving one of these drugs, then healing of the ulcer is usually dependent upon its withdrawal. Patients with peptic ulceration should avoid these substances, as well as reserpine-like drugs which may encourage ulceration by increasing the output of acid.

Drug Treatment of Peptic Ulceration

This is aimed at reducing the secretion of acid and pepsin by the stomach and although it brings about symptomatic relief there is no evidence that such therapy is curative. More recently, it has been shown that some extracts of liquorice will aid ulcer healing.

Antacids. These relieve pain by raising the gastric pH transiently and this has the additional effect of reducing peptic activity. The various antacids differ in their rapidity of action, their neutralizing capacity and the degree to which they are absorbed, with a resulting effect on the extracellular pH. Sodium bicarbonate is a useful antacid if used sparingly because of its immediate action, but if given extensively it will cause metabolic alkalosis and eventually nephrocalcinosis. Of the antacids which do not cause alkalosis, calcium carbonate is the most useful because of its rapid action, but when given over a prolonged period it may cause hypercalcaemia. Because of their opposing actions on the bowel, aluminium hydroxide gel which tends to cause constipation and magnesium trisilicate which causes diarrhoea are often used together.

To maintain the gastric contents above pH 4, antacids have to be given often and in large dosage, because of normal gastric emptying. Thus, to relieve a severe exacerbation of pain, the patient in hospital may be given an intragastric drip of 10 to 20 g. of sodium bicarbonate per litre of milk every six hours for two to three days. Thereafter, antacids may be given hourly in liquid form. At other times, for convenience, antacids should be given in tablet form, the tablets being chewed between meals and when symptoms occur. It is important that a palatable preparation is chosen. A bedside supply of antacids should be available for relief during the night.

Anticholinergics. These act by reducing gastric secretion and motility. In addition to diminishing gastric secretion, they cause a dry mouth, dilation of the pupil and difficulty in accommodating for near vision. They may cause retention of urine and may exacerbate glaucoma and hence must be used cautiously in elderly patients. Care should be taken in prescribing for patients who drive vehicles or work with precision instruments. The commonly used drugs are propantheline bromide (Probanthine), poldine methylsulphate (Nacton) and glycopyrronium bromide (Robinul). They are given four times a day in a dose which is gradually increased until the mouth is slightly dry but because of variable absorption and individual variability of response the actual dose is difficult to define. At night, somewhat larger doses may be given than during the day because any mild side-effects are less important. In these circumstances, the drugs are useful in preventing night pain and they may remain effective for up to eight hours.

AMYLOPECTIN SULPHATE (Depepsen). This synthetic sulphated polysaccharide may reduce peptic activity. Pre-release clinical trials suggest that it may promote the healing of gastric ulcers when given by mouth. Its use is in the experimental stage and optimum doses have yet to be determined.

Carbenoxolone sodium. This promotes the healing of gastric ulcers when given by mouth in a dosage of 100 mg. three times per day. Fifty mg., three times a day, is probably equally effective and causes fewer side-effects. It is claimed that the use of this drug in the patient who is up and about produces the same healing rate as complete bed rest in hospital; it follows that hospital beds should be reserved for patients with severe symptoms or complications. The drug has an aldosterone-like action and can produce sodium and water retention, oedema, hypokalaemia, alkalosis and hypertension. In elderly patients this drug should be given cautiously if at all; its use is contraindicated in patients with cardiac failure. It is unwise to attempt to counteract the side-effects by giving diuretics because aldosterone antagonists inhibit the effect on gastric mucosa and thiazides may accentuate the hypokalaemia. Carbenoxolone may produce muscle weakness and diarrhoea. Physicians hold differing views as to how long a patient with gastric ulcer should receive medical treatment before recommending surgery. Generally, carbenoxolone will be given for at least 4 to 8 weeks, with regular checks on blood pressure and serum electrolytes during this period. When there is no evidence of healing, operation should be considered because there is then a distinct possibility that the ulcer is malignant. In some patients with evidence of healing, conservative measures will be continued. The evidence of healing requires to be examined critically since radiographic healing may represent the disappearance of oedema around the ulcer and therefore gastroscopic assessment is always indicated.

Carbenoxolone sodium has not been shown to be of value in the treatment of duodenal ulcer.

Deglycyrrhizinated liquorice. This is the liquorice residue after removal of the carbenoxolone-like compounds. It has none of the side-effects of carbenoxolone and, as yet, there is no standardized dose for any of the preparations. Preliminary trials suggest that the agent is more effective than a placebo in the healing of gastric ulcers and it may bring about symptomatic improvement in patients with duodenal ulcer.

Sedatives. It is usually important to prescribe phenobarbitone or sodium amytal while the patient is in hospital to allow him to have complete rest without anxiety. A hypnotic at night may be used provided gastric irritants such as chloral hydrate are avoided.

SURGICAL TREATMENT OF PEPTIC ULCERATION

Duodenal Ulcer

Absolute or almost absolute indications for surgery are haemorrhage, perforation and stenosis and the management of these will be discussed later in this section.

The majority of patients undergoing surgical treatment for duodenal ulcer are doing so not on account of any complication of that ulcer, but because of failure to respond to medical management. The decision to offer surgery then becomes a matter of opinion which rests largely on an assessment of the patient, his ulcer and the disability it causes. There are certain useful guides, but none are infallible. A duodenal ulcer which has previously bled or perforated and which is now at a later date causing dyspepsia bad enough to warrant referral to hospital is unlikely to heal permanently or respond adequately to treatment. A high secretion of acid, for example over 50 mEq. per hour as demonstrated on a maximal stimulation test in a patient who is having persistent symptoms, is a finding in favour of operative treatment. Back pain, aggravated by movement or vibration, is significant evidence of a posteriorly placed penetrating duodenal ulcer, and such ulcers are almost certainly untreatable medically. Apart from the severity of symptoms, their general effect on the patient's life must be taken into account. His occupation or his social life may make it imperative that he is able to eat normally. Thus the man who is away from home much of the week on business may find it impossible to arrange a strict diet, as will the person who frequently dines out.

There can be few greater disasters than the selection of the wrong patient for surgery and it is therefore as important to be as aware of the contraindications as the indications. The time-honoured guides of duration of symptoms, age of patient and the degree of work loss are unreliable. The patient with a short history may have an intractable ulcer, whereas the patient with a complaint of many years may have no ulceration. Some stoical individuals lose little work although suffering severe pain, whereas the patient with impressive work loss may prove to be work shy and will remain so with added excuse after operation.

Patients may require a general psychiatric evaluation before surgery is advised. The relevance of their complaints and the probable outcome of operation must be estimated, and this may require nothing more than an interview with the physician and surgeon concerned. If there is any doubt about the patient's personality—if he is depressed or appears to have a low threshold for pain—then more formal psychiatric assessment is required. Given the patient with psychiatric abnormality (and this can be determined relatively easily by simple testing), appropriate psychiatric treatment should precede surgery for the duodenal ulcer. Good results, both physical and psychiatric, are obtainable in such patients by a combined medical, surgical and psychiatric approach. The bad results are from failure to recognize the psychiatric abnormality and to embark on surgery without proper indications and as a venture of despair.

Pulmonary tuberculosis is a contraindication to immediate radical surgery because this would add unnecessary complications to the post-operative management, but well-chosen surgery for an intractable duodenal ulcer, by allowing the patient to tolerate adequate antituberculous chemotherapy may enhance the prospects of his being cured. In the same way, a few patients with rheumatoid arthritis may require surgery for their ulcer in order to permit an adequate regimen of anti-rheumatic drug therapy, but no effort should be spared to deal medically with these problems in the first instance. The weight loss of the so-called ulcer type is not a contraindication to operation if the thinness has developed as a complication of the ulcer. Such patients can be expected to gain weight after operation.

The objections made to the surgical treatment of duodenal ulcer are that it can never guarantee freedom from the possibility of recurrence and that, like all major operations, it carries the risk of death. But these are liabilities of medical treatment, too. The Achilles heel of surgery is that it often involves irreversible mutilation so that an ill-chosen operation in a badly selected patient can give rise to more disability than the original ulcer.

Choice of operation

When the patient's need for surgery has been accepted, it remains to choose the most suitable operation. At present, vagotomy with some form of drainage is in vogue and there are some who claim that it is so effective that no other form of operation need be considered seriously. Others consider that since patients are all individuals, their requirements may consequently differ. In general, it can be said that women require less radical treatment than men. Gastroenterostomy alone, vagotomy with gastroenterostomy or pyloroplasty, and partial gastrectomy with or without added vagotomy are operations that might be selected depending on such factors as acid secretion, the type of ulcer, and the age and general physical condition of the patient.

Gastric Ulcer

In gastric ulcer, the indications for surgery are well defined and again excluding the complications of perforation, stenosis and haemorrhage, the indication for surgery is failure to heal under the conditions already discussed.

Gastric ulcer may be treated surgically by a modified gastrectomy or by vagotomy and drainage, but if the latter type of operation is chosen then excision of the ulcer or at least biopsy is all-important to guard against possible malignancy. Few gastric ulcers may become malignant, but malignant ulcers may seem deceptively benign.

Complications of Peptic Ulcer

Haematemesis and melaena. All patients suffering from haematemesis or melaena should have their blood grouped as soon as possible and an intravenous infusion started. The pulse and blood pressure must be monitored every 30 minutes and any fall in pressure or rise in pulse rate should be followed by transfusion of whole blood. A central venous line is often of value. Any defects in coagulation must be corrected. All patients should receive a sedative such as sodium amytal or sodium phenobarbitone given intramuscularly. Nasogastric suction should not be used and if the patient feels hungry he should be allowed milk and soft foods.

Continued bleeding, bleeding that stops only to start again some 24 to 48 hours later, or repeated small haemorrhages are indications for surgery. Because all patients admitted with bleeding must be regarded as potential candidates for emergency surgery, it is advisable that they be seen by surgeons as well as physicians from the outset. It then becomes easier to decide which patient is in need of operation and to time such intervention with the minimum of delay once the decision for surgery has been reached. In general, older patients stand blood loss badly and bleeding tends to continue because the vessels are more rigid from senile change and from the fibrosis of long-standing ulceration. Operation would be considered earlier in such patients than in the healthy young adult.

It is of value to the surgeon to know the site of the bleeding and an emergency X-ray examination with gastrografin may confirm the presence of an ulcer, define its site and even indicate whether or not bleeding is presently taking place. In some cases, endoscopy may also be indicated. In general, a diagnosis of superficial erosions will favour continuing medical measures rather than resorting immediately to surgical operation.

Once operation has been decided upon, blood transfusion should be at a level sufficient to achieve an adequate blood pressure and peripheral circulation. Full replacement may be impossible before bleeding has been controlled, and in any case it is obtained more rapidly and with the expenditure of much less blood once the ulcer has been treated. In recent years gastrectomy for bleeding ulcer has given way to vagotomy combined with suture of the ulcer or the bleeding vessels through a pyloroplasty or gastrotomy, and there has been a corresponding drop in the operative mortality.

Perforation. Perforation of an ulcer, which is usually duodenal, is an indication for emergency surgery. Rarely the so-called leaking ulcer, of which the diagnosis of perforation is perhaps radiological rather than clinical, can be treated conservatively. The operative treatment of perforation is usually confined to closure of the perforation, with re-assessment of the need for further surgery during convalescence and follow-up. Some surgeons advocate more definitive surgery, as, for example, vagotomy and drainage at the time of closure, but this is to deny the place of medical treatment and the possibility of healing in any such ulcers.

Pyloric stenosis. Established stenosis, as opposed to pylorospasm, is a clear indication for surgery and the one most likely to give a good result. Relief of the obstruction must usually be accompanied by some measure designed to reduce acid secretion, for pyloric stenosis should be regarded as indicating a high potential for ulceration. Thus simple drainage is liable to be followed by recurrent ulcer formation, unless combined with vagotomy or antrectomy. Prior to operation, it is important to correct electrolyte disturbances and dehydration and to clear the stomach of food residue and

secretions. Many patients are alkalotic and sodium and potassium depleted, and replacement may take several days of intravenous therapy. Some fluid may also be allowed by mouth but it is important to avoid gastric distension. The stomach must be washed out with a wide-bore tube on several occasions to remove debris; this allows some improvement in the condition of the mucosa prior to operation.

COMPLICATIONS OF GASTRIC OPERATIONS

In a small number of patients, surgery for peptic ulceration is followed by complications. These may be kept to a minimum by careful selection of the patient for surgery and by the participation of an experienced surgeon: for example, a complete vagotomy is more likely to be achieved in expert hands.

Immediate complications. These may develop hours or days after the operation.

BLEEDING. This may take place from the suture line or from an ulcer which was not removed at operation. The initial treatment is as for any gastro-duodenal haemorrhage (p. 146) but in severe cases, early re-operation is indicated.

LEAKAGE FROM THE ANASTOMOSIS OR DUODENAL STUMP. This is nearly always treated conservatively but, if necessary, drainage to the surface must be accomplished. The amount drained will gradually diminish and cease over a period of weeks. Initially it will be necessary to correct for the loss of electrolytes.

STOMAL OBSTRUCTION. The onset of gastric emptying may be delayed as a result of haematoma, oedema or local leakage developing around the suture line. The site and degree of obstruction can be confirmed by gastrografin. In some patients with mechanical causes such as fibrosis, volvulus and internal herniae, operation will be required. As a guide, oedema or haematoma in the stomach wall can be expected to respond to nasogastric suction and intravenous fluids in 7 to 10 days.

Delayed complications. A number of complications can arise after gastric surgery but though it is important to avoid generating hypochondriasis in these patients it is equally important to carry out a yearly check, using such criteria as weight, haemoglobin level and alkaline phosphatase as well as a review of symptoms. Although the following complaints are noted separately, it is usually difficult to separate the various symptoms into clearly defined syndromes. Occasionally the problem will be mechanical, for example, kinking or twisting of the afferent or efferent loop, and the correction must be surgical, but most of the problems arise from disorders of function or metabolism.

RECURRENT ULCER. This may arise in gastric mucosa, in jejunal mucosa, or at the site of the original ulcer in the duodenum. Benign gastric ulceration after gastric operations should be teated in the same way as any other gastric ulceration. An ulcer in jejunal mucosa is very likely to lead to the complications of perforation or haemorrhage, and the situation must be resolved by revision of the operation. Recurrent duodenal ulcer may be treated medically in the first instance but it is likely that further operation will be required to alleviate symptoms.

Recently the importance of ulcer recurrence at the actual suture line has been recognized. Such an ulcer gives rise to vague dyspepsia, is seldom detectable radiologically but is readily demonstrated by endoscopy. It is due to the use of non-absorbable material as a continuous suture, and its treatment is excision of the suture line and re-anastomosis using catgut.

GASTRITIS AND GASTRIC CARCINOMA. The gastric remnant is prone to progressive gastritis and in some patients carcinoma may develop. The regular follow-up of patients will result in the earlier detection of such cases. In some patients, bile may have a damaging effect on the gastric mucosa, leading to inflammation and bleeding. There is no specific treatment for this disorder but many cases will resolve spontaneously.

DUMPING SYNDROME. Here weakness, tiredness and a sensation of abdominal distension occur a short time after a meal. The exact physiological mechanism is in dispute but the initiating factor is likely to be the presence of substances of high osmolarity in the jejunum; minor symptoms of this kind may occur even in people in normal health. When symptoms are moderate in severity the patient may benefit from avoiding fluid meals with hot soups, etc. and by taking small dry meals, with a short period of rest after each meal. In the most severe cases, it may be necessary to operate again, the procedure to be adopted depending on the mechanics in each individual instance.

BILIOUS VOMITING. Here again the mechanism is unknown but the likely cause is the irritation produced by large amounts of bile in the stomach. The vomiting tends to be periodic and can occur with very little warning. The main method of treatment is dietary; many patients are helped by taking small dry meals. Very severe cases of vomiting should undergo laparotomy as there may be a mechanical cause which can be corrected. If such a cause is not found then a Roux-en-Y anastomosis or other form of surgical revision can be instituted.

HYPOGLYCAEMIA. This response may develop after a rapid rise in blood sugar secondary to dumping, and so it occurs 1 to 2 hours after meals. Treatment involves the ingestion of small amounts of food at short intervals throughout the day.

DIARRHOEA. This is a troublesome feature particularly in some patients after vagotomy and is difficult to treat because of its periodicity. In the occasional case, a remediable factor such as malabsorption may be corrected, but the majority of cases have to be managed symptomatically.

MALABSORPTION. Over the years patients may not absorb iron, calcium or vitamin B_{12} normally, and this may result ultimately in anaemia or bone disease. Any patient developing these disorders should receive the appropriate supplement for life. However, metabolic problems can arise for other reasons. For example, the afferent loop can act as a blind loop giving rise to diarrhoea as well as malabsorption of vitamin B_{12}. Operative correction of this latter disorder may be indicated. Severe malabsorption developing soon after the operation suggests the possibility that the stomach has been anastomosed to the mid- or lower jejunum or even the ileum and the appropriate action should be taken.

Gastritis

This subject has remained confused because the term gastritis has had a different meaning for endoscopists, pathologists and clinicians. In some patients, the development of atrophic gastritis and gastric atrophy is a slow process which is unlikely to be accompanied by symptoms. However, it seems likely that some more acute forms of gastric inflammation are symptomatic. In these cases, the mucosa appears inflamed when viewed through the gastroscope. An example of this is the biliary gastritis which may occur after some gastric operations (p. 233). Acute gastritis can be accompanied by loss of appetite and dyspepsia. There is no specific treatment but symptomatic measures such as antacids together with the avoidance of gastric irritants including aspirin and alcohol may help. Patients with proven gastritis should be kept under review since there is evidence that they have an increased incidence of carcinoma.

Carcinoma of the Stomach

The treatment of carcinoma of the stomach is surgical. Prospects of permanent cure are slender, because most tumours have spread by the time the patient comes to operation. Earlier diagnosis can be achieved by more critical investigation and management of gastric ulcer, and by the greater use of gastroscopic and gastric cytological examinations.

In some cases resection of the tumour and most, if not all of the involved lymph nodes is possible. Careful pre-operative preparation is essential. Anaemia should be corrected by transfusion, and any fluid and electrolyte loss caused by obstruction at the pylorus or cardia made good by intravenous replacement. The nutrition of the patient cannot be appreciably improved in the time available, but after resection a feeding jejunostomy may provide a means of supplementing oral feeding. Before operation and afterwards, care of the chest with physiotherapy and assisted expectoration is important. When there is gastric retention the foul-smelling, blood-containing contents should be aspirated and the stomach washed out with saline in the few days immediately before operation.

When the tumour has spread, as occurs in the majority of cases, local resection if at all possible provides the best palliation by removing the site of chronic blood loss and local infection. Chemotherapy is not indicated. Jejunostomy is to be avoided because it offers no advantage, neither prolonging life nor making the patient's death any easier. With fundal carcinoma which is causing dysphagia, a tube may be inserted through the tumour as a palliative measure.

The patient who has undergone radical gastrectomy will require continual supervision: anaemia will become a problem, first as a result of iron deficiency, and later through depletion of vitamin B_{12} stores. Additionally it is often difficult for the patient to take enough food to maintain his body weight. Advice will frequently be sought about problems of this kind.

INTESTINAL OBSTRUCTION

While this condition often presents as a surgical emergency, it may occur unexpectedly *de novo* in a patient under investigation or treatment for some unrelated complaint. It may also arise as a complication of a variety of so-called medical conditions. In such circumstances the symptoms and signs of obstruction may be obscured or confused and the diagnosis may be difficult. It is of the utmost importance to recognize acute intestinal obstruction, for delay in diagnosis may lead to the development of local complications such as strangulation with gangrene, perforation and peritonitis resulting in shock and toxaemia.

Intestinal obstruction is caused either by mechanical blocking of the lumen or by paralysis of the bowel. Clinically, mechanical obstruction is characterized by increased bowel sounds, visible peristalsis and griping pain. Paralysis of the bowel produces the silent abdomen with general distension, dull pain and effortless regurgitation of intestinal content. While in paralytic ileus, non-operative management is the rule, it is important to realize that paralysis may be the end-result of a mechanical obstruction where the bowel has become exhausted, or it may be due to the toxaemia of a peritonitis, the primary cause of which requires surgery. The distinction between mechanical and paralytic obstruction is particularly difficult in the elderly subject.

In the adult, mechanical obstruction is usually due to herniae, adhesions from previous operations, and carcinoma or diverticular disease of the colon. In the majority of cases, operative treatment is by far the safest course, but when the obstruction is subacute and due perhaps to adhesions or some disease such as Crohn's disease (p. 236), it may be preferable to treat the patient conservatively at least during the attack and until further investigation or definitive medical treatment is complete.

The general principles of non-operative or pre-operative management of intestinal obstruction are to empty the stomach by constant suction through a naso-gastric tube, and to replace lost fluids and electrolytes by the intravenous route. Often a considerable deficit of both fluid and electrolytes has to be corrected; the patient may have had no food or fluid by mouth for a day or two and may have lost water and electrolytes by frequent vomiting. It should also be realized that fluid lying in distended loops of intestine is lost to the circulation as surely as if it had been evacuated. Replacement therapy is guided by accurate charts of fluid balance, and by serial electrolyte estimations. The continuous aspiration of gastric contents by means of a low-pressure electric pump should be carefully supervised and hourly checks for blockage of the tube made by syringe aspiration. Effective suction will relieve much of the abdominal distension if the obstruction is predominantly small intestinal; but it will not materially affect large bowel obstruction, where the continued build-up of pressure in a closed loop with a competent ileo-caecal valve creates a risk of rupture of the caecum. To guard against such possibilities being masked by therapy, periodic straight X-ray films of the abdomen should be used to monitor progress.

In some circumstances it may become necessary to continue gastric suction and intravenous therapy for weeks on end. As a result, considerable strains are put on the patient and his attendants, both medical and nursing. The monotony and discomfort of the intra-nasal tube, the frustration of the cessation of oral intake, the disturbance from the constant monitoring of fluid and electrolyte balances, and the battle to maintain patent veins, combine to exert physical and psychological pressures. It is not surprising, therefore, that ways are sought to cut short the ordeal. In an effort to stimulate the paralysed bowel, purgatives, demulcents and enemas have been recommended, but results do not justify their use unless the bowel is active and the obstruction due to impaction of faeces at a stricture. Occasionally in ileus due to purely nervous factors as in some brain and spinal cord lesions, dramatic relief of distension can be obtained from the use of cholinergic drugs such as neostigmine 0·5 mg. subcutaneously six-hourly. In other instances electrolyte disturbances, particularly hypokalaemia, may be causing or contributing towards the ileus and these must be corrected.

In most cases, however, intestinal obstruction is the aftermath of peritonitis and operation and there are no short cuts in its management, which remains that of patience coupled with the accurate maintenance of a normal fluid and electrolyte milieu, good nursing and constant support of the patient's morale.

REGIONAL ENTERITIS
(CROHN'S DISEASE)

This is an acute or chronic inflammatory disease of the small intestine (especially the terminal ileum) the large bowel and occasionally other areas of the alimentary tract. There is no specific medical treatment and in general, surgery should be avoided unless certain complications of the disease arise. The disease is extremely trying for the patient and much support and encouragement must be given. The disorder is characterized by exacerbations and remissions and the aim of treatment is to tide the patient over the various exacerbations in the hope that eventually the disease will become inactive.

In all patients it is important that a nutritious diet be supplied with supplements of any substances which are not being absorbed normally (p. 346). A low roughage diet may be of value in patients with mild obstructive symptoms, and in others it may alleviate diarrhoea. Antispasmodics (p. 230) and diphenoxylate may be prescribed for colic or diarrhoea.

In the acute phase, some patients benefit considerably from corticosteroids (prednisolone 40 mg. per day) with reduction in the symptoms which are being caused by the acute inflammatory process. Once the symptoms have remitted the dose is gradually reduced and then stopped. There is no evidence to suggest that corticosteroids alter the course of the disorder and indeed there may be dangers in prolonged administration. Sulphasalazine in a dosage of 4 to 10 g. per day is often given on a long-term basis but here too there is no evidence that it affects the outcome of the disorder. In severe cases the use of azathioprine (p. 181) may be justified. The medical management of Crohn's disease of the colon is essentially the same as for ulcerative colitis.

In Crohn's disease, surgery may be required for abscess and fistula formation and for intestinal obstruction. It is undertaken only when all medical measures have failed to resolve or improve the situation, since surgery itself can, on occasions, lead to further exacerbations and fistula formation. Multiple resections of bowel are to be avoided if possible, but on occasion, local resection or by-pass of an affected area may be of value. As in ulcerative colitis, total colectomy for extensive colonic involvement may be required. In other cases where there is extensive fistula formation, especially of the perineum, a defunctioning colostomy may be necessary.

MALABSORPTION

Many alimentary disorders are accompanied by the malabsorption of a variety of substances which include vitamins, electrolytes, minerals, fats, protein and carbohydrate. In general, whatever the cause of the malabsorption, it is correct to supplement the substance that is not being adequately absorbed. However, a precise diagnosis of the cause of malabsorption is necessary in each case so that specific therapy may be given.

The Intraluminal Digestive Phase

Abnormalities of this phase of digestion may occur because of either inadequate lipolysis or inadequate bile salt concentrations. The breakdown of dietary triglyceride is impaired in pancreatic insufficiency, after gastric operations when there may be impaired mixing in the upper intestine, and more rarely when severe gastric hypersecretion causes the pH in the upper small intestine to become too low for pancreatic enzyme activity. A decrease in conjugated bile salts occurs after terminal ileal resection or disease, biliary tract disease, and upper small intestinal overgrowth of bacteria.

Pancreatic insufficiency. Malabsorption of fat and other substances due to chronic pancreatitis and cystic fibrosis may be treated with oral pancreatic enzymes. These preparations must be taken throughout the day, with and between meals. In patients who secrete gastric acid it is wise to give part of the supplement in an enteric coated form, since the enzymes are destroyed at low pH. The total dose is usually 8 to 12 g. per day.

Insufficiency of bile salts. (*a*) In those cases where there is terminal ileal disease or intestinal resection with interruption of the enterohepatic circulation of bile salts, the malabsorption is difficult to treat. The main complaint is of severe diarrhoea which is due, not to the steatorrhoea, but to loss of bile salts into the colon with consequent failure to absorb water and electrolytes at this site. Treatment is aimed at annulling this effect of bile salts on the colon. Cholestyramine, a bile salt binding agent, may be given in an oral dosage of up to 12 g. per day. This may increase the degree of steatorrhoea while at the same time diminishing the diarrhoea. It follows that oral administration of bile salt preparations is contraindicated because the diarrhoea will be increased.

(*b*) Bacterial overgrowth may occur in the afferent loop after some gastric operations, in achlorhydria with stasis, in blind loops, in diverticula and in many other situations in which there may be stasis. It also arises when a fistula allows colonic bacteria to enter the upper small bowel. Here the total concentration of bile salt is adequate but a proportion has been deconjugated by bacteria rendering it ineffective in fat absorption. In addition, malabsorption of vitamin B_{12} may occur due to binding of the vitamin by bacteria. These problems can be corrected temporarily by the administration of broad spectrum antibiotics and indeed this is often a help in diagnosis. In the long term, laparotomy may be necessary with correction of blind loops, relief of partial obstructions or conversion or undoing of an anastomosis.

Problems of gastric resection or hypersecretion. Malabsorption after resection may be alleviated on occasion by conversion of the operation. The rare problems of hypersecretion in the Zollinger-Ellison syndrome are mentioned on p. 252.

Mucosal Cell Transport

Even if intraluminal digestion is normal, disease or abnormalities of the intestinal mucosal cell may result in malabsorption. In gluten enteropathy and Crohn's disease, obvious pathological abnormalities can be seen, but in other disorders, for example, pernicious anaemia and disaccharidase deficiency, there may be specific abnormalities of absorption without histological evidence of cellular dysfunction.

Coeliac disease and gluten enteropathy. Most patients respond to complete exclusion of gluten from the diet. This can result in histological improvement in the intestinal mucosa and marked improvement in absorption. The diet must be regarded as a permanent feature of the patient's life, although after several years it may be possible to relax restrictions in some patients after noting the outcome of a gluten challenge. A gluten-free diet presents many problems, and explicit instruction must be given to the patient as well as to relatives who prepare food. It is usual to provide strict diet sheets together with recipes using gluten-free flour, and these must be adhered to strictly. Most centres keep up-to-date lists of proprietary foods which do not contain gluten, the problem being that gluten is widely used in prepared and proprietary foodstuffs and food additives.

Patients with gluten enteropathy require regular out-patient supervision to check weight, wellbeing and the various biochemical assessments of absorption. Specific replacement therapy is discussed below. In patients who fail to respond to the exclusion of gluten and who continue to deteriorate, the administration of corticosteroids in standard dosage may be necessary. These promote absorption. It is usual to give prednisolone 30 to 60 mg. per day but some patients have responded to the oral administration of β-methasone-17-valerate which is only partially absorbed; this preparation may have the added advantage of a local action on the mucosa of the small intestine. In some patients there may be a response to pancreatic enzyme supplements because of the pancreatic atrophy which can occur as a consequence of malnutrition.

Crohn's disease. Malabsorption may arise for a variety of reasons such as the problems related to bacterial overgrowth (p. 149), fistulae and resections; but when the main cause of malabsorption is generalized involvement of the small intestine, corticosteroids will promote absorption.

Abnormal mucosal cell transport due to bacteria. An abnormal bacterial population within the lumen of the bowel or within the mucosa itself causes abnormalities in mucosal structure and consequently in absorption.

In tropical sprue and Whipple's disease, the infective agents are unknown, but both respond to prolonged administration of broad spectrum antibiotics. In the malabsorption which accompanies the rare disorder of hypogammaglobulinaemia, infestation with *giardia lamblia* may be found and this may respond to quinacrine therapy.

SPECIFIC ABNORMALITIES OF MUCOSAL CELL TRANSPORT

In this group which includes rare disorders such as cystinuria and abetalipoproteinaemia, the only relatively common problem is disaccharidase deficiency. This deficiency may be secondary to widespread mucosal cell disease as in gluten enteropathy or it may occur as an isolated defect. In the latter case, diagnosis is based upon enzyme assay of a jejunal biopsy and the induction of symptoms by means of an oral lactose load. In positive cases omitting the appropriate disaccharide from the diet can be undertaken as a test of the diagnosis.

Abnormalities of intestinal lymphatic transport of fat. These are fairly rare disorders. Impaired lymphatic transport is one of the factors operative in Whipple's disease and in Crohn's disease. Other problems of this type are congenital lymphangectasia and lymphatic obstruction due to lymphoma.

These problems have to be managed by dietary methods (see below).

Malabsorption after intestinal resection. Resection of large amounts of small intestine may be necessary in Crohn's disease or in gangrene after compromise of the arterial or venous blood supply to the bowel. There may then be insufficient mucosal surface for efficient absorption, and if the terminal ileum has been resected there will be low duodenal bile salt concentrations. Many of these patients are difficult to treat and a constant watch on their calorie intake and weight is necessary. Many of the supplements listed below may be required.

GENERAL MEASURES IN TREATMENT OF MALABSORPTION

Diet. A low fat diet may be indicated in some patients in whom the appropriate replacement cannot be given, for example, patients with an interrupted entero-hepatic circulation of bile salts. Very low fat diets are unpalatable and few patients can tolerate a diet containing less than 20 to 30 g.

Medium chain triglycerides. These are absorbed without intraluminal hydrolysis and so may be useful in a variety of pancreatic and bile salt problems and after extensive intestinal resections. In addition they are absorbed mainly via the portal venous system and so they are a valuable source of calories when there is lymphatic obstruction. At the present time, their prime use is in patients with continuing nutritional deterioration when all other measures have proved inadequate.

Supplements

These may be found to be necessary in any of the malabsorptive disorders because of the demonstration of anaemia, coagulation defects or bone problems.

Folic Acid and Vitamin B_{12}. Folic acid is often indicated in gluten enteropathy in a dosage of 5 mg. by mouth three times daily. Care should be taken to see that vitamin B_{12} levels are adequate. In tropical sprue, both vitamins are indicated.

Iron. Iron deficiency is most prone to arise in problems of mucosal transport and indeed iron deficiency may be the presenting problem in gluten enteropathy. An iron supplement in the form of ferrous sulphate 200 mg. once or twice daily should be given regularly in these cases.

Vitamin K_1. Phytomenadione in a dosage of

10 mg. by injection may be necessary in patients with hypoprothrombinaemia who are undergoing investigation, particularly if biopsies are to be carried out.

Vitamin D and calcium supplements are often required by patients with gluten enteropathy who have steatorrhoea. Calcium gluconate 12 g. per day orally may be given together with oral or parenteral vitamin D. Patients on regular vitamin D therapy require measurements of blood calcium levels at regular intervals.

Vitamin B Complex. Oral supplements are often required in gluten enteropathy.

PARENTERAL FEEDING

Parenteral feeding may be necessary in the course of several diseases of the alimentary tract. In some cases, it may be the only method of feeding and therefore life-saving; and in others—for example in patients with increased catabolism—it may be a valuable adjunct to oral nutrition.

Indications. Such feeding may be indicated in conditions in which there is obstruction to the ingestion of food (for example, carcinoma of the oesophagus or tongue), in atresia of the bowel in neonates, in conditions where protein-containing food and body secretions are lost from fistulae or from the bowel wall itself as in ulcerative colitis. In addition, it also has a part to play in the prevention of complications of surgery in the undernourished patient.

Principles. In general, it is not possible to provide an adequate number of calories by giving a solution of 5 per cent. glucose since 1 litre will supply only 180 kcals., and in these circumstances the large volume of fluid required would be harmful in the presence of cardiac or renal insufficiency. Thus, substances must be used which supply a greater number of calories per unit volume. Carbohydrates other than glucose, which are useful, are fructose and sorbitol. Fructose is utilized more efficiently by the liver than is glucose. It tends to have an anabolic action, it is less irritant to veins and is the carbohydrate of choice for parenteral therapy in liver disease apart from hepatic precoma or coma. In patients with normal liver function, it is often given in combination with alcohol because fructose increases the metabolism of alcohol. Alcohol, which provides 7 kcal. per g., may be given in a 3 per cent. solution at a rate of up to 10 g. per hour.

Without a large calorie intake, nitrogen balance cannot be restored satisfactorily, and the administration of fats (providing 9 kcal. per g.) in addition to carbohydrate is thus necessary. Two types of fat emulsion are used, one derived from cottonseed oil and the other from soyabean oil, and from the point of view of mutual utilization one of these forms is best given simultaneously with amino acids. The principle of administration of protein is to provide the necessary amino acids in balanced mixtures so that the body can synthesize its own correct proportions of protein.

Practice. In assessing the requirements of any one patient, individual factors such as weight, catabolic state, faecal and urinary losses need to be taken into account. Requirements per kg. are listed in Table 7, and suggested regimens in

The tables in the following section are modified from those of Allen, P. C. & Lee, H. A. (1969). *A Clinical Guide to Intravenous Nutrition.* Oxford: Blackwell.

TABLE 7

Suggested daily minimum requirements of some nutrients per kg. body weight

	Basal Conditions	Increased Metabolic Rate
Water	25–35 ml.	50–60 ml.
kcalories	25–30	40–60
Protein (amino acids)	0·8–1 g.	1·5–2·5 g.
Carbohydrate	2 g.	4–6 g.
Fat	2 g.	3–5 g.

Table 9. Provided there are no abnormal protein losses from the bowel, the 24-hour urinary urea output can be used to calculate the protein equivalent. For intravenous therapy a proportion of the total calorie intake should always be carbohydrate (probably about 10 per cent.) because of its beneficial effect on protein metabolism, and the simultaneous administration of protein and carbohydrate achieves a better protein retention. These principles are embodied in the use of many commercial preparations, e.g. aminosol. The composition of this and other preparations is shown in Table 8. In the design of any regimen, it should be remembered that the optimum ratio of kcalories to grams of nitrogen for the attainment of nitrogen balance is 200:1 or greater. In making an assessment of a patient's needs, the electrolyte require-

TABLE 8

Composition and caloric value of certain intravenous solutions

Solution	Volume	Water (ml.)	kcal.	Alcohol (g.)	Fructose (g.)	Glucose (g.)	Sorbitol (g.)	Soybean oil (g.)	Amino acid (g.)	N. (g.)	Sodium (mEq./l)	K.	pH
Intralipid 10%	1,000	850	1,100	—	—	—	—	100	—	......	—	—	—
Aminosol-fructose ethanol	1,000	850	875	25	150	—	—	—	33	4·25	54	0·15	5·6
Aminosol 10%	1,000	—	—	—	—	—	—	—	100	12·75	160	0·45	5·6
Trophysan 5	1,000	—	364	—	—	—	48	—	40	6·7	6	8	6·4
Glucose 5%	1,000	950	200	—	—	50	—	—	—	—	—	—	4-5
Fructose 20%	1,000	800	800	—	200	—	—	—	—	—	—	—	4-5
Sorbitol 30%	1,000	700	1,200	—	—	—	300	—	—	—	—	—	6·5-7·5

TABLE 9

Suggested regimens for covering basal and increased metabolic requirements
per average 70 kg. patient by intravenous nutrition

Source	Basal Requirement			Increased Requirement		
	volume (ml.)	g.	kcal.	volume (ml.)	g.	kcal.
20% fat emulsion	700	140	1,400	1,050	210	2,100
20% fructose or glucose	700	140	560	1,750	350	1,400
10% amino-acid solution	700	70	220	1,000	100	320
Total	2,100		2,180	3,800		3,820

ments must also be estimated after taking into account the number of mEq. of each ion given as part of each solution and supplements of magnesium and calcium may need to be added. If the intravenous diet is to be continued for some time, vitamins should be given also. Suggested regimens for two different circumstances are shown in Table 9.

Problems and complications. Thrombophlebitis may develop at the infusion site and this is more likely to occur with a solution of low *p*H (Table 8). Toxic reactions have occurred with fat emulsions but in general the soyabean emulsions (in contrast to the cottonseed oils) do not cause reactions although care must be taken to avoid simultaneous administration of any substance which might destroy the emulsion. Emulsions given over a long period of time may be responsible for the development of anaemia due to marrow depression, and very occasionally thrombocytopenia may be induced. The cottonseed oils have been shown to be hepatotoxic in some patients.

GASTROSTOMY AND JEJUNOSTOMY

One of these procedures may be carried out as a temporary measure to allow feeding when there is an upper gastro-intestinal obstruction. The gastrostomy is not used for the first 24 hours after construction. Then 500 ml. 5 per cent. glucose solution is given in the next 24 hours and thereafter equal parts of milk and water with 100 g. of glucose added to each litre. Two to three litres may be given each day. At a later stage, Complan may be added together with vitamin supplements.

CHRONIC IDIOPATHIC ULCERATIVE COLITIS

The term 'idiopathic ulcerative colitis' is used to describe an inflammatory condition of the colon, characterized by bleeding and ulceration, which is not attributable to any specific organism. Some patients may have more localized involvement of the large bowel, for example proctitis, but there may be progression to more generalized involvement. In other instances, short segments of the colon may be affected. This is often described as segmental colitis and probably represents colonic Crohn's disease.

All grades of severity may occur, from the mildest cases of proctitis to an acute fulminating condition in which the evacuation of liquid, bloody stools occurs 10 to 20 times daily and leads to death within a few days or weeks. Although there is no specific treatment for the condition, it is important that the patient should be strictly supervised since attention to the following brings about symptomatic relief, reduces morbidity and on occasion may be life-saving. The use of any particular measure will, of course, depend upon such factors as the extent, severity and duration of the disease.

Electrolytes. In moderate to severe cases there may be excessive loss of potassium and sodium in the stool and these must be replaced. In some patients, they may be given orally, but in the severely ill case, parenteral therapy is necessary.

Nutrition. Large amounts of protein are lost from the damaged and inflamed bowel wall. Oral replacement is difficult since patients with severe disease feel unwell and nausea is common. Parenteral replacement of calories and protein is thus indicated as described on p. 239. In patients with less severe but chronic disease, a high protein and calorie intake may be given orally with vitamin supplements. Some degree of symptomatic relief may be obtained by avoiding roughage in the diet and an occasional patient seems to benefit from the omission of milk.

Anaemia. In acute cases with frank bleeding from the bowel and a rapidly falling haemoglobin level, the transfusion of whole blood is indicated. In milder cases of proctitis or colitis without a generalized gastro-intestinal disturbance ferrous sulphate may be given by mouth.

Anticholinergic drugs. These may help by reducing the number of stools. Drugs of the morphine group should not be used for their constipating or analgesic effect since they may increase the intraluminal colonic pressure.

Corticosteroids. These drugs are of great value in treatment, particularly of the first attack. They may be used orally or topically. The specific use and dosage tends to vary from one physician to another but the following are generally acceptable indications. For the acute attack, prednisolone 60 mg. per day by mouth will greatly increase the chance of a remission, the dosage being reduced gradually over several weeks once there has been a satisfactory response. The drug may be used again in subsequent episodes. Steroids may also be given rectally as a retention enema, for example, hydrocortisone acetate 100 mg. This can be inserted by the patient night or morning or both and retained in the rectum for as long as possible. In the severe case, in addition to oral therapy, the enema may be used to increase the local concentration of corticosteroid in the rectum and colon, or it may be used without systemic therapy in cases of proctitis.

Sulphasalazine. This drug, taken regularly in a dosage of 4 to 8 g. per day, will reduce the number of exacerbations. It may also be used in maximum tolerated dosage (up to 12 or 16 g. per day) in the more severe case, but its value in such circumstances is not well documented. The main side-effect is nausea. The drug should therefore be taken in divided dosage throughout the day and treatment should start with a small dose which is increased gradually. Sulphasalazine may also cause headache, skin rashes and, on occasion, haemolytic anaemia or agranulocytosis. Suppositories are available for the treatment of proctitis.

General Management

Ulcerative colitis is a particularly distressing disorder and the patient usually requires a considerable amount of support from his practitioner and regular review by a physician and surgeon. The risk of cancer is high in the patient with chronic and extensive disease and for this reason alone, the patient should be seen in hospital at least once per year for sigmoidoscopy and barium enema. Most patients will be seen more often so that the treatment can be reviewed and adjusted. It is also necessary to deal promptly with any complications of the disease or side-effects of therapy.

Surgery

Surgery is indicated in acute ulcerative colitis which fails to respond to medical treatment or which responds only partially and goes on to relapse.

As an emergency, it is the method of treatment in toxic dilatation, and in fulminating forms of the disease. Intensive pre-operative therapy with blood, fluid, and electrolyte replacement is necessary and this is an area where a combined medical and surgical approach is essential.

In the chronic form of the disease where a functionless colon is left, removal of the colon is indicated to abolish chronic diarrhoea, and in subacute forms, particularly when the disease began in childhood or adolescence, to avoid the risk of development of carcinoma. This risk becomes significant when the disease has been present for over 10 years and there is total involvement of the colon. In making a decision on the need for operation, the presence of other complications may be taken into account. Concomitant liver disease or ankylosing spondylitis is unlikely to be improved, but arthritis and some skin lesions which are secondary to the colitis may benefit.

Removal of the entire colon and rectum with permanent ileostomy is the usual method of surgical treatment. In some centres and in selected cases, the rectum is preserved and ileo-rectal anastomosis performed in an attempt to avoid ileostomy. Whether this is desirable is questionable, particularly if there is residual rectal disease. The frequent bowel movements—up to 8 to 10 times per day—and the need for constant supervision to check that the rectum does not develop malignant change are definite disadvantages, while ileostomy has become progressively easier to manage with changes in surgical technique and with improvements in the appliances available for its control (see below).

DIVERTICULAR DISEASE OF THE COLON

It is common to find diverticula in the colon, particularly in elderly patients. If these are asymptomatic, treatment is unnecessary. In those patients who develop minimal or moderate symptoms, it is usually sufficient to keep the stools soft and to ensure regular motions. It is usual to prescribe Isogel or a similar preparation and to treat any episode of constipation with a saline laxative (e.g. magnesium sulphate). More severe episodes of pain, fever or leucocytosis require treatment with phthalylsulphathiazole up to 12 g. per day in divided doses by mouth or ampicillin in a dose of 250 mg. four times a day. Failure to respond leads to consideration of the possible value of surgical treatment.

For obstruction, severe or recurrent bleeding and for perforation, surgery is clearly indicated, as it is in those patients where the presence of a carcinoma is in doubt.

In recent years, there has been an increase in the use of surgical treatment for the primary condition. Local excision of the affected segment, or more often excision of the pelvic colon and pelvi-rectal junction with primary anastomosis is satisfactory. Before operation the bowel should be prepared mechanically and by the use of purgatives, and sterilized by the administration of antibiotics in combinations such as ampicillin (250 mg. four times daily) and framycetin (250 mg. four times daily). Myotomy of the pelvic colon and upper rectum is a lesser procedure which promises good results in selected cases. In severe cases, with pelvic abscess formation, it may be necessary to carry out an initial defunctioning colostomy and then to perform resection at a later date.

CARCINOMA OF COLON AND RECTUM

Resection and anastomosis is the treatment of choice. Emergency surgery is indicated for obstruction caused by tumour and in these circumstances colostomy is usual as the first step. Colostomy will also give worthwhile palliation in some inoperable cases, relieving any tendency to obstruction and reducing the amount of discharge of mucus and blood from the tumour. The best palliation is removal of the primary tumour and this should be practised wherever possible, even if the tumour has to be mobilized, or if there are metastases in glands or liver. Most patients, therefore, will require laparotomy. Carcinoma of the upper rectum can be treated by resection and anastomosis but tumours in the middle and lower parts require total excision of the rectum with permanent colostomy. As with diverticular disease, pre-operative mechanical and antibiotic preparation of the bowel is desirable and will often allow the completion of surgery as a primary procedure.

MANAGEMENT OF COLOSTOMY AND ILEOSTOMY

At the outset the patient should be given a clear description of what to expect after operation. Whenever possible, he should have the opportunity of seeing the colostomy or ileostomy appliances and of talking to someone who has had a similar operation. In many countries there are ileostomy associations which can help in this respect, although most major surgical or medical units can rely on their own resources at this stage.

It is important to emphasize to the patient that colostomy or ileostomy is compatible with normal health and full physical activity, and that in their day-to-day contact with others their operation is undetectable, and that they will be completely independent, being able to manage the stoma by themselves. Thus, in the immediate convalescent period they are shown how to care for the colostomy or ileostomy and are trained to use the prescribed appliance themselves.

Ileostomy. The fluid and irritant nature of the ileal discharge makes the use of an adhesive flange and detachable bag desirable. Care of the skin is important, but is no longer a problem with modern appliances and a well-fashioned stoma. Useful hints and encouragement will be gained from early membership of an ileostomy association, and later, through the means of meetings and publications, information on new appliances and methods will be obtained. The patient will learn from experience what articles of diet cause upset. In general, with the exception of such things as onions, nuts, beans and dried peas, a normal balanced diet can be taken.

A complication of ileostomy that calls for early

and active treatment is diarrhoea. A severe attack rapidly leads to profound fluid and electrolyte loss. Minor cases will respond to the taking of diphenoxylate 2·5 to 5 mg. four times a day and the patient should be encouraged to commence the drugs on his own initiative. All other patients require hospital admission and possibly intravenous fluid and electrolyte replacement.

Colostomy. The usual appliance consists of a disposable plastic bag held in place by an elastic belt and padded flange. The majority of colostomy patients can ensure regular and predictable movement of the bowel by alteration of the roughage content of the diet and by the taking, if need be, of a methyl cellulose or agar preparation. Apart from regular cleansing of the skin with soap and water, no specific care is required. Should excoriation develop as a result of looseness of the bowel or chafing from the appliance, a protective coat of Friar's balsam, or of a plastic spray such as Nobecutane, is helpful. Occasionally some patients find that despite all attempts to regulate it, the bowel remains unpredictable in its action. In them a regimen of daily colostomy lavage may be preferable, but such treatment is time-consuming and requires the exclusive use of toilet facilities of a high standard. A useful guide to the home management of a colostomy is supplied by Harker Stagg Ltd., London, the makers of Celevac granules.

PERITONITIS

The common causes of peritonitis are perforation of a peptic ulcer, an inflamed appendix, a gangrenous gall-bladder or spread of infection from acute diverticulitis or peridiverticulitis. Post-operatively it may follow leakage from an anastomosis or suture line. Other causes of peritonitis such as septicaemia, tuberculosis or ascent of infection from the vagina are rare, and are only safely diagnosed after laparotomy has excluded a local intra-abdominal lesion.

Prevention

In the Western Hemisphere, appendicitis accounts for most cases of peritonitis, but, whatever the cause, both the incidence and severity of this complication are diminishing. The procrastination engendered by the administration of a purgative to a patient with abdominal pain is no longer permissible. Early operation even at the risk of the clinician being wrong, and before the diagnosis is certain, allows removal of the acutely inflamed appendix before perforation has occurred. In other ways, by more active treatment of peptic ulcer, and of gall-bladder and colonic disorders the number of patients at risk from perforation and peritonitis is reduced.

Treatment

The majority of patients with peritonitis urgently require surgery. In them the initial aim of medical treatment is the treatment of shock, sufficient to bring the blood pressure to a level adequate for surgical operation.

The relief of pain by the intramuscular injection of morphine, the passage of a tube into the stomach and aspiration of its contents, and the intravenous infusion of dextran, plasma or saline will in most cases improve the patient's condition sufficiently within an hour or so before operation. Longer delay is seldom useful or advisable. Post-operatively, medical management can be more specific. The intravenous fluid regimen can be guided by clinical and biochemical needs. In the absence of any gross electrolyte imbalance, the intravenous administration of fluid is continued until effective absorption from the bowel is re-established and the patient is taking adequate quantities of fluid by mouth. The return of bowel sounds, the passage of flatus and a drop in the volume of gastric aspirate are indications that the naso-gastric tube can be removed and fluids given by mouth in increasing quantities.

Antibiotics. Antibiotics are not used routinely in all cases of peritonitis. When the cause is perforation of a duodenal ulcer, the peritonitis is sterile initially and only later does it become infected. Operative closure of the perforation within the first six hours or so with local cleansing of the peritoneal cavity is enough. On the other hand, peritonitis which is infective from the onset, as, for example, when it complicates perforation of a gangrenous appendix or acute diverticulitis, merits vigorous antibiotic therapy from the beginning. The responsible organisms usually include *E. coli*, *Streptococcus faecalis* and anaerobes. A broad spectrum antibiotic or combination of antibiotics is required and should be administrable parenterally.

Ampicillin given intramuscularly or intravenously six-hourly in a dosage of 500 mg., or the administration of 1,000,000 units (600 mg.) of benzylpenicillin and 500 mg. streptomycin twice daily is effective. Kanamycin, 1 g. daily, given intramuscularly, is highly effective against the Gram-negative infections derived from the gastro-intestinal tract. Like streptomycin, it must be used with caution in elderly subjects who are liable to eighth nerve damage. Its dosage should be controlled by estimation of the blood level, for in patients with renal disease, or when kidney function is impaired through the hypotension of shock, its delayed excretion may cause dangerously high blood levels.

To be effective, antibiotic therapy in peritonitis should be given in adequate dosage over a period restricted in most cases to four or five days. Prolonged administration is seldom beneficial and often leads to complications such as secondary bacterial and yeast infections and the emergence of resistant strains. Whenever possible, bacteriological control should be undertaken and specimens of peritoneal fluid obtained at operation and subsequently from wound drains should be cultured, both for aerobes and anaerobes.

LOCALIZED PERITONITIS

In localized peritonitis, as occasionally seen in some forms of appendicitis or in the leaking duodenal ulcer or suture line, surgery is not urgently indicated. Each patient must be treated according to his particular needs. The patient with the already well-defined appendix mass and no signs of general peritonitis requires few active measures apart from rest, restriction of the diet and the avoidance of purgatives. The patient with leakage from a suture line may require complete cessation of oral fluids, continuous gastric aspiration and a complicated regimen of intravenous fluid and electrolyte replacement and intravenous alimentation to compensate for loss from the fistula. In every case, medical treatment is controlled by the clinical response. As localization of the peritonitis continues, there will be a progressive fall in pulse and temperature and the abdominal signs of peritoneal irritation will disappear. The appendix mass will become more distinct and its size progressively diminish. Once this resolution is complete, the appendix can be removed some three to six weeks later. The patient with leakage from a fistula will in the same way show diminution of the local signs of inflammation, and the volume of fluid escaping will progressively diminish. However, localized peritonitis may not go on to resolution. A residual abscess may form and, whether or

not antibiotics are given, this will require drainage. Such an abscess may be at the primary site of peritoneal contamination or in one of the peritoneal spaces, usually causing a subphrenic or pelvic abscess.

TUBERCULOUS PERITONITIS

Chronic peritonitis is usually due to tuberculous infection, though the condition is now rare in the United Kingdom—following the decline in the incidence of all forms of tuberculosis. It is attended by loss of weight, low-grade fever and ascites, through which matted masses may be felt within the abdomen. In the adult, it may be confused with malignancy and a hopeless prognosis given without justification. Laparotomy and confirmation of the diagnosis of tuberculosis by biopsy is required in some cases. It responds well to treatment with antituberculous drugs (p. 76).

FUNCTIONAL DISORDERS AFFECTING THE ALIMENTARY TRACT

These disorders are extremely common. The gastro-intestinal tract is richly supplied with autonomic nerves and it may be affected by emotion or stress. It is also affected by hormones, but the part they play in functional disorders is not well understood. Severe stress may, on occasion, lead to pathological changes in the alimentary tract, for example, acute ulceration in the stomach. The alimentary tract of the normal person may respond to less severe stress or anxiety in a variety of ways, for example, with the development of a dry mouth, a sensation of a lump in the throat, dysphagia, anorexia, aerophagy and belching, hiccough, nausea, vomiting, epigastric pain and diarrhoea. In a functional disorder, one or more of these symptoms may become the usual response of a patient to mild stress and eventually the response may occur without the stimulus. These patients usually have a normal personality and no psychiatric abnormality.

Although many of these disorders are often strongly suspected after taking a history from the patient, the diagnosis should be made only after the appropriate clinical and radiological investigations have been performed. This is because the first symptoms of organic disease may occur in a situation of emotion or stress, for example dysphagia with an oesophageal tumour, or diarrhoea with a rectal carcinoma. In addition, the discomfort and worry caused by a functional disorder may convince the patient that a serious disease, perhaps carcinoma, is present and investigation may be necessary to convince the patient that all is well. Such investigation together with the subsequent reassurance may therefore be the first step in treatment.

Psychiatric Disorders

A wide variety of alimentary and abdominal symptoms occur in patients with psychiatric disorders and the patient with an anxiety state may show, in a florid form, some of the symptoms which have been discussed already.

Depression. It is common for patients with depression to have retardation of alimentary function and there may be anorexia, constipation, etc. Other patients may respond by over-eating and develop obesity. Depression may present to the gastroenterologist as an undiagnosed abdominal pain but such a diagnosis should be made only by exclusion since depression may be an early symptom in some cases of alimentary carcinoma. A discussion of the drugs which may be used in such cases will be found elsewhere (p. 425).

Anorexia nervosa. This is a severe disorder which occurs in young women and it is characterized by refusal to eat, severe loss of weight and amenorrhoea. Treatment must be carried out in hospital under strict supervision to ensure that food is consumed and weight gain is occurring. In hospital a regimen of insulin and chlorpromazine is instituted. An initial dose of chlorpromazine of 50 to 100 mg. three times a day is increased daily until improvement in eating occurs. In addition, soluble insulin is given one hour prior to meal times in dosage sufficient to give hypoglycaemia at the meal time. Although a psychiatric problem usually underlies the disorder, psychiatric treatment is not an immediate essential in what is often a life-threatening situation. Discharge from hospital should take place only when there has been definite weight gain and a re-education in eating habits. The relapse rate is high and all patients should be followed up regularly.

Functional Disorders Affecting the Stomach

The most common problems are aerophagy with epigastric fullness and belching, epigastric discomfort and pain due to pylorospasm and psycho-genic vomiting. Some of these symptoms are often termed 'nervous dyspepsia'.

Psychogenic vomiting is characterized by morning vomiting usually without nausea or loss of weight. It is usually associated with anxiety and will respond to reassurance and a tranquillizer taken on awakening.

Aerophagy, belching and epigastric discomfort are all treated symptomatically. Aerophagy is often a response to discomfort arising elsewhere in the alimentary tract and particularly to the irritable bowel syndrome, and treatment of the latter condition brings relief. As far as possible the patients' lives should be ordered so that meals are taken regularly in a relaxed atmosphere. Minor changes in the meal itself may help, for example, small dry meals may be indicated initially. In difficult cases attempts may be made by drug therapy to relieve anxiety and to ensure sleep at night. For patients with epigastric pain dicyclomine hydrochloride, 10 to 20 mg. three times per day before meals may give relief.

Irritable Colon

This disorder is characterized by a wide variety of clinical features and the treatment prescribed depends largely on the symptoms of the individual patient. Some patients suffer from diarrhoea and lower abdominal pain, others pass small amounts of hard stool and mucus, and in others diarrhoea and constipation may alternate. All patients have abnormal colonic muscular activity with high intraluminal pressures.

GENERAL MEASURES. After investigation, the patient should be reassured that no serious disease exists, and told that the symptoms will respond to treatment. The disorder tends to be a chronic one with exacerbations and remissions and the regular support of the practitioner can be very important. If the patient can recognize emotional situations which cause exacerbations, then these should be avoided as far as possible. Measures may need to be taken to reduce anxiety and ensure adequate sleep at night.

DIET. Patients with diarrhoea often recognize foods that precipitate attacks, common ones being tomatoes, salads, spicy foods and beer and other alcoholic beverages. These should be avoided and the majority of patients obtain considerable relief from a low roughage diet together with the avoidance of coffee and hot soups. By contrast, patients with hard stools and the passage of rectal mucus benefit from the gradual withdrawal of all laxatives and the introduction of increased amounts of fruit juices and cooked vegetables into the diet together with the oral administration of methyl-cellulose.

DRUGS. These are often necessary for the patient with diarrhoea. Dicyclomine hydrochloride may be given in a dose of 10 to 20 mg. before meals. The first dose should be given on awakening. An alternative is mebeverine hydrochloride which can be given in a dose of 50 to 100 mg. three or four times per day. Codeine phosphate, 30 mg., may be prescribed as a standby for situations which the patient knows are likely to cause attacks. It should not be prescribed regularly since it tends to stop bowel activity by inducing spasm which may accentuate the condition in the long term. Diphenoxylate hydrochloride is a preferable alternative given in a dose of 5 mg. three or four times per day.

CONSTIPATION

This is not a diagnosis in itself, but it may arise in the irritable bowel syndrome, in depression, in the debilitated and those with faulty eating habits. It is important to realize that one bowel movement every few days can be normal for some patients and there are then no indications for medication. Many such patients have acquired a laxative habit and it is often difficult to withdraw the offending drug.

In certain situations, for example in painful anal or perineal conditions such as fissures, haemorrhoids or after childbirth, there is an indication for the temporary use of agents to soften the stool. Similarly, it may be important to prevent straining in patients with myocardial infarction, pulmonary embolism and after abdominal operations. In bedridden and elderly patients it may be necessary to resort to a more prolonged use of laxatives.

In all other patients treatment should be aimed at the correction of faulty diet, and if a laxative habit has been acquired, every attempt should be made to withdraw laxatives. The diet should be high in roughage with fruit and cooked vegetables. Such a diet may be too expensive for some patients and methylcellulose may be prescribed. It is important for the patient to maintain a good fluid intake. A bowel which has been flogged by laxatives for many years and which has finally subsided into total inactivity is unlikely to respond immediately to the complete change to a high roughage diet. Laxatives must be withdrawn slowly with substitution of less harmful ones such as saline laxatives in place of the muscle stimulants such as senna or cascara sagrada. This process is usually a very slow one and much forbearance is required on the part of the physician and his patient.

DISEASES OF THE LIVER

Viral Hepatitis

A variety of viruses including the infectious mononucleosis virus can be causes of hepatitis but the usual forms are infectious hepatitis and serum hepatitis.

Prevention. There is evidence that both infectious and serum hepatitis may be transmitted by faeces, urine, blood and other body fluids such as ascitic fluid, so that strict precautions are required in hospital to prevent transmission to other patients or members of staff. Excreta and body fluids should be disposed of in an area used only for this purpose. The patient should be barrier nursed in a single room with entry restricted to a minimum of medical and nursing staff. There should be gowning and use of gloves during procedures such as venesection. In suspected cases of serum hepatitis the diagnosis may be made earlier if the test for Australia antigen is positive. Blood transmission of virus can be reduced by screening donors for Australia antigen and by transfusing patients only when strictly necessary. Epidemics of infectious hepatitis are prone to occur in institutions, and gamma globulin has been shown to protect against clinical infection in these circumstances. It is not effective against serum hepatitis.

Treatment. Both infectious hepatitis and serum hepatitis vary in severity from non-icteric forms to acute fulminating cases. In the established case, complete rest in bed should be instituted. Most patients have nausea and loss of appetite and the patient should be encouraged to eat only what he fancies. Drugs of any type should be strictly avoided, and in severe cases particular attention must be paid to any signs indicating the onset of hepatic failure (see below). Once the liver function tests are improving, mobilization can be accomplished gradually, but most cases will require convalescence for several weeks. Treatment with corticosteroids does not affect the rate of improvement or the ultimate outcome. The patient should be followed up until liver function tests are normal and alcohol should be avoided for a year after the attack. The treatment of precoma and coma is discussed on p. 249.

Pyogenic Infection of the Liver

This rare disorder may follow intra-abdominal sepsis or septicaemia, especially portal pyaemia, and there tends to be a diffuse involvement of the liver. Some patients, particularly those less acutely affected, will respond to antibiotic therapy, and in others surgical drainage may be possible occasionally.

Cirrhosis of the Liver

The term cirrhosis covers a wide variety of liver disorders which may be sequelae to viral infection, alcohol or nutritional deficiency. The aetiology is unknown in many instances. In addition there are other rare metabolic disorders such as hepato-lenticular degeneration and haemochromatosis in which cirrhosis may occur.

Prevention. In all these various forms of cirrhosis, prevention of further damage is possible only in the case of alcohol, which, if stopped completely, may bring about a marked improvement even in the most severe case of alcoholic cirrhosis. In haemochromatosis and in hepato-lenticular degeneration there is also evidence that the respective removal of iron and copper from the body will slow or even prevent progression of the disorder.

General measures. Various measures may be required to bring about symptomatic relief.

ABSORPTION. There may be steatorrhoea and malabsorption of calcium and fat soluble vitamins, particularly in biliary cirrhosis. Dietary fat should be restricted and the fat-soluble vitamins D and K_1 given parenterally. Vitamin D, 100,000 units monthly by intramuscular injection together with oral calcium supplements, is adequate.

PRURITUS. An antihistamine such as promethazine hydrochloride, 25 mg. b.d., may be tried but with the severe symptoms which may occur with total biliary obstruction in patients with a limited prognosis, methyltestosterone, 25 mg. per day sublingually, can be prescribed. This drug may increase jaundice. A further method is to bind bile salts in the intestine, thus preventing their reabsorption and causing them to be lost in the faeces. Cholestyramine is used in this way, dispensed in capsules in doses of 6 to 15 g. daily.

ASCITES. Paracentesis should not be undertaken in ascites due to liver disease because it results in the loss of large amounts of protein. The ascites is usually due to lowered plasma albumin levels together with raised portal venous pressure. Sodium retention occurs secondary to these changes. Treatment is aimed at increasing plasma albumin levels and removing sodium from the body. The use of a high protein diet may be limited by impending liver failure, but, if possible, low sodium protein supplements should be given by mouth. A low sodium diet together with bed rest will bring about a response in some patients. Of the diuretics, chlorothiazide in a dosage of 1 g. b.d. on alternate days may be used together with potassium supplements. Such treatment must be given very cautiously since hepatic coma may be precipitated. In patients not responding to the above measures spironolactone is indicated in combination with the thiazide. Spironolactone in a dosage of 50 to 100 mg. per day is usually adequate. Once an adequate response has been attained then the dose of the various diuretics may be gradually reduced to the lowest amount that ensures freedom from ascites. Complications of diuretic therapy are common. Hypokalaemia must be carefully watched for and treated immediately by temporary cessation of diuretics and an increase in oral potassium supplements. Severe hyponatraemia is treated by measures designed to remove water from the body such as mannitol infusion. However, a fast rate of diuresis may precipitate uraemia and the therapy may require suspension because of this.

IMMUNOSUPPRESSANTS. In active chronic hepatitis there is evidence of a marked immunological disturbance, with a high serum gamma globulin, serum antibodies to components of liver cells and marked infiltration of the liver by lymphocytes and plasma cells. Some of these patients benefit symptomatically from the use of immunosuppressants although, as yet, there is no evidence that life is prolonged. Both corticosteroids and mercaptopurine may bring about a reduction in jaundice and the usual feelings of tiredness and malaise. The dosage of drug used requires careful control to the the minimum necessary to alleviate symptoms. Mercaptopurine has the advantage of producing fewer distressing side-effects for the patient, but its use requires strict supervision because of possible actions on the haemopoietic system.

Jaundice due to Drugs

Many drugs and chemicals may produce jaundice by acting upon the liver cell. Carbon tetrachloride and benzene-like compounds may poison the cell, isoniazid and monoamine oxidase inhibitors produce liver damage similar to viral hepatitis, while chlorpromazine and many other drugs may produce a cholestatic type of jaundice.

PREVENTION. Drugs known to have these actions should be used only if absolutely necessary. Halothane should not be used for a second time in patients who have shown an unexplained fever or disturbance of liver function after the first halothane anaesthetic, and it should not be used at all in patients with known liver disease.

TREATMENT. Any suspected drug should be withdrawn immediately and drugs of the same class should not be prescribed again at any time. The various symptomatic measures described above may need to be instituted depending upon the severity and symptomatology of the case. No drugs are of value.

Bleeding Varices

Bleeding may occur from varices situated in the oesophagus, stomach or duodenum. In these cases there is a raised portal venous pressure, usually secondary to chronic liver disease. From the point of view of treatment it is important to establish the diagnosis by radiological and endoscopic methods, since bleeding from peptic ulceration is also common in such patients and the treatment is different. Sedatives must be avoided because they may precipitate hepatic coma.

TREATMENT OF COMA. Many patients lapse into hepatic coma after a severe bleed and measures for the treatment of this should be instituted before it happens.

BLOOD TRANSFUSION with fresh blood should be started and assessments made of the coagulation defects that always exist in these patients. Hypoprothrombinaemia and thrombocytopenia may require correction. Transfusion in the severe case must be regarded as a corrective measure until operation can be arranged.

VASOPRESSIN. This drug lowers portal venous pressure and reduces bleeding from varices. Twenty units may be given intravenously over 10 minutes at hourly intervals. The drug is a coronary artery constrictor, but its use to stem bleeding may warrant the risk of producing side-effects (p. 162).

SENGSTAKEN TUBE. This should be used only as a final measure because, unless the operator is very skilled in its use, there will be a high failure rate. Even when the positioning is correct, there is a high incidence of lower oesophageal damage and inhalation of secretions. In general, a decision on a particular patient should have been reached during the time bought by the above methods.

EMERGENCY SURGERY. The point at which action is taken cannot be defined rigidly but it may be necessary treatment for the patient who fails to respond to the above measures. Operations designed to lower portal venous pressure or to disconnect the area of bleeding varices from the portal system may be carried out.

HEPATIC PRE-COMA AND COMA

This may be the terminal event in cases of long-standing cirrhosis, or it may be secondary to viral hepatitis or poisoning. With the correct supportive therapy the condition can be reversed in many instances, and since there is no means of deciding which patients will recover, all patients with hepatic coma must be actively treated from the outset.

AVOIDANCE OF PRECIPITATING FACTORS. In patients with disturbed liver function who are possible candidates for the development of hepatic coma, certain preventive measures should be taken. All drugs, including alcohol, should be avoided and there is an absolute contraindication to such drugs as morphine and paraldehyde. If diuretics are used, serum potassium levels must be measured and potassium replacements made. High protein diets should be avoided. Any degree of haemorrhage into the bowel must be treated promptly by the measures listed below.

PATIENT MONITORING. Some patients with viral hepatitis must be monitored with daily measurements of prothrombin time. The patient in hepatic coma requires intensive care with regular monitoring of serum electrolytes, pH, coagulation factors and blood glucose levels. The state of the circulation should be assessed with pulse and blood pressure recordings and E.C.G. monitoring may be desirable because of the rapidly changing electrolyte picture.

GENERAL MEASURES. Intravenous fluid replacement is necessary including on average, 2,000 kcals. per day in the form of glucose. Fructose should not be given. Some patients require far greater amounts. Systemic infection must be treated rigorously. Correction of such factors as hypoglycaemia, abnormal coagulation states and disturbed electrolyte patterns must be accomplished as soon as possible.

STERILIZATION OF THE BOWEL. In all cases, whether or not there has been blood loss into the bowel, purgation with a saline osmotic laxative together with colonic lavage is indicated. Neomycin by mouth in a dose of 1 g. six-hourly is the method of choice, and since some of this toxic antibiotic may be absorbed, blood levels should be monitored. An alternative drug in some patients with cirrhosis and chronic pre-coma is lactulose, a non-absorbed sugar which causes osmotic diarrhoea and inhibits bacterial growth by producing a low intestinal pH. The dose varies from 50 ml. to 200 ml. per day.

DIET. Oral nutrition is not used in the patient suffering from coma, but in the recovery phase and in the patient with chronic pre-coma, dietary protein restriction may be necessary. An estimate of the amount of protein permissible in any one patient may be made by E.E.G. monitoring at various dietary protein levels. In addition, care should be taken to avoid constipation in such patients.

DISEASES OF THE GALL-BLADDER AND BILIARY TRACT

Acute Cholecystitis

Obstruction at the neck of the gall-bladder by a stone lodged either in Hartmann's pouch or in the cystic duct is the usual cause of acute cholecystitis. Unrelieved, the obstruction leads to rupture of the gall-bladder and a peritonitis which if generalized is disastrous.

Thus, while the initial management of an attack of acute cholecystitis is medical, the possibility of surgery is ever present. The patient requires analgesics, antibiotics and intravenous fluids. Of the analgesics, pethidine is usually employed and 150 mg. four- or six-hourly may be necessary. A proportion of patients will be suffering from septicaemia secondary to the biliary infection and blood cultures should be carried out before an antibiotic regimen is commenced. Ampicillin, 500 mg. six-hourly by intramuscular injection, is the antibiotic of choice. Kanamycin is an alternative. Initially most patients have nausea and vomiting and it is necessary to supply intravenous fluids. Failure to

improve within 48 hours, as shown by continued tachycardia, pyrexia and persistent or increasing local abdominal tenderness and guarding is an indication for surgery. The usual emergency treatment is cholecystostomy. This is drainage of the distended and inflamed gall-bladder, with, if possible, removal of the impacted stone. Cholecystectomy can be carried out after the acute stage is over and depending on the individual patient may be done from three weeks to three months later. Emergency cholecystectomy is rarely practised in this country because of the fear of damage to a common bile duct that is obscured by oedema and inflammation.

Chronic Cholecystitis

Unless there are strong reasons to the contrary, the treatment of chronic cholecystitis associated with cholelithiasis is surgical. In the patient who is virtually symptom-free, the so-called silent stone remains an unpredictable hazard and may later cause acute cholecystitis, fistula, or rarely carcinoma. An elective operation in a well-prepared patient carries little risk, and is certainly preferable to emergency surgery in an ageing patient. On the other hand, in the great majority of patients such stones do not produce symptoms, and so it is debatable whether operation is indicated. The most frequent complication of calculous cholecystitis is stone in the common bile duct. Pre-operative and operative cholangiography are of value in determining the need for the surgeon to explore the duct. In addition, in patients who have had jaundice for several days or even weeks, there may be prolongation of the prothrombin time and phytomenodione may be necessary to correct this. It should be given parenterally.

Before elective operation on the gall-bladder, it is also important for the surgeon to know if there are other diseases of the upper alimentary tract, such as ulcer or hiatus hernia which should be treated at the same operation. The more general preparation for gall-bladder surgery includes weight reduction, physiotherapy and the abandonment of smoking. In the patient who is not acutely ill it is often advisable to delay operation for three to six months until co-existing medical conditions such as obesity and chronic bronchitis are treated.

Post-cholecystectomy syndromes. Persistence of or the recurrence of symptoms after cholecystectomy occurs in a proportion of patients, but the number is small if cholecystectomy is done only for calculous disease. Further symptoms are then confined almost entirely to patients in whom a stone in the common duct has been overlooked, or in whom a stricture at the ampulla has formed. Rarely, the cholecystectomy has been accompanied by damage to the ducts or bile leakage with subsequent biliary tract stenosis. Otherwise, post-cholecystectomy syndromes are due to failure of diagnosis, the cause of the patient's symptoms being in the pancreas, the bowel or the heart. Coronary ischaemia and cholelithiasis are not infrequently seen in association, and both may give rise to pain of almost identical severity and distribution. Some patients with so-called post-cholecystectomy syndromes have no organic disease and are neurotics or have become drug addicts perhaps as a result of pethidine having been prescribed during an attack of genuine biliary pain before cholecystectomy.

Ascending cholangitis. This is usually associated with obstruction due to stricture, stone, or both, affecting the common bile duct. Persistent infection in the biliary tract in the absence of obstruction is very rare and is confined almost exclusively to fistulae between gut and biliary system. Clinically, cholangitis presents with pyrexia which may be intermittent and regularly recurrent so that it mimics a specific fever, or there may be jaundice which again may be intermittent. Persistent cholangitis leads to liver damage and to spread of infection within the intrahepatic ducts which become filled with debris and small stones. Treatment is surgical to secure drainage and removal of stones. Because many such patients have the propensity to re-form stones, artificial drainage by means of a bypass between duct and duodenum, or a sphincterotomy, may be necessary to avoid further recurrence. The infection in the biliary passages will diminish after establishment of drainage, but long-term treatment with antibiotics is often necessary before the bile becomes sterile, and such therapy is particularly indicated when there is clinical and biopsy evidence of infection in the liver.

DISEASES OF THE PANCREAS
PANCREATITIS

Acute pancreatitis. This is a serious disorder with a high mortality. As with many gastro-intestinal diseases, management is best carried out by a combined surgical and medical approach so that surgical complications can be recognized and treated promptly.

PREVENTION. After a first attack of pancreatitis, it is important to search for possible aetiological factors. Gall-bladder disease must be eradicated. There must be abstinence from alcohol. Metabolic disorders such as hyperparathyroidism and hyperlipaemia must be diagnosed and treated.

TREATMENT. Once the state of acute pancreatitis is established, whether the cause is cholelithiasis, viral disease, alcohol or even trauma, the treatment is the same. It involves careful supportive therapy for the pain, shock, ileus, developing infections and diabetes.

Pethidine should be prescribed for pain; it is less liable than the morphine group of drugs to cause sphincter spasm. Shock should be treated with blood and plasma replacements and all fluid must be given parenterally. Some attempt should be made to reduce pancreatic stimulation by means of constant gastric aspiration and by the use of anticholinergic drugs. Because the patient usually has intestinal ileus, stomach aspiration is necessary for this reason also. Blood sugar levels are measured regularly to recognize and treat a developing diabetic state. In patients with a moderate or severe attack, it is common to see a fall in serum calcium five to seven days after the beginning of the attack. This should be treated with parenteral calcium therapy. In the United Kingdom most cases of acute pancreatitis have concomitant cholelithiasis and biliary tract infection and for this reason it is wise to give ampicillin 500 mg. intramuscularly six-hourly in all cases.

In some patients, the diagnosis of acute pancreatitis is made at laparotomy for 'acute abdomen'. In such cases, and particularly if gall-stones are present, cholecystostomy should be carried out and the patient then be treated as described above. Direct attack on the pancreas or bypass operations are contraindicated at this stage. Complications of acute pancreatitis such as persistent jaundice or haemorrhage, pseudopancreatic cyst or abscess and duodenal obstruction may arise in any patient undergoing medical treatment. In these cases, surgical treatment is indicated, although the precise time at which this is carried out will depend on the exact complication and the condition of the patient.

Relapsing pancreatitis. Recurrent minor or moderate attacks of pancreatitis may occur intermittently in the patient who has recovered from the major attack. Here the main problem is pain, and the amount of pancreatic damage or systemic disturbance suffered at each episode is small. Treatment includes the management of the underlying disorders as described earlier, and the patient must avoid any precipitating causes. In persistent cases there is a high incidence of addiction to narcotics and some attempt must be made to relieve the situation surgically. Treatment is designed to improve pancreatic drainage and to this end sphincterotomy or retrograde pancreatic drainage may be required together with possible resection of the diseased portion of the gland.

Chronic pancreatitis. This may arise after a single severe attack of pancreatitis, as the end-result of relapsing pancreatitis, or in other pancreatic disorders such as fibrocystic disease. Treatment is designed to replace the inadequate exocrine and endocrine secretions of the gland. The diet should be of high calorie value and its fat content should be reduced to a level to control diarrhoea. Pancreatin, B.N.F. is given.

Carcinoma of the Pancreas

Carcinoma of the pancreas when it affects the head of the gland is a common cause of obstructive jaundice in the older age-groups. Usually the tumour is inoperable because of spread to neighbouring structures or because of the frailty of the patient, but the jaundice can almost always be relieved by anastomosis of the distended gall-bladder to stomach or bowel. Surgical palliation is effective in at once relieving the patient of the intolerable itch of his jaundice, and in the longer term it gives a worthwhile period of well-being.

Tumours in the ampullary region cause early jaundice and are slow to spread so that they can more often be treated radically. The duodenum and head of pancreas are resected *en bloc* and continuity of the alimentary tract restored by gastro-jejunostomy. The ends of the pancreas and bile duct are separately implanted into the jejunum. Long-term survival with permanent cure is possible after such operation. Carcinoma of the body and tail of the pancreas is seldom treatable surgically because diagnosis is late.

In both the inoperable cases and those with recurrence after resection, it is usually necessary to prescribe analgesics and to treat symptoms which arise because of pancreatic destruction. Morphine or pethidine may be required regularly. Progressive diabetes and diarrhoea due to pancreatic insufficiency must be treated.

Secreting tumours of the pancreas, producing insulin- or gastrin-like substances are recognizable because of their hormonal effects. The demonstration of unexplained hypoglycaemia, hypersecretion of acid, or the production of gastrin-like substances in high concentration in the blood leads to an exploration of the pancreas. Most secreting tumours are in the body or tail of the gland and can be resected along with the distal portion of the gland. Many are benign so that the prognosis is excellent. If no tumour is found after careful examination of the resected body and tail and if the symptoms continue, then resection of the remaining portion of the gland may be necessary.

10. Disturbances in Water and Electrolyte Balance and in Acid-base Equilibrium

J. S. ROBSON

Disturbances in water and electrolyte balance and in acid-base equilibrium occur in many diseases and contribute significantly to the course of many illnesses; in some they determine the issue between life and death.

In the treatment of these conditions it is essential to define the abnormality in the chemical composition of the body and to assess its magnitude. Unfortunately, major chemical disorders of the body fluids frequently present considerable diagnostic difficulty. They are not often accompanied by specific or pathognomonic signs and dual or multiple disorders commonly occur simultaneously. Furthermore, the features of the underlying disease and the non-specific symptoms of illness such as lethargy, apathy and mental confusion frequently dominate the clinical picture. With few exceptions the information obtained by biochemical analysis of the blood is limited, and if the results are accepted at their face value may even be misleading. A reduction in the concentration of sodium in the blood beyond the limits of normal does not necessarily indicate the presence of sodium depletion, and potassium deficiency may occur in the presence of either an elevation or reduction in the concentration of this ion in the blood.

The major disturbances of water and electrolyte balance described in this chapter are as follows:

Water depletion.
Sodium depletion.
Potassium depletion and intoxication.
Hyponatraemia and water intoxication.
Magnesium depletion and intoxication.
Metabolic and respiratory alkalosis and acidosis.

Water Depletion

Pure or predominant depletion of body water is one of the simplest of these chemical disorders. The total water content of a healthy individual of 70 kg. is about 45 litres. The cells of the body are freely permeable to water and they contain the major part of the total water content, an amount estimated to be about 30 litres. The remaining 15 litres constitute the water of the extracellular fluid, about three litres of which lies within the vascular bed as the water of circulating plasma. In health, water balance is achieved by maintaining equality between the volume ingested and excreted. The renal channel of excretion is under physiological control in the sense that excretion of water can be restricted in the face of inadequate intake. Between 600 and 1,000 ml. of water are lost daily from the body in the expired air and by evaporation from the skin. This daily loss is inescapable and continues irrespective of the state of water balance. Its magnitude is increased to two or three litres with hyperventilation or by fever and may reach as much as six litres in the 24 hours if there is marked sweating. In health the urinary volume usually amounts to 1,500 ml. per day but may be reduced to an amount limited only by the capacity of the renal tubules to conserve water under the influence of the antidiuretic hormone, and the amount of urinary solute. On an average diet the minimum volume of water needed to excrete the urinary solute is about 600 ml. This volume increases considerably in the presence of renal concentrating defects or when fever or severe infection increases catabolism and consequently the amount of urinary solute. Thirst normally regulates the balance between the amount of water required and the volume unavoidably lost from the skin and lungs and needed for the renal excretion of solute.

Causes of water depletion. Pure or predominant water depletion arises most commonly because of inadequate intake. The deficit develops because of the inescapable loss of water from the lungs, from the surface of the body, and in the urine. In this way, water depletion may readily develop in the aged, senile and infirm, in the unconscious or semi-comatose and in all those who are debilitated by disease and who do not communicate their need for water to their attendants. The presence of obstructive lesions in the oesophagus or upper gastro-intestinal tract also leads to the development of progressive water deficit by interfering with normal water intake.

More rarely water depletion develops as a consequence of excessive urinary loss of water. This occurs in diabetes insipidus. In severe forms patients may have difficulty in meeting their urinary loss of water, especially when suffering from inter-current illness. A similar situation may arise in other diseases in which the renal power of concentration is restricted and if the individual is deprived of water, as may occur, for example, after surgical operation. Water conservation is a normal physiological response to surgery or trauma, but its occurrence depends upon the presence of renal tubules capable of responding to circulating anti-diuretic hormone. If this responsiveness is blunted, the liability to water depletion is increased. Such patients include those suffering from many forms of chronic renal disease and renal failure, hyper-parathyroidism and other causes of hypercalcaemia, severe potassium depletion and the recovery phase of acute tubular necrosis. The neonate is especially vulnerable to the development of water depletion, since the ability to produce a concentrated urine is still undeveloped.

Diagnosis and prevention of water depletion. As water is lost from the body, the extracellular fluids become hypertonic in relation to the concentration within the cells. However, osmotic equilibrium is quickly established by the migration of water from the intracellular to the extracellular fluid and the overall water deficit is shared by the entire body water. Because of this, the volume of the blood and of the extracellular fluid is only slightly affected and the blood pressure, haematocrit and serum sodium concentration remain within normal limits until considerable degrees of depletion have occurred. The late development of circulatory inadequacy explains why embarrassment of renal function with consequent uraemia occurs only when water depletion has advanced to a serious degree.

Water depletion should be anticipated in conditions where its development is inevitable, and its prevention should be ensured by giving adequate amounts of water to establish a normal urine flow and to compensate for insensible loss. The normal daily water requirement for an adult of 70 kg. ranges from 1,800 to 2,200 ml. If fever is present or if the patient suffers from a defect in renal concentrating power, as much as four to five litres per day may be required to meet the increased rate of turnover of water. Although many patients express their need for water by thirst, this is an unreliable guide in the very young, in the elderly and in those of any age who are seriously ill.

The diagnosis of established water depletion is best made from the history of a water intake insufficient to meet the metabolic needs. Only in the absence of renal disease or functional tubular defects is the urine output obviously reduced in volume and of high specific gravity.

Treatment of water depletion. For practical purposes it is convenient to consider water depletion in three categories of increasing magnitude:

(*a*) Mild water depletion in which about 2 per cent. of the body weight has been lost. This represents one to three litres of water. Oliguria and thirst may be the only clinical features.

(*b*) Moderately severe water depletion in which about 6 per cent. of body weight has been lost. This represents three to five litres in the average adult. Weakness, mental confusion and slight tachycardia with little change in blood pressure are usually present.

(*c*) Severe water depletion in which up to 12 per cent. of body weight has been lost. This represents seven to nine litres of body water. The patient is collapsed, confused or unconscious. Anuria or severe oliguria is usually present. The concentration of serum sodium may be elevated and the concentration of urea in the blood is increased.

The treatment of water depletion consists of the administration of water either orally or in the form of 5 per cent. glucose 10 per cent. fructose intravenously. Once the assessment of the magnitude of the depletion has been made, the water should be given rapidly within a few hours and allowance should be made for the current daily requirements. Even the mildest case of water depletion requires at least four litres on the first day because of the continued daily need. In the conscious patient suffering from mild or moderately severe depletion much or all of the fluid may be given by mouth. This is frequently not feasible in the seriously ill or elderly and is never possible in severe degrees of water depletion. For such cases the administration of six or more litres of 5 per cent. glucose is necessary within 24 hours or 10 per cent. fructose. In the absence of thirst the best guides to the amount of water required are evidence of improvement in the patient's clinical state and the occurrence of a daily urinary excretion of more than 1,500 ml. In patients with renal disease in whom the ability to vary the concentration of the urine is limited, or in those with severe infection, 1,500 ml. is unlikely to be adequate and a daily excretion of three litres or more may be required, but care should be taken to avoid overhydration and water intoxication (p. 259).

Sodium Depletion

As in the case of water balance, salt balance depends also on equality in the amount of sodium excreted and the amount ingested. In the absence of renal disease the power of the kidneys to conserve sodium in the face of reduced intake is virtually complete and in health salt balance may be maintained with a daily intake of as little as 500 mg. of sodium.

In health, negligible amounts of sodium are lost in the stools and from the skin, and there is no loss of sodium comparable to the obligatory loss of water which occurs through these channels. Whereas the driving force of thirst normally ensures the required daily intake of water, salt intake can vary widely from day to day without ill effect. The kidneys preserve the normal salt content of the body by the simple expedient of adjusting the urinary excretion of sodium in accordance with the variable and unregulated load which dietary inclination imposes.

Because of the intimate relation of salt and water homeostasis, loss of sodium from the body is usually accompanied by a corresponding reduction in its water content. Although pure salt depletion may occur in severe sweating when the loss of water from the body has been made good by the voluntary or forced ingestion of salt-free fluids, more often than not conditions leading to salt depletion are attended by significant degrees of water depletion; the resulting disorder is therefore a mixed one, though salt loss may predominate over water loss.

Causes of sodium depletion. In temperate regions predominant salt depletion arises either as a result of excessive loss of salt in the urine or because of increased loss of sodium-containing fluids in the alimentary tract. The renal causes of salt depletion include such intrinsic diseases as chronic pyelonephritis and the recovery phase of acute renal failure of ischaemic origin. Excessive salt loss also results from inadequate hormonal control of renal excretion of sodium such as occurs, for example, in Addison's disease. In uncontrolled diabetes mellitus, salt is lost because of the osmotic diuresis induced by hyperglycaemia. If diabetic ketosis and acidosis develop, urinary sodium loss is further increased as the hydrogen/sodium ion exchange mechanism in the distal part of the nephron becomes unable to cope with the increasing acidosis. Gastro-intestinal causes of salt

depletion include all conditions involving increased external loss of salt-containing fluids, i.e. diarrhoea, intestinal fistulae and persistent vomiting. In hot climates or in poorly ventilated industrial plants significant degrees of salt loss may occur from sweating alone. The sodium content of sweat is usually about one-third that of the concentration in the blood and in unfavourable conditions of temperature and humidity four to eight litres of sweat may be lost in the 24 hours (p. 557).

Diagnosis of salt depletion. The dominant position of sodium in the extracellular fluids is responsible for the early development of symptoms and signs of circulatory inadequacy. As salt is lost from the body, the blood volume and the volume of the extracellular fluids are reduced. Loss of the normal elasticity of the skin, diminution in intra-ocular tension, tachycardia and fall in blood pressure inevitably follow. The failure to preserve a normal renal blood flow results in the early appearance of oliguria and uraemia.

Treatment of salt depletion. The immediate aim in treatment is the restoration of the volume of extracellular fluid. This is best achieved by the administration of isotonic sodium chloride solution by intravenous infusion. In most instances the magnitude of the salt depletion can be assessed only on clinical grounds, since precise information as to the quantities of sodium or water lost from the body is not available. In general, the serum sodium concentration is not a reliable guide to the degree of salt deficit, since it often remains within normal limits because of the concurrent loss of water from the body. It is convenient to classify salt depletion into three categories of increasing severity.

(a) MILD SALT DEPLETION caused, for example, by vomiting or diarrhoea of one day's duration, is unattended by signs of circulatory inadequacy. This represents a deficiency of about 150 to 300 mEq. of sodium or one to two litres of normal saline (9 to 18 g. sodium chloride).

(b) MODERATELY SEVERE SALT DEPLETION is exemplified by moderately severe diabetic ketosis. There may be a history of some days of vomiting and polyuria. Tachycardia is present and the blood pressure is reduced. There is clinical evidence of water and salt loss, but the patient is conscious. This represents a deficiency of 300 to 600 mEq. of sodium, equivalent to two to four litres of normal saline (18 to 36 g. sodium chloride).

(c) SEVERE SALT DEPLETION. In this case the

I*

patient's history is consistent with the occurrence of considerable acute or chronic loss of body fluid. There is marked circulatory inadequacy, tachycardia and shock. The blood pressure may be unrecordable and all the clinical features of water and salt depletion are present. This degree of severity represents a deficit of the order of 600 to 1,000 mEq. sodium, equivalent to four to seven litres of isotonic saline.

Minor degrees of salt depletion may be made good by the addition of extra salt to the diet with encouragement to drink ample fluids. The salt may be taken as capsules in amounts of about 6 to 10 g. daily for some days. In moderately severe cases of salt depletion intravenous administration of isotonic saline (0·9 per cent.) is necessary and two to four litres of this may be given rapidly over the course of 12 hours. In more severe cases with marked circulatory impairment larger volumes of up to seven or eight litres of isotonic saline may be required. The extent to which treatment has been adequate must be judged in the individual patient, particular attention being paid to the blood pressure, pulse rate, intra-ocular tension and the degree of hydration of the skin. Excessive administration of saline is to be avoided; the veins in the neck should be carefully inspected and the bases of the lungs examined frequently in order to detect crepitations.

Severe salt depletion is almost invariably associated with disturbances in acid-base balance and frequently with superimposed water and potassium depletion. The degree of the deficiency in water should be assessed separately and the appropriate amount of glucose or fructose solution should be given orally or parenterally. When faced with sodium depletion of major severity it is rarely desirable to replace the sodium lost by isotonic saline alone. The extent to which treatment should be modified by the use of sodium bicarbonate, ammonium chloride or potassium is discussed in the appropriate section in this chapter.

Potassium Depletion

Potassium is the major intracellular cation, and abnormalities in potassium balance and distribution within the body occur in a wide variety of diseases. Depending on the daily intake, the healthy individual excretes about 20 mEq. of potassium in the stools daily and about 50 to 100 mEq. per day in the urine. Most of the potassium excreted in the urine is secreted by the distal tubular cells of the kidney. These cells exchange potassium and hydrogen ions for sodium ions filtered by the glomerulus. As might be expected, the rate of excretion of potassium in the urine is influenced by diseases and by drugs which alter the amount of sodium reaching the site of exchange, by the capacity of the renal tubules to reabsorb sodium and by the availability of hydrogen ions.

Causes of potassium depletion. This arises as a result of excessive loss of potassium in the urine or in the gastro-intestinal fluids. Loss of potassium from the gastro-intestinal tract occurs in vomiting, fistulous drainage, diarrhoea due to infection, malabsorption or neoplasm of the small or large bowel and excessive use of cathartics. Renal wastage of potassium on the other hand is more complex in its origin and occurs in any circumstances which lead to an increase in the rate of sodium/potassium exchange in the distal tubules. These include Cushing's syndrome and primary or secondary aldosteronism, the administration of large amounts of sodium-containing fluids, the use of diuretics such as chlorothiazide and its analogues, frusemide and ethacrynic acid. Corticosteroids and carbenoxalone also induce potassium depletion. Since hydrogen ions compete with potassium for exchange with sodium, drugs or diseases which suppress renal hydrogen ion secretion result in excessive potassium loss. These include acetazolamide, chlorothiazide and its derivatives, the Fanconi syndrome and renal tubular acidosis.

Since almost all of the potassium in the body lies within the cells, factors which lower the gradient between the cells and the extracellular fluids are also capable of leading to potassium depletion. These include anoxaemia, impaired oxidation of carbohydrate and acidosis of metabolic or respiratory origin. A combination of all of these appears to be responsible, for example, for the migration of potassium from the cells in diabetic acidosis which is excreted in the urine and this external loss continues for as long as the flow of urine is maintained. When severe water and salt depletion with oliguria supervene, the potassium may then accumulate in the blood and give rise to hyperkalaemia in the face of an overall body deficit.

Diagnosis of potassium depletion. Potassium depletion should be suspected in any of the clinical circumstances described above. If uncorrected, a number of functional disturbances affecting various systems arise. Impaired neuromuscular function ranges from mild weakness to frank paralysis and may interfere with pulmonary ventilation. Gastro-intestinal dilatation with ileus may be a result as well as a cause of potassium depletion. Ventricular extrasystoles, paroxysmal tachycardia with block due to increased sensitivity to digitalis glycosides, abnormalities in renal concentrating power with resulting polyuria and polydipsia, mild uraemia, tetany, oedema and extracellular alkalosis are all consequences of potassium depletion. Very often, however, these features are at least initially obscured by the effects of other electrolyte abnormalities such as water and salt depletion and sometimes become clinically obvious only after these depletions have been ameliorated.

Treatment of potassium depletion. The serious nature of the effects of potassium depletion and the difficulties encountered in replacing large amounts of this ion when considerable external loss has occurred, justifies the prophylactic administration of potassium salts to all patients liable to become depleted. When potassium loss can be anticipated, potassium salts should be given by mouth. This should be routine practice when patients are being treated for long periods of time with corticosteroids, carbenoxolone or diuretics. In general, 3 to 6 g. of potassium chloride daily as tablets are adequate as prophylactic therapy, and are sufficient in patients with chronic mild potassium-losing diseases such as ulcerative colitis and renal tubular acidosis. The higher dose is usually necessary for those with Cushing's syndrome when it is essential to repair at least part of the potassium depletion before undertaking surgical treatment. Occasionally patients are intolerant to oral potassium in this form and it may then be given as slow release potassium chloride wax ampoules (Ciba). Enteric coated potassium preparations should be avoided as they are liable to cause gastro-intestinal erosions. Alternatively, potassium may be given in the form of effervescent tablets such as those containing betaine hydrochloride and potassium bicarbonate, equivalent to 500 mg. of potassium chloride tablets (*e.g.* Kloref).

Once depletion has been allowed to develop, potassium must be given in larger doses and occasionally parenteral administration may be necessary. Deficits in potassium likely to be encountered in clinical practice range from 200 to 800 mEq. (8 to 36 g. potassium), these values representing mild and severe degrees of depletion respectively. Whenever possible potassium should be given by mouth in divided daily doses equivalent to

12 to 15 g. potassium chloride. Depending upon the severity of the depletion and upon the persistence of the loss of potassium from the body this dose may have to be given for several days or weeks. Frequent determinations of the concentration of serum potassium should be undertaken and the dose should be reduced or its administration stopped if the concentration should rise above normal values. It should be remembered, however, that hyperkalaemia may occur in the face of intracellular potassium deficit and especially when factors tending to promote migration of potassium from the cells persist. In severe congestive heart failure, anoxaemia may do so, even in the face of adequate potassium therapy. On the other hand, such a complication is unlikely to arise in the treatment of severe potassium depletion due to gastro-intestinal losses provided any accompanying water and salt depletion has been corrected and circulatory inadequacy abolished.

In severe potassium depletion oral therapy may be impracticable because of prostration, vomiting or continued gastric or intestinal aspiration, and in these circumstances potassium should be given intravenously. This is indicated also in the presence of marked hypokalaemia even when the overall deficit of potassium may not be great. Hypokalaemia may develop very rapidly, an event which is most commonly seen in fulminating diarrhoea or during recovery from diabetic acidosis. In these circumstances it is frequently induced or aggravated by the therapeutic administration of water and salt which not only dilutes the potassium in the extracellular fluids but, by restoring the circulation and improving tissue oxygenation, encourages the movement of potassium into the cells. In such cases of mixed sodium and potassium depletion it is advisable to restore at least in part the volume of the extracellular fluid by giving sodium-containing fluids before administering potassium intravenously even at the risk of producing hypokalaemia. If potassium is administered intravenously before this is done, dangerously high concentrations in the blood may be reached, both because of the effect of water and salt depletion on cellular function and as a result of the oliguria or anuria which accompanies severe extracellular fluid depletion.

Parenteral administration of potassium should be controlled by frequent determinations of serum potassium and the rate of administration adjusted accordingly. In the moderately severe cases, with a serum potassium concentration of about 3 mEq./*l.*

1·5 g. of potassium chloride in 5 ml. of sterile water can be added to 1 pint of 5 per cent. glucose or of isotonic saline. One litre of this solution (40 mEq./*l*.) can be given intravenously within four hours. Further potassium should not be given intravenously until its concentration in the serum has again been determined. Even if this has returned to normal, it should not be assumed that a significant part of the intracellular deficit has been corrected, and intravenous administration should be continued at a slower rate if it is impossible to give the potassium by mouth. On the other hand, if frank hypokalaemia still persists, a second litre of potassium-containing fluid (4 g. KCl/*l*.) may be given within three to four hours.

Potassium Intoxication

An absolute increase in potassium in the body is a rare clinical occurrence, and potassium intoxication is usually the result of an increase in the extracellular concentration of potassium, the cellular content being either normal or diminished. Clinically, hyperkalaemia occurs in those conditions in which the movement of potassium from within the cells is increased and in which its subsequent escape from the body in the urine is retarded by depression of renal function. This combination is liable to develop in acute renal failure, particularly if associated with massive tissue damage, haemolysis, severe infection and acidosis (p. 273). Severe diabetic acidosis, when unrelieved by appropriate therapy, Addison's disease and Addisonian crisis also lead to hyperkalaemia by the same mechanism. A small proportion of patients in the terminal stages of chronic renal failure develop hyperkalaemia.

Hyperkalaemia, although uncommon, is of considerable clinical importance because of the danger of cardiac arrest with levels of serum potassium above 7·5 mEq./*l*. Concentrations of potassium of 10 mEq./*l*. are highly dangerous and demand urgent treatment.

Treatment of potassium intoxication. Hyperkalaemia due to adrenocortical insufficiency is readily corrected by giving adequate doses of corticosteroids and appropriate amounts of 5 per cent. glucose and isotonic saline intravenously (p. 626). In many patients with acute or chronic renal failure, control of a modest rise in serum potassium to 6 or 7 mEq./*l*. can often be achieved merely by restricting potassium intake. If the concentration of potassium continues to rise in spite of dietary deprivation, more stringent measures should be taken. These consist in the use of a suitable ion exchange resin. Resonium A, a resin in the sodium cycle or calcium resin in amounts of 20 to 50 g., should be made into a paste by the addition of water and given by mouth or administered as a retention enema. Serial determinations of serum potassium should be performed and the administration of resin repeated in four hours if necessary. Alternative but sometimes additional methods of value include the intravenous administration of isotonic sodium bicarbonate or the use of 5 per cent. glucose and soluble insulin. The intravenous infusion of up to 1 litre of isotonic sodium bicarbonate reduces the concentration of serum potassium by its effect on the acid-base composition of body cells, but its use is limited to patients who can tolerate salt-containing fluids. An infusion of 30 units of soluble insulin in 500 ml. of 10 to 20 per cent. dextrose solution is also worthy of trial in those patients in whom the use of the resin fails or if sodium containing fluids are contraindicated. This promotes the movement of potassium into cells but its effect is usually temporary. If these measures fail to control the rise in serum potassium and the concentration of potassium rises above 7·5 mEq./*l*. treatment by extracorporeal dialysis (artificial kidney) or by peritoneal dialysis should be carried out with the least possible delay (p. 277).

If there is extreme elevation of the concentration of serum potassium to 10 mEq./*l*. when the patient is first seen, insulin, alkali and glucose should be given immediately as a palliative measure while arrangements for dialysis are being made. An intravenous injection of 10 per cent. calcium gluconate (10 to 20 ml.) should also be given as this diminishes the cardiotoxic effects of hyperkalaemia.

Magnesium Deficiency and Intoxication

Until recently disorders in magnesium metabolism have been difficult to recognize. Rapid methods of determination of magnesium in body fluids have, however, shown that these chemical abnormalities are occasionally responsible for puzzling clinical features and are readily susceptible to therapeutic control. The distribution of magnesium in the body is similar to that of potassium and it is present in relatively low concentration in the blood.

The most frequent cause of magnesium deficiency is prolonged diarrhoea or vomiting in which parenteral fluid and electrolyte therapy without magnesium supplements are given. It occasionally follows long-continued diuretic therapy and is associated with severe undernutrition, such as occurs in kwashiorkor and in the malabsorption syndrome, especially when the latter is treated with medicinal calcium; chronic alcoholism and aldosteronism also lead to magnesium depletion. Clinical manifestations of magnesium deficiency are predominantly neuromuscular with tremor, choreiform movements and aimless plucking of the bedclothes. Mental confusion with hallucinations is common and muscular weakness with areflexia may result. Generalized convulsions occur in severe cases. The diagnosis should be confirmed by finding the concentration of magnesium in the serum to be less than 1·5 mEq./*l*. Patients who are receiving parenteral fluids for long periods can be prevented from developing magnesium deficiency by the addition of 8 to 16 mEq. of magnesium per day (1 to 2 g. of magnesium sulphate) to the intravenous infusion. Established deficits are treated by giving magnesium sulphate by the intravenous route or magnesium hydroxide by mouth. When parenteral treatment is necessary 50 mEq. of magnesium (6 g. of magnesium sulphate) is added to a litre of glucose or saline and infused over a period of 3 to 4 hours. During the remainder of this first day a further 100 mEq. of magnesium is given by continuous infusion (2 litres of fluid each containing 6 g. of magnesium sulphate). On subsequent days 50 mEq. of magnesium is added to the prescribed parenteral fluids. The plasma magnesium should be estimated daily and the amount of magnesium reduced to 8 to 16 mEq./day when the level rises to normal. Magnesium deficits can be restored by giving approximately 100 to 200 mEq. of magnesium per day in the form of magnesium hydroxide by mouth. Milk of magnesia tablets contain 10·3 mEq. of magnesium and may be used, but there is doubt as to how much is absorbed; where a large deficit is suspected parenteral magnesium should be given.

Magnesium intoxication mainly occurs in acute and chronic renal disease and contributes to the central nervous features associated with uraemia. Its treatment is that of the primary disorder and is discussed on pp. 273-281.

Hyponatraemia and Water Intoxication

The low salt syndrome was first described in 1949 when the term was used to describe the occurrence of hyponatraemia brought about by the vigorous application of various therapeutic measures designed to remove salt from cardiac patients with an inadequate circulation and oedema. In such patients, progressive renal failure with uraemia due to reduction in the plasma volume and hyponatraemia occur, often without relief of generalized oedema. They are often in the last stages of congestive heart failure or hepatic cirrhosis and a dramatic if temporary response is sometimes seen after the intravenous administration of 100 to 300 ml. hypertonic saline (5 per cent.).

It is important to recognize other causes of hyponatraemia since the appropriate therapy varies accordingly These are as follows:

(1) WATER INTOXICATION. In health the ingestion of a large volume of water is rapidly followed by a diuresis and water does not accumulate in the body. On the other hand, over-enthusiastic administration of water to patients in whom the renal power to dilute urine is restricted inevitably causes water intoxication. Hyponatraemia and symptoms such as mental confusion, headache, nausea, convulsions and coma may develop. This condition is particularly likely to occur in chronic renal or hepatic disease or in those recovering from acute tubular necrosis, in patients with adrenocortical insufficiency and in the post-operative state. Occasionally, water intoxication develops in cases of bronchial carcinoma in which the tumour secretes an antidiuretic hormone-like substance. This condition subsides if the tumour can be removed surgically. If this is not possible, the severe symptoms of water intoxication may respond to hypertonic saline or to the administration of fludrocortisone, 0·1 mg./per day. In the treatment of water and salt depletion, care should be taken to see that water intoxication does not develop as a consequence of the unbalanced administration of water and salt.

Once hyponatraemia from water intoxication has developed, water should be withheld and loss of water from the body encouraged by inducing sweating with a suitable heat cradle. In severe cases, 100 ml. hypertonic saline (5 per cent.) should be given by intravenous injection and repeated at short intervals until clinical improvement occurs.

(2) POTASSIUM DEFICIENCY. The low salt syndrome due to intracellular potassium depletion is most commonly seen in patients with congestive heart failure who have received treatment which has led to progressive potassium deficiency. This is particularly liable to occur if diuretics are given to

patients who are taking a diet restricted in sodium. Sodium from the extracellular fluids appears to migrate into the cells in place of potassium and the extracellular concentration of sodium ion is reduced. These patients often ultimately develop resistance to diuretics. The serum sodium may rise to normal values with the administration of oral potassium. If oedema still persists, attempts to remove it should then be more gradual. If severe potassium deficiency has been produced, intracellular potassium replacement is limited by the possible development of hyperkalaemia and in some patients this chemical abnormality appears to be irreversible.

(3) REDUCTION IN OVERALL BODY OSMOLALITY (NEW STEADY STATES). The tonicity of the extracellular fluids is almost certainly identical with that of the intracellular compartment and therefore reflects changes which may occur there. In patients who have chronic disease, particularly tuberculosis or malignancy, hyponatraemia is occasionally found without evidence of sodium or potassium depletion or of water intoxication. This is a form of hyponatraemia which probably represents a general body reduction in cell osmolality and it does not respond to any known therapy.

Acidosis and Alkalosis

The limits of the pH of the blood compatible with life lie within the range of 6·9 to 7·8, though in health the variation is very much smaller and the pH is usually between 7·35 and 7·45. Acidosis and alkalosis represent those disorders in which there is respectively an increase or reduction in free hydrogen ions in the blood. In response to these changes in concentration, alterations in the bicarbonate concentration of the blood and Pco_2 are brought about by compensatory renal or respiratory mechanisms.

Acidosis. RESPIRATORY ACIDOSIS arises as a result of impairment in the excretion of carbon dioxide by the lungs and is seen in patients whose ventilation is reduced by such causes as drug-induced depression of the respiratory centre, weakness or paralysis of the muscles of respiration, injuries to the chest, chronic bronchitis and emphysema, bronchial asthma, gross obesity, multiple pulmonary emboli and cardio-respiratory disease. The accumulation of carbonic acid and the fall in blood pH result in the renal conservation of bicarbonate so that the total bicarbonate of the blood increases and the urine becomes acid.

Respiratory acidosis is not a disorder that can be corrected by manipulation of the electrolytes of the body, but it is important not to misinterpret the associated elevated concentration of bicarbonate as being the manifestation of metabolic alkalosis. Therapy is directed towards improving the underlying cardio-pulmonary disease, which includes the treatment of congestive heart failure, pulmonary infection and bronchospasm. Oxygen therapy is also usually indicated, but it should be given with care since an increase in the partial pressure of oxygen in the blood may remove the main ventilatory drive, and severe acute carbon dioxide retention with a precipitate fall in blood pH may ensue (p. 648).

METABOLIC ACIDOSIS results either from the accumulation in the body of metabolic acids other then carbonic acid or from direct loss of the base bicarbonate.

The first category includes diabetic acidosis in which there is abnormal production of acetoacetic and β-hydroxybutyric acids, lactic acid acidosis which develops in shock and in conditions giving rise to circulatory inadequacy (e.g. myocardial infarction), and various forms of renal disease in which a reduction occurs in the power to excrete in the urine the acid produced daily in the body either as hydrogen or ammonium ions. As has already been pointed out, hydrogen ions are normally secreted into the urine by the tubular cells in exchange for sodium ions filtered by the glomerulus. When the tubular excretory power is reduced by parenchymal disease or congenital defect, or when the metabolic production of acid to be excreted is greatly increased, failure to excrete hydrogen ion is necessarily attended by excessive urinary sodium loss. For this reason acidosis is frequently associated with sodium depletion though the sodium loss does not by itself lead to acidosis.

In the second category excessive loss of alkaline intestinal contents in diarrhoea, pancreatic or other fistulae leads to both acidosis and sodium depletion from direct loss of sodium bicarbonate. When metabolic acidosis is fully developed, the pH of the blood and its bicarbonate content are depressed. The alteration in the hydrogen ion concentration in the blood is minimized by extracellular and cellular buffers and also by the response of the respiratory centre; this is stimulated by the change in pH with the result that the ventilatory excretion of carbonic acid is increased and the tension of carbon dioxide in the blood (Pco_2)

is reduced below its normal value of 40 mm. Hg. Some of the hydrogen ions buffered within the cells are exchanged for potassium which migrates from the cells and may be excreted in the urine.

Treatment of Metabolic Acidosis

The oral or intravenous administration of alkali is a logical step in the treatment of metabolic acidosis. In mild cases such as those with chronic renal disease of moderate severity, reasonably normal acid-base balance may be maintained for some years by the daily oral administration of 2 to 6 g. sodium bicarbonate. The amount given and its duration are best judged by determining the bicarbonate content of the blood. In severer degrees of acidosis intravenous therapy is always indicated. Since the patients are commonly suffering from salt depletion, the magnitude of this is best assessed in the first place by the method already described. Once this has been decided, one-third to one-half of the volume of saline needed should be replaced with isotonic sodium bicarbonate (1·3 g. per cent.). It is unnecessary to mix the saline and alkali in the same bottle, separate solutions being given alternately.

Theoretically, when the acidosis is due to excessive acid production as occurs in diabetic acidosis or to gastro-intestinal base loss, the administration of alkali is necessary. Provided that acid production is reduced by the administration of glucose, insulin and water, and that salt loss is restored by isotonic saline, any adjustment that is needed in the acid-base balance of the body would be ultimately accomplished by appropriate renal activity. Although this can be confidently expected in young adults with normal renal function, it is unwise to depend upon this renal physiological co-operation in the elderly, or if there is any doubt about the state of renal function. When acidosis has arisen because of a primary defect in tubular function, the administration of alkali by intravenous infusion with the appropriate amount of saline is essential. As has already been indicated, many of the diseases resulting in acidosis with water and salt depletion are accompanied by varying degrees of potassium loss. The extent of this should be separately assessed and potassium chloride given orally or added to the appropriate solution and given intravenously. In shock resulting, for example, from severe myocardial infarction or cardiac arrest, acidosis due to the accumulation of lactic acid occurs in the absence of water or sodium depletion. This is best treated by the intravenous injection of sodium bicarbonate in as small a volume of water as possible. A convenient and stable concentration of sodium bicarbonate is 5 per cent. (600 mEq./l.). Of this, 300 to 500 ml. should be given intravenously and repeated in four hours depending upon the results obtained by analysis of the blood pH and the concentration of bicarbonate.

Alkalosis. RESPIRATORY ALKALOSIS arises usually as a result of hyperventilation due to emotional causes, though occasionally a lesion in the central nervous system is responsible. It tends also to occur in the course of mechanically assisted ventilation and it is a characteristic complication of salicylate intoxication. The existence of hyperventilation may be clinically detectable and the patient may experience paraesthesiae, numbness and tetany. The renal response to alkalosis of respiratory origin is the rejection of much of the filtrated bicarbonate by the renal tubules, and the urine becomes alkaline. The suppression of hydrogen ion secretion which this involves results in potassium being made available for exchange with sodium in the renal tubules, and potassium loss and depletion may develop.

Treatment of Respiratory Alkalosis. The treatment of respiratory alkalosis is the employment of a method to increase the carbon dioxide tension of the alveolar air and thus of the extracellular fluid. In simple cases of emotional origin this is best done by asking the patient to rebreathe into a paper bag. Sedation may occasionally be needed in addition. With long-continued use of mechanically assisted respiration frequent sampling of blood is necessary to ensure adequate control, and oral or intravenous potassium is indicated if there is evidence of hypokalaemia or potassium depletion.

METABOLIC ALKALOSIS is characterized by an increase in the bicarbonate content of the blood and may therefore arise either because of loss of acid from the body or because of a gain in total base. Vomiting or continued gastric aspiration are among the most common clinical causes of alkalosis and this is due directly to loss of hydrochloric acid. The consequent increase in the blood pH is mitigated by hypoventilation with the retention of carbon dioxide, and by the renal excretion of sodium and potassium bicarbonate. In addition to the loss in the urine, potassium is also lost in the vomitus. Potassium, sodium and chloride depletion are, therefore, quickly superimposed on the acid-base disturbance, and if the vomiting persists and prevents normal water intake, depletion of water also ensues. Alkalosis due to vomiting is thus seen to be a complex chemical disorder.

Treatment of Metabolic Alkalosis

The water depletion usually necessitates the administration of glucose or fructose solution in amounts indicated by the considerations already described. As in the case of metabolic acidosis, restoration of the extracellular volume by the administration of isotonic saline might be expected to go far to correct the acid-base disturbance. Unfortunately, in anything but the mildest degree of vomiting this is not so and the main obstacle appears to be the associated potassium and chloride depletion. The loss of these ions has two major effects. In the first place cellular depletion of potassium results in little being available for sodium/potassium exchange in the renal tubules. Secondly, the chloride deficit promotes the reabsorption of bicarbonate by the renal tubules. For both reasons hydrogen ions are thus excreted in the urine, which becomes acid, and this intensifies the degree of alkalosis in the blood and extracellular fluids.

With these considerations in mind it appears logical to treat the alkalosis of vomiting with a mixture of sodium and potassium chloride. After assessing the degree of sodium depletion on clinical grounds as already described, 1 to 2 g. potassium chloride in 5 ml. of sterile water can be added to each pint of isotonic saline and the total volume estimated to correct the depletion should be given within 24 hours, along with an appropriate volume of 5 per cent. glucose. Although potassium depletion undoubtedly aggravates and perpetuates the alkalosis of vomiting, the primary cause is loss of hydrochloric acid. Because of this, Cook and Crowley devised a solution of ammonium chloride (70 mEq./l.), sodium chloride (63 mEq./l.) and potassium chloride (17 mEq./l.), and this has come to be known as Gastric Solution. Although by present-day standards it probably contains insufficient potassium to meet most requirements, it possesses the advantage that it is directly acidifying. In a patient who is vomiting persistently or in whom there is a need for continued gastric aspiration volume-for-volume replacement of gastric contents with Gastric Solution given intravenously is a satisfactory way to maintain acid-base balance once the deficit of sodium and potassium has been largely made good by the means

already described. In addition, of course, it is necessary to provide water and isotonic saline to balance the insensible loss of water and the water and salt lost in the urine.

Other causes of metabolic alkalosis include overdosage with sodium bicarbonate, excessive administration of diuretics and all conditions associated with potassium depletion. The first usually results from over-enthusiastic treatment of dyspepsia with alkali and may be aggravated by vomiting. Apart from stopping the administration of the bicarbonate, treatment is identical with that given in the case of alkalosis of vomiting. Organic mercurial diuretics given repeatedly in the treatment of oedema frequently give rise to alkalosis by increasing the amount of sodium presented to the site of sodium potassium exchange in the distal part of the nephron. Alkalosis is frequently a cause of resistance to mercurial diuretics and the disturbance is usually overcome by the oral administration of ammonium chloride 1 g. three times a day, care being taken to see that potassium depletion is also remedied. All conditions listed on p. 256 as being capable of leading to potassium depletion are also prone to give rise to alkalosis. This form of alkalosis responds to treatment with potassium chloride.

Special Problems presented by Infants and Young Children

Up to this point disorders in electrolyte balance and in acid-base disturbances have been considered in terms of the needs of an adult of 70 kg. Although these disorders are qualitatively similar in babies and in young children to those present in adults, there are clinically important quantitative differences which arise from certain characteristics of water and salt metabolism in the early months and years of life. The metabolic rate and water content of the infant are relatively higher than that of the adult and the flexibility of renal tubular function matures slowly. The increased respiratory rate and the larger surface area in proportion to the body weight leads to a relatively high rate of insensible water loss. For these reasons infants and young children are liable to suffer severe water and electrolyte depletion in a very short period of time, whenever they are unable to ingest adequate amounts of fluid or in the event of increased gastrointestinal loss from vomiting or diarrhoea. The distinction which has been made in adults between water depletion and predominant sodium depletion is also relevant in infants and careful inquiry into the fluid consumed and lost is necessary in assessing the nature of the depletion. As a guide to treatment it is useful to divide the clinical picture into three stages.

Mild water and salt depletion. The child is cross and thirsty but the eyes and fontanels are not noticeably sunken. Weight loss of as much as 5 per cent. of body weight may have occurred. At this stage the condition is nearly always reversible by oral fluids unless there is vomiting.

Moderately severe water and salt depletion. The child is obviously ill and the eyes and fontanels are sunken. The heart rate is rapid (160 to 180 per minute) and as much as 5 to 15 per cent. of body weight loss occurs (250 to 750 g. in a 5-kg. infant). Parenteral administration of fluid is nearly always necessary.

Severe water and salt depletion. The baby usually appears moribund and is limp, apparently unconscious and in a state of circulatory collapse. The eyes are sunken, the heart rate increased to over 200 per minute and weight loss of 20 per cent. or more of body weight has occurred. Parenteral fluid therapy should be given at once if death is to be avoided.

A normal infant excretes a relatively larger volume of urine than an adult, and a fall in urinary output is an indication of deficiency of either water or water and salt. This may be noticed first by the mother or nurse from the reduction in the number of diapers required. Except in patients with mild depletion, the blood urea is always elevated. Changes in the concentration of serum electrolytes do not occur until the depletion has reached a severe stage. In these circumstances the alteration in the serum concentration of sodium is more reliable than in the adult in revealing the extent to which there has been predominant loss of water or sodium.

Predominant water depletion. A healthy infant of up to 1 year takes about 150 ml. of water per kg. of body weight and in normal infants ranging in weight from 3 kg. at birth to 10 kg. at 1 year this represents about 400 to 800 ml. per day. Moderately severe water depletion may be corrected by an additional intake of one-third to one-half more than the normal until the weight loss has been regained or for as long as undue loss continues. Premature and newborn infants tolerate excessive amounts of water badly and it is best, therefore, to repair moderately severe and severe water depletion

by parenteral administration of 5 per cent. glucose in $\frac{1}{4}$ isotonic saline.

Electrolyte and water depletion. Because deficiencies of sodium and potassium and disturbances in acid-base balance in infants and children arise almost invariably from excessive gastrointestinal loss and are rarely complicated by intrinsic renal disease or by disturbances of the various homeostatic mechanisms, current practice consists largely of prescribing a dilute solution of sodium, potassium, chloride and bicarbonate in glucose water. Provision of these constituents in sufficient amount allows the kidneys to conserve or reject whatever may be necessary to re-establish normal body fluid composition. Infants suffering from mild gastrointestinal loss are satisfactorily treated by the administration of $\frac{1}{3}$ to $\frac{1}{2}$ isotonic saline until oral feeding is resumed. Patients with moderately severe and severe degrees of depletion demand more selective therapy. An intravenous infusion of 5 per cent. glucose containing 70 mEq./l. sodium and 35 mEq./l. each of chloride and bicarbonate, i.e. a mixture of $\frac{1}{2}$ isotonic NaCl and NaHCO$_3$, and to which 1·5 g. KCl/500 ml. (i.e. 40 mEq./l.) has been added is desirable. Darrow's solution was formerly used for this purpose in Britain and North America and is still widely used in the developing countries. However, it suffers the serious disadvantage that it contains lactate and such children may already be suffering from lactic acid acidosis.

In the event of severe acidosis (bicarbonate concentration in the blood of 10 mEq./l. or less), it is best to give a rapid intravenous infusion of 20 to 30 ml. of isotonic sodium bicarbonate per 1 kg. body weight repeating this in six hours if necessary, prior to the giving of half-strength solution of NaHCO$_3$ and NaCl in 5 per cent. glucose.

On the other hand, when dealing with pyloric stenosis, alkalosis is frequently severe and solutions containing bicarbonate are best avoided, at least until the major part of the deficit has been corrected. A 5 per cent. solution of glucose in $\frac{1}{3}$ to $\frac{1}{2}$ isotonic saline is appropriate. Once the greater part of this depletion has been corrected, potassium chloride (1·5 g. to 800 ml. equivalent to 26 mEq./l.) can be added to the infusion.

Intravenous administration of these fluids should be given as soon as possible as in some cases a delay of a few hours in beginning treatment may determine a fatal outcome. The fluids are best given intraperitoneally or by cutting down and inserting a cannula into one of the distal veins of the limbs, preferably either at the ankle or in the forearm or elbow. In most cases an initial infusion of 40 to 60 ml. per kg. body weight should be given in two to four hours, and in an emergency 40 ml. per kg. of this may be injected directly into the vein from a syringe until the infusion is set up. This rate of infusion should be continued until a free flow of urine occurs. When this takes place the rate of infusion can be reduced to 6 to 8 ml. per kg. per hour. As soon as possible, and usually within two or three days after the beginning of treatment, oral feeding should be started, giving increasing proportions of the fluid requirements by mouth, and introducing a milk feed (30 to 60 per kg.) if possible on the third or fourth day.

11. Renal Diseases

J. S. ROBSON

GLOMERULONEPHRITIS

Since 1827 when Richard Bright drew attention to the association between oedema, proteinuria and renal disease, the major unsolved problem of glomerulonephritis has been one of aetiology. For many years classification of this group of diseases depended upon the uncertain correlation of clinical observations of a sometimes chronic illness with the appearances of renal tissue obtained at autopsy. In 1942 Ellis divided the diffuse primary diseases of the kidney into types I and II, each possessing widely different clinical characteristics. Since then the problem has been clarified by the technique of renal biopsy which permits the examination of tissue at every stage of the disease process and allows a degree of clinico-pathological correlation hitherto unattainable. This procedure has enlarged the concepts of glomerular disease and now provides a substantial body of morphological information which partly compensates for ignorance of aetiology.

Of the primary diseases of the kidney which affect the glomeruli diffusely three main types of histological picture are apparent: (1) proliferative glomerulonephritis which is the lesion universally associated with acute post-streptococcal glomerulonephritis; (2) membranous glomerulonephritis and (3) minimal lesion glomerulonephritis both of which are associated with a form of subacute or chronic nephritis which often gives rise to the nephrotic syndrome.

Acute Glomerulonephritis

In its classical form the disease is preceded by infection with a *Group A streptococcus* usually in the throat. The disease is most common in children and adolescents, but occurs at any age. It begins abruptly and is associated with haematuria, proteinuria, hypertension and oedema. Malaise, vomiting, fever and headaches are common. Damage to the glomeruli results in a varying degree of renal failure. The natural history of acute glomerulonephritis depends largely upon the severity of the damage to the glomeruli and the degree of hypertension. In the younger age-groups the illness lasts for two to three weeks in over 90 per cent. of patients and is followed by complete recovery. In adults, however, glomerular damage is more often progressive and death may occur from renal failure usually complicated by hypertension in a matter of a few weeks or after a period of years. Death may also occur in the acute stages from heart failure.

Antibiotic therapy. Infection with *Group A haemolytic streptococci* causes the majority if not all initial attacks of acute glomerulonephritis, and precipitates exacerbations in patients suffering from chronic glomerulonephritis of the proliferative type. Only certain strains of haemolytic streptococci are nephritogenic and this fact accounts for the irregular appearance of the disease and the occasional explosive epidemic within families or small communities. Elevated streptococcal antibody titres confirm recent streptococcal infection in many patients, but do not indicate whether it is still active. The administration of penicillin may not, therefore, be effective once the disease has become established. Although in many patients streptococci may be isolated from the throat when acute glomerulonephritis develops, failure to do so does not necessarily mean that the infection has run its course. Furthermore, continuing infection may influence the severity of established glomerular damage. In addition, some patients who develop the disease continue to harbour streptococci in spite of apparently adequate antibiotic treatment. All patients with acute glomerulonephritis should have cultures taken from the pharynx and tonsils and then be given benzylpenicillin in doses of 600 mg. six-hourly by intramuscular injection. If the patient is a young child the penicillin should be given by mouth after the first day in the form of phenoxymethylpenicillin, 250 mg. six-hourly. Treatment should continue for seven days.

Prompt administration of penicillin to all patients with streptococcal infection may protect them from acute glomerulonephritis. This should be done in acute tonsillitis and pharyngitis when haemolytic streptococci are responsible. Often, however, the disease may follow a sore throat which appears trivial and the complication cannot be eradicated without resort to penicillin therapy for all patients who suffer from infections.

Prompt penicillin prophylaxis effectively aborts the spread of the disease during the course of an epidemic of acute glomerulonephritis. During an epidemic oral penicillin should, therefore, be given to all members of a community with a pharyngeal infection. When a single case of acute glomerulonephritis occurs within a family all its members, and those in close contact with it, should be studied bacteriologically to identify those carrying streptococci in their throats and such individuals should then be treated with penicillin.

There is no satisfactory epidemiological evidence to confirm the effectiveness of long-term penicillin for persons liable to develop infections of the throat in order to reduce the incidence of the disease.

Foci of infection. Tonsillectomy has no beneficial effect upon the incidence, severity or rapidity of healing of acute glomerulonephritis. When streptococcal infection is associated with tonsillitis and has been followed by acute glomerulonephritis, the infection is usually controlled by penicillin. Removal of infected tonsils during the active phase of acute glomerulonephritis frequently leads to an exacerbation of haematuria and proteinuria and should be avoided. If tonsillectomy is thought to be necessary because of persisting enlargement or intractable infection, the operation should be delayed until the features of acute glomerulonephritis have subsided. Search should be made for other foci of infection such as infected sinuses or dental abscesses which should be treated.

General management. All patients with acute glomerulonephritis are best treated in bed, in a warm, well-ventilated room maintained at an even temperature of about 17° C. Exposure to cold or draughts may increase the degree of haematuria in some individuals and delays recovery. Opinions vary, however, as to how long rest should be enforced. In the majority of instances it is best to confine the patient to bed for as long as there is continued improvement in renal function, as determined by the concentration of blood urea or estimations of glomerular filtration rate by creatinine clearance, and by the degree of proteinuria and haematuria. In most patients such an improvement occurs within the first two to four weeks of the onset and recovery is usually rapid and complete. Difficulty arises in those patients in whom recovery is only partial and who continue to show persistent abnormalities in the urine beyond this time. Renal biopsies undertaken in these circumstances show evidence of persisting activity of the disease process

within the glomeruli. If the patient feels well and is free from oedema, if renal function, as judged by the concentration of blood urea or the creatinine clearance, is not deteriorating and urinary abnormalities have reached a constant minimum, it is doubtful whether further rest in bed is of benefit. The few properly conducted trials of the effect of bed rest and ambulation suggest that once the acute stage has been passed further confinement to bed is of no therapeutic value. Proteinuria and microscopic haematuria may persist for months or years in some patients in which case the patient must be allowed to resume normal activities.

Diet and fluid balance. Acute glomerulonephritis causes an acute deterioration in renal function. This results in a diminished capacity to eliminate urea and other products of metabolism and to progressive acidosis. Because of the fall in glomerular filtration the volume of urine excreted is reduced and oedema develops. Potentially fatal consequences such as pulmonary oedema, hyperkalaemia and severe uraemia may, therefore, occur. Appropriate dietary and fluid therapy can influence the rate of development of these complications and provide the optimal opportunity for recovery of renal function.

The single most important factor in the prevention or control of oedema is the restriction of salt and it should be excluded from the diet as far as possible by appropriate selection of food and by using no salt in cooking or at table. The extent to which fluids in all forms should be restricted varies with the severity of the illness and with the degree of oliguria. Many patients with mild or only moderately severe glomerulonephritis continue to excrete almost normal volumes of urine each day. In these subjects modest fluid restriction only should be advised and volumes of up to 1,500 ml. per day can be allowed. Occasionally oliguria is severe and in these circumstances fluids should be reduced to an amount about equal to the volume of urine passed, plus 500 ml. to allow for insensible loss of water from the skin and in the breath. Restriction of protein is advisable to reduce exogenous protein metabolism to near the minimum value. The bulk of the calories should be provided by fats and carbohydrates whose complete oxidation to water and carbon dioxide does not lead to the accumulation in the blood of metabolites which require to be eliminated by the kidney.

From the beginning of the illness most patients should be given a diet containing approximately

20 g. protein, less than 2 g. of sodium chloride and between 1,000 and 1,400 ml. fluid per 24 hours. A sample menu which contains 1,600 calories, made up for the most part from fat and carbohydrate, is shown on pp. 267-268. A variety of exchanges of foods may be introduced in accordance with data obtained from dietetic tables (pp. 318-319). This diet may be maintained throughout the active phase of the disease in most patients. It should be continued until oedema subsides and the concentration of blood urea has fallen to near normal values. If after two weeks, these criteria have not been satisfied and the patient complains of hunger, additional calories may be given in the form of carbohydrate or fat. In most patients, however, clinical and biochemical improvement occurs within this period so that the protein of the diet can be increased to 45 g. per day. An example of this diet is given on p. 268 and contains 1,700 calories. The intake of fluid and sodium chloride should remain unchanged. Additional water may be allowed when the oedema has completely subsided and the daily volume of urine is normal. The point at which further relaxation of dietary restriction is advisable varies. In most patients the concentration of blood urea continues to fall in spite of the rise of protein intake to 45 g. In this event an unrestricted diet may be given thereafter. The persistence of proteinuria or haematuria is not itself a contraindication to such a diet if overall renal function is adequate to cope with a normal intake of salt and protein. In patients in whom the disease is mild and lasts only a few days, a more rapid return to a normal diet can be permitted.

Hypertension and hypertensive encephalopathy. Diastolic hypertension occurs in most patients with acute glomerulonephritis. Usually it is mild or moderate and does not require treatment. When it becomes severe and the diastolic blood pressure remains consistently above 115 mm. Hg. it may be associated with episodes of hypertensive encephalopathy or left ventricular failure. In the majority of patients rest in bed, salt restriction, and the spontaneous occurrence of diuresis with natural recovery, is sufficient to prevent serious hypertension from developing and renders specific antihypertensive treatment unnecessary. If a diastolic blood pressure of above 115 mm. Hg. should develop, however, antihypertensive drugs should be given in accordance with the recommendations on p. 112. When the renal disease subsides it is usually possible to stop this form of treatment.

Hypertensive encephalopathy during the course of acute glomerulonephritis is due to the hypertension and not to uraemia. Its onset is suggested by persistent headache and vomiting in patients whose blood pressure is high. Sometimes a rapid further rise in blood pressure may occur, in which case drowsiness with epileptiform convulsions may be followed by blindness of central origin, hemiplegia or monoplegia. The pathology of this complication is uncertain, but as complete restoration to normal is usual in those who recover, vascular spasm of the cerebral vessels seems probable. Since hypertensive encephalopathy is a curable but potentially lethal condition which does not affect the ultimate prognosis of the renal lesion, the doctor must be prepared to treat the condition promptly (p. 116).

Congestive heart failure. Dyspnoea and pulmonary oedema are frequent accompaniments of acute glomerulonephritis. The distinction between the clinical states caused by severe water and salt retention in primary renal disease and that of congestive heart failure in which the renal circulation is compromised because of a low cardiac output has been the subject of much debate.

DIET FOR EARLY STAGE OR SEVERE FORM OF ACUTE GLOMERU-LONEPHRITIS.

Protein 20 g. Fluids 1,200 ml. Calories approx. 1,600. Sodium approx. 800 mg.

Daily Ration		Prot. g.	Na mg.	Fluids	Cals.
Cream mixture:					
Double cream .	2 oz.	0·8	15	60	262
Water .	5 oz.			150	
Unsalted butter and					
margarine .	1¼ oz.		30		280
Sugar and glucose	2 oz.				224
Jam, marmalade and					
honey .	1½ oz.				115
Bread . .	3 oz.	7·2	444		216
Fruit . .	10 oz.		4		148

Breakfast		Prot. g.	Na mg.	Fluids	Cals.
5 oz. fruit juice with glucose .			3	150	60
¾ oz. cornflakes . .		1·5	224		78
1 oz. bread toasted .					
Unsalted butter . . .					
Sugar and marmalade as					
desired . . .					
Cream mixture . .					
2 cups of tea . .				240	

11 a.m.		Prot. g.	Na mg.	Fluids	Cals.
1 cup of tea or coffee . .				120	
Sugar and cream mixture .					
2 rich tea biscuits buttered .		1·4	46		82

Lunch

1 oz. lean meat or 1 egg .	7·5	22	64
2 oz. grilled tomato or other vegetable (except peas and beans) . . .	0·6	2	8
3 oz. potato mashed or sauté with butter . .	1·2	3	69
Fruit—fresh or stewed or tinned . . .			

Tea

1 oz. bread . . .
Unsalted butter . . .
Sugar, jam or honey as desired
2 cups of tea with cream mixture   240

Supper

1 oz. bread toasted . .
Sugar, jam or honey as desired
2 cups of tea with cream mixture   240
Fruit—fresh, stewed or tinned

                          20·2   793 1,200 1,606

No salt to be used in cooking and none to be added from the tray.

If the cream mixture is not tolerated, omit the meat from dinner and add 8 oz. milk. This increases the Na to 870 mg.

To restrict the potassium, omit fruit juice, supper fruit and 1 oz. potato, and add ¾ oz. jelly to supper. Use only apple, pear or tinned pineapple or mandarins at lunch.

To restrict the sodium further use salt-free bread. This reduces Na to 439 mg.

Diet suitable for Patients with Acute Glomerulo-nephritis or Chronic Renal Disease with Nitrogen Retention.

Approximately: Protein 45 g. Carbohydrate 245 g. Fat 60 g. Calories 1,700.

Breakfast

Fruit (fresh or stewed or tinned), or small glass of fruit juice.
1½ thin slices of bread, which may be toasted.
Marmalade or honey.
Butter and milk from allowance.*
Tea with sugar.

Mid-morning

Tea or coffee with milk from allowance and sugar.
1 biscuit.

Dinner

Small helping of meat or poultry or fish, or 2 eggs scrambled or baked.
Small helping of vegetables.
1 medium size potato.
Milk pudding, using milk from allowance and sugar.
Fruit (fresh, stewed or tinned).

Tea

2 thin slices of bread with jam, jelly or honey, or may be made into sandwiches, using tomato, lettuce, cucumber, dates or banana.
Butter and milk from allowance.

*Allowance for day:
425 ml. (¾ pint) of milk.
37 g. (1¼ oz.) butter or margarine.

Supper

1 thin slice of bread or 2 biscuits.
Jam, jelly or honey.
Fruit (fresh, stewed or tinned).
Butter and milk from allowance.
Tea or coffee with milk from allowance and sugar.

For patients with acute glomerulonephritis some restriction of fluid may be necessary. Only one cup of tea should be allowed on each occasion. Salt should not be used in cooking nor should table salt be allowed.

Patients with chronic nephritis require no restriction of the fluid or salt intake and an increased intake may be needed in some cases.

Although the importance of the renal factor in the causation of the oedema in acute glomerulone-phritis is clear, oedema due to congestive heart failure sometimes also develops. The cause of the heart failure is often obscure but hypertension and myocardial damage due to uraemia itself seem to be the most likely causes. In the great majority of patients, rest in bed and restriction of salt and fluid is effective. In more severe cases of heart failure, dyspnoea, cyanosis, pulmonary oedema and engorgement of liver and neck veins may occur. This emergency calls for the administration of digoxin, 0·5 mg. to 1 mg. intravenously, followed by 0·25 mg. digoxin by mouth six-hourly according to the response obtained. If the patient is distressed, 5 mg. of heroin should be given subcutaneously and oxygen therapy begun. Occasionally peritoneal or haemodialysis may be useful in the control of severe pulmonary oedema (p. 281).

Acute glomerulonephritis with prolonged oliguria. Anuria or prolonged severe oliguria is fortunately an unusual development in the course of acute glomerulonephritis. Its occurrence, however, is unpredictable and it may develop in patients who do not appear initially to suffer from a severe attack of the disease. Renal failure is progressive and uraemia becomes severe; hyperkalaemia and acidosis are the two best known chemical abnormalities in the blood which can prove fatal. Pathologically, glomerular destruction is progressive and usually irreversible. Treatment of this condition is similar to that of any form of acute, severe renal failure (p. 277).

Immunosuppressive therapy and progressive renal failure. There is no evidence from controlled trials that corticosteroid or other immunosuppressive drugs alter the natural history of the disease or reduce the number of cases in whom progressive deterioration in renal function occurs.

Anticoagulant therapy. There is evidence to suggest that intravascular coagulation within the glomerular capillaries may contribute to the development of progressive renal failure. The use of heparin is at present under trial.

MINIMAL LESION AND MEMBRANOUS GLOMERULONEPHRITIS

The outstanding clinical characteristics of these forms of glomerulonephritis are massive proteinuria, hypoalbuminaemia and generalized oedema. Together these features constitute the nephrotic syndrome, a condition which has long been recognized and which is of multiple aetiology. In children the nephrotic syndrome is almost invariably due to primary renal disease which affects the capillary walls of the glomeruli as a result of which their permeability is increased and proteinuria occurs. Originally, because light microscopic examination of renal tissue revealed minimal glomerular abnormalities, this disease was thought to be tubular in origin and was called lipoid nephrosis. Electron microscopic studies have now revealed that the most constant abnormality involves the epithelial cells of the glomerular capillary wall. The delicate architecture of these cells which send fine cytoplasmic processes toward the basement membrane of the capillary is constantly deranged. This pathological appearance is known as minimal lesion glomerulonephritis. In adults minimal lesion glomerulonephritis is also capable of giving rise to the nephrotic syndrome, but in the older age-group the basement membrane of the capillary wall is often thickened and tortuous when the term membranous glomerulonephritis is applied. Until recently these two forms of glomerulonephritis were thought to represent different stages of the same disease. Evidence is accumulating to indicate that this is not so; they are probably two discrete diseases which may give rise to identical clinical features.

Minimal lesion and membranous glomerulonephritis are chronic diseases which run a course of months or years and are usually insidious in onset. The patient generally seeks medical help because of oedema which may become generalized and severe. Even without treatment unaccountable variations in the intensity of the diseases produce fluctuations in the degree of proteinuria and oedema so that the condition may appear to subside and the patient becomes free of oedema for a short time. Proteinuria, however, usually persists though it may cause no clinical distress.

Diet. The primary cause of the oedema in minimal lesion and membranous glomerulonephritis is hypoproteinaemia due to excessive loss of protein in the urine. This results in cellular protein depletion which has a deleterious effect on cellular metabolism and results in migration of water and salt into the intracellular spaces. For this reason patients with the nephrotic syndrome should be given a diet rich in protein and restricted in salt. This regimen should be continued as long as there is no significant reduction in the rate of glomerular filtration or a rise in the concentration of blood urea, and while oedema persists. A suitable diet containing about 120 g. of protein is given below. Foods rich in protein may contain significant amounts of sodium and it is convenient to use a salt-free protein concentrate such as Casilan to supplement the diet. Such a concentrate can be suspended in milk or made up as soup. By use of salt-free bread and unsalted butter or margarine the salt content of the diet may be reduced to less than 2 to 3 mg. of sodium chloride. Salt-free bread is tasteless but is improved by toasting. Salt substitutes which do not contain sodium (Neoselarom) are acceptable to many patients. They contain a significant amount of potassium which may be helpful to the patient who is being treated with diuretics but should not be used in the presence of uraemia. A slight rise in the concentration of blood urea often follows the ingestion of a high protein diet but this occurs in healthy people, and need give no cause for alarm. Provided the concentration does not rise above 60 mg. per 100 ml., the high protein diet can be continued. This regimen should be given indefinitely if proteinuria persists and renal failure does not occur. Very often the serum albumin concentration will rise and this is especially likely to occur if proteinuria diminishes or subsides completely. Sometimes patients with severe proteinuria suffer from a degree of uraemia when first seen. Such individuals may also be hypertensive. These findings are not an absolute bar to a diet rich in protein but it is safer to start with a 20 to 50 g. protein diet and add 10 to 20 g. increments each month up to the maximum that does not cause a further rise in blood urea concentration. Many patients with membranous glomerulonephritis slowly develop progressive impairment in renal function and ultimately serious uraemia. For them the outlook is much more serious. Their treatment is described on p. 277.

Control of oedema. The oedema in the nephrotic syndrome is seldom if ever relieved by the degree of dietary restriction of salt and the high protein diet referred to above. More rigid restriction of salt is difficult to achieve without making the diet extremely unpalatable, and in any case is unnecessary in the great majority of cases in view of recent advances in diuretic therapy. There are now few patients who cannot be rendered free from oedema by a combination of modest salt restriction and diuretic therapy even when severe proteinuria persists. Diuretics depend upon their action in

DIET FOR MINIMAL LESION OR MEMBRANOUS GLOMERULO-NEPHRITIS WITHOUT NITROGEN RETENTION.

Protein 124 g. Sodium 762 mg. Calories 2,200.

		Prot. g.	Na mg.	Cals.
Daily Ration				
Milk . . .	20 fl. oz.	18	300	340
Unsalted butter or margarine	1 oz.	—	24	220
Sugar	1 oz.	—	—	112
Preserve—jam . .	2 oz.	—	—	160
Breakfast				
Orange juice—5 fl. oz. . .		—	—	50
One egg or white fish steamed, 2 oz.		7	70	70
Bread, 2 oz. salt-free (with butter and preserve from ration) .		5	60	140
Tea, 7 fl. oz. (with milk and sugar from ration)		—	—	—
11 a.m.				
Milk, 7 fl. oz. (from ration) with Casilan ½ oz.		13	20	52
Dinner				
Meat, 4 oz.		28	84	280
Potato, 4 oz. . . .		2	4	84
Milk pudding, ½ oz. rice or semolina (made with milk from ration (preserve added) and 1 desertspoonful Casilan)		5	10	35
Fruit, 7 oz.				78
Tea				
Fish, 4 oz., herring fried in breadcrumbs		25	70	260
Bread, 2 oz. (with butter and preserve from ration) . .		5	60	140
Tea, 7 fl. oz. (with milk and sugar from ration) . . .				—
Supper				
Bread or toast, 2 oz. (with butter and preserve from ration) . .			60	140
Milk, 7 fl. oz. (from ration) with Casilan ½ oz. . . .		13		52
		124	762	2,213

reducing sodium reabsorption at various sites throughout the nephron. Their efficacy, therefore, depends upon an adequate level of glomerular filtration which delivers sodium to the tubules and upon a variety of factors which individually influence the sensitivity to the different compounds employed.

Most patients with oedema due to the nephrotic syndrome respond to one or other of the oral diuretics of the thiazide group, to frusemide or to ethacrynic acid. Chlorothiazide (1 g.), hydrochlorothiazide (100 mg.), hydroflumethiazide (100 mg.) and bendrofluazide (10 mg.) are equally potent in their appropriate dosage but tend to increase the potassium loss in the urine and this may lead to serious potassium depletion because of their depressant effect on hydrogen ion secretion. Treatment should begin with a dose given twice daily for three or four days per week and should be supplemented by potassium salts (p. 257). Anorexia, nausea and skin rashes are uncommon complications of the treatment and, if they occur, another type of diuretic should be given. Since insensitivity to thiazide drugs may occur in metabolic acidosis, they should not be given in these circumstances. Chlorthalidone is a diuretic related to the thiazide group and may be given in a dose of 200 mg. per day for two or three days in the week. The fact that it produces a diuresis of longer duration than the other drugs may be an advantage in some circumstances. Frusemide (40 mg. twice daily) or ethacrynic acid (50 mg. twice daily) given three times per week is also effective and is especially rapid in its action. For this reason they are valuable in severe oedema where quick relief is indicated. Potassium supplements are also necessary.

Mersalyl (2 ml.) by intramuscular injection is more potent than any of the more recently introduced oral diuretics. Nevertheless, it should not be used as a first choice as it needs to be given by injection. It may be reserved for occasions when other diuretics have failed or have proved inadequate. It should not be used for longer than four weeks and rarely if ever given more than three times weekly. If there is no diuretic response to an initial dose, sensitivity may be increased by giving ammonium chloride in a dose of 2 g. a few hours before the injection. If mersalyl has been given for some time without ammonium chloride, insensitivity often arises because of the development of alkalosis. Ammonium chloride should then be given in doses of 2 g. four times a day for one to two days before giving the diuretic. A similar potentiating effect can often be achieved by giving an intravenous injection of aminophylline (500 mg.) two hours before the injection of mersalyl. If sensitivity is not established by this means and there is no diuretic response, the drug should be discontinued. Persistence in the use of mersalyl in the absence of satisfactory diuresis may cause serious intoxication and renal damage.

Though the majority of patients can be rendered free of oedema by the use of these drugs combined with modest degrees of salt restriction, very intractable cases are occasionally encountered which prove resistant to all of these measures. Such patients generally suffer from severe proteinuria and have a marked reduction in serum albumin. This abnormality reduces plasma volume and filtration rate and causes an increase in the secretion of aldosterone. Attempts may be made to increase the plasma volume by the use of reconstituted dried plasma used at three or four times its normal strength. The high content of sodium chloride which this preparation contains, however, is a disadvantage and concentrated salt-free plasma albumin dissolved in sterile water is better in this respect. Unfortunately, it is difficult to obtain as only a limited amount is available. Twenty-five grammes may be given intravenously in a concentration of 10 to 20 per cent. and should be repeated as required. Dextran is a synthetic polysaccharide of high molecular weight which may be used as an osmotic substitute for albumin. It is also given by intravenous infusion, 500 ml. being administered over a period of four hours. Two infusions of 500 ml. each are sufficient in one day and may be combined with diuretic therapy. If diuresis occurs it is usually spectacular and is associated with a fall in the haemoglobin level as fluid moves into the blood stream. In the elderly these infusions should be used cautiously as left ventricular failure may occur. Dextran unfortunately gives rise to reactions in some patients: these include fever, nausea, urticaria and dyspnoea. If these occur, the infusion should be discontinued immediately.

Should the oedema prove intractable despite all these measures, the condition of the patient must be carefully reviewed: the adequacy of salt restriction, correction of potassium depletion, bed rest and the effective treatment of intercurrent infection should be assessed. If no satisfactory explanation is found to account for the intractability of the oedema, spironolactone (Aldactone A) should be given in a dose of 100 mg. per day combined with an oral diuretic. Spironolactone has little diuretic power itself. It antagonizes the action of aldosterone in the distal segments of the nephron and permits a full effect of the diuretics which have their main site of action proximal to this site. It requires to be given for several days before it is fully effective. Spironolactone is an expensive drug and the indications for its use in nephrotic oedema are few.

Removal of fluid by aspiration from the pleural or peritoneal cavities is rarely needed nowadays but is indicated if the oedema is extreme enough to embarrass the patient's ventilation. Very rarely long-standing oedema appears to become located in the subcutaneous tissue of the limbs and may need to be removed by means of Southey's tubes. The fluid is drained into the lower limbs by the use of a cardiac bed before the tubes are inserted. The possible drawback to this method is mentioned on p. 91.

Immunosuppressive drugs. The use of corticosteroids in membranous glomerulonephritis was first suggested because of the possibility that this disease is due to an antigen–antibody reaction at the basement membrane of the glomerular capillary. There is no evidence that these agents or other immunosuppressive drugs are of value in this respect.

However, the majority of cases of minimal lesion glomerulonephritis respond dramatically to corticosteroid therapy. This category can only be defined by histological examination of tissue obtained by renal biopsy. Prednisone should be given in a dose of 60 to 80 mg. per day for three weeks, then followed by 20 mg. per day for periods up to six months. In this group of patients a prompt or slightly delayed response is commonly seen and proteinuria usually disappears altogether. Withdrawal of corticosteroid treatment is occasionally associated with relapse and a further course of treatment should be given. Recurrence of the disorder after withdrawal of corticosteroids for a second time occurs occasionally and such patients are often referred to as 'steroid dependent' cases. Because of the adverse effects of prolonged corticosteroid therapy, such patients are best treated with cyclophosphamide 2 to 5 mg./kg. for 2 to 4 months. In the great majority of patients this results in permanent cure. This treatment should be carefully monitored by weekly counts of white cells and platelets.

Since diuretic therapy may occasionally improve renal function and reduce proteinuria as the oedema is relieved, it is best to delay treatment with prednisone for up to two weeks until diuresis occurs. Any water and salt retention which may then follow treatment with large doses of prednisone is less troublesome than it would otherwise be. Potassium supplements should be given during the course of corticosteroid treatment. If mooning of the face or other adverse effects appear, they usually subside when the dose is reduced. Corticosteroids may be used in active tuberculosis provided this is being adequately treated but should not be given in the presence of active ulceration of the stomach or duodenum, psychosis or diabetes mellitus. Antibiotics should not be given prophylactically.

Other Diseases which Predominantly affect the Glomeruli

Involvement of the kidneys and the production of the nephrotic syndrome is an important feature of many general diseases and frequently modifies treatment. These include diabetic nephropathy, lupus erythematosus, polyarteritis, scleroderma, amyloid infiltration and multiple myeloma. In addition, the syndrome may be due to intoxication with mercury, gold or tridione, sensitivity to pollen or dust, or may result from mechanical restriction to renal venous outflow as in renal venous thrombosis, constrictive pericarditis and congestive heart failure. Many of these conditions may be relieved by symptomatic remedies which include in particular the use of diuretics and appropriate adjustments to the diet. Some of them, however, are amenable to specific therapy including the use of corticosteroids and it is important that an exact diagnosis be made before treatment begins. Precise definition of the cause of the syndrome may be obvious from the presence of other features of an underlying disease, but renal biopsy or renal venography may be necessary and the former is particularly valuable in determining the cause of proteinuria of unknown origin.

Diabetic glomerulosclerosis. Diabetic nephropathy may occur at any stage in the course of diabetes mellitus but it tends to give rise to serious symptoms in cases of long duration. Proteinuria may be slight, but when it becomes severe the nephrotic syndrome develops. Although there is no proof that meticulous care of diabetes prevents or postpones the onset of diabetic glomerulo-

nephritis, many physicians consider this to be the case. Urinary infections are also common and require treatment (p. 281). Prednisone should not be used in the treatment of the nephrotic syndrome arising as a complication of diabetes and the principles of therapy are as described for membranous glomerulonephritis. By the time proteinuria is severe and oedema has developed, some degree of renal failure is usual; dietary protein should rarely be higher than 60 g. and may need to be reduced to a lower level.

Renal amyloidosis. The kidneys are involved in about 70 per cent. of patients suffering from amyloid disease. Formerly a common complication of chronic infections, it now occurs much more commonly in association with rheumatoid arthritis, reticuloses or myelomatosis. Proteinuria is ininvariable but the diagnosis can only be made with certainty by renal biopsy. Correct diagnosis is of importance in several respects from the point of view of treatment. Corticosteroids are contraindicated in amyloidosis as they may cause an exacerbation of the disorder. Since renal amyloidosis is a progressive condition which may cause death from irreversible renal failure, the eradication of any causative disease provides the only hope for survival and may determine a less conservative approach to such conditions as chronic pulmonary suppuration or osteomyelitis in a limb. Secondary renal vein thrombosis is liable to occur in renal amyloidosis and the sudden development of acute renal failure in a patient known to suffer from amyloidosis is an indication for anticoagulant therapy.

Henoch–Schönlein purpura. The kidneys are involved in about 50 per cent. of patients with this syndrome. The glomeruli show a focal or generalized proliferative glomerulitis. While treatment with corticosteroids is often useful in relieving the other manifestations of Henoch–Schönlein purpura they seldom affect the renal complications.

The nephropathy of lupus erythematosus. Renal involvement is the cause of death in the majority of patients suffering from disseminated lupus erythematosus though paradoxically the kidneys escape in some individuals with extensive disease. Treatment is described on p. 584. Prednisolone should be given initially in high dosage, e.g. 100 mg. per day or more in some cases.

Polyarteritis. The kidneys are involved alone or in combination with other organs in over 80 per cent. of cases. Glomerular capillaries and arterioles are the seat of a diffuse inflammatory reaction. Clinically the condition is very variable and the patient may present with acute renal failure, massive proteinuria with oedema or a disease resembling acute glomerulonephritis. Renal biopsy is necessary to make a precise diagnosis. While the natural history is one of remission and relapse, corticosteroids very often have a remarkably beneficial effect. Prednisone should be given daily in doses of 40 to 60 mg. for three weeks. The dose may then be reduced to the minimum required to obtain continued suppression of the activity of the disease process.

Bacterial endocarditis. Although the renal lesion in bacterial endocarditis has been called embolic there are doubts as to whether this is a correct description of the pathogenesis. In a minority of patients the diagnosis may be suspected only after finding proteinuria and red blood cells in the urine, and renal failure may occur. Early recognition of the underlying course of the disease with specific antibiotic treatment is the only way of preventing the renal complications (p. 108).

Orthostatic proteinuria. This is a condition in which proteinuria occurs in the upright posture and disappears when the patient adopts the recumbent position. Orthostatic proteinuria is commonly found in applicants for life assurance or in candidates for entry into the Armed Forces. The relationship to posture should be clearly established in each case. If there is no history of glomerulonephritis or hypertension, if renal function is normal and the urine does not contain excessive numbers of red blood cells, a diagnosis of orthostatic proteinuria should be made. It is important to establish this diagnosis as most insurance companies are willing to accept the applicant at normal rates. There is evidence, however, that some individuals with orthostatic proteinuria later develop hypertension and renal failure. Others may represent early or abortive forms of glomerulonephritis. At the present time, however, it is better to regard the condition as benign while reserving final judgment on the renal significance of the abnormality pending more information.

ACUTE RENAL FAILURE

An acute decrease in renal function may arise in many clinical circumstances and this has been mainly responsible for the delay in recognizing the essential unity of the clinical syndrome of acute renal failure. This unity arises from the fact that the syndrome itself is the result of an acute breakdown in the renal contribution to body metabolism, the consequences of which are independent of the cause. The features of acute renal failure are so often clouded by the clinical complexities of the underlying cause that they may be readily overlooked. The excretion of urea and other end products of protein metabolism does not keep pace with their rate of production and they accumulate in the body. The factors responsible for the maintenance of water and salt balance no longer operate and, in the event of unrestricted intake, oedema and hyperkalaemia are inevitable. The renal contibution to acid balance is deficient and metabolic acidosis develops. These metabolic abnormalities, which always accompany acute renal failure, are attended by the clinical features of uraemia and may result in death.

CAUSES OF ACUTE RENAL FAILURE

In the management of patients with acute renal failure the diagnosis of the underlying cause is essential. It is convenient to classify these causes into three categories: (1) pre-renal; (2) renal; and (3) post-renal.

Pre-renal causes. These include all clinical conditions which reduce the renal circulation. The renal share of the cardiac output is normally about 20 per cent. If cardiac output falls, the renal blood flow is disproportionately reduced. As a result filtration rate, urine flow and the rate of elimination of solute are impaired. While systemic hypotension is often present, renal ischaemia may occur in its absence. Regional vasoconstriction is a means by which the blood pressure is maintained in the face of oligaemia and the success of this mechanism deprives the kidneys of a large part of their blood supply. Among the conditions commonly encountered are excessive fluid loss from vomiting, diarrhoea or fistulous drainage, haemorrhage from all causes including in particular uteroplacental haemorrhage, burns and all conditions which lead to shock. General anaesthetics and surgical operations reduce renal blood flow and may precipitate renal failure in those whose blood volume and haemodynamic state is precariously balanced. Acute renal failure often follows crushing injuries to limbs.

Serious infection bears a dual relationship to it. Infection always complicates the treatment of this condition but infection itself may initiate the renal damage. This is particularly liable to occur in major bronchopulmonary infection, in peritonitis and in septicaemia. The offending organisms are usually S*taph. aureus* and *Esch. coli*. It is possible that the endotoxin of some strains of coliform organisms reduces renal blood flow by inducing renal arterial vasoconstriction. Transfusion with incompatible blood is often held to be responsible for acute renal failure but its rôle as a primary cause is doubtful. The haemolysis which follows, however, aggravates the clinical condition by the liberation of potassium from the haemolysed cells and the formation of pigment casts within the renal tubules may contribute to the pathogenesis of the oliguria. Acute severe haemolysis occurring in the course of haemolytic anaemia or induced by drugs such as sulphonamides may cause acute renal failure.

In all these disorders acute renal failure may be a minor complication which lasts only a few days or may constitute a major disaster which threatens and takes life. The need for prompt diagnosis and effective treatment of the underlying disease process is paramount. Where blood loss has occurred transfusion should be prompt and adequate (p. 628), and vasoconstrictor drugs are best avoided. Restoration of salt and water loss should be accurate both in respect of the nature of the fluid given and its amount (p. 253). Osmotic diuretics such as mannitol are unproven in value and are best avoided. Major infection should be treated where possible by specific and preferably bactericidal antibiotics (p. 5). In many patients vigorous, early treatment will prevent the occurrence of significant degrees of acute renal failure. If in spite of such curative measures, oliguria persists and the concentration of blood urea continues to rise, other measures designed to ameliorate the consequences of renal failure itself then require to be adopted (*vide infra*).

Renal causes. These are also numerous and include primary renal diseases, e.g. acute glomerulonephritis, acute pyelonephritis, acute lupus erythematosus, the haemolytic uraemic syndrome, and toxic agents which damage the renal parenchyma. The most important of the latter are carbon tetrachloride, ethylene glycol, mercuric bichloride and sodium chlorate. Hypersensitivity of sulphonamides may also cause acute renal failure. Once failure has developed as result of the action of nephrotoxins little can be offered in the way of antidotes. Provided the patient can be protected from the lethal consequences, however, the renal

tissue shows an astonishing power of regeneration. One specific measure which should be adopted is the use of dimercaprol, a chelating agent in heavy metal intoxication (pp. 559-564). The acute renal failure which develops in the course of primary renal disease also varies greatly in the degree of severity. Apart from the treatment of the primary condition the measures necessary for the amelioration of the renal failure are independent of the cause and are discussed below.

Post-renal causes. These arise from obstruction in the urinary tract. While many conditions which give rise to post-renal obstruction are insidious in onset and lead to chronic renal insufficiency, some of them are capable of causing sudden anuria and of precipitation acute renal failure. Prompt diagnosis of the cause of the obstruction is essential since surgical relief may be curative. These include impaction of calculi in the ureters, carcinomatous invasion of the ureters, periureteric fibrosis, severe urinary tract infection with blockage of the ureters due to inspissated pus, the precipitation of crystals of sulphonamide or uric acid within the renal pelvis and ureters, accidental ligation of the ureter in the course of pelvic operations and prostatic hypertrophy or malignancy.

The diagnosis may be suggested by a history of the occurrence of previous urinary symptoms such as pain in the loin, haematuria, renal colic or difficulty in micturition. It is important to determine whether or not the obstruction is distal to the bladder, and examination should be carried out to determine whether the bladder is distended and if the prostate is enlarged. In this event temporary relief may be obtained by passing a catheter into the bladder, but this should be done under adequate conditions of sterility. If the bladder is not palpable and if the prostate is not found to be enlarged it is usually necessary to pass a cystoscope and investigate the patency of the lower urinary tract by inserting ureteral catheters. A plain radiograph of the abdomen should be taken first to demonstrate the presence of radio-opaque calculi, soft tissue masses and the approximate size of the kidneys. If both kidneys are seen to be of normal size and the history is suggestive of obstructive uropathy, the ureter on the right side is catheterized and contrast media inserted. If no urine is obtained, obstruction can be excluded as a cause of the anuria. If the renal shadow cannot be visualized the catheter should be left in place for a day or two where it may act as a splint to allow urine flow in the event of inflammatory oedema of the ureter being present. If after a few days this does not occur, and obstruction is excluded as a cause of the renal failure and the diagnosis still remains in doubt, the radiograph with contrast media in the right renal pelvis is then available in the likely event of the need to perform a renal biopsy in order to establish the diagnosis.

Cystoscopy and ureteral instrumentation should not be undertaken without careful thought in acute renal failure because of the hazards of infection. On the other hand, the consequences of failing to remove obstruction are so fraught with danger to life that this procedure should be adopted in all patients in whom the history of obstructive uropathy is suggestive or in whom the diagnosis of the cause of the acute renal failure is in doubt.

PRINCIPLES OF MANAGEMENT

Once the physician has assured himself that all steps have been taken to relieve the primary disorder, attempts to force a diuresis by the use of intravenous fluids or diuretics should be avoided. Although the precise intrarenal mechanisms responsible for the prolonged oliguric phase in prerenal acute renal failure are unknown there is no remedy which is known to shorten its duration. The view that 'the body is not analogous to a tank into which water can be forced until it finally bursts through the kidneys' appears obvious, yet it was not generally accepted until comparatively recently. The former practice of giving large amounts of intravenous fluids to patients who are not depleted of water or salt, and the use of osmotic diuretics in those who are, is fraught with danger and merely aggravates the electrolyte disturbances already present. Decapsulation and spinal anaesthesia are also hazardous procedures which should not be used.

In the absence of specific measures which will regenerate tubular epithelium, encourage the reconstruction of damaged nephrons or reverse the process which sustains the suppression of renal function, modern treatment consists in adopting all measures necessary to protect the patient from the potentially lethal consequences of uraemia. In those patients in whom the cause of the renal failure is associated with renal ischaemia, ultimate recovery of renal function may occur in most instances provided the patient can be kept alive in the meantime. The single exception to this rule

is the occurrence of bilateral cortical necrosis, though even here the prospect of some recovery of renal function cannot entirely be excluded. In the case of acute renal failure due to parenchymal renal disease and to obstructive uropathy the recovery of renal function is dependent upon the response to specific treatment and to the extent to which irreversible structural damage to renal tissue has occurred. When severe renal failure arises in the course of acute glomerulonephritis and oliguria persists for several weeks, ultimate recovery of function is unlikely. On the other hand, even severe necrosis due to intoxication with mercury or sodium chlorate is compatible with complete recovery of renal function.

The success of this expectant approach largely depends upon meticulous attention to detail in the metabolic care of the patient, in the extent to which facilities are available to protect the patient from cross-infection, in the judicious selection of patients for some form of dialysis and in the excellence of nursing care.

General care. In all but the milder forms of acute renal failure the patient is best treated in special units by physicians experienced in this disorder and in a single-bedded room designed to protect the patient from extraneous infection. Accurate and detailed information of fluid intake and the volume of fluid lost from the body must be recorded daily. Daily estimations of the serum concentration of sodium, potassium, urea and bicarbonate should be made. The sputum, urine and blood should be cultured frequently during the course of the uraemia. Septicaemia may occur as a complication of acute renal failure and be responsible for an unexpected deterioration in the patient's condition. If active upper respiratory infection develops, knowledge of the organisms determines antibiotic policy. Radiological examination of the chest should also be undertaken as pulmonary infection may be present in patients who are seriously ill long before the lesions are clinically detectable. Antibiotics should not be given prophylactically. If infection occurs it should be treated, preferably with bactericidal antibiotics. Even those antibiotics which are potentially toxic to the kidneys and which are excreted in the urine, e.g. polymyxin or kanamycin, may be given provided blood levels are determined. Suitable attention to hygiene and care of the skin and of the mouth are important. In many instances bed sores may be prevented by such measures combined with the use of a ripple mattress (Talley Surgical Instrument Company).

Uncomplicated, Mild, Acute Renal Failure

When acute renal failure is uncomplicated by major trauma or tissue damage and when the patient is not seriously infected, the uraemia is relatively mild and the period of oliguria usually lasts from one to two weeks. During this period the rate of rise of the blood urea is about 20 mg. a day and the concentration does not exceed 250 mg. per 100 ml. of blood. Thereafter as renal function improves, the patient enters the diuretic phase and the volume of urine passed daily often rises to about three and, on occasions, to four or five litres and the blood urea falls slowly to normal. Under such circumstances the regulation of water and salt intake combined with a degree of dietary restriction is usually all that is required.

Sodium and water balance. In the early stage of acute renal failure, the urine is usually greatly reduced in volume. Water balance can be maintained only by restricting fluid intake to a volume which is equal to that lost from the skin, lungs and through the kidneys. Since it is usually impossible to meet their calorie requirements, these patients tend to oxidize their body fat and so provide themselves endogenously with some water of oxidation, so that 400 ml. per 24 hours is sufficient in the afebrile adult to compensate for insensible loss. Water requirements increase in the presence of fever and up to one litre a day may then be needed. A volume of water equal to the daily volume of urine should then be added to this amount for overall water balance to be attained. The period of oliguria lasts on average for between one to two weeks although it may be much more protracted in severe cases. As renal function improves the daily excretion of urine gradually rises and the intake of fluid should be increased.

During the phase of severe oliguria sodium loss in the urine is minimal and sodium balance is usually maintained without giving sodium chloride. Occasionally hyponatraemia develops. This may be due to slight overloading with water or to the gradual development of sodium depletion from the accumulated small daily losses of sodium, particularly if sweating is prominent. The accumulated loss may be made good by the administration approximately once a week of 500 ml. of isotonic sodium bicarbonate by intravenous infusion. Unless excessive sodium loss has occurred as the result of diarrhoea or vomiting it is rarely necessary to give sodium more frequently than this. As the urine volume increases, the urinary loss of sodium also rises and this should be met by increasing the intake. Ideally, accurate estimates of losses should be made by chemical analysis of urine and appropriate additions made to the intake. If this is impossible, the average need for sodium is met by giving 50 mEq. for every litre of urine passed. Some of this may be given by mouth but it is usually necessary to continue to give some intravenously in the form of isotonic saline.

In most patients fluid can be given by mouth from the beginning of the disease. If this is impossible, the fluid should be given in the form of 10 per cent. fructose through a catheter inserted into a large peripheral vein. The former practice of inserting an indwelling catheter into the inferior vena cava and of infusing 50 per cent. dextrose has been abandoned because of the danger of infected thrombo-embolism. A multivitamin preparation should be added to oral fluids (Multivite) or to fluids given by infusion (Parentrovite).

During the oliguric phase of acute renal failure potassium balance is also maintained without the need to give potassium by mouth or by intravenous infusion. Indeed in most patients the concentration of potassium in the blood tends to rise gradually as potassium is slowly liberated from the body cells. The concentration of potassium rarely rises above 7·5 mEq./l. in this type of patient. If it should reach 6 mEq./l., however, a sulphonic cation exchange resin should be given (p. 258). As kidney function improves, the serum level begins to fall towards normal as potassium is lost in the urine. In many patients in the diuretic phase urinary loss of potassium may become excessive, and if no potassium is given, hypokalaemia may develop. It is then necessary to give potassium either by mouth or intravenously depending on the serum concentration. As in the case of sodium balance, an estimate of potassium loss in the urine should ideally be made by chemical analysis. If the serum level falls below 3·5 mEq./l., it is commonly necessary to give potassium chloride orally or intravenously in a dose of 6 to 10 g. daily. Occasionally larger amounts are needed (p. 258).

DIET FOR INITIAL TREATMENT OF A MILD CASE OF ACUTE RENAL FAILURE.

Protein 10 g.   Fluid 650 ml.   Na 370 mg.   K 400 to 500 mg. Calories 1,100.

Breakfast
½ oz. crustless white bread toasted.
Butter.
Marmalade or honey.
1 cup of tea with sugar.
1 oz. milk.

Dinner
3 oz. tinned mandarin, pear or pineapple, drained of juice;
or 3 oz. appled stewed with sugar and drained of juice.
1½ oz. ice cream.

Tea
2 plain biscuits, such as Rich Tea or Water;
or ½ oz. crustless white bread.
Butter.
Jam or honey.
1 cup of tea with sugar.
1 oz. milk.

Supper
Jelly* *or* cream pudding** with fruit as at dinner.
½ oz. crustless bread *or* 2 plain biscuits.
Butter.
Jam or honey.
1 cup of tea with sugar.
1 oz. milk.

   *Jelly
   ¾ oz. Chivers or other packet jelly.
   4 oz. water.

   **Cream Pudding
   2 oz. double cream.
   3 oz. water.
   1 heaped teaspoonful custard powder or other cereal.
   Sugar.

To reduce the fluid content to 500 ml.
   Omit cup of tea at supper.
   Omit cup of milk at supper.
   Add 1 oz. cream to take with jelly or fruit.

The provision of calories and protein. In patients with mild acute renal failure the concentration of blood urea generally rises by about 20 mg. per cent. per day. This rate of increase occurs in the absence of protein intake and is due to the metabolism of endogenous protein. If protein is given the blood urea rises. It is for this reason that during the oliguric phase some authorities withdraw protein completely from the diet and provide calories exclusively in the form of carbohydrate given orally or intravenously. Nevertheless, a diet containing 10 g. of protein does not influence the uraemia materially and is greatly welcomed by many patients. The calories may be supplemented by liquid glucose (Hycal), which provides about 500 cal. in less than 200 ml. of fluid and is available in several flavours. The patient may also suck barley sugar or mint sweets. When the blood urea concentration begins to fall and the daily excretion of urine increases, a diet containing 20 g. of protein a day (p. 267) may be given. As recovery continues the protein content may be increased to about 40 g. a day within a few days. As sodium and potassium loss may now become considerable salt may be added liberally to the diet and foods which are rich in potassium should be taken. These include fruit juices, jam and meat essences. Suitable diets giving 20 and 45 g. of protein are given on pp. 267-268. With further improvement in renal function a gradual return to a normal diet is made.

Complicated or Severe Acute Renal Failure

In patients in whom acute renal failure is associated with severe infection or major trauma, the catabolism of body protein is greatly increased. During the oliguric phase this is reflected in a daily increase in the concentration of blood urea of about 50 to 80 mg. per 100 ml. per day. Acidosis which occurs slowly in the mild cases also develops more rapidly and in addition serious potassium intoxication is more likely. The latter is especially liable to occur if the acute renal failure has been attended by haemolysis, the giving of incompatible blood or the occurrence of respiratory acidosis from ventilatory inadequacy. In these circumstances conservative measures themselves are not sufficient to control the chemical composition of the body fluids and require to be supplemented by the use of some form of dialysis and by other measures.

This may be achieved either by extracorporeal dialysis using an artificial kidney or by peritoneal dialysis. Except for small children extracorporeal haemodialysis (i.e. the artificial kidney) is most favoured. Any one of the following findings constitutes an indication for its use: (1) Deterioration in the clinical condition and the development of dullness, mental confusion, troublesome vomiting and hiccough. Serious symptoms and signs of uraemia such as gastro-intestinal bleeding, twitching, hypotension and convulsions indicate that the optimal time for dialysis is past. (2) A serum potassium concentration of 7·5 mEq./*l*. or more, a serum bicarbonate concentration of 15 mEq./*l*. or less, and a blood urea concentration rising to above 250 mg. per 100 ml. In the presence of serious infection or severe tissue injury, dialysis is invariably needed in the treatment of acute renal failure. It should be started before the clinical or chemical criteria mentioned above have developed and repeated at intervals of 1 to 2 days for as long as necessary.

DIET FOR SEVERE ACUTE RENAL FAILURE.

Protein 30 g. Fluids 600 ml. Sodium 523 mg. Potassium 890 mg. Calories 900 to 1,100.

Daily Ration	Prot. g.	Na mg.	K mg.	Fluid ml.	Cal.
1½ eggs . . .	9	96·5	97·5		115
1 oz. bread . .	2·4	148	33		72
2 rich tea biscuits .	1·4	46	32		82
¾ pt. milk . . .	14·8	213	690	450	285
1 oz. cream . .	0·4	7·6	22	30	131
¼ oz. cereal . .	0·5	0·5	8		25
¾ oz. packet jelly+4 oz. water . . .	1·5	5·4	5·2	120	55
¾ oz. sugar . .					84
¼ oz. unsalted butter .		6			56
	30	523	888	600	905

Depending upon the general condition of the patient, the above foods may be given according to either one of the two diets given below:

I.

Breakfast

Saps (6 oz. milk, 1 oz. crustless bread and sugar).

Lunch

Jelly with cream and 2 buttered rich tea biscuits.

Tea

Switched eggs (1 egg, 4 oz. milk and sugar).

Supper

Ground rice or other cereal pudding (5 oz. milk, ¼ oz. cereal, ½ egg and sugar).

OR

II.

Breakfast

With addition of ½ oz. unsalted butter and ½ oz. marmalade which adds 150 calories.
½ oz. crustless bread toasted.
Unsalted butter.
1 teaspoon marmalade or honey.
4 oz. milk.

Lunch

Scrambled egg (1 egg with 1 oz. milk, ¼ oz. unsalted butter).
½ oz. crustless bread toasted.
Unsalted butter.
Milk jelly with cream (¾ oz. packet jelly with 4 oz. milk).

Tea

2 buttered rich tea biscuits.
1 cup of tea (4 oz.).
Sugar and 1 oz. milk.

Supper

Ground rice or other cereal pudding (5 oz. milk, ¼ oz. cereal, ½ egg and sugar).

No salt to be used in cooking and none to be added from the tray.

The calorie intake may be supplemented by the use of liquid glucose given orally, and by parenteral amino acids or lipids.

In considering the likelihood for the need for dialysis, it is important that patients be transferred to an artificial kidney unit several days before the above indications are reached if the best results are to be obtained. Such patients may require several dialyses before diuresis occurs and renal function improves. Between dialyses measures designed to maintain water and salt balance as already described do not require to be so rigid as any deviation from ideal balance is readily corrected during the next dialysis. The need for calories and protein in seriously infected or wounded individuals is usually urgent. This is especially the case in those whose illness is protracted and in whom life is preserved by repeated dialyses. If this is not done, patients who survive more than two weeks show the effects of protein deprivation and the concentration of plasma proteins falls. For these reasons it is desirable to give protein in the diet and to give amino acids and lipid parenterally. Amino acids can be given in the form of an aminosol fructose ethanol mixture (Paines & Byrne, Ltd.). Five hundred ml. of this solution contains 900 calories, 16 g. protein hydrolysate and 54 mEq. sodium. Intralipid, a fat emulsion from soyabean oil, provides up to 2,000 calories/litre. If in addition food can be taken by mouth, it is frequently possible to provide 2,000 to 3,000 calories daily with up to 60 g. protein per day over an extended period of recovery from this serious illness.

At the present time there is no evidence that anabolic steroids such as norethandrolone or nandrolone are of value in the treatment of patients with acute renal failure.

While hyperkalaemia remains an important indication for extracorporeal dialysis, it is sometimes possible to reduce the serum level of potassium, at least for a limited period of time, by the use of simpler methods. These may be applied in an emergency and provide time for arrangements to be made for haemodialysis to be carried out. They are described on p. 258. The technique of peritoneal dialysis is described on p. 643.

CHRONIC RENAL FAILURE

Chronic renal failure with uraemia is due to extensive disease of both kidneys and the renal impairment arises from irreversible destruction of nephrons. Chronic renal failure may result from any one of many diseases. These include conditions which primarily affect the renal parenchyma (e.g. chronic glomerulonephritis), the renal vessels (e.g. the accelerated phase of hypertension, polyarteritis nodosa, degenerative disease), metabolic disorders (e.g. diabetes mellitus, hypercalcaemia) and congenital anomalies and obstructive lesions.

Apart from features of the primary disorder causing chronic renal failure, the clinical picture is non-specific. A series of discrete functional disorders, however, can be recognized which can be affected by treatment.

Nitrogen retention. The blood urea concentration is an index of the severity of uraemia. The patient with mild renal failure with a blood urea concentration of 100 mg. per 100 ml. or less can lead a normal life in reasonably good health and take a normal diet. Restriction in protein intake should be applied if the blood urea rises above 100 mg. per 100 ml. A careful search should first be made for factors which increase urea production, notably infection, and for the existence of a pre- or post-renal disorder. Apart from the presence of such obvious factors as water and salt depletion from vomiting or polyuria, mild degrees of congestive heart failure can contribute to renal failure and lead to more severe uraemia than is attributable to renal damage. A diet of 2,000 calories containing 60 g. of protein is of benefit when the concentration of blood urea persists at about 100 mg. per 100 ml. and may be tolerated for years. A more severe restriction of protein to 30 or 40 g. a day may be necessary if the blood urea rises further. When the clinical features of uraemia develop in spite of these restrictions, some relief may be obtained in selected patients by following dietary principles advocated by Giovanetti in Italy. Low protein diets in general are unplanned in respect of requirements of essential aminoacids and contain non-essential amino acids in the protein in vegetables and bread, etc. If the latter are eliminated from the diet as far as possible and the limited protein allowed is given as first-class protein, some of the more troublesome features of uraemia, notably the gastro-intestinal complaints, are temporarily controlled. An example of such a diet is given below.

Anabolic steroids may produce a temporary restoration of the nitrogen balance, but the effect is so transitory that their use is unjustifiable.

Water, salt and acid-base balance and potassium. Loss of ability to vary the tonicity of urine according to the need to conserve or eliminate water

and urinary solute is characteristic of chronic nephron insufficiency. The factors responsible for

MODIFIED GIOVANETTI DIET FOR SEVERE CHRONIC RENAL FAILURE.

Protein 20 g. (18 g. 1st class). Calories 2,200. Na approx. 1·5 g. K 1·5 to 2 g. Food cooked with salt but none added.

Breakfast
   3 to 4 g. fruit fresh, stewed with sugar, or tinned.
   1 oz. gluten-free bread.
   Marmalade or honey.
   Butter.
   Tea with sugar.
   Cream mixture.*

Mid-morning
   3 oz. fruit juice+glucose, *or* Lucozade, *or* Lemonade.

Dinner
   ¾ oz. lean cooked meat, such as roast beef, lamb, pork or chicken, mince or steak;
   or 1 oz. cooked white fish or tripe.
   2 oz. any vegetable except peas or beans } With added
   2 oz. potatoes. } butter or margarine.
   3 to 4 oz. fruit as at breakfast.
   Pudding made with cereal, cream mixture* and sugar.

Tea
   1 oz. gluten-free bread with butter.
   Jam or honey.
   Tea with sugar.
   Cream mixture.*

Supper
   1 egg *or* ¾ oz. cheese *or* ¾ oz. cooked meat *or* 1 oz. white fish.
   1 oz. gluten-free bread with butter.
   Jam or honey.
   Tea with sugar.
   Cream mixture.*

Bed-time
   As mid-morning.

   **Cream mixture*
   4 oz. double cream plus 8 oz. water mixed.
   Use this in place of milk in tea, with fruit, and for cooking.

Take as much as you can of the following foods
   Sugar, jam, marmalade, honey.
   Barley sugar, fruit boilings, peppermints.
   Butter, margarine and cooking oil.
   Spread butter thickly on bread and add to potato and scrambled egg.
   Fry food in cooking oil.

To reduce potassium to below 1 g.
   Omit all fruit juice.
   Omit all fruit except tinned pineapple, mandarin and loganberry, apple and pear raw or cooked with sugar.

To reduce sodium to below 0·5 g.
   Cook food without salt and remove salt cellar.
   Use unsalted gluten-free bread.
   Use unsalted butter or margarine.
   Avoid salty cheese and tinned or salt meat and fish.
   Avoid Lucozade.

K

this are complex. Because of its influence, however, there is an optimum fluid and solute intake for each patient with uraemia. Excessive water or insufficient salt leads to hyponatraemia while inadequate water reduces urine volume and aggravates uraemia. The relative amounts of water and salt required are influenced by the amount of urinary solutes including, in particular, urea. In patients with chronic renal failure salt intake should not be reduced unless oedema is present. Indeed, in the presence of acidosis sodium bicarbonate in a dose of 2 to 10 g. per day may be needed. Occasionally excessive loss of salt occurs in the urine especially when chronic renal failure is due to pyelonephritis. Persistently low values for serum sodium are usually found; the patient often complains of fainting and may be hypotensive. Supplements of sodium chloride and sodium bicarbonate of as much as 10 to 15 g. per day, given in proportions determined by the bicarbonate concentration in the blood, are indicated. In general patients with uraemia should be encouraged to drink three litres per day or more, the volume being reduced if oedema occurs.

Occasionally patients with chronic renal failure become severely depleted of water and salt and develop marked acidosis. This may arise as a result of inadequate attention to the details of water and salt requirement or to some intercurrent illness or infection. Treatment with intravenous fluids as described on p. 254 is then indicated.

Alterations in the concentration of potassium in the blood in chronic renal failure are uncommon. Hypokalaemia may occur occasionally in pyelonephritis or in the malignant phase of hypertension. The concentration of potassium rises spontaneously when the hypertension is controlled but supplements of potassium to the diet may be needed in pyelonephritis (p. 257). Acute deterioration in renal function in patients with chronic renal failure in the terminal phase of the disease are often attended by high serum potassium levels. The treatment of this is similar to that of acute renal failure and is described on p. 273.

Calcium and phosphorus metabolism and renal osteodystrophy. Patients with renal failure suffer from disturbance in phosphorus and calcium metabolism for reasons that are little understood. This manifests itself in hypocalcaemia which may give rise to tetany and in abnormalities in bone structure which are visible radiologically and give rise to bone pain. The disturbance in bone is a complex mixture of osteomalacia, secondary hyperparathyroidism and osteosclerosis. Tetany may be precipitated by over-enthusiastic correction of acidosis and patients with renal failure are better when mildly acidotic. If bone pain is severe or if deformities of rickets are developing in the young patient, symptomatic and radiological improvement may be achieved by giving vitamin D. The dose of calciferol required is, however, unpredictable. It is best to start treatment with 1 to 2 mg. daily, increasing this within a month to levels of 10 mg. per day. It is necessary to control the dose given and its duration by determination of the serum calcium for it is possible to produce severe hypercalcaemia.

Anaemia. This is common in chronic renal failure; it does not respond to iron, folic acid or cyanocobalamin. Most patients become adjusted to their low level of haemoglobin and transfusion is best avoided if the concentration does not fall below 8 g. per 100 ml. When this occurs it is necessary to give a blood transfusion but its effect is usually transient.

Hypertension, oedema and congestive heart failure. These complications in patients with chronic renal insufficiency are bad prognostic signs. Treatment of hypertension as described on p. 112 is indicated. In the milder degrees of chronic renal failure every attempt should be made to control the blood pressure, for good control prolongs life and may even retard progressive renal damage. Diuretics are often of value in oedema in chronic renal failure, provided they are given in large doses. Currently frusemide in doses of 240 mg./day may control oedema in spite of severe renal failure. Since digoxin is normally eliminated in the urine, heart failure is usually controlled by 0·25 to 0·5 mg. of digoxin given on three days a week. If the oedema is associated with hypoproteinaemia, measures which increase the rate of glomerular filtration should be adopted. Aminophylline suppositories at night are worthy of trial and the intravenous administration of salt-free plasma albumin is sometimes very effective (p. 271).

Other Measures

In the advanced stages of chronic renal failure various other measures may be needed. Convulsions may be due to hypertension, hypocalcaemia or both. Treatment of hypertensive encephalopathy is discussed on p. 117. Convulsions due to hypocalcaemia should be treated with the intravenous administration of calcium gluconate (10 ml.

of a 10 per cent. solution) and thereafter with vitamin D by mouth (p. 364). Nausea and vomiting may become troublesome. These may be relieved by cyclizine, 50 mg. intramuscularly twice a day, or by chlorpromazine, 50 mg. per day be mouth.

Intermittent haemodialysis. With attention to detail and to the above measures a great deal can be done to prolong the life of a patient with chronic renal failure in reasonable comfort. When the creatinine clearance, however, falls to below 4 ml. per minute life becomes more precarious and there is chronic ill-health. Dialysis should be considered in patients who have severe chronic pyelonephritis and in whom a temporary exacerbation has occurred which is likely to be lethal. It is frequently possible by dialysis to tide a patient over the ensuing metabolic crisis until the infection is controlled and some effective renal function returns. Dialysis may also be indicated for patients who present in severe uraemia of unknown origin when time is needed to assess the nature or severity of the underlying disease.

Haemodialysis carried out intermittently two or three times a week can be used to maintain life in patients who are devoid of all renal function. This has been made possible by using an exteriorized arteriovenous fistula fitted to either the arm or the leg or by the anastomosis of a suitable artery and vein in the arm. This allows periodic access to blood vessels so that they may be connected to a suitable dialyser. In the United Kingdom this treatment is available on a limited scale but facilities will increase in the course of the next few years. At the present time, patients who might be considered for this treatment should be young and free from systemic disease. This method of treatment is not contraindicated in those suffering from severe or malignant hypertension which can usually be satisfactorily controlled by it. A considerable degree of rehabilitation is achieved and the majority of patients are able to earn a living or to look after their homes and children.

Renal transplantation. The transplantation of fresh renal tissue to the patient dying of chronic renal failure is an exciting development in medicine and dialysis may be necessary to keep the patient alive for some days or weeks during which the possibility of carrying out this procedure is being considered. It is important to inquire about the existence of an identical twin in all patients dying of chronic renal failure. If the patient has a healthy identical twin with two normally functioning kidneys, his survival depends entirely upon the willingness of the twin to give one of his kidneys and the technical success of the surgical procedure. The use of a living donor, however, raises serious ethical considerations. It appears proper to tell a healthy twin of the plight of the other identical twin and to explain the position, including the hazards involved. On no account should persuasion be used to influence a decision once the facts of the situation have been made clear. The healthy potential donor should then be allowed time to come to his own decision regarding his willingness to co-operate in the procedure. In the absence of an identical twin the position is much more complicated. If no special measures are taken to treat the recipient with agents which blockade the reticulo-endothelial system and suppress the immunological response, renal homografts undergo rapid rejection. This reaction may be modified by X-irradiation or the use of a variety of antimetabolites such as actinomycin, 6-mercaptopurine and its derivatives or by prednisolone or antilymphocytic serum. The prospect of success is further complicated by the degree of tissue incompatibility between donor and recipient which at the moment is difficult to estimate. *A priori* histocompatibility is more likely to be favourable when the donor is a close relative and possesses similar or identical red blood cell antigens. Compatibility with white cell antigens, i.e. HLA antigens, is also important. A close relationship between donor and recipient, especially if it is parent to child, also minimizes the emotional tensions which even the discussion of such a procedure is capable of generating within the family. The possibility of carrying out renal transplantation between unrelated persons and from cadavers is also under study. The complexities of the postoperative clinical care of these patients meanwhile limits the frequency with which this procedure can be undertaken. Nevertheless, at the time of writing it is reasonable to consider its practicability in patients under the age of 45 who are dying of irreversible renal failure and who are free from other major disease or infections, widespread vascular degeneration or severe hypertension.

BACTERIAL INFECTION OF THE KIDNEY AND URINARY TRACT

Bacterial infection of the kidneys and urinary tract is common and is associated with considerable morbidity and significant mortality. Acute urinary infection often appears as a trivial and short-lived complaint but evidence suggests that inadequate eradication of a primary infection in the first few years of life or in young pregnant women may be responsible for chronic pyelonephritis later in life. Chronic pyelonephritis itself is the most common cause of chronic severe renal failure and contributes significantly to the occurrence of renal hypertension. Bacterial infection reaches the kidneys either by ascending the lumen of the ureter or by the blood. The susceptibility of the kidneys to infection depends upon a variety of factors which impede the free flow of urine to the bladder and through the urethra. These include prostatic hypertrophy, disorganization of bladder function because of neurological disease, congenital anomalies of the urinary tract, cystocele and the presence of a calculus in the ureter or bladder. Obstruction to the flow of urine within the renal substance itself may also be a factor and is likely to be important in nephrocalcinosis, developmental abnormalities of the nephron and pre-existing renal disease, e.g. chronic glomerulonephritis. Diabetes also predisposes to the development of urinary tract infection. The highest incidence of infection occurs in young women and in female infants. This may be in part due to the short urethra and to the occurrence of vesico-ureteric reflux of urine during micturition. Such a mechanism may exist from birth and be exacerbated by pregnancy. Instrumentation is well known to lead to urinary infection; this is particularly true of catheterization which, as a diagnostic or therapeutic procedure, should be carried out rarely and then only under strict aseptic conditions. Urine for microscopic examination and culture should be obtained as a midstream specimen in both females and males. A satisfactory specimen can be obtained from the female by using plastic disposable cartons.

The common infecting organism is *Escherichia coli* and this is present alone in most cases, particularly in the first acute attack. Other organisms which may cause urinary infections are the *Staphylococcus aureus*, *Streptococcus faecalis*, *Klebsiella pneumoniae*, and *Proteus vulgaris*, while *Pseudomonas pyocyanea* are less frequent. These latter organisms are generally found in individuals with a history of instrumentation when the infections are frequently multiple.

Acute Pyelonephritis

The disease may start with a rigor, fever and backache. There is frequency of micturition, supra-

pubic discomfort and often a burning pain while urine is being passed and immediately after micturition. The patient may notice the abnormal appearance and smell of the urine. Haematuria is not uncommon, but oedema and hypertension do not occur in acute infections of the urinary tract. Microscopical examination of the urine for the presence of excessive numbers of white cells is essential and a specimen must be obtained for culture. Ideally this should be done within 30 minutes or, if this is not practicable, it should be kept in a refrigerator (4° C.) until such time as it can be sent rapidly to the laboratory.

Pyelonephritis may have a more insidious onset: the symptoms are often those of general ill-health such as lack of energy, anorexia and loss of weight; and disturbances referable to the urinary tract may be minimal. Spontaneous urinary infection in pregnancy is usually of this type and is preceded by a long period of asymptomatic bacteriuria. About half of the women who excrete significant numbers of organisms in this way develop acute symptoms later if untreated. In pregnancy the number of bacteria being excreted should therefore be estimated routinely. Counts of organisms of over 100,000 per ml. are regarded as significant and may occur without symptoms.

If there is significant fever the patient should be kept in bed and given the diet recommended on p. 24. After fever has subsided a normal diet is permissible and since renal function is seldom impaired, it is usually unnecessary to order any restriction of protein. Ideally, the concentration of blood urea and the creatinine clearance should be estimated because occasionally acute urinary tract infections give rise to renal failure. The causative organism should be cultured from the urine and its sensitivity to antibiotics determined preferably before specific treatment is begun. These procedures, however, are not always practicable in general practice or when the illness may be so severe as to demand rapid treatment.

The various antibiotics available, together with their dosage, indications and contraindications are considered on pp. 2-23. In domiciliary practice it has been customary to assume that the infecting organism is *E. coli* and to prescribe one of the sulphonamides, which possess the advantage of ease of administration and cheapness. Sulphadimidine is most suitably given in a dose of 1 g. three times daily for 10 days. A combination of trimethoprim (80 mg.) with sulphamethoxazole

(400 mg.), which act synergistically, is available as Septrin or Bactrim, and is effective when given in doses of two tablets twice daily for 10 days. Cycloserine, 250 mg. twice a day for 14 days is also effective, and is non-toxic provided that renal function is normal.

If the bacteriological report indicates that the organism is insensitive to sulphonamides or cycloserine, if blood urea and bacterial sensitivity cannot be measured or if there is no clear indication of a response to therapy, it is necessary to give another antibiotic. Ampicillin (p. 15) is active against many gram-negative organisms including *E. coli* and *Proteus mirabilis* and should be given in a dose of 500 mg. by mouth six-hourly for 14 days. Kanamycin sulphate (p. 14) given intramuscularly, 1 g. daily for 14 days, is very effective against infection with *Proteus vulgaris* and *Klebsiella*. It is also active against many strains of *E. coli* resistant to other antibiotics. It is probably the antibiotic of choice if the infection is very severe and especially if there is associated septicaemia. It has similar toxic properties to streptomycin and should only be given in standard doses when renal function is normal. When renal function is impaired the dosage should be reduced, e.g. about 500 mg. every second day, but the amount and frequency of dosage must be adjusted according to the blood level which should not rise above 30 mcg. per ml. Acute staphylococcal infections of the urinary tract are not common but are best treated with cloxacillin in a dose of 500 mg. orally every six hours, or 250 mg. by injection six-hourly. Alternatively methicillin (p. 6) may be given in doses of 1 g. four-hourly by intramuscular injection. Infections with *Pseudomonas pyocyanea* are fortunately rare and are best dealt with by giving carbenicillin 10 to 30 g. per day by intramuscular injection, or, in severe cases, by intravenous infusion. The sodium sulphomethyl derivative of the polymyxins are also effective, (Thiosporin, 1 to 2 million units daily in divided doses by intramuscular injection, or colistin sulphate, 3 to 6 million units in divided doses by intramuscular injection daily). In the event of septicaemia or severe infection with *Pseudomonas* the polymyxin is best given intravenously as polymyxin B sulphate (Aerosporin), 1·5 million units given as an intravenous infusion over some hours.

Once the acute features of severe urinary tract infection have subsided all patients should be examined by a straight radiograph of the abdomen and intravenous pyelography. Some authorities recommend a micturating cystogram in children. If abnormalities such as hydronephrosis, calculus or a developmental aberration are discovered, the advice of a urologist should be obtained: in many instances cystoscopy and retrograde pyelography will be required to obtain a complete clinical picture. In such cases sterilization of the urinary tract may not be achieved or maintained by chemotherapy alone and appropriate surgical measures should be undertaken as soon as possible. Gynaecological examination should be carried out if there are symptoms suggestive of uterine infection or prolapse.

In pregnancy some dilatation of both ureters is very common and can be regarded as physiological. Compression of the ureter by the foetal head against the pelvic brim is often an additional factor causing stasis and infection. Obstruction ceases after delivery and it is the doctor's responsibility to make sure that infection does not continue since chronic pyelonephritis causing renal failure in later life may often be a legacy of neglected urinary infections acquired during pregnancy. Cycloserine is well tolerated by pregnant women and does not appear in the umbilical blood or liquor amnii at the time of delivery. Trimethoprim affects folate metabolism, so the trimethoprim-sulphamethoxazole combination should not be given during pregnancy.

The prognosis in acute pyelonephritis is not, as a rule, influenced by the severity of the initial symptoms. Only a very small proportion of patients die in the acute stage of renal failure. The prognosis depends largely on the resistance of the organisms to chemotherapy and on the presence or absence of factors causing obstruction in the urinary tract. Some 10 to 20 per cent. of cases relapse for no obvious reason. The criterion of cure is a sterile urine, and samples should be sent to the bacteriologist at the conclusion of treatment, and again at intervals of four days and one or two months. It cannot be too strongly emphasized that a serious attempt should be made to find underlying abnormalities which might predispose to recurrent infections.

Long-term use of suppressive antibiotics is indicated in patients who relapse after a satisfactory course of treatment and in those in whom there is radiological evidence of chronic pyelonephritis. Cycloserine, 250 mg. every second day, is an effective drug, provided renal function is good. Otherwise ampicillin, 250 mg. every second day, should be given for up to six months. Experience with trimethoprim and sulphamethoxazole is not yet extensive.

Chronic Pyelonephritis

Chronic infection in the urinary tract may involve both kidneys to a similar degree or be predominantly unilateral. About one-third of patients present with lumbar backache, persistent pyuria, bouts of fever and dysuria. Another third present with vague ill-health, weight loss and lassitude, while the remainder are diagnosed because of the discovery of hypertension or the occurrence of its complications. Renal failure of greater or lesser degree is invariable and is often attended by defects of tubular function which tend to be disproportionately severe in relation to the fall in glomerular filtration rate.

Investigation and treatment are based on similar principles to those described for acute pyelonephritis. The infecting organism or organisms can be isolated on culture of the urine in most cases. In chronic pyuria, tuberculous infection must be carefully excluded by bacteriological examination of an early-morning specimen of urine on three successive days. Because of renal failure intravenous pyelography is often of little value in demonstrating abnormalities within the urinary tract and recourse has to be made to cystoscopy and retrograde pyelography in the majority of instances. The results of treatment are less successful than in acute pyelonephritis.

If the condition of the patient permits, antibiotics should be withheld until after any necessary urological investigation and ameliorative surgical measures have been performed. Surgery may effect a cure when the lesion is unilateral, e.g. unilateral nephrectomy in extensive disease in one kidney when the function of the other kidney is adequate. In other cases the removal of an impacted stone in one ureter may restore some function even in bilateral chronic pyelonephritis with calculi. Chemotherapy or antibiotic treatment should then be given as indicated by the nature of the infecting organisms.

Cycloserine (pp. 18, 72) is less effective in infections due to *E. coli* when there is poor renal function than it is when renal function is normal even when the organisms isolated are sensitive to the drug. This is because it is often impossible to attain sufficiently high concentrations in the urine owing to impairment of renal concentrating power and the need for an ample intake of fluid because of the renal failure.

In any case it should not be given unless the levels of the drug in the blood can be estimated periodically for there is considerable danger if its concentration in the blood is allowed to rise above 40 mcg. per ml. Kanamycin sulphate (p. 14) is effective in sterilizing the urine for long periods of time but its dosage should also be controlled by blood analysis and it is only suitable for hospital practice. Long-term doses of other antibiotics, e.g. ampicillin and nitrofurantoin may be used as indicated by the changing pattern of the organisms in the urine.

The treatment of chronic renal failure is discussed on p. 278.

Renal Carbuncle, Perinephric Abscess

These conditions may occur in patients suffering from boils or other infected lesions of skin or bone. The condition is usually due to *Staphylococcus aureus* which has reached the kidney by the blood stream. The abscess forms in the renal cortex where healing may occur or it may rupture into perirenal tissue or into the renal pelvis. Usually the patient is acutely ill with a high temperature. Blood culture may reveal the nature of the infection but often this is negative. The urine is also usually sterile and antibiotics may have to be given blindly. Methicillin should be tried first in doses of 1 g. four-hourly by intramuscular injection for 10 to 14 days. Cloxacillin, 500 mg. six-hourly, should be given orally for a similar period. Alternatively cephaloridine or cephalexin may be used with good effect in doses of 500 mg. four times a day. Occasionally surgical drainage is required.

RENAL CALCULI, NEPHROCALCINOSIS AND RENAL TUBULAR DISORDERS

The occurrence of calculi within the urinary tract is common. The factors which promote the formation of stones within the renal parenchyma or in the lower urinary tract are complex and not fully understood. Living in a hot climate or working in hot conditions may be factors of aetiological importance as the amount of water available for urinary excretion is reduced by sweating and this results in a highly concentrated urine in which crystallization is promoted.

Hypercalciuria as a cause of stone formation. A variety of disorders which are associated with hypercalciuria tend to cause stone formation. These include primary hyperparathyroidism, prolonged immobilization, excessive and prolonged ingestion of milk and alkali by occasional patients suffering from peptic ulceration, Cushing's syndrome and the prolonged use of corticosteroids, sarcoidosis, and destructive disease of bone due to primary malignancy or metastatic deposits. It is important that a definite diagnosis of these conditions be made because the appropriate therapy for each condition may prevent the continued formation of renal calculi and the progress of nephrocalcinosis. Hypercalciuria without hypercalcaemia may be part of a syndrome of renal tubular dysfunction, or a genetically determined abnormality.

Renal tubular acidosis. Of the diseases associated with hypercalciuria renal tubular acidosis is the only one due to primary renal disorder and is characterized by a diminution in the ability to establish a high concentration gradient of hydrogen ions between blood and urine. Thus the minimal pH attainable in the urine following the administration of ammonium chloride is usually greater than 6·0 units and metabolic acidosis develops. Although it is rare as an inherited metabolic defect in infancy and in young people, it is more common as an acquired disorder in adults suffering from pyelonephritis. The condition is rapidly improved by the administration of alkali which restores body pH to normal, diminishes urinary calcium excretion and prevents further stone formation. The dose of sodium bicarbonate given should be adjusted to maintain a normal serum bicarbonate concentration and this usually requires 3 g. four times a day by mouth.

Idiopathic hypercalciuria. This condition is probably genetically determined and occurs in young men who appear to be free from other diseases. In areas where the calcium content of the drinking water is relatively low, it is logical to advise a low calcium diet. When the calcium content of the water is high, dietary restriction is of no value, and other measures must be used to lower urinary calcium excretion. Cellulose phosphate (15 g. per day), Sodium phytate (6 g. per day) or bendrofluazide, (5 to 10 mg. per day) may be given; but controlled observations on the long-term value of these drugs in relation to the prevention of stone formation are not yet available.

Certain metabolic diseases which include gout, cystinuria, primary hyperoxaluria and xanthinuria may also give rise to renal calculi.

Uric acid stones. These occur not only in gout but in other conditions associated with elevation in the serum uric acid level, such as various reticuloses and leukaemia following radiotherapy or the use of radiomimetic drugs. Occasionally uric acid stones may form in people who show no elevation of serum uric acid concentration. These appear to be due to a diminished tubular capacity to make ammonia as a result of which an excessively acid urine is always being formed. Urine is supersaturated with uric acid at normal uric acid concentrations when the pH is acid. Uric acid stones can be prevented in patients who are liable to develop them by keeping the pH of the urine above 6·0 units. This is most easily done by giving 3 g. of sodium bicarbonate four times a day by mouth.

Cystinuria. This is a genetically determined defect in the tubular reabsorption of cystine, lysine, arginine and ornithine. Apart from the formation of cystine stones these patients enjoy good health. Dietary restriction of cystine is ineffective and difficult. The solubility of cystine in urine is greatly increased by maintaining the pH of the urine above 7·0 and by ensuring a flow of more than 2 ml. per minute over the 24 hours, i.e. a total of over 3 litres. All relatives of cystinuric patients should be tested for cystinuria and a high flow of urine with alkalization should be maintained in those in whom the test is positive. The successful use of penicillamine in this condition has also been reported, but it is expensive and is best reserved for those who do not respond to more simple measures.

Oxalate stones and hyperoxaluria. Oxalate is a component of large numbers of renal calculi including those in which the underlying cause is hypercalciuria. Most patients with oxalate stones, however, show neither an increased urinary excretion of calcium or oxalate nor any detectable renal tubular abnormality and there is no known means of reducing oxalate excretion below normal values or of increasing oxalate solubility.

Oxalosis and primary hyperoxaluria are two rare genetically determined conditions which occur in children. These patients rarely survive into adult life but the diagnosis should be considered in all children with renal calculi or nephrocalcinosis. At the present time it may be worth while treating them with 10 mg. of pyridoxine and 5 mg. of folic acid daily. This therapy is based on the fact that these substances are co-enzymes in the synthesis of serine from glycine and both conditions are associated with a disturbance in glycine metabolism.

The general management of patients with renal

stones. Stones may cause distress by producing renal colic and by favouring urinary tract infection. All types may be present in the kidney or pelvis for many years without producing symptoms. This is true even of the large staghorn variety. When small stones enter the ureter they cause renal colic. Although morphine causes spasm of smooth muscle, 15 mg. of morphine sulphate subcutaneously with 1 mg. of atropine is effective in controlling pain in most instances. Should symptoms persist after 15 minutes the morphine can be repeated in the same dose. The passage of a stone down the ureter should be followed radiographically. When the severe pain has subsided the patient should not stay in bed and should be encouraged to drink plenty of fluid. The urine should be examined and if the stone is found it should be analysed. When a stone becomes impacted in the ureter it is necessary to obtain urological advice. Surgical removal of the stone is necessary if urinary tract infection occurs or if intravenous pyelography shows hydronephrosis. Infection and obstructive lesions of the urinary tract favour the development of stones of all types and obstruction renders the eradication of infection difficult. Organisms most likely to facilitate precipitation are those which split urea, especially *Staphylococci* and *Proteus vulgaris*. The treatment of these infections is discussed on pp. 2–23.

Other renal tubular defects. While some tubular defects are frequently associated with renal calculi and may present with renal colic, other defects of tubular function are never complicated in this way.

Water-losing renal conditions arise in a variety of diseases which include hyperparathyroidism, myelomatosis, potassium depletion and diabetes insipidus due to vasopressin insufficiency. Polyuria and thirst which often accompany these diseases are usually controlled by treatment appropriate to each disorder. Nephrogenic diabetes insipidus is a congenital failure of the renal tubules to reabsorb water and does not respond to the administration of vasopressin. Some amelioration of thirst and polyuria, however, can be obtained by giving chlorothiazide in a dose of 500 mg. twice a day.

Essential familial hypophosphataemia is a genetically determined defect in renal tubular phosphate reabsorption which leads to rickets. Very large doses of oral calciferol (200,000 to 400,000 units) are needed to cure the condition.

The Fanconi syndrome is an inherited condition characterized by multiple defects in renal tubular function and may give rise to glycosuria, aminoaciduria, phosphaturia and to renal tubular acidosis. Osteomalacia and metabolic acidosis result and are treated with large doses of calciferol and with alkalis as already described for the discrete disorders of hypophosphataemia and renal tubular acidosis.

An exceedingly rare familial defect of tubular function affects amino acid transport and is called Hartnup disease. Apart from its academic interest it is important because patients develop a pellagralike appearance which is believed to respond to the administration of nicotinamide.

12. Hormone Therapy and Diseases of the Endocrine Glands

A. G. MacGregor, J. A. Strong and A. Klopper

THE PITUITARY GLAND

The anterior lobe of the pituitary gland, stimulated by releasing-factors from the hypothalamus, is responsible for growth and the activity of the adrenal and thyroid glands and of the gonads. Disease of the gland may show itself by secretory failure requiring replacement treatment with the hormones of the target endocrine glands. Pressure effects may result from enlargement due to adenoma formation, and overactivity of the anterior lobe may cause gigantism, acromegaly or Cushing's disease. Disorders of the posterior pituitary gland present as a result of interference with the neurohypophyseal tracts leading to diabetes insipidus.

The Anterior Lobe

Adenoma of the Pituitary

Adenomas of the pituitary gland are restricted to the anterior lobe and may be classified as (*a*) chromophobe, (*b*) eosinophil and (*c*) basophil, according to the staining reactions of the cells composing the tumour. The symptoms and signs produced depend upon the pressure exerted on the remaining tissue of the anterior lobe and its surrounding structures, especially the optic chiasma, and the nature of any secretion produced by the cells of the tumour.

Pressure effects, particularly visual field defects, require surgical intervention, but if the optic chiasma is not involved, radiotherapy may be valuable, especially for eosinophil adenomas, and implantation of rods of the beta-emitting isotope yttrium (^{90}Y) can be undertaken when facilities permit.

CHROMOPHOBE ADENOMA. A tumour of the chromophobe cells should be removed surgically before the destruction of surrounding structures is advanced. Operation is urgently required when signs of deterioration of vision occur. Surgical treatment should be followed by a course of radiotherapy. Hypopituitarism frequently accompanies the development of these tumours and usually follows their surgical removal and destruction by radiation. Replacement therapy must be given at the time of operation and subsequently

unless investigation shows it to be unnecessary (pp. 288, 301).

EOSINOPHIL ADENOMA. This tumour causes gigantism or acromegaly, according to the age of the patient. Inactive cases may be encountered which require no treatment unless signs of hypopituitarism are present and it is useful, if practicable, to assess their functional activity by assays of plasma growth hormone. Diabetes, hyperthyroidism, gout and hyperparathyroidism are sometimes associated with this type of tumour and may subside when the acromegaly is controlled. When persistent they require appropriate treatment (pp. 316, 292, 300).

BASOPHIL ADENOMA. The part played by basophilism in the production of Cushing's syndrome and the treatment of the condition is discussed on p. 303.

CRANIOPHARYNGIOMA. Although this is not a tumour of the pituitary gland, it is conveniently considered here. It is usually radio-resistant and requires surgical removal or drainage of fluid from the cyst.

Associated hypopituitarism usually requires treatment.

Pituitary Dwarfism

Pituitary dwarfism, an uncommon cause of retarded growth, generally becomes manifest before the tenth year of life, and may be due to defective production of growth hormone and other secretions. The clinical picture is one of dwarfism with defective development of the primary and secondary sex characteristics. The emotional state generally approximates to the physical development of the child rather then to the calendar age.

Growth hormone obtained from human pituitaries has proved very effective in man, but at the time of writing this is not available commercially and all other preparations have been most disappointing. Androgen replacement is of value in older boys. It has a protein-anabolic effect and usually causes a spurt of growth for from 6 to 12 months, after which time growth ceases altogether, so that these individuals practically never attain a normal height. Nevertheless, such treatment stimulates muscular power and the development of

K*

287

secondary sex characteristics and has a very beneficial psychological effect. Androgen therapy has a similar action in female dwarfs but virilization may occur. Fluoxymesterone in doses of 5 to 20 mg. daily by mouth is the best preparation and has superseded testosterone propionate by intramuscular injection or methyl testosterone by mouth. Implantation of five pellets of testosterone each of 200 mg., under local anaesthesia, into the anterior abdominal wall can provide effective replacement therapy for 6 to 9 months.

Hypopituitarism

Hypopituitarism, characterized by considerable muscular weakness, pallor of the skin and failure of thyroid, adrenal and gonadal functions, results from destruction of the anterior lobe of the pituitary. Thrombosis of the blood supply with infarction of the gland after a post-partum haemorrhage used to be a common cause. Other causal factors include tumour, granulomas, cystic degeneration and embolism, or it may follow the treatment of a pituitary adenoma by surgery or radiation. Panhypopituitarism is not always encountered and selective failure of gonadotrophin, corticotrophin or secretion of growth hormone may occur. Anorexia nervosa and starvation may resemble hypopituitarism in some respects, but the two conditions differ and it is important to make the distinction, since the treatment of each is quite different.

Satisfactory replacement of all anterior pituitary hormones is at present impossible, but cortisone alone can produce remarkable clinical improvement. Theoretically corticotrophin would be ideal, but in practice cortisone is as effective and is more convenient to use. Only small maintenance doses of from 25 to 37·5 mg. daily are required, and with such doses the undesirable side-effects of cortisone are not encountered. This may be the only treatment necessary and it usually transforms the patient within a few weeks. Thyroxine therapy should be withheld until cortisone has been given. It is seldom wise to give more than 0·1 mg. of thyroxine a day. Fluoxymesterone, as androgen therapy, is useful if the patient complains of impotence.

Just as patients with Addison's disease are apt to be precipitated into Addisonian crisis by any form of stress, such as intercurrent illness or the administration of narcotics or anaesthetics, so patients suffering from hypopituitarism may lapse into coma for similar reasons. Hypopituitary coma only occurs in the untreated patient. The clinical features may include profound hypothermia, hypoglycaemia, a low blood pressure, hypothyroidism, water intoxication, and anoxia with acidosis of respiratory origin, all of which may require attention in addition to the chest or urinary infection so frequently associated with the condition. Treatment should be the same as for coma in hypothyroidism (p. 291) together with the rapid intravenous infusion of 250 ml. of 20 per cent. glucose solution followed by a further 500 ml. delivered by slow drip infusion during the next 12 hours.

THE POSTERIOR LOBE

Diabetes Insipidus

Diabetes insipidus, characterized by marked polyuria and thirst, is generally attributed to a lesion in the floor of the third ventricle anterior to the tuber cinereum or in the anterior hypothalamus, an extension of which with the posterior part of the pituitary forms the neurohypophysis. The nature of the lesion varies in different patients and may be the result of injury, an operation on the pituitary or on its surrounding tissues, a tumour or an infection. In addition there is a group of patients with vasopressin-resistant diabetes insipidus in whom the responsible renal tubular defect is probably inherited as a sex-linked dominant characteristic. The condition is closely simulated by polydipsia of psychogenic origin from which it must be differentiated.

If there is evidence of syphilis, vigorous anti-luetic treatment should be instituted. A neoplasm causing this lesion is at present often inaccessible to surgical treatment, although radiotherapy sometimes yields promising results in the rare case of diabetes insipidus due to Hand-Schüller-Christian disease. In most cases treatment should be directed to the relief of the thirst and polyuria for which two methods are available.

VASOPRESSIN. Intramuscular injections of vasopressin as Pitressin Tannate in oil are of great value. Care must be taken to warm and shake the suspension very thoroughly before it is injected intramuscularly. Dosage varies from case to case and at different times in the same patient. An average dose is 0·5 ml. (2·5 units) of Pitressin Tannate injected just before bedtime on alternate days, and this may be reduced or increased as the response demands. The salt intake should be restricted, as salt exacerbates the polydipsia. The patient's ability to lead a normal life by day and night is the test of satisfactory control. With the average dose, retention of water is rare but, when it does occur, is characterized by mental confusion, poor muscle co-ordination, headache, nausea and vomiting. If repeated injections are impracticable, an effective, but less satisfactory, alternative is a nasal spray of synthetic lysine vasopressin (Sandoz Ltd.). The effect of a single application may persist for four hours or more and will keep the patient comfortable till the next injection, but it should normally only be used as a supplement to Pitressin Tannate in oil.

Some patients who have been hypophysectomized because of a tumour of the pituitary or to alleviate metastases from carcinoma of the breast may develop diabetes insipidus when receiving replacement therapy; such patients may well require Pitressin Tannate in addition to cortisone treatment. The diabetes insipidus produced in this way is usually transient.

CHLOROTHIAZIDE. The apparently paradoxical effect of chlorothiazide in relieving the polyuria of patients suffering from diabetes insipidus was first reported in 1959. Since then patients have been treated by a number of thiazide diuretics, which reduce urine volume and thirst by an unknown mechanism, but satisfactory control of symptoms can usually be achieved by the administration of 500 mg. of chlorothiazide by mouth twice daily, or by giving the equivalent dose of one of the newer thiazide diuretics. Some patients seem to become refractory to the treatment after a time, but in others its effect appears to be maintained and this oral form of treatment is then the method of choice.

THE THYROID GLAND

Simple Goitre

Simple goitre is a physiological response to a deficiency of the thyroid hormones, thyroxine and triiodothyronine. Because of this deficiency the output of thyroid-stimulating hormone by the pituitary gland increases, and this in turn is followed by hyperplasia of the thyroid gland and a rise in the concentration of thyroid hormones in the plasma.

The primary deficiency of these hormones may arise by one or more of several possible mechanisms.

(1) DEFICIENCY OF IODINE in the diet is the most important factor in endemic goitre. Absolute iodine deficiency is common in many parts of the world. Relative iodine deficiency may occur when supplies are adequate or marginal, but the ingested iodine is not available for hormone synthesis; for example, because of poor absorption, due possibly to excess of calcium in the water supplies.

(2) ANTITHYROID AGENTS occurring in the diet may inhibit the synthesis of thyroxine in the thyroid gland. Many drugs have this capacity; for example, the thioureas used in the treatment of hyperthyroidism, diazepam derivatives used in the treatment of depression, sulphonamide drugs, para-aminosalicylic acid (PAS) and even iodides, taken in large quantities for long periods may have this effect. Some proprietary asthma remedies containing iodine, such as 'Felsol', can cause large goitres.

(3) INCREASED DEMANDS FOR THE HORMONES at puberty or during pregnancy and lactation, and changes in the protein binding of thyroxine in the plasma in response to the secretion or administration of oestrogens may lead to fluctuations in the size of the thyroid gland. Changes in the renal clearance of iodine may occasionally be important.

(4) CONGENITAL GOITRES develop because of genetic enzyme defects in the thyroid gland leading to impaired ability to synthesize thyroxine.

Sporadic simple goitre may be due to one or more of these various potential causes.

Prophylaxis. The quantity of iodine required per day by an average adult is about 200 microgrammes and this is supplied if iodized salt is used. The Medical Research Council recommends the addition of either 1 part of potassium iodate to 100,000 parts of all common table salt sold, or 1 part to 40,000 parts of all packeted table salt. Legislation to give effect to this simple and harmless measure would do much to control endemic goitre throughout the world, as has been achieved already in Switzerland. The pregnant woman should also receive potassium iodide, but treatment given only during pregnancy will not always prevent pregnancy goitre.

Curative. Whatever be the cause of a simple goitre, a relative deficiency of thyroxine is involved with consequent excess secretion of thyrotrophin.

Treatment, therefore, logically consists in the administration of thyroxine. Thyroid extract should not be used. Synthetic *l*-thyroxine is the drug of choice. It is seldom necessary to give more than 0·3 of thyroxine daily. This treatment is necessary not so much to replace thyroxine, which is already being adequately produced if the patient is euthyroid, but to inhibit the production of thyrotrophin by the pituitary and so to reduce the size of the thyroid gland. In addition, 60 mg. of potassium iodide should be given daily to ensure that any iodine deficiency which may be present is corrected.

The slight enlargement of the thyroid which may occur at puberty and during pregnancy and lactation often responds to treatment with thyroxine and iodine. If the goitre has been present for a considerable time, however, this treatment is usually ineffective. If the swelling is unsightly or if it gives rise to pressure symptoms surgery is required.

Thyroiditis

The forms of thyroiditis which may be encountered are: (1) sub-acute thyroiditis (giant cell thyroiditis); (2) lymphadenoid goitre; (3) fibrous thyroiditis.

Sub-acute thyroiditis. In this condition some non-suppurative inflammation of the thyroid gland occurs, resulting in pain, tenderness, swelling and fever.

The condition usually subsides spontaneously in a few weeks without treatment, but this may be accelerated by the daily administration of 20 mg. of prednisone for two or three weeks, followed by 0·3 mg. thyroxine daily for two or three months. Antibiotic treatment is usually unnecessary.

Lymphadenoid goitre (Hashimoto's disease). This disorder is common and is the most frequent cause of spontaneous hypothyroidism. It may be due to auto-immunization to one or more antigens in the thyroid gland, and should always be suspected when a firm goitre and hypothyroidism coexist. It may, however, present before hypothyroidism develops, or the latter condition may occur without previous thyroid enlargement being detected. The diagnosis is confirmed by characteristic biochemical and serological findings.

Thyroxine should be administered in doses of 0·2 to 0·3 mg. daily, and continued indefinitely, even when clinical hypothyroidism has not developed. Appreciable shrinkage of the gland occurs with treatment.

Chronic fibrous thyroiditis. This is very rare and simulates thyroid carcinoma. Permanent replacement therapy with thyroxine is necessary after surgical removal of the gland.

Hypothyroidism

Cretinism. Hypothyroidism in infancy may be due to a number of causes: in areas of endemic goitre prolonged maternal iodide deficiency may result in the birth of a goitrous cretin; on the other hand hypothyroidism may be due to congenital athyreosis or to a genetically determined defect of synthesis of the thyroid hormone.

The brain of an infant develops with great rapidity during the first year of life, and inadequate thyroid secretion during this critical period will almost certainly result in mental retardation. If adequate treatment is started between the third and sixth months of life the prospect of normal mental development is excellent. Successful treatment of any type of cretinism is dependent on early diagnosis and lifelong treatment with thyroxine. As diagnosis is rarely made early, however, few cretins grow up mentally normal. The majority remain retarded with an intelligence quotient of below 70 per cent., the extent of the mental defect depending largely on the length of time which elapses before the start of therapy. Early treatment is essential for full mental development to result, but a cretin may remain untreated until the age of four or five and then, under proper treatment, may show skeletal growth to almost normal proportions. The administration of thyroxine to untreated cretins over the age of 12 is usually undesirable as it may make a placid imbecile difficult to manage.

The dosage of thyroxine is gauged by the response of the patient. The correct dose is that which will ensure normal growth and development without producing signs of hyperthyroidism. It is usually necessary in a baby to start treatment with a very small dose. The amount required varies with the age and weight of the child from about 0·0125 mg. of thyroxine (one-quarter of a 0·05 mg. tablet) daily in early infancy to doses of 0·1 to 0·3 mg. of thyroxine daily in late childhood. A very small dose of thyroxine is sufficient to banish the grosser stigmata of cretinism and to effect a remarkable improvement, but the practitioner should not be content with the mere disappearance of symptoms, since a dose sufficient to dispel symptoms may be inadequate to ensure satisfactory growth and osseous development. The initial dose should nevertheless be small, since subthyroid cretins are much more sensitive to the hormone than those whose metabolism has been raised to a normal level by appropriate treatment. A large initial dose in an untreated patient may result in alarming toxic symptoms, and the amount should not be increased at intervals shorter than three weeks. The patient's growth and osseous development should be checked by regular measurements, and by a radiological examination of the bones of the hand and wrist every year. Retarded development is usually due to an inadequate dose or irregular treatment. The dramatic improvement which results from properly controlled treatment encourages the belief that permanent cure has resulted, but it must be emphasized to the parents that it is necessary to continue the daily treatment permanently.

Juvenile hypothyroidism. A clear distinction is not always made between sporadic cretinism and juvenile hypothyroidism: in the former the thyroid is deficient from birth; in the latter it becomes deficient after a number of years during which mental and physical development have progressed normally. The prognosis is much better than in cretinism, as permanent damage to the central nervous system is not so likely to result from a deficiency of thyroid secretion in childhood as it is from a similar deficiency during the critical months of infancy. Though this is a rare condition, its recognition and treatment are of great importance as it is one of the few forms of dwarfism capable of being cured. Clinical diagnosis is not always easy as many of the classical characteristics of adult hypothyroidism may be lacking and these children may be quite intelligent.

As in cretinism, dosage with thyroxine should be the maximum consistent with the avoidance of toxic symptoms. From 0·15 to 0·3 mg. will usually suffice for maintenance treatment, but a smaller initial dose is indicated. Treatment should be continued throughout life, and should be regulated during the years of growth, as in cretinism, by frequent measurements and radiological examinations of the hands and wrist to ensure that development is proceeding normally.

Hypothyroidism in the adult. This may be due to a primary atrophy of the thyroid, to therapeutic thyroidectomy, to excessive dosage with radio-iodine or, most commonly, to Hashimoto's disease; it may result from overdosage with antithyroid drugs (p. 294), in which case recovery occurs if the administration of the drug is stopped or the dose is appropriately reduced. Secondary hypothyroidism is due to hypopituitarism (p. 288).

As treatment has to be continued for life it is essential that the diagnosis should be firmly established on objective criteria before it is started. There are few conditions in which the response to treatment is so gratifying as in primary hypothyroidism. The simple oral administration of thyroxine will relieve symptoms entirely : within a week of starting treatment the patient's appearance improves; the speech becomes clearer and cerebration more rapid; intolerance to cold diminishes, the appetite improves and constipation is relieved; some loss of weight occurs, owing to a copious diuresis, but sometimes a gain may occur later as appetite improves; psychotic manifestations, which are not uncommon in untreated hypothyroidism, rapidly improve, though this is not invariable. It usually takes some weeks or even months for the skin, hair and blood picture to become normal.

The aim of treatment is to give a daily dose of thyroxine sufficient to rid the patient of symptoms. Nothing is to be gained by raising the dose if symptoms can be eradicated at a lower level. Elderly hypothyroid patients often develop undesirable cardiac symptoms if their metabolism is raised to normal. There is no way of determining in advance the *exact* dose of thyroxine for an individual patient, but the response to it can usually be predicted. It is seldom necessary to give more than 0·2 mg. a day. It is wise to start with a dose of not more than 0·05 mg. a day when the patient is elderly and suspected of having coronary disease. This can be raised gradually at intervals of a month until a satisfactory response is obtained. In this way there is less danger of producing angina, myocardial infarction or heart failure.

The doctor may have to be content, particularly in elderly patients, to relieve only the grosser features by the prescription of as little as 0·05 mg. of thyroxine daily. If there is a history of angina or of ischaemic heart disease, propranolol or practolol should be given with thyroxine, but with great caution because of the risk of precipitating cardiac failure (p. 101).

MYXOEDEMA COMA. This rare, and usually terminal, state occurs only in patients with very advanced disease and should never arise if the hypothyroidism is diagnosed at an earlier stage and adequate treatment is instituted. Coma may be precipitated by infection, cold or trivial injury. The syndrome results from a combination of heart failure, cerebral ischaemia, adrenocortical failure, hypothermia and—the original factor—absolute thyroid deprivation.

Replacement of thyroid hormone is probably an urgent measure and, although this remains a controversial subject, liothyronine (triiodothyronine) should be given intravenously in a dose of 20 mcg. and repeated in not less than four hours. Oral thyroxine in a dose of not more than 0·1 mg. daily may be adequate if it is absorbed; it is safer and raises the metabolic rate as rapidly as can be tolerated by many patients; should they be unable to swallow, a crushed tablet should be administered by gastric intubation. In addition, the patient will require to be kept warm if hypothermic, but excessive heat from a cage or bath should be avoided. The temperature of the patient may be raised slowly to 92° F. (33·5° C.) by warming, but should thereafter be allowed to rise spontaneously. It is important to give 100 mg. of hydrocortisone sodium succinate intravenously followed by 50 mg. of cortisone intramuscularly twice daily till the emergency is over. Continuous attention must be given to water and electrolyte balance, to respiratory function during the acute phase of replacement therapy, and to the treatment of infection with antibiotics.

Carcinoma of the Thyroid Gland

This condition is responsible for only 0·3 per cent. of deaths from malignant disease in this country and for 0·06 per cent. of all deaths. Its early diagnosis is not always easy, but it should be suspected if a pre-existing solitary thyroid adenoma becomes larger, immobile, hard or tender with enlarged associated lymph nodes, or in any non-toxic goitre of recent origin.

Treatment is usually surgical with radical excision of the primary tumour and of accessible metastases. Anaplastic and undifferentiated tumours may prove to be inoperable, but palliative radiotherapy may be helpful in such cases. The more differentiated and papillary types of adenocarcinoma are relatively radio-resistant and surgery is the treatment of choice with, in rare cases, radioactive iodine (^{131}I) treatment as an ancillary measure. [131]I can be effective only if the tumour and metastases are sufficiently differentiated to be

able to concentrate the isotope. Any normal thyroid tissue must be removed surgically or destroyed by an ablative dose of 80 millicuries of [131]I. The use of ^{131}I in this way is a specialized procedure restricted to a limited number of centres, and although a few spectacular results have been achieved, this treatment has not made any significant difference to the morbidity and mortality of the disease.

A patient who has had a total or partial thyroidectomy for actual or suspected thyroid carcinoma, must receive full replacement treatment with thyroxine (0·2 to 0·3 mg. daily) for the rest of his life, as the high levels of thyroid-stimulating hormone present in hypothyroidism may stimulate residual tumour tissue.

Hyperthyroidism

The symptoms of hyperthyroidism are due to excessive secretion of thyroxine by the thyroid gland. This occurs in primary hyperthyroidism (Graves' disease), the aetiology of which is obscure but is probably due to the presence in the circulation of the long-acting thyroid stimulator. Hyperthyroidism also occurs in toxic nodular goitre and less frequently with a single toxic adenoma.

The condition can be treated effectively by one or more of three alternative methods : antithyroid drugs, partial thyroidectomy or radioactive iodine, for each of which there are indications and contraindications, advantages and disadvantages.

General management. Certain general measures are applicable whichever form of treatment is employed.

REST. Except in mild cases an initial period of restricted activity is desirable, but most patients can be managed effectively as out-patients. In severe cases rest in bed is essential, especially for a week or two at the onset, but unless heart failure is present the patient should be allowed to get up for toilet purposes.

At the outset it is desirable to identify and if possible correct any physical or psychological factors in the patient's environment which may have contributed to the illness.

Mental rest is facilitated by the use of sedatives, of which one of the most effective and probably the most convenient is phenobarbitone. This should be given in doses of 30 to 60 mg. twice or thrice daily, according to the tolerance of the individual for the sedative, which varies greatly.

The diet should be generous, and in most cases

unrestricted in variety, supplemented by additional feeds of egg, milk, fruit juice and glucose or proprietary foods.

A moderate increase in weight is usually a reassuring and satisfactory sign. In active cases an increasing weight is a valuable indication of improvement unless oedema is present ; in quiescent cases a stationary weight is equally reassuring. A fall in weight of even a few pounds, especially if steadily maintained week by week, is disquieting and is the signal for a review of the whole management of the patient. There are, however, occasional patients in whom hypermetabolism has stimulated an appetite in excess of their increased caloric requirements. Such patients may be overweight, and they may require to be dieted as their hyperthyroidism becomes controlled.

Surgical operations, such as tonsillectomy or appendicectomy, in thyrotoxic patients can carry the same risk of post-operative hyperthyroid crisis as thyroidectomy in the uncontrolled case. If possible, therefore, such operations should be deferred until the patient has been rendered euthyroid.

Attempts to convert atrial fibrillation to regular rhythm either by treatment with quinidine or by cardioversion with direct-current shock therapy should be postponed until some weeks after hyperthyroidism has been controlled. In many cases with atrial fibrillation, especially those of recent onset, reversion to regular rhythm will occur spontaneously when hyperthyroidism has been controlled by treatment, but if this does not occur, the procedure described can be adopted at a later date.

Choice of Treatment. The selection of the appropriate definitive treatment must be made from among the following three methods: prolonged use of antithyroid drugs, subtotal thyroidectomy after suitable preparation, or the administration of ^{131}I.

INDICATIONS FOR ANTITHYROID DRUG THERAPY. Antithyroid drugs are not curative but interfere with the synthesis of thyroid hormone and relieve symptoms and signs due to excessive hormone production. They should be the initial form of treatment for children and for young women suffering from moderate primary hyperthyroidism with unobtrusive thyroid enlargement. In such patients an irrevocable interference with the endocrine system by partial thyroidectomy is undesirable if it can be avoided; operation should be considered only if drug treatment is unsuccessful in controlling the disorder, if the patient develops

toxic reactions to the drugs or if relapse occurs following a period of effective control for at least a year.

During pregnancy drug treatment is usually indicated in the control of thyrotoxicosis, for thyroidectomy may be undesirable and treatment with ^{131}I is certainly contraindicated. Provided that the smallest effective dose is used during the latter months of pregnancy, thus avoiding hypothyroidism in the mother, there is little danger that the function of the foetal thyroid will be depressed by the drugs and that the child will be born with a goitre. If control with drugs is unsatisfactory or the gland is large, partial thyroidectomy may be necessary. As these drugs are secreted in the milk, the patient should not be allowed to breast feed her baby. Antithyroid drugs should be used for the very exceptional cases of congenital hyperthyroidism—a self-limiting disorder which remits naturally if the child can be nursed through the critical first few weeks of life.

INDICATIONS FOR SURGERY. In the age-group between 30 and 45 the initial treatment of choice is usually sub-total thyroidectomy after appropriate preoperative preparation, since in this group a sustained remission following antithyroid drug treatment occurs only in about 30 per cent. of patients. This is particularly the case with men, in whom drug treatment is rarely followed by a sustained remission. Operation is indicated under the age of 30 if the patient has been severely toxic, has a large goitre, suffers from pressure symptoms, reacts unfavourably to drugs or has relapsed following a previous course of treatment with drugs.

If an experienced thyroid surgeon is available, partial thyroidectomy is a very satisfactory operation. Even patients over the age of 45 may derive more benefit from surgery than from radioactive iodine therapy, when their general health is good and there are no contraindications to operation.

INDICATIONS FOR ^{131}I THERAPY. Radio-iodine (^{131}I) is the treatment of choice for patients over the age of 50, and for many younger patients, unless the rapid mechanical relief afforded by surgery to a patient with a large gland is necessary. Patients of any age who have a recurrence of hyperthyroidism following a previous partial thyroidectomy should be given ^{131}I as complications often follow a further operation. ^{131}I is, furthermore, the treatment of choice for patients with associated heart disease, and for any patient in whom difficulty is experienced in controlling the hyperthyroidism with drug treatment.

Extensive use for 20 years has shown that the only significant disadvantage of radioiodine therapy is the high incidence of subsequent hypothyroidism, perhaps developing some years after treatment. There is no evidence that this form of radiation therapy is associated with the subsequent development of leukaemia or of thyroid carcinoma.

INDIVIDUAL INDICATIONS. The clinical indications for each specific form of treatment can only be outlined in general, as the particular circumstances of individual patients, their environment, or the medical services available may well determine the selection of one or other method. For example, a somewhat unsightly goitre may be of little importance to an old woman not greatly worried about her personal appearance, but could be one of shattering concern to a pretty girl. Since there is great variation in the number and significance of these factors, generalizations are undesirable.

Antithyroid drugs. These all act by interfering with the formation of thyroid hormone. If used in excessive doses, hypothyroidism, and thyroid hyperplasia and enlargement occur. Methyl and propyl thiouracil and carbimazole prevent the iodination of tyrosine, whereas potassium perchlorate inhibits the capacity of the thyroid gland to concentrate iodide. Carbimazole is the drug of choice, though in terms of toxic effects it is very similar to the thiouracil drugs when given in equivalent doses.

DOSAGE. The degree of inhibition of thyroxine synthesis is directly related to the dose of antithyroid drug used. The aim in hyperthyroidism is to decrease the concentration of thyroxine in the blood to a normal level, but not below.

Antithyroid drugs are given in tablet form. The usual dose of carbimazole for the first six to eight weeks of treatment is 60 mg. a day. As carbimazole is roughly 10 times as powerful as the thiouracil preparations, the equivalent dose of propyl or methyl thiouracil is 600 mg. daily. These drugs are rapidly excreted and should be given eight-hourly, not merely thrice daily. Once a full remission has been produced by this initial treatment, the dose is reduced to a maintenance level. The time required to produce a remission varies, but with optimal dosage usually takes from six to eight weeks. Patients with large nodular goitres are apt to be somewhat resistant to antithyroid drugs and may require more prolonged treatment with large doses to suppress the hyperthyroidism.

The optimum maintenance does varies. A daily maintenance dose of 15 mg. of carbimazole or 150 mg. of propyl thiouracil is usually given, decreasing to 10 or 100 mg. respectively. Should thyrotoxicosis recur or should hypothyroidism be produced, the maintenance dose should be adjusted accordingly. The treatment should continue for at least one year, unless the decision to operate upon the patient has already been taken, in which case treatment is continued only till the immediate pre-operative procedures can be started.

Potassium perchlorate, used in a dose initially of 800 mg. daily and later in doses of 200 to 400 mg. should only be used if sensitivity reactions preclude the use of other drugs. It is inappropriate for pre-operative preparation.

CLINICAL EFFECTS. A normal human subject may be given antithyroid drugs for many months without producing hypothyroidism or goitre. Since the store of thyroid hormone in hyperthyroid glands is very small, antithyroid drugs produce their effect in thyrotoxic patients within a few days; the sweating and flushing of the skin are usually promptly relieved. Thereafter all the thyrotoxic symptoms steadily recede.

The intermittent hyperglycaemia commonly associated with thyrotoxicosis is usually abolished by any measure that controls hyperthyroidism. There are, of course, other patients in whom thyrotoxicosis is associated with true diabetes, and in such patients diabetic control is difficult. In these patients the treatment described on p. 316 must be instituted.

Antithyroid drug treatment in the doses advised does not greatly influence the size of the goitre. Almost invariably it becomes softer in consistency. Occasionally the gland becomes definitely smaller and, in some patients in whom the thyrotoxic tendency has disappeared and it has been possible to give up the drug altogether, the size of the gland may diminish very materially. An increase in the size of the gland, especially when it is associated with signs and symptoms of hypothyroidism, is an indication of overdosage; inadequate control may be due to inappropriate spacing of the doses of antithyroid drugs.

TOXIC EFFECTS. Antithyroid drugs may produce very serious toxic reactions. The recorded signs of toxicity include fever, enlargement of lymph glands and spleen, jaundice, rashes, conjunctivitis, swelling of the legs and feet, leucopenia, granulopenia, thrombocytopenia and acute sensitivity reactions consisting of high temperature and vomiting. Acute sensitivity reactions and the blood dyscrasias require that drug treatment be stopped. Blood dyscrasias occur so rapidly that even frequent white blood counts provide an inadequate safeguard. All antithyroid drugs produce similar toxic effects although potassium perchlorate can produce aplastic anaemia, especially when given in doses exceeding 1 g. daily. Patients should, therefore, be warned to stop taking the drug and to report to the doctor should any untoward symptoms arise and particularly on the first sign of a sore throat.

ULTIMATE EFFECTS OF DRUG TREATMENT. Maintenance dosage must be continued for at least a year. It is unwise to withdraw the drug unless it has been found possible to control the hyperthyroidism effectively for at least four months with a minimum maintenance dose such as 5 mg. of carbimazole daily. When rigid criteria are applied, it appears that in the 20 to 30 year age-group the proportion of patients who achieve permanent remission after drug treatment is little more than 40 per cent.; and in the 30 to 40 year age-group the figure does not exceed 30 per cent. Thyrotoxicosis in men is seldom permanently cured by this treatment alone.

Most relapses take place within two to six months of stopping treatment, and if patients remain well for at least six months a permanent remission may be anticipated with increasing confidence. If relapse occurs, it can be controlled again by further treatment, but this is usually undesirable except as a stage in the eventual management of the patient by operation or by the use of [131]I.

Partial thyroidectomy. The younger patient who has had a course of treatment with antithyroid drugs is likely to relapse when they are withdrawn, usually within a few months. Such patients will require a partial thyroidectomy, but with this and any other type of thyrotoxic patient requiring operation, every effort must be made to ensure that they are euthyroid before the operation. A course of treatment with antithyroid drugs will usually be adequate and for the two weeks preceding operation this should be replaced by potassium iodide. Treatment with iodide should continue for the first week after operation. Potassium iodide can be conveniently given as a 60-mg. tablet, or as a solution containing 100 mg., taken once daily by mouth. Pre-operative treatment with iodide is essential to reduce the size and vascularity of toxic glands, especially in those patients treated previously with antithyroid drugs.

If for some reason operation has to be postponed for more than seven days following preparation on these lines, it is usually wise to withdraw the treatment with iodide and revert to antithyroid drugs. The final preparation with iodide can then be repeated when a new date for operation has been fixed. *Iodide should never be prescribed for the treatment of hyperthyroidism except as an immediately pre-operative measure.*

PRE-OPERATIVE TREATMENT. The regimen described can usually be undertaken before admission to hospital, and this can be postponed until a day or two preceding the operation. The patient need not be confined to bed, but should have an opportunity to get to know the staff and the surroundings. The staff meanwhile must be wholly satisfied that the patient is euthyroid, that her nutrition is adequate, and that she is completely at ease. Phenobarbitone, 60 mg. twice daily, may be required as a sedative.

Patients with congestive cardiac failure associated with hyperthyroidism should normally be treated with radioactive iodine, but if facilities for this are not available, then any evidence of failure persisting after full control of the hyperthyroidism has been established should be treated with digoxin and diuretics (pp. 85-90).

Throughout the day of operation the patient should be under basal narcosis until full anaesthesia is required.

POST-OPERATIVE TREATMENT. The first 48 hours after the operation is a relatively critical period. Heat loss is facilitated by cool air and light coverings. Tranquillity is assured by the hypodermic administration of morphine, which may be repeated as required.

The administration of adequate amounts of fluids is most important. If the patient is dehydrated or unable to swallow, an intravenous drip infusion of isotonic glucose and saline should be continued till the patient is able to take fluids by mouth.

In many cases soreness of the throat is a troublesome post-operative feature. This is best controlled by steam inhalations, rest to the voice and sedatives.

In an uncomplicated case such measures are sufficient to carry the patient over to the third or fourth day, when as a rule rapid improvement occurs. Further progress should be uneventful. The patient can usually get up for a short period within a few days of operation, though severe reaction or the presence of cardiac failure, may delay progress considerably. Convalescence should be gradual and after discharge from hospital a holiday of at least a month advised before a return to work is sanctioned.

Post-operative complications. Mortality from the operation is very rare—certainly well below 0·5 per cent. in experienced hands. About 85 per cent. of patients should become euthyroid after operation. Toxicity recurs in from 2 to 4 per cent. of cases, but demonstrable hypothyroidism *may* be found in at least 10 per cent. of patients. In some series, particularly if the thyroid remnant left at operation has been small, or if there is a degree of round-cell infiltration of the gland and circulating thyroid antibodies are present, a much higher proportion may become hypothyroid. Permanent vocal cord damage or hypoparathyroidism occurs in about 2 per cent. of cases. There are other post-operative complications, such as pulmonary collapse, crisis, tetany, haemorrhage or accumulation of serum in the wound. These demand special treatment and will be considered later. It should be stressed that partial thyroidectomy is a highly specialized procedure and should not be performed by a surgeon not fully trained in its technique.

THYROTOXIC CRISIS. This may occur post-operatively if pre-operative preparation of the patient has been inadequate, or may supervene at any time in severe cases under medical treatment. Its occurrence is usually a reflection on the efficiency of the medical control of the case. A common precipitating factor is a pulmonary infection. In all cases its recognition is only too easy: the high fever, extreme tachycardia and great restlessness present an unforgettable clinical picture. The condition, once it has developed, is very intractable and is attended by a high mortality. The essence of treatment is *prevention*. Crisis arises usually in those patients who have been deteriorating for some time, or who have been toxic for months or years and who, therefore, have not had timely and efficient treatment. It frequently occurs in moderate or severely thyrotoxic patients who have defaulted from medical supervision, and is more common in them than after thyroidectomy. It may also result, with fatal consequences, after ill-timed operations (tonsillectomy, etc.) in moderately toxic patients, and cases of previously unrecognized hyperthyroidism may first become apparent with a thyrotoxic crisis developing after an operation for an unrelated condition.

Established cases of hyperthyroid crisis should be treated on the lines detailed for the management of patients after thyroidectomy. Quiet, seclusion and adequate doses of morphine are essentials. Heat loss and avoidance of hyperpyrexia can be aided by tepid sponging, or, in more desperate cases, cold packs and applications of ice-bags to the trunk and limbs. An electric fan may promote heat loss through evaporation. Chlorpromazine can be used to lower the body temperature and, where the equipment is available, hypothermia can be employed. One to two litres of isotonic glucose and saline to which 100 mg. of hydrocortisone hemisuccinate are added should be administered by intravenous infusion. There is a danger of water-logging and pulmonary oedema if large quantities of fluid are given rapidly intravenously. The rate of administration should not exceed half a litre every 60 minutes. Iodine can be given as 300 to 600 mg. of potassium iodide in the intravenous saline. Antithyroid drugs are ineffective in hyperthyroid crisis owing to the number of days which must elapse before they produce an effect, but they should be started as soon as possible. Sympathetic overactivity can be diminished by the use of adrenergic blocking drugs such as propranolol, which can be given in a dose of 10 mg. intravenously and this may be repeated at two-hourly intervals, provided that its use results in slowing of the ventricular rate. The efficient administration of oxygen is important (p. 647).

TETANY AND VOCAL CORD PARALYSIS. With modern surgical technique these complications are now rare except in the case of a second operation undertaken because of a recurrence of thyrotoxicosis. Recurrent thyrotoxicosis should, therefore, be treated by radioactive iodine (see below). Hypoparathyroidism, usually of minor degree and of a temporary nature, characterized by tetany, may develop post-operatively. The treatment of hypoparathyroidism is dealt with on p. 299.

HAEMORRHAGE. Massive haemorrhage seldom occurs, but causes local tension, and may result in symptoms from pressure on the trachea. It should be remembered that oozing of serous fluid frequently occurs and may cause swelling in the region of the wound. In all cases of doubt as to the nature of such a swelling the opinion of the surgeon should be sought.

HYPOTHYROIDISM. The possibility of this late complication should never be overlooked, for the reasons mentioned above, and any patient who has had a partial thyroidectomy should be reviewed periodically with this in mind for the rest of his or her life.

Radioactive iodine. The overactive thyroid concentrates circulating iodine very efficiently. Radiation delivered by the radioactive isotope ^{131}I can abolish hyperthyroidism by depressing the functional activity of the gland and by inducing cell destruction and radiation fibrosis.

About 60 per cent. of patients treated with ^{131}I become euthyroid after a single treatment with the isotope, and about 30 per cent. require a second dose. The only common complication of this treatment so far encountered is hypothyroidism, which is found to develop in up to 50 per cent. of patients treated with conventional doses if they are followed for as long as 10 years. Transient hypothyroidism may occur, the phenomenon being due to temporary damage to some of the thyroid cells and to subsequent hypertrophy or hyperplasia of the remainder, but in such patients late onset hypothyroidism is also frequent. Most patients who are going to develop permanent hypothyroidism do so within three to five months after receiving ^{131}I. Nevertheless, there is a continuing tendency for hypothyroidism to result irrespective of the dosage and technique used, although the latent period before hypothyroidism develops may be protracted if small doses are used. Hypothyroidism occurs because the regenerative capacity of the cells in the gland is more sensitive to radiation than is the capacity of the cells to make hormone. The frequency with which hypothyroidism develops after treatment with ^{131}I demands the continued supervision of patients so treated to ensure that this iatrogenic hypothyroidism does not go undetected, and all patients treated with ^{131}I must be reviewed periodically for the rest of their lives.

Attempts have been made to diminish the extent or postpone the onset of hypothyroidism by administering half the conventional dose of ^{131}I. This technique undoubtedly does result in a lower incidence of hypothyroidism after five years, but the result is achieved at the expense of very prolonged antithyroid drug treatment for many patients after they have received the ^{131}I.

Although considerable improvement may be observed within a month after the patient has received a dose of ^{131}I, this may not be maximal for two or three months. Thus there may be a considerable time-lag between administering the dose and the abolition of hyperthyroidism. In seriously thyrotoxic patients, therefore, when rapid control of hyperthyroidism is essential, and especially in those showing signs of cardiac failure, it seems wise to use this form of treatment in conjunction with antithyroid drugs. The drugs should be given in the way described (p. 294) until the severe manifestations of hyperthyroidism are controlled. They should then be withdrawn for 48 hours before and after giving the therapeutic dose of ^{131}I. They should be used freely in gradually decreasing dosage to control any hyperthyroidism continuing after ^{131}I therapy.

Treatment with ^{131}I is extremely simple and brings about a euthyroid state in a large proportion of cases without an operation or prolonged drug therapy. Nevertheless, it demands special facilities in properly equipped centres so that it is not as yet as widely available as antithyroid drugs or surgery. It is, nevertheless, the simplest form of treatment for the patient, and is often desirable on that account alone. For example, seriously ill patients such as those with heart disease, can be treated easily and quickly by the administration of a sufficiently large dose of ^{131}I to ablate the thyroid gland. Replacement treatment with thyroxine should be started as soon as the patient is euthyroid without awaiting the development of evidence of hypothyroidism.

The optimal dose of ^{131}I will vary greatly from patient to patient and depends upon a large number of factors—particularly the size and nodularity of the thyroid. Using a tracer dose it is possible to calculate the theoretical therapeutic requirements of ^{131}I by measuring its uptake by the thyroid, the rate of its elimination from the gland and by attempting to assess the volume of gland tissue to be irradiated. Experience has shown, however, that these techniques have not yielded results superior to those based on a clinical evaluation of the size and type of gland to be dealt with and the clinical condition of the patient. The range of dose frequently employed for a first treatment varies from 8 to 20 or more millicuries.

Ocular complications of thyroid disease. Lid retraction and exophthalmos are commonly associated with hyperthyroidism. The former is usually seen only while hyperthyroidism persists and requires no specific treatment. Exophthalmos, on the other hand, varies greatly in severity and it may precede, accompany or follow an episode of hyperthyroidism, or it may occur by itself. Occasionally it appears to be associated with hypothyroidism. At one time it was thought to be due to an exophthalmos producing substance analogous to and possibly chemically related to the pituitary thyroid stimulating hormone. For this reason, the treatment of thyroid disorders tends to be regarded as a factor that might modify the behaviour of exophthalmos, and it would be unwise to ignore this possibility. On the other hand, apart from ensuring that patients with exophthalmos are never allowed to develop thyroid insufficiency, little help can be expected from attempts to suppress exophthalmos by treatment with thyroxine.

Exophthalmos in turn may be complicated by symptoms of conjunctivitis with complaints of 'grittiness', aching, epiphora and photophobia, as well as more striking features such as diplopia and chemosis. Conjunctival oedema may be so severe that the patient may be unable to close his eyes. In these circumstances the integrity of the cornea may be threatened. Diplopia may be suppressed by wearing a shade over one eye at a time, and chemosis may improve a little or develop less rapidly if the patient can manage to sleep in a semi-upright posture. Lateral tarsorrhaphy is a simple procedure and should be considered and discussed with an ophthalmologist before exophthalmos has progressed unduly. In severe cases decompression of the retro-orbital space may be required. Irradiation of the pituitary gland is probably fruitless, but irradiation of the retro-orbital tissues sometimes seems to slow or even arrest the progress of exophthalmos. Corticosteroid therapy has been tried in the past and found useless. Local treatment with 5 per cent. guanethidine drops is often helpful, although it may cause keratitis, and supervision by an ophthalmologist is essential.

The benefit of a simple measure such as wearing dark glasses to reduce photophobia and the discomfort arising from wind and dust should not be overlooked.

THE PARATHYROID GLANDS

Substances acting on Calcium Metabolism

Calcium metabolism depends upon a series of factors serving together to maintain the integrity of the skeleton, and to control neuromuscular excitability so that tetany does not occur. Among these factors must be included the amount of calcium and phosphorus in the diet, the efficiency with which calcium is absorbed from the jejunum, the concentration of the serum proteins to which calcium is bound, and the pH of the blood which in turn determines the proportion of the calcium in serum held in the ionized state and the renal function. Finally, the parathyroid hormone, calcitonin and calciferol (Vitamin D), are further important factors.

In normal circumstances parathyroid hormone is secreted in response to a fall in the concentration of calcium in the blood, and the hormone minimizes this fall by mobilizing calcium (and normally phosphorus as well) from bone. It increases the excretion of phosphorus by the kidney. Calciferol enhances the absorption of calcium, raises its concentration in blood, and facilitates its deposition in bone. Calciferol also increases the excretion of calcium in urine. Deficiency of this vitamin and of the parathyroid hormone, together or separately, may be associated with depression of the concentration of calcium in blood. Either in excess will produce hypercalcaemia which, if severe and not treated vigorously, may lead to death in uraemia. In chemical terms, the parathyroid hormone is a polypeptide extractable from the glands of animals; to be therapeutically effective it must be given by intravenous injection. Its action is short lived and unresponsiveness develops rapidly with repeated injections. For this reason, serum calcium deficiency due to hypoparathyroidism, as well as to other causes, is usually treated with vitamin D or an analogue, in preference to parathyroid extract.

Calcitonin is a peptide hormone secreted by the parafollicular cells of the thyroid gland. Its principal actions include depression of the blood calcium concentration, and in this respect it can be regarded as an antagonist of the parathyroid hormone.

Vitamin D is most appropriately regarded as a group of three sterols with similar pharmacological activities. The most widely used preparation is calciferol or vitamin D_2, providing 40,000 international units of activity per mg. The standard B.P. tablet contains 1·25 mg. or 50,000 i.u., and is widely used for the treatment of calcium deficiency states in the adult. Vitamin D_3 or 7-dehydrocholesterol is found in fish-liver oils, particularly of halibut; it is also the natural vitamin formed in the skin when this is irradiated by sunlight or by artificial sources of ultraviolet light. Vitamin D itself is converted to 25-hydroxycholecalciferol, in which form its potency is enhanced.

Another analogue, dihydrotachysterol, is now available in pure form. It may occasionally have certain advantages over calciferol and can be used as an alternative. It is much more expensive.

Hypoparathyroidism

Acute parathyroid insufficiency with tetany may occur as an emergency after removal of a parathyroid tumour, and should be anticipated when patients have radiological or biochemical evidence of associated bone disease. Tetany will also develop after a total thyroidectomy performed for carcinoma of the thyroid, and it is not uncommon, though usually transient, after subtotal thyroidectomy undertaken for hyperthyroidism. Chronic parathyroid insufficiency may occur spontaneously, or as a sequel to one of the acute forms of the disorder. Tetany is usually due to depression of the blood calcium concentration, or to an alteration in its physical state (a reduction in the proportion present in the ionized form). Nevertheless, when patients fail to respond to orthodox measures, magnesium and potassium depletion or alkalosis should be suspected.

Whatever its origin, severe tetany should be treated immediately by an intravenous injection of 20 ml. of 10 per cent. calcium gluconate. This should be given slowly over the course of 5 to 10 minutes, and should be repeated as often as necessary to relieve recurrent severe cramp, paraesthesiae and carpo-pedal or laryngeal spasm. The need for repeated injections will depend upon the severity of the tetany, the extent of the calcium deficit in the tissues, and the efficacy of other corrective measures, for example, treatment with calciferol (see below). It should be noted that each of the injections recommended provides a dose of 180 mg. only of calcium. The distinction is sometimes made between treating tetany due to a total calcium deficit, and that due to a reduction of the ionized fraction of calcium in the blood. The concentration of ionic calcium in blood depends upon several factors; the most common cause of derangement is the state of alkalosis, a frequent cause of tetany.

If the aetiology of hypocalcaemic tetany suggests that it is likely to be persistent, treatment with calciferol should be started at once in a dose of 1·25 mg. thrice daily. Although a few days' delay may occur before a full response is obtained, there is seldom justification for the use of parathyroid extract. The plasma calcium concentration should be checked daily, and the dose adjusted accordingly, bearing in mind that the response is delayed, and will also persist for several days or even weeks when the dose is reduced or the drug is withdrawn. It is important, therefore, to know whether the concentration of calcium in the blood is rising or falling rather than to depend upon a single observation, since this will make it easier to predict the patient's requirements. As soon as tetany has been abolished or the serum calcium concentration exceeds 9·5 mg. per 100 ml., the dose of calciferol should be reduced to 1·25 mg. daily, and it may then be adjusted according to the symptoms and the biochemical findings. If the serum calcium concentration exceeds 10·5 mg. per 100 ml., the administration of calciferol should be stopped until the blood level is normal, and should then be started again in reduced amount. A final daily dose of 1·25 to 2·5 mg. is usually sufficient. It is important to recognize that a patient's requirements may vary and for this reason the dose of calciferol should be reviewed at intervals according to the blood level of calcium.

Patients who are taking these drugs should be warned of their potential capacity to produce thirst and polyuria, headache, vomiting and diarrhoea, weakness and lethargy, and to report immediately should symptoms of this type appear. The continuance of treatment under such circumstances would involve the risk of death in coma with uraemia, as may occur in fulminating hyperparathyroidism with hypercalcaemia (p. 300).

Milk and cheese, in spite of being rich in calcium, are contraindicated as sources of additional calcium because of their high phosphorus content. Other foods rich in phosphorus such as egg-yolk and cauliflower should also be omitted. Phosphate absorption from the alimentary tract can be diminished by giving 50 ml. of aluminium hydroxide gel three times a day with meals and the calcium intake can be increased by the administration of 2 g. of calcium lactate three times a day which is equivalent to 780 mg. of calcium daily. Calcium gluconate tablets (B.P.C.) contain only 55 mg. of calcium in each tablet of 600 mg., so nearly 20 tablets require to be taken daily to provide 1 g. of calcium. On the other hand, Sandocal Effervescent tablets each contain 400 mg. of calcium.

Hyperparathyroidism

The diagnosis of hyperparathyroidism may be suspected on clinical grounds alone, but confirmation may require protracted biochemical and other investigations. The condition may be due to hyperplasia or an adenoma (very rarely carcinoma) of one or more of the parathyroid glands which may lie in the neck, or occasionally in the superior mediastinum. It is essential that the diagnosis should be established beyond any reasonable doubt before operation is proposed, since once the decision to operate has been taken, the surgeon must be prepared to find and to identify each of the parathyroid glands. The search may occasionally involve opening the superior mediastinum by splitting the sternum. Facilities must be available at the time of operation for the examination of frozen sections of any biopsy tissue removed.

The post-operative treatment is carried out on general lines, but a careful watch must be kept for early signs of tetany. Should these make their appearance, the intensive treatment described on p. 299 must be instituted.

The results of operation are good provided renal calcification or infection has not resulted in uraemia. The serum calcium concentration usually falls to normal or subnormal levels within 24 hours though the serum phosphorus is restored more gradually. A great improvement in health with disappearance of skeletal and urinary symptoms may be expected. When the skeleton has been involved it naturally takes longer for the bones to recover their normal texture, and months may elapse before there is much reduction of the plasma concentration of alkaline phosphatase. This delay serves to emphasize the need for an adequate intake of calcium for a long time.

Hypercalcaemia

Episodic or persistent hypercalcaemia may be a feature of a variety of diseases. While treatment of the primary cause is a matter of some urgency, there is usually sufficient time for full assessment of the patient and to study the response to treatment. Occasionally, however, the serum concentration of calcium may mount rapidly to levels where thirst and polyuria, drowsiness and apathy progress to uraemia, coma and death. Hypercalcaemia then requires urgent and specific treatment. Adequate hydration and promotion of diuresis by conventional methods should be provided. Prednisone,

10 mg. thrice daily, should be given for carcinomatosis, sarcoidosis and vitamin D intoxication, but is not of value in hyperparathyroidism. When daily estimations of serum calcium concentrations show deterioration in hypercalcaemic crisis, sodium edetate may be given in doses of 50 mg. per kg. of body weight by intravenous infusion in 500 ml. of 5 per cent. dextrose solution or isotonic sodium chloride; the infusion should be maintained at a rate of 500 ml. in each four hours until the serum calcium concentration has been lowered appropriately. This treatment may be associated with renal damage, and the urine should be examined regularly for albumin.

Inorganic phosphate has been shown to reduce hypercalcaemia and should be used if other methods fail, but its value is not yet established. Phosphate can be administered either by mouth or, if vomiting precludes this, by the intravenous route. For oral use, either disodium or dipotassium phosphate can be given in quantities sufficient to provide 1 to 4 g. of phosphorus daily. For intravenous use, one litre of a 0·1 molar sterile mixture of disodium phosphate (0·081 mole) and monopotassium phosphate (0·019 mole) will provide a solution of pH 7·4, and this can be given by infusion over eight hours. Careful control of serum electrolyte concentrations must be observed.

Calcitonin, which depresses the serum calcium in hypercalcaemia, is not available for general clinical use.

THE ADRENAL GLANDS

Adrenal Insufficiency

Adrenal insufficiency is not uncommon nowadays. It may be secondary to hypopituitarism or may follow bilateral adrenalectomy performed for Cushing's disease, metastatic mammary cancer and even, occasionally, for hypertension. Defective function may persist for a variable and unpredictable period following corticosteroid therapy. Every precaution should be taken to prevent acute adrenal insufficiency arising, as it is so frequently fatal. It must be treated with speed and intensity.

Addison's disease. This disorder, first described in a classic monograph by Thomas Addison in 1855, is a state of chronic adrenal insufficiency. It may result from *primary* disease of the adrenals due to tuberculosis, or atrophy as a result of an autoimmunizing reaction analogous to lymphadenoid goitre, occasionally to infarction and malignant disease, and very rarely to syphilis, the reticuloses or giant cell granuloma. It is important to diagnose adrenocortical insufficiency before it has advanced to the stage of complete failure which the term Addison's disease implies. In many cases destruction or atrophy of the cortex may be incomplete so that some secretion may persist without, however, allowing for any reserve.

There is excessive loss of sodium chloride and water in the urine and retention of potassium, due to deficient secretion of sodium retaining hormones, particularly aldosterone; as a result, haemoconcentration, hypotension and dehydration occur. The reduced secretion of hydrocortisone causes a tendency to hypoglycaemia and an increased sensitivity to harmful stresses of all kinds. Treatment should aim at redressing these disturbances by suitable mineralocorticoid and glucocorticoid replacement therapy.

Effective substitution therapy has proved lifesaving and enables the patient to enjoy a full and active life and a sense of well-being little removed from the normal. It must, however, always be remembered that maintenance treatment, quite satisfactory for ordinary purposes, may prove entirely inadequate at times of stress. Infections or intercurrent illnesses, injuries and the administration of drugs such as narcotics or anaesthetics may precipitate Addisonian crisis unless replacement treatment is increased. Such crises occur suddenly, are characterized by fever, delirium or coma, vomiting and dehydration, hypotension and peripheral circulatory failure.

MAINTENANCE TREATMENT. For maintenance purposes the dose of cortisone, which is preferable to analogues for replacement therapy, varies from 25 to 37·5 mg. a day (1 to 1½ tablets). Replacement doses of this size never give rise to the undesirable side-effects observed in conditions in which the drug is given in much larger doses. On the other hand maintenance doses are insufficient to restore completely the sodium depletion of Addison's disease and to maintain the body fluids and blood pressure at a normal level. The administration of larger doses or the addition to the diet of 10 g. of sodium chloride a day will have this effect, but the supplementary use of a steroid with a greater sodium-retaining activity than cortisone is preferable.

Fludrocortisone has a sodium-retaining activity approaching that of aldosterone, but a weak glucocorticoid effect. For most patients the ideal maintenance treatment is the combination of 0·1 or 0·2 mg. of fludrocortisone daily with 25 to 37·5 mg. of cortisone.

Doctors should always have a supply of hydrocortisone sodium succinate (B.P.) available for injection. This should be substituted immediately for oral cortisone and fludrocortisone whenever a patient is unable to take and to retain corticosteroids given orally.

Some cases of Addison's disease are still due to tuberculosis. Thus, active tuberculous disease in other parts of the body, particularly in the lungs, bones and genito-urinary tract, must not be overlooked and when present must receive appropriate treatment (see p. 67).

TREATMENT IN CRISIS. Addisonian crisis is a medical emergency which demands the most energetic treatment in hospital where the patient can be given constant skilled nursing and medical care. The general measures employed for the treatment of shock should be initiated.

At least 5 litres of isotonic glucose and saline should be administered in the course of 24 hours, at first rapidly and then, as improvement occurs, more slowly. Hydrocortisone sodium succinate (100 mg.) is given as a single intravenous injection; thereafter it is added to the intravenous infusion and is continued, according to the state of the patient, at a rate of from 50 to 75 mg. every six hours. Crisis is often precipitated by infection and it is then necessary to employ suitable antibiotics. This treatment should be supplemented by intramuscular injections of 10 mg. of deoxycortone acetate twice in the first 24 hours. Sufficient hormonal treatment and glucose and saline should be given to maintain the patient's systolic blood pressure at a level above 100 mm. Hg., or a pulse pressure of 30 mm. Hg., but, on the other hand, care must be taken to avoid inducing pulmonary and peripheral oedema. Should either occur, 40 to 80 mg. of the diuretic, frusemide, should be injected intravenously.

CORTICOSTEROID THERAPY FOR ADRENAL INSUFFICIENCY ASSOCIATED WITH MAJOR SURGICAL PROCEDURES. At the time of any major surgical operation, replacement therapy with full doses of corticosteroids will be required for patients with Addison's disease, for patients undergoing bilateral adrenalectomy or hypophysectomy for any cause and for those who have had such operations previously.

About the time of operation and because of the obvious necessity to avoid oral treatment, corticosteroids should be given by injection. Cortisone is most suitable for this purpose. For elective operations, on the evening before operation a single intramuscular injection of 100 mg. of cortisone acetate should be given, and on the morning of operation a further injection of 200 mg. After operation, these injections should be repeated in doses of 50 mg. at intervals of six hours. Provided the progress of the patient is satisfactory, the dose can be reduced and the oral route of administration can be adopted within 24 hours. If the patient has been accustomed to a high circulating concentration of corticosteroids before operation, for example in Cushing's syndrome, it is essential to continue to use much larger doses of corticosteroid in replacement therapy for considerably longer than would be needed for a patient who has previously had a bilateral adrenalectomy and who has been on normal maintenance doses for some time. Following adrenalectomy, in the absence of post-operative infection, pulmonary complications, or electrolyte abnormalities, the patient can be expected to make an uninterrupted recovery on successive total daily divided doses of cortisone of 200, 150, 150, 100, 100, 75, 75, 50, 50 and finally 37·5 mg. At this stage it may be appropriate to add 0·1 mg. of fludrocortisone once or twice daily, depending on the patient's blood pressure and sense of well-being. Supplements of potassium chloride should be maintained until a normal diet has been resumed. If convalescence is interrupted or delayed, a reduction of the dose of corticosteroid should also be postponed until recovery is again in progress.

Adrenal apoplexy (*Waterhouse-Friderichsen Syndrome*). In the course of fulminating septicaemia—particularly acute meningococcal septicaemia—haemorrhage may occur into the adrenals. The resulting shock, abdominal pain, intense purple cyanosis, ecchymotic haemorrhages and an extremely low blood pressure, create an unforgettable clinical picture. The patient speedily becomes unconscious and quickly dies unless given hydrocortisone. Acute adrenal insufficiency of this type may also occur in other severe illnesses such as acute respiratory failure with CO_2 retention.

Energetic treatment is essential and, apart from the control of the associated septicaemia with antibiotics, treatment is the same as for severe Addisonian crisis.

Adrenocortical Hyperfunction

Many syndromes may result from adrenocortical hyperfunction; thus, Cushing's syndrome is due to an increased secretion of hydrocortisone; the adrenogenital syndrome occurs when there is hypersecretion mainly of the cortical androgens; while the syndrome of primary aldosteronism results from hypersecretion of aldosterone. In congenital adrenal hyperplasia, the patient may actually be suffering from adrenal insufficiency because the glands are unable to synthesize hydrocortisone in spite of the secretion of large quantities of precursors of this steroid. These are not substitutes for hydrocortisone and increase the patient's disability by provoking virilization. Although it is convenient for purposes of description to make such clear-cut distinctions between these conditions, it must be realized that considerable overlapping between them may occur, giving rise to signs and symptoms which are intermediate between the typical clinical pictures.

The rapid development of severe features of Cushing's syndrome, particularly when associated with marked potassium depletion, may be due to the ectopic production of ACTH, by, in particular, bronchogenic carcinoma. Palliative treatment only is possible, as most cases are rapidly fatal.

Cushing's syndrome. This may be due to hyperplasia of both adrenals or to a benign or malignant tumour of one of them with atrophy of the other. Biochemical and radiological examinations may distinguish between the two conditions.

An adrenal tumour should be removed if obvious metastases are not present. As the contralateral adrenal is nearly always atrophic and devoid of function, acute—and probably fatal—adrenocortical insufficiency will result unless careful substitution therapy is undertaken before, during and after the operation (see above). In particular, patients may have profound potassium depletion and a metabolic alkalosis, and these disorders must be corrected by the administration of potassium chloride before operation. Subsequently the administration of cortisone should be reduced very gradually and an attempt can be made to stimulate residual adrenal cortical tissue by injecting 40 units of corticotrophin gel twice daily. The need for this type of treatment can be assessed by appropriate blood and urinary steroid assays. In some patients no response occurs and substitution therapy will have to be continued for life (p. 301).

The results of surgical removal of an adenoma, given adequate pre- and post-operative treatment, are dramatically successful, but the prognosis in carcinoma is poor because metastases to the lungs and liver occur early.

Convalescence following operation in non-malignant cases of Cushing's syndrome is liable to be slow and patients may experience some mental depression, apathy and obscure gastro-intestinal symptoms for many weeks. These symptoms may demand prolonged treatment with high doses of cortisone until a maintenance dosage can be reached. A high protein diet, 4 g. of potassium chloride daily and an intramuscular injection of 25 mg. of testosterone propionate three times a week, will hasten the recovery phase, but 25 mg. of nandrolone injected weekly is a preferable alternative for female patients. Owing to the associated osteoporosis, orthopaedic supports to the spine may be necessary for a time.

When Cushing's syndrome is due to bilateral adrenal hyperplasia, total adrenalectomy is the treatment of choice. Although there is much evidence to suggest that the adrenal hyperplasia is due to excessive secretion of corticotrophin from the basophil cells of the pituitary, the mortality and complications following hypophysectomy are greater than with bilateral adrenalectomy. Irradiation of the pituitary and subtotal adrenalectomy are unsatisfactory.

The adrenogenital syndrome. An increased output of androgenic steroids may cause: (1) in foetal life and in the newborn, female pseudo-hermaphroditism and in males macrogenitosomia praecox; (2) before puberty, sexual precocity with coincident virilization in the female; and (3) at or after puberty, virilism.

Sexual precocity of adrenocortical aetiology is often due to a malignant tumour. An attempt should be made to remove the tumour, but the prognosis is poor.

Bilateral hyperplasia of the adrenal cortex causing the adrenogenital syndrome in the adult may be improved occasionally by suppressive treatment with corticosteroids, the dose being adjusted to reduce the 17-oxosteroid (ketosteroid) excretion in the urine to below 8 mg. in the 24 hours. When the adrenogenital syndrome is due to an adenoma or adenocarcinoma, or when a mixed picture of Cushing's syndrome and virilism exists, the treatment is surgical, with subsequent replacement therapy as described for Cushing's syndrome

(p. 301). In the absence of malignancy the results are good and signs of virilism disappear in the course of a year, though the deepened voice persists as the organic changes in the larynx are permanent.

CONGENITAL ADRENAL HYPERPLASIA presenting in the infant may readily be overlooked, but when recognized can be treated easily and effectively with corticosteroids. It is important that the dose administered should be adjusted to the smallest amount that will suppress production of abnormal steroid metabolites by the hyperplastic adrenals. Suppression can be confirmed by assays of urine for pregnanetriol, 17-oxosteroids or 17-hydroxycorticosteroids at appropriate intervals.

Primary aldosteronism. The isolated hyper-secretion of aldosterone is much more often due to an adrenocortical tumour than to diffuse adreno-cortical hyperplasia. The presenting manifestations are hypertension, severe muscular weakness, tetany, polydipsia and polyuria in association with hypokalaemia, hypernatraemia and alkalosis. Effective treatment is by surgical extirpation of the tumour or, more rarely, bilateral adrenalectomy if adrenocortical hyperplasia is the cause. It may be difficult to correct the hypokalaemia by the administration of potassium before operation as such treatment usually stimulates further aldosterone secretion; large doses should be given immediately before, during and after the operation and may be combined with the use of the aldosterone antagonist, spironolactone, in doses of 100 mg. six-hourly, until the source of the aldosterone has been removed.

If the diagnosis cannot be established with sufficient certainty to justify radical surgery, control of hypertension and potassium depletion may be obtained for prolonged periods with spironolactone in the minimum effective dose.

Tumours of the Adrenal Medulla

Neuroblastoma of the adrenal medulla are extremely malignant tumours usually occurring in children, and are practically never diagnosed in time to permit of their successful removal.

Tumours of chromaffin tissue, producing excess noradrenaline or adrenaline or both, may occur in the adrenal medulla or elsewhere in the sympathetic nervous system. The initial paroxysmal hypertension from such a phaeochromocytoma may later become fixed if removal of the tumour is unduly delayed.

Phentolamine, an antagonist of noradrenaline, may be given to reduce the blood pressure of patients with hypertension, known or suspected to be due to a phaeochromocytoma. It is given intravenously in doses of 5 mg., repeated if necessary, but the effect of this drug is quite transitory. It is primarily used for diagnostic purposes, but it is also particularly valuable at the time of operation in preventing acute pulmonary oedema or heart failure due to the release into the circulation of large quantities of noradrenaline.

Before operation it is also worth considering, as part of the premedication regimen, the use of α and β-sympathetic receptor site blocking agents such as phenoxybenzamine and propranolol.

MALE HYPOGONADISM

The testes have two functions: the production of spermatozoa by the seminiferous tubules and the secretion of androgens by the interstitial cells. Testicular deficiency may result in a complete or moderate loss of one or both functions. Both are regulated by the gonadotrophic hormones from the anterior pituitary, and hypogonadism may be secondary to hypopituitarism or due to primary testicular failure. The signs of testicular insufficiency vary according to whether this commences before or after puberty. In the former case insufficient androgen secretion results in excessive length of the limbs, poor muscular development, high-pitched voice, female type of thyroid cartilage and lack of facial and abdominal hair. When testicular insufficiency occurs after puberty there is no skeletal abnormality, but there may be excessive deposition of fat around the trunk. Sexual activity may be diminished or absent, while there is generally some decrease in the size of the external genitalia. Psychological and emotional disturbances occur.

Primary hypogonadism. The treatment of primary testicular failure consists in replacing the male hormone. It is well, however, to remember that many boys mature late, so that it is unwise and may actually be harmful, to begin the administration of androgens too early, since it may stop growth. If, however, the decision is taken to treat the patient, fluoxymesterone should be given by mouth in doses of 5 to 20 mg. daily until signs of improvement occur. Thereafter the dose should be reduced to the minimum found to be adequate, usually 5 to 10 mg. daily.

Beneficial changes are noted within a few weeks of starting treatment. The genitalia, with the exception of the testes, become larger, while the character of the skin, hair and voice begin to approximate to those found in the normal male. Libido and potency are stimulated and a feeling of well-being develops, due to the improvement in musculature and the acquisition of self-confidence. Epiphyseal lines close in adults in whom they may have remained open beyond the normal time. Sterility, of course, persists.

Secondary hypogonadism. In older patients relief of hypogonadism resulting from hypopituitarism (p. 288) may not be a matter of special concern. It usually becomes obvious that there is no hope of inducing normal sexual function with spermatogenesis and fertility; the indications then are simply to improve the secondary sexual characteristics by androgen replacement therapy in the same manner as for primary testicular failure.

Failure of spermatogenesis. Many males are quite normal in regard to secondary sex characteristics but are deficient in spermatogenesis. This abnormality is usually discovered from sperm analysis or testicular biopsy undertaken during the investigation of a barren marriage. In such patients a careful investigation should be made to exclude systemic disease, and if this is capable of correction spermatogenesis may improve. An obstruction to the efferent duct system may be removed surgically. In many patients, however, no systemic disorders are discovered and, as little is known of the aetiology of azoöspermia or oligospermia, attempts at treatment are unsatisfactory.

It is rational to employ follicle-stimulating hormone when this is available and of proven potency. Paradoxically some success occasionally follows a short intensive course of testosterone. Testosterone propionate is injected intramuscularly in 25 mg. doses three or four times a week for about four months. This results in the total suppression of any spermatogenesis which may be present; but after stopping this treatment a rebound phenomenon may occur and in a few cases the sperm count rises above its pre-treatment level.

It must be emphasized that impotence in the male is usually due to psychological causes. The use of testosterone in such patients is not justified on any sound clinical evidence or by any theoretical consideration; in small doses it may do no harm, but in large doses it will inhibit spermatogenesis.

Klinefelter's syndrome. This syndrome is characterized by failure of spermatogenesis and a high excretion of follicle-stimulating hormone. Barr bodies (sex chromatin) are found in buccal smears, and chromosome studies show the patients to have more than one X chromosome. The hypogonadism may require replacement therapy, and plastic surgery may be necessary for the associated gynaecomastia.

Cryptorchidism. Should cryptorchidism persist to the age of 10 years, an attempt should be made to treat the condition surgically. If this is not done, damage to the seminiferous tubules invariably occurs, and there is a risk of cancer developing later in the undescended testis.

The ultimate functional results in those patients in whom orchidopexy has been technically possible without damage to the blood supply is a matter of speculation. In view of the disparity of opinion and the paucity of long-term follow-up studies a cautious prognosis should be given regarding subsequent fertility in such patients. Androgen therapy is unjustifiable.

Mumps orchitis. This is unfortunately common and results in a variable degree of testicular atrophy in about a third of the patients who develop it. A short course of prednisone has been claimed to be of value in suppressing the inflammatory oedema during the acute phase. Otherwise treatment is limited to rest in bed, the support of the testes by a suspensory bandage and the tapping of a hydrocele should it form.

The male climacteric and premature senility. These may be regarded as occasional indications for androgen therapy. It is doubtful, however, whether any useful effect can be attributed to their treatment with androgens. Reports of clinical trials are not convincing, and it is, therefore, unwise to use androgens as a routine therapeutic measure for these conditions.

The male hormone is of value for its metabolic effect in conserving nitrogen. Even its beneficial effect on eunuchs is to some extent due to the improvement in their musculature consequent on its anabolic action on protein metabolism. Thus it may be used not only in hypopituitarism (p. 288) but to assist in the correction of other conditions associated with a severely negative nitrogen balance, in the preparation of cachectic patients for surgery and in osteoporosis. The value of testosterone in the palliative treatment of metastatic cancer of the breast is discussed below.

HORMONES IN THE TREATMENT OF CARCINOMA

Hormone therapy has been tried in a variety of malignant conditions, but as a measure of established value it is at present largely confined to the palliative treatment of carcinoma of the prostate and of the breast.

Carcinoma of the prostate. Prostatic carcinoma can be favourably influenced by castration, and a similar effect can be achieved by giving oestrogenic substances. One explanation of this is that the oestrogen suppresses the activity of the anterior lobe of the pituitary and thus, by restricting the supply of gonadotrophic hormone to the testes, diminishes the secretion of androgens necessary for the progression of the carcinoma.

Experience has firmly established the value of oestrogen therapy in inoperable prostatic carcinoma, and has shown that stilboestrol, a synthetic analogue, is convenient and effective. With stilboestrol a favourable result may be expected in 80 per cent. or more of cases. Not only is there some increase in the expectation of life, but even in advanced cases there may be striking symptomatic improvement. The duration of the improvement is variable, but may be expected to persist for a year or more in 50 per cent. of cases, and up to five years in 15 per cent.

ADMINISTRATION AND DOSAGE. Stilboestrol therapy should start with doses of 5 mg. three times daily by mouth. The patient should remain on this dose permanently, and this must be impressed upon him. If necessary, it may be raised to 20 mg. or more daily but it may be possible to reduce it if the clinical state remains satisfactory. Clinical improvement is accompanied by a fall in the serum acid phosphate level if this is raised. Castration is also effective in controlling carcinoma of the prostate, and the most satisfactory results occur after combining castration with oestrogen therapy.

SIDE-EFFECTS. Nausea and vomiting may occur and prevent an effective dosage of oestrogens being achieved. Testicular atrophy and loss of erectile power inevitably occur and in most patients enlargement of the breasts, and pigmentation of nipples result. These effects, however, are a small price to pay for the benefits often obtained.

Carcinoma of the breast. Hormones are of value in the management of advanced and inoperable cases of mammary carcinoma, but it must be emphasized that they should in no way be regarded as substitutes for surgery or radiotherapy in patients suitable for these measures. Analogous to the influence of orchidectomy on prostatic carcinoma, ovariectomy or, in the male, bilateral orchidectomy may exert a palliative effect on cancer of the breast. In the pre-menopausal patient this should always be performed either surgically or by ovarian irradiation before hormone therapy is considered. Adrenalectomy or hypophysectomy can also in some instances cause a dramatic temporary arrest of the disease.

OESTROGENS. It has been shown that synthetic oestrogens may cause retardation or even regression of the growth of the tumour. The results are inferior to those obtained in cancer of the prostate, favourable responses being less frequent and of shorter duration. Moreover, in younger women oestrogens accelerate the course of the disease. Oestrogen treatment of mammary cancer should, therefore, be restricted to women who are five or more years beyond the menopause. The older the patient, the more likely is regression to occur. Stilboestrol is the drug usually employed. The dose is similar to that for prostatic carcinoma, and is limited in order to avoid toxic effects.

Recurrent or metastatic carcinoma of the breast in men should be treated by castration, radiotherapy and oestrogens as recommended for women.

ANDROGENS. Androgen therapy may be used as a palliative measure in advanced mammary carcinoma. Considerable symptomatic benefit may occur, both in younger and in older women, but androgens should not be used for this purpose in men. In post-menopausal women, however, oestrogen therapy is preferable to androgen therapy at every decade. Osteolytic metastases may improve, pain and tenderness may disappear, osteolytic lesions may become recalcified and ulcerating lesions of the skin may heal. Relief from pressure symptoms caused by intrathoracic metastases may occur, but substantial improvement results only in about 20 per cent. of cases and may persist for only a few months, although remissions of five years or more have been recorded. Fluoxymesterone is given in the same way as for androgen replacement therapy (p. 304), but a wide range of alternative drugs is available.

Side-effects of androgen therapy include signs of masculinization which may appear after three months. Increased libido may be distressing to the patient. Metabolic effects may occur, some of which may be beneficial, such as increasing alertness, strength and weight, but others like oedema, drowsiness, thirst, headache, nausea and vomiting are obviously undesirable.

CORTICOSTEROIDS. Prednisone and other analogues of cortisone have been used with some success as substitutes for adrenalectomy. Striking remissions may result and the treatment has the advantage of increasing euphoria and causing few serious side-effects. This method of treatment should always be considered along with the others which have been described, but if employed only suppressive doses should be used, such as 5 mg. of prednisone eight-hourly.

FEMALE SEX ENDOCRINOLOGY

Introduction. The reproductive life of female mammals is dominated by a repeated cycle of events, consequent upon the secretion, in an orderly sequence, of a variety of hormones from the brain, the pituitary, the ovaries and, in some cases, the uterus. Endocrine disease arises from an interruption in this series of events: the diagnosis and treatment of the condition depends on identifying the defect and, if possible, setting it right.

There is ample evidence that outside stimuli affect the sex cycle of female mammals. In the human female there is often a clear association between psychological stress and amenorrhoea, and it is likely that many of the aberrations of sex endocrine function presented to the clinician are of psychological origin.

The Female Sex Cycle

Certain areas of the hypothalamus such as the supra-optic or the paraventricular nuclei exert a profound influence on sex endocrinology. They produce releasing factors, or in some cases inhibiting factors, which control the secretion of the anterior pituitary gland. These factors are produced by hypothalamic nuclei and released from nerve endings in the walls of the capillaries which drain directly to the anterior pituitary gland.

Three gonadotrophic hormones are produced by the anterior lobe of the pituitary: the mammatrophic hormone, prolactin, the follicle stimulating hormone (FSH) and the luteinizing hormone (LH). In the male LH is usually called the interstitial cell stimulating hormone (ICSH).

FSH controls the maturation of sperm and, by

virtue of the fact that FSH is more or less continuously discharged, spermatogenesis goes on continuously in the male. Similarly, LH is continuously produced and causes the regular secretion of testosterone from the testes. In the female, gonadotrophins are released in a cyclic fashion and the function of FSH is, as in the male, largely morphological. It causes growth of the Graafian follicle without stimulating hormone production in the ovary. Its clinical application is therefore in the treatment of anovulatory infertility, as growth of the follicle is an essential prelude to ovulation. Steroid formation in the follicle is initiated by LH which is secreted early in the menstrual cycle in a sufficient amount to initiate this process. Luteinizing hormone (LH) is concerned with ovulation, as it is produced in a marked peak, just after the maximal production of follicular oestrogen and immediately preceding ovulation. LH also has a luteotrophic action, but is not available for therapeutic use. Large quantities of a closely related hormone, chorionic gonadotrophin (HCG), can be extracted from human placentae and is widely used in its place. HCG is both immunologically and functionally very similar to LH and will thus cause ovulation of the mature Graafian follicle or prolong the life of the corpus luteum. It is therefore used in the treatment of anovulatory infertility and in recurrent or threatened abortion.

The ovary and the testis are in an endocrinological sense closely related and have a functional kinship with the placenta and the adrenal gland. All four glands share the common property of making steroids from simple acetate molecules or from cholesterol. None of the steroids are unique to a particular gland, and the ovary can make testosterone or the placenta make cortisol. The glands differ, one from the other, in the main pathway down which they direct the biosynthetic process. One gland may make the main product of another as a minor metabolite or may, as the ovary does with testosterone, use it as an intermediate in its own characteristic pathway to its own main hormone.

The Chemistry of Female Hormones

The pituitary hormones. Several teams in different parts of the world are working to discover the structure of the hypothalamic releasing factors and it is probable that some of these will soon be made synthetically. It is evident that their structure is simpler than the protein hormones of the pituitary whose secretion they cause. They are simple peptides, containing less than ten amino acids, and, in the case of LH releasing factor at least, probably consisting of only three amino acids.

In 1949 the first nearly pure sample of FSH was produced by Li and his colleagues in California. They extracted this protein hormone from sheep pituitaries and although this material differs from human FSH, they were able to establish a central fact which was found to hold true for all mammalian FSH. This was that the protein is attached to a carbohydrate moiety which in the case of human FSH was found to contain galactose, mannose, hexosamine and acetyl hexosamine. Like other proteins, FSH is species specific and the only source of the hormone is the human pituitary and menopausal urine.

LH, like FSH, is a glycoprotein, but its carbohydrate moiety is clearly different from that of FSH. There has been much less effort made to prepare LH in a form suitable for administration to man, for human chorionic gonadotrophin (HCG) is an efficient substitute for it. HCG is a glycoprotein with much in common with LH. The hormones have some common antigens and LH will react with antibodies raised to HCG. Their biological actions are also similar and HCG will cause ovulation of the grown Graafian follicle or prolong the life of the corpus luteum. HCG can be prepared from pregnancy urine in a semi-pure state and is readily available commercially. It is widely used as a substitute for LH in the induction of ovulation.

The pituitary gonadotrophins are large complex molecules. It might be possible to make them synthetically if the sequence of amino acids and the spatial arrangement of the peptide chains could be ascertained. Fortunately the number of women suffering from pituitary destruction is small and much more commonly the cause of gonadotrophic inadequacy is a failure on the part of the pituitary to release its hormones rather than an incapacity to manufacture them. The main development in the treatment of pituitary gonadotrophin deficiency is therefore to be sought in means to cause the release of preformed hormone from the pituitary.

The steroid hormones. The steroid molecule is much simpler and is composed of far fewer molecules than the complex polypeptides of the gonadotrophins. There is a basic carbon-hydrogen skeleton common to all the steroids, each individual hormone being produced by additions to or modifications of this framework.

The oestrogens. The first three oestrogens isolated were oestradiol, oestrone, and oestriol. Some potent synthetic oestrogens are derived from minor modifications of the natural oestrogen structure. Ethynyloestradiol has the same structure as oestradiol but with an added ethynyl group at C17. The addition of an ethynyl group is a very common device in the manufacture of synthetic steroids. Oestradiol is normally very rapidly inactivated by metabolism. The enzymes which metabolize oestradiol are unable to attack ethynyloestradiol so easily because the addition of the ethynyl group prevents access of the enzyme to its substrate. The substituted molecule still has oestrogenic activity and continues to circulate unhindered for much longer. Substitution elsewhere in the molecule, notably at C3, is also employed in the manufacture of synthetic oestrogens, and one of the most widely used oestrogens of recent years, mestranol, has substituents at both positions.

The familiar oestrogen skeleton is not essential for oestrogen activity, and the main synthetic oestrogen, stilboestrol, is not a steroid at all.

Progesterone. Progesterone and its related compounds are neutral steroids, not phenols. Consequently, their chemical characteristics and solubility behaviour are different from oestrogens. Progesterone is, for instance, almost completely insoluble in water, but very lipid soluble. As it is inactive by mouth the natural hormone can only be given by intramuscular injection dissolved in oil, but it is rapidly inactivated and it is impossible to attain physiological concentrations at distant target sites.

It is much less easy to produce physiologically active substituted forms of progesterone than is the case with oestrogen. The most successful development along these lines has been to use a related physiological compound, 17-hydroxy progesterone. By far the most commonly used class of physiologically active progestational compounds is not derived from progesterone at all but from *19 nor*testosterone. This is a steroid which lacks the two carbon sidechain of progesterone, and, like the oestrogens with which it has some biological affinity, has no methyl group at C19.

The Disorders of Menstruation

The disorders of menstruation are not disease entities of themselves but the symptoms of a great many diseases. A symptom such as amenorrhoea may be an occasional or a constant concomitant of a disease. It may be transient or permanent. It may be the central feature of a disease or a minor incidental consequence of a pathological process. To classify endrocine diseases by symptoms rather than by cause is to perpetuate confusion. Often enough, however, the cause is not known even where there is general agreement upon the existence of a particular symptom complex such as premenstrual tension. It is necessary in the present description of menstrual disorder to make some compromise between classification by cause and classification by symptomatology. A proper system of disease categorization is essential to the process which leads from symptoms to cause and thence to rational treatment. One of the main criticisms which can be levelled against gynaecological practice today is that it is too often concerned with the haphazard therapy of symptoms rather than the investigation and categorization of causes.

The basis of diagnosis used to be the symptomatic history and such physical signs as could be elicited. With the introduction of laboratory disciplines and of statistical methods more emphasis is now being placed on exact measurement and objective evaluation of data.

Menometrorrhagia. The symptom complex of menometrorrhagia contains two overlapping entities; menorrhagia which is prolonged or profuse menstruation and metrorrhagia which is irregular menstruation. It is a matter of arbitrary definition where either of these begins and normal menstruation ceases. It is proposed to treat them as a single entity as the most prominent symptom of the condition of dysfunctional uterine haemorrhage. Menometrorrhagia may, of course, be associated with gross pelvic pathology such as fibromyomata or endometrial carcinoma, but in the present context consideration will be limited to menometrorrhagia occurring in the absence of such organic disease. It is noteworthy that the incidence of organic bleeding increases sharply with age, while dysfunctional uterine haemorrhage, although it tends to concentrate at the two ends of menstrual life, is not characteristically a phenomenon of older women.

TREATMENT OF MENOMETRORRHAGIA. Naturally, successful treatment of menometrorrhagia is dependent on the cause. So few centres possess adequate facilities for the investigation of the endocrine background of patients suffering from menometrorrhagia that, in general, treatment is based on investigation of the histological state of the endometrium. The treatment has therefore resolved itself into an empirical routine; a number of standard remedies being applied in order. Long periods of remission may occur in nearly all forms of anovular bleeding and where such a spontaneous return to normal menstrual function coincides with the application of a particular treatment it is often given the credit for a cure. The rôle of the physician is to contain the symptoms until spontaneous remission occurs or the menopause supervenes.

One of the most useful forms of treatment is curettage, which in any case is an essential diagnostic procedure. It is not at all clear why a curettage should effect a cure, but a return to normal menstruation follows curettage far too often for this to be an accidental association. Various mechanical explanations, such as the complete removal of hypertrophied endometrium, have been put forward for the beneficial effect of curettage. It is very likely that menometrorrhagia often arises from a functional disorder of hormone secretion by the pituitary. Because of its hypothalamic control, the secretion of pituitary hormones is subject to cortical influence and it is evident that psychological factors have a bearing on menometrorrhagia. Curettage, although directed at the endometrium, may owe much of its value to its effect on the mental state of the woman who finds herself, even if only for a short while, relieved of a burdensome routine and the recipient of attention and sympathy. Psychological treatment has not been notably successful for menometrorrhagia but the inexplicable beneficial effects of curettage suggest the value of simple measures such as the treatment of constipation and iron therapy for anaemia. Many attempts have been made to determine what percentage of success attends curettage. Most publications fail adequately to categorize the menometrorrhagias with which they are dealing. It is hardly likely that the same cure rate will be achieved in all types. It is probable that the better responses to curettage are to be expected in anovular bleeding. Whatever the cause, a reversion to normal menstruation follows curettage sufficiently often in menometrorrhagia for one or two repeat curettages to be justifiable in the majority of cases.

In the past it was often necessary to terminate a bout of severe bleeding with vigorous oestrogen therapy, which often resulted in a resumption of bleeding as soon as the hormone was withdrawn. The introduction of synthetic progestational compounds has transformed the treatment of menometrorrhagia. A suitable compound in high dosage and in combination with an oestrogen very rarely fails to control the bleeding. An organic cause such as endometrial carcinoma should be carefully sought if bleeding does not stop. Compounds such as norethynodrel, norethisterone and ethynodiol diacetate are made up with suitable amounts (50 to 100 μg.) of mestranol or ethynyl-oestradiol added. They will, in effect, produce a medical castration for the period of their use. All endogenous ovarian activity is suppressed and bouts of regular bleeding induced by withdrawing therapy at intervals, thereby removing the direct stimulatory effect of the progestin on the enodmetrium. Such withdrawal bleedings are of much shorter duration than the disordered periods and usually the blood loss is not so heavy. In any case the bleeding can always be terminated by starting a fresh course of steroid. There is no good evidence that such hormone therapy is in fact curative but the courses can be repeated many times and if therapy is withheld every now and then long spells of spontaneous remission often occur.

X-ray or radium therapy to induce the menopause, or a hysterectomy should only be considered in older women and in those whose family is complete. Even in such patients the need for these operative procedures only arises in women who are intolerant of the drug or who revert to severe menorrhagia when it is withdrawn.

Amenorrhoea. This term is applied to an absence of the menses for three months or longer. It often follows oligomenorrhoea from which it is distinguished by the arbitrary definition that in oligomenorrhoea menses are at intervals of six weeks to three months. With a symptom as ubiquitous as amenorrhoea it is possible to name a great many conditions in which it may occur so that many classifications are more notable for wide coverage than for any close applicability to common clinical problems. For the purposes of this discussion it is proposed to ignore the many situations in which amenorrhoea is incidental to another primary disease and to concentrate on those instances where the symptom is indicative of a disorder of the complicated mechanism of the normal menstrual cycle.

It is usual to classify amenorrhoea in two main subdivisions—*primary amenorrhoea* occurring in women who have never menstruated, and *secondary amenorrhoea* in those who, having once menstruated, have not had any period for three months or longer. This distinction serves to emphasize the fact that there is a group of women, for example, those without uteri, for whom menstruation was never possible and who are in a quite separate category as regards therapy and prognosis.

Primary amenorrhoea is said to exist in women who, up to the age of 18 years, have not menstruated. The menarche is a process involving diverse elements and not a single point in physiological time. This arbitrary age limit is widely accepted but in view of the fact that the average age at menarche is falling it would be as well to regard 18 as a maximal rather than a minimal age for the definition of primary amenorrhoea. Thirty to forty per cent. of all cases of primary amenorrhoea are attributable to chromosomal abnormalities and are not amenable to cure. This is also true of congenital abnormalities of the genital tract, which are the next commonest cause. Palliative therapy, such as encouraging breast growth by the administration of oestrogens, should be delayed until no further growth in stature is occurring or desired. Simple delay in the onset of the menarche, another common cause of primary amenorrhoea may be a test of the physician's capacity to exercise restraint. Primary amenorrhoea calls for vigorous investigation, including hormone assays, chromosomal analysis and examination under anaesthesia. If no cause can be discerned and a delayed menarche is the cause, little good is done by premature and meddlesome hormone therapy.

The physiological causes of secondary amenorrhoea (pregnancy, lactation and the menopause) will not be discussed, nor will the great number of situations where secondary amenorrhoea is incidental to other systemic disease. Therapeutic interest centres on those cases of secondary amenorrhoea which are the result of endocrine disorders. These are legion, but they can conveniently be discussed according to the anatomical site of the disorder: the hypothalamus, the pituitary, the ovaries, the uterus. Uterine causes are rarest of all. A refractory endometrium has occasionally been suggested but very little supporting data for such a thesis has been adduced.

THE TREATMENT OF AMENORRHOEA. Normal menstruation often returns spontaneously. Immediate treatment therefore should be restricted to the cure of a specific disease. Patients tolerate this conservative management if they are given a definite regimen to follow. Many of these women are overweight and they should be encouraged to remedy this by means of diet, exercise and physiotherapy. Reassurance and an explanation of menstrual physiology will usually be helpful; and it may be possible to alleviate the adverse effects of overwork and excessive stress.

It has frequently been said that the treatment of amenorrhoea should be dependent on the cause and that treatment should await diagnosis. This is only partly true. Naturally it is preferable to find a cause and apply a specific remedy and, over a considerable range of conditions, it is possible to do so. Sometimes it is possible to apply a remedy when the cause is known only in the most general terms as in the psychological treatment of anorexia nervosa. Some causes, like congenital absence of the uterus, exclude the possibility of effective remedy. In the clinical situation the endocrinologist often has to content himself with having excluded a reasonable range of likely specific causes and to start treatment knowing only in the general area in which the cause is likely to be. In this context it is important to decide whether the basic deficiency is at the hypothalamic, the pituitary, the ovarian or the uterine level.

The rational therapy of *hypothalamic amenorrhoea* would be the administration of the deficient releasing factor at the appropriate stage of the cycle. As no releasing factors are yet available, such therapy is only a hope for the future. In the meantime, treatment of stress factors with reassurance and sedation is the nearest approach to rational treatment.

When the *pituitary* production of gonadotrophins is at fault substitution treatment with FSH and LH would seem to be indicated. The only current sources of FSH are either extracts of human pituitary or of menopausal urine. Such preparations are not readily available and their use is properly restricted to amenorrhoeic patients who wish to become pregnant. The LH component is easier to replace, as HCG is a good substitute. The cases where an isolated LH deficiency exists are rare and as a rule LH acts only on the follicle whose growth has been promoted by FSH.

As regards *ovarian* causes of amenorrhoea, treatment with ovarian steroids is not restricted to those patients who, in spite of adequate gonadotrophin production, do not produce ovarian steroids. In practice this would limit steroid therapy to the most unrewarding subjects such as those with gonadal hypoplasia or endometrial atrophy. Sex steroids are therefore frequently used in patients who have revealed no evidence of defective ovaries. It is easy to provoke an oestrogen withdrawal bleeding provided the uterus is present. Whether such treatment often effects cure, in the sense of a resumption of the normal cycle, is open to question. It is frequently claimed that repeat courses of oestrogens stimulate further growth in a hypoplastic uterus. It is difficult to provide convincing proof of a permanent increase in the size of the uterus, but there is no doubt that growth in secondary sex structures—the breasts and the external genitalia—can be provoked. At worst the induction of an oestrogen withdrawal bleeding can be reassuring to women who are upset by the absence of the menses. This form of therapy has, however, been much abused by physicians who have accepted credit for restoring function without making it clear to their patients that oestrogen withdrawal bleeding is not the same as a restoration of the normal menses. Many dosage schemes for cyclical oestrogen administration have been produced. For the most part they are notable only for their complexity. If an oestrogen only is to be used the synthetic compounds are preferable. An acceptable regimen is a three-weeks' course of 0·5 mg. stilboestrol daily or 50 μg. ethynyl oestradiol. Three or four such courses should suffice with a week's interval between each, during which time the withdrawal bleeding takes place. Although there is no experimental evidence to show that synthetic progestational compounds are superior to the oestrogens, the *nor*testosterone group of progestogens have marked endometrial effects and can be relied upon to produce controlled withdrawal bleeding with minimal side-effects. For this reason three or four courses of a compound such as norethynodrel 10 mg. daily plus 50 μg. of mestranol are to be preferred to simple oestrogen treatment.

Disordered ovarian steroidogenesis. Polycystic ovarian disease, Stein-Leventhal's syndrome and hyperthecosis ovarii are terms applied to the same condition or to very similar ones. The clinical features include some aspects of virilism—hirsutes, clitoral enlargement and breast changes, and also amenorrhoea, infertility and occasionally obesity. It is an inconstant changing state in which none of these features are invariably present. It is commonly but not always associated with a failure of ovulation and the enlarged ovaries have a thick sclerosed capsule and many small cysts of follicular origin. From the functional point of view the underlying cause is a disorder of steroidogenesis. One or other of the enzymes involved in the synthesis of ovarian hormones is deficient, and precursors in steroidogenesis accumulate. The block is generally not complete; the urinary oestrogens are within the normal range but in order to produce these an excess of other steroids is produced. Some of these are androgenic or can give rise to androgenic metabolites which are the cause of the virilization.

Three lines of *treatment* have been used with success in disordered steroidogenesis and each has its place according to the circumstances of the patient. All endogenous ovarian activity can be suppressed by giving a mixture of synthetic progestogen and oestrogen. For this purpose any of the *nor*testosterone derivatives as used in the oral contraceptives is suitable. The usual contraceptive routine of three weeks' treatment with intervals of a week is used. This approach is best suited to young women who do not wish to become pregnant. No form of treatment diminishes the hirsutes which is often a distressing feature of these cases, but ovarian suppression by oral contraceptives usually prevents an increase in facial hair. Resection of a wedge of sclerosed ovarian capsule and puncturing the cysts often causes a return of ovulation and regular menses. A repeat wedge resection is seldom successful so that it is often wise to postpone wedge resection of the ovaries until the woman is ready to start a family. Disordered steroidogenesis has proved to be the form of anovulatory infertility most responsive to treatment with clomiphene, a diphenyl chloroethylene derivative. It is most suitable for women who desire pregnancy but as the drug has few side-effects and the treatment can be repeated at intervals, there is no harm in giving it to single women. Although ovulation can be induced by clomiphene in upwards of 80 per cent. of women with disordered ovarian steroidogenesis, there is no clear evidence as to what proportion continue to have regular ovulatory cycles when treatment is discontinued. The usual course of treatment is 50 mg. clomiphene tartrate twice a day for four days and ovulation most commonly occurs on the ninth day after the start of treatment.

L

There is little point in increasing the dosage in refractory patients as women who do not respond in the first instance seldom do so on prolonged treatment or higher dosage.

Dysmenorrhoea. Pain with the periods is occasionally due to an organic cause such as uterine fibroids but more commonly no lesion can be demonstrated. Sedatives, rest and reassurance are the traditional first lines of treatment for such functional forms of dysmenorrhoea. If more is required a cervical dilatation and curettage is indicated. This may have the effect of relieving cervical spasm or stenosis although the operation often has a salutary effect for no very clear reason. Endocrine therapy should be reserved for the most obstinate cases. It is widely believed that anovular cycles are associated with painless bleeding and for this reason suppression of ovulation with oral contraceptives is often used with success. A more convenient form of therapy is supplementation of the luteal phase with a progestogen such as retroprogesterone. This does not suppress ovulation but dydrogesterone 5 mg. twice daily given from day 10 of the cycle until the onset of the period will often relieve dysmenorrhoea with a minimal upset of the cycle.

Endometriosis. Very severe dysmenorrhoea may be caused by the ectopic implantation of endometrial tissue, commonly in the ovaries. Adhesions form and these, together with the ovarian damage, are responsible for infertility. Endocrine therapy has proved to be of great benefit in endometriosis, the object being to induce a state similar to the amenorrhoea and ovarian quiescence of pregnancy. An oestrogen-progestogen mixture is given continuously and increased to a high dosage which is maintained for 6 to 10 months. Prolonged treatment with progestogens has the effect of causing an exhaustion atrophy of the endometrial glands and it is this, as much as the prevention of ectopic bleeding, which causes the ovarian cysts to shrink. Oral contraceptive mixtures have been used with success and two relatively new compounds appear to be at least as good as the progestins which have been in use for a long time. One, norgestrel, is a nortestosterone derivative and the other, megestrol acetate, is a 17α-hydroxyprogesterone derivative. An early regimen, and still one of the best, is to start norethynodrel or norethisterone in 5 mg. daily doses and raise this by 5 mg. daily every week until a dose of 20 mg. per day is reached. In the commercial preparations of both these compounds mestranol or ethynyloestradiol is added.

Pre-menstrual tension. This designation is applied to a variety of symptoms associated with menstruation. The common complaints are breast tension, restlessness, irritability, insomnia, headache, vertigo and oedema. There are no hormone assay data which show which substances are deficient or in excess, but it is believed that endocrines are involved because pre-menstrual tension is nearly always associated with ovular cycles. Further, the condition often responds to treatment with hormones, and associated phenomena like salt and water retention are part of physiological processes known to be under hormonal control. The psychological state of the patient is also important. The condition is commonest among tense nervous women from the upper social classes. In the belief that the psychogenic element was the dominant one, tranquillizers have been used, and in some trials meprobamate proved to be more effective than either diuretics or hormones. Retroprogesterone can be used as reinforcement of the luteal phase without upsetting the menstrual cycle, but the oral contraceptive regimens are equally rational and successful. If there are signs of water retention, diuretics are helpful.

The rôle of surgery in menstrual disorder. In young women surgical intervention is seldom warranted and even in older women it is a confession of failure. The elucidation of the mechanism by which psychological influences can affect menstrual function has brought recognition of the importance of treating the whole woman and her reproductive functions rather than simply extirpating her uterus and so removing some manifestations of a disease whose primary site may be in the cerebral cortex, the hypothalamus, the pituitary or the ovaries.

The menopause. The age at menopause, like that of the menarche, is subject to social, nutritional and constitutional factors. In European communities the median age lies between 47 and 50 years. Its manner of onset is variable. Most frequently the periods become scanty and occur at longer intervals; sometimes they stop abruptly and occasionally the menopause is signalled by irregular, prolonged bleeding, the so-called menorrhagia of the menopause. This is usually because the menstrual cycle tends to become anovular at the end of reproductive life. Nevertheless menorrhagia at the menopause should always be regarded seriously and investigated by curettage to exclude carcinoma of the cervix or endometrium.

THE MANAGEMENT OF THE MENOPAUSE. The menopause may be accompanied by physical disabilities such as vaginal prolapse which requires treatment, but it is the metabolic and psychological effects that have the most impact on medical practice. The integrated function of the endocrine system is disrupted, and few women are unaffected by the changes. They may express their reaction to it by a variety of symptoms, notably depression, insomnia, restlessness and headaches. Libido does not usually decline with the cessation of the menses. The menopause often precipitates a period of vascular instability manifested by hot flushes or dizzy turns which may be very distressing to a sensitive woman.

The end of their reproductive function may be a cataclysmic event to some women and at the very least medical treatment has a function in dispelling the cloud of mythology that has gathered about it. The physician should, for example, convince his patient that the onset of the menopause does not signal the end of sexual desire or activity. Of course it is possible to perpetuate the menses and to abolish some of the discomforts of the menopause. The prolongation of menstrual life is not necessarily desirable but many women should receive some medicinal support as well as advice. Occasionally sedation is enough, but generally some oestrogen replacement therapy is needed. Doses of 1 mg. stilboestrol or 50 μg. ethynyloestradiol will control flushes or senile vaginitis but in the long run also stimulate endometrial proliferation and may give rise to bleeding. Oestriol, when given in doses of 0·25 mg. three times a day has a beneficial effect on the vagina and on the woman's sense of wellbeing. It does not stimulate the endometrium to the same extent. Such treatment can with good effect be continued for many months, the dosage of oestriol being gradually reduced.

Infertility

There are many causes of infertility in the female. For the most part they are purely the province of the gynaecologist and will not be considered here. A few, however, have endocrine causes and some now have endocrine cures and are therefore relevant; these are related to failures of ovulation. They occur, therefore, mainly in women suffering from oligomenorrhoea or amenorrhoea and in a few who have more or less regular bleeding from a proliferative endometrium. Patients with anovulatory infertility are rare but as they are an example of an advance in reproductive endocrinology they are worthy of consideration. When amenorrhoea is due to a defect at the uterine or ovarian level little can be done to repair it so the treatment of endocrine infertility is confined to the correction of defects of pituitary or hypothalamic function.

Treatment of infertility due to pituitary failure. The indications for substitution therapy include most women with anovulation due to low gonadotrophin secretion, particularly when they fail to respond by ovulation to simple pituitary stimulation with clomiphene

CLOMIPHENE TREATMENT. The induction of ovulation with clomiphene citrate is simpler and less expensive than substitution therapy with gonadotrophins. Further, there is much less chance of overstimulation or of multiple pregnancy. There is a tendency to use the drug on a more or less empirical basis with little control by hormone assay. Such an approach has little to recommend it, although there is something to be said for trying clomiphene first in nearly all patients before embarking on the more formidable enterprise of using gonadotrophins therapeutically. The most favourable group for treatment with clomiphene are those with some evidence of ovarian activity, notably those with disordered ovarian steroidogenesis. The least favourable are the hypogonadal patients with low oestrogens or those with high gonadotrophin excretion levels and findings suggestive of menopause praecox. When the fault is below the pituitary level, the patients are, of course, totally unresponsive to either clomiphene or gonadotrophins. If a woman does not ovulate on 200 mg. clomiphene daily for 4 to 5 days (ovulation generally occurs 9 to 11 days after starting treatment) she will not respond to higher dosages. It is usual to give 100 mg. daily for 4 days.

Clearly the most physiological means of inducing ovulation as long as the pituitary is functionally competent is the use of hypothalamic releasing factors. Already crude extracts of these, made from the median eminence tissue of animals have been used with some success. The chances are good that some of the releasing factors will be synthesized in the near future and they may come to play an important part in the treatment of anovulatory infertility.

GONADOTROPHIN TREATMENT. Presumably, women with a high gonadotrophin excretion stand little chance of being benefited by a further dose of gonadotrophin, although a few women with high gonadotrophin production have been successfully treated. Gonadotrophin assay helps to identify a cause of infertility, not amenable to any treatment, i.e. failure at the ovarian level due to a premature menopause. In clinical practice treatment with gonadotrophins should be reserved for patients who do not respond to clomiphene.

Although pregnant mare serum gonadotrophin is of some value as a dynamic test of ovarian function, its capacity to induce ovulation is small and the only three preparations for human use are those made from human pituitaries, from menopausal urine, or from pregnancy urine. Human pituitary gonadotrophin (HPG) is not available for treatment and for clinical purposes the extract from menopausal urine (HMG) is used. Although intended as substitution for FSH, both the urinary preparations, Pergonal and Humagon, have a considerable admixture of LH which is essential to their function in causing steroidogenesis in the follicles whose growth they stimulate. Human gonadotrophin (HCG) is readily available but its activity is limited to causing ovulation in a follicle whose growth has been stimulated by FSH or in maintaining the function of the corpus luteum after ovulation. HCG is therefore used as an ovulating agent in conjunction with FSH.

The dosage schedule of HMG is complicated by problems of sensitivity. Amounts of HMG which fail to provoke any response in one patient may cause gross overstimulation in another. The technique is to start with a low dose of HMG and work up until a response in terms of increased oestrogen output is obtained. Assays of the urinary excretion of oestrogen and of pregnanediol are a necessary adjunct to the treatment as these are the only certain way to tell whether over-stimulation is occurring, and whether and when any response occurred. They are also required to time the ovulating dose of HCG and intercourse correctly. Providing such steroid assay facilities are available an acceptable routine is to give 75 to 300 i.u. of HMG daily for 8 to 10 days. When ovulatory levels of oestrogen (30 μg. of oestrone or 50 to 100 μg. of total oestrogen per 24 hours) are obtained an ovulatory dose of 5,000 i.u. of HCG is given.

Wedge resection of the ovary in polycystic ovarian disease has been successfully practised for 30 years. Its application now lies, not so much in being a treatment for infertility, as in a measure to cure amenorrhoea and to contain hirsutes.

Abortion and Premature Labour

As a rule the treatment of these is the proper province of the specialist obstetrician but the general physician is apt also to encounter them. Treatment may involve the possible use of progestational compounds, but progesterone itself is inactive by mouth and ineffective when given by parenteral injection or by implanting solid pellets.

When it became possible to use synthetic progestational compounds which were active by mouth it was hoped that they would be effective in preventing recurrent abortion or treating threatened abortion, but it is now known that primary progesterone deficiency accounts for very few abortions. Progestogens, however, have no specific effect, but they are still used and promoted lavishly, without justification.

Premature labour, like abortion, arises from a variety of causes, and no single treatment is uniformly successful. There is no convincing case for the use of sex hormones, although prophylactic suturing of the cervix or the use of muscle relaxants such as isoxaprine is undoubtedly beneficial in suitable cases.

Inhibition of Lactation

In western society, inhibition of lactation is commonplace. This is often achieved by the use of large doses of oestrogen, usually stilboestrol. Disadvantages of this treatment have long been apparent; rebound breast engorgement with occasional abscess formation is common when the drug is discontinued, and its withdrawal may precipitate uterine bleeding. Further, the use of stilboestrol in the puerperium may predispose to thromboembolism. This is unjustifiable for a trivial disorder; and on the few occasions when simple measures such as sedatives, fluid restriction and support are not effective, a single injection of quinestradiol should be given.

Contraception

The first trial of an oestrogen-progestogen combination as an oral contraceptive was in 1956, and twelve years later 14 million women were receiving oral contraceptives. This is mass medication unparalleled in history. Its effects are far reaching both on the individual and on society.

Generally, oral contraceptives consist of a mixture of two types of steroid, an oestrogen and a progestogen. In 1970 there were 17 such preparations on the British market together with a further two consisting of a progestogen only. In all of them only one of two oestrogens was involved, either ethynyloestradiol or mestranol. Seven different progestogens were used, all derivatives either of *nor*testosterone or 17α-hydroxyprogesterone.

The oral contraceptives owe their high degree of efficacy as contraceptive agents to the fact that they act at a number of different points in the process of fertilization and nidation. The principal action of the most successful combinations is the inhibition of ovulation. Patients on such drugs produce no ovarian hormones of their own and shed no ova. The main agent responsible for the inhibition of ovulation is the oestrogen. The purpose of the progestogen is merely to modify the bleeding resulting from oestrogen withdrawal. It is equally probable that untoward side-effects such as thromboembolism are due to the oestrogen. For this reason attempts have been made to dispense

with the oestrogen altogether and, by the action of a progestogen such as chlormadinone acetate, to achieve contraception without the use of oestrogens. Such pure progestogens act mainly on the cervix but they cause irregularities of the menstrual cycle and have a high failure rate.

The compromise of using a progestogen with less than 50 μg. of oestrogen probably results in fewer side-effects, although there are no firm data which establish 50 μg. of oestrogen per day as a threshold level for thromboembolic phenomena.

There is every reason to expect that oral contraceptives are a temporary experiment in the control of fertility. As the endocrinology of the menstrual cycle, of fertilization and of implantation of the ovum become more clearly understood, alternative methods of controlling fertility will become available.

Further Reading

SHEARMAN, R. P. (1969). *Induction of Ovulation.* Springfield, Illinois: Thomas.
GOLDFARB, A. F. (1964). *Advances in the Treatment of Menstrual Dysfunction.* London: Kimpton.
BAIRD, DUGALD (1969). *Combined Textbook of Obstetrics and Gynaecology*, 9th Edition. Edinburgh: Livingstone.

13. Metabolic Diseases—Diabetes Mellitus, Obesity

L. J. P. DUNCAN

DIABETES MELLITUS

The great majority of diabetics can with proper mangement live normal lives. Nevertheless, changes occur in the basement membrane of smaller blood vessels—the so-called specific diabetic microangiopathy—and present clinically as retinopathy, nephropathy or diabetic peripheral vascular disease. These are due to metabolic changes resulting from inadequate action of insulin and occur most frequently and severely in poorly controlled long-standing diabetics. Apart from the probability of accelerating the development of these complications, inadequate control carries with it the dangers of hypoglycaemia and ketoacidosis. It also leads to impairment of general health, undue susceptibility to infections and a lack of personal confidence in being able to undertake normal activities. There is therefore no justification for a *laissez-faire* attitude on the part of the doctor or patient in the control of diabetes.

The purpose of treatment in all diabetics is the relief of symptoms and the attainment and maintenance of a satisfactory body weight. The further degree of control aimed at depends on whether or not the patient already has complications, or if newly diagnosed, is likely to live the ten years or so generally required for them to develop. Thus, for those whose expectation of life, by reason of age or serious organic disease, is unlikely to exceed 10 years, control is adequate if the specimen of urine least likely to contain glucose shows no more than occasional slight glycosuria; any serious deterioration in diabetic control would be reflected by 1 to 2 per cent. glycosuria in this test. For younger patients the aim is to correct the disordered metabolism to the greatest practicable extent and every effort should be made to reduce glycosuria as much as possible in urine tests selected to reflect the blood glucose level before and occasionally after meals.

The quality of the control achieved depends almost entirely on the patient's co-operation, understanding of his disease and knowledge of the principles of diabetic treatment. His education is the doctor's responsibility and demands much time, understanding, experience and patience; a doctor unwilling to undertake this duty properly should refer such patients to a physician who is prepared to do so. It is also essential to begin the diabetic's education as soon as possible after diagnosis, at the time when he is most anxious to co-operate and to learn. When educated, the patient ought to assume responsibility for the assessment and maintenance of his diabetic control. Regular medical supervision at appropriate intervals is nevertheless always necessary, but the doctor's rôle should be essentially that of an adviser. In few other diseases is successful therapy so dependent on a proper doctor–patient relationship. The doctor should not 'treat diabetics'—he educates them to treat themselves and thereafter acts in a supervisory capacity. Regular examinations are also necessary to note the occurrence of complications.

There are many clinical types of idiopathic diabetes: at one extreme is the obese, elderly woman discovered to have glycosuria when she complains, for example, of persistent pruritus vulvae and who suffers from the stable, insulin-independent type of diabetes which will almost certainly be controlled by dietary restriction alone; at the other extreme is the young person who, after a few days or weeks of polyuria, thirst and rapid loss of weight, is likely to develop severe ketoacidosis; he suffers from the insulin-dependent type of diabetes and his life depends thereafter on the regular administration of insulin. Between these two extremes are patients suffering from one or other of the many different permutations of the diabetic syndrome; some may be controlled by diet alone, some may require additional treatment with an oral hypoglycaemic agent and others will need insulin.

Secondary diabetes may be controlled by correction of the primary disorder as in acromegaly or Cushing's syndrome. Diabetes due to pancreatic disease, such as pancreatitis or haemochromatosis, may occasionally be controlled by diet alone or an oral hypoglycaemic agent, but more often such diabetes is insulin-dependent.

THE DIET

All diabetics, irrespective of the type of their disorder, must adhere to some form of dietary regimen. The prescribed diet must: (1) be suited to the patient's finances, domestic circumstances and occupation; (2) be nutritionally balanced— providing enough bulk to satisfy the appetite and sufficient variety to prevent monotony; (3) be simple and easily understood by the patient or the person who prepares the meals.

Unweighed Diets. Many newly diagnosed diabetics, especially the obese, have been accustomed to a diet containing far too much carbohydrate. They usually have mild diabetes and simple limitation of carbohydrate excess is often all that is required to control their diabetes and body weight. The patient is simply given a list of foods showing those which must be avoided, those to be taken in moderation and those permitted without restriction, and is carefully instructed in its use.

A. DO NOT EAT ANY OF THE FOLLOWING:

1. Sugar, glucose, jam, marmalade, honey, syrup, treacle, tinned fruits, sweets, chocolate, lemonade, glucose drinks, Ovaltine, Horlicks, Benger's food, and similar foods which are sweetened with sugar.
2. Cakes, sweet biscuits, chocolate biscuits, pastries, pies, puddings, thick sauces.
3. Alcoholic drinks unless permission has been given by the doctor.

B. EAT IN MODERATION ONLY:

1. Bread of all kinds (including so-called 'slimming' and 'starch-reduced' breads, brown or white, plain or toasted).
2. Rolls, scones, biscuits and crispbreads.
3. Potatoes, peas and baked beans.
4. Breakfast cereals and porridge.
5. All fresh or dried fruit or fruit juice.
6. Macaroni, spaghetti, custard and foods with much flour.
7. Thick soups.
8. Diabetic foods.
9. Milk.

C. EAT WITHOUT RESTRICTION:

1. All meat, fish, eggs.
2. Cheese.
3. Clear soup or meat extracts, tomato or lemon juice.
4. Tea or coffee.
5. Cabbage, Brussels sprouts, broccoli, cauliflower, spinach, turnip, runner or French beans, onions, leeks or mushrooms. Lettuce, cucumber, tomatoes, spring onions, radishes, mustard and cress, asparagus, parsley. Rhubarb.
6. Herbs, spices, salt, pepper and mustard.
7. Butter and margarine.
8. Saccharine or Saxin for sweetening.

Some patients are inadequately controlled by this diet because they continue to eat too much carbohydrate, or occasionally fat; only rarely do patients eat excessive protein. For them the carbohydrate foods given in (*B*) in the diet above can be limited to the desired amount by prescribing them in terms of domestic measures, as listed below, each of which contains approximately 15 g. of carbohydrate and provides about 80 kcalories:

1 thin slice of bread—white or brown (may be toasted).
2 rich tea or digestive biscuits.
2 Ryvita or triangular oatcakes.
3 water biscuits, cream crackers, Macvita or round oatcakes.
Half morning roll or half plain or bran scone.
3 tablespoonfuls of porridge.
1 teacup of cornflakes, rice crispies or other breakfast cereal (not sugar coated).
1 tablespoon of potato, baked beans, sweetcorn or parsnips.
Fresh fruit, e.g. 1 apple, orange, pear, small banana, peach, 1 dozen grapes, 2 plums.
1 teacup of tinned fruit juice.
Small helping of tinned, packeted or thick soup, e.g. broth or lentil soup.
4 tablespoonfuls milk pudding sweetened with Saxin.
2 large or 4 small sausages.
2 squares of packet jelly.
5p. block of ice-cream.

The amount of carbohydrate allowed varies according to the person's age, weight and physical activity. Average requirements are listed in Table 10 p. 318. Thus if 120 g. is to be given, the patient would be allowed one half-pint of milk, which provides 15 g. of carbohydrate, plus 7 portions of these carbohydrate foods (7×15 g. $= 105$ g.) daily. Fat can be limited by specifying the amount of butter or margarine permitted ($\frac{1}{2}$ oz. $= 110$ kcals.).

These unweighed diets are very suitable for obese diabetics who rarely eat too much protein, for non-obese diabetics treated by diet alone or with an oral hypoglycaemic agent and for elderly stable insulin-taking diabetics who do not require strict metabolic control and for the few younger diabetics who have been unable to understand a weighed diet with an exchange system.

Weighed diets. These are required for most insulin-taking diabetics and for a few treated by diet alone or an oral hypoglycaemic agent for whom an unweighed diet has proved unsatisfactory. The system of exchanges must be simple and patients should weigh the foodstuffs for the first few months to recognize the permitted quantities; a set of scales should be provided. Insulin-dependent diabetics are rarely obese at the time of diagnosis and can thus be allowed fat and protein freely, at least initially.

Although most doctors use 10 g. carbohydrate exchanges, we prefer 15 g. exchanges. In general

TABLE 10

Type of Patient	kcals.	CHO (g.)	Prot. (g.)	Fat (g.)	Milk (pints)	Exchanges of		
						CHO	Prot.	Fat
1. *Child aged from 3 to 4 years.	1,300	130	65	60	1	6½	3	1½
2. *Child aged from 7 to 8 years.	1,900	175	86	92	1⅓	9	4	3
3. *Child aged from 11 to 12 years	2,200	220	103	99	1⅓	12	5	3
4. *Child aged from 14 to 17 years	2,400	240	110	109	1	14	6	4
5. *Young female shop assistant.	2,200	225	107	97	1	13	6	3
6. *Woman in latter half of pregnancy.	2,400	240	117	109	1½	13	6	3
7. *Hard working labourer.	2,600	255	121	121	1	15	7	4½
8. *Middle-aged housewife treated with a sulphonyl-urea	1,700	165	80	78	½	10	5	3
9. Middle-aged sedentary man treated with a sul-phonylurea	2,000	180	99	95	½	11	7	3½
10. Elderly, inactive woman treated by diet alone.	1,500	150	68	67	1	8	3	2
11. Obese woman treated by diet alone	1,000	105	52	42	½	6	3	1

* Indicates patients receiving treatment with insulin.

The above are calculated on the basis that 1 CHO exchange contains 0·5 g. of fat and 3 g. of protein.

these are converted more easily to familiar domestic measures and it is simpler for the patient to select a 60 g. carbohydrate meal containing four rather than six exchanges.

SYSTEM OF FOOD EXCHANGES

Carbohydrate Exchanges. Each contains approximately 15 g. CHO, 3 g. protein and from 0·5 to 1·0 g. of fat. The caloric value of each exchange is about 80 kcal.

Cereals
Bread	1 oz.
Toasted bread	¾ oz.
Rice, oatmeal, flour, barley, cornflour, arrow-root, sago, tapioca, semolina, custard powder, macaroni, spaghetti, breakfast cereals (all in dry state)	⅔ oz.
Rice, macaroni, spaghetti (boiled)	2 oz.
Porridge (3 tablespoonsful, cooked)	6 oz.

Biscuits and Scones
Water (3), rich tea (2), cream cracker (3), digestive biscuits (1½), crispbreads (2)	⅔ oz.
White, brown and bran scones; morning rolls	¾ oz.
Oatcakes	1 oz.

Fruit
Dried apricots, currants, dates, figs, peaches, prunes, raisins and sultanas (all in dry state).	1 oz.
Prunes stewed without sugar	3 oz.
Black and white grapes	3 oz.
Bananas (without skin)	3 oz.
Apples, cherries, damsons, green figs, gooseberries, greengages, nectarines, oranges, pears, pineapple, plums, tangerines and peaches.	5 oz.

Apricots, apples, cherries, damsons, gooseberries, greengages, pears and plums (stewed without sugar)	10 oz.
Brambles, blackcurrants, redcurrants, loganberries and raspberries (raw or stewed without sugar)	10 oz.
Grapefruit, melon and strawberries (raw)	10 oz.
Tinned fruit juice (small teacup)	3½ oz.

Vegetables
Dried peas, beans and lentils	1 oz.
Chipped or roast potatoes	1½ oz.
Potatoes raw or boiled, tinned peas, baked beans and sweetcorn	2½ oz.
Parsnip, beetroot, fresh or frozen peas (cooked)	5 oz.

Miscellaneous
Cocoa	1½ oz.
Proprietary milk preparations, e.g. Horlicks, Ovaltine, Bournvita.	⅔ oz.
Ice-cream	2½ oz.
Packet jellies (made up)	3 oz.
Savoury white sauce	5 oz.
Cream, tinned or packet soups	8 oz.

Thus if 240 g. of carbohydrate were to be allowed, this might be prescribed as 1 pint of milk (30 g. CHO) and 14 CHO exchanges (14×15 g. = 210 g.). These exchanges are then distributed between the various meals in a pattern best suited to the times of action of the insulins the patient is taking (Fig. 7, p. 327) and to his work and dietary habits. Patients who become overweight on this diet do so either because they are taking more carbohydrate than allowed or are eating too much fat; in the latter circumstance, the fat can be restricted to 1 to 3 fat exchanges (110 to 330 kcal.) which the patient can select from the following list which in turn can be simply added to the diet.

Fat Exchanges. Each contains approximately 12 g. of fat and almost no CHO or protein. The caloric value of each exchange is approximately 110 kcal.

Butter, margarine, lard, dripping, cooking-fat, olive or corn-oil	½ oz.
Cream . . . single 1 oz., double ¾ oz.	
Salad cream or mayonnaise . . .	¾ oz.
Nuts, except chestnuts (shelled) . .	¾ oz.

The prescription of protein in exchange form is only required for those who do not take sufficient protein, especially children and elderly persons. This can be achieved by prescribing the requisite number of protein exchanges allowed each day from the list given below:

Protein Exchanges. Each exchange contains almost no CHO, and approximately 8 g. of protein and 5 g. of fat. The value of each exchange is about 80 kcal.

Beef, mutton, lamb, pork, veal, bacon, ham, venison, chicken, duck, goose, turkey, pigeon, rabbit, hare, liver, kidney, heart, sweetbreads, tongue and tripe (all cooked)	1 oz.
Corned beef and mutton, tinned meats . .	1 oz.
Meat paste and pâté	1½ oz.
Sausages (cooked)	2 oz.
(includes ½ CHO exchange)	
Fish—white, smoked, cured, fatty, shellfish or tinned (cooked)	1½ oz.
Egg	1
Cheese	1 oz.
Dried peas or lentils—dry weight . .	1 oz.
(includes 1 CHO exchange)	

If, as is seldom the case, an accurate calorie diet containing specified amounts of carbohydrate, protein and fat is required (see Table 10, p. 318) it can easily be calculated and prescribed by the use of the above exchanges.

Patients often ask about alcoholic drinks and the various 'diabetic' foods. Alcoholic drinks should be allowed, but patients must remember that they contain appreciable calories and sometimes carbohydrate. One pint of mild draught ale contains about 15 g. of carbohydrate and one pint of strong ale about 30 g. Spirits such as whisky, brandy and gin contain no carbohydrate although the caloric value is high because of their alcoholic content; these are the most suitable alcoholic beverages for diabetics, but should be taken only in moderate amounts: a single measure of any of these spirits contains little less than 100 kcals. Dry sherries and dry wines can be allowed in moderation, but sweet wines, vermouth, liqueurs and cider should be avoided.

In the so-called diabetic foods the usual carbohydrates are replaced by saccharine, which has practically no caloric value, or by sorbitol or fructose. The latter are not directly metabolized into glucose; their entry into cells is unimpaired in diabetes and they do not raise the blood-glucose level directly. Although sorbitol and fructose

have an appreciable caloric value, the amount contained in diabetic jams, fruit juices and pastilles is so small that they can be taken in moderation. Diabetic chocolate contains a lot of fat and calories, and should not be taken too freely.

Treatment by Diet alone

Approximately a third of all diabetics can be controlled by dietary means alone. Obese diabetics should almost invariably be so treated.

Middle-aged or elderly diabetics who are not much underweight, who have had mild symptoms for some time and who do not show appreciable ketonuria, should also be given an initial trial of dietetic treatment alone, especially if they have at one time been overweight.

Initial treatment. These diabetics can be controlled and educated as out-patients. Each is told, in language and detail suited to his or her intelligence, about the nature of diabetes and why dietary restriction is necessary. A suitable diet is prescribed in accordance with the principles detailed on p. 316. It is easiest to start off with a simple restricted carbohydrate diet, and if this proves inadequate, to limit carbohydrate and fat more strictly by prescribing them in terms of domestic measures, or exchanges if this is desired. No one meal should be much larger than the others.

Diabetic patients should be given a 'Clinitest' apparatus and shown how to use it. The quantity of glucose present in the urine is readily determined by comparing the colour which results with those on the chart. The bottle containing the Clinitest tablets must be kept tightly stoppered and in a dry place; the tablets, normally mottled light blue become uniformly dark blue as they deteriorate and if then used will give falsely negative results. The tablets have a corrosive effect when swallowed and must be kept out of the reach of children. The 'Clinistix' and 'Testape' methods have an advantage over Clinitest in that they are specific for glucose, but should not be used in the assessment of diabetic control because they are too sensitive and give inadequate quantitative readings. The diabetic who is educated in his disease does not regard the testing of urine as being a 'waste of time', but those who are inadequately informed naturally do so, since to them the results are meaningless. They must, therefore, know what the urine test results mean and what change in treatment they indicate. They should show to the doctor at each visit a notebook recording the results of the tests.

L*

If strict diabetic control is desired, the urines to be tested are those passed on rising in the morning (which reflect the overnight blood glucose), before the main evening meal (which indicate the highest blood-glucose level of the day before a meal) and those passed three to four hours after the main evening or largest meal of the day (which reflect the rise in the blood glucose after a meal). Satisfactory control is indicated by the virtual absence of glycosuria in all specimens.

Patients not needing strict control should test only the overnight urines as these are the least likely to contain sugar. If these overnight urines are generally free from glucose and symptoms are absent, control can be considered to be satisfactory. Serious deterioration in diabetic regulation is indicated by a 1 to 2 per cent. overnight glycosuria. It is better for these elderly patients not to test daytime urines as these are likely to show sugar and thus cause unnecessary worry on the part of the patient and relatives. Nevertheless, if symptoms persist despite the absence of overnight glycosuria, then the urinary glucose lost during the day should be assessed by tests of the other two specimens. The response to treatment should also be checked by occasional blood-glucose determinations.

Further treatment. This depends largely on whether or not the patient has adhered to the diet and on the response to it. Initally, patients should report to the doctor every two weeks and then at intervals of four to six weeks until satisfactory control is established. The above specimens should be tested on two or three days each week until the diabetes is controlled.

Obese Diabetics

In the first few weeks of dietary treatment symptoms often disappear quickly and such patients generally lose some weight. The urine tests begin to show less glucose, especially the overnight tests which become negative much earlier in treatment than those done before and after the main evening meal. In some patients glycosuria rapidly and completely disappears within a week or two before there has been any appreciable loss of weight. Final response to treatment becomes apparent within one to six months.

In most patients loss of weight continues in association with reduction in hyperglycaemia and glycosuria. Such patients must persevere with the prescribed diet until they have attained their ideal weight or at least a reasonable one. When this has been reached, the diet may be relaxed a little provided that the extra food does not cause an undue gain in weight or reappearance of glycosuria.

On the other hand, some patients attain their standard weight but continue to show persistent glycosuria and hyperglycaemia. They require treatment with an oral hypoglycaemic agent or, if this fails, with insulin.

A number of patients do not lose enough weight and continue to show considerable glycosuria. This is nearly always due to failure to adhere to the diet, although it is occasionally the result of an excessive diet having been prescribed. Many do not adhere to their diets either because they, or the person responsible for preparing their meals, cannot understand them or because they do not know enough about their diabetes to appreciate the necessity for dietary restriction. Such patients often co-operate when the need for such restrictions is patiently explained to them. Every effort must be made to encourage them to adhere to the diet and they should be seen frequently by the doctor; in certain circumstances he is justified in frightening them a little by emphasizing the risks which they run. Treatment with the prescribed diet must be patiently continued as it may take several months for a completely satisfactory response to be obtained. The temptation to treat such patients with a sulphonylurea or insulin should be firmly resisted as these only aggravate the obesity. Treatment with a diguanide (p. 322) may, however, be justified if symptoms such as pruritus vulvae are intolerable though it must be remembered that persistence of pruritus may be due to local causes and not to glycosuria.

Non-obese Diabetics

The further treatment of these patients is similar to that for the obese. Many patients become well controlled within a few weeks; the diet may then be relaxed a little provided the diabetic control remains satisfactory.

Some lose too much weight although glycosuria and hyperglycaemia have been controlled by dietary restriction. Their diet should be increased; if this causes a return of hyperglycaemia and glycosuria, additional treatment will be needed with an oral hypoglycaemic agent to which they are likely to respond.

Very occasionally continued weight loss in the absence of glycosuria is due to the diabetes being secondary to pancreatic carcinoma.

All diabetics treated and controlled by diet must continue to test the selected specimens of urine on at least one or two days each week. They should show the record of these to their family doctor when they visit him to obtain the prescriptions for their Clinitest tablets, and to the clinic doctor when they visit him at about six-monthly or yearly intervals. They must test the specimens more often should they begin to show glycosuria or during times of intercurrent illness. If glycosuria persists they must report to their practitioner or clinic without undue delay. In this way any deterioration in diabetic regulation, due to dietetic carelessness, increasing severity of the diabetes, intercurrent illness or stress, will be recognized and corrected.

Treatment by Diet and Oral Hypoglycaemic Agents

The Sulphonylureas *Diabenese*

About 30 per cent. of all diabetics in this country are treated with a sulphonylurea. The drugs most commonly used are chlorpropamide (250 mg. and 100 mg. tablets) and tolbutamide (500 mg. tablets). Acetohexamide (500 mg.), tolazamide (100 and 250 mg.) and glymidine (500 mg.) have no advantage over tolbutamide. The most recently introduced is glibenclamide (5 mg.) which, like chlorpropamide, is given once daily; the equivalent dosages have not as yet been exactly determined but 10 mg. is probably equal to 250 to 375 mg. of chlorpropamide.

The sulphonylureas lower the blood glucose only in patients capable of producing endogenous insulin.

Selection of diabetics suitable for sulphonylurea treatment. The age of the patient when diagnosed is most important. Most diabetics diagnosed at an age of less than 40 years have insulin-dependent diabetes. It is usually a waste of time to treat these younger patients with a sulphonylurea since, even if it is initially successful, they soon become secondary failures. Thus, only patients aged more than 40 when diagnosed should generally be considered for sulphonylurea treatment. Most of them will have been tried previously on diet alone and will have failed to be controlled initially or will have become uncontrolled after months or years of satisfactory response. A few may be given a sulphonylurea on diagnosis; they are the thinner patients, with more marked symptoms of shorter duration, and a high spot blood sugar (350 mg. per 100 ml. or more).

Treatment with a sulphonylurea. These patients are unlikely to develop ketoacidosis and should be treated as out-patients.

The choice of sulphonylurea depends on the pattern of glycosuria. Thus, patients who, when treated by diet alone, show appreciable glycosuria in the overnight specimens should be treated with chlorpropamide, or possibly glibenclamide given before breakfast, since the hypoglycaemic effect persists during the night. Such treatment is cheaper than equivalent doses of tolbutamide given more than once daily. Conversely, patients requiring strict control whose overnight urines are free of glucose but who show appreciable glycosuria during the day should be treated with tolbutamide *Tolanase* or one of its equivalents, as the hypoglycaemic effect lasts only for 10 to 16 hours. It may be given as a single dose at breakfast or at both this meal and the midday meal as indicated by the urine tests. For these patients tolbutamide is preferable to chlorpropamide since the more protracted action of the latter is likely to cause hypoglycaemia during the night.

The urines which patients should test are the same as those for patients controlled by diet alone. Satisfactory diabetic regulation is indicated by absence of or only occasional glycosuria in the selected specimens.

The dosage given initially will depend on the severity of the symptoms and the patient's weight, the longer-acting drugs being indicated when significant overnight glycosuria has been present. Those who have lost a good deal of weight and experienced fairly severe symptoms for only a month or two should be given 250 to 375 mg. of chlorpropamide or 5 to 15 mg. of glibenclamide. In general, the maximum daily dose of chlorpropamide is 375 to 500 mg., and of glibenclamide is 15 to 20 mg. Others may be given a smaller dose of chlorpropamide or 1 g. of tolbutamide daily according to which drug the overnight urine test results indicated to be most appropriate. The response to therapy is indicated by the selected urine tests which should be made daily or on alternate days until control is achieved, and their results recorded in a notebook or Clinitest chart. Until satisfactory control is achieved, the patient should report to the doctor at fortnightly intervals.

About 80 per cent. of patients become satisfactorily controlled as indicated by the urine tests, weight change and abolition of symptoms. The time taken for this varies but usually is only a week or two. Some patients continue to show 1 to 2 per cent. glycosuria for several weeks despite significant lowering of blood-glucose levels to normal limits, due, probably, to persistence of a low renal threshold for glucose. Thus, if symptoms have improved it is dangerous to increase the dosage of the sulphonylurea unless the blood-glucose level is known since this might result in hypoglycaemia. When control is achieved, the dosage of sulphonylurea should be decreased and the maintenance dose determined by trial and error. All patients should test the appropriate urine specimens on one or two days each week and record the results in the notebook. This is absolutely necessary to detect loss of control due to stresses or illness, to overeating or to secondary failure. Patients should consult their general practitioners every four to six months when they report for the necessary prescription for the tablets, and the doctor should check the record of their urine tests. Patients must also test more frequently if they begin to show glycosuria or during times of intercurrent illness, and report to the doctor without undue delay if glycosuria persists.

Mild symptoms due to hypoglycaemia occur in about 5 per cent. of patients taking a sulphonylurea. Thus, patients treated with these drugs should take regularly spaced meals and should not fast for any prolonged period.

True secondary failure is nearly always accompanied by loss of weight. It is due to a progressive deterioration in endogenous insulin productive capacity rather than to actual resistance to the drug; in consequence the sulphonylurea, although still exerting its pharmacological effect, can no longer by itself control the hyperglycaemia. The secondary failure rate is probably about 5 to 10 per cent. for each of the first two years of therapy and a smaller percentage thereafter. Other causes of late failure include the use of inadequate doses of the sulphonylurea, failure to take the tablets regularly and the occurrence of intercurrent illness. By far the commonest cause, however, is excessive eating of food in which case there is usually a gain in weight despite increasing glycosuria.

Patients who have never responded satisfactorily (primary failures) and secondary failures may be given a trial of combined treatment with a sulphonylurea and a diguanide.

Toxic and side-effects of the sulphonylureas. Hypoglycaemia will occur if a sulphonylurea is given in excessive dosage, or if a sulphonamide or monoamine oxidase inhibitor is given.

Sulphonylureas can cause allergic skin reactions usually in the first month of treatment, varying from a mild maculo-papular rash to exfoliative dermatitis; the severer reactions are very rare; the milder occur in about 1 per cent. of patients. Another sulphonylurea can be substituted since cross-sensitivity between the drugs is unusual, but if the latter does occur, treatment with a diguanide should be considered.

In perhaps 10 per cent. of patients a sulphonylurea, particularly chlorpropamide, causes undue sensitivity to even small quantities of alcohol resulting in severe flushing of the face, throbbing headache and a feeling of intoxication. Another sulphonylurea may be tried or a diguanide substituted.

The results of prospective study of 8 years' duration carried out in the U.S.A. have been interpreted to show that treatment with tolbutamide, and by implication other sulphonylureas and the diguanides significantly increases the death rate from cardiovascular disease. The American Diabetes and Medical Associations and the FDA have therefore recently advised that these drugs be given only to patients uncontrolled by diet and for whom the addition of insulin is impracticable or unacceptable. There are however many criticisms of the study and the view of the British Diabetic Association is that oral therapy has not as yet been shown to be dangerous and that it, rather than insulin, is the treatment of choice for insulin independent diabetics uncontrolled by diet alone.

Other uses of sulphonylureas. There is no acceptable evidence that sulphonylureas facilitate or improve the control with insulin of patients having juvenile-type diabetes.

It has been suggested that the sulphonylureas may correct abnormal glucose tolerance in asymptomatic pre-diabetic patients and thus delay the onset of overt symptomatic diabetes; this, however, remains very much unproven.

The Diguanides

The two diguanides used in this country are metformin (500 and 850 mg. tablets) and phenformin (25 mg. tablets and 50 mg. slow release capsules).

The mode of action of these compounds has not been satisfactorily elucidated; they do not stimulate the beta cells of the pancreas to produce more insulin but increase peripheral tissue glucose assimilation, reduce hepatic gluconeogenesis, promote lipolysis and potentiate the effect of both endogenous and administered insulin.

Selection of patients for treatment with a diguanide. Although the daily insulin requirement of most insulin-dependent diabetics may be reduced by simultaneous treatment with a diguanide, this rarely leads to improvement in the ease or degree of their control. In this country insulin-independent diabetics, uncontrolled by diet alone, are usually treated with a sulphonylurea. This is because sulphonylureas were available before the diguanides. They have very few side-effects, so that an effective dose can be given initially and the diabetes be quickly controlled. Moreover, treatment with sulphonylureas is cheaper. At present the diguanides are used for primary or secondary sulphonylurea failures and those obese diabetics who, in spite of dietetic treatment, remain uncontrolled and experience persistent and disagreeable symptoms such as pruritus vulvae.

Treatment with a diguanide. In primary or secondary sulphonylurea failures the sulphonylurea must be continued, despite the fact that it does not appear to be having much effect, because it and the diguanide have a synergistic rather than an additive effect in terms of hypoglycaemic action. If failure of sulphonylurea treatment is accompanied by ketonuria and particularly a significant reduction in the plasma bicarbonate—insulin treatment should be given immediately and the temptation to temporize with diguanides resisted. Similarly, patients who develop diabetes when aged less than 40 years rarely maintain satisfactory control on combined treatment which postpones insulin therapy only for a short time and is not without danger since ketoacidosis can develop rapidly.

Treatment is started with 50 mg. of phenformin or 500 mg. metformin given twice daily with meals. These doses are slowly increased at intervals of one or two weeks until control is established or gastro-intestinal side-effects necessitate the abandonment of such treatment. The maintenance daily dose varies from 50 to 300 mg. of phenformin and 1 to 3 g. of metformin. Improvement in diabetic control is assessed by the same criteria in urine testing as are used to control treatment with diet alone or a sulphonylurea (p. 321). About 80 per cent. of primary or secondary failures to a sulphonylurea are satisfactorily controlled by combined treatment with the sulphonylurea and a diguanide. The proportion who eventually become secondary failures to

combined sulphonylurea–diguanide treatment is, however, high—probably about 15 per cent. per year.

It cannot be overemphasized that it is a great mistake to persevere with combined treatment in diabetics who are marginally or inadequately controlled by it. The change to insulin greatly improves their well-being and is better made sooner rather than later.

Combined treatment is also justified in diabetics for whom strict control is desirable and who when treated with a sulphonylurea show glycosuria in the pre- and post-supper but not in the overnight urines. This day-time glycosuria can be abolished by giving a small dose of diguanide with the meals shown to be most appropriate by the urine tests, generally breakfast and lunch.

In obese diabetics who persistently overeat and have marked glycosuria and distressing symptoms, diguanide treatment is initiated as above. In such cases a diguanide is the drug of choice because reduction of glycosuria is not accompanied by the gain in weight which occurs when sulphonylureas are given.

Toxic and side-effects. Gastro-intestinal disturbances occur in about 40 per cent. of patients treated with a diguanide; these include an unpleasant metallic taste in the mouth, anorexia and nausea, dyspepsia, vomiting, diarrhoea and abdominal colic. Such effects are usually transient or are quickly reversed by stopping the drug or reducing its dose for a day or two. Treatment with the diguanides has to be abandoned because of these side-effects in less than 5 per cent. of patients.

TREATMENT BY DIET AND INSULIN

Diabetics who require insulin, especially those needing good control, should be conversant with everything described under this heading.

Diabetic Patients who require Insulin Treatment

About a third of all diabetics require insulin. They can be classified roughly as follows:

(A) All those with severe diabetes, prone to ketosis, whose lives depend on the administration of insulin. Diabetics diagnosed when aged less than 40 years nearly always have this type, except the few who are obese, those fortuitously diagnosed before symptoms have occurred and those who have gone into spontaneous remission. About half of those diagnosed when more than 70 years old also have insulin-dependent diabetes, as do about 10 per cent. of those diagnosed between 40 and 70 years of age.

(B) Patients with moderately severe diabetes who cannot be controlled satisfactorily by oral hypoglycaemic agents. About 15 to 20 per cent. of those diagnosed between the ages of 40 and 70 years have this type of diabetes. In some it may so improve after a period of insulin treatment that they can again be treated with an oral hypoglycaemic agent; nevertheless, sooner or later, they usually again require insulin. Patients with stable diabetes controlled by diet or an oral hypoglycaemic agent may become uncontrolled, and sometimes ketoacidotic if they develop an acute or chronic infection, suffer physical injury, undergo an operation under anaesthesia, or become emotionally upset. Under such circumstances they may require insulin temporarily.

A properly educated insulin-dependent diabetic must: (1) understand the prescribed diet; (2) know how to look after his insulin syringe and how to measure and inject the insulin; (3) know when the insulins are having their effect and how to adjust their dosage according to the urine tests; (4) know which specimens of urine to test and what the results mean; (5) appreciate the symptoms of insulin-induced hypoglycaemic reactions and know how they are to be avoided and treated; (6) know how to adjust the diet or insulin dosage to permit of variations in meals and physical activity; (7) know how to maintain diabetic control during intercurrent illnesses.

Newly diagnosed insulin-dependent diabetics are best admitted to hospital for a short initial education in the principles of self-regulation. In general only a few days are required for this and it is unnecessary to stabilize the diabetes completely before discharging the patient home. Those who have become secondary failures to sulphonylurea or combined therapy and who can visit the clinic frequently can often be educated on an out-patient basis since they are already familiar with the dietetic principles involved and can test their urine satisfactorily.

Dietetic measures in diabetics treated with insulin. The diet is prescribed as described on p. 316. Free protein and fat are allowed, at least initially, and the carbohydrate is prescribed in the form of exchanges. A few additional dietetic principles must, however, be observed by diabetics taking insulin.

As far as possible the corresponding meals each day must be taken at about the same time and contain approximately the same amount of carbohydrate. For example, the diabetic should not take his midday meal at 12 noon on one day and at 2 p.m. on the next; nor should he take a great deal at that meal on the one day and very little on the other. Nevertheless, really well educated diabetics can enjoy great freedom in the timing and size of their breakfasts and evening meals provided they are taking a short-acting insulin before each of them.

Patients should continue to take their meals at their customary times. It is also undesirable to alter drastically the size of the meals relative to one another, although no one meal should be excessively large.

The dietetic habits of every insulin-taking diabetic must, therefore, be thoroughly ascertained and the diet so prescribed and arranged that these habits are altered as little as possible. It is simpler and more convenient for the well-educated diabetic to adjust the dose and times of insulin injection than to alter his dietary time-table.

Care of syringe, measurement and injection of insulin. An insulin syringe BS 1619, and no other type, should be prescribed. These syringes are available in 1 ml. and 2 ml. sizes and are graduated in 20 marks to the ml. without mention of units. Only Luer needles fit these syringes, the size required varying from the smaller 18 to the larger 16. The syringe and needles are kept in surgical spirit, several types of small watertight metal or plastic cases being available. The syringe should be boiled about once a fortnight.

The syringe must be cleared of spirit before use otherwise pain, stinging or a red lump may occur after injection. This can be done by moving the plunger quickly up and down the barrel till it is dry, or by cleansing it with cold water boiled the previous evening.

All types of insulin are supplied in two strengths—40 units and 80 units to the ml. The former should be prescribed when less than 20 units are to be injected, the latter if the amount is larger. One mark on the syringe equals 2 units of 40 strength insulin, and 4 units of 80 strength insulin. It is important to ensure that the needle and syringe are tightly fitted together and that cloudy preparations are well shaken before being drawn up into the syringe.

All diabetics must learn to inject themselves; the only exceptions are very young children, those whose eyesight is too poor, the senile or half-witted and those with hands afflicted by advanced arthritis or tremor. Far too many diabetics rely on relatives, friends or the district nurse. Self-injection is not difficult; it makes the patient independent and saves a great deal of inconvenience later on but often requires patient explanation, encouragement or even a little bullying.

Insulin is given by deep subcutaneous injection. The usual sites are the outer aspects of the thigh, lower buttock, lower abdominal wall and upper arm. The site should be varied from day to day. The skin is cleansed before injection. A thick fold of skin is then picked up and firmly pressed between thumb and forefinger until slight discomfort is experienced and the exposed fold becomes blanched and tense. The sharp tip of the needle is then pressed firmly over several points of the skin until a painless one is found; the needle is then pierced through the tense unyielding skin at an angle of 45 degrees to the surface and the injection made, the plunger being withdrawn a little beforehand to check that the point is not in a venule. The needle is withdrawn and the skin lightly massaged to disperse the injected insulin. This technique makes injection entirely painless. Very nervous patients may find useful one of several makes of spring-injector or hypo-guard, but recourse to these should rarely be necessary.

Some insulin preparations, because of their pH, their type of buffer or the presence of an excess of protamine or zinc, cannot be drawn up with one another in the same syringe as this would alter their normal times of action—for example, soluble insulin and PZI. In such circumstances the insulins are best injected separately at different sites. Alternatively the rapid-acting insulin is injected first, the syringe disconnected from the needle which is withdrawn slightly and pushed in deeper in a different direction and the longer-acting insulin injected through it from a second syringe.

Painful injections are due either to spirit left in the syringe or to an unduly superficial injection. The red, tender lumps and urticarial weals which occasionally appear may be due to local sensitization and are usually troublesome for only a short time. They can be alleviated by the use of antihistamine drugs, but if treatment is persevered with they usually diminish. In about 30 to 40 per cent. of patients local fat atrophy or occasionally hypertrophy of lesser or greater degree occurs at the sites of insulin injection.

There are some patients whose eyesight is too poor for them to measure accurately insulin in the syringe, but who can otherwise inject themselves. They should be given a 'stop insulin syringe'; this special BS 1619 syringe has a threaded plunger stem on which are two small stopper screws. The doctor screws these close together at a point on the plunger stem which allows the plunger to be withdrawn only up to the mark required for the dose of insulin. These screws can be moved only if turned in opposite directions and the stop is therefore firmly fixed. The patient withdraws the plunger to the maximum allowed by the stop, inserts the needle into the inverted insulin bottle, pushes the plunger in and out to its fullest extent about six times to prevent air bubbles remaining in the insulin drawn up, and then withdraws the needle. The required dose of insulin is now in the syringe and ready to inject. The doctor should check the syringe each time the patient reports to ensure that the stop has not moved in position.

Assessment of control. The healthy pancreas continuously secretes a small amount of insulin to regulate endogenous metabolism, and the amount liberated is increased whenever the blood glucose rises as, for example, after meals. At present it is impossible to imitate accurately this physiological secretion by the injection of any of the available preparations of insulin. Nevertheless it is possible to prevent the blood glucose from rising or falling excessively by proper dietetic treatment and by injection of the correct type or types of insulin in correct doses at the proper times. These can be determined only by the accurate assessment of control which is primarily based on the patient's own urine tests and checked by occasional blood-glucose estimations.

The diabetic must know the following about the type or types of insulin he is taking. (1) When the insulin starts to have a hypoglycaemic effect, its time of maximum action and the duration of its effect. These are better understood if they are explained to the patient in terms of meal times and daily activities (Fig. 7). (2) The urine specimens which must be tested for glucose to assess the effect of the insulin so that its dose can be correctly adjusted. Tests of the following specimens (a) to (c) passed before meals give diabetics taking insulin the information from which to assess diabetic control and to regulate the doses of insulin. It is, however, absolutely essential that the patient empties his bladder half to one hour before passing the specimen to be tested because the tests are deliberately timed to exclude post-prandial hyperglycaemia; they reflect the blood-glucose level either before a meal or more than three hours after the previous meal. Thus, if a patient takes his breakfast and does not pass urine until just before lunch then this specimen will contain the glucose which may have been excreted during the temporary hyperglycaemia resulting from breakfast. The blood glucose level, however, may have fallen to normal values by lunch time and yet a heavy glycosuria may be found, giving a misleading indication of the blood-glucose concentration.

(a) The pre-breakfast or true fasting specimen is that passed before breakfast, the bladder having been emptied half to one hour previously. This test reflects the fasting blood-glucose value.

(b) The pre-lunch and pre-supper specimens are those passed just before the midday and the main evening meal—the terms 'lunch' and 'supper' are used to avoid confusion since both may be called 'dinner'. These tests reflect the blood-glucose levels before these meals.

(c) The 'pre-bed' urine is passed as late as possible after supper. If the patient takes a light snack in the late evening, the urine sample is passed immediately beforehand; if he does not, it should be obtained just before he goes to bed. This test indicates the blood glucose value at these times.

Patients who, despite every effort to follow the rules, are prone to rapid and apparently inexplicable deterioration in diabetic control, should be provided with Acetest tablets or Ketostix with which to test the urine for acetone; some may also be given Dextrostix with which to make a rough assessment of their own blood-glucose level.

Preparations of Insulin

These can be classified clinically according to their times of action and miscibility or otherwise. Figure 7 shows the times of action of the insulins commonly used in this country. These depend on the rate of their absorption from the injection site which may vary from patient to patient, on the technique of injection and on the amount given. Doses of more than 40 units have a more prolonged maximal effect and duration of action than those indicated in Fig. 7.

RAPID- AND SHORT-ACTING INSULINS. Soluble insulin is a clear acid solution and cannot be injected from the same syringe with other preparations without altering their times of action except perhaps NPH (p. 328), which has no excess of protamine. NUSO is ox insulin in neutral solution and Actrapid is a clear solution containing recrystallized pig insulin in a neutral acetate-buffered solution.

The effect of an average dose of any of these preparations begins about 10 to 20 minutes after injection, is at its greatest at four to six hours and lasts for about eight to ten hours.

A few diabetics may be controlled by a rapid-acting insulin injected twice daily before breakfast and the main evening meal. However, these insulins are usually used in combination with either an intermediate- or long-acting preparation.

Soluble insulin is, of course, essential for the treatment of diabetic keto-acidosis (p. 334) and may be needed during an intercurrent illness (p. 331).

INTERMEDIATE-ACTING INSULINS. These are IZS amorphous (Semilente) and NPH (Isophane). The latter is perhaps the most commonly used insulin in North America and Australasia and is rightly becoming more popular here. Their effect starts about four hours after injection, is generally maximal at 6 to 10 hours and lasts about 8 to 14 hours. Their use in the achievement of moderate or good control is described later. The medium-acting insulins are also useful in the control of diabetics undergoing surgery with general anaesthesia (p. 335).

DELAYED AND LONG-ACTING PREPARATIONS. PZI (protamine zinc insulin) contains excess protamine and cannot be mixed with any other preparation. IZS crystalline (Ultralente) can be injected together with IZS amorphous. Their effect begins about six hours after injection, is greatest at 10 to 18 hours and lasts for 24 to 32 hours. They are also generally used in combination with other preparations.

INSULIN MIXTURES. IZS Lente is a mixture of Semilente and Ultralente insulins in the proportion of three to seven. Rapitard is a mixture of Actrapid and an intermediate-acting ox insulin in the proportion of one to three.

Except where specified, any of the above preparations may contain insulin derived from the ox or pig, or from both. There is some indication that pig insulin is less antigenic in man and that smaller doses of it may be needed than of ox insulin.

Achievement of fair or moderate control. Many older patients can, if they were previously treated by an oral hypoglycaemic agent, be educated on an out-patient basis. The choice of insulin depends on

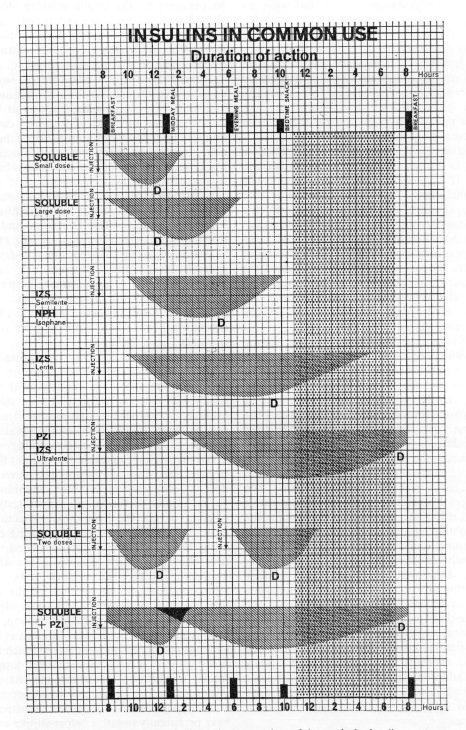

FIG. 7.—The urine tests used to indicate the correct dose of the particular insulin are shown
by D.

the doctor's own preference and the following are three examples of satisfactory regimens.

Patients who on oral therapy had overnight or true fasting specimens relatively free from glycosuria but had persistent day-time glycosuria with symptoms, may be controlled by the daily injection of an intermediate-acting insulin (NPH or IZS Semilente) given before breakfast. The dose required is that which keeps the pre-supper tests showing traces of glucose.

Most patients will, however, have considerable glycosuria in the true fasting or overnight urines. For them IZS Lente injected before breakfast is usually satisfactory. The dose required is that which keeps either the before supper or true fasting urines showing little or no glucose; since IZS Lente is a mixture of intermediate- and long-acting preparations it may have its maximal effect either before the main evening meal or during the night so that the urine test selected to determine dosage is that which shows the least glycosuria.

Adequate control can also be obtained by the single injection before breakfast of PZI (or IZS Ultralente) in a dose that keeps the true fasting urines showing occasional glycosuria. However, many elderly patients cannot pass two specimens of urine before breakfast: they should adjust the insulin dose to that which keeps the overnight or first urine passed on rising showing about $\frac{1}{4}$ to $\frac{3}{4}$ per cent. glucose. The results will vary from 0 to 2 per cent. depending on whether and when the patient urinated during the night. Any attempt to keep these overnight urines persistently glucose free will certainly result in night-time hypoglycaemia. The writer prefers this regimen because the overnight or true fasting urines are the most convenient for the patient to obtain and test, they ordinarily show the least glycosuria and any serious loss of diabetic control results in their showing persistent heavy glycosuria. Moreover, because no short- or intermediate-acting insulin is being given, there is little or no danger of day-time hypoglycaemia and the very simple diet (p. 319) suffices. Some patients may, however, have persistent symptoms due to gross day-time glycosuria even though the true fasting and overnight tests are negative. They require an additional injection of soluble or other rapidly acting insulin before breakfast in a dose sufficient to keep the pre-lunch tests showing a little glucose.

Achievement of good control. In the writer's experience, good control of diabetes can only rarely be obtained by the insulin mixtures Rapitard or IZS Lente. Their predetermined proportions deprive the patient of that flexibility of dosage which is so essential to the day-to-day control of the disorder and it is impossible to get all four daily specimens showing little or no glucose without very considerable changes in the distribution of food. The proportion of both components of IZS Lente can be altered but that of Rapitard can only be adjusted by giving more Actrapid since the medium-acting ox insulin component is not commercially available. The best results can usually be obtained by one of the following regimens.

COMBINATION OF A SHORT- AND LONG-ACTING INSULIN. These may be PZI and either soluble or Nuso, or IZS Ultralente and Actrapid injected separately. The dose of PZI or its equivalent is adjusted to keep the true-fasting tests generally glucose-free, and the dose of the morning soluble insulin, or its equivalent, to keep the before-lunch urine tests usually glucose-free. When the appropriate doses of these two insulins have been determined, tests of the before-supper and before-bed urines must be made.

Persistent glycosuria in the before-bed tests indicates the need for a second injection of soluble insulin before the main evening meal in a dose which will keep the before-bed tests showing, on average, $\frac{1}{4}$ to $\frac{1}{2}$ per cent. glycosuria—these should not be kept always glucose-free because of the danger of night-time hypoglycaemia. An additional precaution to prevent reactions at this time is to reduce the dose of PZI until the correct evening dose of soluble insulin has been determined.

The results of the before-supper tests indicate whether or not the hypoglycaemic action of the morning soluble insulin has lasted long enough to cover lunch and the afternoon period. If these tests show too much glucose in the absence of glycosuria in the before-lunch tests, the mid-afternoon snack can be omitted. If this is ineffective the dose of morning soluble insulin can be increased in order to prolong its action, in which case extra carbohydrate must be given at breakfast and mid-morning to prevent before-lunch reactions. A few patients, usually those taking a large dose of soluble insulin in the morning, may have marked glycosuria before lunch and yet experience occasional hypoglycaemic reactions in the afternoon and have persistently negative before-supper urine tests. This is due to the more prolonged action of larger doses of soluble insulin and the urine test required to determine its dosage is the before-supper one. In such patients carbohydrate can be shifted from breakfast to lunch and the mid-afternoon snack increased.

In this combined regimen the patient requires to test urines passed before each of the four main meals on about two days a week. The significance of these tests is illustrated in Fig. 7, p. 327. Expected or unanticipated extra exercise in the morning can be allowed for by reducing the morning dose of soluble insulin or by eating extra carbohydrate. Similarly, exercise in the evening can be covered by reducing the evening dose of soluble insulin or by increasing the carbohydrate at supper. Extra food taken at breakfast or at supper requires an increase in the appropriate dose of soluble insulin.

COMBINATION OF A SHORT- AND INTERMEDIATE-ACTING INSULIN. Such combinations may be soluble and NPH, Nuso and NPH or Actrapid and IZS Semilente, injected twice daily. NPH and soluble insulin may be injected together provided they are not mixed in the syringe and are injected within a minute of being drawn up. The doses of soluble and NPH (or their equivalents) given before breakfast should respectively be adjusted to keep the pre-lunch and pre-supper tests generally free of glucose. The doses of the short- and intermediate-acting insulins which should be given before supper are respectively those which prevent there being more than traces of glucose in the pre-bed and true fasting tests.

Sometimes the renal threshold for glucose is reduced during the first few weeks of treatment and this must be taken into account when adjusting insulin dosage according to the urine tests. On the other hand the insulin requirement may fall very appreciably shortly after the start of treatment, especially in younger diabetics. About two-thirds of these younger patients need very little or no insulin during the 'honeymoon' period of partial remission which may last for months or even years before the insulin requirement increases. The temptation to treat these patients with an oral hypoglycaemic drug should be strongly resisted (p. 323).

Most insulin-dependent diabetics should be admitted to hospital for initial instruction in the principles of diabetic self-regulation. These should be clearly written down and the patient must understand them before he is discharged. It is unnecessary to have the diabetes completely controlled before discharging the patient from hospital, since the circumstances prevailing at home are those to which the diet and insulin must be adjusted in terms of satisfactory urine tests. When the patient has eventually determined the necessary doses of insulin, the appropriate tests need only be done about twice a week. Nevertheless, he must test more frequently during times of illness or should there be persistent glycosuria, and should not hesitate to seek medical advice whenever loss of diabetic control occurs.

The majority of diabetics can control themselves satisfactorily by one of the regimens described above. It must be confessed, however, that some, because of their occupation, changing shift work, dietary habits or diabetic pattern need highly individualized regimens. Thus, a hard-working coal-miner should not take a short, strongly acting insulin just before going to work, since a reaction occurring underground might have serious consequences; it is better for him to inject himself on getting home from work when he will usually take his largest meal.

Hypoglycaemic Reactions

All insulin-taking diabetics should be deliberately given a hypoglycaemic reaction at the beginning of treatment to know what are the symptoms. They should know why such reactions occur and how to prevent and treat them. Hypoglycaemic reactions may be due to the injection of too much insulin, to delay in taking or to missing a meal, to taking too little food or to extra physical activity. The well-educated diabetic will, of course, reduce the dose of the appropriate insulin should he anticipate unusual exercise or reductions in diet and will take sugar or other carbohydrate to cover them if they are unexpected. Reactions do, however, sometimes occur even in the best-regulated patient. Sometimes this may be due to failure to shake properly a bottle of cloudy, usually long-acting preparation; this results in more concentrated and larger doses being injected as it becomes emptier. Very occasionally they may also occur when insulin-taking diabetics are given a mono-amine oxidase inhibiting drug which potentiates the effect of insulin. Lastly, reactions may result in those changing from an ox to a pig insulin since the latter is unaffected by antibodies formed to the bovine preparation.

The level to which the blood glucose must fall before hypoglycaemic symptoms occur varies considerably. In normal people a blood-glucose concentration of below 40 mg. per 100 ml. is usually necessary to produce symptoms. They may occur, however, at higher levels in diabetics who have become accustomed to a high blood-glucose concentration.

Hypoglycaemia due to short- and medium-acting insulins may begin with a feeling of weakness and emptiness in the stomach. Tremor, tachycardia and blurring of vision are common and diplopia occasionally occurs. The person feels faint and dizzy and often experiences a strong desire for food. Clammy sweating is almost invariable and, as the condition becomes more pronounced, mental symptoms are common, the patient sometimes becoming hysterical—laughing, crying, shouting and struggling. Many of these are due to adrenaline secreted in an effort to raise the blood glucose. Diabetics, while hypoglycaemic, may run amuck in the streets and be apprehended by the police as drunk and disorderly. At other times irritability or lassitude and somnolence are most marked features, especially in children. The advanced stages of hypoglycaemia are characterized by muscular twitchings, deepening coma and eventually by cerebral oedema and death.

Mild reactions due to long-acting insulin are often characterized by headache, drowsiness, failure to wake in the morning or by night sweats.

Any doubt regarding the diagnosis of hypoglycaemia can be confirmed or refuted very quickly by the use of Dextrostix, the instructions in the use of which are printed on the container.

The more severe hypoglycaemic symptoms seldom manifest themselves for several minutes after the initial sensations have been experienced. Thus the patient usually has time to rectify them. Treatment consists in raising the blood glucose by the administration of carbohydrate. All patients who are taking insulin must therefore carry with them several lumps of sugar, or preferably tablets of glucose which can be obtained from most pharmacists. After taking sugar the patient should remain inactive till the symptoms have disappeared. If the symptoms do not quickly subside or become worse, more sugar or glucose should be taken: it is far better to take too much than too little. When sugar is not at hand, as it always should be, any other carbohydrate food—such as orange juice or bread—can be taken. The latter, however, being more slowly absorbed, is much less effective than sugar or glucose in dealing with the emergency of hypoglycaemia.

In the great majority of cases these measures are rapidly effective. Occasionally, however, patients are encountered in deep coma and unable to swallow. Glucagon is an important advance in the treatment of hypoglycaemic coma and has greatly simplified treatment. It is a hormone secreted by the pancreatic α cells which rapidly raises the blood glucose concentration by stimulating the conversion of hepatic glycogen to glucose, and causing it to be released into the blood. Glucagon is available in sterile vials containing 1·0 mg. in powder form which has to be dissolved in 1 ml. of a special diluent which is also supplied. This dose should be injected either subcutaneously or intramuscularly and will arouse most patients sufficiently from their coma to enable them to take sugar by mouth. Unlike adrenaline, glucagon is safe and produces no undesirable consequences, even when excessive doses are given. Thus, in an emergency it can be injected by an intelligent friend or relative, and it is also much more convenient for the doctor than giving intravenous glucose. Its more frequent use would greatly reduce the dangerous delay which so often attends the treatment of patients in hypoglycaemic coma. A few patients, particularly those unconscious for several hours as the result of hypoglycaemia due to a long-acting insulin, fail to respond to glucagon. In these circumstances 25 g. of glucose, or more if necessary, should be injected intravenously as a 20 to 50 per cent. solution. The giving of rectal glucose-saline is a very inadequate method of raising the blood-glucose concentration and is not to be recommended in such emergencies. Patients recovered from severe reactions due to a long-acting insulin often relapse into coma unless given sufficient glucose at intervals for several hours; in severe cases it is often best to give an intravenous infusion of one litre of 10 per cent. glucose solution over the next few hours. When the patient has been successfully treated it is imperative to ascertain the reason or reasons for the occurrence of the hypoglycaemic reaction. In most instances these will be obvious and must be thoroughly explained to the patient.

In many of these patients severely hypoglycaemic for a long time, even large doses of parenteral glucose do not restore consciousness in spite of the blood glucose having been raised to high levels. This is due to cerebral oedema which may be fatal; it requires treatment by the intravenous infusion of mannitol to induce diuresis.

All patients taking insulin should carry a card

giving their name and address, the telephone number of their doctor or diabetic clinic, the type and dose of insulin which they are receiving and instructions to give them sugar if they are discovered in a faint or ill condition. Many doctors overstress the dangers of hypoglycaemia, causing their patients to become unduly alarmed about it. This is often responsible for inadequate insulin dosage, or even for insulin administration being withheld or stopped, with disastrous consequences. Thus the slightest, and often imaginary, feelings of discomfort are sometimes made the excuse by the patient for taking sugar. Nevertheless, frequent and prolonged episodes of hypoglycaemic coma may cause irreversible damage to the brain and must be avoided by the proper education of the patient.

Treatment with a sulphonylurea in excessive doses will also cause symptoms of hypoglycaemia. These are insidious in onset and usually consist of lightheadedness, mental confusion and drowsiness which may progress to coma.

Causes of Deterioration in Control

In diabetics who are not taking insulin the most usual cause of deterioration is eating too much carbohydrate; this is readily detected, however, since the patient usually gains weight or at least does not lose it despite the glycosuria. Quite commonly a chronic infection is responsible, particularly pyelonephritis. The use of certain drugs, such as the thiazide diuretics, may also impair control of diabetes. The recurrence of hyperglycaemia and glycosuria is, however, not infrequently due to increasing severity of the diabetes, or occasionally to the development of hyperthyroidism. Diabetic control will, of course, deteriorate whenever the patient has an acute infection, such as a common cold, or an emotional stress.

Deterioration of control in insulin-treated diabetics is often caused by one of the above factors. However, leakage of insulin either at the junction of needle and syringe or backwards past an ill-fitting plunger is a common cause which must always be excluded. In the previously well controlled woman, pregnancy may cause the reappearance of glycosuria (p. 337).

A few diabetics develop true insulin resistance. This can be due to one of several factors and results in a very marked increase in insulin requirements. Such patients require investigation by special techniques which necessitate their admission to hospital.

If tests demonstrate the presence of antibodies to insulin, treatment with corticosteroids is justified.

In many cases of apparent insulin-resistance the cause is the injection of too much insulin—the so-called Somogyi phenomenon. Usually a considerable reduction of the dose re-establishes control.

As mentioned on p. 337 the deterioration of control of diabetics treated by oral hypoglycaemic agents may be due to the development of secondary failure.

Diabetic Control during Illness

Doctors often become unduly alarmed when an insulin-treated diabetic develops a minor illness, such as gastritis, which prevents the patient from taking his normal diet. The educated diabetic should be able to handle the situation himself. The most common error is to assume that because less food is being taken little or no insulin is required so that the insulin is stopped and the patient develops severe diabetic ketoacidosis.

If the patient is able to eat solid foods, he can maintain the normal balance of his diet by selecting the appropriate carbohydrate exchanges in the form of lighter foods from his diet sheet or fluid feeds from those tabulated below. Each of the latter contains about 30 g. CHO and is equivalent to two exchanges. The insulin must still be injected and the dose required is that which allows the appropriate urine tests to show a trace of glucose. In this way the danger of hypoglycaemia is avoided.

If, however, the patient is unable to tolerate any solid food he must then take at least 120 g. of carbohydrate daily in the form of the fluid feeds given below. These should be taken slowly at three- to four-hourly intervals and the dose of insulin adjusted according to the urine tests. It is seldom necessary to resort to the administration of soluble insulin thrice daily and it is usually better to continue with the insulins with whose actions the patient is familiar. Patients who have been vomiting for some time and who have considerable glycosuria and ketonuria should be admitted to hospital where glucose can be given intravenously (p. 627).

FLUID FEEDS OF APPROXIMATELY 30 g. CHO
1. $\frac{1}{4}$ tin of fruit juice (15 oz. tin).
2. 1 pint of milk.
3. Teacup of Lucozade.
4. $3\frac{1}{2}$ tablespoonsful of Ribena.
5. $\frac{1}{2}$ oz. of cereal $+\frac{1}{3}$ pint of milk $+\frac{1}{2}$ oz. of sugar or glucose.
6. 4 tablespoonsful of porridge $+\frac{1}{3}$ pint of milk.

SEVERE METABOLIC DECOMPENSATION

Although the primary consequences of marked metabolic decompensation in the diabetic are hyperglycaemia, metabolic ketoacidosis, dehydration and electrolyte loss, these need not develop simultaneously nor parallel each other in severity. Thus, it is essential that blood is immediately obtained for estimation of glucose, potassium and bicarbonate (or another parameter of acidaemia) since the correct form of treatment can only be determined by the interpretation of these results considered in relation to the patient's clinical history and state. The response to therapy can never be confidently predicted so that the continued services of a biochemist are needed until such time as the physician considers the metabolic situation to be sufficiently corrected. Although there are several forms of metabolic decompensation, each can be managed initially in a fairly routine way.

Initial Management

A practitioner should immediately send to hospital any patient whom he suspects to have diabetic ketoacidosis or coma. Provided he is sure of the diagnosis he should give about 50 units of soluble insulin intramuscularly.

As soon as the patient arrives in hospital, blood is withdrawn and the biochemist asked to make the necessary analyses without delay. The most urgently required are the blood-glucose, serum-potassium and plasma-bicarbonate values, but the sodium, chloride and urea should also be determined as they may help in assessing the degree of fluid depletion. Except in the mildest cases, 100 units of soluble insulin or an appropriately modified dose if insulin has been given by the practitioner should be administered intramuscularly or added to the first bottle of the intravenous infusion of normal saline which should be started without delay. 'Cut-down' drips should be avoided since they may destroy the vein and prevent its subsequent use. Even in severely collapsed patients a suitable vein can usually be found if a tourniquet is applied to the arm after immersion in hot water, or if the arm has been made ischaemic a minute or two before by compression with the sphymomanometer cuff to above systolic pressure for a minute or so and then released.

The biochemical results should be available within half an hour. While waiting for them, about a litre to a litre and a half of saline should be given and the doctor should try to assess, from the history and physical examination, the cause and severity of the metabolic disturbance. Treatment should be started for any infection which may have been found after the necessary specimens, including blood, have been obtained for bacteriological examination. Other precipitating causes may also require specific therapy, but surgery should be deferred until the ketoacidosis has been at least partially corrected.

The comatose patient needs special care to prevent respiratory obstruction and aspiration pneumonia. If vomiting has occurred, careful gastric aspiration may prove beneficial.

A chart should be kept on which is recorded, as treatment progresses, the patient's blood-pressure, pulse and respiration rate; the route, volume and nature of the fluids administered and lost; the dose of insulin and its method of administration; the blood-glucose, serum-electrolytes and plasma-bicarbonate values; the relevant clinical observations and urine glucose and ketone content. The bladder, however, should not be catheterized as the sequelae of this procedure outweigh its potential value.

Further Management

The following paragraphs outline the further treatment of the three main forms of diabetic ketoacidosis or hyperosmolarity. Only brief consideration can be given to some of the problems that individual cases may present initially and/or during treatment.

Hyperglycaemic ketoacidosis. Inadequate insulin activity reduces tissue glucose assimilation and utilization and accelerates lypolysis and hepatic gluconeogenesis. Excessive protein and fat catabolism result; more ketone bodies are formed than can be utilized so that ketonaemia and later true metabolic acidosis develop. Impaired glucose uptake by the tissues and excessive gluconeogenesis lead sequentially to hyperglycaemia, glycosuria, osmotic diuresis and variable but usually considerable loss of water and electrolytes. The latter may be aggravated by vomiting, diarrhoea, fever or previous diuretic therapy. These changes are responsible for the glycosuria, ketonuria, hyperglycaemia, metabolic acidosis, acidotic breathing, clinical features of intra- and extracellular fluid depletion and symptoms of thirst and polyuria. Marked depletion of the extracellular fluid may cause circulatory collapse and the reduction of glomerular filtration may cause extreme hyperglycaemia. The resultant hyperosmolarity aggravates the intracellular dehydration and this, rather than the degree of ketonaemia or metabolic acidosis, is probably responsible for the clouding of consciousness and coma.

The principles of treatment are: (1) to correct ketoacidosis by giving insulin and, later, glucose to promote tissue utilization of glucose and to reduce gluconeogenesis and lipolysis; and (2) to replace fluid and electrolyte loss by appropriate therapy. The details of management vary from patient to patient.

The patient will usually be conscious. The biochemical results anticipated in a moderately severe case are usually about: blood glucose 650 mg. per 100 ml., HCO_3 8 mEq. per litre, K 6 mEq. per litre, Na 145 mEq. per litre, Cl 104 mEq. per litre, blood urea 55 mg. per 100 ml.

Fluid replacement. Because of the continued fluid loss during treatment the patient will require to be given more fluid (6 to 10 litres) than the initial deficit. About half should be extracellular, i.e. sodium-containing, and half intracellular, i.e. isotonic dextrose. Thus, after the initial 1 to $1\frac{1}{2}$ litres of normal saline has been given, infusion can be continued with two bottles of 5 per cent. dextrose to one bottle of saline, or dextrosaline if the blood glucose has fallen satisfactorily. The rate of infusion depends on the clinical state, but in general 1 to 2 litres should be given hourly for the first two to three hours and then somewhat less as rehydration occurs. Care should be taken to ensure that signs of overhydration do not develop.

Insulin. The amount of insulin to be given varies considerably and very large doses may be needed as ketoacidosis and the rise in fatty acids may cause insulin resistance. Soluble insulin should be injected intramuscularly or added to the intravenous infusion. If the initial blood glucose level was greater than 700 mg. per 100 ml. an additional 100 units should be given. Blood should be taken 90 minutes after the initial injection of insulin for determination of glucose, potassium and bicarbonate. Further specimens should be obtained at similar intervals until the clinical and biochemical state of the patient is satisfactory. Further insulin dosage is determined from these serial blood-glucose results and depend as much upon the rate of change as the absolute level. Once the blood-glucose level has fallen to 300 mg. per 100 ml., about 12 to 24 units of soluble insulin should be added to each bottle of 5 per cent. dextrose or dextrosaline but if it falls below 150 mg. per 100 ml.,

insulin should be discontinued. When rehydration is completed the intravenous infusion is stopped and the patient given small doses of soluble insulin subcutaneously before each 25 g. carbohydrate feed. The insulin requirements are thereafter determined on the basis of the urine and blood tests for glucose. In some cases little insulin is needed for several days following an episode of severe ketoacidosis.

Although a fall in the blood glucose concentration indicates that the insulin is being effective, it does not express the extent to which the ketoacidosis is being corrected. The latter is reflected by an increase in the plasma bicarbonate. In severely ketoacidotic patients four to six hours generally elapse before there is any real rise in bicarbonate because this does not occur before the ketone bodies have been utilized or excreted. In some patients, however, the bicarbonate level remains dangerously low after several hours of effective treatment. Such patients require treatment with more intravenous glucose and insulin as described for those with ketoacidosis without marked hyperglycaemia. The question of giving alkali intravenously is considered later.

Potassium. The serum-potassium level is initially often high due to shift of potassium from intracellular into extracellular fluid, this being roughly proportional to the severity of keto-acidosis and dehydration. Effective rehydration, sodium administration and restoration of the intracellular glucose utilization reverse this shift and reveal the overall deficit of the ion due to urinary and possibly gastrointestinal losses. Potassium should be given intravenously if its serum level is below 5 mEq. per litre provided urinary output is satisfactory. Potassium chloride ($\frac{1}{2}$ to 1 g.) should be added to each litre of fluid infused, the aim being to keep the level between 4·5 and 3·5 mEq. per litre as revealed by the serial biochemical estimations. If the serum potassium falls below 3 mEq. per litre the rate of administration should be doubled and, if necessary, redoubled; it should be appreciated that very large quantities of potassium may have to be given and it is safe to do so provided biochemical control is available. In less severe cases and in patients who are improving, the potassium can be given orally in effervescent form in a dose of 2 g. every two to four hours for 24 to 36 hours or until the body deficit has been made good.

Alkali. The metabolic acidosis should be corrected by administration of sufficient insulin and, as required, exogenous glucose to restore carbohydrate utilization. More rapid correction of the acidosis can be achieved by infusion of isotonic sodium bicarbonate or lactate in the place of saline. It may be more physiological to administer one part of sodium bicarbonate or lactate to every two parts of saline as the latter contains more chloride than is present in the extracellular fluid. In practice, however, alkali administration merely confuses the situation by artificially elevating the plasma bicarbonate and arterial pH and may thus lull the clinician into misplaced optimism.

Circulatory failure. This is rarely central in type and is usually due to gross dehydration. This results either from a prolonged osmotic diuresis or gross hyperglycaemia and hyperosmolarity. The latter is usually corrected by adequate replacement with isotonic fluids. When there is extreme hyperglycaemia, intravenous administration of hypotonic fluid is required.

Severe Ketoacidosis without marked Hyperglycaemia

This occurs in insulin-treated diabetics who for some days are unable to take carbohydrate by mouth because of gastric upset but who continue to inject insulin. The latter prevents excessive gluconeogenesis and gets the limited amount of glucose that is available into the cells. Thus, gross hyperglycaemia, glycosuria and osmotic diuresis do not occur but the relative inadequacy of intracellular glucose utilization leads to excess protein and fat catabolism with resultant ketonaemia and metabolic acidosis. The clinical manifestations are marked ketonuria, acidotic breathing and biochemical evidence of metabolic acidosis in the absence of thirst or polyuria, marked glycosuria, hyperglycaemia, electrolyte loss and dehydration. As there is little or no intracellular dehydration the patient is alert and fully conscious. Typical biochemical results might be levels of blood glucose of 200 mg. per 100 ml., potassium 7·5 mEq. per litre, sodium 140 mEq. per litre, chloride 98 mEq. per litre, bicarbonate 4 mEq. per litre, blood urea 40 mg. per 100 ml. Such patients require large amounts of glucose, sufficient insulin to ensure its assimilation and utilization by the cells and, if there has been much vomiting, fluid and electrolyte replacement. The response to therapy is assessed very largely by the serum bicarbonate which, after four to five hours of therapy, should begin to rise fairly rapidly. Dehydration if present is corrected with 5 per cent. dextrose or, when the patient is fully hydrated, by 10 per cent. dextrose; into each bottle 40 to 60 units of soluble insulin can be added and this dosage should be subsequently adjusted to the patient's response as indicated by the biochemical results.

Sometimes this syndrome is associated with renal tubular acidosis and such patients benefit from the administration of about 25 ml. of 8·3 per cent. sodium bicarbonate added to alternate bottles of intravenous dextrose.

Extreme Hyperglycaemia without Ketoacidosis (*hyperosmolar coma*)

Gross hyperglycaemia, glycosuria, dehydration, electrolyte depletion and altered consciousness can occur without metabolic acidosis or significant ketonuria. This is seen in elderly or middle-aged, often previously undiagnosed diabetics sometimes receiving a diuretic, who have had thirst and polyuria for several weeks; it may be that they have sufficient atypical endogenous insulin to maintain glucose utilization by liver and fat tissue but not enough typical insulin to maintain adequate glucose assimilation elsewhere. The resultant and increasing hyperglycaemia leads to glycosuria, osmotic diuresis, increasing hyperosmolarity, intracellular dehydration, clouding of consciousness and coma—all in the absence of significant ketoacidosis. Such patients are hypotensive and have impaired renal function. Typical biochemical results might be blood-glucose levels of 1,200 mg. per 100 ml., sodium 158 mEq. per litre, potassium 4 mEq. per litre, chloride 116 mEq. per litre, blood urea 98 mg. per 100 ml. and the serum osmolarity 380 m.u. osm per litre or more. The plasma bicarbonate value might vary from about 17 to 26 mEq. per litre.

Insulin should be given at a rate of 80 units per hour or more if needed until the blood glucose has fallen below 500 mg. per 100 ml. when the dosage can be reduced. Vasopressor drugs, corticosteroids and blood transfusion have all been advocated to correct hypotension but the rational and correct treatment is proper rehydration. The amount of fluid required is considerable and about 1 to 2 litres should be given hourly for six hours. Following the initial administration of normal saline, patients require rapid infusion of 2 to 3 litres of hypotonic solutions, half of which should be sodium containing and half given as 2·5 per cent. dextrose. These should be replaced by isotonic fluids when the blood-glucose concentration has fallen to about

500 mg. per 100 ml., unless the patient remains severely hypernatraemic, in which case hypotonic infusion is continued.

Potassium replacement is always needed; many patients have profound depletion and require massive replacement therapy, especially if the initial level is low. Occasionally 8 g. or more of potassium chloride per litre of infused fluid has to be given.

Summary. It must be emphasized that severe metabolic decompensation in a diabetic is a medical emergency. The causes of this condition, its metabolic development, the initial degree of hyperglycaemia, ketoacidosis, dehydration and electrolyte depletion do not necessarily parallel one another. Thus, the initial treatment and the response to it must be determined by an accurate assessment of the clinical and biochemical picture by an experienced physician who has the assistance of a biochemist and competent nursing staff.

Diabetes in Children

Less than 5 per cent. of diabetics develop the disease in childhood. This is fortunate, for the control of the diabetic child is usually more difficult than that of the adult, for several reasons: all diabetic children have insulin-dependent juvenile-type diabetes and very readily develop ketonaemia; they are often extremely sensitive to small changes in insulin dosage; moreoover, it is difficult to enforce strict dietary disciplines on children and marked variations in their daily activities and emotions are unavoidable.

These difficulties are nevertheless not insurmountable and there is no reason why diabetes in children should not be satisfactorily controlled without undue interference with their normal life. It is important to treat the child as an intelligent person and to give him a sense of responsibility in regard to his own health. Children respond well to this approach and often become the best diabetic patients.

The prescription of a diet for the diabetic child differs in several respects from that for the adult patient. It is important to give adequate but not excessive calories for growth and activities; overfeeding results in the child becoming unduly fat, particularly if the insulin dosage is large. Sufficient protein, vitamins and minerals are required for growth. Sweets, jams and sugar should be avoided; the child soon forgets their taste and his desire for them abates; in addition the likelihood of dental caries is much diminished. Suitable dietary prescriptions for diabetic children are given on p. 318; these may have to be increased or decreased according to individual needs.

The principles upon which control of the diabetes by insulin is based are the same as for adults. Perhaps the most suitable regimens are the daily injection of PZI and soluble insulin before breakfast and the administration of a second dose of soluble insulin before the evening meal or the twice daily injection of soluble and NPH insulins. Urine tests for ketones and blood-glucose estimations by 'Dextrostix' are useful adjuncts to the assessment of diabetic control by the child's parents. The parents must also know what steps to take during periods of digestive upsets, infections and minor illnesses to which children are so prone; they should also have glucagon for treating hypoglycaemic reactions.

The Care of the Surgical Diabetic

The discovery of insulin and the improvement in anaesthetic techniques have made surgery as safe for the diabetic as for the non-diabetic. Nevertheless, an operation is a considerable risk if the patient falls into inexperienced hands. Successful treatment depends upon close co-operation between surgeon, physician and, if possible, a nurse who has been trained in the care of diabetic patients.

The risks involved are those of ketosis on the one hand and of hypoglycaemia on the other. Ketosis may result from administration of an unsuitable anaesthetic, from prolonged starvation, from vomiting or from inadequate diabetic control; hypoglycaemia during or after operation is caused by the injudicious administration of insulin.

The routine testing of every patient's urine before operation is imperative. The overnight or prebreakfast specimens of urine of many patients having mild untreated diabetes maybe glucose-free; the specimen which ought to be tested by Clinitest is that passed two to three hours after a meal. If this post-prandial urine contains glucose, the patient should be considered to be diabetic until proven otherwise. The fasting blood-glucose concentration is also an unreliable criterion of diabetes as in many mild diabetics it is less than 120 mg. per 100 ml.; the blood glucose should be determined two hours after a meal. It is quite common for diabetics to be diagnosed for the first time post-operatively, sometimes because of the development of severe diabetic ketoacidosis or even coma; their urine was either never tested pre-operatively or only an overnight or pre-breakfast specimen was examined.

It is impracticable to outline a routine to be followed for all surgical diabetic patients. Experience is the only sure guide to treatment, but the following are the guiding principles: (1) to ensure that the diabetes is well controlled for the days preceding elective operation; (2) to prevent the patient from becoming hypoglycaemic when under the anaesthetic but *to give nothing orally* for at least eight hours pre-operatively; (3) to prevent keto-naemia and acidaemia post-operatively by giving sufficient glucose either by mouth or intravenously and, when required, by ensuring its utilization by the administration of adequate doses of insulin; (4) to maintain the patient in proper fluid and electrolyte balance. The method of preparing the patient will vary according to whether the operation is undertaken as an emergency measure or whether the patient can be prepared for surgery at leisure. It will also depend on whether the patient is being treated with insulin, a sulphonylurea or by diet only and on the nature of the surgical procedure.

Elective surgery. The patient should be admitted to hospital two or three days before the operation for assessment and if necessary rectification of the diabetic control. He is allowed his usual diet and, if treated with insulin or a sulphonylurea, is given his ordinary dose of either. Diabetic control is assessed on the results of the appropriate urine tests and the fasting blood-glucose concentration determined on the day preceding, and the day of the operation.

Patients correctly treated by diet or a sulphonyl-urea will have a fasting blood-glucose concentration of between 110 to 160 mg. per 100 ml. They should be given nothing by mouth on the morning of the operation. After they have regained consciousness light feeds may be given or, if this is impossible, 5 per cent. glucose solution by intravenous infusion. Insulin is rarely required.

In the case of insulin-treated diabetics, the dose of the long-acting insulin given on the morning, or that of the medium-acting insulin given in the evening of the day before operation which ought to be timed for mid-morning—is adjusted to bring the fasting blood-glucose level to between 120 and 180 mg. per 100 ml. The practice of giving the patient about 25 g. of carbohydrate orally and an injection of soluble insulin four to six hours before operation is to be deplored since a large proportion of the feed may remain in the stomach due to suppression of gastric motility by anxiety or pre-operative medica-

tion. Two serious consequences ensue; firstly, when anaesthesia is commenced the retained glucose feed may be vomited and inhaled into the respiratory tract; secondly, the glucose is not all absorbed and the insulin—the dose of which is in any case arrived at by pure guesswork—is liable to cause hypoglycaemia while the patient is under the anaesthetic. It is thus undesirable to give anything by mouth pre-operatively.

The insulin-taking diabetic undergoing a surgical operation which is not going to be excessively pro-longed should be prepared according to the fasting blood-glucose value: if this lies between 120 and 250 mg. per 100 ml. neither insulin nor glucose is given; if it is less than 120 mg. per 100 ml. then an intra-venous infusion of 5 per cent. glucose should be started and continued throughout the operation; if it exceeds 250 mg. per 100 ml. about a third or a quarter of the usual daily dose of insulin may be injected as NPH or IZS semilente. These are preferable to soluble insulin because the onset of their hypoglycaemic effect is delayed for three or four hours. There is, therefore, no danger of hypoglycaemia occurring while the patient is unconscious and any post-operative hyperglycaemia is effectively covered. The maximal effect of soluble insulin on the other hand may occur whilst the patient is under anaesthesia so that there is a danger of hypoglycaemia at that time.

This technique of pre-operative diabetic care is exceedingly simple, safe and satisfactory: the patient comes to the theatre with an empty stomach, usually with no intravenous infusions to incon-venience the surgeon and there is no danger of hypoglycaemia developing while he is under the anaesthetic. Though it is ideal for the operation to be done at mid-morning, the technique can be adapted for operations in the afternoon. In the latter circumstance a normal breakfast is given and covered with a small dose of soluble insulin; the blood glucose is determined an hour before opera-tion and the appropriate measures taken as described above.

The operation will usually be completed at latest by early afternoon. The blood-glucose concentra-tion may, if needed, then be determined and the patient can usually take 100 to 120 g. of carbo-hydrate in the form of three or four fluid feeds (p. 331) before midnight. These may be covered by appropriate doses of soluble insulin which involves repeated injections; it is far better to give the patient when he has regained consciousness about half to two-thirds of his usual daily dose as NPH or Semilente insulin whose time of action is ideally suited to cover the three feeds given at about 4 to 5 p.m., 7 to 8 p.m. and 10 p.m. to midnight. If oral feeding is not possible, about 125 g. of glucose can be given by intravenous infusion lasting until next morning and equal amounts of soluble insulin added to each bottle to provide about half the usual daily dose.

The insulin-treated diabetic undergoing very prolonged surgery will require to be 'covered' during the operation by an intravenous infusion of 5 per cent. glucose solution (not glucose saline) to which the requisite dose of insulin is added.

On the day following operation the patient is given his usual meals and insulin; the diet can be made more easy to assimilate by choosing appropriate exchanges from the list on p. 318. If food cannot be taken orally the intravenous infusion of insulin and glucose must be continued and the usual steps taken to prevent or remedy any water or electrolyte imbalance.

If a minor operation is carried out under local anaesthesia, no insulin will be required, except post-operatively in the case of those normally receiving insulin.

The patient who has had a lens extraction for cataract should, for the first week post-operatively, be given a diet in such a soft form that little mastication is required.

Emergency surgery. For the diabetic undergoing emergency surgery no rule-of-thumb routine can be given. The administration of either glucose and/or insulin will depend on the time when the patient last had a meal, on the dose and types of insulin taken, the times of their injection and on the metabolic situation. The blood-glucose, plasma-bicarbonate and electrolyte values should be determined in diabetics taking insulin and those showing ketonuria or gross glycosuria. If the surgeon is in any doubt as to what to do he should seek the advice of a physician experienced in diabetes.

Diabetes in Pregnancy

Although insulin treatment made pregnancy safe for the diabetic mother, the foetal loss rate remained for a long time exceedingly high at about 40 per cent. This, however, can be reduced to between 15 and 20 per cent. if the child is delivered electively prior to full term, if the mother is meticulously supervised during pregnancy and if close co-operation between physician, obstetrician, anaesthetist and paediatrician is obtained. The diabetic woman should be admitted to hospital for a few days not later than the 10th or 12th week of her pregnancy. This ensures that she knows how to control her diabetes to the best possible extent. The renal threshold for glucose is not usually lowered at this stage. The diet prescribed should be that suitable for the pregnant patient (p. 339). The blood Wassermann, haemoglobin and Rhesus group should be ascertained and the obstetrician should become acquainted with the patient.

Thereafter, up to the 24th week of pregnancy, she should be seen each fortnight and then at weekly intervals; it is ideal that she be interviewed by both physician and obstetrician in combined consultation. The patient must test regularly and sufficiently often those specimens of urine required for the type or types of insulin she is taking (p. 325) and must bring a record of the results. If the renal threshold for glucose is much lowered, the patient may be guided in respect of insulin dosage by occasionally checking the blood-glucose value before meals, using Dextrostix. In many patients the dosage of insulin will have to be progressively increased as pregnancy advances.

If the renal threshold for glucose is low, it is not unusual for acetone to be present in the urine in addition to glucose, especially in the before-breakfast urines, despite relatively normal blood-glucose levels. The carbohydrate of the diet will then have to be increased; a 40 g. carbohydrate feed during the night may also be needed, and the dose of insulin raised. Lactosuria may occur in the later weeks of pregnancy but is of no significance.

The patient should be readmitted to hospital not later than the 34th week. She should not be confined to bed and should take a moderate amount of gentle exercise. During this time diabetic control must be strictly maintained, the insulin dosage being based on the daily urine tests and the blood-glucose profile obtained every three to five days.

The incidence of toxaemia of pregnancy and hydramnios is increased in diabetic women.

In general, delivery towards the end of the 37th week gives the best results. Earlier delivery should be effected in patients who have lost a child in a previous pregnancy following intra-uterine death prior to the 36th week and in those with significant toxaemia or a rapid increase in hydramnios.

It is also indicated if there are signs of impending foetal death; this may be heralded by a fairly rapid decrease in insulin requirement or in urinary oestriol excretion. Each case presents its own particular problems and the decision as to when delivery should be made is the joint responsibility of obstetrician and physician.

Caesarean section is certainly indicated when the child is very large, in patients who in the past have had prolonged or difficult labours, in those who have had a previous section and in those—particularly primigravidae—who have failed to deliver themselves after a reasonable number of hours following induction of labour.

The patient must be properly prepared for elective surgery. The dose of insulin given the previous day should be adjusted so that the blood-glucose concentration on the morning of operation lies between 120 and 180 mg. per 100 ml.; no insulin, food or fluids should be given on the morning of operation, and the administration of sedative drugs likely to depress the respiratory centre of the child is to be avoided. It should rarely be necessary to give any premedication to allay anxiety in the patient if a confident relationship has been established with her medical attendants including the anaesthetist. Spinal analgesia avoids any respiratory depression in the infant, and thereby reduces the risk of neonatal pulmonary complications. General anaesthesia can, of course, be used in place of spinal anaesthesia if the patient so desires. Delivery is effected by lower segment Caesarean section. Vomiting may occur within a few minutes after delivery. This is probably related to the intravenous injection of ergometrine, and the intramuscular injection of oxytocin is preferable.

The mother's blood-glucose concentration should be determined two or three hours after delivery and, according to the result, a small dose of medium-acting insulin given to cover the feeds which she should be able to take in the late afternoon. If she cannot eat, an intravenous infusion of glucose should be given, to which is added appropriate small quantities of soluble insulin. On the following day her ordinary pre-pregnancy diet can usually be tolerated. It is particularly important to remember that the insulin requirement falls dramatically after delivery, so that the dose should be drastically curtailed. Diabetic mothers should not be encouraged to nurse their babies as they seldom secrete sufficient milk.

In recent years delivery *per vaginam* has become more popular, since babies so born are thought to be less liable to develop pulmonary hyaline membrane disease and have better prospects of survival. An attempt to induce labour by rupture of the membranes in the late evening followed next morning by oxytocin infusion intravenously can be made provided there is no obstetric contraindication; analgesics which depress respiration must be used sparingly. The patient is prepared as for Caesarean section and the intravenous infusion of oxytocin started as early as possible in the morning. During the day she may be given either small snacks or 25 g. CHO drinks at three- to four-hourly intervals, these being covered by injections of soluble insulin, the doses of which are based on blood-glucose estimations. The onset of labour, however, may be associated with nausea and vomiting and it is generally safer and easier to give the glucose by continuous intravenous infusion to which insulin is added.

In most cases delivery will occur by early evening, with or without the aid of forceps; if the patient can take food by mouth, the glucose infusion is then stopped, and the mother's further care is as described following Caesarean section. If no obvious progress toward delivery has been effected by early evening, the oxytocin should be stopped and the mother delivered by Caesarean section.

Ideally the care of the baby is supervised by a paediatrician. It cannot be too strongly emphasized that the babies of diabetic mothers, in spite of the fact that they may be very large, are physiologically premature, exceedingly prone to the respiratory distress syndrome, and that their first few days are critical; the infant should therefore be carefully nursed for the first 48 hours by the trained staff of the premature baby unit. During this time feeds may be given and controlled oxygen administration may be required. Neonatal hypoglycaemia is seldom a cause of death in these babies and the practice of giving them parenteral glucose has largely been abandoned. In the first few days the babies of diabetic mothers catabolize a great deal of fat which, together with the resultant diuresis, causes a considerable loss of weight.

A few mildly diabetic women can be treated with a sulphonylurea or diguanide during pregnancy. Tolbutamide should be substituted for chlorpropamide or glibenclamide after the 35th week; babies delivered from mothers treated by chlorpropamide have developed profound, prolonged and occasionally fatal neonatal hypoglycaemia due to the passage of the long-acting sulphonylurea through the placenta.

Diabetes itself does not constitute an indication for therapeutic abortion apart from the presence of severe diabetic nephropathy or retinopathy. Nevertheless, in respect of ultimate longevity, pregnancy constitutes a hazard to the diabetic mother and sterilization is justified after the second or third delivery—or earlier if the patient is no longer young and exhibits degenerative diabetic complications.

Although glycosuria is common in non-diabetic pregnant women owing to lowering of the renal threshold for glucose, many true diabetics are missed because the glycosuria is ascribed to this benign cause; the presence of fasting glycosuria is almost certainly due to diabetes. In unrecognized diabetic patients the foetal loss rate is exceedingly high. Women who show repeated post-prandial glycosuria in pregnancy should be screened for diabetes by appropriate tests—particularly if they have a family history of the disorder, or have given birth to large babies, or have lost them on account of late intra-uterine deaths in previous pregnancies. The most practical method is for the patient to take a breakfast containing 100 g. of carbohydrate, i.e. one containing six or seven carbohydrate exchanges (p. 318) and to have a blood sample withdrawn two to two and a half hours later. Should this contain more than 120 mg. of glucose per 100 ml., a full glucose-tolerance test must be undertaken.

COMPLICATIONS OF DIABETES

Ocular changes. Many diabetics, when first treated, complain of failure of near vision or blurring of vision, which result from osmotic changes in the lens due to rapid lowering of the blood glucose. They should be warned that this is likely to occur and that it will disappear once diabetic control has been established for a few weeks. On no account must they be sent for spectacles until the diabetes has been controlled for two or three months.

The specific type of diabetic cataract, which is extremely rare, can be reversed if control of the diabetes is established at a very early stage, for it occurs in young patients who are very poorly controlled. Senile cataract probably occurs no more frequently in diabetics than in non-diabetics and its treatment is conducted along the usual lines.

Once diabetic retinopathy has become established, it is doubtful whether better control of the diabetes will improve it although it may prevent further deterioration. Visual impairment is nearly always due to hard exudative type retinopathy or vitreous haemorrhage and fibrosis secondary to primary capillary neovascularization or venous changes.

Patients showing deep waxy retinal exudates should be treated with clofibrate, 500 mg. four times daily. This does not accelerate removal of established exudates by phagocytosis, but in about two-thirds of patients it reduces or prevents fresh exudation. Since the retinal tissue is irreparably damaged by pre-existing exudates no improvement in any loss of visual acuity can be anticipated, but deterioration can largely be prevented by this prophylactic therapy.

Diabetics showing evidence of primary neovascularization or venous changes should be referred to and checked regularly by an experienced diabetician or ophthalmologist. Serious haemorrhage may be largely prevented by light coagulation or pituitary ablation, the choice of therapy being determined by the nature and site of the lesions. In patients with hypertension, reduction of the blood pressure may reduce the frequency and severity of bleeding.

About one in every 40 diabetics is registered as blind. This number could be greatly reduced if the retinae were examined at yearly intervals and therapy instituted before the retinal changes had advanced sufficiently to cause irreversible visual impairment.

Diabetic nephropathy. In most cases the course of this disorder is that of slowly progressive chronic renal failure. In only a few patients is it characterized by the nephrotic syndrome that includes proteinuria, low plasma albumin, oedema, hypertension and diabetic retinopathy—sometimes erroneously called the Kimmelstiel-Wilson syndrome. In the latter cases treatment with a suitable diuretic is desirable and the protein and salt content of the diet adjusted as required.

Diabetic neuropathy. The painful peripheral neuropathy associated with poor diabetic regulation is usually reversed when the disorder is satisfactorily controlled. In the interim period, analgesics should be given. The commonest diabetic neuropathy is the painless peripheral type affecting legs and feet; the accompanying loss of the sense of pain in the feet, associated with the presence of peripheral diabetic microangiopathy, makes the patient particularly prone to traumatic and infective lesions. The absence of pain often leads to delay in seeking advice. The most important treatment of such trophic ulcers is rest and the administration of antibiotics if there is infection. When surgery is required, local measures often suffice.

Diabetic myelopathy or amyotrophy affects mainly the proximal muscles of the legs. Vigorous physiotherapy to restore power to the quadriceps and adductors is usually effective though it may be many months before the patient can walk unaided.

Diabetic autonomic neuropathy is not uncommon and presents most frequently as impotence, bladder disturbances, diabetic diarrhoea or postural hypotension. It must never be diagnosed unless the appropriate physical signs are present. Treatment is unsatisfactory. Diarrhoea can sometimes be combated with anticholinergic drugs such as benzylonium bromide. Symptomatic treatment also includes the use of codeine phosphate (60 mg. three times a day). The diet should be altered to reduce fat and high-residue foods. Occasionally an attack responds to 250 mg. of tetracycline given twice or thrice daily.

Peripheral microangiopathy in the limbs. This, in association with painless neuropathy, leads to local areas of necrosis resulting from trauma or infection. Its treatment is as described above.

Non-specific complications. Although diabetics are no more susceptible to tuberculosis than non-diabetics, it is wise to have all newly diagnosed diabetic children tested with tuberculin and to vaccinate negative reactors with BCG.

Ordinary atherosclerotic or obliterative peripheral vascular disease is more common in diabetics than in non-diabetics, although its incidence in this disorder may be more apparent than real because the majority of diabetics are middle-aged or elderly. Patients having peripheral vascular disease should be instructed in the care of their feet (p. 139) and, if possible, should attend a chiropodist at regular intervals.

Pruritus vulvae which fails to respond to adequate control of the diabetes is probably due to local causes. When moniliasis has been excluded these patients should be referred to a gynaecologist. Conversely, gynaecologists and doctors should not consider pruritus vulvae to be due to a local cause until a post-prandial urine has been tested for glucose.

Spontaneous Hypoglycaemia

This condition may be considered conveniently in this section of the book though it is, of course, the direct opposite of diabetes mellitus. Some patients suffering from hypoadrenocorticism or hypopituitarism experience hypoglycaemic symptoms when deprived of food for some time, particularly on waking in the morning. Correct replacement therapy with corticosteroids restores the capacity of the liver to release glucose into the blood. Fasting hypoglycaemia also occurs in patients with severe hepatic insufficiency, in idiopathic hypoglycaemia of childhood which may or may not be leucine sensitive, and in a few patients suffering from neoplasia, usually of mesothelial origin. Treatment consists of sufficiently frequent carbohydrate feeds, avoidance of leucine-containing foods when indicated and of alcohol, which can certainly induce hypoglycaemia in those with hepatic insufficiency.

Patients who have had a total or subtotal gastrectomy sometimes experience hypoglycaemic symptoms about an hour or so after a meal, particularly if it is rich in carbohydrate. Treatment consists of the avoidance of large quantities of carbohydrate and of the attempt to delay gastric emptying by the inclusion of ample fat in the diet.

Benign or malignant tumours or hyperplasia of the beta-cells of the pancreatic islets also give rise to both fasting and post-prandial hypoglycaemia. Treatment consists of the removal of the small tumour or subtotal pancreatectomy if it cannot be distinguished at laparotomy. Persistent hypoglycaemia due to inoperable tumour or metastases may be treated by diazoxide.

Hypoglycaemia three to four hours after food may be a feature of early diabetes or prediabetes. Excessive alcohol may precipitate it in cirrhotics.

In an appreciable number of patients who experience post-prandial or fasting hypoglycaemia no cause can be found. This syndrome is termed functional, spontaneous or idiopathic hypoglycaemia. It is believed to occur most frequently in anxious, agitated or depressed persons, but these attitudes may be due to the inconvenience and misery produced by the symptoms. The majority respond to redistribution of the diet so that moderate amounts of carbohydrate are taken at not unduly long intervals, but if this is unsuccessful, corticosteroid or diazoxide treatment may be tried.

OBESITY

Quite apart from aesthetic considerations, long-continued obesity has as its sequelae more or less grave disturbances of most of the systems of the body. Thus the statistics of Life Assurance Companies all show that mortality rates rise steadily in proportion to the extent people are overweight. Flat foot, varicose veins, osteoarthritis of the knees and hips, backache, herniae, cystocele, prolapse, cholecystitis and gall stones, diabetes, degenerative changes in and overstrain of the myocardium, angina of effort, hypertension, bronchitis and post-operative complications are all more frequent in the obese than in the lean. The more specific treatment of these aliments is likely to be unsuccessful if associated obesity is disregarded. Indeed, reduction in weight is sometimes the only treatment necessary for the milder forms of such conditions.

The immediate cause of obesity is the prolonged consumption of a diet containing more calories than are needed to provide for the body's tissue repair, vital functions and physical activities. In modern society, foods have become very plentiful and attractive, and the physical effort demanded by many occupations has diminished. Most people in civilized communities eat more than they require and it is surprising that obesity is not more common than it is. It is difficult to escape the conclusion that there exists some unknown fundamental mechanism by which the body is enabled to dissipate the surplus calories which would otherwise be stored as fat. If there were not such a mechanism, obesity would be much more common, for a daily intake of 200 kcalories in excess of actual requirements, such as would be represented by an extra glass of milk or two slices of bread, would increase the body weight by some 12 kg. a year. This is what does occur in certain unfortunate people who do not seem to possess this undefined ability to deal with excess calories. Conversely an obese person must burn up about 6,000 kcalories of his own fat to lose 1·0 kg. in weight.

The actual cause or causes of overeating in man are obscure. Appetite and satiety seem to be controlled by distinct areas in the hypothalamus, and, in animals, experimentally produced lesions in this region can result in either voracious appetite or complete anorexia. In man, however, these areas seem to be dominated by the higher cortical centres and there is little doubt that overeating is almost always due to habit, to the pleasures associated with eating or to the need for sublimating an emotional want or dissatisfaction. Indeed overeating—like alcoholism or drug taking—is often a symptom of emotional disturbance.

The general public—particularly the obese—tend to blame obesity on heredity. In man obesity does often tend to occur in families, and farmers have for years recognized and utilized a genetic determination of obesity in animals. Nevertheless, obesity in humans is seldom entirely due to genetic inheritance and is more often the result of the habit of overeating inculcated in childhood at the family table.

It is also commonly believed that obesity often results from endocrine disturbances, but in fact this is exceedingly rare, apart from hyperinsulinism, occasionally hypothyroidism and possibly Cushing's disease; Fröhlich's syndrome is due to hypothalamic and not to pituitary dysfunction. The obesity which so commonly starts after pregnancy or the menopause has probably little or no endocrine connection.

Lack of exercise is also a frequent cause of obesity and adequate exercise is important in weight reduction. Regular muscular work is, however, necessary if a significant increase in the expenditure of calories is to be attained; a man of average size burns only about 200 extra kcalories an hour while walking on the level. Further, owing to the disabling effects of obesity it is rarely possible, and sometimes dangerous, for a very fat person to take really hard or prolonged physical exercise.

Drastic purgation by hypertonic salt solutions and the encouragement of profuse sweating by Turkish baths still have their vogue as treatments of obesity. However, their effects are transient and shortlived, being due to a temporary loss of water from the body.

Since the immediate cause of every case of obesity is the eating of more food than is—or was—required, the important practical procedure in treatment is dietetic restriction using rationally constructed subcaloric diets. Nevertheless, an attempt should also be made to determine and, if possible, to correct any emotional or other cause of overeating and to encourage regular exercise.

DIETETICS

In this country the majority of obese patients are fat because they eat too much food containing starch or refined carbohydrates. For many of these, a simple restricted carbohydrate diet (p. 317) will suffice. Those who do not respond can then be given a diet in which the carbohydrate exchanges are prescribed either as domestic measures or weighed exchanges (p. 318) and the fat limited by restriction of milk and butter or margarine (p. 319).

TABLE 11

Approximate Caloric Value	Carbohydrate	Protein	Fat	
1,000 kcal.	100 g.	50 g.	45 g.	=½ pint milk, 5½ CHO, 3 Protein and 1 Fat exchange.
1,200 kcal.	120 g.	65 g.	50 g.	=½ pint milk, 7 CHO, 4 Protein and 1 Fat exchange.
1,400 kcal.	135 g.	75 g.	65 g.	=½ pint milk, 8 CHO, 5 Protein and 1½ Fat exchange.
1,600 kcal.	150 g.	85 g.	75 g.	=1 pint milk, 8 CHO, 5 Protein and 1½ Fat exchange.

INEXPENSIVE		EXPENSIVE	
Menu	Exchange Value	Menu	Exchange Value
Breakfast 1 oz. bread Tea; butter and milk from allowance.	1 CHO	**Breakfast** 5 oz. grapefruit ¾ oz. toast. Tea; butter and milk from allowance.	½ CHO 1 CHO
Mid-morning 1 tea biscuit Tea with milk from allowance.	½ CHO	**Mid-morning** 1 water biscuit Coffee with milk from allowance.	⅓ CHO

Dinner
Clear soup.
½ oz. bread.
2 oz. corned beef.
Cabbage and carrots.
5 oz. stewed apple.
	—
	½ CHO
	2 Prot.
	—
	½ CHO
		Lunch
		Salad containing:
		  ½ boiled egg,
		  ½ oz. grated cheese,
		  Lettuce, tomato, asparagus and celery.
		1 crispbread
		5 oz. melon.
		Coffee with milk from allowance.
			
			½ Prot.
			½ Prot.
			—
			½ CHO
			½ CHO

High tea 1 boiled egg. 1½ oz. bread. Tea; butter and milk from allowance.	1 Prot. 1½ CHO	**Afternoon tea** 1 oz. bread as cucumber sandwich. Tea; butter and milk from allowance.	1 CHO
Mid-evening snack 1 oz. bread. Tomato Tea; butter and milk from allowance.	1 CHO —	**Dinner** Tomato juice. 2 oz. chicken. 2½ oz. parsnips Carrots and spinach. 5 oz. fresh pineapple. Coffee with milk from allowance.	— 2 Prot. ½ CHO — ½ CHO
Bed-time 1 tea biscuit. Tea with milk from allowance.	½ CHO	**Bed-time** 2 water biscuits. Tea with milk from allowance.	⅔ CHO
Allowance for day of one half-pint of milk and 1 fat exchange.			

Failure to respond to either of these two diets generally means that the patient needs a full exchange system diet containing the selected number of calories. It is very important to take a reasonable dietetic history and to suit the diet to the patient's finances and domestic circumstances.

In constructing a detailed weighed diet for the treatment of obesity the most important consideration is its total caloric value, taking into consideration the height, age and nutrition of the patient concerned (p. 344). For most patients the prescrip-tion of a diet of 1,000 or 1,200 kcal. is all that is necessary although, occasionally, a hard-working man may require one of 1,600 kcal. and a grossly obese person of sedentary habit as little as 600 kcal. It must be remembered that unless patients are under close supervision in hospital, it is safe to assume that they will tend to be liberal in the inter-pretation of their diets.

The doctor's responsibilities are not liquidated by the mere prescription of a suitable subcaloric diet: the patient must be made to realize why dietetic restriction is necessary and must have the diet patiently explained so that she thoroughly understands how to convert the exchanges allowed at each meal into terms of actual foodstuffs. She should be allowed to take her main meal when she is most hungry. Patients given a weighed diet should be given a set of scales and, for a few weeks, should weigh all food. No food is allowed other than that prescribed in the diet. All foods are fattening to a greater or less extent and there are no such things as 'slimming' foods. Many patients think quite erroneously that brown bread or toast is less fattening than white bread.

Some success may be obtained by giving patients a list of meals containing 500 or 200 kcalories of which they may eat either two or five respectively each day. In this way a 1,000 kcal. diet may be adhered to the more easily.

A recent form of dietetic treatment, commercially instigated, is the complete substitution of normal foodstuffs by an artificially prepared powder, biscuits or other foodstuffs containing a balanced mixture of carbohydrate, fat and protein and adequate quantities of minerals and vitamins. Although these are occasionally successful short-term expedients it is better to try to alter radically the patient's faulty habits of eating.

Drugs

THYROXINE. The treatment of obese persons with small doses of thyroid hormones is useless; large doses are dangerous.

APPETITE-REDUCING DRUGS. The spontaneous food intake of experimental animals is reduced by drugs which either depress the appetite centre or stimulate the satiety centre in the hypothalamus. Those in common use are the amphetamines and chemically related compounds. Because of the dangers of addiction or dependence it is most inadvisable to prescribe an amphetamine or phenmetrazine; both drugs also cause insomnia. Diethylpropion, phentermine, chlorphentermine and fenfluramine do not seem to have these disadvantages. The last named is not converted in the body to amphetamine and often has a mildly sedative effect.

The prescription of an anorectic drug is rarely justified at the beginning of the dietary treatment. It may be useful if the patient, despite efforts to adhere to the diet, is unable to do so and does not lose weight. Nevertheless, it should be recognized that the effect of an anorectic agent is transient

and any one course of treatment should not last for more than two or at the most three months.

Anorectic agents are used excessively nowadays: too often their prescription is evidence of the doctor's unwillingness or inability to instruct the patient properly in the principles of a well-designed subcaloric diet. The aim of treatment should be to alter fundamentally and permanently the food habits of the patient rather than to inhibit appetite by artificial and temporary means.

DIURETICS. The excessive deposition of fat in adipose tissue is accompanied by retention of water. The aim of the treatment of obesity is to cause loss of fat, not of water, and the use of diuretics is therefore valueless and misleading unless oedema is present due to cardiac or other causes.

DRUGS WHICH INCREASE THE BULK OF FOOD. Methylcellulose is a substance which is not absorbed from the alimentary tract and which swells in water. It has been claimed that, when administered with water before meals, it increases the bulk of the gastric contents and so gives rise to a feeling of satiety, leading to a decreased food intake. Controlled clinical studies have, however, shown that this compound is valueless as an adjunct to the dietary treatment of obesity.

OTHER DRUGS. An astonishing number of preparations are widely advertised to the public as possessing remarkable properties in causing weight reduction. They can all be dismissed as being valueless and the doctor should quite bluntly tell his obese patients that this is the case, thereby preventing them from wasting their money.

Starvation

For grossly obese patients who have been refractory to all out-patient attempts to reduce weight, complete starvation in hospital may be justified. This treatment is not without danger and should be restricted to patients who are aged less than 40 and who have no evidence of heart disease. Only coffee, tea, water and other non-caloric drinks are allowed; vitamins, salt and potassium supplements should also be given. Although some ketonuria may develop, there is no significant reduction in the plasma bicarbonate, and it is remarkable how few patients experience hunger. The rise in serum uric acid which occurs may be controlled by allopurinol. Nevertheless, such patients usually put on weight again quickly when exposed to conditions in the outside world; this, however, is less likely in those starved until they have been reduced to within 25 per cent. excess of their standard. For those, however, who have sufficient determination, complete fasting on one or two days each week may result in a surprisingly satisfactory and maintained loss of weight. There is some evidence that patients subjected to this form of therapy can adhere to a low caloric diet as outpatients much more readily than previously.

The Control of Treatment

Patients trying to lose weight should be seen frequently by the doctor. Their dietetic enthusiasm wanes unless they receive constant encouragement and occasionally mild bullying. It is important to warn them against taking sweets, fruit, sweet drinks or indeed any food between meals. Many patients take these oddments quite innocently, thinking that there is little or no food value in them. Again, it is common for patients to become careless about their diet when they go on holiday, or they may be unable to observe it accurately in hotels or lodgings. In this way the labour of months may be undone in a few weeks.

Patients should be weighed weekly and the aim should be an average loss of about 2 lb. (about 1 kg.) a week. If the loss of weight is constantly more rapid than this, the diet, if thought desirable, may be slightly increased. When the loss averages less than 2 lb. a week, the patient should be carefully questioned regarding strict observance of the diet as slackness in this respect is nearly always the cause of failure to lose weight satisfactorily. Occasionally, however, it may be necessary to modify the diet still further from perhaps 1,200 to 800 kcal.

During the first few days of dieting there is often a rapid fall in weight—sometimes as much as 5 or 6 lb.—which is largely due to fluid loss. The rate of loss thereafter is less rapid but varies considerably from day to day. Such fluctuations are of little importance, though they occasionally make it difficult to ascertain the real rate of loss over a short period and make it unnecessary to weigh the patient more often than once a week. Some of these fluctuations may depend on the wearing of different clothes and on whether or not urine or faeces have been evacuated before weighing, but changes in water balance probably account for most of them. In addition to these daily variations, a disturbance in the rate of weight reduction often accompanies menstruation: for two or three days before the period, weight loss usually ceases and a slight gain

may occur, to be followed about the middle of the period by an increased rate of loss.

With very rare exceptions all patients who adhere to a properly prescribed subcaloric diet lose weight satisfactorily though they vary considerably in the

TABLE 12

Desirable Weight for Men and Women, according to Height and Frame, ages 25 and over

HEIGHT (in shoes)	WEIGHT IN INDOOR CLOTHING		
	Small Frame	Medium Frame	Large Frame
MEN			
ft. in.	lb.	lb.	lb.
5 2	112–120	118–129	126–141
5 3	115–123	121–133	129–144
5 4	118–126	124–136	132–148
5 5	121–129	127–139	135–152
5 6	124–133	130–143	138–156
5 7	128–137	134–147	142–161
5 8	132–141	138–152	147–166
5 9	136–145	142–156	151–170
5 10	140–150	146–160	155–174
5 11	144–154	150–165	159–179
6 0	148–158	154–170	164–184
6 1	152–162	158–175	168–189
6 2	156–167	162–180	173–194
6 3	160–171	167–185	178–199
6 4	164–175	172–190	182–204
WOMEN*			
ft. in.	lb.	lb.	lb.
4 10	92– 98	96–107	104–119
4 11	94–101	98–110	106–122
5 0	96–104	101–113	109–125
5 1	99–107	104–116	112–128
5 2	102–110	107–119	115–131
5 3	105–113	110–122	118–134
5 4	108–116	113–126	121–138
5 5	111–119	116–130	125–142
5 6	114–123	120–135	129–146
5 7	118–127	124–139	133–150
5 8	122–131	128–143	137–154
5 9	126–135	132–147	141–158
5 10	130–140	136–151	145–163
5 11	134–144	140–155	149–168
6 0	138–148	144–159	153–173

*For girls between 18 and 24 years, subtract 1 lb. for each year under 25.

rate at which this occurs. Those who are initially grossly obese often lose weight more rapidly than those in whom the initial excess weight was only moderate. There is generally no difference in the response to treatment between those who have been fat for a long time and those who have been fat for only a few years. Long-standing obesity is, therefore, no drawback to successful treatment.

Unfortunately, once the weight has been satisfactorily reduced, there is often a tendency for the patient to start overeating again if treatment is discontinued altogether. A slightly modified diet is usually sufficient to counteract this tendency since the patient has learned dietetic discretion and is generally able to maintain the weight at the new low level by the exercise of a little care so that very strict dieting is no longer necessary. In a few unfortunate people, however, the slightest relaxation in dietetic care is followed by a renewed gain in weight. Indeed, the greater the original obesity and the greater the response to dieting, the greater must be the care in relaxing treatment.

It is important to distinguish between average weight and the desirable weight which is given in Table 12, that is, between what people *do* weigh on the average and what they *should* weigh by the criterion of greatest longevity. On the whole

desirable weights past the age of 30 are 15 to 25 lb. below *average* weights. Nevertheless, no single value can be designated as desirable for all persons of a specified height since people vary in many respects. The tables given of desirable weights constructed by the Metropolitan Life Assurance Company take into account body frame in addition to height.

In conclusion it may be said that there are few therapeutic measures in medicine so certain to restore health or to prevent disability as the controlled weight reduction of obese persons. It must again be emphasized, however, that the subcaloric diet must be carefully explained to the patient who must be made to understand its principles and the permitted food exchanges. There is no easy road, nor even a short cut, along which an obese person may travel safely to an ideal weight, but only along the thorny path of dietetic restriction, for drugs have little place in the long-term correction and control of obesity.

14. Nutritional Disorders

Sir Stanley Davidson and Ronald H. Girdwood

By definition, nutritional disorders are those which are due to faulty diet: the patient has received too much or too little food, or not enough of the right kind. Too much food results in obesity, discussed on p. 340. Simple lack of food is now an uncommon cause of ill-health in Britain. Yet for mankind as a whole, deficiency of calories often combined with an insufficient intake of protein (the protein-calorie malnutrition syndrome, p. 349) is far more important as a cause of ill-health than all the vitamin deficiencies put together. The population of the world is steadily increasing through the expanding application of medical science and the refusal by the great majority of men and women to practise birth control; unfortunately the application of agricultural science has failed to keep pace with this increase. Consequently, today at least one-third of humanity is not getting enough to eat.

Even in countries where the total supplies of food are sufficient, nutritional disorders may arise through poverty, prejudice, ignorance or bad housekeeping aggravated by bad housing. The children of large families living in industrial cities or on impoverished farmland, and the old and solitary, dependent on their own resources, are most frequently affected.

Finally, there are those patients who, despite every advantage of nationality, income, education and standard of living, develop a nutritional disorder because they suffer from some other disease which 'conditions' the disorder, by interfering with the absorption, digestion or utilization of their food, or by increasing their nutritional requirements so that their usual diet becomes insufficient. Alcoholism may be a factor.

THE COMPONENTS OF AN ADEQUATE DIET

Calories. The quantity of food necessary to provide an individual with sufficient calories cannot be predicted from published tables of 'requirements'. Energy expenditure varies enormously from one individual to another, even among people of the same age, sex, size and habits. In fact, tables like those published in 1969 by the Department of Health and Social Security, UK are not intended to express *requirements*; they are recommended allowances or intakes. The intake suggested for a moderately active man is 3,000 kcal. and for most women 2,000 to 2,200 kcal. Slightly lower figures are recommended by the Food and Nutrition Board of the USA. It is important to remember that such recommendations apply to large groups of people and that individual requirements may vary considerably. In the vast majority of instances the daily energy expenditure ranges from 2,400 to 4,000 kcal. per day for men and 1,700 to 2,900 kcal. per day for women.

Official recommendations are stated in terms of 'intake' calories—the energy value of the food actually eaten. Food administrators more often deal with 'retail' calories or the value of the food at the time that it is sold in the shops. No comparison between retail calories and recommended allowances can be made without some deduction for wastage.

Carbohydrates. Though carbohydrates provide the greatest part of the calories in most normal diets, no single carbohydrate is indispensable to health, in the sense that the body has a special metabolic use for it and cannot make it from other nutrients.

Fats. Fats have a caloric value and are useful in good cooking. They therefore help to make a diet appetizing and small in bulk. Nevertheless it has yet to be shown that fats in themselves have unique chemical virtues for the maintenance of satisfactory nutritional health. Recently the quantity and quality of dietary fats have been the subject of much anxious appraisal in relation to the incidence of atherosclerosis and its sequelae in the heart, brain and peripheral vessels. This problem is discussed on p. 103.

Proteins and amino acids. The proteins of food are the only important source of nitrogen, sulphur and essential amino acids. An adequate diet must contain sufficient protein to satisfy the body's need for these essentials. There must be enough to maintain a positive nitrogen balance, so that the nitrogen lost in the urine is replaced. Of the 23 known amino acids, only 10 seem to be 'essential' for man, in the sense that the human body is incapable of making them for itself and must obtain them from food. These 10 are: lysine, tryptophan, phenylalanine, leucine, isoleucine, threonine, methionine, valine, histidine and arginine; the last two are probably indispensable for maintaining growth in infancy. Their names are given here because some of them are now available in synthetic form and may prove to have therapeutic uses.

The remaining non-essential amino acids, which the body makes for itself when given an adequate supply of the others, are nevertheless important contributors to good human nutrition; they all provide nitrogen. One of them, cysteine, together with methionine, is practically the only source of sulphur in human diets; another—glutamic acid— has a strong meaty taste that has given it a marketable value as a flavouring agent.

Some proteins are notably deficient in certain amino acids; e.g. zein, the chief protein of maize, contains no lysine or cysteine. On the whole, individual animal proteins have better 'biological value' than plant proteins, in that they supply a more varied mixture of amino acids. This has been used to argue the need for abundant meat (by those who enjoy their beef steaks)—an argument that did much to lose the 1914-18 war for the Germans, who used their limited land to raise beef rather than cereals and potatoes. Though some animal protein is certainly desirable and probably essential, there is good evidence that satisfactory nutrition can be sustained on proteins derived almost entirely from vegetable sources; but in such circumstances it is most important to ensure that a sufficient variety of plant foods are eaten in order that any amino acid missing from one may be supplied by another.

Whether a diet is adequate in protein is generally best decided by calculating the contribution that the proteins make to the total calories consumed. A satisfactory diet for a healthy person should contain sufficient protein to provide not less than 11 per cent. of the total calories, or 14 per cent. in the case of a lactating woman. When, for any reason, the diet is restricted in calories, this general rule may break down; the daily intake of protein for an adult should not be less than 50 g. There is no evidence that hard physical work increases the rate of utilization of protein.

In addition to calories, carbohydrates, fat and protein, adequate amounts of water, minerals and vitamins must be consumed otherwise the various deficiency disorders discussed below may develop.

GENERALIZED UNDERNUTRITION
(*Disorders due to Quantitative Dietary Deficiency of Calories*)

The prolonged consumption of too little food results in loss of weight in adults and restricted growth in children. It is not always easy to diagnose undernutrition on simple clinical inspection; some people are thin by nature, though in excellent nutritional health. Repeated measurements showing loss of weight or failure to grow provide important evidence of undernutrition. One of the most useful things that a doctor can do towards keeping his patients in health is to weigh them regularly. The appearance of loose folds of skin may also give evidence of recent loss of weight. People partly adapt themselves to an insufficient caloric intake by restricting unessential bodily movements.

A good example of conditioned undernutrition is provided by the thin diabetic whose fall in weight is due to loss of calories in the form of glucose in the urine. Conditioned undernutrition may also arise as a result of any gastrointestinal disorder that sufficiently impairs appetite or interferes with digestion or absorption. Prolonged fevers raise the metabolic rate and so increase the need for calories, but the patient may be disinclined to eat, and so develops undernutrition; this is especially true if the patient is a child, who should be actively growing. A clinical state of undernutrition may result from pulmonary tuberculosis or malignancy.

In simple underfeeding it need hardly be said that the essence of treatment is to give the patient more to eat. But unfortunately in many lands it is beyond the power of the physician to provide this except indirectly, by persuading farmers, economists and statesmen to provide more food. Fortunately some countries now have well-developed Maternity and Child Welfare Services, through which milk and school meals are supplied. Full use should always be made of such services in the treatment of underfed children. Similarly, the 'meals on wheels' scheme, run by the Women's Voluntary Service in Britain, for delivering hot, ready-cooked meals to old people living by themselves, is an invaluable service for maintaining the nutrition of this vulnerable group and keeping them out of hospital. Unfortunately the need for hot meals from a mobile service by large numbers of old people living alone greatly exceeds the numbers of voluntary workers able and willing to undertake this work. Some churches supply facilities for old people to meet and have a daily meal together. When under-nutrition arises as a direct result of poverty, the physician should see to it that full advantage is taken of any existing organizations—local, national or charitable—for financial assistance. When the chief fault lies in the disorganized feeding arrangements of a slum home, the local housing authority can sometimes help, and the doctor should approach the Medical Officer of Health. Simple parental ignorance or neglect may some-times result in children being given unsuitable food; in such cases the physician, aided by the health visitor, must educate and admonish. An important therapeutic means of combating nutri-tional disorders of all kinds is good cooking; the art of a good cook is of more value than any number of 'tonics' or other supposed stimulants to appetite. The physician should do all he can to ensure that his patients receive appetizing food, both at home and in hospital.

Starvation and Famine

Starvation may conveniently be defined as under-nutrition of sufficient severity to require in-patient treatment in hospital. The starving patient is emaciated and may have lost 25 per cent. or more of his original weight. Except for the nervous system and skeleton, all the organs of the body are reduced in size, including the heart. Oddly enough, the total body water is not reduced, so that with the wasting of tissues, oedema ultimately ap-pears, not necessarily associated with any reduction in plasma protein concentration; this is the iso-hydric type of famine oedema (p. 349). The oedema is usually most obvious in the face and lower limbs.

The agricultural, political or social conditions that created this desperate condition must be over-come—if possible. The patient should be removed to an entirely fresh environment, with good nursing and a new hope in life. If the cause is a famine, he should be transferred to an emergency hospital as near as possible to his home. Starving people do not readily recover without new hope.

Food is obviously the next consideration, but what food? Many starving people have died because they were given anything that well-meaning relief workers happened to have available: tins of bully-beef, baked beans or brown bread. Diar-rhoea, from eating unsuitable food, may result in dehydration and death. The paper-thin walls of the wasted intestine are intolerant of coarse foods, and the lack of digestive enzymes, particularly, impairs the absorption of fats.

Dietetic Treatment. In starvation the single most important therapeutic agent is skimmed milk (fresh or reconstituted from dried milk powder to give a mixture of 10 to 15 per cent. strength). In times of famine its supply should be controlled by the medical officer and it should be distributed as a medicine. Gravely ill patients should be fed at first on frequent small feeds of skimmed milk (100 ml.) as often as the patient is willing and able to take them. This demands constant and personal attention and nursing care. The appetite is usually fickle and may be completely absent. Variation of flavour—vanilla, chocolate or straw-berry—may help to stimulate it. Predigested (hydrolysed) protein by mouth has no apparent advantage over skimmed milk.

If semi-solid foods are tolerated without digestive upset, these should be allowed. They should include foods containing protein of good biological value, such as junket, custard made from milk and eggs, pounded fish, minced lean meat or chicken. It is important that the diet should also contain adequate carbohydrate to 'spare' the proteins, so that they are used to replenish the plasma and tissues and are not used exclusively as a source of calories. Milk puddings, mashed potatoes and sweetened fruit juice will provide this. In the preparation of such foods, salt should be restricted or excluded, since feeding with ordinary foods cooked with salt may increase famine oedema. The degree of restriction must depend on whether there is, in addition to protein deficiency, a defi-ciency of sodium chloride, in which case a moderate amount of salt should be allowed as this is bene-ficial in the relief of asthenia and the improvement of appetite.

As the patient's appetite and digestion gradually improve, more solid foods may be given, though it is best to avoid those high in roughage, such as coarse bread, stringy vegetables and the skins and pips of fruit. It is important to see that the diet remains well-balanced, providing adequate amounts of the protective foods, particularly dairy produce, meat, fruit and vegetables. A sudden increase in the caloric intake of an underfed patient, as for instance by an increased ration of polished rice or by large amounts of glucose given by mouth or vein, may precipitate an acute state of vitamin depletion. Recovery may take many months, but is usually complete provided there are no complications, such as tuberculosis, which is a frequent aftermath of famine.

The prognosis is very grave when a patient suffering from severe starvation, though still rational, refuses all food. Skimmed milk may be slowly dripped through a tube passed into the stomach through the nose. This provides the only hope, but at subsequent autopsy the milk may be found lying in the stomach.

Parenteral feeding is usually of little help and has dangers. The small brown-atrophied heart does not readily tolerate any additional load, which may precipitate pulmonary oedema.

Infections of various kinds occur frequently in the starving, but they often go undetected because a pyrexial reaction may not occur. Apart from the great epidemic diseases of famine (typhus, cholera, smallpox, influenza and malaria) tuberculosis is particularly common. The spread of these diseases among a starving people is the result of the collapse of general hygiene rather than of increased susceptibility to infection; consequently proper attention to hygiene is an essential part of treatment.

Finally, it should be remembered that the starving patient often suffers from important psychological changes which show themselves in irritability, sensitivity to noise, liability to take affront, ill-temper, inability to concentrate, depression and apathy. The physician must be reconciled to this situation and must not expect to be rewarded with thanks. It is also unrealistic to expect strict racial prejudices or taboos about articles of diet to be overcome even by starvation. In underdeveloped countries the most straightforward of Western foodstuffs may be totally unacceptable, perhaps merely because of suspicions about the manner in which it has been prepared.

Oedema associated with Undernutrition or Malnutrition

So far, the term undernutrition has been used to mean prolonged lack of intake of sufficient food. Malnutrition (pp. 349-350) is a word used to indicate that there has been insufficient consumption of particular nutrients such as amino acids, minerals or vitamins. Undernutrition and malnutrition may coexist.

There are at least four possible dietary causes of nutritional oedema which should be distinguished: (1) *beriberi*, with or without cardiac failure (p. 355); (2) *famine oedema*, the isohydric type already described (p. 348), in which oedema appears in starving people through wasting of tissues without any change in the volume of body water; the level of plasma proteins may be within normal limits; (3) *oedema associated with protein deficiency*. This is a classical feature of the protein-calorie malnutrition syndrome. Its aetiology prevention and treatment are discussed on pp. 349-352. The plasma proteins are reduced, and the consequent reduction in osmotic pressure of the plasma contributes to the oedema.

Oedema is more likely to occur in protein-calorie malnutrition than in general calorie restriction, and it is found particularly when people subsist for long periods on a diet providing less than 1,000 kcal. and less than 50 g. of protein daily. The oedema is usually most evident in the face if the patient has been lying down. However, when the patient gets up and walks about, it shifts quite rapidly to the feet and legs. It may be so extensive as to conceal the underlying emaciation.

Protein depletion occurs in the nephrotic syndrome (p. 269) and protein-losing gastro-enteropathy (p. 236) through losses in the urine and faeces, and sometimes in cirrhosis of the liver (p. 248) because of interference with synthesis.

(4) *epidemic dropsy*. Epidemics of this disease have claimed many victims in India and Pakistan. It has also been reported in Mauritius and South Africa. The cause of the oedema appears to be damage to the capillaries, with increased permeability by a toxic alkaloid, sanguinamine, that has been isolated in crystalline form from the seeds of the poppy-like plant, *Argemone mexicana*. Seeds of this weed find their way, by accident or design, into mustard seed from which cooking oil is extracted. They may also contaminate bread grains. Treatment obviously consists in withdrawing the contaminated food. There is no known specific antidote.

MALNUTRITION
(*Disorders due to Qualitative Dietary Deficiencies*)

1. PROTEIN-CALORIE MALNUTRITION

The concept has recently been advanced that protein-calorie malnutrition (PCM), especially in early childhood, should be regarded as a spectrum of disease. At one end there is kwashiorkor in which the essential feature is a qualitative and quantitative deficiency of protein. Calories are often restricted but may even be in excess of requirements. At the other end is nutritional marasmus (p. 352) which is a total inanition of the infant and is due to a severe and continuous restriction of calories and protein as well as other nutrients. In the middle of the spectrum is marasmic kwashiorkor in which children have the clinical features of both disorders.

PCM is the most important nutritional disorder in the world at the present time, affecting millions of children wherever the dietary conditions described below are present.

Kwashiorkor

First described in Ghana in 1933, kwashiorkor is now known to occur in many developing countries. Although the disease may occur at any age, it particularly affects children between 1 and 4 years whose mothers wean them from the breasts on to a diet which is mostly composed of starchy gruels containing little protein and usually providing too little energy.

The onset of clinical kwashiorkor is often conditioned by an acute infection, e.g. measles, malaria or gastroenteritis, which increases the breakdown of tissue proteins and may decrease the dietary intake of protein. The clinical features are of failure of growth, muscular wasting, oedema, mental irritability or apathy and anorexia. In addition, pigmentary changes in the hair and skin and a liability to hepatic damage are frequently present in chronic cases and diarrhoea may cause important losses of potassium and magnesium. Many patients die from lack of adequate treatment.

Prevention

Ignorance and poverty are the two main factors responsible for kwashiorkor. Obviously these causes must be removed. Education in nutrition, the introduction of improved farming methods and the development of food industries whereby protective foods may be made available at a reasonable cost to the consumer, are all important. In each country careful thought must be given to the provision, from local crops, of protein-rich foods which are suitable both for infant feeding and for supplementing diets low in protein. For this purpose concentrates of vegetable protein made from oil-seed cakes and from flours made from edible pulses are valuable supplements to cereals such as wheat, sorghum and other millets.

Even small amounts of foods of animal origin such as dried milk or concentrates of fish protein, which are not readily available and are expensive in countries where kwashiorkor is prevalent, are of great value when mixed with high protein vegetable foods. A mixture of one part of casein and 10 parts of groundnut flour is effective in the prevention and treatment of kwashiorkor.

Education of parents, particularly mothers, in regard to the value of foods and the best methods of preparing them, especially at the time of weaning, is invaluable. Much could be done to alleviate this disorder by the establishment or extension of Child Welfare Clinics and Health Centres where free or subsidized skimmed milk powder is supplied, advice on diet given, and where diseases which are liable to lead to kwashiorkor can be prevented or treated.

Treatment

Several aspects merit detailed consideration.

General measures. An easily digested diet which provides sufficient calories and adequate amounts of protein of good biological value, together with sufficient minerals and vitamins, is essential. Dried skimmed milk is the most useful form of protein for hospital patients and should be used in treating serious cases in the early stages. Calcium caseinate is also of great value for this purpose, but is more expensive than dried skimmed milk powder. If neither of these preparations is available or the cost of maintaining the supply of milk becomes prohibitive, protein-rich preparations such as one of those described above should be used as these have been shown to be effective substitutes for milk for such patients.

Severely ill children are often unable to maintain their body temperature even in warm climates. Hence heated rooms or electric blankets or heat cradles are essential for such cases. Parenteral therapy, if used at all, must be given with great caution. If dermatosis is severe, the skin should be cleaned and carefully protected. During the first days of treatment the child's weight may fall due to loss of oedema fluid. The initiation of cure is indicated by increasing appetite and a gain in weight.

Dietetic measures. For the first day or two, if the child is unable to feed from a spoon, a polythene tube passed into the stomach through the nose will be necessary. The following recipe for a baby food based on skimmed milk powder has been widely used in Jamaica:

Ingredients: 60 g. (2 oz.) skimmed milk powder
15 g. (1½ teaspoons) butter
20 g. (2 teaspoons) flour
250 ml. (½ pint) water

250 ml. (½ pint) of this mixture contains about 22 g. protein and 250 kcal.

Method: Add skimmed milk powder to cold water gradually while stirring. Pour mixture through a strainer. Melt butter in saucepan and add flour to form a smooth paste. Add 2 to 3 tablespoons of liquid skimmed milk. Stir and cook for two minutes. Add remaining milk and continue to cook and stir until the flour and butter mixture is well distributed throughout the milk and the flour is cooked.

This recipe was constructed after it had been demonstrated that skimmed milk powder alone is unable to meet a child's needs for growth and moreover is liable in excessive amounts to cause diarrhoea. The mixture should be given in divided doses four to six times a day so as to provide the patient with approximately 5 g. of protein for each kg. of the ideal weight of a child of the same age. On the second or third day it should be possible to start on a banana/milk or cereal/milk diet. In countries such as Uganda and Jamaica, where bananas are a staple article of diet, they should be used because they mix better with skimmed milk powder than do flours made from cereals or roots (cassava) and the mixture is very palatable.

The following instructions for a banana/skimmed milk diet are based on the experience of Trowell, Davies and Dean in Kampala, Uganda:

1. Take 400 g. of peeled sweet bananas, mash with a fork, spread out in a shallow dish and allow to stand for six to eight hours.
2. Take 200 g. of dried skimmed milk powder, stir into a smooth paste with a little cold water, add hot water to a final volume of 500 ml. and heat to boiling. Allow to cool.
3. Mix the banana and the reconstituted milk thoroughly, if possible in an electric blender, adding up to 70 g. sugar.
4. Divide the mixture, which represents one day's ration, into six equal amounts. Feed with a spoon.

M*

This diet, which provides in one day's ration about 75 g. of protein and 1,200 kcal., will lead to an improvement in appetite, digestion and strength. Where bananas are not available, as is the case in many countries where kwashiorkor is endemic, a flour made from semolina, rice, cassava or cereals will have to be used. In this case it is strongly recommended that an ounce of some fat (butter or margarine) or an edible oil such as that made from sunflower seeds, should be added as it makes the mixing of the flour and milk powder easier and the mixture is more palatable, digestible and of higher caloric value.

Anorexia may be serious, but often can be overcome by feeding the child very slowly in the mother's lap and not in bed. Food may be taken better cold than hot. Sometimes Marmite or Bovril as flavouring may be acceptable.

As the clinical condition improves, the food consumption should be increased gradually. Whole milk powder can be substituted for skimmed milk powder, and eggs, fish and bean flour added until the child is eating a satisfactory diet of local pattern, including adequate amounts of easily digested protein-rich foods. Mild cases may be treated on an out-patient basis from the start, and it is essential that the mother of a child with kwashiorkor should be given instructions in regard to hygiene, cooking and methods of feeding.

Infants may lose 1 to 4 g. of potassium chloride (13 to 52 mEq.) in the stools in one day if there is severe diarrhoea. The effect of the resulting potassium depletion on the myocardium may cause sudden death. Potassium should be given by mouth as a routine to all infants admitted with kwashiorkor. Depending on the age and weight of the child and the severity of the diarrhoea, the dose should be from 500 mg. to 1 g. of potassium chloride dissolved in water and added to three or four feeds each day. There is little or no danger of potassium intoxication when the mixture is given by mouth in the doses recommended.

Parenteral therapy. For very ill patients who are suffering from marked dehydration, hypoglycaemia, acid-base disturbances and electrolyte imbalance, parenteral therapy with appropriate solutions (p. 239) may be a life-saving measure which should be started prior to the beginning of dietetic treatment. Likewise, for severe anaemia from any cause, repeated slow transfusions of packed erythrocytes is of the greatest value. Unfortunately, in underdeveloped countries, facilities for treating the majority of severe cases of PCM by such measures are not available.

Vitamins. Therapeutic diets based on skimmed milk and plant proteins are unlikely to be seriously lacking in any of the B group of vitamins and it should be necessary to prescribe them only in exceptional circumstances. Such diets are more likely to be deficient in vitamin A and ascorbic acid, which are present in insignificant amounts in dried skimmed milk powder. The treatment and prevention of these deficiencies are discussed on pp. 354-364. Large doses should be avoided, 400 i.u. of vitamin A and 20 mg. ascorbic acid being sufficient. Megaloblastic anaemia, when it occurs, is usually due to folate deficiency. It is advisable to give folic acid (p. 149) routinely in treatment, Vitamin B_{12} depletion is much less likely to occur.

Lipotropic factors accelerate the mobilization of fat deposited in the livers of experimental animals as a result of the ingestion of defective diets or poisoning with a variety of toxic agents. Choline, methionine and preparations of pig's stomach, all known lipotropic agents, have been tried in kwashiorkor. Most workers have found them valueless and their use cannot be recommended as part of routine treatment.

Treatment of infections and infestations. This is important. If a respiratory infection or skin sepsis is present, a course of penicillin is advisable. Tetracycline or some other suitable antibiotic should be given for infections of the gastro-intestinal tract. Most of these children suffer from infection with worms and require treatment (p. 532). However, all anthelmintics are potentially toxic and treatment must be postponed until convalescence is established. If anaemia from hookworm is so severe as to endanger life, blood transfusions should be given and will probably restore the child's condition sufficiently to permit appropriate treatment later. Iron-deficiency anaemia is frequently present as a result of dietary deficiency, infections and infestations, and requires appropriate treatment (p. 143). Antimalarial drugs in both prophylactic and therapeutic doses are well tolerated. The possibility of tuberculosis being present should always be considered, particularly if the child does not make the expected progress to recovery. Tuberculosis, if not too far advanced, responds well to streptomycin combined with other antituberculous drugs (p. 68).

It is important to realize that kwashiorkor is an advanced form of protein-calorie malnutrition and

that nutritional dwarfing is a very real entity in underdeveloped countries.

Nutritional Dwarfing (Growth Retardation)

Prolonged mild to moderate protein-calorie malnutrition may result in a syndrome called nutritional dwarfing, in which children are light in weight and short in stature with relatively normal body proportions and subcutaneous fat. This is a form of preclinical PCM which occurs in millions of children in underdeveloped countires. Its clinical recognition is very important, since the children are liable to develop marasmus or kwashiorkor if they suffer from gastro-intestinal or respiratory disease or infections such as measles or malaria.

This, however, is not the full story and in Fig. 8

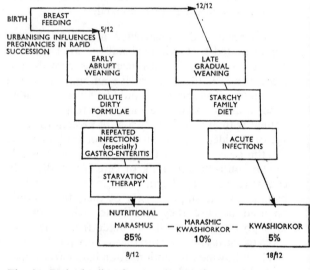

Fig. 8.—Paths leading from early weaning to nutritional marasmus and from protracted breast feeding to kwashiorkor.
    Numbers represent approximate age in months. Percentages of types of malnutrition are based on figures for Jordan but are typical for many other countries. (By courtesy of D. S. Maclaren, *Lancet*, 1966, **2**, 486.)

there is reproduced an analysis by Professor D. S. McLaren of Beirut of protein-calorie malnutrition in his experience.

In kwashiorkor the essential feature is a qualitative and quantitative deficiency of protein. Calories are often restricted, but may even be in excess of requirements. Where there is total inanition of the infant due to a severe and continuous restriction of calories and protein as well as other nutrients the condition is named nutritional marasmus.

Oedema is not a feature and if it occurs the term marasmic kwashiorkor is frequently used.

Nutritional Marasmus

The importance of marasmus as a cause of mortality and morbidity in infants at the present time has not been adequately appreciated. In parts of some underdeveloped countries marasmus is of greater clinical importance than kwashiorkor. It affects principally infants under 1 year of age in contrast to kwashiorkor which is chiefly encountered in the pre-school child (1 to 4 years). Marasmus is more likely to occur in poor people in underdeveloped countries who live in cities, while kwashiorkor occurs more frequently in people living under tribal conditions in rural areas. The urban influences which predispose to marasmus are a rapid succession of pregnancies, and early and often abrupt weaning, followed by dirty and unsound artificial feeding of the infant with very dilute milk or processed milk products given in inadequate amounts because of the expense involved. In addition the unsatisfactory conditions existing in most homes of poor people in underdeveloped countries make the preparation of uncontaminated feeds almost impossible. Thus, repeated infections develop, especially of the gastro-intestinal tract which the mother often treats by starvation for long periods, the infant receiving water, rice water or some other non-nutritious fluid.

The most important aetiological factor in marasmus, namely early weaning, is in contrast to the late weaning, often extending over two years, which is characteristic of kwashiorkor. The mother may be induced to stop breast feeding for various reasons, including the presence of infections in herself or in the infant. Unfortunately she may have been influenced unwisely by advertisements in the press or on the radio which advocate, for commercial reasons, the advantages of artificial food products. The most frequent reason for stopping breast feeding is the beginning of another pregnancy. There appears to be a widespread belief among poor, uneducated women in underdeveloped countries that the milk of a pregnant woman is bad for her child.

Prevention and Treatment

This is a complex and difficult problem. Education of mothers so that they will continue breast feeding for as long as possible is of the greatest importance.

Further research is urgently needed into improved methods of feeding both healthy and ill infants in underdeveloped countries. The epidemiology of the failure of lactation and the control of infection in infants are other important matters requiring further investigation. In the acute stage of marasmus survival depends primarily on the efficiency with which measures can be applied to combat dehydration and hypoglycaemia and restore electrolyte balance. In addition the child must be given a satisfactory diet such as the skimmed milk diet used in Jamaica. Even when these objectives have been successfully accomplished the death rate may be much higher and the morbidity greater than in equivalently severe cases of kwashiorkor.

In summary, it may be concluded safely that in the future marasmus will become of increasing clinical importance in underdeveloped countries as a consequence of a continuing decline in breast feeding, the urbanization of uneducated families, socially insecure and living in poor, insanitary houses with insufficient money to buy adequate supplements of milk or expensive milk substitutes.

2. WATER AND ELECTROLYTES

The normal concentration of ions, both in the intravascular and extracellular fluid, is preserved by a balance between the intake of water and electrolytes in the diet and the output in the excertions. In Britain a healthy adult takes from $1\frac{1}{2}$ to $2\frac{1}{2}$ litres of fluid and 10 to 15 g. NaCl daily. In tropical countries this intake will have to be increased considerably to make up for the loss in sweat. Disturbances in water and electrolyte balance and in acid-base equilibrium are discussed on pp. 253-264.

3. MINERALS

Of the mineral elements present in the human body and known to have physiological activity, potassium, magnesium, manganese, zinc, copper and cobalt are never deficient in man *solely* as the result of an inadequate diet. Iron deficiency is a very common cause of ill-health among women in all parts of the world especially during their menstrual life; it is discussed on p. 145. Nutritional needs for sulphur are supplied by the sulphur-containing amino acids, methionine and cysteine. Provided that a diet contains sufficient calcium, it will normally provide sufficient phosphorus; deficiency of calcium is inseparably connected with the problem of rickets and osteomalacia (p. 360). Iodine deficiency is discussed in relation to simple goitre (p. 290). Clinical signs of deficiency of potassium (pp. 256, 258) and magnesium develop only if there is an excessive loss from the gastrointestinal tract or in the urine.

Fluorine is of interest in connection with dental caries. If the drinking water in a locality contains more than 1 part per million (p.p.m.) of fluorine, dental fluorosis will be found among its inhabitants; such teeth are softer than normal and yet are unusually resistant to caries, probably because of the bacteriostatic properties of fluorine which is deposited in the enamel. Fluorine in excessive amounts (over 10 parts per million) is toxic, producing a form of spondylitis and other changes in bone. In many cities, particularly in North America, fluorine is now deliberately added to the water supply to bring the level to one part per million, as a prophylactic measure against dental caries. It has been repeatedly shown that provided this level is not exceeded, the incidence of dental caries is markedly reduced and no undesirable effects are produced.

4. VITAMINS

Although gross vitamin deficiency disorders are now rare in Britain and other affluent industrialized countries they deserve consideration in some detail because they are still widespread in some parts of the world. Laboratory workers have discovered and described many vitamins, but deficiency states which have *clinical significance in man* have so far been demonstrated in relation to only 10 of them. These are:

Fat-soluble:
  Retinol (vitamin A), cholecalciferol (vitamin D), and vitamin K.

Water-soluble:
  Ascorbic acid (vitamin C) and six components of the vitamin B complex: thiamine, nicotinic acid, riboflavine, folic acid, cyanocobalamin (vitamin B_{12}) and pyridoxine.

The aetiology and treatment of vitamin K deficiency and its sequelae of hypoprothrombinaemia and a tendency to bleed are described on p. 188. The parts played by folic acid and vitamin

B_{12} in haemopoiesis are discussed on pp. 149–150 and by pyridoxine on p. 154.

Two other components of the vitamin B complex have been reported to have therapeutic effects: pantothenic acid ('burning feet' syndrome, p. 365) and biotin. The only known case of human biotin deficiency was that of a man who had subsisted on an extraordinary diet of raw eggs and red wine.

Fat-soluble vitamin E occurs in human tissues and has interesting biological properties as an antioxidant; but there is no indisputable evidence that ordinary mixed diets are ever deficient in vitamin E or that it has any therapeutic application.

Those three vitamins will not be discussed further.

Recommended Intakes of Vitamins

There has been much confusion in the use of terms to define the amounts of vitamins in the diet to maintain health, e.g. minimum requirements, optimum requirements, recommended allowances, etc. Hence the importance of the World Health Organization Technical Report Series, No. 362, published in 1967. This contains the recommendations of a joint FAO/WHO group of nutritional experts on the requirements of vitamin A, thiamine, riboflavine and nicotinic acid. 'Recommended intake', which was chosen as the most suitable term for this purpose, was defined as 'the amount of the vitamin considered sufficient for the maintenance of health in nearly all people'. It was not expected to cover additional needs which may result from such conditions as infections, malabsorption or metabolic abnormalities. In addition the recommended intake is applicable only when the requirements for calories and other nutrients are met. The Committee states that in view of the well recognised rôles of thiamine, riboflavine and nicotinic acid in energy expenditure, it seems reasonable to relate these requirements to energy expenditure. Therefore the recommended daily intakes should be expressed in terms of mg./ 1,000 kcal. Vitamin requirements vary with factors such as body weight, physical activity and the presence of infections, but only to the extent that calorie expenditure is related to these factors. Hence the advantage of expressing vitamin requirements in terms of milligrams per 1,000 kcal. ingested as this enables the same value to be used for adult (male and female), pregnant and lactating women and children.

The recommended daily intake per 1,000 kcal.

ingested is 0·4 mg. for thiamine, 0·55 mg. for riboflavine and 6·6 nicotinic acid equivalents for nicotinic acid. The term 'nicotinic acid equivalents' is used because it enables the calculation of the combined effects of nicotinic acid and tryptophan in preventing the symptoms of pellagra (p. 357). One nicotinic acid equivalent is defined as being equal to either 1 mg. of nicotinic acid or 60 mg. of tryptophan.

The Committee states that in view of the availability of crystalline retinol (vitamin A_1 alcohol) and crystalline cholecalciferol as reference standards, the practice of expressing vitamin A and vitamin D values in terms of international units (i.u.) is no longer necessary or desirable. Hence recommended intakes should be described in units of weights, namely micrograms. The conversion factor for vitamin A is 1 i.u. = 0·3 micrograms of retinol or, in the case of the provitamin, 0·6 micrograms of β-carotene. For vitamin D the conversion factor is 1 i.u. = 0·025 micrograms of crystalline cholecalciferol (1 microgram of crystalline cholecalciferol = 40 i.u.).

The recommendations of the Joint FAO/WHO Committee have received universal acceptance.

The British National Formulary (1968) contains the following instructions for prescribing:

(1) When fractional doses are prescribed, liquid preparations will be diluted with a suitable vehicle to a dose-volume of 5 ml. or multiples thereof.

(2) The unit dose for children is 5 ml. and for adults 10 ml. A 5-ml. spoonful is officially recognized.

(3) Micrograms should be written in full and the symbol μg. should not be used.

(4) No medicine should be put into an infant's feeding bottle with milk.

DISEASES CAUSED BY EXCESSIVE DEPENDENCE ON CEREALS

The cultivation of cereal grains has enabled the human species to survive and multiply. Cereals provide most of the calories and much of the protein for the vast majority of mankind. But whenever people have to rely exclusively on one kind of grain, not only for their calories but also for their qualitative dietary needs, troubles develop.

Although cereals are traditionally regarded as the staff of life', in general they have certain qualitative defects. Their protein is poor in some essential amino acids, and though the germ and outer coats of the grain contain satisfactory amounts of the vitamin B complex, these are usually largely removed in modern milling and sold to feed animals. Cereals provide no ascorbic acid. Though they contain useful quantities of the two nutritionally important minerals—iron and calcium —these are partly unavailable because of their insoluble combination with phytic acid, which is present particularly in the outer layers of the grain. Because of this, it is advisable that calcium carbonate should be added to flour by the millers in amounts sufficient to neutralize the phytic acid.

BERIBERI

Beriberi is a nutritional disorder formerly widespread in South and East Asia. It has almost disappeared from prosperous Asian countries such as Japan, Taiwan and Malaysia and from big cities such as Hong Kong, Manilla and Singapore. The frequency with which absence of knee jerks and the presence of tenderness of the calf muscles has been noted in nutritional surveys undertaken in regions where the disease is still endemic, suggests that a mild to moderate deficiency of thiamine is not uncommon. Beriberi is caused by eating diets in which most of the calories are derived from highly milled rice. The disorder is often precipitated by infections, hard physical labour or pregnancy and lactation. The clinical picture usually suggests the presence of a multiple nutritional disorder, although lack of thiamine produces the predominant clinical changes.

Three forms are described: (1) wet (cardiovascular) beriberi in which oedema and cardiac failure occur, (2) dry beriberi, a nutritional polyneuropathy, and (3) infantile beriberi. Thiamine is life saving in the treatment of cardiovascular and infantile beriberi and Wernicke's encephalopathy as discussed below, but has no clear-cut effect on the neuropathy (p. 365). Wet and dry beriberi differ greatly in their clinical features, yet they are closely associated epidemiologically. Though caused by the same types of diet, the biochemical lesions responsible may differ in degree or in kind.

Wet (Cardiovascular) Beriberi

This disease is practically confined to rice-eaters who can afford few other foods. The disease rarely occurs among thin people who are markedly underfed. Much more important is the gross disproportion between the amount of carbohydrate in the diet and the quantity of thiamine available to ensure its complete metabolism. Hence the disease may be precipitated by an increase in the ration of rice or other foods rich in carbohydrate. Thiamine is required by the human body because it is an essential component of the enzyme systems concerned with the utilization of carbohydrate. Insufficient thiamine leads to an accumulation in the tissues and blood of pyruvic and lactic acids—intermediate catabolites of glucose.

The first symptom of cardiovascular beriberi is usually pain and tenderness in the calf muscles on walking and it is probably due to inability of the muscles to eliminate with sufficient speed the products of carbohydrate catabolism. These products are vasodilators and may cause extreme dilatation of the peripheral vascular bed; in consequence oedema develops though the plasma proteins may be unaltered at this stage. Because of the vasodilatation the swollen legs are hot to the touch and there is an unusually rapid circulation time. This places a burden on the heart which is already working at a disadvantage, since the myocardium cannot catabolize carbohydrate normally. Cardiac dilatation and failure ultimately result and may cause sudden death; hence it must be recognized that the patient with beriberi heart disease is seriously ill and it is never wise to offer more than a guarded prognosis.

Treatment. Immediate bed rest is essential and thiamine should be given at once. Thiamine hydrochloride has been shown to have a rapid and dramatic effect in the majority of cases. This is because the cardiac condition is due to a reversible biochemical process and not to structural alterations as is the case in dry beriberi.

For a case of average severity thiamine should be given intramuscularly in amounts of 25 mg. daily for three days. In critically ill patients the initial dose should be increased to 50 or even 100 mg. and should be administered intravenously very slowly; a dose of 50 mg. should be given intramuscularly for the next two or three days. Thereafter oral treatment with thiamine should be continued in a dose of 10 mg. two or three times a day until convalescence is established.

To ensure that in such a dangerous disorder as cardiovascular beriberi the body's depleted stores of thiamine are rapidly and completely made good, the large doses mentioned above are recommended by many authorities today because the drug is in plentiful supply and is cheap and non-toxic. It is probable that considerably smaller amounts would be adequate since many prisoners of war in Malaya during the Second World War responded excellently to a daily dose of thiamine as low as 5 mg. which was all that could be allotted in view of the severe shortage of supply.

With relief of the cardiac emergency, the patient may still be incapacitated as a result of other deficiencies in his former diet. These may include protein, vitamin A, nicotinic acid and riboflavine. A good mixed diet with less emphasis on rice is needed. Whole wheat, millet or some other cereal should, if possible, be substituted for part of the rice in the diet. Pulses have a well-deserved reputation for curing and preventing beriberi; 120 g. (4 oz.) of beans or lentils are a useful daily addition to the diet. Any foods of animal origin that are available should be included. The diet can be supplemented usefully by natural sources of the entire vitamin B complex such as yeast or yeast extract, wheat germ or rice polishings. Half an ounce or more of dried yeast daily is a valuable remedy for aiding recovery.

In both wet and dry beriberi, preoccupation with dietary treatment should not divert attention from the necessity of good nursing, management of associated infections, physiotherapy and subsequent rehabilitation.

Sometimes patients with cardiovascular beriberi suffer also from nutritional polyneuropathy, traditionally called dry beriberi.

Dry Beriberi

This and other neurological features of thiamine deficiency are considered on p. 355.

Infantile Beriberi

This is a special form of beriberi, common in endemic areas. It occurs in breast-fed infants, usually between the second and sixth months. Although the mothers of such infants must have been eating a diet and secreting milk with a low thiamine content, classical signs of beriberi are stated to be absent in 50 per cent. of them. The clinical features differ somewhat from the adult disease, and infantile beriberi exists in acute and chronic forms. In the former, the mother may have noticed that the infant is restless, cries a lot, is passing less urine than normal and shows signs of puffiness. The infant may then suddenly become cyanosed with dyspnoea and tachycardia and may die from cardiac failure within 24 to 48 hours. Other serious signs are convulsions and coma. In the chronic form, a state of marasmus develops due to a general failure of nutrition often associated with anorexia, vomiting and diarrhoea, and there is little evidence of structural disease in the nervous system.

Infantile beriberi was formerly the chief cause of death in infants between 2 and 6 months of age in regions where the disease was endemic, and it may still be an important cause in certain isolated rural areas in South-East Asia.

The simplest way to treat infantile beriberi is through the mother's milk. The mother should receive 10 mg. thiamine hydrochloride twice daily—in severe cases by injection. Thereafter she should take a good diet, supplemented if possible by yeast or rice bran. In addition, the infant must be given thiamine. In cases of mild to moderate severity 10 to 20 mg. of thiamine should be given intramuscularly once a day for three days. This should be followed by oral treatment with 5 to 10 mg. of thiamine twice a day for several weeks. For patients critically ill with severe heart failure or convulsions and coma the initial dose of thiamine should be increased to 25 mg. or even 50 mg., given intravenously very slowly. Thereafter treatment is by intramuscular injection followed by oral therapy as described above.

PELLAGRA

Pellagra is a nutritional disease which commonly occurs all over the world among poor people who subsist chiefly on maize (Indian corn). In recent years pellagra has disappeared from many countries where it was endemic, and in areas where it remains, the incidence is much less than formerly. An exception is South Africa where big outbreaks occur in the spring and summer in certain Bantu reserves. It may lead to the patient being admitted to a mental hospital.

Maize is a good food if included in a well-balanced diet. Nevertheless, when it is relied upon as the principal source of calories, it produces nutritional failure because it is short of certain essential amino acids, notably tryptophan, and the nicotinic acid it contains is bound in such a way that it is not available.

Isolated cases of pellagra occur among people who are not dependent on maize. It is a well-recognized complication of chronic alcoholism. Any chronic disease of the gastro-intestinal tract, leading to malabsorption, may result in the development of one or more of the clinical features of the disease but rarely does so.

The human body uses nicotinic acid as an essential part of one of the enzyme systems concerned with tissue oxidation. In normal circumstances it can make at least a substantial part of its requirements for this nutrient from the amino acid, tryptophan. An old clinical observation is that milk is good for pellagrins; milk contains little nicotinic acid though considerable amounts of tryptophan. This observation was forgotten in the excitement that attended the discovery that nicotinic acid would abolish the florid signs of pellagra.

The typical clinical features are loss of weight, increasing debility, mental changes, red swollen tongue, gastro-intestinal disturbances, often with persistent diarrhoea, and an erythematous dermatitis brought on by the first sunshine of spring. Pellagra has been called the disease of the three D's: 'dermatitis, diarrhoea and dementia'.

Treatment. *Specific vitamin therapy.* For quick relief of symptoms, nicotinamide is invaluable. This preparation is better than nicotinic acid, not only because it is the form in which the vitamin is actually utilized in the body, but also because it does not cause the unpleasant flushing and burning sensations that often result from taking nicotinic acid. These sensations are harmless and transitory but many embarrass or alarm the patient. A suitable dose for either nicotinamide or nicotinic acid is 100 mg. four- to six-hourly by mouth, although a smaller dose is likely to be effective. The vitamin is very rapidly absorbed from the stomach and small intestine, despite the most severe digestive disorders. There is, therefore, no indication for giving it by intravenous or intramuscular injection, although perparations can be obtained for this purpose. The immediate response to nicotinamide is usually dramatic; within 24 hours the erythema of the skin diminishes, the tongue becomes paler and less painful and the diarrhoea ceases. Often there is also striking improvement in the patient's behaviour and attitude. Nicotinamide alone is usually insufficient to restore health. The orogenital syndrome, peripheral nerve and spinal cord changes, anaemia and hypoproteinaemia are clinical features which may be present and are clearly due to deficiencies other than of nicotinic acid. Appropriate treatment is required. The administration of yeast, yeast extract, liver or wheat germ is a valuable aid to treatment, supplemented if necessary by riboflavine, thiamine, folic acid and vitamin B_{12}.

Diet. The first aim should be to compensate for the qualitative and quantitative deficiencies of the previous diet. If possible, the food should provide 100 to 150 g. of good protein, supplied by milk, eggs, meat or fish. Plenty of carbohydrate and fat is also desirable, sufficient to provide up to 3,500 kcal. per day, to restore the patient to normal weight. The food should be low in roughage at first in order to avoid further irritation to the inflamed intestines and consequent continued diarrhoea. When the diarrhoea ceases, fruits and green vegetables are useful for preventing the constipation that sometimes follows. The diet may be poorly tolerated at first, because the mental state of the patient may result in his rebelling against the unaccustomed food. Furthermore, the sore mouth may make eating difficult, and extra food may temporarily intensify the diarrhoea

General Measures. Rest in bed and sedation are necessary if the patient is severely ill. Troublesome behaviour must be tolerated with objective understanding of its cause. If the dermatitis is associated with much crusting or secondary infection, gentle washing with a bland solution is indicated followed by the application of a cream containing vioform (3 per cent.) and hydrocortisone (1 per cent.). If the diarrhoea is severe enough to interfere with sleep or to cause electrolyte disturbances, preliminary treatment with tincture of opium or codeine phosphate should be given until is is brought under control with nicotinamide.

Prevention. The dramatic disappearance of pellagra from the Southern States of the U.S.A. is clear proof that the disease can be prevented. Its disappearance has sometimes been attributed to the fortification of bread with nicotinic acid, but this is only one of several factors which have produced this satisfactory result. A marked fall in the incidence of pellagra occurred many years before this procedure was adopted. It is more likely that the rarity of the disease is the natural consequence of an improved standard of living due to a reduction in the incidence of poverty, better education, especially on nutritional matters, and a change in the traditional methods of farming and feeding in

rural districts. It is to be hoped that in the near future pellagra will be abolished in those regions of underdeveloped countries in South America, Africa and Asia where maize is the staple cereal consumed and the disease is endemic.

From the standpoint of agricultural policy, it is clearly wise to avoid too much dependence on a single cereal crop, such as maize, or to devote an excessive acreage to the cultivation of cash-crops, such as cotton or tobacco. Animal husbandry should be encouraged in areas where pellagra is endemic so that the production of milk and milk products and meat is increased.

For the medical practitioner in such an area, without direct influence in matters of agricultural policy, the best advice that he can give to his patients is to take as much milk, eggs and meat as they can afford. He will also do well to prescribe yeast extract for the families of his pellagrinous patients.

DISEASES DUE TO AN INSUFFICIENT CONSUMPTION OF FRUIT AND VEGETABLES

SCURVY

Scurvy is a nutritional disease which results from prolonged subsistence on diets practically devoid of fresh fruit and vegetables. Such diets are likely to be deficient also in other nutrients such as iron, folic acid, vitamin A and sometimes protein. Its characteristic features are due to lack of ascorbic acid. Scurvy has been recognized as a clinical entity since mediaeval times. It came into prominence when sailing-ships began to open up the great oceans of the world to regular traffic. Over 200 years ago (1753) James Lind, a naval surgeon, wrote a classic work *A Treatise of the Scurvy*. He provided the first experimental proof that scurvy could be relieved by the juice of citrus fruits.

As a consequence of the acquisition of knowledge of the chemistry of food in the nineteenth century, various preserved and artificial milks were manufactured which provided an adequate substitute for the protein, fat and carbohydrate of human milk but which contained little or no ascorbic acid. Hence, infantile scurvy became an important disease by the end of the nineteenth century. In Britain and other highly developed countries it is now rare. This satisfactory position is partly due to the increased production of citrus and other fruits and green vegetables and to their distribution in the canned or frozen state in which the ascorbic acid content is retained. This makes them available at all seasons of the year. Infantile scurvy still occurs occasionally as a result of poverty, ignorance and maternal neglect as is clearly indicated in recent reports from Australia, Canada and the USA. Sporadic instances of scurvy occurring in adults are encountered particularly at the extreme of life because an increasing number of old people live alone and do not have the opportunity or the aptitude to feed themselves properly. Scurvy appears to be a rare disease in infants and children in most subtropical and tropical countries though it may occur in arid parts of the world in times of drought, as in Arabia and in India after failure of the monsoon rains.

Treatment. The normal human body when fully saturated with the vitamin contains about 5 g.; treatment should, therefore, aim at achieving saturation by giving 250 mg. of synthetic ascorbic acid by mouth four times a day for a week. It should be given orally because by this route it is more slowly absorbed and better retained. There should be no delay in starting treatment, as sudden death without warning, apparently due to cardiac failure, may occur in severe scurvy. If the pure vitamin is not available, natural sources of it (fresh fruit or vegetables) should be used; of particular value are citrus fruits, blackcurrants and extracts of rose hips. Ascorbic acid, as it occurs naturally or as the synthetic preparation, rapidly brings to an end the characteristic bleeding into the tissues and the consequent pain. Once the haemorrhagic manifestations are under control a liberal diet including fresh fruit and properly cooked vegetables should be given. It remains for the physician to remedy so far as he can the social, and economic circumstances that originally deprived his patient of foods providing ascorbic acid, and to attend to the other dietary deficiences which are almost invariably present. In particular, if the patient is anaemic, ferrous sulphate tablets by mouth are indicated.

Prevention. It has already been said that in Britain at least, scurvy tends to occur at the two extremes of age: infancy and old age. The prevention of scurvy in infants has been accomplished by the better education of mothers and safeguarded by the regular distribution of cheap, concentrated orange juice of standard ascorbic acid content, now being withdrawn on dentists' advice.

Routinely infants should be given the equivalent of 20 to 30 mg. of ascorbic acid daily, starting with small amounts during the second or third month. This daily requirement is present in 1 to 3 oz. of fresh orange juice. Concentrated orange juice issued through the British Welfare Food Service contained 60 mg. ascorbic acid to the fluid ounce and hence had to be diluted. Black currant juice or syrup of rose hips in lesser amounts is a satisfactory substitute if the infant does not like orange juice. It is advisable to continue giving a supplement of ascorbic acid in its natural form to children until the age of 2 years. It can then be discontinued provided the child is taking a good diet containing fruit and vegetables.

So far, however, the Welfare State has failed to find any simple administrative means of preventing scurvy among the old and solitary, who are largely unresponsive to education. It is a pity that the orange juice once provided for infants is not available for the elderly.

Should the physician be unsuccessful in achieving the dietetic aims discussed above, he should at least insist on the patient taking one 25 mg. tablet of synthetic ascorbic acid daily. Alternatively, a massive dose can be given at longer intervals—say 500 mg. on the first day of every month. This method is justified only by the fact that patients who are careless about diet are nearly always defaulters when daily medication is called for.

Special provision against scurvy is desirable for any group of people living on packed, preserved rations for any length of time. The problem may arise with explorers of inaccessible lands and oceans, or armed forces operating in a barren territory. In such circumstances the bulk of the rations is a prime consideration, especially if airlifts are involved and tinned fruit and vegetables provide few essential calories in proportion to their weight. Synthetic ascorbic acid tablets are, therefore, invaluable under such conditions. In default of such supplies antiscorbutic remedies can often be prepared from green herbs on the spot. Scurvy grass (*Cochlearia officinalis*) which grows on seashores and infusions of pine and spruce needles are traditional remedies.

In times of drought and famine, when fresh vegetables are not available, ascorbic acid can be obtained by the germination of pulses or cereals. This is accomplished by spreading pulses under wet cloths.

Night Blindness, Xerophthalmia, Keratomalacia and Allied Disorders

The importance of fruit and green and yellow vegetables in the prevention of diseases due to deficiency of vitamin A is not sufficiently appreciated by the laity. Retinol is found only in foods of animal origin, namely milk, butter, cheese, egg-yolk, liver and some of the fatty fishes. These products are in very short supply among many poor people in underdeveloped countries. Hence they have to rely on the carotenoids of fruits and vegetables which man and certain animals can convert into retinol. However, this conversion is always incomplete and hence involves considerable losses of vitamin A activity (p. 355). It is therefore not surprising that the disorders due to deficiency of vitamin A mentioned above are liable to occur in poor people in Asia, Africa and South America, whose diet consists mainly of a single cereal such as rice or maize and whose intake of daily products is very small. This is particularly the case in hot arid countries where great difficulty is experienced in growing adequate crops of fruit and vegetables and pasture for animals. Deficiency of vitamin A affects the epithelial surface of all parts of the body which undergo squamous metaplasia; as a result the sebaceous glands and hair follicles of the skin and tear glands of the eye became blocked with horny plugs of keratin so that their secretions are diminished. This causes the clinical features due to vitamin A deficiency of the skin and eye. Their prevention and treatment are described on pp. 367-368.

DISEASES DUE TO DEFICIENCY OF VITAMIN D AND CALCIUM

(*Rickets, Osteomalacia, Osteoporosis*)

Vitamin D is necessary for the formation of normal bone and the calcification of rachitic bone. It probably has a direct effect on bone but the mechanism underlying this action is uncertain. In addition it promotes the absorption of calcium and phosphate from the gut, thus ensuring a sufficient supply of these minerals at the growing points of the bones where the calcium comes in contact with inorganic phosphates liberated from organic phosphates under the influence of the enzyme phosphatase. Thus calcium phosphate is formed and used by the osteoblasts to make new bone.

Dietary sources. The sources of the natural vitamin are all fat-containing animal products. The richest sources are fatty fish and their oils, some of which contain many thousands of international units of vitamin D per 100 g. edible portion. Vitamin D is also present in dairy products such as milk, eggs, butter and in vitaminized margarine in much smaller quantities. It is important to remember that milk has a very small content of vitamin D. Cereals, vegetables and fruit grown in temperate climates contain no vitamin D and meat and white fish insignificant amounts.

Recommended intakes. As already noted on p. 355, vitamin D is now measured by weight. One mcg. of cholecalciferol is equal to 40 i.u. The recommended daily dietary intake for infants and children up to 5 years of age and for pregnant lactating women is 10 mcg. (400 i.u.). For older children and adults about 2·5 mcg. (100 i.u.) is adequate.

Infantile Rickets

Rickets is a nutritional deficiency disease occurring mainly in infancy and early childhood. It is due to a disorder of calcium and phosphorus metabolism which occurs when infants are weaned on predominantly cereal diets and receive insufficient vitamin D. In addition, the intake of calcium is usually low because of insufficient milk in the diet. Vitamin D can be synthesized in the skin on exposure to sunlight; hence rickets rarely occurs in young children who can run naked out of doors in sunny climates; yet those in such climates who are clothed and confined may develop the disease. Rickets has been rightly called a disease of poverty and darkness. Lack of calcium affects the nerves and muscles and especially the bones, resulting in characteristic rachitic deformities.

Rickets is still an important clinical problem in some underdeveloped countries, especially in infants under one year of age living in large towns and cities. It is now a rare disease in Britain and other highly developed countries as a result of a variety of measures which have been introduced during the last 40 years and have led to greatly improved standards of nutrition and housing. Of particular importance are the various schemes which have resulted in a satisfactory supply of milk, the organized distribution of cod-liver oil and other sources of vitamin D and the fortification with vitamin D of preparations of dried milk, margarine and some proprietary cereal foods. That it would be rash to suggest any of these measures is now redundant is clearly indicated by recent reports of limited outbreaks of clinical rickets in coloured immigrant children in Glasgow, London and Birmingham, and occasionally in underprivileged white children living in slum areas in Glasgow and other big cities in many countries. Although clinical rickets is rare in Britain there is good evidence to show that it is not uncommon for poor children below the age of 5 years to have a daily dietary intake of vitamin D of less than 2·5 mcg. (100 i.u.). Such children may be said to have hypovitaminosis D and if growth continues without an increased intake of vitamin D or if gastro-intestinal infection occurs, they are in danger of developing clinical rickets.

The Treatment of Rickets

The two essential of treatment are the provision of a supplement of vitamin D and an ample intake of calcium.

Vitamin D preparations. A therapeutic dose of vitamin D varies from 25 to 125 mcg. (1,000 to 5,000 i.u.) daily, depending on the severity of the disease and the age of the child. In contrast, the prophylactic dose is 10 mcg. (400 i.u.) or less daily depending on the intake of vitamin D from other sources. The B.P. preparation of cod-liver oil contains approximately 10 mcg. (425 i.u.) per 5 ml. which is the official standardized volume of the 5-ml. plastic spoon supplied with the medicine.

When the vitamin content of a preparation is contained in 1 ml. of a solution or less as in the case of B.P. Calciferol Solution (see below), the pharmacist must make the necessary dilution with an inert oil so that the quantity of the vitamin ordered by the doctor is contained in 5 ml., i.e. one standard spoonful.

Children who find cod-liver oil unpalatable can be given halibut-liver oil in a very small dose since its concentration of vitamins A and D is approximately 20 to 40 times that of cod-liver oil. Each B.P. capsule of halibut-liver oil contains slightly more than 10 mcg. (400 i.u.) of vitamin D and 4,000 to 5,000 units of vitamin A. One capsule on four or five days in a week would be adequate for prophylaxis. The advantages of giving natural sources of vitamin D, e.g. fish-liver oils, is that they contain valuable amounts of vitamin A. This is of particular importance in underdeveloped countries where a dual deficiency of vitamins A and D is frequently present. For severe cases needing 125 mcg. (5,000 i.u.) or more daily, synthetic calciferol

is useful because the volume of cod-liver oil required to provide this dose may be excessive. For such patients the B.P. Calciferol Solution is satisfactory. It contains 75 mcg. (3,000 i.u.) of vitamin D per ml. Alternatively the dose of vitamin D can be given as drops. For this purpose Adexolin (Glaxo Laboratories Ltd.) is particularly suitable as it contains 1 mcg. (40 i.u.) per drop as well as 150 mcg. (400 units) of retinol, and is sold in specially designed bottles which ensures that only drops of the correct size are delivered. This bottle has replaced the use of droppers. For prophylaxis, up to 10 drops of Adexolin should be given daily and the number of drops should be reduced to four or five daily according to the amount of vitamin D the child is getting from other sources. In times of social upheaval, such as may be occasioned by war, floods or pestilence, when an infant or young child may be seen once by an emergency medical service and perhaps not again for months, a single massive dose of vitamin D, e.g. 3·75 mg. (150,000 i.u.), can be given by mouth with reasonable safety and curative effects. For this purpose three Strong Calciferol Tablets B.P. each containing 1·25 mg. (50,000 i.u.) are suitable. A single dose of 3·75 mg. (150,000 i.u.) can be given by intramuscular injection (Calciferol Injection B.P.) but this has no proved advantage over the oral route. The daily administration of small doses is the method recommended for normal practice, because of the danger of overdosage (p. 362).

Calcium preparations. Rachitic infants and children require an ample supply of calcium in addition to vitamin D, and the best source of this is milk. At least half a litre (about 1 pint) should be taken daily by a young child with mild rickets. For a severe case a supplement of calcium should also be given. For this purpose calcium gluconate is more acceptable for oral administration than calcium chloride or lactate since it is tasteless, odourless and does not irritate the stomach. The dose is one to two tablets of Calcium Gluconate B.P.C. three times a day. Each tablet contains 600 mg. of calcium gluconate (53·5 mg. of elemental calcium). The tablets should be well crushed and chewed before being swallowed. Alternatively, and preferably, one to two tablets of Calcium Gluconate Effervescent B.P.C. can be given dissolved in a glass of water three times a day. Each tablet contains 1 g. of calcium gluconate. When much larger amounts of calcium are required as may be the case in resistant rickets (see below), malabsorptive disorders or osteoporosis, the Sandoz preparation of calcium gluconate effervescent (Sandocal) can be given dissolved in a glass of water. The dose is one tablet three times a day. Each tablet contains 4·5 g. of calcium gluconate (400 mg. of elemental calcium) as compared with 1 g. of calcium gluconate in each B.P.C. effervescent tablet.

For emergency treatment, e.g. tetany, Calcium Gluconate Injection B.P. in 5-ml. and 10-ml. ampoules can be given by slow intravenous injection or intramuscularly in a dose of 10 to 20 ml. This solution contains 1 g. of calcium gluconate in 10 ml. of water. For infants and young children the dose should be reduced to 300 to 600 mg. of calcium gluconate.

Vitamin D and diet are not the whole solution to the treatment of rickets. An attempt must be made to improve the hygienic environment of the child. This often requires the tactful education of the mother in better feeding practices and general care. Unnecessary clothing should be removed and, if the child was previously confined indoors, he should be allowed out as much as possible to enjoy the sunshine. This is particularly important in countries where supplements of vitamin D are not provided. An adequate intake of iron and ascorbic acid is needed.

The earliest evidence of healing in rickets is provided by radiological examination of the growing ends of the bones. The levels of calcium and phosphorus in the serum provide an inconstant and unreliable guide. A more constant change is a decrease in the raised serum alkaline phosphatase level, but as a rule this does not occur for several weeks after treatment is initiated. The normal value for alkaline phosphatase in adults is around 3 to 12 King Armstrong units, but in children about 3 years of age it varies from 10 to 20 units. When rickets is present the figure is from 30 to 40 units. The therapeutic dose of vitamin D should be continued so long as the phosphatase level remains elevated; thereafter it may gradually be reduced to the prophylactic dose of 10 mcg. (400 i.u.) daily.

Occasionally, cases of rickets are encountered which are resistant to ordinary therapeutic doses of vitamin D. The disease persists into late childhood ('late rickets') or even adult life, producing the the clinical appearance of osteomalacia, unless adequately treated. The cause of this resistance is not understood, though in some cases it is due to a defect in the reabsorption of phosphate by the renal tubules, e.g. the Fanconi syndrome. A similar state may sometimes arise as a conditioned deficiency resulting from malabsorption or renal failure. Whatever the cause, treatment consists in giving large doses of vitamin D by mouth in the form of strong calciferol tablets B.P., together with calcium salts, e.g. one effervescent Sandocal tablet dissolved in a glass of water three times a day. The initial dose of calciferol may be 1·25 to 3·75 mg. (150,000 i.u.) daily (one to three strong calciferol tablets B.P.), but it should be reduced at the first suspicion of toxic symptoms. These include nausea, vomiting, diarrhoea, drowsiness and signs of renal failure; metastatic calcification in the arteries, kidneys and other tissues may occur.

Prophylaxis

The provision of adequate milk for children, the clearing of industrial city slums, the building of new housing estates and the attack on the smoke nuisance are basic prophylactic measures which must be continued at all costs. In addition, mothers must be educated in the need to keep their infants and children in the sunshine as much as possible. Nevertheless, for reasons already stated, and particularly in northern countries, the supply of the vitamin from this source is uncertain and attention must be paid to the dietary supply. It must be remembered that none of the common foods in a child's diet is a good source of vitamin D. Practical experience shows that the majority of children benefit by receiving a daily supplement of about 10 mcg. (400 i.u.), preferably in the form of some natural source such as cod-liver oil, which provides useful amounts of vitamin A in addition. This is also advisable in sunny tropical countries if the mothers insist on keeping their infants wrapped in swaddling clothes during the first year of life. It seems reasonable that the supplement should be started within four weeks of birth because human and animal milk has a negligible content of vitamin D.

Before deciding on the prophylactic dose of cod-liver oil or other fish oil, it is necessary to consider how much vitamin D the infant is getting from other sources. Thus, if he is being brought up on a preparation of dried milk 'fortified' with vitamin D the supplement of cod-liver oil should be small. Furthermore, it should be remembered that some proprietary cereal foods for infants are 'fortified' by the manufacturers with vitamin D.

All brands of British margarine are fortified with vitamin D and contain about twice as much vitamin D as butter. This may help to secure a good calcification of the bones during the growth of older children.

Not only is there no advantage in giving infants and young children more than 400 i.u. of vitamin D daily from all sources for prophylactic purposes, but there is a distinct possibility that higher doses given over a long period may have harmful effects. The potential dangers of overdosage with vitamin D have been emphasized by the discovery that infantile hypercalcaemia is not such a rare condition as was formerly believed. It may produce metastatic calcification in the arteries, kidneys and other tissues.

It should be noted, however, that the prophylactic dose of vitamin D for premature infants should be twice that for full-term infants and the supplement should be started within two weeks after birth. There has been divergence of view among paediatricians in the past about the length of time that the prophylactic adminstration of vitamin D should be continued. Obviously such features as the social and economic status of the parents and the climate in which the family lives are matters of importance. It seems reasonable to suggest that in temperate climates at least, a daily intake of about 10 mcg. (400 i.u.) should be continued summer and winter for the first five years of life.

OSTEOMALACIA

Aetiology

Osteomalacia is the adult counterpart of rickets. In its fully developed form as it occurs in women in purdah in oriental countries, it causes great deformity and suffering. It is found in women of child-bearing age who live on poor cereal diets devoid of milk, who are kept indoors all day and seldom see the sun and who by repeated pregnancies become depleted of calcium. At the present time in Europe the disease is not uncommon in old people, especially women. It may be due to malabsorption from any cause including previous gastro-intestinal operations, or to direct dietary deficiency of vitamin D. Chronic renal disorders are a less important cause of the disease.

Diagnosis

The early symptoms may be mistaken for those present in osteoporosis or rheumatic disorders.

The clinical examination must be supported by a careful inquiry into adverse social, economic and dietary factors which may be present. In addition biochemical tests, including alkaline phosphatase determinations and radiological examination of the skeleton should be undertaken, and histological examination of bone, obtained by biopsy, may be required. Radiological examination shows rarefaction of bone and commonly translucent bands (pseudo-fractures, Looser's zones), often symmetrical, at points submitted to great compression stress. Common sites are the ribs, the axillary borders of the scapula, the pubic rami and the medial cortex of the upper femur. Looser's zones are diagnostic of osteomalacia. It has been referred to in the past by radiologists as 'Milkman's syndrome'. Correct diagnosis is essential, as the results of treatment with vitamin D are excellent if undertaken prior to the establishment of gross deformities, and it is also necessary for the assessment of dosage of vitamin D.

Treatment

This is essentially the same as for rickets when osteomalacia is primarily due to a defective intake of vitamin D, namely 25 to 125 mcg. (1,000 to 5,000 i.u.) daily. If there is evidence of malabsorption the dose should be 1·25 mg. (50,000 i.u.) daily. If the disease is secondary to renal disorders the dose may be 2·5 mg. (100,000 i.u.) or more. In addition a good diet should be given which includes milk, eggs, butter or margarine. This may be difficult or impossible under the conditions in which the disease arises in the East. Maintenance treatment with vitamin D will be required for cases of osteomalacia in which the cause cannot be removed. In all cases of osteomalacia a supplement of calcium should be given orally, namely 1 to 2 g. in the form of calcium lactate or, preferably, two calcium Sandoz effervescent tablets each containing 380 mg. of elemental calcium. Within four to eight weeks of starting treatment the pain and weakness has usually disappeared. The decision to reduce or discontinue the dose of vitamin D and calcium is based on the improvement in the clinical features and the disappearance of biochemical and radiological abnormalities. The dangers of vitamin D intoxication should be kept in mind (p. 362).

Prevention

Once major deformities are established they cannot be corrected by diet or drugs, but only by an orthopaedic surgeon. Hence the great importance of early and correct diagnosis and proper treatment. Free access to sunshine and an adequate intake of dairy produce, supplemented when necessary with fish-liver oil, will prevent nutritional osteomalacia. With improved education and better standards of living the disease is now rare in many Asian towns where previously it was common.

Secondary Rickets and Osteomalacia

The clinical picture of rickets or osteomalacia is occasionally seen as a result of other diseases which 'condition' the calcium deficiency. These diseases are of two kinds.

1. *Malabsorptive disorders.* If the intestinal absorption of fat, and, therefore, of fat-soluble vitamin D, is impaired, the body is deprived of a sufficiency of this vitamin to promote the normal absorption of calcium. In the adult, secondary osteomalacia may result. Of particular interest is the frequency with which osteomalacia alone or in combination with osteoporosis has been reported as a sequel to the Polya-type operation for partial gastrectomy. Treatment should include both vitamin D and calcium salts by mouth (p. 239).

2. *Renal disorders.* In renal failure with uraemia and in a variety of disorders of the kidney with disturbances in tubular function, including the Fanconi syndrome, renal rickets may occur in children and osteomalacia in adults. These disorders are probably due to defective absorption of calcium secondary to the development of resistance to the action of vitamin D on the absorption of calcium and on the metabolism of bone. Patients with renal rickets and osteomalacia may derive great benefit from treatment with large doses of vitamin D and calcium. For further information see pp. 280-281.

Osteoporosis

With the possible exception of Paget's disease, osteoporosis is the disease of bone most frequently encountered in clinical practice. It may be a localized or generalized disease, the cause of which is uncertain.

The view that senile osteoporosis is an endocrine disorder has long been held and was supported by the fact that its clinical features could often be relieved by hormonal therapy. It has also been claimed that if patients with senile osteoporosis are given large amounts of calcium (2 to 3 g. per day) the majority retain 0·5 to 1 g. calcium daily, while healthy controls retain little or none of the extra mineral. This suggests that osteoporosis may develop as a result of a long period of negative calcium balance due in part to inadequate intake, in part to diminished alimentary absorption, and in some cases to increased urinary excretion of calcium. For further information see p. 462.

NUTRITIONAL ANAEMIAS

Nutritional anaemias arise in people subsisting on predominantly cereal diets and are fully discussed on pp. 143-145.

NUTRITIONAL DISORDERS OF THE NERVOUS SYSTEM

Clinical knowledge of the dietary neuropathies was greatly advanced by the bitter sufferings of prisoners in Japanese hands during the Second World War, but delay in treatment to permit investigations to be done after their release was rightly considered to be unethical. A convenient classification is as follows:

Group I—where the lesion is predominantly in the peripheral nerves.

   (*a*) The polyneuropathies of beriberi, alcoholism and pregnancy.

   (*b*) The 'burning feet' syndrome.

Group II—where the lesion is predominantly in the central nervous system.

   (*a*) Wernicke's encephalopathy.

   (*b*) Nutritional amblyopia.

   (*c*) The cord syndromes—spinal ataxia; spastic paraplegia and lathyrism; subacute combined degeneration.

NUTRITIONAL POLYNEUROPATHY

This is a disease characterized by signs of bilateral and usually symmetrical lesions involving the peripheral nerves, both sensory and motor, with a dietary history indicating a failure in nutrition as the primary cause. The polyneuropathy of oriental dry beriberi is the classic example. It arises from the consumption of a poor diet composed chiefly of polished rice. In countries outside the tropics an essentially similar disease occurs not infrequently in chronic alcoholics. Alcohol provides calories but none of the other essential materials needed for metabolism of the nervous system. Rarely during pregnancy and in malabsorptive disorders polyneuropathy may arise.

The patient is usually unduly thin, in contrast to the common appearance of patients suffering from cardiovascular beriberi. The earliest symptoms are weakness and paraesthesia in the legs. Hypoaesthesia, nocturnal cramps, ataxia (due to loss of proprioceptive sensation) and foot-drop frequently follow. Degeneration of the motor nerves results in muscular wasting and loss of tendon reflexes. The disease is essentially chronic, developing slowly and leading to gradual incapacity so that the patient needs the aid of sticks to get about, and eventually may become bedridden. It is important to remember that certain drugs and chemicals (e.g. arsenic, isoniazid) may produce a syndrome that mimics nutritional polyneuropathy.

Treatment

This demands immediate attention to the patient's diet both in quantity and quality. The neurological lesions will not improve until the patient regains his strength, so every effort should be made to restore him to his original body weight. Plenty of protein —milk, eggs, meat, fish—is desirable, supplemented by natural sources of the vitamin B complex— yeast or yeast extract (e.g. Marmite), liver extract, rice bran or wheat germ. This may be difficult to provide for poor, rice-eating sufferers from beriberi and unacceptable to alcoholic patients with gastritis, or pregnant women who have been vomiting after every meal. The physician's art must be adapted to find the best means of supplying the needs of the individual patient.

The value of synthetic thiamine is disputed, but it certainly should be given a trial in the oral dosage suggested for cardiovascular beriberi (p. 354).

Prevention

The disease as it occurs among rice-eaters can be prevented by the same general measures described for the prophylaxis of cardiovascular beriberi. Its occasional occurrence in alcoholics and sufferers from chronic vomiting (of whatever cause) can be prevented only by attention to the malady that conditioned the nutritional failure.

BURNING FEET SYNDROME

Outbreaks of this distinct clinical syndrome, characterized by aching, burning or throbbing in the feet, have occurred at various times in Europe, Central America, Africa and India among people living on very poor diets. It became very trouble-some among European prisoners in the Far East during the Second World War.

The syndrome results from the prolonged consumption of a diet deficient in protein and the B group of vitamins, but precisely which factor is missing is uncertain. Patients who suffer from it may develop in addition the oro-genital syndrome (p. 366) or nutritional amblyopia (p. 367), or frank beriberi. Patients improve when given yeast, Marmite, rice polishings, soya beans and other foods rich in the vitamin B complex.

WERNICKE'S ENCEPHALOPATHY

This disease is caused by an acute biochemical lesion in the brain through lack of essential nutrients to maintain normal metabolism. The principal deficiency concerned is almost certainly lack of thiamine; indeed, the disease may be considered to be the human counterpart of the encephalopathy produced in animals by acute deprivation of this vitamin.

The majority of patients described in Europe and the USA have been alcoholics, although the disease occasionally occurs as a result of carcinoma of the stomach, pregnancy toxaemia, prolonged vomiting, diarrhoea or other causes of gross digestive failure. The condition occurred not infrequently in Japanese prisoner-of-war camps in association with beriberi.

The disease is characterized by diplopia, mental changes (Korsakoff's psychosis) and peripheral polyneuropathy.

Dramatic therapeutic responses have been obtained in early cases by the parenteral administration of thiamine. When ample supplies are available it is best to give large doses parenterally as described on p. 354, until the major clinical features are relieved. Treatment should then be continued with a well-balanced mixed diet (if possible) and some natural supplement of the entire vitamin B complex, e.g. yeast extract, rice polishings or wheat germ. When treatment is started early, recovery is usually complete, but if delayed the mental changes may persist.

NUTRITIONAL AMBLYOPIA

(See p. 367).

NUTRITIONAL SYNDROMES INVOLVING THE SPINAL CORD

Signs of involvement of tracts in the spinal cord occasionally appear in pellagra and other disorders associated with deficiency of the vitamin B complex. The pyramidal tracts may be chiefly affected, producing a spastic paraplegia, which is seen in its most striking form in lathyrism, a disease that occurs in epidemics during famines, especially in India. Lathyrism is due to excessive consumption of the lathyrus pea; this contains a toxic substance which selectively damages the pyramidal tracts of underfed people. The possibility of the existence of a poisonous factor in the diet should always be kept in mind in cases of nutritional spastic paraplegia. Thus the cause of the spastic paraplegia which has been intensively studied in Jamaica may be a toxic factor in 'bush teas'. There is no specific treatment for these forms of spastic paraplegia. Sometimes the principal lesion is in the posterior columns of the cord, producing a spinal ataxia resembling subacute combined degeneration of the cord, but not necessarily associated with anaemia or achlorhydria. In such cases it would seem reasonable to administer hydroxocobalamin (pp. 149–150) as a supplement to a good general diet.

The treatment and prevention of subacute combined degeneration of the cord is discussed on p. 151.

NUTRITIONAL DISORDERS OF THE SKIN

Various changes may be seen in examining the skin of patients who are undernourished or malnourished. The thin, dry, inelastic, pigmented skin of the starving person is extremely characteristic. The loose skin-folds, lacking subcutaneous fat, of the underfed patient are familiar. Simple atrophy, in which the skin appears thin and tightly stretched, especially on the legs, is sometimes seen in malnourished people. When vitamin A deficiency is present for a considerable time, there may be dryness of the skin (xeroderma) in association with an appearance as though a layer of lacquer had been painted on and then had dried, leaving a crazy-paving design (crackled skin). This is often accompanied by a fine, branny desquamation. The most common site for this lesion is the shins. There may be thickening and roughening of the skin over the elbows, knees, insteps and other bony prominences (elephant skin). The follicles may be blocked with horny plugs of keratin (follicular keratosis, sometimes called 'toad skin'). In cases of vitamin C deficiency there may be swelling round the margins of the follicular orifices (folliculosis), but without

the projections of horny plugs, producing the appearance of permanent goose flesh. This is sometimes associated with twisted, unerupted hairs. It is around these swollen follicles that the perifollicular haemorrhages, characteristic of the disease, commonly first appear. In protein-calorie malnutrition the hair may be dry, lustreless, depigmented and inflexible (staring hair). Nutritional failure can affect the colour of the skin in many different ways. The dirty brown pigmentation of the skin in chronic subnutrition, as well as the patchy hyperpigmentation and depigmentation often associated with kwashiorkor, is well known. In pellagra there is typically an erythema of exposed surfaces, whilst in anaemia the skin may be unduly pale.

All these changes are familiar to students of nutrition but few with experience would care to state categorically that any one of them results *invariably* from the lack of one particular nutrient. They are merely indications of malnutrition and should draw attention to the patient's diet. In this way they are useful signs; they emphasize again that the aim of medicine is to treat the patient as a whole individual.

Angular Stomatitis, Cheilosis and the Orogenital Syndrome

Angular stomatitis is an infection of the skin at the angles of the mouth, characterized by heaping-up of greyish-white sodden epithelium into ridges, giving the appearance of fissures radiating outwards from the mouth. Secondary infection and staining by food may give the lesion a yellowish colour.

CHEILOSIS. This is the name given to a zone of red, denuded epithelium at the line of closure of the lips. Both lesions are considered to be due to riboflavin deficiency, but vitamin deficiency states are frequently multiple. In Britain the most common cause of angular stomatitis is ill-fitting dentures and failure to wear dentures following total extraction of teeth. In malnourished persons the lesions have been reported to respond rapidly to large doses of riboflavin (10 mg. daily by mouth), but also equally well to pyridoxine.

OROGENITAL SYNDROME. This syndrome has been reported in many parts of the world and is apt to appear wherever diets are seriously deficient in the vitamin B complex. In addition to the genital features there is usually angular stomatitis, cheilosis and glossitis. There may be a scaly, greasy dermatitis around the sides of the nose, on the lips and often behind the ears. The eyelids may be affected and sometimes there is photophobia. The diagnosis may be missed if the genitalia are not examined. The scrotum or labia often shows a dry, itching, erythematous eczema, and this was particularly noticed by prisoners in Japanese camps. Later, secondary infection may produce a wet, weeping sore, extending to the anus and along the inner sides of the thighs. The syndrome presents itself in many forms, and its protean manifestations suggest a multiple deficiency disorder.

Treatment. In addition to riboflavine, 5 mg. three times a day, it is generally agreed that natural preparations of the vitamin B complex such as yeast extract (e.g. Marmite) are beneficial and often curative. A teaspoonful (4 g.) taken four times daily, mixed with the food or spread on bread or biscuits is a suitable dose. Simultaneously a good mixed diet containing meat, eggs, milk, fruit and vegetables must be prescribed.

Tropical Ulcers

These affect chiefly the lower limbs and occur in hot damp climates among people whose tissues are vitiated by malnutrition. They are often induced by minor injuries, but in well-nourished people they rarely if ever occur. They are much less frequently encountered at the present time than formerly. Their presence in any community or labour force is a certain indication that the diet and hygiene conditions are unsatisfactory. The aetiology is still in doubt and it cannot be said that any specific deficiency predisposes to the occurrence of this lesion. The lesion is unlikely to heal satisfactorily unless the patient is given a liberal diet with ample protein. Rest in bed with elevation of the limb is important. Local treatment consists in thorough cleansing of the ulcer with hypertonic magnesium sulphate. Procaine penicillin in oil, containing 2 per cent. aluminium monostearate (300,000 units) intramuscularly, repeated in 48 hours, or oxytetracycline, 2 g. daily for seven days, gives good results. In very chronic cases, after cleansing and treatment with antibiotics, excision of the ulcer and scar tissue may be required, to be followed by skin grafting.

Ambulant treatment, with the ulcerative area supported with strips of adhesive plaster, may be effective when rest cannot be enforced. The dressing is changed at intervals of about five days. Antibiotics should also be given.

Impetigo, Furunculosis

These and other infections of the skin are particularly common among the malnourished and local treatment may be unavailing unless attention is also paid to the diet. Vitamin A in therapeutic doses (see below under Xerophthalmia) is often especially useful in treating such infections among people living on poor diets in hot, dry climates.

The dermatitis of pellagra is mentioned on p. 357.

NUTRITIONAL DISORDERS OF THE EYE

There are probably more than 10 million blind people in the world. Nutritional disorders of the eye are only one of several causes of blindness. The six other main causes are trachoma, smallpox, onchocercosis, venereal disease, accidents in the home or at work and cataract and glaucoma. If one-tenth of the money spent to support unnecessary blindness was devoted to its prevention there would be a tremendous economic gain, not to mention the improvement of the happiness and welfare of tens of thousands of people.

Nutritional Amblyopia (*Retrobulbar Neuropathy*).

This distinct clinical entity was first fully studied by Fitzgerald Moore among West Africans. It became extremely troublesome among prisoners in Japanese hands during the Second World War. Blurred vision, often with photophobia and aching at the back of the eyes, associated with central or paracentral scotomata may result in irreversible optic atrophy if the disease remains untreated for a year or more.

All the patients appear to have one feature in common—a period of many months on diets grossly deficient in respect of many essential nutrients. Lack of one or more components of the vitamin B complex was almost certainly responsible. The disease has been reported in association with beriberi and pellagra, though it often occurs quite independently. Vitamin A, synthetic thiamine and nicotinic acid have all been tried and found to be useless in its treatment. On the other hand, good results have been repeatedly obtained with yeast extract (Marmite). The probability of a toxic factor, such as tobacco, contributing to the disorder should be kept in mind in individual cases.

Night Blindness, Xerophthalmia and Keratomalacia

These disorders are due to a dietary deficiency of vitamin A which arises only when there is an insufficient supply of dairy produce, fish and vegetables.

Night blindness has several causes unconnected with nutrition (e.g. retinitis pigmentosa). It may, however, arise under the same conditions that produce xerophthalmia and often precedes it. Retinol is an essential component of the retinal pigment, visual purple, on which vision in dim light depends. Retinol 25,000 mcg. (75,000 i.u.) for a week by mouth, is generally curative if the cause is nutritional, which in Britain is seldom the case.

Xerophthalmia is very common among rice eating people in Asia and it also occurs in Arabia, Africa and Latin America. The ducts of the tear glands become blocked with keratin and consequently the anterior surface of the eye is dry. The scleral conjunctiva takes on a 'ground glass' appearance and becomes thickened and easily thrown into folds by the gentle pressure of a finger. There may be small clear-white flecks of altered epithelium fixed to the sclerae (Bitôt's spots).

A good diet and attention to any associated infection is essential for the treatment of xerophthalmia. In severe adult cases 25,000 mcg. of retinol (75,000 units) daily, in the form of halibut-liver oil or some equally potent preparation (0·6 ml. of the B.P. concentrated solution of vitamin A contains about 8,000 mcg.) by mouth for one or two weeks is usually sufficient to bring about rapid improvement, while in early mild cases 3,000 to 7,000 mcg. retinol (10,000 to 20,000 i.u.) daily suffices.

Keratomalacia. This is a grave disease which may threaten both sight and life. It occurs most commonly in children raised on grossly deficient diets and is sometimes seen in association with kwashiorkor. It can also occur in adults. Xerophthalmia and frequently night blindness precede it. The cornea becomes opaque, ulcerates and may finally perforate, leading to total blindness. This is probably a multiple deficiency disease. The best empirical treatment is a good diet supplemented by retinol 25,000 mcg. (75,000 i.u.) by mouth daily for a period of several weeks. Riboflavine, 5 mg. three times a day by mouth, should also be given. An antibiotic should be instilled into the eye for the prevention or treatment of secondary infection.

The essential needs for prevention are the education of mothers, better maternal and child health services and an improvement in food production. The prime objective is to make sure that infants and young children obtain adequate amounts of vitamin A in their diet or as a supplement. In countries where vitamin A deficiency is endemic the distribution of a national concentrated source of vitamin A is desirable, especially for children. For this purpose cod-liver, shark-liver or red palm oil can usefully be given according to which is most easily available locally. A satisfactory prophylactic intake of retinol is 300 mcg. (1,000 i.u.) for infants and young children, 500 to 600 mcg. of retinol (1,500 to 2,000 i.u.) for children of 9 to 15 years and 750 mcg. of retinol (2,250 i.u.) for adolescents and adults daily. For lactating women, 1,200 mcg. of retinol daily is advised.

Vascular Cornea

The cornea, which is normally avascular, sometimes becomes invaded by minute capillary vessels, visible with a slit-lamp. This change, generally attended by photophobia and lachrymation, sometimes occurs in association with the oro-genital syndrome (p. 366). At one time is was regarded as a specific sign of riboflavine deficiency. Though it has been reported to respond to riboflavine (e.g. 5 mg. three times a day by mouth) in patients whose diet has been deficient in this vitamin, in other cases this treatment has proved disappointing.

Trachoma

Most sufferers from trachoma are malnourished, but as yet there is no evidence that deficiency of any specific nutrient predisposes to this infection which is now known to be caused by a virus.

DISEASES DUE TO
POISONOUS SUBSTANCES IN FOODS

Food poisoning may be due to natural poisons, to infective agents or to chemical products.

Natural poisons. Before the advent of the synthetic drug industry early in this century, most of the physician's drugs were either simple chemical substances or galenicals derived from plants. Many drugs are toxic if taken in excessive dosage and many common plants contain potentially harmful substances. For instance, rhubarb and spinach contain oxalic acid as oxalates, and one type of cassava plant from which tapioca is prepared contains cyanide. The traditional methods of selecting and preparing such plants for eating usually result in the elimination of the poisonous factor. The fruit of the deadly nightshade, the seeds of the common yellow laburnum and the fruit of the akee tree in Jamaica may all cause serious illnesses, while death can result from eating certain poisonous toadstools and tropical fishes.

Recently a new class of poisons in food has been discovered, namely the anti-vitamins. An example is dicoumarin in spoilt sweet clover which causes a haemorrhagic disease in cattle. When rye was widely cultivated in Europe ergotism was not uncommon; this illness resulted only when the grain was infected by the fungus *Claviceps purpurea*. One species of tare (*Lathyrus sativus*) when eaten in excessive amounts, is responsible for a severe disease of the spinal cord called lathyrism (p. 366).

Infective agents. Food and water can be contaminated by a wide variety of bacteria, viruses, spirochaetes, protozoa and worms. In Great Britain and America by far the most important bacterial agents are salmonella and staphylococci; the latter produces a heat stable exo-toxin in the infected food. Milk, meat and many made-up dishes are the principal examples of foods in which infection occurs in temperate climates. In addition in tropical and subtropical countries infected vegetables, fruit and water commonly give rise to a variety of illnesses due to the ingestion of pathogenic bacteria, spirochaetes, protozoa and worms. Wherever the sanitation is primitive, and particularly in hot climates, it is wise to assume that all food is contaminated unless proved otherwise, and to adopt a few simple rules to avoid possible dangerous consequences.

Choice of food. Select foods of local origin that are produced under the best conditions that circumstances will permit, e.g. vegetables grown in one's own garden are safer than those bought in the bazaar or market.

Storage of food. All food should be stored in the coolest place available, free from flies and vermin. The modern process of refrigeration and the ancient processes of drying, salting and pickling all help to discourage the growth of pathogenic organisms.

Kitchen staff. Those who handle food should be taught rigid rules of personal hygiene and should be under medical supervision to see that they do not suffer from worms, staphylococcal skin infections, open tuberculosis or are carriers of the organism of typhoid fever or other infections.

It is an essential duty of all those responsible for the handling and preparation of food to see that their staff have proper, fly-free lavatories or latrines, and that clean water, soap and towels (preferably disposable paper towels) are provided near by so that hands may be washed routinely after defaecation.

Preparation of food. Water used for cooking, drinking or for washing food should be sterilized by boiling if its purity is in doubt. All foods that are eaten raw, such as fruit and salads, should be carefully washed immediately before consumption.

Chemical products. These have been deliberately used for many years for the prevention of infection and purification, and for the improvement of texture, flavour, appearance and preserving qualities of food. In recent years antibiotics have been used as food preservatives, and ionizing radiation for the sterilization of processed foods. Insecticides, fungicides and weed killers containing arsenic, copper and various organic compounds are used in very large quantities as sprays for crops. Clearly the addition of chemical products to food is a potential menace to future health, the more so because the possible consequences are likely to develop slowly and insidiously.

The addition of chemical agents to food has come to stay, for it is the only solution to some of the problems of feeding the modern city dweller who is now divorced from the land that raised his ancestors. Manufacturers eager to satisfy public demand may add agents to preserve, colour, sweeten, flavour or stabilize foodstuffs. Moreover, pesticides, weed killers and antibiotics are widely used by arable and stock farmers. Many of these substances are a potential hazard to man. Hence the need in every country for a strong body, such as the Committee on Food Additives of the Ministry of Agriculture and Fisheries in Britain and the Food and Drug Administration in the USA, to keep the whole subject under constant review. This has been repeatedly stressed by responsible people in recent years.

Radioactive material in food. Food can become contaminated with radioactive material. This may be brought about by the testing of nuclear weapons and also by accidents at atomic power stations. This is a subject which has generated much emotion, but it has also led to careful and thorough investigation of the resulting hazards.

Radiation hazards. Ionizing radiations may have harmful effects on living tissues and can lead to sterility, malformations, leukaemia and other forms of malignant disease.

Irradiation of foods. This can be done deliberately to sterilize and preserve foodstuffs by destroying bacteria and other micro-organisms. There is no danger to health if this method of preservation is correctly carried out and carefully controlled.

Fall-out consists of radioactive materials which are released as a cloud of dust at a great height consequent on the explosion of nuclear devices. The dust drifts in the stratosphere and the upper atmosphere and then settles slowly and is dispersed widely over the earth's surface.

Vegetables, fruits and cereals can be directly contaminated. A more serious danger to man could arise from drinking milk and eating meat from cattle which have been feeding on contaminated herbage, and have concentrated the radioactivity into their tissues and secretions. The most dangerous elements in the fall-out are strontium-90 (^{90}Sr, half life 28 years), caesium-137 (^{137}Cs, half life 30 years) and iodine-131 (^{131}I, half life 8 days).

Foods which can be packaged and stored can be protected quite easily against fall-out. Complete protection can be achieved by the use of air-tight tin cans or jars, which are preferable to single-layer wrappers of paper, cellophane or polythene which may not be sealed satisfactorily and are not always impervious. If the outside of such containers is known to have been contaminated they should be washed thoroughly with uncontaminated water before opening. Most fruits which have a protective skin, such as oranges or bananas, can be eaten with safety provided they are well washed before peeling.

A close watch is being kept by governments and international agencies on the extent to which food-stuffs are becoming contaminated by fall-out and especially on those grown in the vicinity of atomic plants. In Britain the milk supply is analysed every two weeks for radioactive strontium, iodine and caesium, as well as for stable calcium and potassium.

The medical profession must be on its guard against undue panic on the one hand and undue complacency on the other. There is little that the doctor can do as an individual to prevent the poisoning of food with radioactive material except to express publicly such indignation and distress as he may feel.

NUTRITIONAL DISORDERS IN WESTERN MEDICAL PRACTICE

The disorders mentioned above that are relieved (though rarely completely cured) by pure synthetic vitamins occur chiefly among people living on grossly deficient diets consisting of little else but cereals. Consequently, they are rarely seen nowadays in Britain except when conditioned by some other disease. Examples of such conditioned disorders are: rickets resulting from steatorrhoea, polyneuropathy following chronic pyloric obstruction and manifold nutritional disorders attending chronic alcoholism. People who habitually rely upon alcohol to provide the chief portion of their daily calories lack other nutrients; they may develop scurvy, pellagra, beriberi or polyneuropathy, depending on their habits and, perhaps, constitution.

In all such cases of conditioned nutritional disorders, treatment should first be directed to removing the underlying cause; thereafter it should proceed along the lines indicated for the relief of the same disorders arising primarily from faulty diet.

'Sub-clinical' nutritional disorders. Ever since the first introduction of synthetic vitamins, a great deal of propaganda has been pressed on the medical profession to encourage the belief that any patient who is tired or 'out of sorts' may be suffering from a mild vitamin deficiency. In fact, serious vitamin deficiency disorders are extremely rare in Britain and, by inference, minor deficiencies must be uncommon; whoever heard of an endemic disease that manifests itself solely as *formes frustes*? Analysis of the diets of the people in Britain usually shows that they provide a fair supply of the essential vitamins, with the possible exception that some individuals do not obtain enough fresh fruit and vegetables during the long winter, and so may run short of ascorbic acid in the spring.

The indiscriminate prescribing of synthetic vitamins as general, non-specific tonics is poor and slipshod practice. Pills and capsules containing various mixtures of pure synthetic vitamins are no substitute for food. The shot-gun prescription of such preparations is deplorable; for one thing it is unnecessarily expensive; further, it lulls the physician into a complacent sense of having done all that is necessary to safeguard his patient's nutrition.

The proper treatment of subnutrition and malnutrition continues to rest on attention to the patient's diet. When the diet has been deficient in some important respect, the first line of treatment is to supply the food that is lacking. Thereafter, special shortages may be replaced by the following: proteins, by dried milk or milk products; fat-soluble vitamins, by fish-liver oils; ascorbic acid, by orange juice, black-currant or rose-hip syrup; the vitamin B complex, by yeast or yeast extract (e.g. Marmite), liver, rice polishings or wheat germ. The synthetic vitamins are of real value for the imme- diate relief of the classic nutritional diseases— pellagra, beriberi, rickets and scurvy.

Reference

DAVIDSON, Sir STANLEY & PASSMORE, R. (1969). *Human Nutrition and Dietetics*. 4th ed. Edinburgh: Livingstone.

15. Diseases of the Nervous System

J. A. SIMPSON

In the treatment of patients suffering from diseases of the nervous system, the general principles are identical with those which apply to other systems of the body. For example, by means of drug therapy it is possible to influence disturbances of function; but drugs cannot confer new functions upon tissues, nor can they restore activity to structures which have perished as a result of disease. In general, physicians are disposed to be pessimistic about the results of therapy in neurological disorders, but it should not be forgotten that many of the infections that involve the nervous system are now amenable to chemotherapy; and the surgical treatment of compressive lesions of the nervous system is often highly successful. Again, though the degenerative diseases of the nervous system are usually incurable they are often compatible with long life.

Some of the body tissues—notably the liver and the endocrine glands—are endowed with the capacity to undergo cellular proliferation. Thus compensation may be achieved for loss of functioning tissue by the recurring assaults of disease, and the patient may be pronounced 'cured'. Unfortunately this phenomenon does not occur in the nervous system; here there is no regeneration of new nerve cells to compensate for loss of tissue by degeneration or other pathological change. At the same time a remarkable plasticity of function is exhibited. This is highly important because it enables patients to utilize a reserve of function and to *reduce the degree of disability*, notwithstanding that the underlying disease is incurable. Physiotherapy, occupational therapy and speech therapy all play an important rôle in exploiting residual capacity in order to minimize disability. The outcome is undoubtedly affected by the skill and resourcefulness of the therapist and by the rapport established between the therapist and her patient. It is also important to recognize the limitations of such therapy in cases where there has been extensive damage to the brain and spinal cord. The physical forms of treatment are necessarily prescribed on the basis that certain functions have been lost. The indications for physiotherapy in its various forms are determined not by the nature of the underlying disease (for example, poliomyelitis, syringomyelia, etc.) but solely by defining the patient's loss of function and the procedures necessary to help him to overcome his disability. The general principles of management of patients with disabilities due to neurological lesions are discussed in the following pages.

PARALYSIS

A patient may lose the ability to contract a muscle (or a group of muscles) because of disease of the muscle itself or because of involvement of its nervous control. Failure of transmission at the neuromuscular junction creates special problems, and these will receive attention in a later section.

Lower Motor Neurone Paralysis

The paralysis due to disorder of lower motor neurones results in an inability to use the affected muscle as a prime mover or as a synergist in active or postural contraction. Characteristically the muscle undergoes rapid wasting; and because of lack of reflex innervation it is also flaccid. It is, therefore, highly vulnerable to stretching by more powerful muscles or even by the effect of gravity; it follows that the first aim in management should be the prevention of overstretching. If the patient is confined to bed this is best achieved for the lower limb by the use of sand-bags or pillows suitably arranged. The weight of the bedclothes should be supported by a cradle. Weak muscles of the upper limbs may be protected by splinting with the wrist dorsiflexed 20°, the fingers slightly flexed and the thumb flexed and opposed (the position for holding a tumbler).

Splints and calipers. The type of splint used depends on the nature and degree of the paralysis. In acute lesions such as poliomyelitis and peripheral neuropathy the immobilization need only be maintained during sleeping hours. At other times the splints should be removed for passive movement of joints and to exercise any surviving muscles. A very satisfactory compromise is a splint of 'lively' type in which the desired position is maintained by springs which are just powerful enough to control the position at rest and yet can be extended by the contraction of the weak muscles, thus providing exercise against resistance. This form of splinting is particularly valuable in acute lesions of peripheral nerves. When recovery is improbable (as in the later stage of poliomyelitis) or when the affected muscle is too weak to act against springs, the opposite principle may be adopted of providing a mobile splint in which the action of the paralysed muscle is assisted by means of springs, or in which stops are so placed as to prevent stretching the muscle beyond its natural limits. Examples of this principle are walking calipers with toe-raising springs or drop-foot stops.

Physiotherapy. As soon as possible (pain may prevent it in poliomyelitis) the weak muscles should be exercised. This is best supervised by a physiotherapist so that overstretching of the paralysed muscle may be prevented. In order to determine the appropriate exercises some knowledge of anatomy is necessary. For instance, the traditional hand exercise of squeezing a ball is futile if only the interosseous muscles of the hand are paralysed. Careful functional analysis is followed by suitable exercises against resistance, and this is increased gradually as recovery takes place. Resistance may be provided by springs or pulley-cords supporting weights. Either of these may be attached to specially designed machines in an occupational therapy department.

At this stage further treatment depends on the nature of the lesion. If recovery is possible (as in disease of peripheral nerves or nerve roots), it is desirable to prevent the patient from adopting 'trick' movements to achieve his object, since these may prejudice recovery of normal function after re-innervation has occurred. If recovery is improbable as in late poliomyelitis, or the disease is progressive as in motor neurone disease, alternative methods should be encouraged. The circumstances often provide a challenge for patient, doctor and therapist. For instance, a patient who cannot step on to the pavement because of weakness of hip flexion may be able to step on backwards.

Orthopaedic operations. The logical extension of this principle is the use of muscle transplants and prostheses. A strong muscle may be transplanted by an orthopaedic surgeon to a position where its contraction will reinstate the impaired function. Orthopaedic surgery of this type and stabilization of joints by arthrodesis have been widely used in the rehabilitation of patients with poliomyelitis or peripheral nerve injuries. They should also be considered in other chronic paralyses of lower motor neurone type. Prosthetic devices to increase the range of movements possible to weak muscles are being developed. Their use is at present limited by cost, and by the necessity for individual design and fitting.

Upper Motor Neurone Paralysis

The voluntary control of movement requires the normal functioning of the motor areas of the cerebral cortex and their projection systems, the corticospinal (pyramidal) tracts. Damage to these upper motor neurones causes complete or partial loss of certain movements, but the affected muscles are still capable of other movements, voluntary or involuntary. As some corticospinal fibres are inhibitory to the reflexes which maintain muscle tone, damage to these fibres leads to spasticity and this can prevent the full utilization of surviving movements. In addition, the uninhibited withdrawal reflexes of the lower limbs result in painful spasms. If these contractions are not prevented, deformities may develop and may become permanent because of contracture of muscles and tendons. Treatment of paralysis of upper motor neurone type has five aims: (i) to increase the power of affected muscles; (ii) to use remaining movements for the requirements of daily life; (iii) to reduce hypertonicity; (iv) to limit or abolish flexor spasms of the lower limbs; and (v) to prevent contractures of muscle and secondary disorders of joints. The order of priority depends on the type of disease.

Where there is a slow development of upper motor neurone damage (whether due to disease of the brain or the spinal cord) the main disability at first is loss of power and, progressively, loss of the ability to perform certain movements—notably the finer skilled movements of the fingers and the apparatus of speech. Treatment should aim at increasing the power of the affected muscles and promoting their skilled use. If this is not possible other muscles should be recruited to achieve the same functional end.

Physiotherapy. Provided some power remains, it is always possible to increase it by active exercise. When the affected limb can be moved against gravity, the work to be done should be increased progressively. The physiotherapist uses weights or springs suitably positioned to be moved by the muscles under treatment. By appropriate grading, the work done by the muscle is increased progressively. With a little consideration of the anatomical position and the action of the paretic muscles, a practitioner can easily improvise similar graded exercises which the patient can perform at home.

Where some voluntary movements are absent, the affected muscles may be exercised by taking advantage of the fact that they may contract synergically in other movements (in this respect paralysis of upper motor neurone type differs from the lower motor neurone type). For instance, a hemiplegic patient may be unable to dorsiflex his ankle voluntarily and hence he tends to walk with circumducting gait, but if he flexes his thigh against resistance or lifts his knee as high as possible when walking, the ankle will dorsiflex as part of the movement pattern. This reflex facilitation of movements which are not under voluntary control is a procedure that is widely used by trained physiotherapists. It is a valuable means of increasing the power of paralysed muscles, but it has yet to be proved that it enables the patient to perform movements which cannot be evoked by voluntary command.

The ability to make muscles contract with adequate power is the basic essential, but recovery is less than satisfactory if the patient cannot perform *useful* movements. If his lower limbs are strong enough for him to stand, it is also possible for him to walk. Even if he cannot flex his hip and knee joints, he can be taught to walk 'from the waist' if his legs are stabilized by muscular spasm or by the use of calipers. With upper motor neurone lesions affecting the upper limbs, movements of the shoulder and upper arm are less seriously affected. The patient may be able to open and close the hand with a reasonably strong 'power grip' but discrete movements of the fingers and the prehensile 'precision grip' are severely disturbed. These are the movements required for developing skills such as writing, shaving, and using cutlery or tools. Without these movements the hand is little better than a prop.

Occupational therapy. When the physiotherapist has developed as much power as possible in the muscles of the hand by exercising the fingers, using a rubber ball, a spring grip-developer or, best of all, silicone putty, the occupational therapist retrains the patient in the performance of accurate movements. She may have assisted in the previous stage of graduated exercise by the use of treadle-driven apparatus to exercise the legs, specially designed looms for shoulder and upper arm movements, and simple crafts or games for the hands—the apparatus being loaded to provide resistance in a manner acceptable to the patient. Now the emphasis is changed to craft work requiring specific precision movements such as basket-making and leather work or, when possible, a modified version of the patient's own work.

At this stage it is usually obvious if full recovery cannot be expected or if the disability is progressive. The practitioner must recognize the situation and take advantage of the remaining functional capacity in order to teach the patient how to adapt himself to his new circumstances. There is no veto on 'trick' movements; where recovery of neurones is impossible, the end justifies the means. The occupational therapist is specially trained to assess the patient's ability to perform the acts of normal daily living (dressing, feeding, toilet, housekeeping, etc.) and to train the patient in alternative methods of performing them, with or without the provision of special gadgets. The occupational therapist can also advise how to modify the patient's environment so that he may resume independent living. The alterations in the bedroom, bathroom or kitchen, or to the doors and steps are usually simple and inexpensive. It may seem unnecessary to delegate them to a therapist, but experience shows that they are often ignored if the patient does not have this assistance. It should be noted that the Local Authority has statutory powers to undertake appropriate alterations in a patient's home when requested to do so.

Spasticity

Hypertonicity in spastic paralysis is caused by increased activity of postural and protective (withdrawal) reflexes. It is desirable to distinguish between these two mechanisms since hypertonicity due to overactivity of postural (mainly stretch) reflexes is not necessarily harmful. Though it may hamper voluntary movement, it may be beneficial by providing a firm basis of postural tone in the lower limbs.

Dominance of postural tone is promoted by encouraging the standing posture or, if this is impossible, by nursing in the prone position. Regular passive stretching of spastic muscles is helpful and may be easier if the limb is first cooled by ice packs.

Increased activity of protective reflexes in the lower limbs results in flexor spasms which may be painful and serve no useful purpose in the conscious subject. It is the latter type of spasticity which constitutes the main indication for treatment though reduction of postural tone may also release an unsuspected reserve of voluntary movement.

Spasmolytic drugs. These are disappointing in clinical practice. Given by slow intravenous injection, mephenesin, 30 mg. per kg., produces considerable relaxation of muscle tone which may be valuable in permitting passive stretching of the muscles by a physiotherapist. Diazepam (up to 30 mg. a day in divided doses) or chlordiazepoxide (up to 100 mg. a day in divided doses, but usually 15 mg. four times a day) taken by mouth reduce hypertonicity in some patients but the lyssive action is slight and its continued administration is not justified if no significant relaxation has occurred after three weeks. Unfortunately the same reservation applies to mephenesin, tigloidine, orphenadrine, carisoprodol and chlorpromazine. The occasional favourable result may be associated with the mild psychotropic effects of these drugs.

Intrathecal phenol. A more effective method of reducing muscle tone may be used to prevent flexor spasms when these are painful or prejudicing the nursing of a bed-ridden paraplegic patient. Briefly, it consists of the intrathecal injection of a corrosive substance at suitable levels to disrupt the appropriate reflex arcs. Solutions of phenol in 5 per cent. strength in anhydrous glycerol or myodil may be used.

Surgical methods. In some circumstances the operation of anterior rhizotomy may be preferable if extensive destruction of anterior roots is required with sparing of bladder function. The surgeon may also assist by carrying out muscle-sliding operations to reduce the mechanical efficiency of spastic muscles; and arthrodesis of the knees may be performed to stabilize the lower limbs.

DISORDERS OF SPEECH

About 1 per cent. of schoolchildren stutter and a further 3 to 5 per cent. have other defects in speech. Subjected to mimicry from schoolmates and unfeeling relatives, the sufferer may become a creature of retarded progress and warped personality. Adults may be victims of speech defect continued from their youth or acquired in maturity. Their lot is scarcely less difficult; they are hampered in all self-expression by word of mouth.

Too often in the past the sufferer has been exploited by quacks. Today, however, the speech therapist is an officially recognized medical auxiliary; her special training in normal and disordered speech, in the relevant anatomy and physiology, and in psychology and educational method are all conducive to efficient handling of the problem. Speech therapy clinics have now been established at many hospitals and where necessary treatment is available as part of the school health service.

The selection of patients for training by the speech therapist depends on the cause of the defect and the outlook for the individual. Cases of dysarthria from bulbar paralysis and also dysphasia from progressive disease of the brain must be excluded. On the other hand, sufferers from cleft palate, stuttering or impediment from cramping of the muscles of articulation, dysphasia following head injury or from static lesions of the brain are all candidates for treatment. Speech therapy should be complementary to the medical or surgical alleviation of the causative disease. The practitioner who refers a patient to the speech therapist should send an adequate case history. This enables the therapist to co-operate constructively in the interests of the patient and also to supply helpful reports from time to time.

The methods used by the therapist vary with the cause of the defect. In deformity of the upper respiratory tract, treatment is directed towards producing the best articulate sound consistent with the deformity by exercises in the use of a limited speech equipment.

The spasms and tics of stuttering demand exercises in progressive relaxation of the whole voluntary musculature. These exercises combat spasm in the muscles of articulation and rid the patient of that general muscular tension which is the result of emotional strain. When complete muscular relaxation has been achieved, for some unknown reason, there is a corresponding reduction in psychological tension and the mind responds more readily to suggestion and instruction. Because the dysphasic patient is made worse by emotional stress, relaxation therapy becomes an important means of helping him.

Language difficulties caused by lesions of the dominant hemisphere make greater demands on the skill and experience of the therapist. She has to use educational technique to facilitate activity over such associative pathways as remain intact. The patient is made to associate various sensory experiences of one object with another and with the appropriate word symbol. Patients who have seriously limited intellectual powers present a major

N

challenge to the therapist for they are virtually obliged to learn to speak *ab initio*.

Writer's Cramp

In the past, insufficient emphasis has been laid on the fact that stuttering and writer's cramp belong to the same group of disabilities. Writing and speaking are motor forms of expression in language. Writer's cramp and stuttering are muscular spasms which interrupt the normal flow of writing and speaking and may postpone or prevent the initiation of these acts. Exactly the same kind of treatment is required in both—clearing the distorted emotional background, correcting posture and bad patterns of motor activity, and exercises in progressive muscular relaxation. The speech therapist's training is admirably suited to providing these requirements and she should be encouraged to accept the responsibility of dealing with the condition.

EXTRAPYRAMIDAL DISORDERS

Diseases of different parts of the basal ganglia interfere with the ability to initiate voluntary movement but do not cause paralysis in the usual sense; power is substantially normal. Muscle tone may be increased as in Parkinsonism, decreased as in chorea, or vary from one to the other as in dystonia and athetosis. More or less abrupt changes in the distribution of postural tone between antagonistic groups of muscles cause spontaneous movements of various types—tremor, chorea, or athetosis. All these disorders of function depend on the site rather than on the nature of the lesion. Thus Parkinsonism and chorea are not disease entities but clinical syndromes. The primary cause may be treated in rheumatic chorea and in Wilson's disease (p. 406), but the management is otherwise symptomatic and unrelated to the aetiology.

Parkinsonism

The syndrome is common to paralysis agitans, arteriosclerosis of the basal ganglia, and to the later effect of virus encephalitis as well as to other rarer pathological processes. It is characterized by widespread rigidity of skeletal muscle, difficulty in initiating voluntary movements and rhythmical tremor which is most obvious at rest. Tremor is more prominent in paralysis agitans, and rigidity in the post-encephalitic and arteriosclerotic types. The post-encephalitic type may show in addition intellectual and personality deterioration; inver-

sion of the sleep rhythm is characteristic of the early acute stage. Post-encephalitic patients also suffer from various kinds of *crisis*—oculogyric, sweating, respiratory, etc.—and in some cases visceral disturbances such as severe constipation are found. These episodic crises are unusual in the other types though mild dementia or focal neurological signs other than extrapyramidal may be found in arteriosclerotic Parkinsonism. Dribbling of saliva, especially during sleep, occurs in all types because of the sluggish swallowing reflex and true hypersalivation may be caused by encephalitis.

Of the three cardinal symptoms, rigidity can be improved by antispasmodic drugs and tremor by sedatives, but the difficulty in initiating voluntary movements remains a serious handicap. It may be alleviated by L-dopa (see below). Nevertheless, the reduction of rigidity may restore a large measure of voluntary function though it may unfortunately allow the involuntary movement to increase and thus the improvement that might be expected from spasmolytic drugs is limited. Emotional disturbance, including natural apprehension and anxiety, increases the tremor; when associated mental changes occur, diminished awareness may lessen emotional and muscular tension. Sedation may be helpful but should be used with caution, as barbiturates and the phenothiazine tranquillizing drugs may exacerbate the Parkinsonian syndrome. The sedative action of diphenhydramine, used primarily to diminish rigidity, may be of incidental value.

Post-encephalitic patients differ in other ways. They may be remarkably tolerant to cold which increases the rigidity of the patient with paralysis agitans. By avoiding worry and embarrassment and by altering the routine of daily life in many small ways the individual patient may be helped. The replacement of trouser buttons by a zip-fastener, the discarding of loose mats and carpets from the home, the provision of toilet paper in cut sheet packs instead of in a roll may enable the afflicted patient to continue in his normal environment.

Although drugs which relax muscle are the most useful form of therapy, activity designed to widen the range of joint movement is to be encouraged, mainly by direction of the daily routine of life and occasionally by physiotherapy. In severe cases precautions must be taken to safeguard the patient when he walks, for rigidity of muscles so interferes with the execution of body reflexes that he may trip over the edge of a carpet and fall headlong. The grossly disabled person may have to be turned in bed and helped out of a chair. A special chair with a spring-locked seat to assist rising is available.

Special treatment may be required for dysarthria (p. 376).

Drugs. In many cases, regardless of aetiology, the rigidity and disorder of voluntary movement of Parkinsonism are alleviated by L-dopa (L-3, 4-Dihydroxyphenylalanine) given by mouth (3 to 8 g. daily). Side-effects sometimes noted are nausea, vomiting, postural hypotension, cardiac arrhythmia, psychic disturbances and choreiform or athetotic movements, but the frequency of side-effects is low. Other drugs used to relieve rigidity of voluntary muscle fall into two categories: (1) the atropine group—including preparations of belladonna, stramonium, hyoscine and atropine itself; and (2) synthetic preparations which have some of the virtues of drugs in the atropine group, but also possess mild antihistamine effects. Drugs of the atropine group are undoubtedly valuable if they are ordered in gradually increasing doses until substantial amounts are being given daily. A convenient official preparation is the dry extract of stramonium, prescribed as a tablet. Its effectiveness is due to the hyoscyamine and atropine which it contains. The initial dose of 60 mg. thrice daily should be gradually increased at intervals of a few days up to the patient's limit of tolerance, which is often eight times the initial dose. Sialorrhoea is also alleviated and any resulting dryness of the mouth is usually accepted by the patient. Paralysis of ocular accommodation is more disturbing, but can be alleviated by instilling once daily into the conjunctival sacs 0·5 per cent. physostigmine salicylate eye-drops (B.P.C.). The dosage of stramonium need not be reduced unless more serious side-effects such as agitation, confusion, and vomiting occur. Side-effects are less prominent with therapeutic doses of one of the synthetic drugs, such as benzhexol. In addition these drugs often have the additional advantage of creating a sense of well-being; they may reduce tremor, but this action is less constant and conspicuous, and indeed tremor may become greater as rigidity is reduced.

The patient's assessment of the value of a drug is largely but not entirely subjective—he bases his conclusions on the relief of general disability, increased agility of movement, greater exercise tolerance, improvement in mood, and control of salivary secretion. As response to treatment is so individual a matter, a variety of drugs either alone or in combination should be tried for an adequate period in an amount just short of the toxic level. There is a tendency for each drug to lose its effect in time, but further response can often be obtained by changing to another in the group listed below. When it in turn becomes ineffective the original drug may be found to be potent once more. Sometimes a combination is most effective such as one from the atropine group with one from the synthetic spasmolytic series. No sudden intermission of therapy or rapid change from one drug to another should be permitted; abrupt cessation of all treatment may be fatal.

Of the synthetic compounds used in the long-term treatment of Parkinsonism, benzhexol hydrochloride and orphenadrine hydrochloride are particularly notable because they often give considerable relief from muscular rigidity and also create a sense of well-being; they may reduce tremor to a limited extent. Benzhexol hydrochloride is available in tablets containing 2 mg. or 5 mg. At the start of treatment one tablet may be given thrice daily after meals, but the dose should be increased at intervals of about three days until the patient is receiving 16 to 20 mg. daily according to his response and tolerance. Orphenadrine is started in doses of 50 mg. (one tablet) thrice daily, and the dose is increased as already described. Its euphoriant and antihistaminic actions are greater than those of benzhexol which has atropine-like effects on sialorrhoea and visual accommodation. Alternative preparations are ethopropazine hydrochloride, procyclidine hydrochloride, benztropine methane-sulphonate and methixene hydrochloride, each of which may have its own merits in the individual case. All drugs with atropine-like actions should be avoided if the patient also has glaucoma. Antihistamine drugs such as diphenhydramine and promethazine have a place when sedation is desired though they are less powerful spasmolytics.

Regular medication with one of these drugs may in some measure prevent crises (oculogyric, sweating, psychological). These rarely occur except in the post-encephalitic type of Parkinsonism and may be further limited by adding dexamphetamine, 5 to 10 mg. once or twice daily, to the antispasmodic treatment. Large dosage of amphetamine, especially if combined with a drug which restricts sweating, may cause heat stroke in hot climates.

General management. The management of Parkinsonism varies with the type and is largely influenced by the mental state. Depression is common and its relief (p. 425) may release unexpected powers of movement. The sufferer is usually able to continue at work unless this involves manual activity beyond his skill. The arteriosclerotic subject with mild dementia should consider retiral and the enjoyment of a restricted life at home. The unfortunate sufferer from post-encephalitic Parkinsonism with intellectual or personality disturbances may require institutional care.

Activity short of undue fatigue should be encouraged. General supervision by a physiotherapist raises the patient's morale; this is particularly important when advancing disability results in segregation and loneliness. Diversional therapy is also often a boon for, despite their laborious movements, many post-encephalitics retain remarkable competence in games of skill such as billiards.

In the later stages of the disease when post-encephalitics become seriously disabled, bedridden and perhaps show signs of mental deterioration, nursing becomes particularly exacting. Frequent change of posture is necessary to prevent severe discomfort and pressure sores in the immobile; occasional gross deformities of the hands and feet make it difficult to avoid ulceration of the skin and the attendant infection but the use of lamb's wool between the fingers and in the palms keeps the skin dry and prevents maceration of the epidermis. Progressive constipation and abdominal distension (often with spurious diarrhoea) necessitate the giving of preventive enemata. Help is often needed with feeding.

Stereotaxic surgery. None with any experience of extrapyramidal disorders will deny the dramatic benefit to be gained from the neurosurgeon's attack on the disease. In skilled hands the operation of pallidotomy or thalamotomy is so successful as to merit its consideration in terms of precedence. What then are the criteria and contraindications? Whenever the disability is severe enough to interfere with work—and capacity for work cannot be restored by L-dopa or antispasmodic drugs—the operation should be contemplated. The disability must be severe enough to ensure that relief by surgical means is eminently worth while. Nothing is gained by operating on patients whose lives are reasonably normal under the influence of drugs. Vascular disease and degenerative change are contraindications. Surgeons prefer the patient who

is under 50, but will not hesitate to operate on a 'young' 60-year-old. Operation must not be undertaken in ignorance of the risks such as hemiplegia and aphasia and the patient should be told of the chances of such complications. Surgery, however, is never the first approach to treatment: part of the justification for operation lies in recognizing the limitations of drug therapy in the individual patient; but it is nearly always desirable to continue the use of drugs after operation—usually in small doses.

Chorea, Hemiballismus, Athetosis, Dystonia

None of the drugs at present available has much effect on any kind of involuntary movement. Although sedatives are not selective, given in substantial doses they may reduce activity. Formerly chloral hydrate or phenobarbitone were the drugs of choice for chorea, but nowadays one of the phenothiazine group of drugs is usually preferred; in *Huntington's chorea* the drug of this type commonly used is thiopropazate, 10 mg. three times a day. Neither sedative nor spasmolytic drugs have any obvious effect in patients suffering from athetosis or dystonia; in such cases relief is often achieved by pallidotomy or thalamotomy. These operations are rarely indicated for chorea; an exception is the type called hemiballismus, in which the continuous and violent involuntary movements result in profound exhaustion, carrying a threat to life.

Myoclonus

Myoclonus occurring as a manifestation of epilepsy is treated with anticonvulsant drugs (p. 381). Similar myoclonic jerks may be caused by disease of the cerebellum or upper brain stem and occasionally of the spinal cord. Mephenesin carbamate, 500 mg. to 1·0 g., or diazepam, 5 to 20 mg., may be effective in suppressing them.

ATAXIA

Incoordination of movement may result from lesions in many parts of the nervous system, but the principal types of ataxia are cerebellar and sensory.

Cerebellar ataxia. This is characterized by tremor of voluntary movement, staggering gait and faulty balance which are not materially improved by the use of vision. It occurs in patients with multiple sclerosis, cerebellar tumour or abscess, and in Friedreich's ataxia and other hereditary types of ataxia. Where there is progressive loss of cerebellar connections as in the hereditary ataxias and delayed cerebellar atrophy associated with carcinomatosis, the prognosis is poor and treatment of little value. There may, however, be surprising recovery of co-ordination after removal of a cerebellar tumour or abscess. In multiple sclerosis the position is intermediate. Physiotherapy may be very valuable until progression of the lesion makes functional compensation impossible.

The ataxic patient should be taught exercises designed to encourage accurate positioning of the hands and feet. With constant practice the defect may be minimized. If the patient is confined to bed the compensation rapidly breaks down and gait deteriorates. This is a much more severe handicap than most motor disorders. The use of a stick or crutch to aid walking may be impossible if the upper limbs are ataxic. It may be necessary to prescribe a walking-frame or, at worst, a wheel chair.

Sensory ataxia. This is a failure of co-ordination due to interruption of proprioceptive information from the muscles and joints to the central nervous system, caused by lesions of peripheral nerves, dorsal nerve roots, dorsal columns of the spinal cord or a parietal lobe of the brain. It occurs in peripheral neuropathy, tabes dorsalis, subacute combined degeneration of the cord and in parietal lobe lesions. Sensory ataxia differs from the cerebellar type in that the visual sense can largely replace the proprioceptive so that ataxia is minimal when the eyes are open but severe when they are closed.

Treatment is along the same lines as for cerebellar ataxia but the patient is trained to use vision to assist placement of hands and feet. Recovery is possible if the sensory fibres are damaged peripherally but unlikely with lesions central to the dorsal root ganglia.

DEAFNESS

It is essential to establish the cause of deafness. Conductive deafness, due to obstruction of the external auditory meatus or derangement of the middle ear requires appropriate treatment. Wax or a foreign body in the meatus are removed by careful syringing with warm (37° C.) water, or wax may first be softened with liquid paraffin or paradichlorobenzene instilled twice daily for 2 to 3 days. Children sometimes push seeds and dried peas into the auditory canal. These should not be moistened with water because they may swell and

become firmly impacted. Acute otitis media is treated by antibiotics. Most of the causative organisms are penicillin sensitive. Immediate injection of 0·1 to 0·5 mega-unit of benzylpenicillin, according to age, should be followed by four-hourly administration of 250 mg. of phenoxymethylpenicillin by mouth for at least seven days. Analgesics and sedatives are usually called for during the first 1 to 2 days. If full hearing is not restored, or aural discharge persists after a week, the patient should be referred to a specialist for otological investigation. This course is also advised for chronic otitis media and other chronic types of conductive deafness. There may be underlying structural disease such as cholesteatosis, or otosclerosis, requiring surgical treatment. Posterior or attic infections of the middle ear and chronic mastoiditis may lead to lateral sinus thrombosis, labyrinthitis or meningitis (p. 44). Perceptive ('nerve') deafness, due to lesions of the inner ear, the cochlear division of the 8th nerve, or certain brainstem lesions, is not directly amenable to treatment.

Hearing aids. These are valuable in bilateral deafness of conductive type or incomplete perceptive deafness, but will not restore perfect hearing. Skilled prescription is essential to match the amplification characteristics to the audiogram of the patient. The Medresco aids are efficient instruments. Smaller proprietary aids may be equally effective, but the reduction in size involves some reduction in amplification. Whatever type is used the patient must be prepared to persevere with its use to obtain maximum benefit. Some auditory rehabilitation is necessary. A person with normal hearing habitually concentrates his attention on speech or other sounds of interest, and disregards irrelevant sound. The amplifier of an aid is not discriminative in this sense, and the patient has to relearn this faculty. In older people the old-fashioned speaking-tube may prove more effective and less confusing to the patient. The deaf should be encouraged to learn lip reading. Severely deaf children should have the benefit of training by a qualified teacher of the deaf.

Tinnitus. Tinnitus is a sensation of noise caused by abnormal excitation of the acoustic apparatus or of its afferent paths or cortical areas. It is frequently associated with deafness and sometimes with vertigo. Any primarily otological disorder should receive appropriate treatment. There is no specific treatment for tinnitus due to organic disease of the nervous system, but phenobarbitone makes the symptoms tolerable. However, this type of tinnitus is rare. It is more often a manifestation of depression, particularly in elderly people, and this type responds well to treatment of the depression (p. 429).

EPILEPSY

There are many causes of epilepsy, and it would be more correct to refer to 'the epilepsies'. The origin of the neuronal discharge and its mode of propagation within the brain determine the nature of the epileptic fit. Thus the different types of seizure—grand mal, petit mal, psychomotor epilepsy, etc.—are simply indications of the neuronal systems involved. A seizure is a physical sign. It is no more a diagnosis than is hemiplegia; its significance depends on the underlying cause, and only when this is known can a diagnosis be made. Thus, it is not sufficient to diagnose 'grand mal epilepsy' without further specifying the cause. This may be genetic (or idiopathic) or the result of a structural or biochemical lesion of the brain (and hence symptomatic). The first step in the treatment of a patient who has recently had a seizure is to search for the cause and remove it if this is practicable. The treatment of cerebral tumour, abscess or vascular disease, hypoglycaemia, etc., is discussed in the appropriate sections. The further symptomatic treatment for prevention of recurrent seizures is common to idiopathic and symptomatic forms of epilepsy; it depends only on the site of origin and hence on the clinical pattern of the fit.

With the exception of true petit mal, fits of all types may be treated with the same range of anticonvulsant drugs. The different therapy for petit mal makes it essential to distinguish, clinically or by electroencephalography, between true petit mal and other minor types of epilepsy which may resemble it. The practitioner should make it a rule not to diagnose petit mal if attacks start in adult life, for it invariably starts in childhood, though it may continue into adult life. Minor fits starting after adolescence are more likely to be one of the other forms of minor epilepsy for which the appropriate treatment is to use one of the anticonvulsant drugs.

Petit Mal

In the majority of cases—where the spells start earlier than 7 years of age—an initial trial may be made of belladonna in conjunction with phenobarbitone. A suitable preparation is the B.P.C. tablet which contains 50 mg. phenobarbitone and 25 mg. of the dry extract of belladonna. An initial dose of one tablet twice daily may be increased to four tablets daily. If this fails the drug of choice is ethosuximide in doses of 250 mg. four to six times daily. Some children are unable to tolerate it because of nausea, hiccup or vomiting, but it is relatively free of serious side-effects. Also valuable but more toxic is troxidone, 300 mg. three to six times daily. The patient taking troxidone sometimes notices that light seems unpleasantly bright, but this effect is not intolerable and it has no sinister significance. If necessary tinted spectacles can be worn. More serious toxic effects, which are fortunately comparatively uncommon, are agranulocytosis, nephrosis and exfoliative dermatitis. An effective drug which is unfortunately too toxic for general use is phenylacetylurea. It causes toxic hepatitis too frequently to justify its use except in the case of the child with so many attacks of petit mal that normal life is virtually impossible (200 to 300 attacks per day). A less toxic drug which is sometimes effective when others have failed is mepacrine. Given in a dose of 50 mg. twice daily this (and other antimalarial drugs) may be surprisingly effective, but after a few months of use the turns often recur. Amphetamine (2·5 to 5 mg. twice a day) or acetazolamide (250 mg. three times a day) are sometimes useful adjuvants in the treatment of petit mal but rarely effective as the sole treatment.

Some general principles of dosage with ethosuximide and troxidone should be followed. If there is good evidence that the daily number of attacks has been reduced though not eliminated when dosage of the selected drug has been raised to the maximum indicated above, the dose may be further cautiously increased by one or two capsules or tablets daily. Medication for petit mal should be continued for two to three months after attacks have ceased. When it is withdrawn it is rare for this type of epilepsy to recur. If, on the other hand, the recommended maximum dose has caused no appreciable reduction in the number of attacks it is unlikely that a higher dosage will be effective. The question obviously arises whether it is desirable to continue the use of a drug which may prove toxic. There is no evidence that withdrawal of treatment affects the prognosis. Ethosuximide and troxidone may potentiate any tendency a patient may have to develop major seizures. If a child under treatment for petit mal has a grand mal seizure, it is advisable to give phenobarbitone in addition. Many physicians consider that it should always be given.

Grand Mal

As with petit mal, the plan of drug therapy involves a compromise: the dose must be high enough to suppress the fits but it must also fall short of the toxic dose. Probably all fits could be prevented by giving a sufficiently large dose of modern anticonvulsants, but the acceptable dose is determined by the onset of side-effects—especially drowsiness and ataxia. The converse of this—that all hypnotics are anticonvulsants—is not true. Only *barbiturates* with a phenyl group in the molecule (phenobarbitone or methylphenobarbitone) have a significant anticonvulsant effect; and indeed other barbiturates and the phenothiazine group of drugs may provoke seizures. Withdrawal of a barbiturate after prolonged administration may induce a fit in a patient who has no history of overt epilepsy.

Because of its low toxicity, *phenobarbitone* is the sheet-anchor in the treatment of major epilepsy and minor forms other than petit mal. It has the further advantages of being effective and inexpensive. An initial dose of 30 mg. twice daily in childhood may be increased steadily until the fits are controlled. Increments of dosage should be made at intervals of a week until the daily dose is 180 mg. At this dose level drowsiness may be troublesome. If fits have been reduced in frequency it may be worth pushing the daily dose up to 240 mg. even though amphetamine (2·5 to 5 mg.) must be taken after breakfast and after the midday meal to abolish drowsiness. This does not significantly reduce the anticonvulsant action of phenobarbitone. Children may show a paradoxical increase of motor activity and aggressiveness while taking phenobarbitone. In these circumstances, or if phenobarbitone proves ineffective, it is advisable to prescribe a different anticonvulsant. When a change of drugs is made it is essential that one anticonvulsant should be withdrawn gradually as the other is introduced. An anticonvulsant should never be withdrawn abruptly as this procedure may precipitate status epilepticus.

Phenytoin causes drowsiness less often than phenobarbitone but ataxia and nystagmus are more troublesome. These side-effects may develop rapidly after an increase of dosage but subside equally quickly if the dose is reduced by one capsule (100 mg.). The ataxic signs are, therefore, like drowsiness, rather a manifestation of overdosage than of true toxicity. Vomiting, agranulocytosis, megaloblastic anaemia or dermatitis occur rarely. An average dose of phenytoin is 100 mg. three times a day, but most patients can tolerate twice this dose. Many develop unpleasant hypertrophy of the gums. This may be treated by a dental surgeon and need not cause withdrawal of phenytoin if the anticonvulsant effect is satisfactory. If the patient cannot tolerate an effective dose of phenytoin, the drug may be prescribed with phenobarbitone and sometimes the combination acts better than large doses of either drug alone. On this assumption pharmaceutical manufacturers have produced capsules containing both phenytoin and barbiturate. It is strongly recommended that these expensive combinations should not be used. This advice is given for two reasons: it is simple to alter the dosage of either drug when that dose is known and when the drugs are given separately; and it is very easy to forget the amounts of each drug in any given combined preparation. Phenytoin Mixture (BNF) is available for children; up to five years the initial dose is 4 ml. (30 mg. phenytoin), increasing to 8 ml. three times daily.

Primidone is a very effective anticonvulsant and only its greater toxicity prevents it from being the drug of first choice. A single isolated dose of 250 mg. may cause intense giddiness, vomiting and drowsiness. These symptoms may disappear with persistent administration, but if adaptation to the administration of primidone has not occurred within a period of three days it may be assumed that the patient will never tolerate it. This type of response may be avoided if the drug is first introduced in a dose of 125 mg. or less by using the syrup instead of the tablet. If the patient tolerates primidone, the drug should be gradually substituted for the previous one or added to it. If the introduction is gradual, a combination of primidone and phenytoin is usually well tolerated. Contrary to earlier belief, phenobarbitone and primidone may also be given simultaneously. In many cases primidone alone is quite satisfactory. The daily requirement of 750 mg. to 2 g. should be divided into three or four doses. Although it may be desirable to give a major part of the dose before the period of the day when the individual patient is most liable to have fits (usually within an hour of waking in the morning or during sleep), it is necessary to adjust the dose schedule in order to maintain a suitable blood level of the drug. If the frequency of fits is significantly reduced, an attempt is made to find the optimum dose by increasing it gradually until the side-effects of drowsiness or ataxia prevent further increase. Blood dyscrasias, notably megaloblastic anaemia, may develop from the prolonged use of primidone—a hazard common to all anticonvulsant drugs.

Sulthiame may be of value. Its dose is 200 mg. two to four times daily. The frequency of side-effects such as confusion, amnesia, hyperpnoea and tingling of the face and fingers, is higher than with the drugs already described and its clinical value is lower. Nevertheless, when a patient with grand mal has proved unresponsive to phenobarbitone, phenytoin, or primidone alone or in combination it is advisable to try other drugs such as sulthiame or *pheneturide* as individual patients may respond better to one of these though, in general, they are less valuable than the three drugs already described. There is a natural pressure from patients and their relatives or employers to try some other drug in the hope that fits will be abolished. It should be remembered, however, that if the maximum tolerated dose of phenytoin or primidone does not achieve this object it is most unlikely that any other drug will do so. Each drug should be given an adequate trial (about three months) in dosage as high as can be tolerated before it is rejected in favour of another (by gradual transfer as described above). The best compromise between reducing fits and preventing toxic effects must be accepted until the resourcefulness of the pharmaceutical industry produces even better anticonvulsants. Unless a new drug proves particularly efficacious it is best to revert to phenobarbitone alone or in combination with phenytoin, since this is the least toxic drug. There is strong evidence that a series of major convulsions is detrimental to the brain. It is, therefore, necessary to take an anticonvulsant drug regularly even though it fails to suppress all attacks.

The need for regular administration must be stressed. It is quite useless to prescribe an anticonvulsant drug for a few weeks following a fit and then to withdraw medication until a further fit occurs. Such a course may be justifiable after a single seizure when the diagnosis of epilepsy is in doubt, but once the diagnosis is established by recurrence of seizures or by electroencephalographic (E.E.G.) investigation, the appropriate drug should be taken regularly for a prolonged period. How long this should be continued is debatable. It should certainly not be stopped until the patient has been free from attacks (major or minor) for at least two years. Most neurologists prefer to continue medication for a period of three years after the last seizure. At the end of that time an electroencephalogram should be taken. If it provides evidence of a continuing convulsive tendency the drug should be continued. If the E.E.G. is normal it does not unfortunately mean that the tendency has disappeared, but it is then reasonable to withdraw medication gradually over a period of two to three months. Many patients will remain free from further fits. If convulsions recur, the previous medication should be resumed and preferably maintained for life, or at least until another three years have passed without fits.

Focal Epilepsy

The classical signs of both petit mal and grand mal are the sudden loss of consciousness and the involvement of muscles on both sides of the body. These signs are thought to prove that the paroxysmal neuronal discharge originates in the grey matter of the upper brain stem. Fits may also occur when there is a spontaneous discharge from groups of neurones in other parts of the brain, particularly the cortex and subcortical white matter. The clinical manifestation of these discharges is naturally determined by the neuronal system involved—motor, sensory or psychical; consciousness may be retained but thought processes are often disturbed. The fit may remain focal. Alternatively it may spread to neighbouring areas of cortex causing Jacksonian signs or extend rapidly to the deep midline structures and culminate in a major convulsive seizure. The nature of the local seizure preceding it, formerly called an aura, differentiates this type of attack from true grand mal.

Focal epilepsy arising in or near a temporal lobe may be manifested by disorders of behaviour with partial or complete amnesia. The resulting automatism is sometimes termed psychomotor epilepsy. Hallucinations or illusions of visual, auditory, gustatory or olfactory type may occur. The automatisms and hallucinations must be differentiated from those of the hysterical fugue, toxic states or psychoses. Diagnosis is simple in the florid case but the attack may consist of a fraction of the whole temporal lobe syndrome with only a brief lapse of consciousness. Such fits are readily confused with true petit mal. The differential diagnosis cannot be discussed here, but the distinction is important as minor fits of this type are resistant to troxidone and the suxinimide drugs.

The drug treatment of focal epilepsy, including the temporal lobe type, is similar to that of grand mal. Primidone is often the most effective anticonvulsant. Sulthiame is sometimes very effective in psychomotor epilepsy.

Surgical treatment. It is in the case of focal epilepsy that surgical treatment should be given serious consideration. The focal fit is likely to result from localized organic disease of the brain, and this may warrant excision—quite apart from the treatment of the fits. Benign tumours such as meningioma or angioma may be removed. The decision to operate is not always straightforward. Removal of a scar caused by trauma or meningitis in earlier life may not influence the incidence or severity of fits, and no operation on the brain is free from risk. Thus, unless it is necessary to remove a life-threatening tumour, operation should be advised only when the most vigorous medical treatment, carried out for a period of two years, has failed to make life tolerable for the patient. If fits are infrequent there is seldom any justification for operation. Occasionally some act of violence by an epileptic patient (usually with a temporal lobe lesion) results in his appearing in the criminal courts, though the case is unlikely to be heard until medical reports have been submitted. Such patients may require to be under restraint in a mental hospital. In these circumstances there would be greater justification for advising a surgical attack on an epileptogenic focus in the temporal lobe.

The Convulsion

It is unnecessary to treat a single convulsive seizure in an adult apart from ensuring that his airway is not obstructed and that he is protected from injury by traffic, fire or other dangers. If he is a known epileptic and under close observation, it may be possible to recognize the onset of a fit at a sufficiently early stage to allow insertion of the traditional padded spoon between the teeth. More often the tonic or clonic phase has already started and there is nothing to be gained by forcing an object between the clenched teeth—with the possibility of causing injury to them or to the gums. If, however, the patient is wearing dentures, it is advisable to remove these if this can be done without risk of breakage. Neck-ties, belts or other articles restricting respiration should be loosened. No further action need be taken until the motor

N*

discharge is finished. This is frequently followed by a stage of muscular flaccidity. At this time there is a danger that respiration will be embarrassed by inhalation of saliva or by the tongue falling backwards in the pharynx. To prevent this the patient should be turned semi-prone and his tongue pulled forward. A pharyngeal airway may be inserted if available. The patient should then be supervised and kept warm until full consciousness is restored.

In the young child the fit should be treated along similar lines, but there is more urgent need to terminate the fit in order to prevent cerebral hypoxia. The child should be placed in the semi-prone position, secretions sucked out of the pharynx and a pharyngeal airway inserted as soon as there is adequate muscular relaxation. If the fit has not stopped by the time the airway has been assured, it is advisable to inject soluble phenobarbitone intramuscularly in a dose of 30 mg. for a child under one month, 60 mg. between one month and one year, 120 mg. between one and three years, and 120 to 180 mg. over 3 years of age. If there is no previous history of convulsions, it is advisable to arrange admission of the child to hospital because the most common cause of convulsions in childhood is meningitis. After 10 years of age this is less likely and no emergency admission to hospital need be considered unless status epilepticus develops.

Status Epilepticus

In dealing with this dangerous condition there is no place for half measures. The following schedules are for adult patients. Diazepam, 10 mg., should be injected intravenously or intramuscularly. Fits are often controlled in 2 to 10 minutes. If they recur the dose may be repeated or 50 mg. in 500 ml. saline may be given by slow intravenous drip. The traditional remedy, paraldehyde, is also valuable and safe: 4 ml. is injected into *each* buttock (upper and outer quadrant) and the part massaged to disperse the fluid in the tissues. Few patients fail to respond to this treatment. Alternatively sodium phenobarbitone 200 mg. may be injected intravenously, but if convulsive movements make this difficult or dangerous the drug can be given intramuscularly. A solution of sodium phenytoin (5 per cent.) is available for intravenous injection and the dose is 5 ml. Extravasation into the tissues must be carefully avoided as the preparation is extremely irritant (pH 12). A relatively easy way of bringing status epilepticus under control is to inject thiopentone sodium intravenously (100 mg.

as a 5 per cent. solution). However, for the single-handed general practitioner coping with the problem in the patient's home this method is not recommended: the dangers of thiopentone are greatest in the partially asphyxiated anoxic patient; and even under relatively favourable conditions thiopentone may induce laryngeal spasm—which calls for immediate intubation. If status epilepticus proves resistant to paraldehyde and to sodium phenobarbitone parenterally, it is best for the practitioner to resort to chloroform. The patient should not be allowed to emerge rapidly from the narcotic state therapeutically induced: after emptying the rectum by lavage an enema of paraldehyde should be given, the dose being 0·5 ml. per kg. of body weight in 10 times its own volume of physiological saline; the total quantity of paraldehyde should not exceed 25 ml. The onset of hyperpyrexia is a real danger in status epilepticus. The greatly increased metabolism resulting from the seizures raises the temperature to such a degree that the thermal regulatory functions of the hypothalamus are impaired. The management of hyperpyrexia is discussed elsewhere (p. 389). Chlorpromazine is best avoided as it may aggravate seizures in the epileptic.

The care of a patient in status epilepticus extends far beyond the use of drugs: it is imperative to deal with the needs of the unconscious patient and these include the maintenance of efficient respiration, skilled nursing, adequate hydration of the tissues, maintenance of normal bladder function, checking of electrolyte balance, the prevention of infection, and so on. The patient should, therefore, be transferred to hospital when the convulsions and asphyxial state have been relieved; there the advice of an anaesthetist should be obtained immediately so that the plan of general management and special forms of treatment can be carefully surveyed in relation to the needs of the individual. The treatment of status epilepticus necessarily lowers the level of consciousness and may abolish the reflex activity of the throat. Care has to be taken to ensure the patency of the upper respiratory pathway. Further, as a natural result of prolonged coma, dehydration supervenes unless measures are taken to prevent it.

Occupation

For the patient's own safety and for the safety of other people, prohibitions have to be imposed on the epileptic. If a patient is liable to have an epileptic seizure during the day he must not drive a car. The legal position with regard to this is ill-defined. Many epileptics apply for driving licences and obtain them largely because specific inquiry into their fitness to drive is loosely worded and underemphasized in the application form.

It is extremely difficult to know where to draw the line. When applying for a driving licence, the epileptic, having admitted the occurrence of bouts of unconsciousness, may, after seeking professional advice, be considered capable of driving because adequate treatment and the infrequency of attacks have rendered remote the risk of a seizure while driving. It is now permissible to drive if fits occur only during sleep, and the prophylactic use of anticonvulsants is no longer a bar to driving. If the doctor says the patient is capable of driving, there is no onus placed on the Licensing Authorities to challenge his opinion and responsibility lies with the doctor. The view has been held, with some justification, that the history of an epileptic seizure should debar the patient from driving for life. If this view is pushed to its ultimate conclusion, then the history of convulsions in infancy would disqualify the potential driver. When a man, having had an epileptic seizure, depends on driving a car for his livelihood, a certain amount of hardship is caused by preventing him from continuing. Nevertheless, if the possibilities in most instances are appreciated, the prohibition for those who do not fulfil the legal requirements should be absolute in spite of all attempts at persuasion. This prohibition should not, however, be final. If a man has been free of epileptic seizures for a period of six or seven years, the risk of accident in driving a car is minimal. Indeed, the risk is much less than from the intoxicated or drugged motorist or from one severely physically handicapped, whether the disability be due to trauma, to primary disease of the nervous system or to cardio-vascular disease.

Occupations which involve potential danger to the individual and to others should be forbidden the epileptic: he should not work in heavy industry among unguarded machinery; he should not risk working at a height if this carries the danger of a serious fall; nor should he be entrusted with the control of any mechanical device such as a crane, in the operation of which serious damage could occur if consciousness were suddenly lost. Perhaps the most important prohibition so far as recreation is concerned is in swimming, which should be forbidden except under the most stringent expert supervision.

Marriage

Prevention of epilepsy must depend on some understanding of its aetiology. Sometimes there is a definite inheritance of the epileptic reaction. Advice against marriage and the procreation of children should be given to the individual in whose family there is a strong hereditary tendency to the disorder; and the doctor should be most emphatic in advising against the marriage of two such people. On the other hand, when epilepsy occurs as an isolated instance in one member of a family, the chances of that individual producing an epileptic child by a normal person with no family history of epilepsy are no greater than that of two normal persons having an epileptic child. Sometimes advice against marriage rests primarily upon economic circumstances, depending upon employability and earning potential. Frequent attacks, difficult to control by anticonvulsant drugs, and the presence of mental deterioration in spite of treatment, are further contraindications to marriage. When epilepsy is a manifestation of trauma, vascular disease, syphilis, inflammation or tumour of the brain, it does not, of course, carry with it a hereditary stigma.

Narcolepsy

This condition, sometimes a sequal to encephalitis, is to be carefully distinguished from hypersomnia. Narcolepsy is paroxysmal; sleep may overtake the patient in spite of all efforts to remain awake. Unless the condition is adequately controlled by appropriate treatment, the limitations imposed on the patient are not unlike those of epilepsy. There is, however, no real connection between epilepsy and narcolepsy. There is an association between paroxysmal overwhelming sleep and cataplexy— a disorder which, without loss of consciousness, causes the patient to fall into a state of muscular atonia whenever he is amused enough to laugh.

Dexamphetamine is the drug of choice: it should be given in 5 to 10 mg. doses up to 40 mg. a day. Its use should be avoided within a period of five hours before the usual time of retiring to bed at night. The pharmaceutical industry now provides elegant preparations in capsule form (spansules, 15 mg.) which are said to prolong absorption time: thus, the initial dose may be larger and the taking of tablets at inconvenient times may be obviated. Other drugs which may be used are methylamphetamine, 2·5 to 10 mg., and methylphenidate hydrochloride, 10 mg. It is claimed that the latter is less likely than other drugs of this type to cause loss of appetite. Insomnia is often troublesome and can be overcome by a suitable hypnotic dose of a short-acting barbiturate such as pentobarbitone, 45 to 90 mg. Amphetamine should never be prescribed without attention to the risk of addiction. This is not so widely realized as it should be; drugs of this type should not be allowed to fall into the hands of an alcoholic.

CARE OF THE UNCONSCIOUS PATIENT

The management of the unconscious patient is essentially the same whatever may be the cause of coma; but some therapeutic procedures are determined by its depth and duration. The deeper the coma the greater is the loss of protective reflexes such as coughing, swallowing and the withdrawal of a limb from a noxious stimulus. Thus the patient's most pressing need may be simply protection from physical injury. In the management of coma that is expected to be of short duration (e.g. in the post-epileptic state) attention to nutrition is not a matter of importance, but in those patients who do not regain consciousness for two days it becomes a highly important part of the therapeutic plan.

No matter how brief the loss of consciousness, respiration must be maintained by clearing the airways of surplus secretion, using a sucker if available. A pharyngeal airway should be inserted to prevent the tongue from falling back. If there is no contraindication to the posture, the head should be lower than the chest and turned to one side to allow secretions to escape. If coma is likely to be of short duration, the patient should be nursed in the semi-prone position with a soft pillow under one shoulder and one hip. When coma lasts for more than six hours it may be necessary to use other positions including the recumbent in order to protect the skin from excessive pressure. If there are signs that coma will persist for more than a few days, it is important to estimate the degree of reflex failure, because if there is a poor cough reflex it is advisable to perform a tracheostomy and to maintain respiration by a positive pressure ventilator (p. 652). Prophylactic use of antibiotics is not recommended. It is preferable to be on the lookout for the development of respiratory tract infection, and to intervene when necessary with specific treatment according to the organism isolated from the bronchial aspirate.

Pressure sores must be prevented by the methods used for the nursing of the insensitive patient (see below), and contamination by faeces and urine avoided as far as possible. As the bladder and rectal reflexes are usually intact, it should not be necessary to catheterize a male patient; the urine may simply be led through a condom and polythene tube to a drainage bottle. Women may be nursed for short spells with pads of material suitably placed to absorb the urine, but in prolonged coma catheterization becomes necessary (p. 387). Faecal soiling is prevented by regular use of the enema aided if necessary by digital evacuation of scybala.

The reflexes controlling body temperature (vaso-motor, sweating, and shivering) may be impaired in deep coma. It is important to prevent body temperature from falling excessively. Blankets should be used; but the application of heat should be avoided owing to the dangers of burning the skin and promoting loss of salt and water by sweating. Dehydration is one of the serious hazards of prolonged coma. If coma has persisted for four hours, it is advisable to pass a nasal tube into the stomach to facilitate the maintenance of fluid and electrolyte balance (p. 641). It is then also a simple matter to provide adequate calories by suitable fluid nutrients (p. 239).

LOSS OF SENSATION

Cutaneous anaesthesia resulting from lesions of the thalamus or spino-thalamic tract, as in syringo-myelia prevents the patient from detecting stimuli which would normally be painful. Provided, however, that peripheral reflex arcs are intact and control of voluntary movement preserved, the skin may be protected if the patient is instructed how to avoid obvious hazards such as burns from a cigarette or contact with a hot-water bottle, protruding nails in the shoes or amateur attempts at chiropody.

When the withdrawal reflexes are abolished, as in lesions of the cauda equina or peripheral nerves, or the absence of sensation is associated with paralysis of movement, it is difficult to avoid these dangers and, in addition, pressure sores may develop over bony prominences because of failure to change posture sufficiently often to avoid tissue necrosis from ischaemia. The patient's position in bed must

be changed every two hours. It is essential that the undersheet should be free from wrinkles, crumbs or other objects which might cause local points of pressure if the patient lies on them. In addition to these precautions, the resistance of the skin to ischaemic necrosis is increased if standard nursing procedures are meticulously observed; the pressure points are dabbed with spirit every time the patient is turned and then powdered with fine talc or smeared with a silicone cream. The effect on the skin of the individual patient must be carefully noted: sometimes repeated application of silicone cream produces a hard skin which is liable to crack, and it may be preferable to use zinc and castor oil ointment which provides protection against maceration and also keeps the skin soft and pliable. In addition to the obvious pressure points over the heels, malleoli and buttocks, similar treatment should be applied to the shoulder blades, points of the shoulders, elbows, occiput, knees, iliac crests, sternum and if necessary the forehead, according to the positions adopted in quadriplegic or unconscious patients. When a paraplegic patient becomes capable of co-operating with his nurses he may be taught to vary the position of his pelvis and lower limbs by raising himself in bed by means of a suspended stirrup, and to move his lower limbs with his hands. By suitably placed pillows the weight of the body may be distributed over a large area instead of being concentrated on the bony prominences. Foam rubber mattresses have rendered obsolete such awkward devices as the water-bed and the air-bed. For long-term care of paraplegic or quadriplegic patients a ripple mattress is available in which alternate sections are rhythmically inflated and deflated by an automatic pump to vary the distribution of pressure. For the adult patient a rubber mattress should be of suitable thickness and consistence (there is an optimum degree of resilience to ensure the patient's comfort and to facilitate nursing). For those who are incontinent the outer layer of the mattress must be impervious to excreta so that it may be easily and rapidly cleansed.

The frequent turning which is so essential if the paralysed or unconscious patient is to avoid pressure sores is readily achieved in a ward generously staffed with well-trained attendants: it is difficult or impossible in the home or in a poorly staffed ward. In these circumstances it is more satisfactory to nurse the patient in a specially designed frame such as the Stryker, in which at the correct times the patient can be fixed firmly and safely and then turned with ease by one attendant.

CARE OF THE NEUROGENIC BLADDER

Incontinence must be regarded as irremediable when it occurs in a demented patient or one who has a lesion of the frontal lobes; only the skill and devotion of the nurse can minimize the unfortunate consequences. Lesions of the spinal cord and cauda equina disturb bladder function by abolishing the reflex control of the detrusor muscle and sphincter or by interfering with the supraspinal control of these reflexes.

Incontinence of urine is extremely disagreeable and complicates the care of the skin; but there are even more important sequelae to it which may, if uncontrolled, endanger life. These are chronic cystitis, with retrograde pyelonephritis and possible hypertension as long-term sequelae, and the effects of backward pressure on the urinary tract.

The atonic bladder. Regular emptying of the bladder is the obvious way to prevent the effects of backward pressure and the methods used depend on the exigencies of the particular case. If the lesion involves the conus medullaris or cauda equina and there is loss of the reflexes controlling the bladder and the voluntary musculature of the pelvis, the atonic bladder will distend passively and overflow dribbling of urine and stress incontinence will ensue.

The flaccid bladder may be stimulated to contract by administration of carbachol. A test dose of 0·5 ml. of Carbachol Injection B.P. is given subcutaneously and, in the absence of untoward effects such as fall in blood pressure, the drug may then be injected in doses of 2 ml. as required. For regular treatment carbachol may be taken orally in doses of 1 to 3 mg. It is rarely effective if there is gross denervation but is valuable for partial lesions in which there is diminished bladder tone, and its use may delay the onset of urinary infection. Alternatively, distigmine may be used, 0·5 mg. by injection or 5 mg. by mouth. Emptying of the bladder may also be effected by manual compression applied through the anterior abdominal wall. It is necessary to catheterize the patient from time to time after this manœuvre to estimate the volume of residual urine. If a pool of stagnant urine remains after abdominal compression and injection of carbachol, the patient must be catheterized. For the first week catheterization should be carried out three times a day with full aseptic precautions. After this the urethra should be conditioned to tolerate a fine polythene indwelling Gibbon's catheter which should be tied in place and led to a sealed collecting bottle. If leakage past the catheter is excessive, a large self-retaining catheter of the Foley type must be substituted (No. 14–16). The Foley catheter should be taped to the abdomen or attached to an abdominal belt or binder in order to straighten out the peno-scrotal angle and to minimize the risk of peno-scrotal fistulae and diverticulae. The catheter is provided with a clip which is released every hour. This procedure is as effective as tidal drainage in ensuring that the bladder fills regularly to a suitable capacity without becoming overdistended. Before changing the catheter, about 100 ml. chlorhexidine gluconate solution should be gently injected through it into the bladder. The patient should be encouraged to drink at least three litres of fluid a day. If, in spite of this regimen, the patient with an atonic bladder is unable to pass urine, his ability to do so may be restored by transurethral resection of the vesical neck.

The spinal reflex bladder. If the lesion is above an intact lumbo-sacral cord, there is hope that an automatic bladder may develop. The disorder of function depends on the extent of the damage to the cord and the rate of its development. In diseases of slow onset without complete transverse cord block (for example, multiple sclerosis) the disorder may be of two types and both may be present in one patient. The most common is failure of inhibition of the bladder reflexes, resulting in precipitancy or urgency of micturition. Less common is hesitancy of micturition, but both disorders may coexist. The hyper-irritability of the bladder can be significantly lowered or completely eliminated for some hours by administration of anticholinergic drugs. A mixture containing 0·3 to 0·6 ml. of tincture of belladonna or a tablet of atropine sulphate (0·6 mg.) may abolish vesical irritability for from two to four hours. Occasionally a better response is obtained from propantheline bromide, 15 mg. three to six times a day according to the reaction of the individual patient. As an alternative the tone of the urethral sphincter may be increased by ephedrine sulphate given orally (30 mg.) two or three times daily. The last dose should not be given later than 5.00 p.m. as it may cause insomnia.

Hesitancy. There is no effective treatment for hesitancy of micturition. When this proceeds to retention, carbachol may be tried as described above for the atonic bladder, but it is often necessary to resort to catheterization—at first intermittently and later, if retention persists, with an indwelling catheter. When recurrent retention of urine is a problem, as in some cases of multiple sclerosis, the operation of transurethral resection of the vesical neck may restore satisfactory micturition by reducing resistance to the outflow of urine. Operative treatment should not be considered until conservative management has been tried for at least a year, as spontaneous recovery may ultimately take place. In persistent flaccid paralysis of the bladder (lesions of the conus medullaris or cauda equina, as in tabes dorsalis and diabetes mellitus) this operation may be the treatment of choice enabling the patient to dispense with his catheter, thereby reducing the danger of urinary infection. It is undesirable to operate if there is no significant urinary reflux and the decision must be reached only after consultation with a urological surgeon.

Incontinence. Once a patient has reached a catheter-free state it is necessary to collect the urine in some suitable manner: male patients may wear a portable urinal strapped to the thigh if ambulant or to the leg if in a wheelchair. For the patient in bed condom drainage to a collecting-bottle is efficient if properly managed. The condom should be changed daily. It is fixed to the penis by a special cement. Failing this, a one-inch elastoplast tape may be used, applied in such a way as not to obstruct the urethra. No satisfactory receptacle has been developed for use by women: most of them require permanent catheters, though some are able to remain reasonably comfortable by wearing absorbent pads in plastic pants. Stimulation of the muscles of the pelvic floor by electronic stimulators is a technique that is being developed.

Every effort should be made to manage the neurogenic bladder without prolonged catheterization, as urinary infection is inevitable in such circumstances. The use of antibiotics (pp. 2-23) may postpone but will not prevent infection and the author does not recommend their prophylactic administration. These should be withheld until infection occurs. The further treatment then depends on the nature of the infecting organism. For many of these patients, long-term care is a matter for the urological specialist.

The care of the neurogenic bladder has been described in some detail as there is a general failure to appreciate its importance. In chronic disease of the spinal cord the complications of urinary retention and infection are the most common causes of death, yet they may be prevented or at least postponed by careful treatment.

VENTILATORY FAILURE

Many patients with neurological disease have respiratory difficulties due to inadequate ventilation of the lungs. This may be due to central causes (for example, head injury, intracranial haemorrhage, cerebral tumour) or peripheral (polyneuropathy, myasthenia gravis or other neuromuscular disease). Provided incurable progressive disease is not present, it is necessary to support respiration passively. Details of the management of the artificially ventilated patient will be found on p. 651. Here it is only necessary to outline the main indications for the alternative methods.

Respiratory paralysis. The main differences between neurological causes of ventilatory failure and respiratory insufficiency due to pulmonary or cardiac disease should be noted: in patients with neurological lesions the lungs and circulation are usually normal, at least in the initial stages, but there may be associated dysphagia due to paresis of the tongue and nasopharyngeal muscles. If there is no difficulty in swallowing, pulmonary ventilation may be readily maintained by a tank type of respirator. This complicates the nursing care of the skin, bowel and bladder, but saves the patient from the risks of tracheostomy. It is a suitable method for the management of the long term case but, except in skilled hands, is unsuitable for the patient whose respiratory reserve is too limited to permit his being removed from the respirator at intervals.

Bulbar paralysis. If there is disturbance of swallowing, however slight, with pooling of saliva in the nasopharynx, or if the cough reflex is absent, it is dangerous to use a tank respirator since foreign matter will be aspirated into the lungs. This is usually the case in myasthenia gravis and acute polyneuritis and often in acute poliomyelitis. It is then essential to ventilate the patient by positive-pressure inflation of the lungs through a cuffed tracheostomy tube (p. 652). In addition to preventing reflux of the air pumped into the trachea the inflatable cuff round the tracheostomy tube prevents aspiration of nasopharyngeal contents. It is, however, essential that the latter should be cleared regularly by suction, and in any event before deflation of the cuff which must be carried out every two hours to minimize the risk of pressure necrosis of the trachea.

Management by artificial ventilation is a matter requiring special experience and it is advisable to send the patient to a special centre. Every doctor should be skilled in the emergency ventilation of the lungs by mouth-to-mouth breathing or by the use of a portable inflator (p. 652) as this may be life-saving in many neurological emergencies.

Cough paralysis. A neglected aspect of the management of patients with weakness of the diaphragm and abdominal muscles is their inability to cough. If the patient is able to cough actively but with insufficient expulsive force, he may be helped by the application of a tight abdominal binder or by an assistant applying firm manual pressure over the abdomen during active coughing. The bed-ridden patient may be helped by a physiotherapist carrying out vibratory movements to the thorax during the act of coughing. This should be preceded by firm percussion over the lung bases to loosen mucous plugs in the bronchi; the foot of the bed should be raised during both procedures.

BODY TEMPERATURE

Hyperpyrexia. Some intracranial diseases affect the thermoregulatory centres of the hypothalamus and brain stem, either directly or by interference with circulation to these parts. This may lead to hyperpyrexia which is always a threat to life and demands urgent treatment. A few elementary points are germane to the understanding of the basic problem of hyperpyrexia. The patient may be pallid, his skin cold and dry, yet his blood temperature may be above 41° C.—an expression of the failure of the body to lose heat by radiation and evaporation. In the periphery the skin vessels are tightly constricted and the sweat glands have ceased to act. Rational treatment must, therefore, attempt to bring about peripheral vascular dilatation and sweating or its equivalent. Artificially produced vascular dilatation in the periphery can be achieved by mechanical means. The patient should be stripped of his clothing and bedclothes. His skin should be subjected to rough friction until it is red. Sweating does not follow, but the erythematous skin should be kept wet by spraying or washing

continuously with cold water, and a constant stream of air from electric fans should be directed on to the body surface. In addition, ice may be applied to the reddened skin. Recourse should only be made to stomach or rectal lavage with ice-cold water if the temperature does not fall as the result of these measures. The indications for starting these vigorous measures depend on the rapidity of rise as well as the absolute level of the rectal temperature. (The 'core' temperature of the body is more accurately measured at the aural tympanum, but rectal thermometry is more usual). When the rectal temperature has been lowered to 39° C., cooling treatment should stop, but it must be taken hourly during the next few days—a period of instability inevitable after the breakdown of such a fundamental biological mechanism as thermostatic control. These physical expedients designed to make the body lose heat are facilitated by giving chlorpromazine and pethidine; the former is administered intramuscularly in 100 mg. doses four-hourly during the time when the patient is receiving physiotherapy and until the emergency is over.

Heat stroke. This may also be a danger during hot weather in patients who are unable to perspire because of loss of sweating reflexes (for example, quadriplegia from high cervical lesions and polyneuropathy). Such patients should avoid the sun and maintain a high fluid intake during the summer. The same danger may be present in patients taking large doses of drugs of the atropine group used in Parkinsonism (p. 377); and if amphetamine is prescribed it is advisable to avoid strenuous exercise in hot climates.

Hypothermia. This is less common in neurological disease, but it should be remembered that shivering and voluntary contraction of muscles play important rôles in maintaining body temperature, so that many patients with muscular dystrophy, polyneuropathy or spinal cord disease require extra clothing. While in bed it is better to rely on a thermostatically controlled electric blanket or a good quality down-filled quilt for warmth, as the paretic patient is unable to tolerate the weight of the blankets necessary to keep him warm and it is dangerous to use hot water bottles.

PAIN

Pain may be abolished by removal of the cause; it is often reduced by giving analgesic drugs (p. 440) and by the application of heat—an empirical procedure which is nevertheless comforting to the patient. The use of drugs to produce reversal of the mechanism causing pain may also prove effective. Many headaches are caused by dilatation of extra-cranial vessels and may be relieved by administration of a vasoconstrictor drug which has no analgesic action in itself. Few neurological diseases cause pain by direct stimulation of sensory nerve fibres or their endings, but secondary pain—associated with muscle spasm—is common. The appropriate treatment is the removal of the cause of reflex spasm or the alleviation of spontaneous spasms in upper motor neurone disorders (p. 373).

Deafferentation may be used as a last resort when pain is severe and cannot be alleviated by other means. For pain localized to the distribution of a single nerve or nerve root, the injection of a local anaesthetic into the nerve or root is an essential preliminary to further procedure in order to confirm the localization of the disturbance. This sometimes has a surprisingly prolonged effect, suggesting the interruption of some cyclical process responsible for the perpetuation of the pain. In certain circumstances it may be possible to make the analgesia permanent by injecting absolute alcohol into the nerve which has been identified in this way. Destruction of posterior nerve roots by intrathecal injection of phenol in glycerin has a limited rôle in the treatment of pain due to malignant disease in the lower limbs and pelvis. The technique is essentially the same as for the treatment of spasticity but the patient is postured differently so that the sensory roots are blocked instead of the motor ones (p. 375). For higher lesions such as are caused by intra-abdominal, thoracic or spinal tumours and for disorders of the upper limbs, it is desirable to section the contralateral spinothalamic tract of the spinal cord at a level several segments above the highest entered by the sensory nerves from the painful lesion. The resulting analgesia is not always acceptable to the patient and the operation requires a skilled neurosurgeon to avoid damage to the pyramidal tract. If the pain is bilateral in origin, requiring bilateral tractotomy, there is the additional danger of interference with the control of micturition. For these reasons its use is restricted in general to the control of severe pain due to malignant disease. Selective lesions of the thalamus by stereotaxic surgery have been made in an attempt to avoid these disadvantages, but the control of pain achieved in this way is at present uncertain.

FACIAL PAIN

Successful treatment of pain in the face demands accurate diagnosis. The majority of patients referred to a neurologist with a diagnosis of trigeminal neuralgia do not have this disorder. It is essential to search for and apply appropriate treatment to the sources of pain in the superficial tissues of the face and the structures below it, bearing in mind that some deep-seated lesions sharing a common nerve supply from the trigeminal nerve will cause pain referred to the face.

Local and Referred Pain

Such disorders are inflammation of the antral, ethmoidal or sphenoidal sinuses, dental disease and malignant disease of the nasopharynx. Glaucoma or inflammatory lesions of the orbit may present as pain in the face. Perhaps the most common cause other than toothache is pain referred from a temporo-mandibular joint. This may be due to arthritis of the joint or it may result from overclosure of the bite when molar teeth have been lost. The pain may resemble that of tic douloureux in its lancinating explosive quality and in its precipitation by eating or speaking, but its duration is usually longer and it is not triggered by cutaneous stimulation. The pain may be referred to the face or may be experienced deep in the ear and radiate into the throat and tongue. The cure is the prosthetic procedure of supplying dentures of sufficient depth to avoid traumatization of the mandibular joint and backward pressure on the thin tympanic plate.

Psychogenic Pain

Depression is an important cause of facial pain which may be missed, and it is important to recognize and treat its psychiatric origin. Possibly related to this is the condition given the unsatisfactory name of 'atypical facial neuralgia'. There is a severe facial pain which comes in spells, lasting for a few days but not in brief paroxysms like true trigeminal neuralgia. Such pain is not confined to the distribution of the trigeminal nerve or one of its branches and is unrelated to stimulation of trigger areas. It usually occurs in women with an emotional disturbance or an obsessional state but without true depression. Analgesic drugs are without effect but chlorpromazine or chlordiazepoxide may be helpful. The patient usually attributes the pain to disease of teeth, sinuses or to some other local cause. It is important to recognize its true nature so as to prevent unnecessary extractions of teeth, and operations on the nose, sinuses, throat or ears.

Trigeminal Neuralgia

Paroxysmal trigeminal neuralgia, or tic douloureux, is characterized by attacks of pain within the distribution of one or more branches of the trigeminal nerve, usually the maxillary or mandibular, but rarely the ophthalmic division. Each attack lasts for only a few seconds, during which the pain is extremely severe and often compared to touching a live electric wire. It is stabbing in quality, shooting from a point where it may be triggered by a light touch on the skin towards the ear or outer canthus of the eye on the same side. Attacks may also be precipitated by eating or speaking. Trigeminal neuralgia is often succeeded by aching discomfort, less severe but more prolonged. These diagnostic points are emphasized because this type of facial pain is amenable to specific forms of therapy. Assessment of the value of drug therapy or surgical operation must take into account the well known tendency for remission to occur for months or years. Again, drug therapy (see below) carries considerable disadvantages in terms of side-effects and even serious toxic effects; and in a patient severely disabled by trigeminal neuralgia and also susceptible to the toxic actions of the drugs in current use, there would be a strong case for surgical intervention (see below).

Drug therapy. When these patients are first seen by the physician analgesics such as aspirin and paracetamol have usually been tried and found to be unsatisfactory or useless. The anticonvulsant drugs carbamazepine or phenytoin sodium are the alternatives, used individually or together. Carbamazepine is given in doses of 100 mg. twice daily gradually increasing to 200 mg. three or four times daily as required. The great majority of patients obtain relief within 48 hours of starting treatment. Side-effects are common and include giddiness, nausea, anorexia, vomiting and skin rashes. Serious toxic effects have been reported—aplastic anaemia, lupus erythematosus and the Stevens–Johnson syndrome. Adverse effects are most likely to occur when high doses of the drug are required. Phenytoin sodium is much less effective than carbamazepine, but as its side-effects are less serious it is reasonable to give it a trial first (300 to 600 mg. daily in divided doses). If this is unsatisfactory, supplementary doses of carbamazepine can be added—say 100 mg. three times a day. These regimens of drug therapy are also effective in glossopharyngeal neuralgia.

Surgical treatment. Drug treatment may be repeated during relapses, but in later life remissions become shorter and the pain may be so frequent and intolerable as to drive the patient to suicide. Pain of such appalling intensity justifies radical measures. If it is limited to the region of the infra-orbital foramen or the mandibular foramen, the respective nerves may be destroyed by injection of absolute alcohol after confirmation of the site by injecting a local anaesthetic as described on p. 390. Pain of wider distribution requires to be blocked more centrally by differential section of the sensory root of the trigeminal nerve. This operation and others of like nature are remarkably free from risk in the hands of a competent neurosurgeon and the results are gratifying. Hypertensive patients over the age of 70 do not tolerate the operation well and it may be desirable to use the less satisfactory technique of injecting alcohol if drug treatment does not prevent attacks.

Herpes Zoster of the Fifth Cranial Nerve

This depressing condition may give rise to much disfigurement and pain. When the eruption develops, the skin should be kept dry and dusted with a simple dusting powder. Aspirin or paracetamol usually alleviates the pain in the acute phase, though occasionally it is so severe as to require morphine. Post-herpetic neuralgia is a sequel which often presents a baffling problem. The physician may be obliged to resort occasionally to the use of analgesics which are drugs of addiction—a potentially perilous situation. Again the nature of the pain is so disagreeable and dominating that it often generates in the sufferer a neurosis as intractable as the pain itself.

Application of cinchocaine ointment 0·5 per cent. is a simple procedure which is worth a trial: the objective is to make the skin in the affected area less sensitive to stimuli that precipitate exacerbations. Operations on and injections into the Gasserian ganglion or its roots are ill-advised; the condition usually subsides spontaneously in the course of time. The most intractable post-herpetic neuralgia usually occurs in the first division of the trigeminal nerve. The site of pain suggests to the sufferer that some serious disease is present within the skull itself; he believes the gravity of the disturbance must equal the severity of the symptom. Assurance must go hand in hand with any physical or medicinal treatment. Ulceration of the cornea is another unfortunate sequel of the acute attack of herpes of the first division of the fifth cranial nerve, and this complication calls for immediate consultation with the ophthalmologist.

Migrainous Facial Neuralgia

Pain confined to the face may occur as a variant of migraine. It may resemble tic douloureux in its distribution and severity, but does not have its brief paroxysmal quality and trigger spots are absent. Ergotamine and other measures advised for migraine should be used (p. 393).

HEADACHE

The treatment of headache depends on the diagnosis of its cause. The most common is a psychological disturbance and the emotional state must not, therefore, be neglected. In addition to pain as a psychosomatic manifestation or a hysterical conversion symptom, headache may be caused by worry about the possibility of intracranial damage after head injury or by the unjustified fear of a cerebral tumour. Reassurance and explanation, with the temporary prescription of a sedative, may suffice in such cases. When headache is more persistent, it should be recognized that psychological tension may produce pain by physical means, either by vasodilatation or by tension of the scalp and neck muscles. Indeed it is difficult to define the borderline between 'psychogenic headache', 'tension headache' and 'true migraine'. It is inappropriate here to discuss the differential diagnosis of the various types of headache, but the following disorders illustrate the main pathological mechanisms and their treatment.

'Simple Headache' and 'Psychogenic Headache'

Occasional headaches, occurring during or after periods of stress or frustration, respond best to sympathetic handling by an understanding doctor prepared to give time to listen to a worried or unhappy patient. Aspirin or paracetamol given on two or three occasions, and a short-acting hypnotic for two or three nights to ensure refreshing sleep, may be all that is required. Long-acting barbiturates should be avoided as they may exacerbate headache on the following day.

If headache persists for more than a week after such treatment, the practitioner should review the diagnosis. If there are no other symptoms or signs of intracranial disease and the ocular fundi are normal, the need for a psychiatric opinion should be considered. It is particularly important to recognize a depressive state masquerading as headache. If a major psychiatric disorder is excluded, a valuable method of treatment is to combine a simple analgesic such as aspirin with chlordiazepoxide. This treatment may be very successful but it must be recognized that long established psychogenic headache may resist all forms of treatment.

Sinusitis and Referred Headache

Acute and subacute infection of the frontal sinuses may cause intense throbbing frontal headache. Local tenderness, nasal discharge and often pyrexia indicate the diagnosis. Aspirin or paracetamol may be required for a few days, but the pain subsides as the infection is brought under control with antibiotics. A diagnosis of chronic sinusitis as a cause of headache is more difficult to sustain. It should be accepted only on the advice of a specialist. Pain may be referred to the head when there is a lesion of one of the other paranasal sinuses, the teeth, the mastoids, the cervical spine, and on rare occasions it results from hypotension complicating myocardial infarction. Treatment directed to the cause often suffices. In some cases, however, pain appears to be perpetuated by spasm of muscles which is caused reflexly and requires appropriate treatment.

Tension Headache

Prolonged contraction of the muscles of the scalp, jaw and neck may cause headache. It is associated with emotional disorders or reflex spasm as described above. Treatment with aspirin or paracetamol may need to be supplemented with meprobamate or chlordiazepoxide. Physical forms of treatment such as hot baths, light massage, and relaxation exercises may be beneficial and the psychiatric or physical management of the underlying cause should not be ignored.

Raised Intracranial Pressure

The headache associated with hydrocephalus or an expanding intracranial lesion, such as tumour or abscess, is due to traction on the great vessels at the base of the brain. It is increased by lying down and so is often most severe in the morning, or following coughing or straining at stool. The patient should therefore be nursed with a high pillow and the bowels kept loose. Dehydration by avoiding excessive fluid intake and by the use of frusemide

(p. 89) will help to minimize the rise in pressure within the skull. It is dangerous to attempt to do this by lumbar puncture. If decompression is required because of increasing drowsiness, the fluid must be removed by ventricular cannulation. In an emergency the intravenous injection of hypertonic fluids may be undertaken (p. 400).

Aspirin or compound codeine tablets may be given for pressure headache, but stronger analgesics should not be used unless death is inevitable. The more potent analgesics depress respiration and cause a secondary rise in intracranial pressure which may endanger life.

Vascular Headache

Many headaches are due to dilatation of extra-cranial blood vessels. Headache associated with pyrexial disorders, the post-epileptic state and some forms of psychoses may be caused in this way. If it is not severe, the traditional cold compress on the forehead may constrict the vessels sufficiently to relieve pain. Headache associated with hypertension may be of this nature. Intra-cranial aneurysm and arteriovenous anomalies are usually painless but may be associated with migraine. Temporal arteritis causes severe localized pain which is throbbing in type. Local excision of the painful segment of the temporal artery gives rapid relief, but corticosteroid therapy in high dosage (40 to 60 mg. of prednisolone daily) is usually effective and should be started immediately to avert the danger of blindness.

Migraine

As with epilepsy, the migraine syndrome may be either idiopathic or symptomatic. If the headache and visual disturbance (or other symptom of localized cerebral ischaemia) remain confined to one side in successive episodes, it may be due to an intracranial aneurysm or arteriovenous anomaly; alternatively it may be caused by ischaemic attacks secondary to carotid or vertebrobasilar insufficiency (p. 395). Migraine starting in later life may be caused by cerebral atherosclerosis, polycythaemia vera or hypertension. These examples of sympto-matic migraine serve as a reminder to consider the treatment of an underlying cause. Nevertheless, the treatment of the headache itself is similar to that used in idiopathic migraine.

In true migraine, which is often hereditary, the initial symptoms (visual, sensory or motor) are due to constriction of retinal and cortical vessels, and the subsequent throbbing headache is caused by dilatation of extracranial vessels. Pain is prolonged by secondary muscular contraction of the scalp and probably by other factors such as cerebral oedema following the local extravasation of polypeptides. The whole process is initiated by some triggering mechanism which is commonly psychological, the patient often being tense, obsessional or worried. No single form of treatment is effective against all these factors and the successful management of the migrainous patient requires consideration of them all.

General management. The patient (usually a young woman) should be advised to regulate her life to avoid as far as possible the tensions or obsessions which may be recognized as precipitating factors. Many migrainous patients are highly intelligent professional or artistic people, and their headaches are manifestations of the intellectual commotion that is inseparable from creative work in a civilized community. Over-fatigue (physical and nervous) and indiscretions of diet should be avoided. Specific articles of food such as chocolate or bananas are blamed by some patients. The content of tryptamine may be important but there is no evidence that allergy is important as a causative factor. Factors such as nasal disorders, errors of refraction, gall bladder disease or menstrual disturbances may be of minor importance as 'triggers' in the predisposed subject, but the emotional factor is much the most important. Indeed it is sometimes difficult to decide whether headache should be classified as psychogenic, tension, or migrainous. If migraine is intensified by taking an oral contraceptive drug, an alternative method of contraception should be used. This is imperative if paraesthesia accompanies migraine, as the risk of a stroke is then increased.

Prophylaxis. Phenobarbitone and drugs of the phenothiazine series may be used to reduce the frequency of attacks. A tranquillizer with anti-emetic properties such as prochlorperazine (10 mg. once or twice daily) may be useful if taken regularly. Amitryptiline, prescribed for associated depression, may achieve striking reduction in the number and severity of migraine headaches. The prophylactic use of ergotamine is undesirable because of the danger of ergotism, but it may be necessary in severe cases. The risk is much smaller with methysergide which is the most effective prophyl-actic at present available. It is given in a dose of 1 to 2 mg. two or three times daily. Retroperitoneal fibrosis is a rare complication of this treatment. The risk is much reduced by withdrawing the drug for one month after each six months' period of use. Restriction of fluid and salt may be valuable, and the regular administration of urea as a diuretic may reduce the incidence of attacks.

Drugs. For the acute attack ergotamine is the most effective drug, but because of the risk of ergotism its use should be restricted to patients for whom no other therapy will suffice. Ergotamine is contraindicated in pregnancy and hypertension. Pethidine or morphine-like drugs should never be used owing to the danger of drug addiction.

Infrequent attacks of migraine are best treated with paracetamol, aspirin, caffeine, codeine or mixtures of these drugs. The patient should lie down in a quiet darkened room, if this is possible, until the attack subsides. If attacks are moderate but occur as frequently as once a week, it is advisable to use prochlorperazine or methysergide prophylactically and to take an extra dose at the earliest warning of an impending attack. More severe attacks may be treated by ergotamine administered orally. A tablet of ergotamine tartrate (1 mg.) should be allowed to dissolve under the tongue; the dose may be repeated in one to two hours. Nausea or vomiting—fairly frequent symptoms in migraine —may prevent the patient from swallowing and retaining ergotamine. The addition of an anti-emetic drug such as prochlorperazine or cyclizine is often effective, and some proprietary preparations of ergotamine are combined with cyclizine. Ergotamine is a vasoconstrictor drug and others with a similar activity on the cranial circulation—such as caffeine— may be used. One preparation containing both substances (Cafergot—Q) is prepared as a tablet for oral administration, and as a suppository which may be useful if vomiting is troublesome.

Another effective method of administration of ergotamine is to disperse it as an aerosol by means of a small nebulizer (Medihaler). This is a valuable method for ensuring rapid absorption. Few patients now require subcutaneous injection of ergotamine tartrate, but this is sometimes the only effective method. The patient should then be taught to give himself an injection of 0·25 to 0·5 mg. of the drug as soon as the attack begins.

In a few sufferers from migraine the symptoms do not progress beyond the phase of vasoconstriction. For such patients and for some resistant cases of the classical syndrome, a trial of nicotinic acid is worth while. An initial dose of 25 mg. should be increased

in successive attacks until a dose is reached which causes facial flushing. Thereafter this dose should be taken immediately there is a visual aura of an impending attack. Frusemide (p. 89) may also be taken at these times to promote diuresis. The prevention of cerebral oedema or hydraemia provides the rationale for this treatment, but there is no justification for the use of hormonal preparations.

VERTIGO

Dizziness is a common symptom of cerebral disturbances—some innocent, others serious. It does not have a localizing value. A sensation of rotation of the environment or of the patient's head is termed vertigo. This is indicative of a disorder of the labyrinthine mechanism in the ear or of its central connections. A sensation of falling in one direction without rotation has a similar significance. Both types of vestibular disturbances may be associated with organic disease of the ear, auditory nerve, or brain stem, or with Ménière's syndrome. Treatment of vertigo is symptomatic. Cyclizine tablets, 25 mg., three times a day, are often effective in controlling symptoms. Unfortunately the rapidity of onset of vertigo makes it virtually impossible to treat each attack as it arises and these drugs must be used regularly twice or three times daily if vertigo recurs frequently. Regular sedation with phenobarbitone may be effective.

Many sufferers from migraine find that their symptoms disappear about the age of 40, only to be replaced by labyrinthine vertigo. For this type, a trial of ergotamine tartrate—as in the treatment of migraine—is worth while. Conversely, the vasodilator drug nicotinic acid may be effective.

MÉNIÈRE'S DISEASE. Hydrops of the labyrinth is believed to be present in Ménière's syndrome. Mild progressive perceptive deafness is associated with brief paroxysms of severe vertigo, vomiting and, occasionally, transient loss of consciousness. The symptomatic treatment of vertigo is described above. When attacks are frequent it is justifiable to adopt procedures which tend to dehydrate the tissues. Thus, it is customary to prescribe a low-salt diet, and a diuretic such as chlorothiazide (500 mg. to 1 g. every second or third day) and ammonium chloride (500 mg. three times daily at meal times) may be given in alternating periods of three days.

In intractable cases of Ménière's disease the surgical procedure of sectioning the eighth nerve in the posterior fossa may be carried out, provided the disturbance can be traced to one internal ear and provided the other ear is intact. Selective ablation of the labyrinth with sparing of the cochlea may be achieved by an ultrasonic applicator.

VESTIBULAR NEURONITIS (*Epidemic Vertigo*). This disease is distinguishable from Ménière's disease by the absence of deafness. Sporadic cases are common. Epidemic occurrence suggests a viral origin. Treatment of vertigo is symptomatic. The disorder is usually self limiting but if imbalance persists, Cooksey exercises are helpful.

POSITIONAL VERTIGO. Vertigo and nystagmus which appears when the head is in a critical position may be due to a brainstem or labyrinthine disorder. Either form may occur after head injury. There is a benign form of unknown aetiology which tends to disappear gradually. Phenobarbitone provides symptomatic relief.

CEREBROVASCULAR DISEASE

Cerebral atherosclerosis. Generalized or local atrophy of the brain due to chronic ischaemia results from atherosclerosis of the cerebral vessels. Seizures, paresis, incontinence and dementia are common symptoms which should be treated as described in the previous sections. There is no effective method of increasing cerebral blood-flow.

STROKES

The treatment of acute cerebrovascular accidents is complicated by the difficulty of determining the exact nature of the underlying lesion. For this reason the practitioner may approach the subject empirically, differentiating cerebrovascular accidents into transient ischaemic attacks, a 'stroke-in-evolution', and a completed stroke.

Transient Ischaemic Attacks

This description is applied to episodes lasting from a few minutes to an hour due to temporary ischaemia of some part of the brain followed by full recovery. The particular symptoms and signs depend on the part of the brain which is temporarily deprived of sufficient blood to maintain its function. The common causes are embolism, stenosis of a major blood vessel such as carotid or vertebro-

basilar artery, hypertensive encephalopathy and, rarely, migraine.

Cerebral embolism. Recurrent cerebral embolism with transient ischaemia of a limited region of the brain may originate from platelet emboli separating from a thrombus attached to an atheromatous plaque in the internal carotid artery. Other sources of emboli are the left atrium in cases of mitral stenosis and of atrial fibrillation, especially when these two conditions are associated. A mural thrombus in the left ventricle following myocardial infarction is another common source.

If the source of emboli persists, anticoagulant treatment (p. 185) should be instituted immediately and continued indefinitely if the source cannot be removed. The danger of producing haemorrhage in the zone of cerebral infarction is minimal.

Carotid and Vertebrobasilar stenosis. Transient ischaemic attacks associated with stenosis of the carotid or vertebrobasilar artery, though often embolic, may also be precipitated by circulatory insufficiency in states of traumatic or post-operative shock, massive haematemesis, recent myocardial infarction and other causes of hypotension, including the administration of hypotensive drugs. Haematemesis may precipitate a stroke by inducing hypercoagulability of the blood. Early recognition of the neurological disturbance and correction of the hypotensive state may prevent permanent cerebral damage.

If the transient ischaemic attack has terminated, the further management to prevent recurrence must be considered. Transient cerebral ischaemia due to severe stenosis of a carotid artery should be treated by endarterectomy or an operation by-passing the affected segment of the artery, provided that full angiographic exploration shows adequate patency of the other extracranial arteries and the site of the lesion in the brain is in the area of distribution of the occluded artery. In patients with slight stenosis it is unlikely that such operations will be beneficial as the cerebral attacks are probably embolic in nature. Anticoagulant therapy (p. 185) is preferable. Its value is supported by careful clinical trials, but it is marginal and many physicians consider that the potential benefit does not justify the risk of cerebral or subdural haemorrhage. Logically anticoagulant therapy should be continued for life. In practice it can be discontinued six months after the last ischaemic attack. Withdrawal should be gradual over a period of six weeks to avoid rebound thrombo-embolic phenomena. The relative merits of radical and conservative measures are debatable when angiography reveals stenosis which is moderate in degree, but at present the results of operation are probably inferior to conservative management with anticoagulants.

The presence of hypertension complicates the management of transient ischaemic attacks. It is dangerous to give anticoagulant drugs until the blood pressure has been lowered by means of a hypotensive agent (p. 112). If the diastolic blood pressure is not allowed to fall below 100 mg. Hg. the combination of hypotensive and anticoagulant drugs is probably beneficial though the necessity for careful control of both forms of treatment simultaneously is difficult in practice.

Hypertensive encephalopathy. The treatment of hypertensive encephalopathy as a cause of transient ischaemic attacks is dealt with on p. 116.

Other causes. Less frequent causes of transient ischaemic attacks such as severe anaemia or polycythaemia require appropriate treatment. There is no evidence that vascular spasm, other than that associated with hypertensive encephalopathy, is a factor to be reckoned with. Contraceptive tablets containing oestrogen should be discontinued after a transient ischaemic attack.

Stroke-in-Evolution

When the patient still has signs of a neurological deficit such as hemiplegia or dysphasia when first seen by the doctor, it is important to decide whether the stroke is already complete or is still in evolution. This may be difficult; it calls for a comparison of the extent of the paralysis with what would have occurred if occlusion of the affected artery had been complete. Nevertheless, careful attention to the history and especially a comparison of the physical signs with those recorded earlier by colleagues may enable the physician to recognize that the loss of cerebral neurones is still proceeding. This is the only type of stroke requiring emergency treatment, the results of which in patients under the age of 60 (constituting half of all cerebrovascular accidents) may be very rewarding.

It is in these circumstances that the differential diagnosis of the cause of the stroke is particularly important. The prevalent belief that the slowly progressive stroke is always due to thrombosis is mistaken; and the routine use of anticoagulant therapy based on this assumption will have unfortunate results.

Cerebral infarction is the most common cause of a stroke-in-evolution. Some of the later clinical deterioration is due to cerebral oedema, causing brain stem compression and this is amenable to treatment (p. 400). Clinical trials of anticoagulant therapy in patients with evolving strokes indicate that cerebral damage is limited compared with those untreated. Nevertheless, there is a real risk of cerebral haemorrhage which is only minimized by careful laboratory control of the prothrombin level of the blood. The present consensus of opinion is against the use of anticoagulants within three weeks of non-embolic infarction.

If the stroke has a 'stuttering' onset or is accompanied by loss of carotid pulsation, a bruit over the artery, or Horner's syndrome contralateral to the hemiplegia, it is likely that the infarction is due to progressive stenosis of the internal carotid artery, probably with secondary thrombosis. In these circumstances it is necessary to consider endarterectomy.

Cerebral haemorrhage is a less common cause of a slowly progressive stroke than is infarction, but the possibility should be considered before prescribing anticoagulants. If there is neck stiffness or a blood-stained cerebrospinal fluid they should certainly not be given, though the absence of these signs does not exclude intracerebral haemorrhage. Echo-encephalographic or radiological evidence of a pineal shift may be valuable clues where these investigations are feasible, but without angiography a firm diagnosis may be impossible.

Steadily progressive neurological signs are not due to rupture of nerve fibres by continuing bleeding. The osmotic effect of a small haematoma causes it to attract fluid and expand by displacement of nerve fibres. Aspiration of the liquefied clot by a cannula inserted through a trephine opening in the skull may lead to gratifying recovery from such serious symptoms as aphasia and hemiplegia.

Subdural haematoma. When the history suggests that an injury to the head may have been the cause rather than the result of the stroke, the possibility of subdural haemorrhage must be considered. If the diagnosis is confirmed, aspiration is immediately indicated. If, after a head injury, there has been temporary recovery of consciousness followed by deterioration and the onset of unconsciousness, a clinical diagnosis of extradural haemorrhage due to fracture of the skull is inescapable. The findings call for an immediate radiograph of the skull and the advice of a surgeon, otherwise the patient may die within a few hours.

Completed Stroke

Assessment of the situation at the onset of a stroke has been considered at some length because the correct management at that time may determine the degree of subsequent disability or even the survival of the patient. This does not apply to the patient who, when he is first seen by the doctor, already has a completed stroke. In this instance, the first step is to nurse him into a suitable state for rehabilitation. The second is to take any necessary action to prevent further strokes in other vascular territories; but at this stage it is useless to try to deal surgically with a completely stenosed carotid artery or to institute anticoagulant therapy for an acute non-embolic infarction already involving the whole distribution of the thrombosed vessel. Evacuation of an intracerebral haematoma may reduce disability; but the decision to undertake this may be postponed for careful evaluation; there is not here the element of urgency which is inseparable from the management of the progressive stroke (p. 396).

General Management

If the patient is conscious he should be placed in bed in the position which he finds comfortable, a paralysed limb being supported with pillows to prevent subluxation of the shoulder and other joints. Headache, which is commonly present, should be treated with aspirin or paracetamol, but no stronger analgesic should be used as it is necessary to note spontaneous changes of consciousness during the first one or two days. If he is unconscious he should be nursed in the semi-prone position with the head lowered to ensure drainage of fluid from the mouth and pharynx. Since many of these patients vomit, it is necessary to aspirate all foreign matter from the pharynx with a sucker or, failing this, with a gauze swab. The tongue must be prevented from falling back. An airway, preferably of cuffed type, should be inserted; and if this is not sufficient to permit unobstructed breathing, there should be no hesitation in carrying out tracheostomy if the prognosis is reasonably good. The measures already described for the management of the unconscious patient should then be instituted (p. 385).

Physiotherapy for the paralysed limbs should be started at once. Every joint should be moved passively through its full range of movement at least twice a day in order to prevent subsequent development of 'frozen shoulder' and similar syndromes. These movements are continued until active movement becomes possible. When the patient is able to sit up in bed he should be taught to use his unaffected hand to carry the paralysed one round behind his back and up behind his head, and to extend the paralysed fingers. Later he should be provided with a sling and pulley, fixed to the wall behind his bed or chair, by which he can raise the paralysed arm by pulling on a cord with his good one. This is a simple but valuable device readily assembled in his own home. The further management of the hemiplegic patient is described on p. 372. When the patient is able to sit up in bed unsupported and without undue giddiness he should be encouraged to get into a chair for increasing periods, and then to walk with assistance. These activities should be embarked upon as soon as possible. Speech therapy may be valuable for the dysphasic patient as soon as he becomes alert and aware of his environment. If it is possible for the therapist to establish communication with the patient, some restoration of speech may be hoped for, although full recovery is only possible when the speech mechanism is not directly involved by necrosis of cerebral tissue.

If a patient survives a stroke he should be capable of a reasonably active life after a few months but only if rehabilitation is started early and in this the occupational therapist plays an important rôle.

Subarachnoid Haemorrhage and Intracranial Aneurysm

Bleeding into the subarachnoid space occurs in many cases of intracerebral haemorrhage, and a clinical stroke due to rupture of cerebral tissue is not uncommon in haemorrhage from intracranial aneurysms. Nevertheless, the management of haemorrhage from a ruptured aneurysm within the skull is sufficiently distinctive to justify separate treatment. If an aneurysm is suspected and confirmed by angiography, it may be desirable to ligate the artery supplying it if this can be done with impunity. The decision to operate depends on a balanced assessment of the risks of potential haemorrhage as against the technical difficulties of surgery and the possible ill-effects of ligation of a major artery. The decision is never a simple one, and a diagnosis of intracranial aneurysm is not necessarily followed by a recommendation for surgical treatment.

When an aneurysm bleeds into the subarachnoid

space or brain tissue the immediate treatment is that of intracerebral haemorrhage, coupled with the management of the comatose patient (p. 385). There is no indication for emergency surgery to stop the bleeding. The special feature of bleeding from an aneurysm is the liability for recurrent haemorrhage during the following two weeks; and the mortality rate from a second haemorrhage is high. The aim of treatment is to minimize this risk. After three weeks the chance of recurrent haemorrhage is much less and after six weeks it is so slight that surgical treatment is unnecessary. Aneurysms, however, are often multiple. If angiography shows this to be the case, preventive surgery may still be desirable at a later date.

Most of the problems calling for careful judgment and decision are likely to present themselves during the first two weeks. Surgical intervention in the first 48 hours carries a high mortality; and if the patient is in coma operation should rarely be considered. If the patient regains consciousness, angiography should be undertaken forthwith. When the aneurysm can be localized the appropriate surgical measures should be adopted as soon as possible. Clinical judgment is crucial to success: premature operation is undoubtedly dangerous, but at this stage postponement carries the risk of a further haemorrhage and this is likely to be fatal. Conservative (non-surgical) management should not be regarded as the treatment of choice in the three weeks following the haemorrhage. After this time the risk of further bleeding diminishes rapidly and by the sixth week the risk is remote. Not all of the patients investigated during the first fortnight are considered suitable for operation; in particular cases the technical hazards create risks equal to, or greater than, those of conservative management. The surgical risk may be diminished by cooling the patient to hypothermic levels, but even so the mortality from ruptured aneurysm of the anterior communicating artery or the proximal part of the anterior cerebral artery is not reduced by surgical operation.

If conservative management is preferred for technical reasons or because it is impossible to get skilled neurosurgical treatment, the patient should be nursed in bed as advised in the section on the completed stroke. The bowels should be kept loose to avoid straining at stool. The patient may be allowed out of bed for increasing periods in the third week, followed by convalescence for three or four weeks. If a significant degree of arterial

hypertension is discovered it is advisable to institute long-term hypotensive therapy after the first week (p. 112), as hypertension is a common aetiological factor.

Cerebral Venous Thrombosis

Thrombosis of the intracranial venous sinuses and cerebral veins is associated with (i) a thrombophlebitis, spreading from an infection of the middle ear, accessory nasal sinuses, face and scalp; (ii) thrombotic and dehydrated states such as occur in polycythaemia, the puerperium, and cachectic conditions in infancy and old age; (iii) head injury without penetration of the skin. The signs vary according to the site of the thrombosed vessel but include lesions of the 3rd, 4th, 6th, 7th and 8th cranial nerves, unilateral or bilateral cortical damage, focal epilepsy and raised intracranial pressure.

Thrombophlebitis associated with infection should be treated with the appropriate antibiotic, and rehydration should be achieved with all possible speed. Anticoagulant therapy should be started except where haemorrhagic infarction of the brain has occurred—indicated by a blood-stained cerebrospinal fluid on lumbar puncture. In patients suffering from thrombosis of the lateral and sagittal sinuses the main problem arises from raised intracranial pressure; this is due to interference with absorption of the cerebrospinal fluid and it may progress to hydrocephalus (communicating hydrocephalus). This is one type of benign intracranial hypertenstion and its treatment is outlined below.

HYDROCEPHALUS

There are four types of hydrocephalus. (i) The first is a sequel to cerebral atrophy, whatever its aetiology. Intracranial pressure is not raised and no treatment is required. (ii) A more serious condition is obstructive hydrocephalus due to blockage of cerebrospinal fluid drainage. The intracerebral ventricles are passively distended, the intracranial pressure rises (sometimes rapidly), the patient lapses into coma, and death is inevitable unless the fluid is allowed to escape from the ventricles. This type of hydrocephalus is caused by a cyst or tumour within the third or fourth ventricle, by blocking of the aqueduct of Sylvius (congenital stenosis or compression by a tumour of the brain stem), or by adhesions around the foramina by which CSF drains from the fourth ventricle into the subarachnoid space. Adhesions of the meninges at the base of the brain may similarly obstruct the flow of CSF in the subarachnoid space; this is commonly a complication of meningitis due to pyogenic infection; it illustrates the importance of giving prompt curative treatment before the meningeal inflammatory exudate can undergo organization.

The effect of obstructive hydrocephalus depends on the age of the patient. In infancy, before the cranial sutures have firmly fused, the result differs from that produced by comparable lesions in later life. The younger the patient, the greater is the characteristic ballooning of the skull above the level of the eyes and ears and the smaller the absolute increase in intracranial pressure. If the sutures have not united, gradual expansion of the volume of the skull may occur with little or no impairment of intellect and cranial nerve function. Increase of intracranial pressure may cause incompletely united sutures to separate and compensate slightly for the increase. If the cranial vault is unyielding, the rise in pressure soon interferes with cerebral function; medullary coning may occur and may constitute a serious surgical emergency. When hydrocephalus expands the ventricular system, spontaneous cure may sometimes follow rupture of the lamina terminalis; the free communication between the intraventricular system and subarachnoid space thus established may restore hydrostatic equilibrium. Careful measurements of the cranial dimensions should be recorded monthly in the case of the hydrocephalic child.

The neurosurgeon's advice should be sought in all these cases, because he may be able to re-establish the cerebrospinal fluid circulation by the operation of third ventriculostomy, or by draining the lateral ventricles into the jugular vein by a one-way valve such as the Spitz-Holter or the Pudenz type. The operation devised by Torkildsen of draining the ventricles into the cisterna magna should probably be restricted to cases of hydrocephalus caused by non-inflammatory blockage of the aqueduct of Sylvius. In communicating hydrocephalus the spinal theca may be anastomosed to the peritoneal cavity. One word of warning should be given: when the brain is expanded and the cortex is a mere shell, sudden collapse of the ventricular system may tear the small veins which traverse the subarachnoid space from the brain to the superior longitudinal sinus, with the formation of a subdural haematoma.

Mechanical stretching of the cerebral hemispheres may impair function and give rise to a picture resembling congenital cerebral palsy (p. 373). In some cases intellectual capacity is preserved and development continues—very necessary requirements for co-operation in treatment. Owing to prolonged pressure on and thinning out of the infundibular region of the third ventricle, endocrine imbalance may follow. Thus some hydrocephalics become giants and some dwarfs. The writer does not know of any rational or useful treatment for these complications.

(iii) The third type of hydrocephalus is due to failure of resorption of cerebrospinal fluid. Since there is no obstruction to the circulation of the fluid it is named communicating hydrocephalus. The Pacchionian corpuscles may be blocked by exudate after meningitis or by blood clot after a severe subarachnoid haemorrhage (the latter cause is too rare to warrant repeated spinal drainage in the treatment of subarachnoid haemorrhage). Absorption of CSF is temporarily impaired when thrombosis occurs in the upper chamber of the superior sagittal sinus—sometimes a sequel to the spread of clot from a lateral sinus which is thrombosed because of adjacent infection in the middle ear. This kind of hydrocephalus is, therefore, called otitic hydrocephalus.

It is doubtful if anticoagulant therapy alters the course of the illness. Fortunately the raised intracranial pressure is rarely severe enough to cause drowsiness or coma; drainage eventually re-establishes itself and spontaneous recovery is the rule. This type of intracranial hypertension is classed as benign, but it does cause headache and papilloedema, and if allowed to persist permanent loss of vision may occur. It is permissible to wait for the condition to subside while treating the primary otitis media and the headache, provided that the visual fields are charted carefully at intervals of not more than a week. If the blind spot in one of the visual fields begins to enlarge, the intracranial pressure must be reduced. Although as a general principle a lumbar puncture is contraindicated in the presence of papilloedema, it is in this instance the treatment of choice. It should be carried out daily with a fine needle and the cerebrospinal fluid allowed to escape slowly until the pressure measured with a manometer has dropped to 100 mm. of water. When the papilloedema has subsided the interval between the lumbar punctures is gradually increased. The supervision of the visual fields must continue for at least a further month. If deterioration of vision continues despite daily taps, or if these are still necessary after three weeks, it may be advisable to carry out a decompressive operation.

There is an important type of hydrocephalus in which the cause of malabsorption of CSF is unknown: it is associated with dilatation of the ventricular system, minimal cortical atrophy, but little or no rise in intracranial pressure. The principal clinical signs are progressive dementia and extrapyramidal signs. Recognition is important as these signs rapidly resolve if cerebrospinal fluid drainage is carried out by one of the surgical methods described above.

CEREBRAL TUMOUR

All cerebral tumours whether benign or malignant, primary or secondary, cause three groups of symptoms, differing in detail according to the site and type of the tumour.

(i) Destruction of neurones causes contralateral upper motor neurone paralysis, sensory loss or hemianopia, and a lesion of the dominant hemisphere may cause dysphasia. Change of personality or progressive dementia may be due to a frontal lobe tumour. The loss of function does not differ from that caused by other types of lesions and the management of these symptoms has already been discussed.

(ii) Epilepsy is often an early manifestation of a malignant cerebral tumour, or a continuing symptom of a benign one such as a meningioma or an angioma. This may be *focal* in type, including the Jacksonian seizure, or *diffuse* (grand mal). Cerebral tumour must always be considered as a cause of epilepsy occurring for the first time after the age of 25. The fits are treated symptomatically as described on p. 381. Removal of the tumour may abolish epilepsy, but unfortunately it does not always do so.

(iii) The third group of symptoms is due to raised intracranial pressure. Headache is often most noticeable on waking, since pressure increases in the recumbent position. In the early stage it responds well to aspirin or paracetamol, but in the later stages the simpler analgesics are inadequate. Opium derivatives and other drugs which depress respiration should be avoided until it is certain that no cure is possible, as hypercapnia causes a further rise in intracranial pressure.

Dehydration therapy. The only effective treatment of pressure symptoms such as vomiting, visual failure due to papilloedema, and progressive drowsiness is to lower the intracranial pressure. This must never be done by lumbar puncture as this may cause a 'pressure cone' with fatal consequences. If it is necessary to lower the intracranial pressure while awaiting operation, intramuscular injection of betamethasone, 10 mg., followed by 4 mg. orally every six hours is valuable. In more urgent circumstances, frusemide, 40 mg. or a hypertonic solution can be injected intravenously to produce rapid diuresis and to dehydrate the brain. The most satisfactory substances are urea and mannitol. Urea is injected as a 30 per cent. solution in 10 per cent. glucose. The dose is 1 to 1·5 g. per kg. of body weight. During the injection none of the fluid must be allowed to escape around the vein. Many neurosurgeons now prefer to use mannitol, 0·5 to 1·0 litre of a 25 per cent. solution intravenously. If neither of these substances is available, glucose (50 ml. of 50 per cent. solution) may be used with the same precautions, but it carries the disadvantage that its action is brief and may be followed by an exacerbation of the cerebral oedema. The only

justification for the use of dehydration therapy is to gain time so that essential investigations may be completed or preparations made for surgical operation.

Surgical treatment. There is seldom any point in dealing surgically with a metastatic tumour of the brain but it may be worth while to remove a solitary metastasis in the cerebellum or in the frontal lobe. In most cases of metastasis and in all cases of malignant glioma, treatment is palliative unless a complete lobectomy is possible. A short history and extensive focal signs of tumour diminish the prospect of surgical relief. This hope is further reduced if mental confusion and general emaciation accompany the rapid development of neurological signs. Such patients should not be submitted to operation. Dysphasia and weakness of the limbs controlled by the dominant cerebral hemisphere are bad prognostic signs and deep tumours involving the thalamic region or infiltrating the brain stem defy a surgical approach.

Once it has been decided that a full neurosurgical investigation of a tumour should be undertaken the onus of care lies with the neurosurgeon. The growth may be removed or it may be investigated further by arteriography or ventriculography. Some tumours so investigated are found to be unsuitable for operation.

Radiotherapy, however, may still be possible. Irradiation undoubtedly has its place in the treatment of certain cerebral neoplasms, and some are too vascular to remove. Glioblastoma multiforme will shrink with radiation, but relief from symptoms is so short-lived that it is inexpedient to irradiate this type of growth. Certain meningiomas respond well to deep radiotherapy, and this form of treatment should be applied when surgical removal would sacrifice the intellect and motor power. Results from irradiation of ependymal, pineal and oligodendroglial tumours are varied; although opinion is divided, radiotherapy is frequently the only therapeutic weapon worthy of trial. Before it can be undertaken, localization may have to be proved by ventriculography, and decompression of the brain carried out. Reactive oedema to radiotherapy is common in the treatment of tumours in other sites, and presumably neoplasms of the brain do not differ in this respect from those elsewhere. Further increase of intracranial pressure from irradiation may have disastrous results unless room for expansion has been assured. Although the radiation of a cerebral tumour may be brilliantly successful, overdosage may occasion post-radiation necrosis and transform the patient's life into a vegetative existence. The methods used in decompression operations are matters for the neurosurgeon.

SEQUELS TO HEAD INJURY

Generally speaking, the treatment of traumatic lesions is the concern of the surgeon. After surgical treatment—or when no surgery has been necessary—it falls to the physician to deal with residual disabilities. At no time has the importance of clear thinking about head injuries been greater than at present. The risks in industry and on the highway are increasing and legal actions for reparation do not diminish in a welfare state. Genuine claims are often justified, but frequently demands for compensation spring from cupidity. Unfortunately the malingerer has prejudiced the attitude of medical, legal and insurance experts to the general problem of head injuries, with the result that many a genuine victim is given short shrift by all three. Satisfactory settlement through the agencies of law and insurance is a part of treatment to which the physician must make his contribution. There is no uniform principle involved, so great is the variety of sequels to a head injury. After trifling injury the psychological consequences may be of major significance even in the absence of residual organic damage. After very severe injury resulting in prolonged unconsciousness, psychological overlay may be entirely absent in spite of a profound organic psychosis. The anxiety of those who face the prospect of litigation is aggravated by their having to wait a long time (often years rather than months) before their cases are heard in the Courts. The outcome in these circumstances is often deplorable. Post-concussional symptoms of any severity and duration are unlikely to improve pending the process of legal proof, and it is inadvisable to attempt psychotherapy until final settlement is made, for while waiting there is every reason for the patient to remain ill. A sense of grievance engenders self-pity, which is followed by the development of a post-traumatic neurosis, the magnitude of which must match the size of the sum claimed. Every effort must be made for a true assessment as soon as possible, and not the least important part of treatment is to expedite ultimate settlement in so far as the physician is able.

Post-concussional syndrome. The term concussion is an arbitrary one and is best restricted to signify brief loss of consciousness immediately following a head injury. No one will put a time limit to the duration of loss of consciousness in defining the term concussion. It is, therefore, difficult to mark the point in time beyond which continued loss of consciousness denotes cerebral contusion. By definition the post-concussional state is a sequel to loss of consciousness from head injury. It is surprising, however, to note the wealth of symptoms which may occur after a head injury not accompanied by loss of consciousness, the symptoms of which bear a strong resemblance to the generally accepted description of the post-concussional state. No doctor can be in a position to help such patients unless he appreciates this. Light-headedness, giddiness on stooping or alteration of posture, intolerance of heights, and headache resist the doctor's most emphatic reassurance to his patient that these symptoms are of no morbid significance. In the early days after concussion such assurance is very important when head movement exercises are given and may prove uncomfortable.

Extradural haemorrhage. Apart from the common picture of the post-concussional state, other residua may follow head injury either as immediate, late or remote manifestations. The most immediate threat, apart from the effects of contusion, is extradural haemorrhage from tearing of the middle meningeal artery. This constitutes a surgical emergency. With progressive deepening of unconsciousness and dilatation of the pupil on the side of the haemorrhage prompt operative treatment is indicated. Decerebrate rigidity resulting from 'coning' is a sign that treatment is a matter of extreme urgency if the patient's life is to be saved.

Subdural haematoma. Operation is required, but less urgently, when there are indications of subdural haematoma from rupture of veins which traverse the subarachnoid space. The correct treatment of this condition depends entirely on accuracy of diagnosis. Too often subdural haematoma is wrongly diagnosed as cerebral thrombosis, uraemia or diabetic ketosis. Coma may occur in all these conditions, but subdural haematoma in common with cerebral thrombosis may cause palsy; and albuminuria occurs with uraemia, and glycosuria with diabetes. If the possibility of subdural haematoma is not considered in the diagnosis of coma of obscure origin, mistakes will be made occasionally and life may be endangered. It must be remembered that subdural haematoma may follow comparatively slight head injury without any loss of consciousness at the time of injury and is more liable to occur in the aged, in the arteriosclerotic and in cases of cerebral atrophy from whatever cause. The insidious march of symptoms such as headache, personality change, disorientation, dilatation of the pupil on the side of the haematoma, contralateral hemiparesis and later decerebrate rigidity are indications for exploration by trephining. Fluctuation in the mental state, variations in the depth of coma and the history of a head injury two or three months previously suggest the possibility of subdural haematoma when a clinical picture is present with any combination of the signs and symptoms described.

Late sequels. The later and permanent sequels to head injury—dementia, aphasia and epilepsy—are considered elsewhere. It is good practice in cases of head injury to give maintenance doses of phenobarbitone sufficiently large to prevent convulsions.

INFECTIONS OF THE CENTRAL NERVOUS SYSTEM

The parenchyma, coverings and blood vessels of the nervous system may be invaded by various microorganisms—bacterial, viral, fungal or protozoal. The specific treatment does not differ from infection by these organisms in other parts of the body. There is, however, a special difficulty in obtaining an adequate therapeutic level of many drugs at the site of infection because of the blood–brain barrier. For convenience of description it is customary to divide the syndromes produced according to the chief site of involvement, though few infective processes are confined to one tissue.

With the exception of infection introduced directly as the result of open injury to the skull or spinal column, infection of the central nervous system is blood-borne. Thus meningitis or cerebral abscess may be secondary to septicaemia or to bacteraemia originating in a septic focus elsewhere in the body, notably in the lungs. Loculations of pus anywhere are a potential source of danger, no matter how well encapsulated they may be. Infections within the drainage area of veins entering the skull or the paravertebral plexus of veins are particularly dangerous. Osteomyelitis of the skull or spine, paranasal sinusitis and infections of the face and middle ear, cause intracranial infection by the spread of thrombophlebitis to the brain rather than by the more obvious route of direct spread. Pelvic sepsis, though seemingly remote from the nervous system, has similar dangers.

Bacterial Infection

Leptomeningitis. This is due to infection by bacteria and is readily treatable if an appropriate antibiotic is given in adequate dose by the proper route as soon as possible. Treatment is described on p. 2. Failure to give such treatment may result in permanent damage to the brain, spinal cord, and cranial nerves by encephalitis, myelitis, infarction or adhesions at the base of the brain. The last of these may interfere with the free circulation of cerebrospinal fluid and cause hydrocephalus (p. 398). The effectiveness of corticosteroids and PPD tuberculin in preventing adhesions in tuberculous meningitis has not yet been fully assessed.

Suppurative encephalitis (*Cerebral Abscess*). Acute suppurative encephalitis is treated by immediate intramuscular injection of benzylpenicillin, two million units followed by one million units four hourly. Surgical assistance should be sought early and the abscess which soon develops must be localized by electro-encephalography and angiography. A cerebral cannula should then be introduced to aspirate pus and instil antibiotics. Most surgeons favour initial intramuscular injection of a mixture of crystalline penicillin and streptomycin, but antibiotic therapy is subsequently determined by the bacteriological findings and the sensitivity of the causal organism.

Myodil, a radio-opaque iodine compound, is also instilled so that progress may be followed by serial radiography. Measures to reduce intracranial pressure may also be required (p. 400). Excision of the abscess may be necessary, but the indications and contraindications for this are technical matters for the neurosurgeon which need not be discussed here. There is a high incidence of symptomatic epilepsy during the phase of acute pyogenic encephalitis, and this may persist even after excision of an abscess. All patients should, therefore, be given phenobarbitone prophylactically (30 mg. three times daily) for a minimum period of two years after the acute phase. During this time the patient should be under close surveillance since recurrence of infection is not uncommon and may be delayed.

Cranial or spinal epidural abscess. This is treated on similar lines. It is an emergency in which early treatment may prevent permanent paraplegia. Once transverse myelitis has appeared with spinal epidural abscess, the prognosis for recovery is poor since the cord is softened as a result of secondary thrombosis of the spinal vessels. Treatment must start as soon as suspicion is aroused by the onset of fever and by pain in the back or in the distribution of a spinal nerve root in a patient who has recently had an infection of the skin or other part of the body. Two million units (1·2 g.) of benzylpenicillin should immediately be given intramuscularly followed by one million units 600 mg.) four-hourly. The patient must be transferred to the care of a neurosurgeon at the earliest possible moment for surgical drainage by laminectomy.

Neurosyphilis. Syphilis of the nervous system gives rise to the well-known clinical syndromes of meningovascular syphilis, dementia paralytica, tabes dorsalis and primary optic atrophy, but these divisions are not absolute. Parenchymatous damage, characterizing the last three groups, is irreversible and treatment can only be symptomatic. Endarteritis obliterans, lepto- and pachy-meningitis, and gummatous granuloma can be arrested or reduced in extent by vigorous anti-syphilitic treatment (p. 600).

Fungal, Protozoal and Rickettsial Infection

Fungal infection. Although these are rare in Britain, fungal meningitis, cerebral abscess or granuloma are becoming more common—perhaps on account of the increasing use of antibacterial agents and corticosteroids which promote the proliferation of pathogenic fungi. The most common of these is *Cryptococcus neoformans*. Fungal infection should be considered as a possibility if a patient suffering from chronic meningitis or cerebral abscess deteriorates progressively during antibiotic therapy; the diagnosis should also be considered when meningitis supervenes in patients with diabetes mellitus or a reticulosis. Anti-fungal agents such as amphotericin B are worth a trial. An initial dose of 1 to 5 mg. in 500 ml. of 5 per cent. dextrose is given intravenously over a period of about six hours. Injections are repeated on alternate days with gradually increasing doses until a total of 3 g. has been given. The course may be repeated if there is a relapse. Nausea and fever are common toxic reactions. The addition of heparin to the drip has been recommended to prevent thrombophlebitis at the site of injection. A less toxic drug which may be equally effective is 5-fluorocytosine; the dose is 100 to 200 mg. per kg. body weight given by mouth for 6 to 8 weeks.

Cerebral malaria. The possibility of cerebral malaria arises in a patient who, after returning from a malarial country, develops an acute illness complicated by cerebral symptoms, drowsiness and coma. Its treatment is described on p. 511.

Toxoplasmosis. Toxoplasmosis is endemic in this country though symptomatic forms are rare. Congenital and acquired forms are seen, involving the eyes, central nervous system, muscles, liver and spleen. The neurological lesion is an encephalitis which may be associated with disseminated small foci of calcification in the brain, demonstrable radiologically. A combination of a sulphonamide, 1 g. six-hourly, with pyrimethamine, 25 mg. daily for two weeks, may be effective in the treatment of both the congenital and the acquired forms, but the prognosis is poor in children and survivors show persistent mental and neurological defects.

Cysticercosis. The brain and meninges may be the seat of cysticercosis. This disease is the result of encystment in the tissues of the larvae of a tapeworm, *Taenia solium*, derived from infested pork. The cysts may be the cause of symptomatic epilepsy which should be treated in the usual way (p. 381). Hydrocephalus may also require treatment (p. 398). Single cysts can sometimes be removed surgically. There is no effective treatment for the larval infestation.

Rickettsial infection. Most rickettsial infections such as typhus fever, scrub typhus, and Q fever cause meningo-encephalitis. Their treatment is described on pp. 520–21.

Viral Infections

Some viruses are naturally 'neurotropic' and invade the nervous system causing necrosis of cells with reactive inflammation and perivascular cuffing. Each virus has a predilection for a particular type of nerve cell, for example the anterior horn cell in poliomyelitis and the posterior root ganglion cell in herpes zoster; but occasionally the invasion is widespread and results in meningo-encephalitis of various types. It is doubtful if a true infection of peripheral nerves by viruses occurs. Other viruses which characteristically attack viscera may occasionally invade the nervous system, such as the viruses of mumps and infective hepatitis. More commonly, inflammatory disease of the brain. spinal cord, or peripheral nerves may be associated with viral disease elsewhere; in such circumstances there is loss of myelin of the central or peripheral nervous system due to delayed allergy, whereas a primary virus disease of the nervous system destroys nerve cells.

Viral meningitis. In Britain this is now the most common type of meningitis. Alternative names are acute lymphocytic choriomeningitis and benign lymphocytic meningitis, emphasizing the good prognosis and the nature of the cellular reaction in the cerebrospinal fluid. There is no specific treatment; headache can be relieved with aspirin. The patient should be kept at rest in bed until the temperature has returned to normal.

Viral encephalitis. In this country the viruses responsible for encephalitis are usually those of herpes simplex, influenza, ECHO or poliomyelitis. The virus is seldom isolated from patients, but the diagnosis is established by serological studies. In other parts of the world, rabies (p. 528), yellow fever (p. 527), and other locally endemic diseases may be the cause. Symptoms vary according to the relative extent of the inflammation of the cerebral cortex and of the grey matter in the brain stem.

There is no specific anti-viral treatment for most of these infections, but for encephalitis due to herpes simplex early intravenous infusion of idoxuridine (500 mg. per kg. in dextrose saline) may be valuable. Skilled nursing is required during the pyrexial phase and especially if the patient is delirious or comatose. Aspirin or paracetamol may be required for headache and sedatives may be needed for restlessness. If the sleep rhythm is interrupted, it may be necessary to prescribe amphetamine during the day as for narcolepsy (p. 385) and a hypnotic drug at night, but these measures should be postponed until it is obvious that spontaneous recovery is unlikely. If the basal ganglia are involved, it may be necessary to treat a Parkinsonian state at this time, but more commonly the symptoms of postencephalitic Parkinsonism emerge months or years later (p. 376). Hyperpyrexia due to damage of the thermoregulatory centres may endanger life if it is not treated (p. 389), and attention must be directed to the maintenance of normal water and electrolyte balance.

Acute anterior poliomyelitis. The prophylaxis and management of this disease are described on p. 45

Herpes zoster. The zoster virus, which is antigenically identical with chickenpox virus, invades the cells of posterior root ganglia and, less commonly, the grey matter of the spinal cord and brain. The symptomatic treatment of the condition is described on p. 583.

The virus of herpes zoster may invade the central nervous system causing myelitis or encephalitis; but when focal signs or diffuse symmetrical polyneuropathy (motor as well as sensory) develop late in the course of the disease, these should be regarded as manifestations of delayed allergy. Corticosteroids may be helpful for this type of complication, but their use should be postponed until the rash has disappeared. It should also be remembered that 'symptomatic herpes' may develop when a posterior root becomes involved in a reticulosis or is the site of a primary lesion such as a neuroma.

THE DEMYELINATING DISEASES

The myelin sheath of axons within the central nervous system may be damaged as a secondary result of disease of the nerve cells or their axons. The primary demyelinating diseases are those in which myelin breaks down while the axon is intact and the latter is only secondarily affected. It is uncertain whether the diseases so grouped have anything in common other than the primary demyelination which is their pathological characteristic.

Acute Disseminated Encephalomyelitis

This is a disease in which areas of inflammation with demyelination occur in the white matter of the brain and spinal cord. It may occur spontaneously or after one of the exanthematous diseases such as measles, rubella, or chickenpox. An apparently identical disease may follow primary vaccination against smallpox. It is considered that the postexanthematous and post-vaccinial types are due to a sensitivity reaction. A similar disorder may occur in serum sickness. The spontaneous type is probably of the same nature and may be the result of viral infection of the respiratory system. Headache, vomiting, pyrexia, delirium and meningism are common features calling for symptomatic treatment.

Transverse myelitis may occur and is often associated with bilateral retrobulbar neuritis. This syndrome is known as neuromyelitis optica (Devic's disease). Retention of urine is a frequent complication in the spinal type of this disease; it should be treated as described on p. 387. Paraplegia or quadriplegia are treated as described on pp. 372-375.

Acute disseminated encephalomyelitis and its variants may respond to treatment with corticotrophin (80 to 120 units intramuscularly), or prednisolone by mouth, 60 mg. daily for one week and reduced to a maintenance dose for two or three weeks. The response to treatment is often disappointing but this may be because it is often started too late. In the cerebellar type of encephalomyelitis which is characteristic of chickenpox, corticosteroids should not be used until the rash has subsided as they may cause the skin lesions to become confluent and haemorrhagic. If neurological signs persist after three weeks, they are likely to be permanent, and the continued administration of corticosteroids is valueless. In some cases of the spontaneous disease, especially in Devic's syndrome, evidence of further demyelination may occur at a later date. These cases are indistinguishable from disseminated sclerosis.

Disseminated Sclerosis

This is the most common type of demyelinating disease. Its aetiology is unknown but some clinical and pathological resemblances with acute disseminated encephalomyelitis have suggested that there may be an immunological factor. For this reason, and to inhibit the gliosis following inflammation which is the main reason for permanent loss of function, there has been widespread use of similar forms of therapy. There is now general agreement that corticosteroids are valueless; but corticotrophin seems to have a limited use in acute relapses of the disease. A relapse characterized by retrobulbar neuritis, spasticity, or vertigo appears to remit more rapidly if corticotrophin is given in large doses. The response of brain stem signs such as diplopia and nystagmus is less favourable and ataxia is seldom diminished. Indeed the remission of spasticity of the lower limbs may aggravate the disability attributable to ataxia. It is doubtful whether treatment with corticotrophin alters the end results of the disease, but the shortening of the period of acute disability during relapses is worth while and justifies the use of the drug. There is no evidence that long-term treatment is of any value. It is necessary to give high doses for a short period followed by a gradual reduction. A suitable regimen is 60 units of corticotrophin gel intramuscularly twice daily for one week, followed by 40 units twice daily during the second week, and 60, 40 and 20 units daily for periods of three days. A maintenance dose of 10 units daily is then given for two or three weeks. No other form of drug therapy is effective in disseminated sclerosis. Cyanocobalamin is useless.

The patient may be made more comfortable by judicious use of symptomatic forms of treatment for spasticity (p. 374), ataxia (p. 378), and defective control of the bladder (p. 387). The avoidance of urinary infection is particularly important as an exacerbation of spasticity may be the sequel to cystitis and not to a sudden extension of demyelination. The general management of the patient is also important. Regular exercise (not necessarily formal physiotherapy) is valuable provided the patient avoids fatigue. Emotional stress, extremes of heat and cold, and infections of any sort are harmful and may precipitate a relapse. The patient should never try to 'fight off a cold' but should at once go to bed until the infection has subsided. Normal activities should then be resumed within a few days, as rest in bed has the undesirable effect of increasing ataxia if this is present. The patient with disseminated sclerosis must steer a middle course between too much activity and too little. The best guide is his own sense of well-being. He should be encouraged to undertake quite vigorous exercise when he feels well, providing he stops short of fatigue, and to restrict his activity when he feels exhausted. These states may well alter from one day to another.

Pregnancy should be avoided (p. 314) until the disease has been quiescent for a period of two years. The risk of aggravation by pregnancy is, however, not so great as was previously thought and, if contraceptive methods fail, the need for therapeutic abortion must be determined on the merits of the individual case.

Some patients do not experience remissions, and in such circumstances the burden of continuous disability is apt to produce a feeling of hopelessness. In the past patients were allowed to become bedridden and to develop contractures, bed sores and urinary infection. There is no doubt that under such conditions, death was often a welcome relief. This state of affairs can be postponed and life may be made tolerable if modern methods are adopted for the care of the paraplegic patient (p. 373) and especially for the control of the neurogenic bladder. Though it seems that in warm climates there is a lower incidence of disseminated sclerosis, there is no evidence that the condition is alleviated in any way when a patient removes to a subtropical country. He would be better advised to conserve his financial resources for the time when he may require extra help or comforts at home. Enthusiastic physiotherapy and training by an occupational therapist in the methods of daily living available to the handicapped patient will enable some patients to continue in active employment or in the management of a household for many years. Unfortunately the facilities available for this purpose are not commensurate with the size of the problem.

BIOCHEMICAL AND DEGENERATIVE DISORDERS OF THE CENTRAL NERVOUS SYSTEM

There is a large group of neurological disorders in which the name is descriptive of the functional deficit or the anatomical site involved without indicating the nature of the pathological lesion. Examples of these are paralysis agitans (p. 376), Huntington's chorea (p. 378), dystonia musculorum deformans, hereditary ataxia including Friedreich's ataxia (p. 378), motor neurone disease, muscular dystrophy (p. 414), and idiopathic epilepsy (p. 380). In the majority of cases there is a genetic determinant and it is very probable that some biochemical disorder of neurones underlies the functional or structural abnormality. In the present state of our knowledge it is unrealistic to expect such diseases to be curable. Reference to the appropriate pages of this chapter will, however, show that much can be done to compensate for the functional disability.

In other cases the genetically determined biochemical disorder is known with some precision. The group of cerebral lipidoses and the glycogen storage disorders are now well understood but no treatment has yet emerged from this fundamental knowledge except in the case of Parkinsonism (p. 376). Hydroxocobalamin may be valuable in Leber's hereditary optic atrophy (p. 152).

Acute porphyria. This inborn error of metabolism is a cause of convulsions, mental symptoms, polyneuritis, colic and hypertension, but no treatment is known to correct it. Nevertheless, it is important to recognize that attacks may be precipitated by barbiturates or sulphonamides. Thus hydantoinates are to be preferred for the treatment of fits due to this disorder and phenothiazine drugs for its psychotic symptoms. Peripheral neuropathy (p. 372), oliguria (p. 273) or hypertensive crises (p. 113) may require treatment.

Amino-aciduria. A group of genetically determined disorders of amino-acid metabolism have

recently become amenable to treatment. The better-known types are phenylketonuria, maple syrup disease, and Hartnup disease. All are associated with oligophrenia or progressive dementia in infants, and often with seizures and focal neurological abnormalities. All these signs are arrested and may disappear if a child with phenylketonuria is given a diet low in phenylalanine from a sufficiently early age until the fifth year of life. In Hartnup disease, which is due to abnormal metabolism of tryptophan, the attacks of cerebellar ataxia, psychosis and pellagroid rash may be arrested by the administration of nicotinamide.

Hepatolenticular degeneration. Amino-aciduria is associated with abnormal metabolism of copper in the genetically determined hepatolenticular degeneration (Wilson's disease), in which progressive symptoms and signs of damage to the basal ganglia occur in adolescence. Cirrhosis of the liver is also present, and may indeed be the only clinical manifestation. The principles of treatment are to reduce copper absorption from the bowel by the use of potassium sulphide, 10 mg. thrice daily. By means of penicillamine it is also possible to promote mobilization and excretion of the copper which tends to accumulate in the liver, basal ganglia and other tissues. Penicillamine is a chelating agent which has a strong affinity for heavy metals. It is given orally in capsules containing 300 mg. four times a day which may be administered over long periods if care is taken to avoid producing a loss of calcium and iron from the body. An immediate excretion of copper in the urine follows its use, but clinical improvement may be delayed for a month or more.

If treatment is started before serious cerebral degeneration and sclerosis have occurred, the patient may become symptom free. Symptomatic treatment for Parkinsonism or dystonia should follow the principles outlined on p. 376 and treatment may be required for cirrhosis of the liver (p. 248).

NUTRITIONAL DISORDERS OF THE NERVOUS SYSTEM

The central and peripheral nervous system may be damaged by deficiency of vitamins because of insufficient dietary intake or malabsorption. Since these diseases are largely preventable by corrective measures they are described elsewhere in this book (p. 365). The outstanding example is subacute combined degeneration of the spinal cord, with its associated neuropathy due to lack of cyanocobalamin in pernicious anaemia (p. 149) or certain malabsorption states (p. 236), notably tropical sprue (p. 523). In the established case neurological signs seldom disappear completely and residual symptoms often remain; these are mainly the result of loss of proprioceptive sensibility. The treatment of the sensory ataxia which this causes is described on p. 378.

The treatment of pellagra, beriberi and other types of nutritional neuropathy and of Wernicke's encephalopathy is described on p. 365. These diseases rarely occur as primary conditions in this country but may result from malabsorptive states, alcoholism or from the administration of a drug such as isoniazid which competes with the B group of vitamins. In these conditions there is urgent need to administer the appropriate vitamins in large doses, but there is no evidence that they have any therapeutic value in similar neurological disorders not caused by vitamin deficiency.

COMPRESSION OF THE SPINAL CORD

When a clinical diagnosis of spinal cord compression has been made, it is imperative to complete essential investigations without delay to ensure immediate surgical decompression or removal of the causative lesion. If the diagnosis has not been considered until lumbar puncture shows evidence of spinal block, the neurosurgeon should be notified immediately as rapid deterioration of function may occur and this may become irreversible if decompression is not carried out at once. Thus, it is desirable to postpone lumbar puncture and myelography until a surgeon has been consulted if the diagnosis seems probable on clinical grounds.

The likelihood of improvement as the result of operation depends on the nature of the lesion and its site. Thus, compression may be due to injury, Paget's disease, extradural abscess (p. 403), herniated intervertebral disc (p. 408) or neoplasm. Naturally there is less chance of full recovery if the cord is damaged by a malignant tumour than by a benign lesion, but the site of the lesion is almost as important. Provided no irreversible vascular changes have occurred in the spinal cord, the prognosis is good for extradural lesions and fair for extramedullary causes of compression within the spinal theca. Intramedullary lesions are rarely amenable to operation. Thus the removal of a

primary or secondary neoplasm from a vertebral body or from the extradural space may cause a gratifying return of function, especially if the operation is followed by local radiotherapy. This form of treatment is recommended for spinal cord compression due to myelomatosis and other neoplastic diseases in which survival for more than six months is considered possible.

Cervical spondylosis. This is frequently associated with damage to the adjacent cord, leading to progressive paraplegia. Decompression of the cord followed by internal fixation of the cervical vertebrae may allow neurological signs to disappear if this is done at a sufficiently early stage. Immobilization of the neck by a plaster Minerva-type collar or by similar devices is a less effective procedure, but it is not to be despised if operation is rejected; the bony bars associated with degenerated intervertebral discs continue to compress the tissues, but immobilization may allow oedema of the cord to subside.

Extramedullary tumours. Meningiomata or neurofibromata may be removed by the neurosurgeon with complete restoration of function if the diagnosis has not been too long delayed. Removal of a tumour composed of anomalous arteriovenous communications is less satisfactory for, though the tumour is not malignant and there is no compression, it is often impossible to remove it without seriously damaging the blood supply of the cord.

Intramedullary tumours. These are unsatisfactory to treat. The residual defect may be tolerable after removal of an ependymoma and the attempt is certainly justifiable, but tumours of glial tissue are not amenable to surgery. Radiotherapy has been used but its value is doubtful.

Syringomyelia. Some consider syringomyelia to be a developmental anomaly, others regard it as a slowly growing tumour. From the therapeutic point of view it may well be grouped with the intramedullary tumours. Operations designed to tap the fluid encysted in the cavity have been abandoned except when there is gross dilatation of the cervical canal. Radiotherapy aimed at the supposed site of the cavity is widely used if physical signs are progressive or if there is pain in one or other arm. The value of this treatment is debatable, but its use is justified because of the not unusual development of a glioma in relation to the capsule of the cavity.

The urgency of the assessment for surgical decompression should not lead to neglect of other forms of care required by the paraplegic patient. These are

o

detailed in earlier sections and include the care of the skin (p. 386), bladder (p. 387), bowel, paralysed limbs (pp. 372-374) and eventual rehabilitation. The collaboration of an orthopaedic surgeon may be invaluable at this stage.

SCIATICA, BRACHIALGIA, ACROPARAESTHESIA AND NEUROPATHIES

There are many causes for this group of disorders with the common symptoms of pain, paraesthesia and weakness of an upper or lower limb. Separate consideration of them is desirable because of the way the clinical problems present themselves to the practitioner.

Sciatica. Among the causes of sciatica, retropulsion of an intervertebral disc takes first place. Long before the relationship between lumbago and herniated discs was recognized, most of these patients recovered spontaneously, and this fact is not without importance in the modern therapeutic approach to patients suffering from herniation of the nucleus pulposus. Once the diagnosis has been established rest in bed should be ordered. Fracture boards are placed under a hair mattress and only one pillow is allowed. The patient may be permitted to roll on to either side. He is not permitted to sit up; his spine must be kept as nearly horizontal as possible. The use of bedpans and urinals is part of the routine. After or during the third week of this treatment hyperextension exercises in bed are ordered; these are graduated and the patient is allowed up at the end of the third or during the fourth week. The whole object of treatment is to prevent movement between the herniated disc and the affected nerve root. The affected root is oedematous, and oedema and pain are perpetuated as long as movement occurs in the surrounding structures. With rest, the oedema disappears and the root adapts itself to the deformity. After the period of rest has been completed, the carrying or lifting of weights with the spine flexed is forbidden for some further three to six weeks. The importance of prevention of flexion must be emphasized because this movement precipitates the condition.

The initial exquisite pain of lumbago and sciatica is sufficient to immobilize the patient. Any movement causes pain and reflex spasm at the site of damage. Morphine should not be given, even though the pain may appear to demand it. Tablets of aspirin or paracetamol given frequently in full doses are usually effective.

The small percentage of patients who fail to respond to this conservative treatment should be dealt with surgically by removal of the offending protrusion. This also applies to the small number who suffer from florid paralysis. When paralysis is extensive, the earlier the operation is undertaken the better.

Sciatica is a symptom which is often associated with a psychological overlay. Not only does the sufferer have to contend with recurring excruciating pain but with the fear which his symptom engenders. The layman may be left to explain his disability as best he may. This he does in terms of something happening to his spine. Anything which aggravates his pain also provokes fear. This emotion has its physical counterpart in increased muscular tension. The patient avoids all movement of the spine, imagining that this will cause permanent damage to it or to his nerves. Assurance must be given of the stability of the spine and of the forces which protect it against damage. Much residual pain also is caused by local spasm of muscle brought about by fear, and that fear must be allayed.

Brachialgia. Although the relationship between sciatic pain and protrusion of an intervertebral disc is now widely accepted, it is comparatively recently that a similar mechanism causing severe pain in the upper limb has been recognized. The term cervical spondylosis is usually restricted to the syndrome caused by chronic compression of the spinal cord (p. 407) or cervical nerve roots by osteophytes.

Acute protrusion of a cervical intervertebral disc into the intervertebral canal causes stiffness of the neck with pain radiating to the cutaneous and deep distribution of the affected spinal root, usually along the axis of the upper limb. As in the case of sciatica, there may be localized sensory loss or paresis of lower motor neurone type, usually involving the small muscles of the hand. The acute syndrome is treated by rest in bed or by intermittent neck traction carried out by a physiotherapist. For the best results it is important that the neck should be placed in a suitable posture during traction—usually slight flexion—and application of a heated pad to the neck encourages muscular relaxation. Between treatments the neck is immobilized in slight flexion with a light metal or plastic collar. Some form of immobilization should be maintained for at least three months. Surgical treatment is rarely necessary.

Acute brachial neuritis (*Neuralgic Amyotrophy*). With the increasing recognition of cervical disc as a common cause of brachialgia, there has been a tendency to discard the older concept of brachial neuritis. This is unfortunate as the syndrome of acute brachial neuritis is a distinct entity with well-defined indications for treatment. One form occurs following the injection of serum or vaccine, suggesting an allergic basis. It is probable that there is a similar mechanism for the majority which occur without obvious cause or during convalescence from infection, injury, operation or childbirth. Pain affects the shoulder girdle on one or both sides, and is soon followed by lower motor neurone paralysis of muscles supplied by C5, 6, 7 spinal roots. Prednisolone in full dosage shortens the duration of pain and may hasten recovery. It is usually necessary to give analgesics for the first fortnight and a hypnotic may also be required. The weak muscles waste rapidly. They should be treated along the lines described for a lower motor neurone type of paralysis (p. 372). Massage and electrical stimulation of the paralysed muscles are valueless.

Acroparaesthesia. Acroparaesthesia is an unpleasant tingling sensation affecting some or all of the digits of one or both upper limbs. It is a symptom of irritation of sensory nerve fibres, usually due to compression of one or more nerves or their roots. Treatment must be aimed at the causative lesion. Accurate diagnosis is essential since the symptoms disappear rapidly if pressure is removed. Common causes are cervical spondylosis (p. 407), thoracic outlet compression syndrome, carpal tunnel syndrome, 'tardy ulnar palsy' (see below), and Raynaud's phenomenon (p. 139). The sensation of acroparaesthesia usually develops during the night when posture, diminished movement and venous stasis combine to increase the compression in the various sites. This factor may be alleviated by resting the arm on a pillow. A sedative drug may be necessary to allow the patient to sleep.

Thoracic outlet compression syndrome. The neurovascular bundle to the upper limb may be compressed between the clavicle and first rib if defective muscular tone allows sagging of the shoulder. It is aggravated by carrying weights or by the presence of an accessory cervical rib. If symptoms are severe, treatment should be started by resting the arm for a short period in a sling. As soon as they can be tolerated, exercises should be prescribed to increase the tone of the shoulder girdle muscles and to improve posture. Aggravating factors should be avoided including the wearing of unnecessarily heavy clothes such as a fur coat. Clothing should be suspended from the waist rather than by shoulder straps and a strapless brassière should be used. Occasionally, it is necessary to undertake operative treatment when an anatomical abnormality of the thoracic outlet such as cervical rib has been demonstrated, but this should only be done after conservative treatment has failed or if weakness develops in the muscles of the hand.

Carpal tunnel syndrome. A more common cause of paraesthesia of the fingers in middle-aged women is compression of the median nerve in the carpal tunnel. The usual precipitating factor is obesity, but others are fluid retention in pregnancy, myxoedema, rheumatoid arthritis, myelomatosis and other bony abnormalities. When possible the primary condition should be treated and this is especially valuable in myxoedema. The effect of fluid depletion by means of a diuretic should be determined. The affected hand should be rested, avoiding trauma such as that caused by wringing dish cloths or scrubbing floors. It is helpful to place the hand in a padded splint at night with the wrist in the mid position. This treatment may be continued when the causative lesion is self-limiting, as in pregnancy, but in other cases if symptoms have not subsided in two weeks 50 mg. of hydrocortisone should be injected under the flexor retinaculum of the wrist. If there is motor involvement, as shown by weakness and wasting of the abductor, short extensor, and opponens muscles of the thumb, early operation is preferable. This should also be the treatment in patients who do not respond favourably to rest and hydrocortisone, since the operation is simple and highly satisfactory.

Traumatic median and ulnar lesions within the hand. Traumatic median and ulnar nerve lesions in the hand may occur from occupational causes such as wielding a pick-axe or operating automatic riveting machines. The first essential in treatment is cessation of manual work. Rest to the affected part, by splinting if necessary, should follow. Complete restoration of function after rest can usually be ensured by remedial exercises. Sometimes chronic irritation causes development of a ganglion which compresses the nerve and these cases respond admirably to surgical removal of the ganglion.

Ulnar neuropathy. Workers in certain occupations are liable to develop slowly progressive paralysis of the ulnar nerve. In the past this has been attributed to pressure on the nerve at the elbow where the ulnar nerve, if mobile, might be dislocated from its bed in the epicondylar groove. Subjects with a wide carrying angle were considered to be particularly susceptible. It is probable that the critical factor is full flexion of the elbow causing pressure on the nerve as it passes through a tunnel between the humeral and ulnar heads of the flexor carpi ulnaris muscle (the cubital tunnel). Treatment is directed to removing the cause by instructing the patient about these postures which render the ulnar nerve liable to compression. Further treatment may be unnecessary. Surgical transposition of the nerve to the anterior aspect of the forearm is less commonly carried out than previously, but many orthopaedic surgeons advise dividing the fibrous arch of the cubital tunnel. Weakness and atrophy of the intrinsic muscles of the hand should be treated by exercises and appropriate occupational therapy.

Musculo-spiral paralysis (*Saturday-night palsy*). This is best treated by resting the extensors of the wrist and fingers in a cock-up splint. If the paralysis is profound, electrical stimulation of the affected muscles may prevent wasting if carried out assiduously. As soon as voluntary power begins to return, remedial exercises can be started.

Bell's paralysis. The majority of patients recover spontaneously without any special treatment. Counter-irritation applied over the region of the stylomastoid foramen is futile. It is probably unwise to recommend decompression of the facial nerve by operation because spontaneous recovery is the general rule. The writer does not believe that operation has any real advantage over the administration of corticosteroids, which mitigate the inflammatory reaction in the nerve itself and prevent the adverse effects of prolonged pressure within the canal. For the milder case with little loss of muscle tone and showing early signs of recovery, exercises in front of a mirror are sufficient. Lax and grossly paralytic facial muscles require splinting. The splint takes the form of a rubber-covered wire bent to form a 'U' at one end and a spectacle leg at the other. The 'U' bend hooks into the angle of the mouth on the paralysed side and the spectacle leg fits over the ear to exert traction on the angle of the mouth and so to restore facial symmetry. If the patient wears a suitable denture, this may be modified to carry a plastic device to retract the angle of the mouth. Contracture sometimes occurs because of random regeneration of the facial fibres after a pathological process has destroyed the fascicular pattern of the nerve. Nothing can be done to correct the results of random regeneration. Should no regeneration occur, medical treatment is unavailing and the patient should be referred to a plastic surgeon for the insertion of a fascial sling.

Meralgia paraesthetica. Some of the neuropathies just described are caused by chronic pressure on a part of the nerve passing through a musculotendinous canal. Meralgia paraesthetica is a common symptom with a similar cause. There is dysaesthesia in the cutaneous distribution of the anterior division of the lateral cutaneous nerve of the thigh. It is usually unilateral and is more frequent in men. Spontaneous compression may occur where the nerve pierces the fascia lata. Increasing obesity and pressure from corsets or other underclothes are all possible causative factors. The symptoms may persist for periods of up to five years but almost invariably disappear spontaneously. It is, therefore, rarely necessary to split the fascia lata at the point of emergence of the nerve or to correct the angulation of the nerve at the iliac spine. The use of sedatives may be necessary to make the symptoms tolerable while awaiting recovery.

Mononeuropathy. A non-traumatic lesion of a single nerve may be due to entrapment, polyarteritis nodosa or one of the other diseases associated with arteritis, diabetes mellitus or, in some countries, leprosy—perhaps the most common cause of all. The appropriate chapters should be consulted for the treatment of polyarteritis (p. 458), diabetes (p. 316), and leprosy (p. 524). Entrapment neuropathy should be treated by rest in the first instance, followed if necessary by surgical decompression of the nerve. The lower motor neurone palsy is treated as described on p. 372. With femoral or lateral popliteal neuropathy it may be necessary to prescribe a caliper or foot-drop appliance until recovery takes place.

Polyneuropathy. Symmetrical polyneuropathy may be due to one of many causes. It is rarely a 'neuritis' in the true sense of the word. Treatment may be considered under the headings symptomatic and specific.

Symptomatic treatment involves all the considerations already described for the nursing of the incontinent patient (p. 387) and the management of lower motor neurone palsy involving possibly all the limbs (p. 372). Paralysis of bladder and bowel may occur, but the disability is rarely as severe as in paraplegia. The paralysis of the bladder will be of the atonic type (p. 387). The most serious aspect of polyneuropathy is involvement of the muscles of respiration and of swallowing. These may develop very rapidly and prove fatal if not recognized early. Artificial respiration is life saving. It may be required for many months but must be employed with the most meticulous attention to detail even in what may seem a hopeless case because eventual recovery is more probable with peripheral neuropathy than with any other cause of paralysis of comparable severity. If the swallowing reflexes are completely normal and the patient is conscious the most suitable form of ventilator may be a tank type ('iron lung') though the management of the respirator and the problems of nursing call for a specially trained team. If paralysis is spreading rapidly or if the muscles of swallowing are already involved, positive pressure ventilation through a cuffed tracheostomy tube is essential to prevent inhalation of foreign matter from the pharynx. The management of such a patient and the methods of weaning him from the respirator are described on p. 652. When he has recovered sufficiently to sit up in bed it is important to remember that many diseases resulting in polyneuropathy also affect the heart muscle. The patient should not, therefore, be allowed to sit up without assistance until the physician is certain that there is no significant myocardial disease.

Specific forms of treatment are available for the minority of cases of polyneuropathy in which a causative factor can be identified. Thus diabetes mellitus, vitamin B_{12} deficiency, myelomatosis, and carcinoma of the bronchus are susceptible to therapy with consequent benefit to the neuropathy. Aneurine is of therapeutic value if beriberi is diagnosed, but is useless in other types of polyneuropathy. A possible exception to this dictum is alcoholic neuropathy in which there may be a conditioned nutritional deficiency. Certainly aneurine is of no value in the most common type of acute polyneuropathy—acute infective polyneuritis (Guillain-Barré syndrome). This is almost certainly not directly due to infection but may have an allergic aetiology like the demyelinating encephalo-myelopathies discussed on p. 404. Here the use of corticosteroid therapy is justified. Prednisolone is recommended in a dose of 60 mg. daily for 2 days, then 40 mg. daily for 2 days, followed by 20 mg. daily for as long as may be necessary. In severe cases with bulbar and respiratory involvement treatment may be started with intravenous hydrocortisone hemisuccinate, 100 mg. twice daily for two or three days.

Many neuropathies are the result of ingestion of a toxic substance. All drugs should be stopped at once and measures taken to promote excretion of potentially toxic substances. Heavy metals such as lead, arsenic, gold, mercury, zinc, bismuth, antimony, and thallium may enter the body in contaminated food, medicaments or cosmetics, or from an industrial hazard. Infantile acrodynia ('pink disease') is an example of toxic neuropathy due to ingestion of mercury. Teething powders containing mercury are no longer sold in Britain, but calomel can still be bought by the public and used as baby powders. Heavy metal poisoning is treated with chelating agents such as penicillamine or disodium calcium edetate (p. 559). The majority of toxic hydrocarbon compounds have no effective antidotes, but neuropathy usually recovers gradually after the offending substance is removed, provided that death from respiratory failure is prevented. The neuropathy associated with ingestion of isoniazid (p. 69) is believed to be due to a conditioned deficiency of pyridoxine. Toxic polyneuropathy may be caused by insecticides and other chemical substances used in agriculture (p. 540). There is no specific antidote for these, but it is important to differentiate the paralysis of peripheral neuropathy from that due to blockage of neuromuscular transmission which may be caused by some organophosphorus insecticides. The cholinergic poisoning which they produce may be rapidly fatal but efficient treatment is available. It is described on p. 541.

DISORDERS OF MUSCLE AND NEUROMUSCULAR TRANSMISSION

Myasthenia Gravis

In this disorder there is failure of transmission at the myoneural junction, and this can be corrected by the use of anticholinesterase drugs such as physostigmine (eserine) or its synthetic analogues. Inhibition of cholinesterase by such drugs prevents rapid hydrolysis of acetylcholine and the consequent accumulation of acetylcholine facilitates neuromuscular transmission. Excessive dosage, by permitting prolonged depolarization of muscle endplates, may in itself cause transmission failure (cholinergic crisis). Effective therapy, therefore, calls for careful and intelligent use of these potent drugs. For this reason, though many anticholinesterase drugs are now available, the practitioner is advised to restrict his prescribing to the three preparations mentioned below, since response to treatment is very variable.

Drugs. The drug which is most generally useful is *pyridostigmine bromide*. One or more of the 60 mg. tablets are given as often as necessary to control symptoms. This varies from three to six hours or even longer in individual patients. Pyridostigmine gives a very satisfactory smooth control with few parasympathomimetic side-effects, and the long action without sudden withdrawal effects makes it particularly suitable for treatment during the night. If, however, bulbar symptoms are troublesome or if the patient is very weak on waking in the morning, it is advisable to rouse him for a dose at an appropriate time during the night.

Neostigmine bromide, 15 mg., has an equivalent potency to 60 mg. of pyridostigmine given by mouth. Its duration of action is little if at all shorter than that of pyridostigmine, but the anticholinesterase action diminishes more rapidly so that the patient is more acutely aware of the necessity for further dosage. On the other hand, the therapeutic effect of the oral tablet is more rapidly felt and the peak effect is somewhat greater. Thus the average patient prefers pyridostigmine for the smoother control it gives. However, a few need the extra 'boost' of neostigmine and for them these drugs may with advantage be prescribed together. The dose required varies from 2 to 20 tablets of either preparation daily, distributed throughout the day according to the effective time shown by preliminary trial. When the patient has difficulty with chewing and swallowing it is desirable to arrange for a dose to be given half an hour *before* meals so that the exertion of eating coincides with restoration of normal muscle power.

In severe cases it may be necessary to give neostigmine by injection. A subcutaneous injection of 1 mg. has a dramatic effect in alleviating the myasthenic condition; sometimes the disability is completely abolished within 15 minutes. When given by this route, neostigmine should be administered with atropine sulphate, 0·5 mg., to prevent vagal effects—intestinal colic, sweating and bradycardia. If possible the atropine should be injected 15 to 30 minutes before the dose of neostigmine. Parasympathomimetic effects are rarely troublesome with oral medication, but can be countered by the use of atropine sulphate, 0·6 mg. orally, or one of the other anticholinergic drugs such as propantheline bromide (15 mg.) or tricyclamol (50 mg.). The routine use of atropine is not recommended as it may prevent recognition of the onset of a 'cholinergic crisis'. If the increasing weakness resulting from overdose by anticholinesterase drugs is mistaken for 'neostigmine resistance' and more neostigmine is given, the patient may die.

Neostigmine methylsulphate (1 to 1·5 mg.) may be given subcutaneously or intramuscularly, with atropine, as a therapeutic test which is a valuable aid in the diagnosis of myasthenia gravis. It should not be given intravenously because of the danger of cardiac arrest. This prohibition does not apply to edrophonium, a drug of similar action. Its brief effect renders it useless for treatment of myasthenia but makes it a valuable diagnostic aid as its intravenous injection causes relief of symptoms in about half a minute, and any unpleasant parasympathetic effects are soon over. A trial dose of 2 mg. intravenously should be given in case of hypersensitivity, and a further 8 mg. half a minute later if no undesirable reactions (fasciculation, sweating, colic) occur. The effect of edrophonium is additive to that of neostigmine and pyridostigmine: thus it may be used to determine whether the dose of the latter drugs is optimal, and whether a patient who is becoming weaker requires still higher dosage or has developed cholinergic blockage. In the first case there will be temporary improvement immediately after an intravenous injection of edrophonium and the dose of the anticholinesterase drug may be increased with safety. If parasympathetic overactivity occurs, especially with the initial small dose of edrophonium, or if weakness is increased, the patient is already having too much of the anticholinesterase drug. The brief action of edrophonium makes this test possible, but the dangers should be recognized and preparations should be made in advance to give artificial respiration. An important consideration is that some of the patient's muscles may be at the stage of cholinergic block while others require still more neostigmine. Hence the test should be directed to the respiratory muscles. In some cases the edrophonium test is equivocal or no clinical response may be seen in the short period available for observation. It should be a firm rule that this 'null response' must be interpreted as a warning of incipient cholinergic block. No further long-acting anticholinesterase drugs should be given until the edrophonium test, repeated hourly, shows a 'myasthenic' response.

Notwithstanding some response to treatment, a number of patients suffering from myasthenia gravis retrogress and ultimately develop atrophic changes in the affected muscles. These patients are extremely resistant to even the most generous administration of neostigmine. Adjuvants to neostigmine are potassium citrate (1·3 g.) and ephedrine (30 mg.) three times a day. In the resistant case the use of these drugs in combination is desirable while the administration of neostigmine continues. Corticosteroids are helpful occasionally, but must be used with caution as they may cause temporary increase in weakness. Aldosterone inhibition by spironolactone (400 mg.) increases the sense of well-being and may potentiate the action of neostigmine.

Sedatives are also potentially dangerous if they produce depression of the respiratory centre. Curare, quinine, quinidine, morphine, chloroform and ether are absolutely contraindicated. Myasthenics should not receive enemata as this form of treatment has occasionally resulted in prostration and death.

Thymectomy. Most patients with myasthenia gravis have an abnormality of the thymus. It is usually a disorder of lymphadenoid type but 15 per cent. of patients have a thymoma; and the presence of a tumour is often associated with a particularly severe form of myasthenia resistant to all forms of treatment. When the thymus is not malignant its removal may be of great therapeutic value. It is unfortunately not possible to select those patients likely to benefit from thymectomy, but young women with myasthenia of not more than five years' duration usually respond best. Patients in this category should be operated on as soon as possible unless myasthenia is confined to the extra-ocular muscles when the prognosis may be good. Men and women over 40 years old, and also any patient who has had myasthenia for more than five years, should all be treated medically; but if response to drugs is unsatisfactory and the patient is fit for operation it is certainly worth while. In experienced hands the risk is not great and the improvement is sometimes remarkable. Operation for thymoma is occasionally indicated when it is suspected that the tumour is malignant, but excision is rarely beneficial

to the associated myasthenia. The gland should always be treated with radiotherapy before operation for a malignant thymoma, but this treatment is not otherwise indicated.

General management. It is important to review the patient's daily activities. Fatigue and stress (physical and emotional) should be avoided. Ptosis may be prevented by a lid crutch attached to an eyeglass frame. If there is diplopia, an eye patch may be worn but should be changed from eye to eye to prevent suppression of vision. Surgical correction of ptosis or strabismus should be postponed until it is certain that no further variation is likely to occur. Orthopaedic appliances have limited value in myasthenia and rarely justify the extra burden imposed on the patient. Persistent dysphagia may cause starvation with rapid loss of weight. A fluid diet with concentrated protein supplements (p. 239) should then be given by gastric tube which the patient or a relative may be taught to pass. Respiratory embarrassment must be detected early so that artificial respiration can be started without delay. Positive pressure respiration by a cuffed tracheostomy tube is advisable. This may be life-saving and frequently tides a patient over a crisis which would otherwise be fatal. Such an episode does not affect the prognosis, and a complete remission may still occur. Hence this form of treatment must not be classed among the desperate remedies or regarded as a last resort.

Cholinergic crisis. When increasing neostigmine resistance or the edrophonium test indicates the onset of a cholinergic crisis the safest procedure is to stop anticholinesterase drugs and to use an artificial ventilator to maintain regular breathing while muscle cholinesterase regenerates. Atropine sulphate 2 mg. should be given intravenously every 60 minutes until the patient is obviously fully atropinized or is improving.

POLYMYOSITIS AND OTHER
ACQUIRED MYOPATHIES

A group of diseases of muscle produce a final clinical picture closely resembling hereditary muscular dystrophy. These, however, are not determined genetically; they are liable to spontaneous arrest; and they may recover fully with or without treatment. Clinically, five types are recognized: (i) polymyositis, primary and secondary; (ii) carcinomatous myopathy; (iii) infections and infestations of muscle; (iv) endocrine myopathy; and (v) toxic myopathy.

Polymyositis. Polymyositis, whether primary or associated with dermatitis (dermatomyositis, p. 459), rheumatoid arthritis, systemic lupus erythematosus and other connective tissue diseases, responds favourably to treatment with corticosteroids. The low dosage appropriate to uncomplicated rheumatoid arthritis is inadequate. Long-term maintenance therapy may be required with a temporary increase of dosage during exacerbations. In the first few weeks, polymyositis may resemble myasthenia gravis as muscle power decreases with exercise and recovers with rest. There may be a response to neostigmine or edrophonium but this is less striking than in myasthenia gravis and it does not last for more than a few weeks. Anticholinesterase drugs are of no value in treatment and their use is best avoided because of the danger of increasing weakness by overdosage.

Carcinomatous myopathy. This is very similar to polymyositis. The tumour which most commonly produces it is carcinoma of the lung, but the primary lesion may be in any organ. A myasthenic phenomenon with temporary response to anticholinesterase drugs may also be found in this disorder. An unusual syndrome, also found in other acquired myopathies but most characteristically in the carcinomatous type, is progressive increase of power with repeated contraction of the muscle. These patients may benefit from guanidine hydrochloride, 25 to 50 mg. per kg. body weight, divided into three doses, and from gentle exercise. The condition is incurable but may improve temporarily with corticosteroid treatment.

Myositis. This may be due to infection by viruses of the Coxsackie group (Bornholm disease). It is a self-limiting disorder without specific treatment. Analgesics may be necessary for the severe pain. Other viruses may cause epidemic myalgia. Myositis due to Weil's disease, or to infection with known pathogenic cocci is rare. Any organism identified from pus should be destroyed by the appropriate antibiotic. Trichinosis is a painful type of myositis due to infection with *Trichinella spiralis*; there is no treatment for the muscular disease.

Endocrine myopathy. Weakness and wasting of proximal muscles may also be found in association with many endocrine diseases. The most common is thyrotoxicosis but an apparently identical disorder may occur in myxoedema, Cushing's syndrome, Addison's disease, hyperparathyroidism, hyperinsulinism and occasionally in diabetes mellitus. Treatment of the endocrine disorder is sufficient to arrest and often to reverse the muscular disease.

Toxic myopathy. A disorder resembling endocrine myopathy may be seen in patients treated with triamcinolone and dexamethasone. A toxic myopathy of the lower limbs may also be caused by the use of chloroquine in the treatment of rheumatic disorders. Both types of myopathy recover slowly when the toxic drug is withdrawn.

The physical care advised for patients with muscular dystrophy is also appropriate for the acquired myopathies.

Hereditary Muscular Dystrophies

There is no satisfactory specific treatment for the muscular dystrophies. The therapeutic use of glycine arose from the idea that ingestion of amino acids might spare muscle by providing readily available protein. There is no evidence that such treatment can either reverse or arrest the dystrophic process. Anabolic steroids, preparations containing nucleotides and nucleosides and a-tocopherol (vitamin E) have also been tested and found useless. Deformities and contractures should be prevented by exercise as long as the patient is able to execute the necessary movements, and by passive movement when the limbs become immobile. The care of these slowly deteriorating patients presents many problems. The best form of treatment is to provide them with work under protected conditions suited to their limited capacity. Any superfluous weight creates an unnecessary handicap for them and obesity must be prevented. Dystrophic patients require to be protected against cold. The weight of ordinary woollen blankets may cause discomfort and obstruct movement of the limbs. Open weave blankets such as Lanaircel are to be preferred. An electric blanket is also a boon to these patients.

Dystrophia myotonica (*Myotonia atrophica*). No specific treatment can arrest or modify the course of this disease. Any influence exerted by drugs is purely symptomatic in effect. The delayed relaxation of skeletal muscle can be reduced by procainamide, 250 mg. to 1 g. four times daily or phenytoin sodium 100 mg. three times daily by mouth. If they are not tolerated, quinine bisulphate, 600 mg. orally once a day, is a less effective substitute. Restriction of potassium by diet or the use of prednisolone or ion exchange resins are less effective and difficult to maintain in practice. It must be emphasized that each of these treatments influences only the myotonic after-contraction and has no influence on muscular strength. Lenticular cataract, an early accompaniment to the muscular disorder, is appropriately treated by operation if there is no further abnormality in the refractive media or in the retina.

Myotonia congenita. This is a muscular disorder similar to that of myotonia atrophica; it is treated in the same way.

Familial periodic paralysis. This is a rare disease. There is no specific cure, but by proper management attacks may be prevented or symptomatic relief given if they occur. The patient must avoid fatigue, and his carbohydrate intake should be restricted—particularly at the evening meal. If this regimen does not prevent attacks, he should be given 3 g. of potassium chloride before he goes to bed. A paralytic attack is treated with 5 g. of the same drug orally. It should be given intravenously only in emergency—when there is respiratory and pharyngeal muscle paralysis: it is infused well diluted in normal saline (1 g. in 250 ml.) and given by very slow drip. An excess of potassium in the blood stream is toxic to the heart and may cause cardiac arrest. Should potassium overdose occur, calcium gluconate (10 to 12 ml. of 10 per cent. solution) should be injected slowly intravenously.

Clinically identical attacks occur in aldosteronism (Conn's syndrome, p. 303). Some patients with the same clinical syndrome do not have hypokalaemia during the attacks and administration of potassium is unhelpful and may be harmful. For this reason biochemical confirmation of hypokalaemia is virtually indispensable before administering potassium salts.

In the hyperkalaemic type there may be myotonic disorders in the family. Spontaneous attacks of weakness are usually brief in this type, but if they are prolonged calcium gluconate should be injected intravenously (1 to 2 g.). Potassium excretion may be promoted by means of the thiazide diuretics e.g. bendrofluazide, 5 mg. after breakfast.

16. Psychiatry in General Practice

T. F. RODGER

INTRODUCTION

Health and disease are manifestations of a complex process of adjustment to many factors both internal and external, and what the patient thinks and feels is never entirely irrelevant and may often be crucial to the understanding of illness. The experienced doctor is constantly aware of, and treats psychological effects in all kinds of illness. Even in the infectious fevers, where the physical findings may follow a standard pattern, the patient's emotional response and consequently the real significance of the illness to him will be determined by his personality, his responsibilities and his social environment.

We owe a great deal to Freud. His main ideas have gained acceptance because they accord with facts and give meaning and order to clinical observations in the neuroses. The symptoms of the neuroses are not haphazard, incoherent and irrational, but with patience they are capable of being understood and their sources identified; our personality is affected by our upbringing and the parental care we receive; we have learned that we can be influenced by conflicts which are unrecognized by us and occur below the level of consciousness. We have, therefore, come to seek an understanding of a neurosis in the life-history of the patient, in the cultural influences to which he has been exposed and in the current emotional stresses which he is facing.

Our understanding of psychological factors in disease is not entirely due to the work of psychiatrists; it has emerged also from the clinical studies and research within general medicine. Success in dealing with harmful factors in the environment characterized the first sanitary phase of modern medicine, and then followed the great advances in immunotherapy, chemotherapy and the correction of hormone and vitamin insufficiencies. These discoveries gave a satisfactory explanation of the aetiology of the majority of diseases, but some remain, as the textbooks say, 'of indefinite or unknown pathology'. A number of the latter conditions are now called stress diseases or psychosomatic disorders because the general adaptation of the individual appears to play a part, and emotional as well as physical factors are considered to be relevant to their aetiology.

In many countries there has been a great increase in the number of people suffering from stress diseases. The fact that this has occurred only in industrialized communities with a complex and rapidly changing environment seems to confirm the view that difficulty in adaptation is a factor in these illnesses. Specific environmental causes, however, have not yet been identified. Many believe that in peptic ulcer, chronic rheumatic conditions and hypertension, to mention only a few representative 'stress diseases', it is often possible to demonstrate characteristic emotional reactions which appear to be aetiologically relevant—though this does not imply that psychiatrists maintain that such factors are the only ones concerned in the pathogenesis of such disorders.

It is therefore safe to predict that, until such time as a new preventive medicine emerges to deal with these problems, practitioners will perforce be concerned more and more with illness in which thought and emotion play a significant part and which will demand that they should exercise psychotherapeutic skill.

Finally the family doctor must take note of such circumstances as social class, educational attainments and religious beliefs. People who adhere to certain conventions of behaviour or strive to attain prescribed standards of proficiency—and equally those who repudiate such formulae—are beset with psychological problems which they must try to resolve, because the individual can never escape from the awareness that he is constantly being judged by the herd or 'community'.

THE DOCTOR-PATIENT RELATIONSHIP

It is only in comparatively recent times that the doctor has attempted to assume a purely technical rôle in the diagnosis and treatment of disease. His traditional rôle was much more that of a psychotherapist. In primitive societies, as the medicineman, he was invested with magical powers which allowed him to exercise powerful therapeutic effects by suggestion; as the priest-physician through prayer and by exorcising feelings of guilt he was able like-wise to relieve his patients of mental distress and so contribute to their recovery. The doctor still retains much of his traditional status, but in his newer more competent technical rôle he sometimes finds it irksome to be regarded irrationally as a purveyor of magic or to be burdened with confidences and intimacies which often seem irrelevant to his task and which he would gladly see his patients take elsewhere.

The doctor–patient relationship is the essential tool of psychotherapy. It is often assumed that the psychotherapeutic process is necessarily based on the uncovering of repressed material, but as Freud showed, the emotional relationship between doctor and patient is at least as important. In psycho-analysis this relationship is described as *the transference situation* because in the course of psycho-analysis emotions formerly attached to other persons are transferred to the doctor, who becomes the object of fluctuating emotions which are both positive and negative. Something very like the transference situation plays a part in all treatment although the handling of this relationship is specially important in the case of neurotic persons. All sick patients need psychotherapy in the sense that the emotional significance of the doctor–patient relationship can never be neglected. It is this broad meaning of psychotherapy that is considered here.

The emotion which patients feel about their doctors is always, at least potentially, *ambivalent*, that is, compounded of opposite feelings of respect and contempt, gratitude and ingratitude, love and hate. Even if many patients 'think the world' of a doctor, there are usually a few who would not return to him at any price; and there are many patients who, although they are constantly complaining of their doctors—their neglect, their lack of patience and so on—nevertheless continue to rely on them and are dismayed by the suggestion that they should seek advice elsewhere.

To the patient the doctor is necessarily someone of prestige and wisdom, and when the patient approaches him he is usually afraid and bewildered and sometimes guilty. He looks to the doctor for more than mere technical skill and he expects that the doctor will give him not only the remedy he needs but understanding and friendliness in an atmosphere of privacy and secrecy. Approaching the doctor as he does in an anxious, dependent state, he expresses towards him some of the emotional attitudes which as a child he felt towards his parents. The doctor assumes for the patient the psychological characteristics of a 'father-figure', and just as children differ in their attitudes to their parents so patients differ in the emotional demands which they make of their doctors. It is important that the doctor should realize the nature of these demands and should exercise skill and judgment in the manner that he chooses to satisfy them.

He should recognize the patient who resembles the anxious insecure child who clings to the parent for support and refuses to grow up. Such a patient will often be anxious to prolong a dependent relationship which has originated in illness; he will be sensitive to the doctor's suggestions and anxious to please him, but he will also be reluctant to abandon his symptoms. Another patient will resemble the aggressive badly behaved child who objects to parental authority; he will be resentful of his illness, challenge the doctor's diagnosis, refuse or simply fail to co-operate in treatment and, just as the rebellious child plays off one parent against another, he will go from doctor to doctor or from one hospital to another seizing on inconsistencies and contradictions in what he has been told.

The doctor will recognize, too, the greedy child who wants more and more from the parent and is never satisfied, who will demand tonics and remedies that have been given to other patients or recourse to hospital facilities which others are enjoying. Among his patients there will also be those who quite sincerely 'don't wish to bother him'; they are like those apparently self-contained children who play for hours alone bearing their misfortunes in silence but who inwardly feel unworthy of love and attention.

There are several ways in which the doctor in turn can react to the emotional attitudes of his patients, not all of them therapeutic.

The doctor should respect his patient's confidences and should never appear shocked by what is revealed to him. He should refrain from moralizing. His attitude should be one of accepting the patient for what he is, good and bad together; and he should not suggest a punitive attitude in what he says or in the treatment he prescribes or administers. Moral lecturing will do no good at all, nor is there any therapeutic value in exhorting the patient 'to snap out of it'; accusations of malingering and bald statements that there is nothing the matter with him will have no influence on a patient whose sufferings, albeit neurotic, are real to him and not imaginary. An authoritarian attitude to such patients is usually to be deprecated, for it will often serve only to stiffen the patient's resistance and thereby thwart the doctor's efforts to understand his problems. On the other hand, if the patient feels accepted, he will feel secure enough to abandon his defences and express the emotions which determine his illness or impede his recovery.

But the doctor need not and should not feel that he must identify himself with the patient's problems and feel the same concern. The patient expects detachment and the emotional wisdom that pertains to that detachment. If the doctor begins to appear anxious and involved in his problems, the patient will lose the feeling of security which comes from being able to approach someone who is himself secure and stands outside of his difficulties. But he must feel that his physician has a human interest in him and can give him emotional understanding. To strike the right balance between over-detachment and over-involvement is the main problem of the doctor–patient relationship; fortunately, the conscientious doctor who tries to serve all his patients without favouritism is likely to arrive at an attitude which is more or less appropriate.

Emotional dependence is not difficult to endure when it is positive. It is easy to like and appreciate and do our best for patients who like us and show us respect, but we should contrive also to give of our best to those who are negative towards us. Positive and negative attitudes expressed towards the doctor are usually not personal attitudes expressed towards him as a real person, but accrue to him in his capacity as a symbolic figure. In other words, it is helpful to realize that the doctor does not usually earn the negative feelings which some patients display towards him even if it is salutary for him to remember that positive feelings and respect are often unmerited and unreasonable.

Transference acts in two directions and the doctor has to be alive to his own emotional response to a patient's display of respect and affection. A likeable dependent patient should be saved from over-dependence and continued invalidism even at the risk of the doctor falling somewhat in the patient's regard.

When the patient is negative that attitude can be challenged too, and the doctor should ask—not aggressively but in a way which the patient realizes is intended to increase the doctor's understanding of his problems—why he appears hostile and unco-operative. The doctor must be prepared to hear a few home truths and to accept them in unruffled

fashion, but the upshot may well be and usually is a reduction of hostility, increased co-operation, and the realization that what the patient has expressed had very little to do with what the doctor had actually done.

The doctor should strive to recognize his own blind spots and prejudices. If he observes his own behaviour in the doctor–patient relationship and consistently tries to avoid a moralistic and critical attitude he will not only learn a good deal about his patients but in course of time he will come to learn a good deal about himself.

THE PSYCHOTHERAPEUTIC INTERVIEW

Theory. Psychotherapy is carried out mainly by means of the interview. How a psychiatric interview is conducted is determined by what is known about the aetiology of the neuroses.

It is useful, for example, to remember that neurotic symptoms have a significance comparable with that of pain, tenderness, rigidity and vomiting in physical disease; that is to say, they are warnings of things going wrong and at the same time they are defensive. Pain is physical unease, and for its psychic analogue, mental unease, we use the term *anxiety*. Anxiety occurs whenever there is a threat to the functioning of the organism; if it comes from without, the anxiety has the character of fear, whereas when the danger threatens from within, in a conflict between desire and conscience, it may have the quality of worry, guilt or remorse depending on the precise internal situation which creates the anxiety. Anxiety is the commonest symptom of neurosis, and many other neurotic symptoms arise out of it as a means of avoiding, dispelling or absorbing anxiety. In the healthy person anxiety can be removed by taking appropriate action unless, as sometimes happens, there is no escape from the situation which provokes it. When, however, anxiety is neurotic there is either no obvious situation to which the individual is responding or his reaction to the situation is inappropriate or out of proportion to the threat it holds for him. There is no hard and fast line between neurotic and normal anxiety. Emotional situations always stir up reverberations from similar situations in earlier life, so that emotional reactions are seldom, even in the healthy person, entirely appropriate to the circumstances which arouse them.

In interviewing, it is important to discover in the

first place whether there is any current situation which appears to be provoking anxiety. The patient, especially if he feels guilty, may be reluctant to disclose such a situation or to acknowledge its significance—he would often rather believe that he is suffering from a physical illness than face up to his emotional problems. We know from lengthy psychotherapeutic procedures of an analytic or uncovering type that neurotic anxiety arises from repressed infantile situations which are touched off by current happenings, the connection being unrecognized by the patient. In the childhood situation there may have been overwhelming anxiety and guilt due to an intolerable conflict between instinctual demands seeking gratification and opposing attitudes of the personality conforming to social, conventional, moral and realistic aims. This neurotic attitude persists unrecognized (in the *unconscious*), allowing some gratification of the forbidden impulse while, at the same time, in obedience to the censoring attitudes of the personality, exacting punishment in the shape of severe guilt and anxiety. The patient who tortures himself with the fear that he may have syphilis is an example of this type of reaction. His syphilophobia may follow gratification of an impulse or it may arise merely because he has entertained a forbidden wish. In the life-history of such a patient, evidence may be found of the same kind of maladjustment in a repeated tendency to experience undue guilt after minor misdemeanours. It is important to review the patient's emotional reactions and to seek such characteristic patterns. By discussing these patterns of behaviour the patient will achieve emotional insight. It is not enough for the doctor to perceive the neurotic pattern in the patient's behaviour and to point it out in the expectation that he can thus be given insight in a purely intellectual way; the insight which the patient needs is one which he must achieve for himself and which he must feel through the actual ventilation of the related emotion. This can occur when a good personal relationship has been established between doctor and patient.

When anxiety shows itself, quite irrationally, in certain situations in which there is no apparent danger, as is seen very commonly in *phobias* of closed places such as cinemas or churches, we are usually dealing with a very deep-seated source of anxiety. Such anxiety is not easily modified by psychotherapy, although the patient can receive a great deal of support from his physician. Here the danger arises from an inner conflict, but the device of projecting it outwards to specific situations in the form of a phobia allows the patient to deal with it by avoidance as if it were an external danger.

In *hysteria* the typical symptom is one of a physical disturbance without physical disease. The symptom is an attempt to solve an emotional conflict by translating it into physical terms and so reducing anxiety.

A middle-aged woman, attempting to carry out her mother's unreasonable death-bed command to take an imbecile sister into her home and thereby finding herself in serious conflict with her husband and children, solved her problem by developing a paralysis of her legs which attracted the attention and concern of her family and also prevented her from obeying her mother's command.

The hysteric by exploiting this mechanism often succeeds in avoiding anxiety altogether, presenting a picture of smiling indifference in spite of severe disability. This evasion of anxiety is fundamental to the personality of hysterics.

Since neurotic symptoms arise out of and have relevance to enduring traits in the personality, an important part of the life-history interview both for diagnosis and treatment lies in an assessment of personality and an understanding of its dynamics. Hysterics, for example, are often impressive characters, sure of their own virtues and superior to the failings of others, skilful in manipulating the emotions of those around them—sometimes even including those of the doctor—and contriving always to present themselves in the best possible light. They are usually women and can be recognized by their capacity for self-dramatization and the profession of emotions which they do not feel; they are flirtatious but sexually cold. They seek to dominate every relationship and use feminine wiles and histrionic artifice to achieve this end. Their spite and revengefulness may be perceived only by their few immediate victims who often prefer to remain silent, doubting their own judgment and blaming themselves, rather than challenge the good opinion held by others. When the doctor listens to a life-history in which there are few shortcomings and which seems to be unusually devoid of blame, this in itself suggests hysteria, for it is characteristic of the life-pattern of hysterical patients that they avoid imputing blame to themselves.

The *obsessional* personality should also be recognized from the life-history even in the absence of overt manifestations of the obsessive-compulsive neurosis. The following traits can be regarded as typical. There is obvious concern about the control of the inanimate environment with emphasis on orderliness, cleanliness, neatness and method. There is scrupulous attention to detail: obligations involving the welfare of other people are discharged with meticulous care. In human relationships there is an ill-concealed desire for power and a fear of losing self-esteem. Justice and fair play are of special emotional significance, but underlying these attitudes there are concealed aggressive trends towards significant persons. Ambivalence towards love objects is a special problem for obsessionals and is seen in their difficulty in the choosing of a marital partner and in their constant indecision and inability to terminate tasks. Interest in vague humanitarian concepts implying altruism and love for all mankind may represent a retreat from more intense personal relationships in which the obsessional is afraid of his aggressive impulses. The obsessional personality is analogous to—and tells us a great deal about—many personalities seen in the stress diseases or psychosomatic disorders; in these, tension translated into somatic dysfunction may arise from an inability to express freely emotions of love or hostility.

It is true to say that nearly all neuroses have their roots in disturbances of personal relationships whether we are considering the early primary family relationships or the traumatic situations of adult life which precipitate the neurosis. Even in the extreme case of the war neurosis there is not only fear of death but also fear of disgrace in the eyes of the group; and it is this fear which precipitates the conflict and gives rise to the neurosis. The infantile conflicts which determine the form of later neurosis are concerned with the most significant persons in the child's environment, his parents or parent substitutes, brothers and sisters. The ways in which he adjusts to the family, the first group of which he is a member, modify and characterize his relations with those he meets in all later groups, and insight into this fact is an important aim in therapy. Of these early relationships that with the mother is most crucial for emotional development. Later feelings of insecurity and incapacity in forming affectionate relationships often appear to arise from separation from the mother in infancy or from attitudes of rejection on her part which deny the child the experience of a warm affection.

Procedure. To start the patient talking he should be asked about his *complaints* and everything he says should be carefully noted. In considering these complaints the doctor should make due allowance for the patient's tendency to minimize the expression of emotion while emphasizing any somatic disturbance which he experiences; if the patient does try to describe his tension or his feelings of anxiety, he should be encouraged to expand his description. No attempt should be made to switch the patient away from his complaints until the doctor is satisfied that he fully understands them.

The patient should next be asked to describe the history of his present illness, describing in detail when and how the symptoms began. The doctor should note any indications of possible emotional situations which might have a bearing on the symptoms. If the patient has sustained an accident, inquiries about insurance and compensation may provide relevant data.

When the history of the illness has been brought up to the present, the interview should go on to take account of the patient's *life-history*. It is necessary to get to know the patient as a person, and this aim can be conveyed by asking 'Where were you born and brought up? Where do you come in the family?' If the patient begins to talk of the family situation and his early relationships with his parents, so much the better, but, at this stage in a first interview, direct questioning about sibling rivalry, attitude to parents or parental attitudes to the patient, may arouse resentment and should be avoided. It is better to come back to these points later when the patient has gained confidence and through discussion of his contemporary situation has developed insight into his basic emotional attitudes.

The usual medical inquiries about illnesses in childhood should precede questions about nervousness and childhood fears, which should be made as concrete as possible as, for example: 'Most children fear the dark; did you have any special fears of that kind? How did you get on at school? Did you have any special worries about your school work? How did you get on with your teachers?' Such inquiries may lead the patient to describe other significant fears or upsets related to his family.

The age of the patient at the time of the death of a parent or a near relative should be carefully noted along with any indications of emotional disturbance related to the death. The sequence of events is specially important and questions should be put so that any relationship between significant events and developments in the life situation of the patient is clearly established.

It is important to assess the patient's intelligence and the best indicator is usually the school record. A careful note should be taken of the ages at which the various educational levels were achieved.

The work record often provides clues to personality difficulties in the reasons given for leaving a job or for choosing a new occupation. It is also important to inquire into the patient's prospects of promotion and any disappointments he has suffered in this respect.

The importance of sexual experience in determining psychological attitudes should not be forgotten, and some attention should be devoted to the sex life of the patient. It is possible in a first interview to ask questions about the sex life, but these should be factual and more or less confined to such conventional inquiries as the patient would expect from the doctor. He can be asked about courtship, when he married, and the number and ages of the children. Direct questions about marital relations should be avoided at the start unless the patient is obviously forthcoming and wishes to talk, as he usually will when there is marital discord and overt emotional stress. Women patients usually talk more readily about their sex life than do men and are more apt to grasp the significance of the doctor's inquiries in this field.

Questions about the financial position of the household, housing difficulties, relationship with in-laws, etc., are often of special importance, and the doctor should satisfy himself that he has a clear picture of the patient as he now lives in respect of his family situation, work, friends and recreation.

Personality is best assessed by considering the life-history and also the clues which the patient gives in the interview, for instance, the things he stresses, his attitude towards the doctor, his mannerisms and his emotional reactions. Some inquiries can be made directly; for example, his sociability can be assessed by questions regarding his leisure time pursuits, whether he seeks the company of others or prefers a solitary hobby. Knowledge of his habits and likes and dislikes may indicate the unduly methodical personality of the obsessional which in turn may suggest further investigation into his relationships with others.

In taking the *family history*, it is as well to avoid too direct inquiries into the presence or absence of mental illness in the family. Patients suffering from neurosis are often afraid of insanity, and if the doctor makes a special point of this question it will suggest to the patient that the doctor suspects that he is liable to become insane. The importance of a family history of mental illness is, in any case, for the individual, not so much the hereditary factor as the effect it has had on the patient's upbringing, and this should emerge incidentally in the account that the patient gives of his life-history.

In all cases the doctor should carry out a careful *physical examination* and, in doing so, he should remember the neurotic fears which the patient may have and the need to reassure him. If he finds it necessary to linger over the auscultation of an area in the chest, he should remember the consequent fear that may arise in the patient's mind and try to allay it immediately. He should keep to himself any doubts he may have and so avoid implanting the idea—widespread among neurotic patients—that they are puzzling cases of physical illness.

When he has covered the life-history and made a physical examination, the doctor should be in a position to decide whether the patient is suffering from a neurosis or whether the diagnosis needs to be completed by special investigations such as a radiograph of the skull, blood and C.S.F. examinations, electroencephalography or examination by a specialist. If the doctor has no reasonable doubt, and especially if he has positive findings of an emotional disturbance to account for the patient's complaints—which will usually be the case—he should be quite positive in explaining the patient's symptoms on an emotional basis. Because patients are apt to think there is only one kind of real illness, namely, that with a physically detectable lesion, the explanation should be full enough to prevent the patient from gaining the impression that the doctor is accusing him of malingering or of having imaginary pains, and this may involve giving the patient a simple account of how emotions may produce bodily disturbance. For instance, if the patient has pain and stiffness in muscles, the doctor can point out that heightened emotion is often accompanied by a tense bodily state and that this could account for his symptoms. The patient can also be made to understand how headache, tachycardia, nausea, diarrhoea or constipation can be produced in a like manner.

An interview such as has been described, especially if it has given the patient an opportunity to vent his emotions, has in itself great therapeutic value. It will be noticed that the doctor has been called upon to do little more than adopt the attitude of an interested listener and no interpretation of the patient's emotional attitudes has necessarily been undertaken. Premature interpretation and re-assurance have to be avoided; there is usually resis-tance on the part of the patient to gaining insight into his own emotions, and he therefore discloses his fears and his guilt only by instalments. If the doctor rushes in with an interpretation of the patient's attitudes before they are fully disclosed, it will diminish the patient's confidence in the doctor's wisdom and will effectively block, at least for a time, any further disclosure which he had been willing to make. The patient may well react negatively in such a situation and the doctor may become aware of his hostility. He should take it in an unruffled fashion which will effectively reassure the patient and reduce his resistance, because it will have demonstrated to him that the doctor accepts him for what he is, good and bad together, and that the doctor's aim is to understand how he has become what he is and not to sit in judgment on him.

Each interview will leave some questions un-answered and suggest topics for further interviews. This material should be noted and raised again when a suitable opportunity occurs.

LIMITATIONS OF PSYCHOTHERAPY

If the practitioner's psychotherapy is to be effective and rewarding, he must try to avoid under-taking the treatment of those *deep-seated neuroses* which require techniques beyond his scope. In deciding what treatment the patient requires he should bear in mind the following rough guides:

1. Acute neuroses respond more readily than chronic neuroses.

2. Neuroses which arise in a clearly traumatic way, for example, from an accident or an intolerable situation, are of better prognosis than those which occur without any obvious cause.

3. Anxiety states with marked phobias (fear of closed spaces, fear of being out alone, etc.) are more difficult to treat than those in which the anxiety is unrelated to specific situations.

4. Obsessional neuroses, which are usually very chronic, are notoriously difficult to treat radi-cally even by the most expert and lengthy

procedures: patients do, however, benefit from supportive therapy given by their practitioner (see below).

5. Patients suffering from neuroses accompanied by a profound personality disorder, or in whom there is a psychotic element such as morbid suspicion, are not good subjects for psychotherapy.

6. When hysterical symptoms arise out of severe acute anxiety states, for example, in acute neuroses following trauma where loss of speech and hysterical paralysis of the limbs is not uncommon, the prognosis is good. Generally, however, in cases of hysteria, where the symp-toms are exploited to deal with long-term emotional difficulties, only the most intense and lengthy treatment is likely to be effective. The success of superficial procedures, e.g. suggestion, hypnotism, etc., in temporarily removing a symptom is no indication that the underlying condition is significantly affected.

PSYCHOPHARMACOLOGY

Psychopharmacology, the study of drugs which influence behaviour, is an increasingly important subject, and the physician now has available to him large and increasing numbers of psychotropic drugs. These compounds are divided into two main groups: the tranquillizers, used in dealing with symptoms of anxiety and agitation, and the anti-depressant drugs, used in the management of depressive symptoms. Before dealing with their indications and use, some general points should be noted.

While many of these drugs are potent and valuable, some have not yet been adequately assessed, and all of them have side-effects and occasionally prove toxic. In evaluating the usually overoptimistic claims that are made for newly introduced drugs, it is important to remember that a drug trial in this field can be misleading unless a large number of factors are taken into account which would not ordinarily affect the trial of a remedy for physical illness. The placebo effect, the variability in the occurrence of spontaneous remission, the lack of physical signs and the subjective nature of the disability are some of the factors which often bedevil analysis of the findings. It is wise, therefore, to be guided only by the results of carefully devised and controlled trials which have taken such variables into account. Even then unforeseen toxic effects may come to light only after the drug has been in use for a considerable time.

Before prescribing any new remedy in this, as in any, field the doctor should ask: Am I reasonably certain that it is effective and if so for what symptoms? Is it safe and has it been in use long enough to be proved safe? If it is effective, is it an improvement on existing remedies? If it costs more, do its advantages justify the extra cost?

TRANQUILLIZERS

The simplest classification is into major and minor tranquillizers. The major tranquillizers are phenothiazine derivatives which are used predominantly in psychoses to control excitement, agitation and overactivity in patients in hospital. The minor tranquillizers (chemically, a diverse group) are used for the control of psychoneurotic symptoms, mainly tension and anxiety in ambulant patients.

Phenothiazine derivatives. The introduction of this group of compounds had an immediate and lasting effect on psychiatric hospital practice because of their effect in controlling disturbed psychotic behaviour. Symptoms of acute schizophrenia such as delusions and hallucinations with accompanying excitement and overactivity yield most readily but the phenothiazines are also of great value in enabling many chronic schizophrenic patients to leave hospital and lead useful lives in the community. They may require maintenance doses of phenothiazines continued indefinitely over many years under the supervision of their family doctor. States of delirium associated with head injury, toxaemia and senility respond well to this group of drugs.

In the dosage required, side-effects are frequent. The calming effect may be accompanied by drowsiness, especially when the drug is first prescribed and while the dose is being increased; but even with large doses patients become tolerant to the drug within a short time and it is unusual for drowsiness to persist. In the early stages of treatment, tachycardia, dizziness and postural hypotension may be troublesome. Dry mouth is a frequent complaint and if oral hygiene is neglected a raw, painful tongue results and, occasionally, a monilial infection may be superadded. With many compounds, when high doses are reached, extrapyramidal symptoms supervene. These are akin to the clinical

features of Parkinsonism, but more unusual neurological effects can occur with dystonic and dyskinetic reactions. Extrapyramidal symptoms can be satisfactorily controlled with the drugs used in Parkinsonism and do not call for the withdrawal of the phenothiazine. Dermatitis may occur through contact with the drug and can be a hazard to the nurse and the doctor as well as to the patient. Photosensitivity is common, and in the summer months all patients on phenothiazines should be warned of this possibility and advised to avoid long periods of exposure to sunlight. Jaundice of an obstructive type is seen occasionally. Agranulocytosis occurs very rarely and major epileptic seizures sometimes develop in non-epileptic patients.

Many phenothiazines are available. There are three main groups, according to the type of sidechain that is attached to the phenothiazine nucleus: (a) those with a dimethylaminopropyl side-chain, e.g. chlorpromazine and promazine; (b) those with a piperazine side-chain, e.g. perphenazine and trifluoperazine; (c) those with a piperidine sidechain, e.g. thioridazine.

Chlorpromazine, the first to be introduced, is the most widely tested of these drugs. It is available in 10 mg., 25 mg., 50 mg. and 100 mg. tablets and in ampoules containing 50 mg. in 2 ml. for intramuscular injection. In acute schizophrenia treatment should begin with a dosage of 150 to 300 mg. daily, increasing over a week or two to 500 mg. to 1 g. daily. The maintenance dose in chronic schizophrenia is usually of the order of 150 to 300 mg. daily. The most frequent toxic effects are jaundice, contact dermatitis and photosensitivity. Parkinsonism can be expected with doses above 300 mg. daily and when the first symptoms appear it is usual to add benzhexol hydrochloride 2 mg., orphenadrine hydrochloride 50 mg., or another drug of this type. The doses of these drugs should be gradually increased in accordance with the patient's needs. Chlorpromazine is useful in the treatment of restlessness, in delirium or in senility in doses of 25 to 50 mg. four times daily.

Promazine is similar to chlorpromazine in structure but less likely to lead to jaundice. For this reason it is widely used in the management of the withdrawal phase of alcoholism, in drug addiction and in delirium tremens; 100 to 200 mg. three times a day is usual in such cases. The drug is also helpful in the management of restlessness in senile patients in doses of 50 to 100 mg. four times daily.

Tablets of 25, 50 and 100 mg. strengths are available and ampoules for injection.

Trifluoperazine and *perphenazine* are representative of the phenothiazines with a piperazine side-chain. They are more potent weight for weight than chlorpromazine and less hepatotoxic, but more liable to produce severe and even alarming neurological side-effects. They are used mainly in the management of schizophrenia. Trifluoperazine is given in doses of 10 to 30 mg. daily with a maintenance dose of 2 mg. thrice daily. Tablets of 1 mg. and 5 mg. are available. Perphenazine, available in 2, 4, and 8 mg. tablet strengths, is used in doses of 8 to 16 mg. thrice daily with a maintenance dose of 2 to 4 mg. thrice daily.

Fluphenazine has the advantage of being available in the form of a long-acting injection—fluphenazine enanthate or fluphenazine decanoate (25 mg. in 1 ml.). Many chronic schizophrenics who require maintenance therapy do not take oral medication regularly because of their mental state. In such cases a long-acting preparation has a place in management. Unfortunately side-effects are very common, especially extrapyramidal reactions, which require regular oral medication with anti-Parkinson drugs, thus limiting the scope of this approach to maintenance. Small test doses are essential and establishing the correct dosage may require hospital admission. Maintenance injections are given at two- to four-week intervals.

Thioridazine is representative of the phenothiazines with a piperidine side-chain. The drugs in this group have fewer extrapyramidal effects. It is available in 10, 25, 50 and 100 mg. tablets, the average daily dose varying from 30 to 300 mg.

In selecting a phenothiazine for clinical use, the doctor should confine himself to one compound and learn to use it well. He should avoid the use of proprietary preparations containing phenothiazines in combination with other drugs.

Minor tranquillizers. In contrast to the previous group the compounds in this class are chemically diverse but similar in effect. They reduce anxiety and are, therefore, widely used in the management of symptoms of anxiety occurring in psychoneurosis or arising out of stress. Patients, however, need to be reminded from time to time that anxiety is not always abnormal and indeed is useful in appropriate circumstances. This applies not only to the patient who asks for a tranquillizer when about to face a driving test or an examination but to some patients who have more serious and lasting prob-

lems in their life. The progress made in psychotherapy may depend on the level of anxiety shown by the patient. If this level is unnecessarily reduced by tranquillizers, he will have less incentive to co-operate in facing and discussing his difficulties. This problem is not peculiar to the misuse of tranquillizers. It has existed for a very long time in the use and abuse of sedatives and hypnotics. Patients with anxious and inadequate personalities quickly become dependent on both drugs and doctors for support. The drug dependency may be physical or psychological. In the latter the drug is being used as a placebo. If medication over months and years is ever necessary for these patients a placebo will usually be as effective as an active drug.

Over the years many minor tranquillizers have been introduced, some of which have had only a brief period of fashion before vanishing into the limbo of forgotten drugs. A short-acting barbiturate is at least as effective in reducing anxiety as a minor tranquillizer but since the tranquillizer is less likely to produce drowsiness and, more important, is less likely to produce habituation and addiction, it should be preferred to the barbiturate. The relief which a tranquillizer gives to a patient suffering from psychoneurosis is restricted to diminishing anxiety, and psychotherapy is still the treatment of choice.

Chlordiazepoxide, diazepam, and *meprobamate* are representative of this group. They are relatively safe and, in addition to their effect on anxiety, have mild anticonvulsant properties. They may be used in simple anxiety states, in states of tension associated with organic disease, and in psychosomatic disorders as well as in the management of drug or alcohol withdrawal. Individual response to these drugs varies considerably. As they have sedative effects, they may impair concentration, and since they are likely to be given to ambulant patients the dose should be adjusted carefully and the patient warned about possible drowsiness in relation to work and to driving vehicles. These drugs may also potentiate the effects of alcohol and this may be both embarrassing and dangerous. Chlordiazepoxide is available in 5 and 10 mg. strengths for oral use and in ampoules of 100 mg. for injection. The usual dose range is 15 to 40 mg. daily. Diazepam is available in 2, 5 and 10 mg. tablets. The dose varies from 15 to 40 mg. daily. Meprobamate can be prescribed in 200 or 400 mg. tablets in a dose of 600 mg. to 1·6 g. daily.

ANTI-DEPRESSANT AND STIMULANT DRUGS

Three main groups of drugs are used in the treatment of depression: the iminodibenzyl derivatives, the amines, and the mono-amine oxidase inhibitors.

The *iminodibenzyl derivatives* are at present the most effective drugs for the treatment of depressive symptoms. The first to be introduced was imipramine. The other compound in wide use is amitriptyline. Imipramine gives its best results in the treatment of retarded patients. Amitriptyline, which has a more sedative effect, is useful in the treatment of the patient with agitated depression.

The full effect of these drugs does not appear until ten days to three weeks after administration has begun and too often they are withdrawn before an adequate amount has been given. The patient should be encouraged to persevere and warned that side-effects may precede improvement. The sedative effect of amitriptyline is immediate and helpful in the interval before anti-depressant effects appear. Treatment should be started with 25 mg. three or four times daily and increased to 50 mg. three times daily after a week. In resistant cases the dose may be increased to 200 mg. daily but the duration of therapy is usually more important than the dosage. On this regimen side-effects are to be expected, especially dryness of the mouth and drowsiness. In the elderly, retention of urine may occur or sudden falling attacks which may have serious consequences. Because of this it is usual to start with a smaller dose in patients over 60 and to increase it cautiously. Jaundice and agranulocytosis have been reported. Peripheral neuropathy and oedema may occur and abnormalities may appear in the E.C.G. The combination of these drugs with the mono-amine oxidase inhibitors is potentially toxic and must be avoided: at least a week must elapse between stopping one type of drug and starting the other.

The *amines* comprise amphetamine and related compounds such as dexamphetamine and methylamphetamine. All have sympathomimetic effects: they increase energy, and produce euphoria or anxiety in the normal subject. They may lead to transient improvement in patients with a depressive illness but have no true anti-depressant effect. All are likely to lead to habituation and addiction and, as this is a problem of increasing gravity, most psychiatrists feel that this group of drugs has no place in the management of any kind of psychiatric illness.

The *mono-amine oxidase inhibitors* are divided into hydrazine derivatives, e.g. phenelzine, nialamide and isocarboxazid; and non-hydrazine derivatives, e.g. tranylcypromine. They have sometimes been shown in controlled trials to be more effective in treating depression than a placebo, but the results are not striking and only a minority of patients are helped. Despite their name there is no definite proof that the effectiveness of these drugs is related to their ability to inhibit amine oxidase.

Serious side-effects are liable to occur including jaundice and agranulocytosis. They also potentiate morphine and other analgesics and sedatives. Tranylcypromine especially increases the effect of tyramine and other sympathomimetic amines and patients on these drugs who take cheese or other foods containing a significant quantity of these amines are liable to develop paroxysms of hypertension which may be slight but have been fatal.

If these drugs were of obvious value in the treatment of depression, their side-effects and the rare fatalities which result from their use, could be regarded as a justifiable risk. As it is they should at best be reserved for patients who have failed to respond to other and safer means of treatment.

To summarize: when prescribing anti-depressant drugs it should be borne in mind that, although effective, they are potentially toxic and they should not be used without a clear indication. Not every patient complaining of depression has a depressive illness. When there is a suicidal risk the patient is probably better treated in hospital in view of the prolonged period that elapses before the drug takes effect. In cases of this kind electrical treatment is usually preferred because it is more rapidly effective.

PATIENTS REQUIRING A SPECIALIST OPINION

Some patients require to be referred to a psychiatrist for further investigation and treatment. It is important to recognize such cases as early as possible but the need for a second opinion may, of course, become apparent only when it is obvious to the family doctor that the patient is not responding to treatment.

Before sending a patient to a psychiatrist it is usually necessary to pave the way by explaining very carefully to him why he is being sent; if this is not done, the patient may be resentful and suspicious towards his doctor and hostile and unco-operative to the psychiatrist. This can happen even when the patient himself has already come to the conclusion that he should see a psychiatrist. His objection arises from the fact that he suspects he is being sent for the wrong reason; he may believe that the doctor thinks he is going insane or that he is malingering. An adequate history is invaluable to the consultant. If the doctor has already been taken into the patient's confidence and knows his patient's intimate problem, he should obtain his consent to include this information in the letter of introduction, which will save the patient the embarrassment of having to break into the subject himself and will smooth the process of communicating the history to the specialist.

The specialist's advice will take the form of recommending how the practitioner can continue to treat the patient or he may advise treatment in hospital or as an out-patient. It sometimes happens that the patient refuses to co-operate in the line of treatment which has been suggested and, in rejecting the advice which has been offered, he may criticize the psychiatrist and demand to be sent elsewhere. The doctor's duty in such a case is to try to persuade the patient to return to the psychiatrist, offering to convey to him the substance of the patient's criticism; the patient's feelings about the psychiatrist may well be an example of the negative transference already described, which, in this case, has been provoked by a therapeutically directed interview. The alternative is to expose the patient to the risk of making a fruitless pilgrimage from one specialist to another, accumulating negative attitudes on his way, and in despair at his journey's end falling into the clutches of the quack.

The closer the practitioner works with the psychiatrist the better, and he should try to know him personally so that informal exchanges on the telephone can help to smooth out difficulties as they arise. The doctor should not hesitate to ask advice about social services which might be available to help patients. It is in the nature of his work that the psychiatrist should have a special knowledge of such facilities and the doctor should profit from his knowledge so that he himself can make the best use of all the services and agencies which are available.

Certain groups of patients will almost always have to be referred to specialist facilities.

Acute psychotic patients. These cannot as a rule be handled in general practice and the doctor's main duty is early recognition. In such cases the relatives will emphasize the change in behaviour and personality which indicates not the part-reaction of the neurosis, in which the personality is preserved, but the whole-reaction of the psychosis, where the personality change is conspicuous. Seclusiveness, bizarre behaviour and utterances, grotesque, hypochondriacal complaints and un-accountable impulsive actions suggest *schizophrenia*. Modern treatment (electroconvulsive therapy and the transquillizers), combined with the facilities for rehabilitation in the modern mental hospital or general hospital psychiatric unit, offers the best chance of recovery, and if admission to hospital is advised it is the doctor's duty to do his best to influence the patient's relatives to follow this advice.

Sometimes the patient suffering from a psychosis is seen as an acute emergency in a state of great restlessness or excitement, and rapid sedation is necessary. In these circumstances the most effective method is to administer chlorpromazine, 50 to 100 mg. intramuscularly, or alternatively hyoscine hydrobromide, 1 mg. hypodermically, or an injection containing morphine, 15 mg., and hyoscine, 0·5 mg.

The management of a patient who complains of *acute depression* raises a number of problems requiring careful consideration. The doctor will wish to know whether the danger of suicide is great, necessitating the patient being placed in a mental hospital even against his will. Surveys of attempted suicides show that while in all cases there is some degree of psychiatric abnormality before an attempt is made, the motive for suicide is frequently an escape from threatened scandal and exposure, and consequently a number of would-be suicides do not regard themselves as being ill and do not seek a doctor's help. But while it is statistically true that suicide is frequent in the absence of a complaint of psychiatric illness, the risk of suicide is always to be taken seriously when a patient does complain of depression. Unfortunately there are no precise criteria by which the danger of suicide can be judged, but there are some guiding principles which will help the doctor in forming an opinion. The first guide is to be found in the diagnosis. Patients can be divided into three groups: (*a*) those suffering from endogenous psychoses (the depressive phase of the manic-depressive psychosis, and involutional melancholia); (*b*) the reactive depressions in which the depression is clearly connected with an event in the patient's life which has produced great disappointment, financial loss, humiliation or disgrace, to which group we may conveniently add the depressions which are incidental to a neurotic illness such as an anxiety neurosis, hysteria or obsessional state; (c) depressive reactions occurring in organic conditions such as G.P.I., arteriosclerotic disease of the brain or cerebral tumour.

The danger of suicide is probably greatest in the first of these three categories, i.e. those suffering from endogenous psychoses. In these psychoses there is not merely a desire to escape from life but an aggressive attitude to self-destruction arising from strong feelings of unworthiness and self-hate. This is manifest in the ferocity with which some of these patients attempt suicide—for example, a patient suffering from manic-depressive psychosis committed suicide by thrusting a red-hot poker down her throat. Some patients never relent in their desire for self-destruction, and by sheer cunning they succeed even where the greatest care is taken under the conditions of a mental hospital.

In coming to the opinion that the patient is suffering from a severe endogenous psychosis we are often guided by the history of previous spells of depression or mania. If the patient has previously attempted suicide, this should serve as a warning that the danger is likely to arise again. In the endogenous psychosis the mood of depression is usually more intense than in other conditions and this can be estimated by the patient's demeanour; the depression is often worse in the morning and improves as the day goes on. In older patients suffering from involutional melancholia the picture is often one of extreme agitation with great restlessness; the patient wrings his hands and picks at his skin. In those suffering from manic-depressive psychosis, the emphasis is on inactivity; the patient sits motionless with downcast head, his answers to questions are slow and come after a pause and he complains of feeling changed and of things around him appearing to be different. When depression is as intense as this, the need for care and supervision is undeniable. It is possibly true that when the patient is very inert and in the acute phase of his illness he will display less initiative even in attempting suicide, but this is no real safeguard and he may well seize any opportunity which presents itself. Other indications of the severity of the depression are to be found in the somatic symptoms; severe insomnia with early morning wakening, loss of appetite, constipation and loss of weight all point to a dangerous condition.

If the practitioner has come to the conclusion that the patient is seriously depressed, the risk of suicide should be regarded as being great even if the patient does not mention it. Sometimes, however, the doctor can also be guided by what the patient himself says. If the patient describes depression and says that life is not worth living, he can usually be asked whether he has contemplated suicide and he may well give an accurate account of any such preoccupations. The common belief that those who talk of suicide never carry out their threat is quite untrue, although, of course, there are patients who talk glibly about suicide without having any suicidal intention. Most patients who do commit suicide have usually mentioned their intention to someone.

In the reactive depressions the danger of suicide is less easy to gauge. If depression is constant and is maintained unrelieved for days or weeks at a time, the risk is greater. But in many cases, although the patient complains of depression, he experiences it at most only for a day or two at a time and in the intervals his spirits are normal; in these cases the danger of suicide is much less. In addition, in the reactive depression there is a need to estimate the gravity of the external situation and the possibility that the patient may respond to a serious dilemma by attempting suicide. Occasionally it is advisable to recommend admission to a psychiatric unit even when his response appears to be a normal one.

A young man had started a business and had received advances of capital from several friends. Owing to the defalcations of a partner the money had been lost. In the face of this situation the patient was contemplating suicide. He agreed to come into a psychiatric unit and after a short time he was discharged able to face the situation in a more realistic way.

Generally speaking, the more intense the depression the more likely it is to respond to electro-convulsive therapy; and if the doctor is in any doubt about the danger of suicide he should suggest in-patient treatment, knowing not only that the patient's life will be safeguarded but that treatment is likely to be effective. In some cases the doctor may come to the conclusion that the danger of suicide is slight or non-existent and may wish to try the effect of an anti-depressant drug before having recourse to hospital facilities for treatment by E.C.T.

Imipramine or amitriptyline may be used. Starting with a dose of 25 mg. thrice daily, this should be raised after four days to 50 mg. thrice daily (occasionally still further to 75 mg. thrice daily) and continued at that level for at least two weeks before deciding that the treatment is ineffective. If the treatment proves successful, it should be continued for another month before the withdrawal of the drug is begun, and this should be done gradually, stepping up the dose once more if signs of depression reappear. During treatment agitation may be increased especially with imipramine and may require the exhibition of chlorpromazine, 50 mg. twice or thrice daily, or promazine, 100 mg. twice or thrice daily.

The much commoner minor degrees of depression necessarily fall to be treated by the practitioner and are dealt with later (p. 429).

Organic Psychoses. These are characterized in the acute reactions by delirium and confusion and in the more chronic reactions by change in personality and loss of memory. Acute delirium is easily recognized, and if it is due to an infection or alcohol, the duration of the illness is likely to be short and the patient should be admitted to a general rather than to a mental hospital. Organic cerebral disease should be considered as a possibility when any patient over the age of 40, in the absence of great stress, develops neurotic symptoms for the first time; it was mentioned above that depression may be the leading symptom in such a case. A careful physical examination is necessary to exclude especially cerebral tumour, arteriosclerotic brain disease and G.P.I. All patients suffering from organic cerebral disease should be seen by a specialist.

Mental deficiency. If the practitioner has reason to believe that a young child is suffering from serious *mental deficiency*, he should advise that the child should be taken to a specialist in mental subnormality as early as possible. It sometimes seems kinder to wait for a time in the hope that the parents will learn more gradually the true extent of the child's disability, but where there are other children it is in the interest of the mental health of the family that the best solution should be found and this may well mean institutional care. Equally, when it is an only child the doctor has to think of the lifetime of painful adjustment, increasing attachment, and sacrifice which the mother has to face, and he should use all his skill and emotional understanding to help the parents to a correct decision.

Until recent years the only solution appeared to be to provide institutional accommodation for all patients unable to compete for jobs in industry or to lead a normal life. It is now realized that many can be helped while remaining at home and this policy should be pursued wherever possible. Developments in industrial therapy have demonstrated that even quite severely handicapped patients may, through practice, acquire simple, yet valuable, skills. Occupational centres for subnormal patients of all ages are now being provided by local authorities, and sheltered workshops are being set up in which patients can earn wages. Those so trained may eventually become sufficiently well adjusted and skilful to be accepted as normal workers in open industry. Increasing tolerance on the part of employers and the community at large is providing more opportunities for the mentally handicapped to obtain work. The spread of these progressive social measures through the Mental Health Acts should mean that fewer patients will require institutional care in future.

Sexual maladjustments. When patients with these are seen by the practitioner they are commonly of a kind in which his therapy is likely to be effective. There are others, however, which require lengthy investigative techniques if, indeed, they can be treated at all.

Homosexuality, which is accepted by the patient, and which he does not desire to change, will probably be unaffected by treatment; it is for the practitioner to advise the patient to this effect and to give him what support he can in coming to an adjustment which will enable him to avoid antisocial activity. Homosexuals are, however, more prone to suffer from neurosis than those with normal sexual attitudes, and these patients should be referred to the psychiatrist.

Fetishism is a deviation in which sexual gratification and excitement are associated with the sight or possession of certain objects, for example, women's shoes, furs, underclothing, long hair, the naked foot, etc. *Transvestitism* is a condition in which sexual gratification is associated with wearing the clothes of the opposite sex. These are sexual deviations which should always be referred to a psychiatrist. Fetishists and those who suffer from transvestitism are prone to overwhelming attacks of anxiety and depression which may lead to suicide, and since they are likely to consult the doctor only when their anxiety becomes great, this danger should be recognized.

Nowadays child guidance or child psychiatry clinics are available in many places for the treatment of *children with behaviour disorders*. When the disturbance constitutes more than a passing phase in development it is probably better to refer the child for treatment to one of these centres. Minor disturbances are discussed below.

PSYCHIATRIC TASKS WITHIN THE SCOPE OF THE GENERAL PRACTITIONER

Mild depressions. In the previous section the importance of recognizing the more severe states of depression was emphasized. There are other patients who either complain of mild depression or who may present themselves with minor physical complaints. Not all of these need specialist treatment. Indeed, depression arising out of modern stresses is among the commonest of all complaints, and for this the general practitioner can do a great deal. The patient will often feel a need to unburden himself about his disappointments, his frustrations and his sense of failure. This need not be a lengthy affair, and if the symptoms seem clearly to be those of a minor depressive reaction, not interfering noticeably with work or concentration or leisure-time pursuits, the doctor can proceed to reassure the patient. The patient may require to be taken in hand and helped to organize his work and his leisure in such a way that he obtains more satisfaction from them. Occupational therapy is useful, and in general practice this may amount to advice on a hobby, taking into account the patient's personality and previous interests.

If he is sleeping less soundly than usual the patient should be given a hypnotic. For this purpose the practitioner should not be reluctant to use sodium barbitone, 300 to 500 mg. The slight continuance of the effect noticeable after waking is usually no disadvantage to the patient, who is apt to feel anxious and depressed when he first faces the cares of the day. Chloral hydrate, 1·3 to 2 g., well diluted with water, flavoured with syrup of orange, is a reliable and harmless sedative. Phenobarbitone should be avoided because in some patients a hypnotic effect is not obtained, except with an unduly large dose. The more rapidly acting barbiturates should, if prescribed at all for psychiatric patients in practice, be used only for very short periods and in small dosage because they can produce habituation and addiction and a troublesome withdrawal syndrome.

It is of special importance to keep in frequent touch with the mildly depressed patient; the interest shown in him will help to counteract his own feelings of unworthiness and the doctor will be able to keep watch lest more severe depression develops. Treatment with anti-depressant drugs is described on p. 425.

Patients with slight mental defect. Patients who are mentally inadequate, but not sufficiently so to be classed as mental defectives, constitute a largely unrecognized psychiatric problem. They are specially prone to psychiatric disorders of all kinds, psychoneuroses, psychoses, sexual deviations and delinquency. Although, because of their inadequate intelligence, they are unable to co-operate in formal psychotherapy, their neurosis is often less deep-rooted than in more intelligent patients so that they respond to simpler therapeutic aid.

The main problem of their lives lies in the extreme difficulty which they experience in coping with tasks which are well within the powers of the average person. This was seen in their reaction to military training. When subjected to normal programmes these men reacted with acute anxiety states often characterized by tremors, fainting, dyspepsia and vomiting; when, however, they were given simplified training and duties they became fit and enthusiastic soldiers. The doctor, if he recognizes a mentally handicapped patient from the account he gives of his school record and his lack of educational attainments, should provide help in dealing with environmental difficulties. The work situation is important. The job should be within the patient's powers and the employer should be understanding. In larger concerns the patient may become the butt of his workmates; in smaller groups protective attitudes are more likely to be developed towards him. The doctor should seek the help of social service agencies and official personnel officers in dealing with these problems. Often the patient prospers if a social worker makes a good contact with him and his family and the patient knows he can readily turn to her whenever he is in a difficulty.

Childhood problems. Concern about the behaviour problems of children has become so earnest and so fashionable that the slightest deviation is apt nowadays to give rise to serious anxiety on the part of the parents. The effect of parental behaviour in developing personality probably needed emphasizing, but the lesson has been so well learned that parents are too ready to feel guilty and overanxious. Usually all that is required is normal warm affection and tolerance.

Since many problems of childhood are transient, the doctor's task is often to ensure that the parents do not take too serious a view of the child's deviation and are able to treat him with understanding and patience. It has been said that there are no problem children, only problem parents, which is largely, but not entirely, true. Problem parents have often had difficult childhood experiences themselves, and without the background of a happy upbringing they are frequently at a loss to know what to do with their own children. Commonsense support and advice from the doctor can in these circumstances be of great service. It is well to remember also that there are inevitable conflicts and anxieties connected with growing up and surrendering the gratification of instincts in response to social demands; and it is not within the power of the parents to prevent such conflicts. It is even helpful to inform some parents that discipline, including some punishment, is necessary for the mental health of the growing child who cannot be reared in a state of nature but must, like his parents, conform to certain social conventions.

A view propagated by authorities a generation ago is still held by some mothers who believe it is possible to train a child in *sphincter control* from the earliest months. It is possible to achieve a brief and spurious success at the age of six months or even earlier by placing the child on the pot soon after he has been fed. The mother's pride in this achievement is soon dashed when after a short time the inevitable failure occurs. These failures tend to be regarded as naughtiness, and the mother persists in her efforts at training but with heightened emotion and greater determination. Antagonistic reactions usually follow; the child stubbornly refuses to perform while on the pot but gives way immediately afterwards while he is being dressed. It is when this stage is reached that the parent is apt to consult the doctor. Such difficulties are easily avoided if parents are made to realize that the child is not equipped, neurologically or psychologically, to respond to habit training until he is well into his second year, and that occasional failures are normal and to be expected for another year at least.

For her convenience alone, a mother may begin to place a baby on the pot at eight or nine months and, by careful strategy based on observation of the rhythm of the child's activities, benefit from the reflex activity which occurs after feeding or after waking up from sleep, but she should not deceive herself into believing that she is likely to succeed in permanently solving the problem at this stage. It is important to deal with the anxiety of parents in regard to sphincter training, because, if they believe that they are failing or that the child is playing up, they may respond by punishment which is likely to make things worse. A severe attitude on the part of parents during habit training, producing anxiety in the child, is a common cause of bowel incontinence (*encopresis*) in later childhood. The state of anxiety and insecurity which a child may experience on the arrival of a new baby, when he has to take second place, may cause a regression to infantile behaviour and soiling so that he can obtain more of his mother's attention. A simple explanation of the emotional reasons for the child's failing, which avoids blaming the mother who is probably already overanxious, is the correct line of treatment. If soiling occurs in children of school age, however, this is evidence of a severe maladjustment for which the child should be referred to a clinic.

Constipation in young children in the absence of physical causes is more often a symptom of maternal anxiety than of an emotional disturbance on the child's part. The mother who complains of the child's constipation is usually one who has been brought up to believe that there is something wrong if the bowels do not move with absolute regularity. They have usually had recourse to enemas, suppositories and laxatives before consulting the doctor. Again it is the mother who requires re-education and emotional understanding.

What has been said of encopresis is true also of *enuresis*; overanxiety and in a few cases, parental neglect and carelessness, are the chief causes. Control of the bladder is not usually achieved until the child is well into his second year and, again, accidents are frequent for the next year or so, especially in boys. By the time a child is established as a bed-wetter there is usually already a long history of parental nagging, scolding, punishment and shaming, and the child has come to regard himself as wicked or very abnormal. The doctor has to handle the parents very carefully to obtain all the co-operation he can from them. It is usually difficult for them to give up the punitive and hostile attitudes which they have developed towards the child: they may look upon themselves as being morally in the right and believe that they punish the child more in sorrow than in anger. The best results are often achieved by the doctor assuming the rôle of the good parent; adopting a permissive attitude to counterbalance the parent's severity, reassuring the child that he is not bad and promising to see him once or twice a week so that he can report progress.

Eating difficulties are another source of parental anxiety and overprotectiveness, trouble often beginning in early infancy when the mother interprets too literally and too slavishly the amount of milk prescribed in the baby-book and a struggle commences to make sure that the child takes enough on each and every occasion. The problem becomes more acute when the child starts to take solid food and is able to show his likes and dislikes. The mother may then take refuge in all kinds of manœuvres to 'get him to eat', including bribes, threats and distractions. Refusal to eat may be exploited by the child as a means of dominating and attracting attention.

Feeding difficulties are often most acute when the child is two or three years old: he then begins to show his emerging independence in his desire to feed himself; he eats what he wants and not what his mother insists on his having because it is good for him. The first step in treating a difficulty of this kind is to allay the mother's anxiety by conducting a careful physical examination to assure her that the child has come to no harm. It may be as well also to discover whether the mother has any special reason to fear that the child may not grow up into a vigorous adult; as may be the case if, for example, there is a family history of tuberculosis. Otherwise, the doctor should aim at reducing the mother's anxiety, guiding her in allowing the child more freedom in choosing what he will eat and not insisting on his eating too much of what he dislikes.

Most parents know nowadays that *thumb-sucking, nail-biting and masturbation* are deviations which are of little emotional significance and should be treated with tolerance and without anxiety. If, however, such deviations are persistent over a long period of time, the child should be referred to a clinic for further investigation.

Occasional *temper tantrums* are normal in childhood. They may represent outbursts of anger against a thwarting parental authority, jealousy towards a sibling or, in later childhood, difficulty in adjustment to the tensions engendered by beginning to mix with playmates. If the child is usually happy and the parents are otherwise satisfied with his behaviour, nothing needs to be done about the tantrums. They should be regarded as a healthy and natural protest against encroachments, albeit inevitable, on his rights and satisfactions as an individual.

Psychoneuroses. *Anxiety neuroses* form the bulk of the neuroses seen in practice. The more general principles of treatment have already been dealt with, but there are some special points to be borne in mind in dealing with these conditions. The process of mental *catharsis*, that is to say the discharge of emotion in the presence of the doctor, is especially helpful in anxiety neurosis. Often all that the patient needs is a sympathetic and understanding listener, and if the doctor is able to assure the patient of his interest and does not hasten to interrupt with premature explanations or reassurance, the patient may be relieved of his tension even in a single session. At one time it was believed that the anxiety neurosis was an *actual* neurosis, that is to say, that it was due to accumulated tension producing direct physical effects. It was also believed that tension was always due to sexual excitation in the absence of sufficient discharge. This is now regarded as an extreme view, but the doctor should bear in mind the possibility that the patient's symptoms may, at least in part, be due to the practice of coitus interruptus. It is certainly true that improvement often occurs when intercourse is accomplished in a more satisfactory fashion, and this is especially so in women when unsatisfactory coitus has been accompanied by anxiety connected with the fear of pregnancy. In some cases a doctor may decide to give contraceptive advice or to refer his patient to a Family Planning Clinic.

There is a special form of anxiety neurosis which has been called *traumatic neurosis* and which follows severe trauma. While it is seen typically in war, it occurs also after accidents in civil life. This neurosis is characterized by attacks of anxiety of the usual kind, broken sleep, terrifying dreams, headache, and irritability, especially towards members of the patient's family. In more severe cases there is tremor of the head and limbs. There may be amnesia for the actual traumatic incident, especially in the war neurosis. The feature of the trauma which precipitates the neurosis is an apparently inescapable situation threatening the life of the patient. At the time of the trauma there is no way in which the patient can master the situation and the overwhelming anxiety aroused cannot be dissipated by action. The repetition of the incident in the waking thoughts and the dreams of the patient may be an attempt to relive the situation and achieve control over it.

> Working on a railway line a man had to throw himself down between the rails on the unexpected approach of a freight train. As the train passed over him he saw a broken brake-rod projecting downwards. He felt that death was certain but somehow managed to throw himself outwards between the wheels. He developed a traumatic neurosis.
>
> Another patient was helping to lower, down a lift shaft, a large counter suspended by ropes. He was standing at the bottom to receive it when the rope slipped and the counter fell towards him. By an extraordinary chance he escaped by flattening himself against the wall. Following this he had terrifying dreams in which the incident was repeated and as he walked on the street he had a constant feeling that the buildings were about to fall on him.

When feelings of tension and anxiety are great, they may be treated by the use of a tranquillizing drug such as chlordiazepoxide, 10 to 20 mg. thrice daily, diazepam, 15 to 40 mg. per day, meprobamate, 400 mg. thrice daily, chlorpromazine, 25 to 50 mg. thrice daily or promazine, 50 to 100 mg. thrice daily.

When the neurosis persists unrelieved it is usually necessary to go more deeply and to discover, for example, whether the incident was interpreted by the patient as a punishment associated with a previous feeling of guilt. Where there is amnesia or impaired memory for the event the best treatment may be a complete and repeated recall, a virtual reliving of the incident. This technique is known as *abreaction* and it entails the recovery of the memory and the expression of the emotion associated with the incident. A patient may be led to this if he is put into a relaxed state and taken over the events up to the point where the amnesia began. It may be necessary to do this several times before he begins to abreact. The process can be facilitated by making the patient drowsy with an intravenous injection of thiopentone or by giving him light ether anaesthesia. If a narcotic or an anaesthetic is used the incident recalled has to be gone over again when the patient is fully conscious. These methods are not suitable for general practice. During the abreaction the patient may become very excited, shouting and screaming, and may remain in an excited state for some hours afterwards.

In traumatic neurosis recovery may be hampered by the existence of a legal action against another party for damages or compensation. In some cases the patient is quite conscious of the desirability of maintaining his symptoms so that he will obtain a favourable financial settlement, but perhaps more frequently the persistence of symptoms in such a situation is determined by emotional factors of which he is not fully aware. Resentment towards an employer may be part of a lifelong pattern of resentment arising from a feeling that he was rejected by his parents and enjoyed fewer privileges than his siblings, or the patient may have a need to demonstrate to himself and to others the justice of his cause in the face of an underlying sense of guilt and a conviction of his own culpability. It is necessary to try to deal with these attitudes, but the doctor will often find he is playing a losing game, and that conferences with lawyers and trade-union officials and the pressure of the patient's friends and relatives will only too readily neutralize the effects of the psychotherapy. The patient should, of course, be told that it is in the interests of his future health to obtain an early settlement of the dispute so that he can then devote himself in a whole-hearted fashion to his rehabilitation.

The fact that *hysteria* usually arises out of a personality not readily accessible to psychotherapy renders the prognosis unfavourable for superficial treatment. The patient will often respond to placebos and to the demonstration of attention on the part of the practitioner, but this usually prepares the ground for the fabrication of a new disability. The doctor must be shrewd in dealing with the hysterical patient and endeavour to assess the meaning of the symptom in relation to the total life situation, including the manipulation of relationships with close friends and relations, not excluding the doctor himself. He should try to adopt the attitude of a firm and rather strict parent who, nevertheless, does not thereby threaten rejection but who remains positive. Hysterical outbursts must certainly be treated in this way, and while superficially the patient may appear to resent the doctor's attitude, it will on a deeper level provide much-needed security and reassurance; it will also help the family and perhaps relieve them to some extent of the guilt aroused by the resentment they at times feel towards the patient.

The *obsessional neurosis* is exceedingly difficult to treat in a radical fashion and the practitioner must not expect striking therapeutic results; he should, however, aim at giving support and reassurance.

The patient is always aware of the unreasonable nature of his doubts, compulsions and obsessions, but he is, nevertheless, unable to withstand the impulse to give way to them. He often feels ashamed of his actions and thoughts and may believe that his illness amounts to insanity. It is for this reason that he may hesitate to approach the doctor about his symptoms, but his relief is correspondingly great when he finds that his illness is one which is recognized by his doctor. It is in the nature of the complaint that the patient should continually struggle against his compulsions, and it is helpful for him to be assured that it is better not to make these strenuous efforts. When the patient is obsessed by the fear of harming someone and has, for example, developed an obsessional phobia of knives so that he feels upset when he sees them and cannot handle them, it is necessary to assure him that he will never give way to the act he fears. Reassurance of this kind may have to be given again and again and it may seem to be quite useless, but in fact it may provide for the patient the necessary support to see him through an acute attack. Obsessional symptoms sometimes accompany a psychosis and the practitioner should always have in mind the possibility of a patient developing an attack of depression. When symptoms are acute the tension from which the patient suffers may be reduced by the use of a tranquillizer (meprobamate, 400 mg. twice or thrice daily; chlordiazepoxide, 10 to 20 mg. thrice daily), but drugs should never be given to those who suffer from a chronic condition without obvious tension.

The practitioner may sometimes have to accept the fact that there is little that he can do for some of his patients who are suffering from neurosis, and that his therapeutic task must be restricted to persuading the patient to accept his neurosis and the limitations it imposes upon him so that he can live a full life within those limits. In some patients the cure may indeed be worse than the disease. It may be better that a woman should carry the burden of her neurosis rather than have to face the intolerable character of her marital situation. Such a patient not only needs her neurosis: she has a right to it. The visit to the doctor may be for her an assertion of her dignity and of her rights as an individual, which should be respected and which it would be cruel to deny her.

Psychosomatic illness. It is barely possible to enumerate all the physical symptoms in which emotional factors may and often do play a part. The most obvious and the most frequent is *headache*. In common speech and universal experience the connection between headache and tension, especially frustration, is recognized. Discussion of current emotional problems may be exceedingly effective and should always be considered when symptomatic treatment by analgesics does not quickly bring relief. *Pains and stiffness in the back, neck and shoulders* are worth investigating in the same way before attaching the label rheumatism or fibrositis. Such pains are often symptoms of mild depression or of acute resentment, and the truth of this may not be difficult to elicit.

These are the conditions which are probably most readily treated, but spastic constipation with or without the passage of mucus and persistent diarrhoea will often repay simple psychological investigation. The more serious diseases in which an emotional factor is probably relevant—such as peptic ulcer, some skin conditions and hypertension—are frequently associated with a rigid, often overconscientious and inhibited personality which readily reacts to occupational stress and domestic discord. In these cases the practitioner should inquire carefully into the patient's routine of work and his periods of rest and recreation; with the support of his doctor he may learn to relax and with firmness he may be induced to delegate work or obtain the holidays he needs. Hobbies and sports may be useful to the patient, but it is not enough to prescribe these and expect the advice to be taken automatically. It is necessary to show an interest in the patient's progress with his hobby or his sport, and continue to support him until his own enthusiasm has ensured that he will continue to practise it. In some illnesses it is possible to relate acute phases to the existence of a particular emotional situation; for example, a young man suffered from asthma while at home but was well while doing his period of National Service, and, again, when he left home for a short time to do a job elsewhere. In such a case it may be advisable to draw the obvious conclusion and arrange that the patient should go off on his own and avoid the home situation which upsets him.

Chronic psychotic patients. For every psychotic

patient who is in a mental hospital there is probably another living in the community. Some of the latter are very disordered in their thought and occasionally also in their behaviour. There are many middle-aged women with florid delusions of persecution about their neighbours who, nevertheless, contrive to live peaceably beside them. When the practitioner is convinced that such a psychotic patient is harmless and incurable, and after he has sought a second opinion if necessary on the subject of possible treatment, he should try to look after the patient at home. Fortunately there is usually a great deal of domestic tolerance for such patients, although the family may require the doctor's support and encouragement to maintain their morale in such a long-term task. The help of a social worker should be sought in finding suitable employment; if the patient cannot take a job it may be possible with the aid of a hospital Occupational Therapy Department to have him taught some simple pursuit which will keep him occupied in a satisfactory fashion. The same care and supervision are required for those schizophrenic patients who are now discharged from mental hospitals when they have responded favourably to tranquillizing drugs.

Sexual problems. Patients increasingly turn to their doctors to help them when difficulties occur in sexual life, and it is, therefore, necessary for doctors to be well informed in these matters and to be able to act as educators as well as therapists. Many patients nowadays read books on sexual adjustment and marriage problems, and the practitioner is recommended to make himself familiar with a few representative texts on the subject.

Some of the most intractable psychotherapeutic problems lie in the field of sexual behaviour. The doctor should, therefore, not expect to be uniformly successful either as an educator or as a therapist. Sometimes when it seems that only a little enlightenment is required he may be faced with an unexpected persistence or worsening of symptoms, but in other cases he will as surely be gratified by the improvement which follows on the advice he gives. Difficulties and abnormalities in sexual performance are almost always of a neurotic kind, constitutional and physical factors entering into the genesis of symptoms only to the extent which they do in other neuroses. They should be treated in the same way, remembering that an inquiry into disturbances in general personal relationships may have relevance to the sexual problem.

Competence in the sexual act is apt to be regarded as a measure of virility, and fears of impotence are widespread in our society. In early adolescence many boys begin to show anxiety of this kind when they develop the idea that they have an unduly small penis. Arising out of this they may develop feelings of inferiority or shyness, and *masturbation* may be resorted to largely from a need to reassure themselves about the integrity of their sexual functions. Guilt about masturbation is reinforced by theories of the harm which it may cause, and the adolescent may come to believe that he has in some way damaged himself so that he will be unable to perform the sexual act as an adult. Those occasions when he has to undress in front of others, especially medical examinations, are feared because he believes his sexual inferiority will be noticed and ascribed to his guilty habit. This type of anxiety is so frequent in adolescence that wherever possible the doctor, in conducting a medical examination, should endeavour to allay it by making a forthright statement about the patient's physical fitness. He should also, when he feels that this course is indicated, give the patient an opportunity to talk to him about any worries he may have about himself. This is equally true of the youth who comes to be treated for his acne but who may be more worried by the nagging idea that his pimples are the result of his masturbation. Masturbation occurs in such a large proportion of males during adolescence with no noticeable effect on sexual performance in marriage that it can be held to be sufficiently proved that it produces no impairment of sexual capacity. This is the kind of reassurance which patients require who are worried about masturbation. The doctor may be tempted to feel that fear of the consequences may be a help to the patient in abandoning the habit, but experience suggests the opposite. Guilt and self-loathing may drive the patient to repeated masturbation in the belief that, since the act is harmful, giving way to it will bring in its train the punishment he deserves. Masturbation during adolescence and homosexual tendencies in Service personnel may be treated by diversion of the sex urge into physical activities such as athletics, swimming and climbing.

This is the background to many of the fears which arise before marriage or during the early months of marriage, and these fears are in turn the chief cause of impaired performance or total *impotence*. It is true that in a narrow biological view coitus is an act which need not be learned and which should, in marriage, come quite naturally, a belief which most patients have derived from their observations of animals. Since, however, sexual behaviour in man is affected by the taboos and restraints of the society in which he lives, it is usually necessary for some instruction to be given. In most marriages a consistently adequate performance is not achieved before a year has passed. The patient who complains of an inadequate performance should be reassured and advised to give up his strenuous attempts and his intense preoccupation with his failures in the assurance that, as many other men have discovered, his difficulties will disappear with time.

The whole subject of sexual relations in marriage is bedevilled by traditional beliefs and attitudes which are now becoming obsolete. Whereas formerly virtue on the part of the wife was associated with submissive frigidity, it is now almost universally recognized that satisfaction for the woman is a reasonable aspiration in the marital relationship. As yet, however, and in spite of this knowledge, a considerable proportion of women are unable to achieve any marked degree of satisfaction. It is possible, indeed, that some women are constitutionally unable to achieve true orgasm although the sexual act is pleasurable to them, because of a more diffuse excitement which is followed by relaxation. In such cases, where there is no dissatisfaction, it is as well not to be too perfectionistic and to explain that this is a common and quite healthy response to coitus. Women often suffer from ideas of sexual inferiority, believing unreasonably that the vagina is too small or too large for satisfactory coitus. Consequently, where there is dyspareunia it is usually more important to discuss the patient's fears and thus relieve anxiety than to proceed to surgical measures. Associated with the idea that the vagina is too small there is often also a carry-over from adolescence of the fear that in defloration serious damage may be caused—an idea which may also be tackled psychotherapeutically. The doctor should remember too that guilt over masturbation, and a belief that incapacity in the sexual act may thus have been caused, may require to be discussed with female patients. Although dyspareunia may be mainly attributable to psychological factors, some immediate relief may be obtained from physical means including the use of suitable lubricants, adjustment of posture during coitus and, if necessary, digital stretching of the introitus.

Since coitus is a mutual act, mutual adjustment is necessary and co-operation is required from both partners. The frigidity of a wife may arise from precipitate orgasm (ejaculatio praecox) on the part of the husband. Normal coitus requires an erection sustained for three to five minutes, and if orgasm in a male habitually occurs in a shorter time his partner may well have difficulty in obtaining satisfaction. It is often assumed that the natural duration of coitus tends to be shorter in the male than in the female. While there is no real evidence to support this view, it is true that some consideration is often required on the part of the husband to ensure that the act is sufficiently prolonged for his wife's satisfaction. Impotence due to ejaculatio praecox may be amenable to mild sedation. The bromides —though now obsolete as hypnotics—have the advantage in these circumstances that they depress spinal reflexes; sodium bromide, 1 g. thrice daily, may be given and the effects assessed after two to three weeks. Ejaculatio praecox may also be attributable to prolonged abstinence or associated with physical fatigue.

The pattern of intercourse varies greatly between one culture and another and in different individuals. The way in which sexual satisfaction is achieved is dependent on factors in the upbringing similar to those which determine the personality. Domination and submissiveness, aggressiveness and tenderness, the pleasure derived from stimulation of extragenital as compared with genital areas; all these are components which may vary from one person to another. The fact that their sexual behaviour may seem to deviate from an imaginary norm is a cause of concern to many patients. It should be pointed out that there is no normal or standard pattern and that behaviour is perverse only when it is persisted in despite the protests of the marital partner, or when instead of being a preliminary to the normal completion of the act it takes precedence over and is a substitute for it. If there is *perversion* defined in this way, the patient requires psychotherapy which is probably beyond the resources of the practitioner.

From what we know of human sexual behaviour it would appear that we are all bi-sexual to some extent. In a very high proportion of both men and women we can find some evidence in the life-history of at least transitory attachments to members of the same sex, and in many cases there has also been some overt expression of homosexual activity. It is very important, therefore, not to overestimate the prognostic significance of a homosexual episode in a life-history; a good marital adjustment can occur even when there has been a quite persistent pattern of homosexual activity, provided, of course, that the individual concerned has sufficient heterosexual feeling to make such an adjustment possible. The practitioner's own prejudices may create a barrier to the full investigation and understanding of these patients; he should, therefore, try to be as objective as possible. In assessing the depth and significance of a homosexual relationship the factor of privation has to be taken into account. When men live isolated from women, as for example, in the fighting services, it is well known that homosexuality is more liable to occur. It should also be remembered that neurotic factors may isolate an individual from the opposite sex; a feeling of inferiority because of a deformity, a speech defect or a chronic skin lesion, may reduce the individual's capacity to meet the opposite sex and lead to homosexual behaviour as a substitute outlet. Cases of this kind provide the practitioner with considerable scope for treatment. He should encourage the patient to take up social activities by carefully graduated stages, while the energetic treatment of any handicapping condition may give the patient more hope and confidence and the doctor's positive attitude and reassurance may help his self-esteem.

ALCOHOLISM AND DRUG ADDICTION

It is difficult to define precisely what should be included under the term 'drug addiction'. Addiction may be said to exist when a state of dependence has clearly become established. This condition of dependence is seen when the use of the drug is discontinued: the addict then develops *abstinence symptoms* characterized by various constitutional disturbances and the phenomenon called *craving*. If these criteria are applied to the use of alcohol and tobacco, it is obvious that most people who drink or smoke are not addicts; on the other hand it cannot be denied that there are many alcoholics and also heavy smokers who are undoubtedly addicts.

As already pointed out, with most drugs of addiction there are two types of dependence which have to be clearly distinguished: (*a*) *a physical dependence* which exists when the drug is being taken and is demonstrated, following abstinence, by *withdrawal symptoms* of a severe nature which are relieved by a resumption of the drug; (*b*) *a psychological craving* which is not a dependence on the drug as such, but is a desire for the effects it produces, the addict aiming to achieve the euphoria which the drug is capable of producing or has produced for him in the past and this aim is pursued even when his addiction is long past the point where the desired condition can be achieved.

Treatment has to be directed, therefore, in the first place to diminishing or abolishing the physical dependence on the drug, but when this phase is over and complete withdrawal has been effected the much more difficult problem of handling the craving remains, and this requires psychotherapy of some kind. Treatment which stops at physical measures can only lead to relapse. Nor should it be assumed that when one euphoriant drug is replaced by another any degree of success has been achieved; the patient is still, and perhaps more deeply, in the clutches of his craving while a new addiction in the form of a new pathway to his desired euphoria has been provided for him. Obvious examples of this error in treatment can be provided from the past. As is well known, Freud was enthusiastic for a time about the virtues of cocaine as a cure for morphinism: it is possible to repeat this error today by using a new drug pronounced safe by its manufacturers before its true character has become known. Up to the present no such safe substitute has emerged and all such claims should be viewed with suspicion.

The euphoriant effects of amphetamine compounds and of barbiturates, especially the short-acting type, are conducive to addiction. Their illicit use has created a formidable problem, second only—in terms of numbers—to that associated with alcoholism; and this is true even in countries where the control of drugs is otherwise strict. Chronic barbiturate intoxication is shown in unsteady gait, disinhibited behaviour, nystagmus, and withdrawal fits. When an unexplained major seizure occurs in a patient, barbiturate addiction should always be considered. Amphetamine and related compounds such as dexamphetamine, methylamphetamine and phenmetrazine used to be widely prescribed as appetite suppressants. They readily give rise to dependence and addiction. An acute psychosis with delusions is not infrequently seen in amphetamine addiction and may be mistaken for paranoid schizophrenia. Addicts often forge and steal prescriptions and in many cities these drugs are black-market commodities primarily because there are virtually no medically justifiable indications for prescribing them.

ALCOHOLISM

Various stages in the development of alcoholism can be distinguished which require different kinds of treatment.

Early alcoholism. Propaganda in recent years is leading to a changed attitude, and as a result, drinkers who are beginning to find that their drinking has become a problem to them are more readily turning to their practitioners for help. At this stage, psychotherapy of a supportive type can succeed, aimed at reinforcing the motivation of the alcoholic to stop drinking. The attitude of the doctor should be the same as is described in dealing with neurotic problems although only a minority of alcoholic patients show any signs of neurosis. It should be explained to the patient that indulgence in even small quantities of alcohol will lead to relapse and that total abstinence is imperative. It is at this stage that patients who are genuinely anxious to be helped can be tried on disulfiram. This drug, when taken over a period, results in an unpleasant reaction in the patient when alcohol is subsequently consumed. Its use should be avoided in patients who show obvious abnormalities of personality or who have reached the reckless, self-destructive stage of alcoholism; in such cases its administration constitutes a real danger. The drug should also be avoided in patients suffering from hepatic or circulatory disorders and in diabetics who are not adequately controlled by diet and insulin. When the patient has to receive a general anaesthetic, the drug should be stopped for some days previously.

Treatment begins with the oral administration of two 500 mg. tablets on the evening of the first day and one tablet on each of the following five to six days. Thereafter a maintenance dose of half a tablet (250 mg.) can be given every day, and in some cases even this dose can be reduced to 250 mg. every other day. At the end of the first week's treatment it is usual to administer alcohol to demonstrate to the patient that he can no longer tolerate even a small quantity and that the effects are not only very distressing but even dangerous. A small dose, e.g. 3 teaspoonsful of whisky (12 ml.) or a glass of beer, should be given and the patient should be kept under observation for two or three hours afterwards lest there should be a delayed reaction. The symptoms which normally ensue are pronounced tachycardia, dyspnoea and intense flushing of the face; these are accompanied by a fall in blood pressure. Subjectively there is great uneasiness and fear accompanied by drowsiness. The patient should be warned that this reaction will develop whenever he takes alcohol and that if he takes a large quantity it is likely to be much more serious and might be very dangerous. He should also be warned not to take paraldehyde, which has the same effect as alcohol, paraldehyde being the hypnotic preferred by many alcoholics. Severe reactions can occur even with a test dose and, for this reason, the test should be carried out in circumstances in which the doctor is prepared to deal with them by the use of oxygen inhalations and respiratory stimulants such as nikethamide, 5 ml. of a 25 per cent. solution intravenously. Provided the patient avoids the risks which have been mentioned, there are seldom any obvious side-effects from the use of disulfiram, but a few patients complain of tiredness and diminished sexual potency.

It is obvious that this treatment is not likely to succeed with an unwilling patient, and even with a willing patient it should be regarded only as ancillary to the main form of treatment, which is psychotherapeutic.

In all stages of alcoholism, when the patient has expressed his need of help, the doctor should certainly consider advising him to get in touch with the group of Alcoholics Anonymous (A.A.) in his neighbourhood. This organization is now in existence throughout Western Europe, North America and in many places elsewhere and has done more in a few years to reclaim alcoholics than has ever been done by purely medical endeavour. As a rule, however, medical treatment must precede successful rehabilitation by A.A.

Established alcoholism. At this stage the alcoholic's situation has usually become very involved; he has neglected or lost his employment and he has often created intolerable difficulties in his home. His bouts are prolonged and uncontrollable, his physical condition has deteriorated and in-patient treatment in a suitable nursing home or hospital has become necessary. He should be informed that a period of some months may be required to effect recovery and that thereafter further efforts on his part and usually the help of A.A. will be required to keep him well.

Aversion treatments using apomorphine or emetine are falling into disfavour; they appear to have little lasting effect in eliminating the craving, especially if psychotherapeutic measures are neglected. These methods may be of value in some cases, but the treatment is most suitable for in-patients.

In the later phases of alcoholism deteriorating mental illness can result, e.g. Korsakoff's psychosis. The problem is then one of permanently impaired capacity requiring psychiatric care. More important in ordinary practice are withdrawal symptoms.

Treatment of Alcohol Withdrawal

Judgment as to whether a patient should be admitted to hospital during the withdrawal period depends partly on the severity of his symptoms and on whether he has had a previous history of delirium tremens or withdrawal fits. The decision must also be influenced by whether he has a family who can look after him and an interested A.A. sponsor who will visit him. If the general practitioner can keep an eye on him in these favourable circumstances out-patient withdrawal of alcohol is feasible.

Mild or moderate withdrawal symptoms, usually clear fairly quickly. Although the benefits conferred by tranquillizing drugs probably are often only marginal they are useful. Chlordiazepoxide is widely used and on the whole the evidence is that it is effective. Chlormethiazole can also be tried.

Treatment of established delirium tremens is a very different matter, however, and a proper regimen must include a thorough search for medical complications. Good nursing care is imperative. Other requirements are: correction of fluid and electrolyte loss and sometimes of hypoglycaemia; a careful watch on pulse rate, temperature and blood pressure; immediate symptomatic treatment of hypothermia or circulatory collapse. Cardiovascular complications may supervene rapidly and are a common cause of death. For these reasons admission to hospital is to be preferred.

In delirium tremens, paraldehyde in doses of 10 to 12 ml. in orange juice is perhaps the drug of choice. It should be withdrawn as soon as the delirium has subsided because addiction even to this unpleasant drug has been known to occur. High potency vitamin injections, especially of B vitamins, may be necessary for the correction of coexisting vitamin deficiency.

DRUG ADDICTION AND ABUSE

Drug addiction in Britain has changed radically in the last decade. Ten years ago addiction to the so-called 'hard drugs' (opiates and cocaine) was a small problem. Most addicts were middle-aged and either in positions allowing them access to dangerous drugs (doctors, nurses, pharmacists and their relatives) or had become addicted by the prescription of drugs for severe pain in chronic illness. Now new addicts are adolescents or young adults and their number has been rising so alarmingly that new legislation was introduced in The Dangerous Drugs (Notification of Addicts) Regulations, 1968. The regulations restrict the authority of doctors to prescribe or supply heroin or cocaine to addicts, although the drugs may be prescribed for the relief of pain due to injury or organic disease. Only doctors expressly licensed under the regulations may prescribe these drugs for addicts (usually psychiatrists employed in hospitals). Units and hospitals throughout the country have been designated as treatment centres for addiction and the regulations provide for notification of addicts.

Emergency treatment of heroin addicts. Young addicts may approach the non-specialist for help in an emergency. Such patients are seriously disturbed people, awkward, difficult, demanding, untruthful and sometimes violent; and even emergency management can be time-consuming. The addict is often on the move and may give a false name. If he is having regular supplies he will be registered with the Home Office where the inspectors will be able to give information about him (in U.K. telephone no.—01-930 8100, exts. 326 and 420). The signs to look for which indicate acute withdrawal symptoms are sniffing, lacrimation, restlessness, sweating, abdominal cramps, irritability, and self-absorption, pallor, goose-flesh, diarrhoea, vomiting, shivering, yawning and muscular weakness. Subjective complaints are difficult to verify. Heroin can be prescribed only by a specially licensed practitioner and in an emergency, methadone should be given instead, 20 mg. in the form of the linctus swallowed in the doctor's presence and repeated in 1 to 2 hours if necessary. If he is showing definite withdrawal symptoms then 10 mg. of methadone should be given by intramuscular injection and 10 mg. taken orally; it should not be given intravenously.

Treatment of morphine addiction. Although treatment centres were established under The Dangerous Drugs Regulation in 1968, to deal with heroin addiction, the practitioner, although not obliged to do so, would be well advised to refer any morphine addict he encounters to a treatment centre for care and management. *Sudden withdrawal* of the drug is an exceedingly unpleasant and possibly dangerous process. Although it can be effective, on a long-term view it is unwise to subject the patient to a procedure which he will recall with loathing and horror. Relapse is always to be expected in morphine addiction, and if the patient then has cause to shrink from a repetition of the treatment, nothing has been gained. Nowadays *rapid withdrawal* over a period of two weeks is common practice. The dosage on which the patient is stabilized without developing abstinence symptoms should first be ascertained. This is likely to be less than the dosage which the patient declares he has been getting; he is naturally anxious to postpone the effects of withdrawal as long as possible. Once ascertained, the dose should be reduced by one-fourteenth per day, but the patient should not be informed that withdrawal has begun until a day or two later and he should be told that it is complete when one or two of the final doses are still to be given. In this way the anxiety of expectation can be reduced. To mitigate the effects of withdrawal promazine, 100 mg., or chlorpromazine, 50 mg., orally or intramuscularly three times daily, are valuable. With the help of these drugs withdrawal can now be safely carried out in an even shorter time (five to seven days).

Abuse of other drugs. Associated with the rise in heroin addiction among adolescents and young adults there has been widespread experimentation with other drugs. Fashions change rapidly, but currently the smoking of marihuana ('Pot'), and the use of intravenous methyl-amphetamine and lysergic acid diethylamide (LSD) are most often encountered. The dangers of marihuana have been exaggerated—it is a mild drug whose effects are rarely alarming, and it is doubtful whether true addiction occurs although prolonged abuse probably leads to loss of drive and to personality changes. Its main danger lies in its possible rôle as a precursor to heroin experimentation.

Amphetamine injected intravenously may result in states of extreme excitement and even psychosis with paranoid symptoms. It should be considered as a possibility in any excited state in an adolescent; it is usually accompanied by tachycardia and flushing. A phenothiazine, such as chlorpromazine 50 to 100 mg. should be given, but hospital admission may be necessary.

LSD is an extremely potent and dangerous drug. It produces a psychosis with anxiety, fear, unreality feelings, illusions and visual hallucinations. Aggressive and suicidal acts may occur. In some cases a more prolonged psychosis may be precipitated, but usually the symptoms can be controlled by chlorpromazine 100 mg. given orally or parenterally. Glue sniffing, eating ground nutmeg, and other experiments occur from time to time, some more dangerous than others.

Prophylaxis. Physicians should regard their therapeutic task as being mainly prophylactic and since non-habit-forming local anaesthetics are available as substitutes for cocaine (except perhaps for direct application to the eyes, ears, nose and throat), no problem of creating addiction to cocaine need ever arise. In the case of opiates care has to be exercised. It should be remembered that no person is immune to opiate addiction. Prolonged administration will be followed by abstinence symptoms in everyone, and this stage can be reached in the case of heroin after only 10 to 12 injections. For this reason the risk of addiction should always be kept in mind, although the physician should not be so cautious as to avoid the use of opiates when they are clearly indicated. The following are useful principles. Opiates should not be administered when other analgesics are adequate. When morphine is used, the smallest effective dose should be given to avoid the euphoriant effects of a larger dose; this is of special importance when repeated doses have to be given. Opiates should never be used as pure hypnotics (they are in fact poor hypnotics) and should never be given in the treatment of alcoholism or any other form of drug addiction. For suppressing cough, morphine and heroin can, in most cases, be replaced by methadone.

Many middle-aged women and some men abuse amphetamines and barbiturates, initially obtaining prescriptions for weight reduction or insomnia. A number of them become addicted and resort to obtaining prescriptions from different doctors in a partnership, forging prescriptions or obtaining black-market supplies. Abuse can be spotted and arrested forthwith; addiction will require hospital admission. The responsibility for prophylaxis rests firmly with the doctor; he should never lose sight of the possibility of abuse of these drugs.

The young addict nowadays frequently adopts illegal means to obtain supplies, notably forgery and theft. It is more than ever essential to write prescriptions with great care, ensuring that alterations or additions to the script cannot easily be made. Prescription pads, and supplies of drugs, whether in surgery, home or car, should always be carefully safeguarded.

P

17. Analgesics and Hypnotics

S. Alstead and T. J. Thomson

ANALGESICS

Introduction. Pain, as a symptom of disease, rarely exists as an isolated phenomenon sharply defined by the sensorium. Beyond it there is the penumbra of distress, and this may be more disabling than the pain itself. The emphasis to be placed on this component varies greatly from one patient to another. Its existence, however, serves to remind the physician of the need to take a comprehensive view of therapy and to avoid a mechanistic attitude towards the use of analgesics. These general considerations, bearing upon the relief of suffering, are not the least important part of the doctor–patient relationship. There is undoubtedly a place for explanation and reassurance. But it is also true that for patients who are in the throes of the agonizing pain of peritonitis, acute pleurisy, myocardial infarction and certain other diseases, the situation calls for the immediate use of drugs which are known to be powerful analgesics. It is only when the crisis has passed that such patients are receptive to appropriate explanation and reassurance. Current opinion regarding the mode of action of morphine lends support to the view that pain is an unstable complex of sensory and psychological components.

In the absence of analgesics which block the pain receptors in the thalamus and sensory cortex, the alternative is to use drugs of the morphine group. These greatly alleviate the severest pain and induce a state of tranquillity which creates indifference towards residual discomfort. It is this dual action of morphine that makes it indispensable, for it was apparently contrived by providence to meet the needs of the intellectual animal racked by severe physical pain.

The state of detachment induced by drugs like morphine—though important for its bearing on analgesia—is apt to merge into euphoria, which is a state of intellectual pleasure bordering on ecstasy. Herein lies the well-known danger of addiction to opiates. However, the circumstances in which these powerful analgesics are used and the limited number of doses ordinarily required make it unlikely that the patient will develop dependence or addiction. The risk is, of course, greater when the patient is a doctor or a nurse who, having access to drugs, may later resort to self-medication. When morphine is being used in the terminal stages of a mortal illness it is occasionally apparent that the patient has become highly dependent on medication and perhaps addicted to the drug, but in these circumstances the matter is of little importance.

Many chapters in this book include references to the use of analgesic drugs. Recommendations are made here regarding choice of drug, doses and routes of administration. These are matters which are also profitably reviewed in relation to the general management of the particular disease under discussion. In the paragraphs that follow, attention is focused on the particular aspects of pharmacology which are important in medical practice.

Morphine

For the rapid relief of severe visceral pain, morphine or its derivative diamorphine or certain synthetic drugs akin therapeutically to morphine (for example, methadone or pethidine), are virtually indispensable. Unless there is some clear contraindication to giving morphine, for example, respiratory depression or hepatic failure, the doctor must ensure that the patient receives the full benefit of the drug; timid medication is a disservice to a patient genuinely distressed and certainly brings no credit to his attendants. The appropriate dose is that which relieves pain, and not infrequently the pharmacopoeial maximum dose falls short of the needs of the individual patient: for example, patients suffering from severe pain are remarkably tolerant of full doses of morphine. It has been well said that 'a painful deathbed is a reproach to the doctor'. Where the needs of the patient are met by giving three or four doses of morphine, fear of producing addiction should not be allowed to affect the doctor's judgment. Certainly in Great Britain, addiction can rarely be attributed to experience of the drug at the hands of a competent practitioner. The state of surgical shock is not a contraindication to the use of this drug.

Conditions modifying the use of morphine. Oligaemia of the superficial tissues may seriously retard absorption of morphine injected subcutaneously, and in these circumstances the solution should be injected intravenously; but not more than half of the usual dose should be given by this route, and it must be injected *slowly*. Although the presence of organic heart disease does not *per se* constitute a contraindication to the administration of drugs of the morphine group (and indeed they are the mainstay of treatment in myocardial infarction and cardiac asthma), it should be used with great care if the presence of cyanosis is interpreted as a sign of depression of the respiratory centre; and in cor pulmonade morphine is absolutely contraindicated. When morphine is given to infants the dose should be determined on the basis of body weight. In old age the amount should be 5 to 10 mg.—about half the usual dose for an adult. Again, patients suffering from hypothyroidism, Addison's disease and hypopituitarism are intolerant of morphine as they evidently detoxicate the drug very slowly; but thyrotoxic patients may need relatively large doses to produce adequate analgesia. When morphine is given with other depressants of the nervous system, summation of effects is to be expected. The result may be valuable if it is the outcome of a therapeutic plan. For example, the simultaneous administration of morphine and hyoscine is a time-honoured practice —though here analgesia is usually less important than the relief of agitation and restlessness. On the other hand, when combined therapy with cerebral depressants occurs fortuitously and without due regard to the circumstances of the individual patient, there are serious hazards. The main danger lies in causing excessive depression of respiration through the simultaneous action of morphine and certain hypnotics (especially the barbiturates) on the respiratory centre. Idiosyncrasy to cocaine and (more rarely) to cocaine substitutes may cause excitement and convulsions: here the use of morphine as a sedative is strictly contraindicated as, in these circumstances, the signs of cerebral stimulation are often accompanied by depression of the vital centres in the medulla— making the use of opiates dangerous or even lethal.

Nalorphine as an antagonist. The most dangerous toxic effects of morphine can usually be relieved by using the antagonist nalorphine hydrobromide. This drug is closely akin to morphine in its chemical structure. It is an analgesic, but its therapeutic value depends upon actions that are entirely different from those of morphine. Pharmacologically it competes with morphine for certain receptor sites in the central nervous system, and it actively displaces morphine that is already affecting the respiratory centre and the higher centres in the cerebrum. Thus nalorphine abolishes morphine narcosis and signs of respiratory depression caused by morphine poisoning. These remarkable effects are obvious within a minute of injecting the drug intravenously; the dose is 10 mg., but it may be necessary to give further doses of 10 mg. at intervals of five minutes; the total dose of nalorphine should not exceed 40 mg. Nalorphine is also effective in poisoning due to other opiates related to morphine, and it abolishes the effects of overdose of synthetic analgesics such as methadone and pethidine. Excessive doses of nalorphine result in exaggerated anticholinesterase activity: in consequence there is excitement, restlessness, pallor and sweating; and the blood pressure falls.

Potentiation of analgesia. At the beginning of this chapter it was emphasized that severe pain creates anxiety and this in turn aggravates the distress of pain. On this assumption it is logical to combat the two components in the pain syndrome by a more selective pharmacological attack at the appropriate levels in the brain. This special type of adjuvant action is in fact demonstrable and can be applied therapeutically. Thus in patients receiving promazine relatively small doses of morphine suffice to relieve symptoms. This finds useful practical applications when repeated doses of powerful analgesics are needed, and particularly in patients who are in continuous pain during the terminal stages of incurable disease. On the other hand it would not be justifiable to use promazine routinely in all cases where morphine and similar drugs are prescribed as analgesics; in the majority of patients only one or two doses of morphine are needed and therefore an adjuvant is not required. When morphine and similar drugs are used for a period of only a few days, such combinations of drugs are unnecessary.

Side-effects. When all the possible side-effects of a therapeutic dose of morphine are enumerated, the list is indeed formidable. However, if the drug is used with skill and discrimination the complications that actually occur in the great majority of patients are not unbearable. This is partly because administration is continued for a limited period of time; and although alimentary upsets are common, serious side-effects elsewhere are exceptional. Many of the actions of morphine are rightly regarded as unwelcome side-effects when the drug is being used simply as an analgesic; but in other circumstances they are obviously useful pharmacological actions—as for example in the symptomatic control of diarrhoea, the suppression of a useless cough, or in allaying the anxiety and agitation that may accompany acute illness.

Various side-effects of morphine are attributable to its power to increase the tonus of involuntary muscle. In the bowel this causes constipation; if the biliary tract is in an irritable state as in chronic cholecystitis there may be severe spasm in the bile ducts causing distressing pain in the right hypochondrium; in acute pancreatitis spasm at the sphincter of Oddi induced by morphine increases the risk of pancreatic necrosis (p. 251); occasionally ureteric colic is intensified by the use of morphine; and in men there may be retention of urine if there is incipient obstruction due to prostatic enlargement. Atropine, hyoscine or some other preparation in the belladonna group of drugs is often given with morphine to counteract its tendency to cause spasm in involuntary muscle. It cannot be assumed, however, that this corrective action always occurs. When morphine and atropine are injected together, the effects of the two drugs do not appear simultaneously: the actions of morphine are nearly always seen within a minute of intravenous injection, but those of atropine may be delayed for five to ten minutes. If, therefore, it is considered to be important to give atropine or hyoscine when morphine is being used as an analgesic, the spasmolytic should be injected first and sufficient time should be allowed for its effects to become established. Hyoscine hydrobromide (0·5 mg. intravenously) is particularly valuable because its atropine-like effects, including a spasmolytic action, though powerful are not excessively prolonged. Hyoscine also promotes drowsiness and amnesia—effects which are often desirable in drugs used in association with morphine to abolish severe pain. More specifically hyoscine is effective in preventing excessive nausea and vomiting during morphine therapy. These actions of hyoscine are undoubtedly useful, but the limitations of this drug should also be noted. Repeated administration on consecutive days is liable to cause troublesome hallucinations. Hence not more than three doses of hyoscine should be given in the course of 48 hours, and its use should

then be discontinued. If a sustained anti-emetic effect is required over a period of several days, promazine is preferable to hyoscine: the first dose of 50 mg. is best given by subcutaneous injection, and subsequently oral administration (25 mg. twice daily) usually suffices.

When the respiratory centre is already depressed or is likely to be excessively sensitive to the action of opiates, extreme caution is necessary. In chronic bronchitis with emphysema, patients are more or less intolerant of morphine; and cor pulmonale constitutes an absolute contraindication to the use of this drug or its congeners. In patients who suffer from head injuries the respiratory centre is often very susceptible to the depressant action of morphine; and the fact that morphine tends to raise the cerebrospinal fluid pressure provides a further reason for avoiding drugs of this group after concussion and in convulsive states. Many old people react adversely to morphine, and doses should be conservative. Further, when severe constipation occurs in older patients following the use of morphine there is a special danger of intestinal obstruction from impaction of faeces in the rectum and descending colon.

The parenteral injection of morphine gives much better analgesia than oral administration. The contrast is attributable to the slowness of absorption of morphine from the alimentary canal. On the other hand, pethidine and methadone are well absorbed when given by mouth, and the effectiveness of oral medication is obviously an advantage when repeated administration is necessary.

PAPAVERETUM. This is a combination of the alkaloids of opium in the form of their soluble salts. As it contains about 50 per cent. of morphine, its dose is about twice that of morphine. It appears to have no special merit therapeutically. The dose of papaveretum is 20 mg. by subcutaneous injection.

Diamorphine hydrochloride (*heroin*). The analgesic potency of diamorphine is about twice that of morphine. Small doses (5 mg.) administered subcutaneously promote euphoria and relieve pain without causing conspicuous side-effects such as nausea and abdominal distension. For this reason some surgeons prefer diamorphine to morphine in the post-operative management of abdominal cases. It is also recommended in the treatment of patients suffering from the pain of myocardial infarction. Here it is particularly desirable to relieve pain with a small dose of analgesic and so reduce the risk of subsequent retching and vomiting. Another important use of diamorphine is deliberately to create euphoria and to abolish pain and distress in patients who are dying from malignant disease; here it can be given as an elixir containing diamorphine hydrochloride 2·5 mg. and cocaine hydrochloride 5 mg. in 5 ml. of brandy or other suitably flavoured vehicle. Heroin is readily absorbed from the intestine, and oral administration may give satisfactory results if dosage is adequate. Thus when cancer of the lung is accompanied by a troublesome cough the diamorphine and terpin elixir B.P.C. is a very effective cough suppressant; 5 ml. contains 3 mg. of diamorphine hydrochloride.

Pethidine. This synthetic preparation has pharmacological actions akin to those of both morphine and atropine. Although the analgesic action of pethidine is more transient and less powerful than that of morphine, the quantitative difference can be overcome by giving the drug in appropriate doses at intervals of two to three hours. There can then be no doubt that pethidine is correctly placed in the morphine group of analgesics, and this is further confirmed by the occurrence of euphoria, which is sometimes even more intense than that produced by morphine. The usual dose of pethidine is 50 to 100 mg. by intramuscular injection or 100 mg. by mouth; an intravenous injection (25 to 50 mg.) can also be given, but this is rarely necessary and as it is more likely to cause euphoria it is not recommended. During a course of treatment with pethidine patients often develop tolerance—which necessitates increasing the dose to ensure adequate analgesia. The depressant action of pethidine on the respiratory centre is relatively weak. It therefore has a special place in the practice of midwifery when analgesics are required. At the onset of labour, 100 mg. of pethidine is injected intramuscularly, and this may be repeated in about two hours: analgesia is achieved without significant interference with the force of uterine contractions. On the other hand, as the cough centre is hardly affected by ordinary doses of pethidine, this drug is practically useless as a cough suppressant. For the same reason it is a safer analgesic than morphine in the post-operative management of patients suffering from bronchitis and asthma; and here the mild spasmolytic action of pethidine on bronchial muscle is an advantage. Elsewhere in the body the atropine-like actions of pethidine are not conspicuous. The effect of this drug on the biliary tract resembles that of morphine. Consequently pethidine, like morphine, may inten-

sify spasm occurring in the bile ducts and at the sphincter of Oddi.

Methadone. This is remarkable for its selective action at two sites—the pain receptors and the respiratory centre. In full doses (10 mg. intramuscularly) it is at least as potent as morphine in relieving severe pain and its effects last as long (about six hours). Methadone is not a hypnotic and it rarely causes drowsiness. Euphoria, however, is common enough to justify the inclusion of this preparation among the drugs of addiction. Although the depressant effect of methadone on the respiratory centre limits its usefulness—and even debars it in the practice of obstetrics—it enhances its value when a selective action on the adjacent cough centre is required. In the short-term management of painful and unproductive cough, small doses of methadone often prove invaluable—even ranking with heroin—and it can be conveniently given in the form of linctus of methadone, B.P.C.; 4 ml. of this preparation contain 2 mg. of methadone hydrochloride. In order to combat severe pain, it is best to give 5 to 10 mg. by intramuscular injection, though local discomfort is usual at the site of administration. If these large doses are given by mouth, patients often complain of nausea, but constipation is unusual. Intravenous injection is rarely necessary and it is hazardous because of the increased risk of depression of respiration. Few patients develop tolerance to methadone; and in this respect the drug has an advantage over pethidine.

Pentazocine. Pentazocine is a powerful analgesic which has also weak narcotic antagonist properties; it is chemically related to morphine. It can be prescribed for the relief of pain which does not respond to aspirin or similar analgesics. Pentazocine may cause repiratory depression, but this is less marked than with other narcotic analgesics, and it is mildly sedative. Pentazocine does not lower the blood pressure and this has been found to be of value in the treatment of patients suffering the pain of myocardial infarction.

When given by subcutaneous or intramuscular injection (30 to 60 mg.) the analgesic effect of pentazocine is about one-quarter that of morphine. This drug may also be given intravenously, but this has been followed by a rise in pulmonary arterial pressure. The dose of pentazocine by mouth is 25 to 100 mg. four-hourly. When side-effects occur they are similar to those of morphine— nausea, vomiting, drowsiness and lightheadedness.

Exceptionally there may be tachycardia, palpitation and a rise in blood pressure. There have been reports of hallucinations and sensations of depersonalization in patients receiving pentazocine, but the risk of drug dependence appears to be slight compared with drugs of the group. At the present time (1970) pentazocine is not subject to the D.D.A. regulations (p. 619) but there have been reports suggesting that true physical dependence to this drug may develop in some patients. It should be remembered that being a weak narcotic antagonist, pentazocine should not be given to a narcotic addict, as this may produce a withdrawal syndrome.

As with morphine, pentazocine should be used only with extreme caution when there is depression of the respiratory centre, as in head injuries or in the presence of severe pulmonary disease. Where there is impaired renal or hepatic function, cumulation of drug metabolites may occur. The sedative effects may be increased by alcohol or other drugs which depress the central nervous system. Pentazocine is not antagonized by nalorphine and the treatment of overdosage is symptomatic.

Codeine. The status of this drug as an analgesic has been obscured by the practice of combining it with aspirin and phenacetin—as in the official compound codeine tablets. If codeine (or codeine phosphate) were prescribed alone for the relief of pain, its serious limitations would soon become apparent. It is credited with a cough-suppressant action, but in the doses usually given (15 to 30 mg.) it is greatly inferior to opium (Camphorated Opium Tincture, B.P.), nor can it compare with methadone (tablets or linctus). Codeine phosphate is remarkably effective in causing constipation, and this action is of potential therapeutic value; but as a side-effect to analgesia, obstinate constipation is altogether undesirable. In brief, though codeine is not without therapeutic uses, it takes a lowly place among the analgesics.

Dihydrocodeine bitartrate. This is a much more effective analgesic than codeine and is less liable than pethidine to cause euphoria. Given by mouth in doses of 30 mg. it is worthy of trial in patients who ordinarily require full doses of aspirin; and when given intramuscularly in doses of 50 mg. it usually gives adequate relief from post-operative pain for two to four hours. Large doses cause euphoria and depress the respiratory centre, showing that pharmacologically it is closer to morphine than to codeine.

Aspirin (*acetylsalicylic acid*). This is the analgesic which is most widely used throughout the world. There are at least four reasons for this: it is undoubtedly effective; it gives relief in those very common musculo-skeletal disorders (including myalgia, arthritis, neuritic pain and headache) in which pain is usually mild to moderate in its severity; it is also an antipyretic and often abolishes the muscular discomfort that accompanies the febrile state; and aspirin produces neither addiction nor habituation. Aspirin is of little use in severe pain associated with acute visceral disease and especially inflammation of the serous sacs: here morphine or a drug of similar potency is needed. Aspirin is a more potent analgesic than sodium salicylate, but in the treatment of rheumatic fever the latter has a special place—based on tradition rather than therapeutic advantage.

There is an extensive literature on the possible toxic effects of aspirin and other preparations derived from salicylic acid. In so far as the toxic effects are directly related to overdose, the subject belongs to toxicology rather than therapeutics. Aspirin has been used as a domestic remedy since 1899, and the annual world consumption is now measured in tens of thousands of tons. The conclusion derived from this massive experiment by the lay public is in keeping with the results observed by physicians, namely that the frequency of untoward effects is relatively very low. The manifestations of *idiosyncrasy* are sometimes distressing—commonly urticarial skin rashes, angioneurotic oedema and asthma.

Among the most serious side-effects of aspirin is gastric haemorrhage. Haematemesis or melaena may occur, accompanied by the constitutional effects of sudden blood loss. Alternatively, the symptoms may be those of persistent oozing haemorrhage, with anaemia developing insidiously over a period of months. The underlying lesion is erosion of the gastric mucosa; it is not prevented by using 'soluble aspirin', but on general principles patients should be advised to crush aspirin tablets and to take them during meals or immediately after meals. Aspirin is a constituent of many proprietary preparations, though this is rarely apparent from their trade names. The public is thus exposed to a hazard which could be avoided.

Phenacetin. Aspirin and phenacetin are of similar potency as analgesics, but as they are entirely different in their chemical structure there is a *prima facie* case for giving a compound tablet containing these two preparations in small doses

(200 mg. of each). In practice, however, no advantage has been shown clinically in giving phenacetin as an adjuvant to aspirin. This makes it difficult to justify the continuing use of phenacetin, for it has been recognized for a long time that this drug's harmful effects, if used daily for weeks or months, include sulphaemoglobinaemia, methaemoglobinaemia and haemolytic anaemia and, if grossly abused for years, it may cause renal papillary necrosis. Further, the use of phenacetin has been made unnecessary since its breakdown product N-acetyl-*p*-aminophenol (paracetamol B.P.) became available as an analgesic.

Paracetamol. This drug is widely used as a useful alternative analgesic to phenacetin because it does not produce abnormal blood pigments, and to aspirin because it rarely causes gastric irritation and has not been reported as a cause of gastric bleeding. The dose is 1 g. (two tablets) every four hours, but up to 2 g. may be needed.

Phenylbutazone. This antipyretic-analgesic has actions and toxic effects comparable with those of the obsolete drug amidopyrine. It is not a 'general purposes analgesic' such as aspirin, but it has limited uses in the symptomatic treatment of acute arthritis and other fulminating types of musculo-skeletal disease. In acute gout, 600 to 800 mg. of phenylbutazone may be given daily for the first three days if necessary. The best results are obtained from intramuscular injection; dosage is then reduced to the minimum required to prevent relapse. There is no doubt about the value of phenylbutazone, but because of its toxicity in high doses it is reasonable to reserve this drug for those patients who have failed to respond to indomethacin or to colchicine (p. 459). Phenylbutazone is also a valuable analgesic in other acute and subacute musculo-skeletal diseases, including rheumatoid arthritis and bursitis. Here again this drug should be held in reserve until it is clear that full doses of aspirin have failed to give relief. There is a long list of possible toxic effects—rashes, gastro-intestinal upsets, hepatitis and blood dyscrasias. If long-term therapy is attempted with this analgesic, only the minimum effective dose should be employed—say 100 mg. twice or thrice daily.

Indomethacin. This drug is an indole derivative and is chemically unrelated to the salicylates, phenylbutazone or the corticosteroids. Its mode of action is not yet understood. Indomethacin is a powerful analgesic and appears to be particularly effective in relieving pain in osteoarthritis and ankylosing spondylitis. Its anti-inflammatory action is superior to that of phenylbutazone; in active rheumatoid arthritis and in acute gout reduction of tissue swelling is often seen within two days. The dose is 25 mg. twice daily, increasing to three doses per day after 3 to 4 days. At this level of dosage, side-effects are slight and may be diminished or prevented completely by giving the drug as a suppository containing 100 mg. The commonest side-effect is generalized throbbing headache, but tinnitus and vertigo may occur. Some patients complain of epigastric pain, nausea and vomiting; there may be gastro-intestinal bleeding. This drug should, therefore, not be given orally to patients who have a history of gastric or duodenal ulcer.

INSOMNIA

General management. The cause of insomnia may be obvious. Pain, anxiety, bereavement, change of surroundings, an excessively hot or cold bedroom, lack of out-door exercise, dietetic indiscretions, and many other circumstances may produce restlessness and broken sleep. As the physician's objective is to restore a physiological sleep rhythm, such causative conditions must, if possible, be eliminated or their effects mitigated. Plans for dealing with the various situations range from prompt and vigorous intervention to cope with a medical emergency (incipient left ventricular failure or the onset of a psychosis) to a leisurely consultation aiming at giving firm reassurance and sound advice about work and exercise. Whatever may be the original cause of insomnia, the disability nearly always tends to perpetuate itself; most patients are convinced that sleeplessness will culminate in permanent illness—mental or physical. In a genuine case of insomnia it is important to break the vicious circle by resorting at once to the use of hypnotics. This may succeed more than anything else in restoring the patient's self-confidence; and it provides time in which to initiate such general measures as may be appropriate (work, exercise, diet, etc.). It should be made clear to the patient that this is a temporary expedient, and that after about a week on a hypnotic drug, treatment will be gradually withdrawn.

Hypnotics. A hypnotic is a drug that produces sleep resembling natural sleep. A large number of such preparations are available. None of them conforms to the ideal. The physician should make a small selection of these drugs and try to acquire experience and skill in their use. A few general principles of prescribing may be mentioned. A single drug should be used—usually as a tablet or a capsule. It should be taken by the patient just before he goes to bed and three to four hours after his evening meal; absorption is more rapid if the stomach is empty. At the start the maximum dose should be ordered. Smaller doses can be given on the third or fourth night—when the patient has been fully convinced of the effectiveness of the drug. Combinations of several hypnotics in one preparation are to be avoided. The depressant effects of hypnotics may be notably increased by taking them after fairly heavy indulgence in alcohol; self-medication with hypnotics in such circumstances carries obvious dangers.

It is customary to classify hypnotics into two groups: barbiturates and non-barbiturates. This has perhaps led to some misunderstanding about the relative values of the drugs in these groups. The barbiturates have been the most popular hypnotics in general use for many years and indeed they provide the standards against which new hypnotics are assessed by controlled clinical trial. The therapeutic effects of the barbiturates are the result of their characteristic pharmacological action, namely cerebral depression. Not surprisingly, in gross overdose they produce coma and serious depression of the respiratory centre. A great deal of effort has therefore been devoted to the search for a potent non-barbiturate hypnotic. It is obvious, however, that all hypnotics are by definition depressants of the central nervous system, and when taken in excessive doses they inevitably result in coma and depression of the vital centres in the medulla. The following is a useful grouping of the hypnotics for clinical purposes: (*a*) the barbiturates, such as butobarbitone, cyclobarbitone, pentobarbitone, and amylobarbitone; (*b*) the chloral hydrate group; (*c*) other hypnotics.

Barbiturates. There is little to choose between the barbiturates mentioned above as regards potency and duration of action. The hypnotic effect begins in about half an hour and lasts for four to eight hours. For an adult a suitable oral dose is 100 mg. but at the start of treatment the full dose of 200 mg. should be given. In some patients there may be a hang-over effect with drowsiness and confusion on waking. The physician should take particular note of after-effects during the early stages of treatment with a barbiturate. Phenobarbitone is often given as a hypnotic, but for this purpose its prolonged action makes it compare unfavourably with the preparations mentioned above.

The undesirable effects of the barbiturates call for brief comment. *Tolerance* may occur, and if the patient is gradually increasing the dose in order to maintain the hypnotic effect, it is wise to discontinue the drug and use a non-barbiturate preparation. Similarly, *psychic dependence* may necessitate a change of therapy. *Addiction* is much less common; but treatment of the barbiturate addict consists in withdrawing the drug gradually under careful medical and psychiatric surveillance. The commonest side-effect is *idiosyncrasy* to barbiturate and it is more likely to occur in patients with a history of allergic upsets such as asthma, urticaria and kindred disorders. The chief sign is puffiness of the face, and this may be accompanied by erythema, urticaria or even a frank dermatitis.

In elderly patients barbiturates may cause mental confusion and disorientation. This is particularly obvious when they are in strange surroundings (hospitals, etc.). The symptoms may be mistaken for those of cerebrovascular disease.

There are several *contraindications* to the use of barbiturates. The occurrence of any serious side-effect would justify immediate withdrawal of the drug. Barbiturates should not be given to patients suffering from mental depression with suicidal tendencies. Again as the respiratory centre is depressed by toxic doses of the barbiturates, it is wise to avoid using them (even in therapeutic doses) if there is evidence of severe respiratory insufficiency; and as the barbiturates that are used as hypnotics are metabolized in the liver, signs of poisoning readily occur when these drugs are given to patients with gross impairment of liver function.

See also Interaction of Drugs, p. 553.

The chloral hydrate group. Chloral hydrate, given in full doses, is a powerful and reliable hypnotic. Unfortunately it has an unpleasant taste and may also cause epigastric discomfort and nausea because of gastric irritation. It should, therefore, be given in dilute solution with flavourings such as orange squash or syrup of ginger. The hypnotic dose of chloral hydrate is 2 g. but this can be decreased to 1·5 g. after the first two or three doses. It is largely reduced in the body to trichlorethanol, itself a powerful hypnotic. New preparations incorporating chloral hydrate are available. They are to be preferred because they rarely cause gastric irritation. One of these drugs is triclofos; it is available as a tablet which is palatable and well tolerated. A suitable hypnotic dose is four tablets, each containing 500 mg. (500 mg. triclofos approximately equals 300 mg. chloral hydrate). Like chloral hydrate, it is changed in the body to trichlorethanol. For children and elderly patients, the drug may be more suitably dispensed as triclofos syrup, which contains 500 mg. in 5 ml. Drugs of the chloral hydrate group should not be prescribed with other cerebral depressants such as alcohol or barbiturates because the combined effect is apt to result in deep narcosis. In therapeutic doses hypnotics of the chloral hydrate group produce sleep lasting six to eight hours, and there are no untoward effects on the cardiovascular or respiratory systems. Skin rashes occur occasionally and prolonged medication may result in mild blepharitis. Elderly patients often tolerate these drugs better than barbiturates. Chloral hydrate or triclofos are useful substitutes in any patient who has shown sensitivity to a barbiturate.

Other hypnotics. Paraldehyde has been used as a hypnotic for many years. Although it is safe when given in therapeutic doses, it has a burning taste and a pungent unpleasant odour—and these are major disadvantages. There seems little justification for retaining it as a hypnotic now that so many effective drugs are available.

In recent years, many synthetic non-barbiturate hypnotics have been introduced. These include glutethimide, methyprylone, methaqualone, ethchlorvynol and nitrazepam. Each of these drugs in appropriate dosage produces a hypnotic action lasting for six to eight hours but none has been proved to be therapeutically superior to the barbiturates or chloral hydrate. Nevertheless, when a patient exhibits sensitivity to the barbiturates and to the chloral hydrate group of drugs (e.g. by development of skin rashes) one of them can often be used safely and effectively.

The search for the ideal hypnotic will continue, but it is unreasonable to expect that a drug which is an effective depressant of the sensorium—an action essential to its hypnotic effect—will not inevitably carry the risk of producing medullary depression and even death when dosage is grossly excessive. Claims for the complete safety of any new hypnotic must, therefore, be treated with reserve. A final opinion must await the results of controlled therapeutic trials and also the critical assessment which emerges from experience in clinical practice over a long period of years.

Further Reading

Analgesics:

Today's Drugs (Editorial)—Pentazocine (1970) *Br. med. J.* **1**, 409.

Today's Drugs (Editorial)—Narcotic Analgesics (1970). *Br. med. J.* **1**, 587.

Today's Drugs (Editorial)—Aspirin and Alternatives (1970). *Br. med. J.* **2**, 89.

Hypnotics:

MILLER, R. R., DE YOUNG, D. V. & PAXINOS, J. (1970). Hypnotic Drugs. *Postgrad. med. J.* **46**, 314.

18. Chronic Rheumatic Diseases

J. J. R. DUTHIE

INTRODUCTION

The rheumatic diseases, both acute and chronic, constitute a serious menace to the health and well-being of the community. Only within recent years have statistics been compiled which indicate the magnitude of the problem. It is officially admitted that one-sixth of the total annual invalidity of insured persons in Britain is due to rheumatic disease in one or other of its forms. Population surveys reveal that approximately 1,740,000 persons are affected by rheumatoid arthritis in Britain. Osteoarthrosis is responsible for some degree of disablement in nearly 4,000,000 people over the age of 65. Such figures give some indication of the economic loss resulting from the ravages of this group of diseases, and of the amount of pain and misery produced.

Considerable progress has been made in providing better diagnostic and therapeutic facilities for this group of diseases. Only by accurate diagnosis in the early stages of the more severe forms, and by the immediate institution of the proper lines of treatment, can the regrettably common legacy of permanent incapacity be reduced or avoided.

From the point of view of treatment it is convenient to consider the rheumatic diseases in three main groups: (1) rheumatoid arthritis and its variants, ankylosing spondylitis, the diffuse diseases of connective tissue (collagen diseases) and gout. In this group symptoms are inflammatory in origin; (2) osteoarthrosis, intervertebral disc degeneration and osteoporosis. Symptoms arise as a result of degenerative changes in articular structures; (3) nonarticular rheumatism which includes a miscellaneous group of conditions of diverse aetiology causing pain and stiffness of extra-articular origin.

Before any scheme of treatment is adopted for an individual patient the diagnosis must be clearly defined. It is also essential to assess the degree of activity of the disease in the affected tissues. This is done by using conventional clinical methods, but much importance is also placed upon serial estimations of the erythrocyte sedimentation rate.

The first consideration in the treatment of chronic rheumatic disease is to secure the co-operation of the patient. It should be explained that dramatic results must not be expected and that reliance should be placed on the judicious application not of one form of treatment but of a combination of methods which have been carefully thought out. His confidence won, his co-operation secured and the fundamental principles underlying correct treatment observed, a prospect of progressive improvement lies before the patient. Treated early and adequately, the outlook in the severe forms of chronic rheumatic disease is far from being as gloomy as has been formerly held by the laity and the profession.

The treatment of all forms of chronic rheumatic disease is summarized thus: (1) the improvement of the general health of the patient; (2) the elimination or correction of aetiological factors; (3) treatment of the local manifestation of the disease.

PROPHYLAXIS OF THE CHRONIC RHEUMATIC DISEASES

Rheumatoid arthritis. Recent surveys of the incidence of rheumatoid arthritis in the general population reveal no evidence that the disease affects one social class more than another, or that the type of employment is of aetiological importance. The impression that thin, visceroptotic people are more prone to develop rheumatoid arthritis than those of sturdier build is probably erroneous. Research has not as yet shed any light on the aetiology of the disease. In these circumstances it is not possible to recommend any specific measure to reduce the general incidence or to prevent the onset of the disease in the individual.

Osteoarthrosis. Osteoarthrosis is a degenerative condition and an accompaniment of the ageing process. There are many circumstances that predispose to the onset of osteoarthrosis and some of them are preventable. They are gross injuries leading to dislocations of joints, fractures of bones which involve the articular surfaces, and excessive or long-continued strains. When a bone is fractured, a seconday osteoarthrosis will result in adjacent joints unless proper alignment of the fragments is procured. When a fall or injury results in trauma of the joint structures and contusion of the overlying tissues, proper treatment by rest followed by heat and movement may delay and minimize the effect of the trauma in conditioning the occurrence of osteoarthrosis. Long-continued trauma from occupational strains is a common cause of osteoarthrosis. It is well recognized that certain trades produce arthritis in particular sites. For example, stone-masons commonly suffer from osteoarthrosis of the wrist, elbow or shoulder, whereas in agricultural labourers the spine and hips are more usually affected. The question arises, when early signs of osteoarthrosis are noted by the doctor, whether a change of occupation should be advised before the affected joints become hopelessly crippled. The decision in such a case will depend on the circumstances, but for economic reasons advice to change a patient's occupation in middle age is seldom practicable.

More hopeful fields for the reduction of osteoarthrosis in industry lie in the province of public health administration. Improvement of working conditions in factories, workshops, mines, etc., would help to lower the incidence of this disease.

Another factor which leads to continuous joint strain and undue pressure on the articular surfaces is obesity. Its correction by dietetic restriction (p. 340) is a preventive measure of great importance.

Postural defects predispose to the development of osteoarthrosis for the same reason as does obesity, and their correction by special exercises or orthopaedic measures is important in its prevention. The commonest faults are lumbar lordosis and scoliosis, genu varum or valgum, and pes planus.

RHEUMATOID ARTHRITIS

The treatment of rheumatoid arthritis is governed by the stage of the disease and the degree of activity present when the patient is first seen by the practitioner. We have arbitrarily divided the disease into three stages, although in practice no sharp dividing line exists.

THE ACUTE STAGE OF RHEUMATOID ARTHRITIS

Empirical therapy must necessarily be directed to the relief of discomfort and disability. In rheumatoid arthritis treatment, therefore, aims at providing skilled supervision for a patient who may be febrile, exhausted and worried and for the relief of pain, stiffness and muscular wasting.

General Treatment

It cannot be too strongly emphasized that treatment embraces the management of the patient as well as measures which aim at relieving the disease. Accordingly the physician must secure the intelligent co-operation of the patient by taking him into his confidence, by explaining in simple language the nature of the disease and the principles on which the treatment to be adopted is founded, and by assuming an optimistic attitude regarding the results to be expected.

REST, both physical and mental, is the first object to be achieved. In the acute stage rest must be complete, and this means that the patient must stay in bed, for several weeks if necessary, until signs of active inflammation have begun to subside. It is advisable to explain to the patient that the prescription of rest must be considered as only the first step in an organized scheme of treatment. Recumbency affords the opportunity of correcting faulty posture and, as Goldthwait says, 'enables the physician to remodel the body no longer handicapped by the unfavourable influences of gravity'. Good posture should be maintained while the patient is in bed. A firm mattress or fracture boards should be used. Only one firm, low pillow should be allowed at night. A cage should be used to remove the weight of the blankets from the legs and feet. A support for the feet should be provided in the shape of a sandbag or foot-board, and the spine should be kept in good alignment during the day by a back-rest. An important factor in securing rest is the control of pain, which impairs appetite, causes insomnia and increases physical and mental fatigue. For this purpose analgesic and anti-inflammatory drugs must be prescribed in adequate quantities.

After a week or two of complete rest, when the more acute symptoms may have abated, other measures of value in increasing the feeling of well-being should be employed. *The care of the skin* is an important feature in the treatment, because of the defective peripheral circulation and the marked tendency for these patients to sweat excessively. Accordingly, tepid sponging of the whole body, followed by gentle rubbing with a soft towel, should be carried out at least once a day. Even at this early stage *exercises* should be prescribed for the purpose of improving the circulation and correcting faulty posture. They are carried out in the recumbent position, and their frequency and amount graduated to suit each individual patient in accordance with the degree of asthenia present. Breathing exercises are designed to teach the patient to use his diaphragm and abdominal muscles more efficiently. Postural exercises are given for improving the tone of the spinal and gluteal muscles. We are satisfied, from daily experience of these measures, that the claims made by Goldthwait and Swaim regarding the beneficial effects produced are justified, and we strongly recommend their adoption in every case of rheumatoid arthritis. Details of the exercises for use in the acute stage are given in the Appendix (p. 465).

FOCAL SEPSIS. The belief that foci of infection play an important part in the aetiology of rheumatoid arthritis is no longer tenable. It has been shown that the incidence of such foci in patients with the disease is the same as in people of the same age, sex and social status without evidence of arthritis. Obvious sepsis should, of course, be dealt with in patients with rheumatoid arthritis, but it should be made clear to the patient that removal of teeth or tonsils will not cure this disease, but constitutes part of the plan to improve his general health.

DRUGS

The majority of drugs claimed to have a specific effect in rheumatoid arthritis have proved valueless and have now been discarded. Used intelligently, however, some of them can make a useful contribution to treatment.

Anti-inflammatory and analgesic drugs. These drugs are of particular importance, since pain must be abolished if the other measures recommended are to have their maximum effect. *Aspirin* is the safest and most useful anti-inflammatory drug and should be given in the maximum dose tolerable to the individual patient. Common toxic effects are tinnitus, deafness, gastric discomfort, and bleeding from the alimentary tract. In the majority of adults, the daily dose will lie between 4 to 6 g. Many patients tolerate soluble *calcium aspirin* better than plain aspirin. If gastric intolerance persists an equivalent dose of enteric coated tablets should be prescribed. When pain is inadequately controlled by aspirin alone, one or two tablets of *codeine phosphate* (B.P.) twice or thrice daily

should be prescribed in addition. If aspirin causes persistent side-effects, other analgesics must be used. *Paracetamol* can be used as an alternative in doses of about 1 g. six times a day; this is a derivative of phenacetin, but it is much less likely to have the toxic effects of phenacetin on the kidneys. A drug of the barbiturate group, such as amylobarbitone, 100 to 200 mg., should be used if sleep is disturbed. In proved cases of iron-deficiency anaemia, iron should be prescribed (p. 143). The anaemia of rheumatoid arthritis, however, is usually normochromic and fails to respond to iron given by mouth, but the majority of patients respond to administration by intravenous or intramuscular injection (p. 144). A total of up to 3 g. may be needed according to the severity of the anaemia and the patient's tolerance. The response is markedly enhanced by the concomitant administration of corticotrophin 20 units daily for two weeks and 10 units daily for a further two weeks. Additional calcium is not required if the patient is able to drink plenty of milk. Provided the diet is well balanced and adequate in amount, the addition of synthetic vitamins is unnecessary. The claims that muscle relaxants are of value in treatment has not been substantiated and their use is not recommended.

Phenylbutazone. This drug, a pyrazol derivative, is a powerful analgesic. Patients may be started on 200 mg. daily. If this proves inadequate, the amount may be increased by 100 mg. to a maximum of 300 mg. daily. If adequate subjective improvement has not occurred after three or four days on this dose, the drug should not be continued, as the incidence of toxic effects increases sharply above this level.

Toxic effects occur in 40 to 50 per cent. of patients, most commonly during the first few weeks of treatment. Gastro-intestinal disturbances in the form of stomatitis, dyspepsia, nausea and vomiting, oedema due to sodium retention, skin rashes and albuminuria are the most frequent. More serious, though much rarer, complications are haemorrhage or perforation of peptic ulcers, jaundice, agranulocytosis, aplastic anaemia, thrombocytopenia, optic neuritis and toxic psychosis. The drug should not be given in the presence of cardiovascular, renal or hepatic disease, or to patients with a history suggestive of peptic ulcer.

Oxyphenbutazone. This drug is a derivative of phenylbutazone, and is equally effective. A few patients intolerant of phenylbutazone can take it without ill-effect. The dose should be limited to 300 mg. daily.

Indomethacin. This drug is now widely used, but controlled trials have shown that it is no more effective than phenylbutazone or aspirin. Side-effects are common and include headache, vertigo, depression, nausea, peptic ulceration and haemorrhage. It may mask signs of infection in children. The dose is 25 mg. three or four times daily. The drug is not recommended for long continued use in the treatment of rheumatoid arthritis.

Other analgesics. A number of new analgesic and anti-inflammatory drugs have been used in the treatment of rheumatic arthritis in recent years and require brief mention. *Dihydrocodeine* tablets, 30 mg. thrice daily, and pentazocine, 25 mg. three or four times daily, are valuable analgesics and may be useful when pain persists. *Mefenamic acid*, 250 mg. four to six times daily, and *flufenamic acid*, 100 mg. four to six times daily are claimed to be as potent anti-inflammatory agents as aspirin, but both can cause troublesome diarrhoea. *Ibuprofen*, 200 mg. three or four times daily, has been shown to be effective. It causes no gastric bleeding and is relatively free from other side-effects. None of these drugs has proved consistently superior to aspirin.

Chrysotherapy. Gold was first used in the treatment of rheumatoid arthritis as a result of the belief in its value in the treatment of pulmonary tuberculosis. The mode of action of gold preparations is unknown. The lack of any immediate dramatic response, the undoubted psychological value of a weekly injection combined with regular supervision, and the fact that between 50 and 60 per cent. of patients improve on a conservative regimen of treatment, have made it very difficult to reach a definite conclusion as to the value of chrysotherapy. Nevertheless many authorities still believe that benefit follows its use in a worthwhile proportion of cases (50 to 70 per cent.). It is generally accepted that in those patients who respond, the first course is the most effective; the results of subsequent courses are often disappointing. Satisfactory remissions following its use occur more frequently in early cases, but this can be truthfully said about all forms of treatment. The exhibition of gold salts must be considered merely a part of and not a substitute for a general plan of treatment carefully arranged for each particular patient.

The course of chrysotherapy generally recommended consists of 20 weekly intramuscular injections of 50 mg. sodium aurothiomalate (B.P.) over a period of six months totalling approximately 1 g. Thereafter the course may be repeated for a second, third or fourth time, depending on the clinical response. Gold should be discontinued for at least eight weeks between courses. Others have stated that better results are obtained if the effects of the first course of treatment with 1 g. of gold are maintained by a monthly injection of 50 mg. for periods up to a year, but there is no clear proof of this and there is a risk that unnecessarily large amounts of gold may be given. When the weekly dose is 50 mg., complications are uncommon. It is advisable for the physician to explain the dangers to the patient or his relatives before beginning treatment. Gold treatment should not be recommended if serious organic disease is present, particularly if it affects the liver, kidneys, haemopoietic tissues or skin. Before each weekly injection, careful questioning and clinical examination, including testing the urine for albumen, should be undertaken to elicit the earliest signs of damage to these organs and tissues. General skin reactions, purpura, leucopaenia, jaundice, albumen, casts and blood in the urine are findings of grave significance and are indications for complete cessation of gold treatment. A trace of albumen in the urine by itself is not a contraindication to continued treatment but indicates the need for careful urine analysis prior to each subsequent dose of gold.

The most effective drug in the treatment of gold poisoning is dimercaprol (p. 561). It is given in doses of 3 mg. per kilogram of body weight every six hours for three or four days. The calculated quantity is injected intramuscularly. Smaller doses will be found effective for less severe toxic reactions. In gold hepatitis the dose should never exceed 3 mg. per kilogram of body weight given at six-hourly intervals and should generally be less, since it has been shown that in cases with hepatic damage the toxic effects from dimercaprol may be severe.

Corticosteroids have proved valuable in the treatment of toxic reactions to gold. Prednisolone, 15 to 20 mg. daily, should be given for some days and then the dose should be gradually reduced. The simultaneous administration of two potentially toxic drugs such as gold salts and phenylbutazone should be avoided.

In conclusion, we feel that the use of gold salts in the treatment of rheumatoid arthritis is unsatisfactory in view of the frequency of toxic reactions and the fact that a substantial proportion of patients derive no benefit from their administration. The circumstances which may justify the use of this drug have been discussed and the dangers and limitations of chrysotherapy have been stressed.

Chloroquine and hydroxychloroquine. In recent years a number of workers have reported favourably on the use of anti-malarial drugs in the treatment of rheumatoid arthritis. Good results have been claimed in some 70 to 80 per cent. of cases. Mild or moderate toxic effects occur in 40 to 50 per cent. of cases and include pruritus, skin rashes, gastro-intestinal upset, headache, mental confusion and leucopenia. Visual disturbances have also been reported resulting from corneal opacities or, less commonly, from retinopathy and macular degeneration. Although it cannot be claimed as yet that these drugs are both effective and safe, they may be of some value as an adjunct to the conservative treatment of rheumatoid arthritis. The dose of chloroquine should not exceed 250 mg. daily. Hydroxychloroquine is claimed to be less toxic, and 400 mg. daily has been given for more than one year without the occurrence of serious toxic effects. Routine examination of the eyes of patients taking these drugs should be carried out at intervals not exceeding six months. In long-term treatment, these drugs should be withdrawn for four to six weeks each year both to assess their clinical effects and to minimize excessive accumulation in the tissues.

Corticosteroids. Considerable experience in the use of corticosteroids in the treatment of rheumatoid arthritis has been gained since the dramatic effects of cortisone were first reported by Hench and his colleagues in 1949. The synthetic analogues of cortisone and hydrocortisone, *prednisone* and *prednisolone* have now been shown to be superior to the parent steroids in the treatment of rheumatoid arthritis. They are relatively free from salt-retaining effect and are about five times more potent, weight for weight, in controlling symptoms and signs. In a clinical trial conducted under the auspices of the Medical Research Council and the Nuffield Foundation, the effect of prednisolone was compared with that of aspirin or other analgesics such as phenylbutazone. At the end of one year and two years, patients on prednisolone had maintained a significant advantage over the control group. However, at the end of three years' treatment, the difference between the two groups was less marked.

The optimum daily dose of prednisone or prednisolone is 10 mg., and it should never exceed 15 mg.

except in an emergency. The hormones are best prescribed in the form of 1 mg. tablets as this allows maximum flexibility in their administration; 2 mg. thrice daily and 4 mg. at night is a regimen which suits the majority of patients. Others find it more helpful to take the larger dose first thing in the morning or after their midday meal. Tablets should always be crushed and taken with food or a glass of milk.

If there is no satisfactory response within two to three weeks on a daily dose of 10 mg., it may be increased by 1 to 2 mg., but should never exceed a total of 15 mg. If the response is still inadequate at this level, it is unwise to persist with this form of treatment. In these circumstances the dose should be reduced by 1 mg. every three to four days. In patients who show a marked response to 10 mg. daily, the dose may be reduced by 1 mg. each week until the minimum dose required to achieve satisfactory control of symptoms is reached.

Triamcinolone is slightly more potent than prednisone or prednisolone, but holds no other advantage as far as is known at present. In addition to the side-effects common to all corticosteroids tested up to the present time, it may cause severe weakness and wasting of muscles, from which recovery may occur only after a long time.

Methylprednisolone is equivalent in potency to triamcinolone, but possesses no other advantage and is much more expensive. Marked spontaneous bruising commonly occurs during its administration.

Dexamethasone is the most potent corticosteroid yet produced: 0.85 mg. is equivalent to 5 mg. of prednisolone. The results of clinical trials have not supported the initial claims that the incidence of side-effects is reduced. In a proportion of patients it causes a rapid and undesirable gain in weight.

Other analogues, betamethasone, paramethasone and fluprednisolone, have become available, but all these share the undesirable features of earlier corticosteroids, without significant advantages over them.

Prednisone or prednisolone are the corticosteroids of choice at the present time in the long-term treatment of rheumatoid arthritis. With the doses now recommended serious side-effects have become less common, but still constitute a real risk. The most common is dyspepsia, which occurs in about 30 per cent. of patients. In the majority it is mild and can be controlled by the prescription of alkalis and strict adherence to instructions never to take uncrushed tablets on an empty stomach. Enteric-coated tablets of prednisolone are now available and are worthy of trial in patients with persistent dyspepsia. Peptic ulceration occurs in 10 per cent. of patients having corticosteroid therapy and in half of these cases it is complicated by haemorrhage or perforation. Hypertension of moderate degree has been recorded in about 13 per cent. of patients, but rarely reaches a dangerous level. The incidence of infections is not increased by moderate doses of corticosteroids, but symptoms may be so mild that they may not be reported. Patients should be instructed to inform their doctor immediately of any new symptoms which may arise during treatment. In those with severe disease and in post-menopausal women, prolonged administration of corticosteroids may lead to marked osteoporosis, collapse of vertebral bodies, or fracture of long bones. The value of non-virilizing anabolic steroids in preventing these complications has not been confirmed. Psychotic illness is a rather rare complication of corticosteroid therapy, but a past history of mental instability should be regarded as a contraindication to their use.

Only about 10 to 15 per cent. of patients with rheumatoid arthritis become severely crippled and dependent on others, but it is difficult to forecast the course which the disease will run in a patient seen for the first time. Experience gained from a study of the course of the disease over a number of years in a large group of patients treated on conservative lines suggests that the following are the main indications for the use of corticosteroids: (1) patients under 50, not yet irreversibly crippled, with continuing economic and social responsibilities, with disease of more than one year's duration running a progressive course, and who have failed to improve significantly following an adequate period of conservative treatment in hospital; (2) patients with progressive disease who cannot, for domestic or economic reasons, undergo an adequate period of conservative treatment, and who are in danger of losing their employment or becoming unable to look after home and family; (3) patients who have become severely incapacitated and dependent on others may justifiably be treated with corticosteroids when other methods have failed to restore personal and social independence.

In an individual case the decision to use corticosteroids may be influenced by a variety of factors, but it must be emphasized that, when given in effective doses, they suppress adrenal function. Further,

this suppression persists as long as the patient is receiving corticosteroids, and during this time his capacity to withstand the sudden stresses of illness or injury is reduced. It follows that such therapy must never be terminated abruptly. If withdrawal becomes necessary on account of persistent side-effects, the dose must be reduced very slowly over several months. A reduction of more than 1 mg. weekly is inadvisable. In the face of stress the maintenance dose must be increased during the period of emergency and slowly reduced to its former level when the need is passed. A patient should always carry a card indicating the preparation in use, the daily dose, and the name and telephone number of his doctor.

Corticotrophin (ACTH). The dose of this hormone required to produce adequate clinical suppression of symptoms in rheumatoid arthritis varies. The initial dose of corticotrophin gel recommended is 20 International Units every 24 hours. If response is satisfactory, the dose is reduced by 5 units every two to three days until the maintenance level is found. Side-effects and complications are similar to those produced by corticosteroids, but disturbance of the electrolyte balance with fluid retention may be more marked. These considerations, combined with the need for a daily injection, have markedly restricted the use of corticotrophin in rheumatoid arthritis. It has been noted, however, by a few workers that sustained remissions of the disease have followed the use of corticotrophin over a period of months. This is in contrast to the almost invariable recurrence of symptoms which rapidly follows the withdrawal of corticosteroids. It may be that the greater advantage to both patient and doctor of giving corticosteroids orally has led to a premature loss of interest in the use of corticotrophin. A synthetic form of corticotrophin (tetracosactrin) with a more prolonged action has been produced. If this results in giving patients less frequent injections the number of cases of acquired resistance will also be reduced. In the depot form the recommended dose is 0·5 to 1 mg. by intramuscular injection every second or third day according to response.

DIET. The diet should be well balanced and should contain sufficient calories to restore the body weight to normal in patients underweight, while for obese patients it should be designed to ensure the necessary reduction in weight. Small frequent meals attractively served will help to stimulate appetite. The need for an adequate intake of protein and an ample supply of vitamins and minerals is based on the general physiological principles which govern the dietetic requirement of a patient suffering from a chronic wasting disease in which metabolism may be further increased by fever.

Local Treatment

During the acute stage of rheumatoid arthritis the affected joints are swollen and tender. Movement is accompanied by severe pain and the muscles moving the joints are in spasm. The patient soon discovers that the flexed position gives the greatest ease for the affected joints, and conditions are created which culminate in permanent deformity. Such a patient lies with flexed knees, flexed hips, flexed elbows. The forearms and hands are laid on the chest, the wrists in a position of palmar flexion, and the feet are allowed to remain plantar flexed for lengthy periods. As the disease progresses, peri-articular and intra-articular adhesions form and movement becomes progressively more limited.

From the outset there are two objectives: the prevention of deformity and the maintenance of function. As a result of the long-maintained position of flexion, the flexor groups of muscles undergo compensatory shortening and thus still further limit the range of movements. Pain, therefore, must be relieved. Analgesics and anti-inflammatory drugs in adequate dosage are essential, but this alone will not suffice. The affected joints must be completely immobilized in order to avoid stretching of the inflamed structures, and this is most satisfactorily obtained by application of properly fitting splints. The relief obtained by support and fixation in such splints is of great therapeutic value, as it allows the patient to sleep without the large doses of sedatives previously required, with consequent improvement in the mental outlook.

Light, easily removable, perfectly fitting splints can be made quickly and simply with muslin bandages impregnated with plaster of Paris. The technical details for their manufacture are given on pp. 466–68. Whenever possible, the splints should be skin-tight, to ensure complete immobilization of the joints, since the slightest movement within the splint will lead to the return of pain and spasm. In very thin patients it may be necessary to pad the bony-prominences. This is best done by means of small pieces of chiropodist's felt, which are easily cut to shape and adhere to the skin. Before applying the plaster the skin should be oiled or the limb encased in stockinet, which forms an effective lining to the splint. The splint should hold the joint in the position which will produce the best functional result, should ankylosis occur.

Although we believe that splints made by the plaster technique are ideal, their application requires some degree of technical skill, and other materials may be found more convenient. Plastic materials, malleable on heating, are now available which can be used for the manufacture of light waterproof splints. These should be used when splints of a more durable character are required.

Some authorities believe that the danger of fibrous ankylosis is most likely to be avoided if splints are removed daily and gentle active movements are encouraged. Others feel that this danger has been exaggerated and that in the acute stage symptoms will subside more rapidly if complete immobilization is maintained for two to three weeks. After this initial period, splints are removed once or twice daily for active exercises (pp. 468–69). Active exercises should be preceded by heat because of its value in easing pain and relaxing muscle spasm. Portable radiant heat cages or lamps can be used for this purpose. Moist heat in the form of simple hot fomentations or kaolin poultices is also valuable as a preliminary to exercises. When the joints of the lower limbs are involved, a resumption of walking must be delayed until muscular control has been restored by the systematic use of carefully graded exercises. The more strenuous forms of physical treatment should not be given until the activity of the disease has diminished. They are discussed in the next section.

Intra-articular corticosteroids. Hydrocortisone acetate in suspension can be injected intra-articularly and has proved a useful means of controlling inflammation locally. Following injection, pain is reduced and effusions may subside. The duration of relief varies from a few days to two or three weeks. This treatment is particularly useful when progress is retarded by persistent pain and swelling in one or two joints, particularly the knees. Effusions, if present, should be aspirated before the injection is given. Strict asepsis must be observed, as invasion of the joint by bacteria may be facilitated in the presence of hydrocortisone. For the treatment of large joints, such as the knee, 25 to 50 mg. should be given; 2 to 5 mg. may prove adequate for the small peripheral joints in the hands and feet.

The interval between injections will vary according to the duration of relief obtained. It has been claimed that, in patients receiving corticosteroids by mouth, local treatment of one or two persistently painful joints may enable the daily dose to be reduced.

There is no doubt that the intra-articular injection of hydrocortisone is of value in the local treatment of the joints in rheumatoid arthritis. Nevertheless, there are reports of disorganization of the joint occurring after a prolonged course of injections. They should therefore not be given more often than once a month and repeated only if relief of pain is maintained for at least three weeks.

Painful extra-articular lesions can also be successfully treated by the local use of corticosteroids. The injection of painful ligamentous attachments, tendon nodules and inflamed bursae is often followed by relief of pain and improvement in function.

SUBACUTE STAGE OF RHEUMATOID ARTHRITIS

The patient may reach the subacute stage after weeks or months of treatment in the acute stage. Alternatively the disease may commence insidiously and the patient presents for treatment in the subacute stage. Characteristically one or more of the joints is swollen and painful, a considerable degree of asthenia and muscular wasting is generally present, fever is absent, but the sedimentation rate is raised to 30 to 50 mm. in one hour. In such cases the investigations and general management which have already been described must be undertaken. If the disease has passed from the acute into the subacute stage, the transition from recumbency to active movements and weight-bearing must be made gradually.

Rheumatoid arthritis is a general disease, and even if the weight-bearing joints are affected slightly or not at all, this in no way invalidates the need for general bodily rest for considerable periods in the day in order to counteract the general fatigue invariably present. Busy housewives treated at home are at a serious disadvantage as they rarely obtain enough rest. The benefit derived from resting the swollen and painful joints in splints is as great in the subacute stage as in the acute, but the number of hours per day during which the joints are immobilized should be reduced according to the degree of activity still present. Rest splints should always be worn in place during the night.

Physiotherapy. In the subacute stage physiotherapy plays a more important part in treatment than it does in the acute stage. The measures for the application of heat locally, e.g. radiant heat, wax baths or mud packs, are as useful in this stage as they are in the acute one. In addition, hydrotherapy may be valuable as a means of improving the function of the skin as well as for its effect in helping to restore movements to stiff joints. Accordingly, it is only in the subacute and chronic stages of the disease that it is advisable to send patients to spas for treatment, and this should be done early rather than late. A full report of the patient should be sent by the family doctor to the spa physician.

Hydrotherapy. In a hot bath pain is relieved and muscular spasm is largely eliminated; non-weight-bearing movement is facilitated.

In the deep pool the patient can stand or sit in water at a temperature of from 35° to 39° C. It is of a sufficient size to allow of free movement of all the joints and of sufficient depth to reduce the action of gravity to a minimum.

Following any form of hydrotherapy the patient should be allowed to cool down slowly in a warm room, at least one hour's rest being prescribed. Immersion baths cause considerable exhaustion to debilitated patients. They should not exceed 15 minutes in duration, and in general should not be given more than three times a week. On alternate days the joints should be treated by local applications of heat in the form of mud packs, wax baths, kaolin poultices or radiant heat.

Electrotherapy. Electrical treatment may also be of service. The interrupted current (faradism) is used to improve the condition of wasted muscles in the neighbourhood of arthritic joints. When the patient can adequately contract the affected muscles, faradism should be replaced by active exercises carried out for short periods twice or thrice daily.

Massage. Massage, when applied by a skilled physiotherapist, improves the local circulation and induces relaxation of muscles. Its value in easing pain may depend on a combination of these effects, but its mode of action is not clearly understood. It no longer occupies such a prominent place in the treatment of rheumatoid arthritis. Its effect in easing muscular pain and stiffness may be helpful as a preparation for active movement of the affected joints.

Exercise. Active movement and re-educational exercises are of the greatest value in the restoration of function. In the subacute stage movement of the joints under water is particularly beneficial. Re-educational exercises, under the guidance of a properly trained physiotherapist and devised according to the individual patient's needs, play an important part in the prevention and correction of deformity and the restoration of function.

Physiotherapy at home. Many simple but effective forms of physiotherapy can be used by the patient at home. These methods can be taught during the patient's stay in hospital or while attending as an out-patient. Simple means of applying heat to painful joints are described on p. 466. Heat should be followed by appropriate remedial exercises, and those prescribed in hospital should be continued at home (p. 466). The importance of following a regular regimen of rest and exercise must be strongly emphasized. Local rest is attained by splints worn at night and, if necessary, for periods during the day. Patients should lie down for an hour in the middle of the day, if possible, and be encouraged to go to bed early. The household bath can be used to provide a form of hydrotherapy little inferior to the more elaborate methods used in spas. Patients should spend 10 to 15 minutes fully immersed at a temperature between 37° and 40° C. This should be followed by an hour's rest in towels. In the case of housewives rearrangement of kitchen and household equipment and the provision of a number of suitable aids can do much to take the load off damaged joints. The regimen of physiotherapy in the home should be adjusted and controlled by regular review of the patient's progress.

CHRONIC STAGE OF RHEUMATOID ARTHRITIS

If all cases of rheumatoid arthritis were correctly treated in the acute and subacute stages, deformities would be met with much less frequently. However, much can now be done to improve the lot of those patients in whom the active phase of the disease has passed but in whom marked deformities have arisen.

In addition to the physiotherapeutic methods already described, special procedures are required for the correction of deformities and restoration of function, which are wholly orthopaedic in nature and may include surgical intervention in a proportion of cases (p. 465).

Treatment of deformities. The commonest deformities are fixed flexion of the hips, knees and

elbows, limitation of abduction and rotation in the shoulders, limitation of movement or ankylosis of the wrists in palmar flexion and of the ankles in plantar flexion, subluxation of the metacarpophalangeal joints with ulnar deviation of the fingers, subluxation of the interphalangeal joints, flat foot and hallux valgus. The joints usually become fixed in the position which is most comfortable to the patient during the acute stage. The maintenance of the joints in these positions for long periods leads to the formation of intra- and extra-articular adhesions, destruction of the cartilage becomes complete, and in the more progressive cases bony ankylosis may ensue.

Serial plasters. One of the most valuable methods available for the correction of deformities is the use of serial plasters. It is of particular value for the correction of flexion deformities of the knees, but can be used for any joint which is accessible to the application of plaster (p. 466). The advantages of serial plasters are that no strain is thrown on the articular structures, the muscles are put at rest, spasm is overcome and pain is relieved.

Peri-articular infiltration and intra-articular injection. When minor degrees of pain and disability are present, local infiltration of the peri-articular structures on one or more occasions with 1 per cent. solution of procaine according to the technique described on p. 641, followed by heat and movements, may be sufficient to banish pain and restore full function.

The intra-articular injection of hydrocortisone (p. 454) has proved as useful in the more chronic phases of the disease as it has in the acute stage, so long as symptoms are due to persistent inflammation rather than to structural changes in the joint structures. The technique employed is similar to that already described.

SPLINTS AND CRUTCHES. In more severe cases the damage to weight-bearing joints may be of such a degree that appliances are necessary to supplement the impaired function before the patient can regain the power to walk. The simplest of these is crutches, which serve a useful purpose in the transitional stage between recumbency and unaided weight-bearing. It is important that they should be the correct length for the individual patient, otherwise they may be the cause of further deformity, especially of the spine and hips. Walking cylinders, made of plaster of Paris or fibre-glass are valuable in the treatment of unstable knees. Another simple method of supporting an unstable joint is the application of a firm crêpe bandage. This will serve the double purpose of lending support and preventing excessive movement, especially in the knees and ankles. When the knees are incapable of supporting the patient's weight it becomes necessary to fit a walking caliper splint. This should be furnished with a locking device at the knee which permits flexion when the patient wishes to sit down. Similar splints are used to take the weight off a damaged hip, but they must be fitted with great care by a skilled technician, otherwise they will prove more of an encumbrance than a help. For less severe degrees of disability in the knee, laced elastic kneecaps are useful when the objects are to provide light support and to prevent excessive movement. These should be provided with jointed metal side-pieces if additional stability is necessary. Anklets of a similar type are available.

When a marked degree of flat foot is present, special shoes are necessary. They should not cause constriction and the heels should be carried forward 1 to 2 cm. farther on the inner than on the outer side, and should also be raised on the inner side of the sole ('crooked' shoe). When collapse of the transverse arches of the feet causes metatarsalgia the provision of insoles with a metatarsal raise will relieve pain by removing pressure from the heads of the metatarsal bones.

In the chronic stage of rheumatoid arthritis it is of paramount importance to prescribe a carefully planned scheme of exercises, both for the improvement of faulty body mechanics and for the restoration of function after deformity has been corrected. Details of exercises for these purposes will be found on p. 468.

Occupational therapy. One of the most difficult aspects of the treatment of rheumatoid arthritis is the rehabilitation of the patient once the active stage of the disease has passed. Re-educational exercises, physiotherapy, etc. (pp. 468–69), may do much to improve movement and muscular tone, but restoration of full function in the affected limbs may be very difficult to obtain. The selection of the occupation is determined by the degree of incapacity present and the particular joints involved. In addition to its therapeutic use in restoring function, occupational therapy provides a psychological stimulus of great value. The patient's interest is aroused and his mental outlook improved.

For patients with permanent impairment of function, a wide variety of simple aids is now available which enable them to become independent of help in their toilet and dressing. These cost only a few shillings and can be made in the occupational therapy department or splint-maker's shop. Similar appliances may enable a patient to resume work which he could not otherwise perform. In the case of crippled housewives, a variety of adjustments can be made in the home to render daily tasks easier and to enable them to resume family responsibilities.

This section can be summarized by emphasizing that the correction of faulty body mechanics, the restoration of muscular tone and movement and correction of deformity in various joints constitute an essential part of the co-ordinated plan of treatment. The physician in charge of the patient should enlist the assistance of the orthopaedic surgeon, whose special training and experience in these fields will enable him to give invaluable help.

STILL'S DISEASE

A type of rheumatoid arthritis occurs occasionally in children below the age of 10. It is accompanied by fever, leucocytosis, glandular enlargement and splenomegaly. There is a tendency for the infantile proportions of the limbs to persist, due to interference with normal growth by the disease. The findings in the joints do not appear to be specific for the disease but are similar to those of rheumatoid arthritis. The disease tends to run a prolonged course but the prognosis is good in some 60 per cent. of cases. Corticosteroids are effective in suppressing the symptoms of Still's disease, but their use in treatment is limited by the same considerations already discussed in relation to rheumatoid arthritis (pp. 452-53).

ANKYLOSING SPONDYLITIS

This is a disease mainly of early adult life and is much more common in males. Its incidence is relatively small, but when it arises it is a serious condition which may completely incapacitate the sufferer. The pathology is so similar to that of rheumatoid arthritis in the peripheral joints that it has been called rheumatoid arthritis of the spine, although in the opinion of most observers it is an entirely different disease. In the early stages patients are ambulatory, with the result that, owing to decalcification and softening of the vertebral bodies, the spine assumes a kyphotic position, and unless treatment is instituted early this deformity will become permanent owing to ossification of the ligaments and capsules of the joints.

General treatment. Although the cause of the disease is unknown, a scheme of treatment similar to that described in the section on rheumatoid arthritis must be adopted (p. 449), including application of all the measures already detailed to raise the general resistance and improve the health of the patient. In active cases, with marked systemic symptoms, an initial period of rest in bed may be required, but movements of the spine and thoracic cage must be maintained by daily active exercises. Experience shows that movement is better preserved when these patients are ambulant.

Drugs should be used with discretion as in rheumatoid arthritis, analgesics again being the most valuable. Phenylbutazone is claimed to be particularly effective in relieving pain in this disease (p. 450). Similar considerations to those discussed in connection with rheumatoid arthritis on pp. 452–54 govern the use of corticosteroids.

Radiotherapy. The results of radiotherapy in this disease are very satisfactory. The small risk of leukaemia developing is outweighed by the benefit obtained. The best results follow a course of daily treatment lasting two weeks. Treatment is applied to the whole spine and sacro-iliac joints. Even in very early cases it should never be confined to the lumbar spine and sacro-iliac regions. The skin dose on all fields is 1,500 r. The course should not be repeated except in special circumstances, but if the hips or shoulders become painful at a later date, further radiation may be applied to these joints. In young women, the sacro-iliac regions should be avoided in view of the danger of causing sterility.

Rest and exercise. In early cases with no deformity, the disease process may be completely arrested and full movement may be regained. The maintenance of good posture must be ensured. When radiological changes are confined to the sacro-iliac joints, rest in bed may be unnecessary, but postural and breathing exercises must be performed daily. In more advanced cases, where radiological examination shows no ossification of the spinal ligaments, but where posture is already poor, a period of two to three weeks' rest in bed combined with postural exercises is necessary. Fracture boards should be placed under the mattress. On getting up, these patients should be fitted with a spinal brace, which should be worn until muscular power has been completely restored. The brace is removed several times daily and active exercises performed. In advanced cases with established deformity, the relief of pain and stiffness

following radiotherapy greatly facilitates the restoration of good alignment by the use of serial plaster shells. In cases with a marked kyphotic deformity which cannot be corrected otherwise, spinal osteotomy may be used to improve postural alignment. These patients may have to wear some form of orthopaedic support permanently. Recognition of the disease at an early stage, followed by adequate treatment, will effectively prevent the occurrence of such late manifestations. Even in patients in whom the disease appears to be completely arrested, medical supervision should be continued to ensure the maintenance of good posture.

DISEASES OF CONNECTIVE TISSUE (COLLAGEN DISEASES)

In the group of conditions defined by Klemperer and his colleagues in 1942 as diseases of collagen, a widespread lesion of connective tissue is the common factor linking disorders with diverse clinical features and very different prognoses. The lesion affects all components of extracellular connective tissue and for this reason diseases of connective tissue is a more accurate description than collagen diseases, which suggest a specific lesion of collagen alone. The diseases in which the lesion is always present are rheumatic fever, rheumatoid arthritis, polyarteritis nodosa, systemic lupus erythematosus, scleroderma and dermatomyositis. The aetiology of these conditions is unknown, but all show evidence of systemic disturbances as well as the local lesions upon which the diagnosis is based. Symptoms referable to the joints may be present at some time in all members of the group and, with the exception of rheumatic fever, the course of the disease tends to be prolonged. Rheumatic fever and rheumatoid arthritis have been dealt with elsewhere (pp. 106, 449). The other members of the group are relatively uncommon, but are important since they may present a difficult diagnostic problem when joint symptoms are also present.

Polyarteritis Nodosa and Systemic Lupus Erythematosus

Until the advent of corticosteroid therapy, treatment for these two conditions was entirely symptomatic and the outcome was invariably fatal. A dramatic response to corticosteroids regularly occurs, and their administration may be life saving. Acute manifestations can be suppressed and a fair measure of health restored. It is now clear, however, that these hormones are in no way curative. Continuous maintenance therapy is essential. The presence of impaired renal function before treatment, common in both diseases, is of serious significance as these patients frequently deteriorate while receiving the hormones. Large doses are often required to control acute symptoms. Prednisolone in daily doses of 60 to 80 mg. by mouth may be necessary. The dose is gradually reduced until a satisfactory maintenance one is reached which is frequently about 10 to 15 mg. daily. Moderate or marked signs of hyperadrenalism will occur in many patients so treated, but this disadvantage must be accepted if control is to be maintained. This policy is justifiable in diseases which otherwise end in death. It is not yet certain that life can be prolonged by this treatment, but the great increase in comfort which accompanies it fully justifies its continued use.

Scleroderma and Dermatomyositis

The results of corticosteroid therapy in these two diseases have been disappointing. In scleroderma little alteration in the skin condition has been observed. This disease does not as a rule cause marked systemic upset and the use of high doses of corticosteroids is not justified by the results obtained.

In dermatomyositis, acute exacerbations with marked weakness of the muscles, not infrequently involving the respiratory muscles, may endanger life. In these circumstances the use of prednisolone may tide the patient over the crisis. Adequate doses must be used initially. Slow reduction with a view to withdrawal should be started when acute symptoms have been controlled.

GOUT

Gout is a disease characterized by recurrent attacks of acute pain and swelling of sudden onset, affecting one or more joints, and by a marked increase in the production of uric acid. Recent evidence suggests that precipitation of microcrystals of uric acid in the joint is the cause of the acute inflammatory episodes. It has now been clearly demonstrated that the prolonged use of uricosuric agents, by ridding the body of excess uric acid, may substantially reduce the number of attacks. The disease is familial in the majority of cases. Raised levels of plasma uric acid in relatives who have never suffered

from gouty arthritis suggests that factors other than the abnormality of purine metabolism are concerned in the production of clinical gout. The almost complete immunity of women before the menopause suggests that the sex hormones may play some part.

Prevention. With modern methods of management much can be done to reduce the number of acute attacks, shorten their duration and prevent the later complications of the disease such as the development of osteoarthritic changes in affected joints and progressive renal failure. It is doubtful if the imposition of dietetic restrictions is justifiable in males with a family history of gout unless the blood uric acid is shown to be above normal on more than one occasion, but these men should be advised to live temperately and avoid excesses in eating and drinking.

Treatment of acute stage. During the acute attack of gouty arthritis, pain in the affected joints may be excruciating. Some degree of systemic upset in the form of fever, malaise, leucocytosis and a raised E.S.R. is almost invariable. The patient should be confined to bed and the joints should be protected from pressure by a cradle. Phenylbutazone is the drug of choice in the treatment of the acute phase. It should be prescribed in a dose of 600 mg. daily until pain is controlled, usually within 24 hours. The dose is then reduced to 300 mg. daily for another two to three days. Fluids should be drunk freely (4 to 5 pints) and the diet should consist of eggs, fruit, milk and cereals (see below). Prompt treatment along the lines described will give rapid relief in the majority of cases.

Both the corticosteroids and corticotrophin can be used to control acute gout. Corticotrophin is the more effective, but must be given in conjunction with colchicine if relapse on withdrawal of the hormone is to be avoided. This method of treatment is not recommended for routine use, as only exceptional cases will fail to respond to phenylbutazone in the doses specified.

Treatment between attacks

Investigations of the metabolism of uric acid in normal persons and sufferers from gout, using isotopically labelled uric acid, have shown that there is a large increase in the total quantity of freely exchangeable uric acid in the body fluid of gouty subjects. Treatment between attacks is based upon partial control of uric acid production by dietary measures and increased excretion of uric acid by the kidneys induced by the administration of uricosuric drugs.

Diet. In view of the formation of uric acid from many components of the diet and from endogenous sources there is no justification for *severe* restriction of purines and protein. In general, the diet should be low in purines and fat and should not exceed the caloric needs of the patient. Foods with a high purine content should be forbidden, namely sweet-breads, liver, kidney, brain, heart, anchovies, sardines, meat extracts, herring roe, white-bait, sprats, smelts. Fatty foods, cream, butter and margarine should be restricted because of their caloric value and because of the evidence that fat influences adversely the excretion of uric acid. The treatment and prevention of obesity is of prime importance. Occasionally patients find that certain articles of food or drink have a specific effect in precipitating an acute attack, and these must obviously be omitted from their diet. Alcohol is best avoided. Nevertheless, total prohibition is not easy to justify as teetotallers can develop classic gout, and only a few alcoholics ever suffer from the disease.

Drugs. A number of drugs increase the excretion of uric acid by the kidneys. The drugs of choice are probenecid and sulphinpyrazone which can be administered over long periods without ill effect.

Probenecid in doses of 500 mg. three or four times daily or sulphinpyrazone in doses of 200 to 400 mg. daily increase uric acid excretion by 30 to 50 per cent. in gouty subjects. Over a period of months the blood uric acid may return to normal levels and tophi decrease in size. Neither drug prevents acute attacks, but these can be reduced in frequency by the administration of colchicine 0·5 mg. two or three times a day. Occasional toxic reactions from probenecid have been reported, in the form of gastrointestinal symptoms and skin rashes. The clearance of excess uric acid from the body may well prove of great value in diminishing the frequency of renal damage, the most serious complication of chronic gout. Ample fluids should be drunk to prevent deposition of urates in the kidneys.

Salicylates inhibit the action of probenecid, and should not be used during treatment.

Allopurinol is now being widely used. This drug reduces the level of the serum uric acid by inhibiting the enzyme—xanthine oxidase—responsible for the formation of uric acid from xanthine and hypoxanthine. The daily dose is 300 mg. This

treatment may be particularly valuable in patients with pre-existing impairment of renal function, or who have a history of renal stone formation. Colchicine should also be prescribed along with this drug to reduce the possibility of acute attacks.

Treatment of Chronic Stage

Local treatment of damaged joints should be along similar lines to those described for osteoarthrosis. Where tophi have become large and unsightly, or have ulcerated through the skin, they can be removed surgically. General management on the lines indicated has improved the outlook for patients with chronic gout. The late complications of the disease in the form of progressive renal failure and grossly damaged joints may be prevented in the majority of cases, but it must be made clear to patients that treatment must be continued indefinitely if relapses are to be avoided.

OSTEOARTHROSIS AND DISC DEGENERATION

For the prophylaxis of osteoarthrosis see p. 448.

Treatment of the established disease is palliative. This is inevitable as degenerated cartilage or bony outgrowths cannot be repaired or removed by drugs or physiotherapy. Treatment may be divided into (1) general, which includes the removal or correction of aetiological factors, and (2) local.

General Treatment

If severe pain in a weight-bearing joint such as the hip or knee is being experienced the best method of taking the strain off the joint and relieving the pain is to confine the patient to bed for a week or two. During this period, active non-weight-bearing exercises should be prescribed. Patients with severe pain have frequently reached this state by accepting the advice of their friends or medical attendant that the best treatment is to 'walk it off' lest the joint should become stiff. For patients with less severe pain, modified rest should be ordered to meet the individual requirements of the case. Short walks on level turf may be encouraged, but walking on hard or uneven surfaces for any distance must be discouraged. Exercise that leads to an increase in pain or stiffness must be regarded as excessive, and the distance allowed must be reduced. If the patient is unable to accept this advice because of his occupation, the mechanical devices discussed below may be of value in relieving the strain of weight-bearing in an individual joint. The occupational factor may be of great aetiological importance in osteoarthrosis (p. 449), and the doctor must discuss with his patient the question of whether it is possible to change or modify his occupation should it be unsuitable.

Obesity may be present in individuals with osteoarthrosis, and reduction of weight is of great importance (p. 340). If the obesity affects the abdomen particularly, the patient tends to assume a posture which throws still greater strain on the weight-bearing joints, and exercises for the correction of faulty posture (p. 468) should be carried out regularly.

Drugs play only a small part in the treatment of osteoarthrosis. Analgesics (p. 444) are prescribed when necessary for the relief of pain. When the safer drugs such as aspirin and paracetamol are ineffective, phenylbutazone is worthy of trial (p. 450).

Local Treatment. Physiotherapy and not drug therapy is the sheet anchor of treatment. Its rationale is discussed on p. 455. If a single joint is affected, such as the knee, considerable relief may be obtained from the local application of heat. Any of the methods described on p. 455 may be used. In deep-seated joints such as the hips or spine, the analgesic effects of heat may be best attained by means of diathermy or short-wave therapy.

Where wasting of muscle is present, active exercises of the non-weight-bearing type should be prescribed.

Hydrotherapy (p. 455) is of great value in osteoarthrosis, particularly the deep-pool bath in which the patient can move his limbs under warm water. This relaxes spasm and eliminates the effect of gravity, thus enabling movements to be carried out with the minimum of pain. For those unable to visit a spa, a hot bath and the other measures described in the section on Physiotherapy at Home (p. 456) are useful substitutes in enabling the patient to obtain the benefits of heat and movements.

Peri-articular and intra-articular injections. Good results have been claimed to follow the injection of a variety of substances into the joint cavities in osteoarthrosis. Controlled clinical trials have shown that, if improvement follows such treatment, it bears no constant relationship to the material injected.

Intra-articular injection of a 1 per cent. solution of procaine combined with infiltration of tender areas in the peri-articular soft tissues is a useful method of treatment worthy of trial in cases of osteoarthrosis in accessible joints. The amount required will vary from 2 to 3 ml. in smaller joints to 15 to 20 ml. in the case of the hip or shoulder. If relief of reasonable duration is achieved, the injection can be repeated as required. Hydrocortisone suspension should be reserved for trial in cases where procaine has been ineffective. The results achieved have not been so impressive in this disease as in rheumatoid arthritis. It has been reported that worthwhile relief of pain is most likely to be obtained in cases where radiological changes are not marked. Methods of puncturing the cavities of joints are described on p. 641.

Orthopaedic procedures. Manipulation under a general anaesthetic may be a valuable procedure, but it must be employed with great caution and only in selected cases: typically there is considerable pain and limitation of movement, but only moderate bony changes. In such a case, peri-articular adhesions and capsular thickening are believed to be largely responsible for the disability which is present and benefit may be obtained from gently manipulating the joint under full surgical anaesthesia. This must be followed by daily movement of the joint preceded by heat.

Mechanical appliances for the relief of weight-bearing joints may be necessary if the measures already outlined fail to give relief. The types most frequently used are caliper splints constructed to take the weight off the knee or hip or a steel brace to support the spine. These appliances are expensive and should be ordered only on the advice of a competent orthopaedic specialist and should be fitted by a trained technician. The indications for surgical treatment are discussed on p. 465.

Osteoarthrotic spondylitis. Degenerative changes in the spine occur in two situations: the intervertebral disc and the posterior articulations. Changes in both are frequently present in the same patient. The osteophytes arising from the edges of vertebral bodies, often the most prominent abnormality seen on radiological examination, are now considered to be the result of primary degeneration of the intervertebral disc, with consequent narrowing of the space between the vertebral bodies. The osteoarthrotic changes which affect the posterior spinal articulations may also be a consequence of disc degeneration, which alters the anatomical relationship of the articular facets. Both conditions are commonest in those whose occupation throws a heavy strain on the spine, e.g. miners working at the coal face. Radiological changes are frequently present before symptoms appear. Pain may arise from abnormal stresses and strains falling on the spinal ligaments and posterior articulations. It may also arise from pressure on nerve roots caused by narrowing of the vertebral foraminae or protrusion of the intervertebral disc. It is probable that many cases of brachial neuralgia and sciatica (pp. 409, 408) and a proportion of cases of acute lumbago are caused by lesions of the intervertebral discs.

In the majority of cases of backache due to the changes described, pain is intermittent in character, but attacks tend to increase in frequency as age advances.

In milder cases, the application of hot packs over the affected area will give relief. At this stage the various forms of baths already described are valuable. In more severe cases, where pressure on the nerve roots is causing pain, the patient should be put to bed and the spine kept flat by the insertion of fracture boards under the mattress. Where arthrosis of the cervical spine is giving rise to brachial neuralgia, relief may be obtained by applying weight extension. The weights are attached to a cord running from a head sling through a pulley at the top of the bed. Ten to fifteen pounds weight is usually sufficient. Complete immobilization of the cervical spine in a plaster cast for several weeks may be the only form of treatment which gives relief in more intractable cases. The fitting of a spinal support may be of value in the more chronic cases.

In cases of osteoarthrosis of the spine which fail to respond to these measures, it may be necessary for the patient to change to a less strenuous form of employment.

OSTEOPOROSIS

The term osteoporosis implies a reduction in bone mass without change in its chemical composition. Local osteoporosis follows prolonged immobilization after soft tissue injury or fracture. It occurs in the neighbourhood of joints in inflammatory arthritis. Treatment is that of the primary cause. Generalized osteoporosis may complicate a number of metabolic and endocrine disorders, such as Cushing's syndrome, hyperparathyroidism, thyrotoxicosis, acromegaly and diabetes mellitus. It is a well-recognized hazard of the prolonged administration of corticotrophin or corticosteroids. Pri-

mary osteoporosis is common among the elderly—particularly post-menopausal women. It occasionally arises in younger subjects in the absence of any other signs of disease. Bone mass may be reduced by 40 to 50 per cent. before symptoms or signs of the disease become evident. The usual complaint is of pain in the back, radiating round the trunk and down the legs. Compression fractures of vertebral bodies are common and often multiple. Fractures of bones of the lower limbs may follow trivial injuries. Recent investigations have suggested that the main aetiological factor is a prolonged deficiency of calcium resulting from inadequate intake, diminished absorption from the gut or increased excretion in the urine.

Treatment. A high protein diet should be provided, including an extra pint of milk daily, and the prescription of calcium in the form of calcium gluconate (effervescent tablets), 3 to 4 g. three times daily. It now seems doubtful if the use of androgens, oestrogens or anabolic steroids conveys any additional benefit.

In younger patients with osteoporosis absorption of calcium from the gut may be impaired, even in the absence of steatorrhoea. In these cases the combination of vitamin D, 30,000 to 50,000 International Units, by mouth with a high calcium intake may be effective.

It may be possible to delay or avert the development of the disease in older people by ensuring that they continue to eat a well balanced diet, including 1 pint of milk daily. They should be encouraged to lead an active life for as long as possible. Periods of prolonged immobilization on account of intercurrent illnesses or injury must be avoided because the sedentary state promotes the loss of calcium from bone and muscle. Even when symptoms develop, regular daily exercise should be continued to prevent undue deterioration in postural control. A firm corset or light spinal brace may help to relieve backache.

NON-ARTICULAR RHEUMATISM
('FIBROSITIS'—MUSCULAR RHEUMATISM—MYALGIA)

Introduction. No satisfactory classification has ever been devised of the various disorders which give rise to pain and stiffness, but which are not associated with obvious changes in the joints. A number of authorities now hold the view that many painful conditions included in this group are in fact due to primary changes in joints or their immediately related structures, although radiological examination may fail to reveal any deviation from normal. This change in outlook is well illustrated in the case of painful conditions arising in relation to the spine, formerly believed to be due to fibrositis (lumbago, sciatica, cervical fibrositis, brachial neuritis, etc.). The opinion is now widely held that the majority of such complaints are due to degenerative changes in the intervertebral discs, or the posterior spinal articulations (p. 408).

Aetiology. Although the aetiology of non-articular rheumatism is still unsettled, common experience has shown that certain factors are of particular significance.

Cold. Exposure to cold and damp are universally recognized as factors which commonly precipitate an acute attack, especially in those people with a predisposition to the disorder.

Physical fatigue. Fatigued muscles are peculiarly prone to become the seat of an attack. Chronic fatigue brought on by continued over-use of specific muscle groups is more important in this respect than general fatigue following excessive physical exertion.

Trauma. The effects of trauma and fatigue cannot be clearly separated. Fatigued muscles are prone to injury, and the effect of continued use of exhausted muscles may result in rupture of individual fibres.

Posture. Poor posture is associated with muscular imbalance, which results in chronic local fatigue of certain muscle groups. Such local fatigue is accompanied by dull aching pain, often diagnosed as fibrositis.

Infection. Muscular pain and tenderness are prominent features in the acute phase of many general infections. It has been stated that tender areas in the muscles may persist after such infections and form a basis for future attacks of fibrositis. Epidemics of stiff neck have been reported in this country among industrial workers. This form of epidemic myalgia is believed to be due to a virus infection.

A few words must be said at this stage about certain conditions where a diagnosis of fibrositis is only too commonly made and where such a diagnosis may lead to marked prolongation of disability.

Psychoneurosis. Many patients complaining of muscular pain and stiffness have no local organic basis for their symptoms, which are an expression of emotional tension or mental conflict.

Referred pain. Lesions in deep structures can give rise to pain and spasm in anatomically related muscles and in muscles distant from the lesion but with a nerve supply from the same segment of the cord. These symptoms may mask the presence of the primary lesion and lead to an erroneous diagnosis of non-articular rheumatism.

Polymyalgia rheumatica. In this condition there is severe pain and stiffness mainly affecting the muscles of the shoulder, trunk and pelvic girdle. There are signs of systemic disturbance such as mild fever, moderate anaemia and a raised E.S.R. It is not infrequently associated with signs of cranial, giant cell arteritis, commonly involving the temporal arteries, and less frequently the internal and external carotid, ophthalmic and occipital vessels. When signs of arteritis are present, treatment with large doses of prednisolone, 30 to 40 mg. daily, should be instituted at once in view of the dangers of thrombosis. When symptoms are controlled the dose should be reduced very slowly. A maintenance dose (10 to 15 mg.) may be required for as long as two years.

Summary. From what has been said above, the term non-articular rheumatism used in clinical medicine covers a variety of lesions of known and unknown aetiology which give rise to pain, stiffness, aching and limitation of movement.

The diversity of the causes of such symptoms emphasizes the need for a careful history and a complete physical examination in every case. The application of a rigid clinical discipline will reveal causes capable of correction in many cases. In addition it will eliminate cases of functional origin which would otherwise be labelled fibrositis and relegated to the physiotherapy department, a procedure harmful to both the patient and the physician in charge of the case.

Treatment of Acute Stage

If pain and spasm can be relieved, active movements can be started earlier, and disability may be cut short. General and local measures should be combined to achieve this object. Analgesics should be prescribed in full doses (p. 444). Aspirin in doses of 1 g. six-hourly will suffice in most cases. Tension should be removed from the painful structures by arranging the patient in bed in the position of greatest comfort but which permits the application of local remedies. Heat should be applied locally by any of the methods described on p. 466 In many cases these measures will give marked relief within a few hours, and it may become possible to locate the acutely tender areas which are believed to be the trigger points or primary 'myalgic lesions'. These areas should be infiltrated with 2 to 5 ml. of 1 per cent. procaine in normal saline. As soon as the pain has been relieved and spasm relaxed, gentle active movements should be encouraged. A thorough inquiry into possible aetiological factors should be made and commonsense advice given as to how their effects can be mitigated.

Treatment of Subacute and Chronic Stage

A number of patients continue to complain of residual symptoms after the acute attack has subsided. Others never experience an acute attack but suffer from continuous or recurrent pain and stiffness of a less intense degree. Disease of deep structures giving rise to referred pain and tenderness must be excluded by a complete physical examination supplemented by radiological or biochemical investigation when indicated.

Analgesics, heat, massage, local infiltration of painful nodules and exercise are the principal methods of treatment. Accurate localization and infiltration of tender areas is as valuable as in the acute phase, but injections may have to be repeated on several occasions and should be followed immediately by heat, vigorous deep massage and active exercises.

Obesity must be corrected. Otherwise there is no indication for the institution of dietetic measures.

Rehabilitation following a severe attack of non-articular rheumatism should be thorough. Complete restoration of general fitness is required in those patients returning to heavy work. This may best be carried out in a residential or day-to-day rehabilitation centre where graduated physical training and games can be used to restore the capacity for hard physical exertion.

It is now proposed to discuss briefly the treatment in certain sites where diagnosis may be difficult or where special forms of treatment should be employed.

Occipital and cervical regions. Pain in the occipital and cervical regions is frequently referred from the cervical spine, where osteoarthrotic changes and narrowing of the disc spaces are very common (p. 408), but in a proportion of cases examination will reveal the presence of tender points in the region of the occipital ridge. Careful localization and infiltration of these trigger areas, followed by a short course of heat and massage, will usually give complete relief.

Shoulder. If acute traumatic conditions are excluded, the common causes of painful shoulder are: (1) supraspinatus tendinitis; (2) subacromial bursitis; (3) adhesive capsulitis.

Supraspinatus tendinitis. The aetiology of this condition is unknown, but minor repeated traumata probably play an important part. In the early stage of the disease it is possible to move the shoulder passively through a full range of movement, but active abduction causes acute pain, which may disappear when the arm has been abducted beyond a right angle. Treatment consists of the injection of 20 to 30 mg. of hydrocortisone into the area of maximum tenderness, followed by heat and active exercises. In early cases this may lead to complete cure. In long-standing cases there is almost invariably an accompanying subacromial bursitis.

Subacromial bursitis. Radiological examination may show deposits of calcium salts in the tendon and bursa. Abduction and rotation in the shoulder will be limited to a greater or lesser degree. The injection of 50 mg. of hydrocortisone into the bursa followed by heat and graduated exercises may lead to cure, but in a few cases more radical measures are required. Radiotherapy gives relief in some cases. Good results have been obtained by washing out the bursa with saline. In cases which fail to respond to these measures surgical removal of the calcareous deposits may be required. Whichever method proves necessary, function must be restored by graduated exercises.

Adhesive capsulitis. Progressive limitation of movement in the shoulder is a common complication of the above conditions. It may arise independently following trauma. In the elderly it is a common complication of fractures of the arm, forearm or hand, when active movements of the shoulder have been neglected during immobilization of the injured limb in plaster. Movement is best restored by a series of manipulations under general anaesthesia. The condition can best be avoided by early and adequate treatment of painful lesions in and around the shoulder.

Lumbar region. It is now generally accepted that the majority of cases of *acute lumbago* are due to lesions of the intervertebral discs, even though sciatic pain may be absent. Radiological examination is not infrequently negative, and simple treatment in the form of analgesics, local heat and rest in bed on a firm mattress supported by fracture boards is usually effective in controlling the acute attack. This should be followed by exercises for the extensor muscles of the spine, and the patient should receive instruction in those methods of lifting heavy weights which are least likely to cause a recurrence of symptoms. The most important cause of *chronic backache* is degenerative changes in one or more of the intervertebral discs with or without secondary osteoarthrosis in the posterior intervertebral articulations. Rest, including immobilization in plaster when necessary, should form the basis of treatment in these patients in the first instance. Surgery should be reserved for those in whom conservative measures have failed (see below).

In chronic backache every effort should be made to correct bad posture, as this factor alone will tend to perpetuate symptoms. (For suitable exercises see p. 468).

Sciatica. Although sciatica is most commonly due to lesions of the intervertebral discs, it may be a symptom of a number of other conditions. The problem of sciatica and its treatment is dealt with in the section on Neurology (p. 408).

THE ROLE OF SURGERY IN THE CHRONIC RHEUMATIC DISEASES

Experience gained in recent years has clearly shown that surgery has much more to offer than was hitherto believed in the treatment of chronic rheumatic diseases at all stages in their development. This is particularly true in the case of rheumatoid arthritis. The idea that the orthopaedic surgeon should be consulted only in the late stages of the disease when fixed deformities require correction by operation or when unstable and painful joints require to be treated by arthrodesis has been discarded. The main reason for this change of attitude on the part of both physicians and surgeons has been the demonstration of the therapeutic value of early removal of inflamed synovial tissue from both tendon sheaths and joints: pain has been relieved, function improved and the morbid process seems to have been arrested locally for long periods which implies that surgical intervention will be most successful when it is performed before serious damage to articular structures has taken place. This prophylactic rôle requires close collaboration

between rheumatologists and orthopaedic surgeons if the optimum time for surgery is to be chosen.

This approach has been particularly successful in treatment of the hand. Pain and weakness of grip are often due to involvement of the synovial lining of the flexor tendons in the carpal tunnel, palm and fingers. Signs of median nerve compression are not infrequently present. Extensor tendons are similarly involved on the dorsum of the wrist. Results suggest that early synovectomy may prevent invasion of the substance of the tendon and its subsequent rupture. Early synovectomy of the metacarpo-phalangeal joints has been shown to check ulnar drift.

This re-appraisal of the rôle of surgery has led to improved techniques in the treatment of other joints commonly involved, particularly the hips, knees and feet. Similar progress has been achieved in the surgical treatment of osteoarthrosis especially of the hip joint. As yet only a few centres in this country have developed the necessary hospital facilities for detailed pre- and post-operative care of these patients and an expansion in this field will require an increase in the hospital beds available and a larger number of surgeons prepared to devote a substantial portion of their time to these problems.

Recommended Reading

COPEMAN, W. S. C. (1969). *Textbook of the Rheumatic Diseases*, (4th edn.) Edinburgh: Livingstone.
DIXON, A. ST.J. (1965). *Progress in Clinical Rheumatology*. London: Churchill.
HILL, A. G. S. (1966). *Modern Trends in Rheumatology*. London: Butterworth.
HOLLANDER, J. L. (1966). *Arthritis and Allied Conditions*, 7th edn. London: Kimpton.

APPENDIX

The Organization of a Rheumatic Clinic

As has already been emphasized, a prolonged stay in hospital is often essential for the treatment of arthritis, especially of the rheumatoid type. On discharge from hospital the patient has to readjust himself to a mode of existence demanding the resumption of a certain degree of independence and responsibility and too often finds himself unequal to the task. If the best results are to be obtained from institutional treatment, provision must be made for the supervision of such patients on their return to home and occupation. Accordingly, an important function of a hospital or clinic for the treatment of chronic rheumatic disease is the provision of a social service department to undertake the care and supervision of patients after their discharge. This service is particularly required for those patients who, for medical or financial reasons, are unable to report at the clinic at regular intervals for medical and ortho-paedic overhaul. Certain members of the social service department must receive special instruction in the various problems peculiar to the chronic rheumatic diseases. They must visit these patients at regular intervals and report progress to the physician in charge of the case. It is also their duty to improve home conditions where these are unfavourable and to help the patient find employment which will not predispose to exacerbations of the disease.

It has long been recognized that severe mental shock, profound emotional disturbance and long-continued states of worry and anxiety appear to be of aetiological importance in initiating the onset or precipitating a relapse in patients suffering from rheumatoid arthritis. The psychological aspect is also of importance in patients who, after months or even years in bed, have lost the desire to assume once more the responsibility of independent existence. The correction of this mental attitude is essential and requires the most careful consideration of the medical and social service. It is only by close co-operation and prolonged supervision that the full benefit of treatment can be ensured.

Methods of applying Local Heat

Dry heat. Hot-water bottles of the rubber-bag variety can be applied to a painful area or moulded to a joint and are available in the majority of homes. They should be held firmly in place by a bandage or a flannel binder. Electrically heated pads which can be plugged into any electric-light socket can be purchased cheaply. These pads can be kept in position for two to three hours. Radiant heat and infra-red lamps form clean and efficient sources of heat. An electric radiator or gas fire can be used if the patient cannot afford a portable lamp, and are satisfactory. Exposure to radiant heat or infra-red rays should not exceed 15 to 20 minutes at a distance of 2 ft.

Moist heat. A convenient method of applying local moist heat is the use of a kaolin poultice. The material is packed in tins and is heated by placing the tin and contents in a pan of boiling water. When thoroughly hot, the contents are spread on calico or linen and applied to the affected joint or muscle. It should be left in position for two to three hours.

Paraffin-wax baths. One of the best methods of applying local heat is by means of paraffin-wax baths. The wax can be obtained in bulk from oil merchants or from any pharmacist. A double boiler or steamer is used to melt the wax, the melting-point of which is around 38° C. The receptacle should be of sufficient size to permit the immersion of a hand or foot. A large biscuit-tin may serve the purpose. When the limb has been immersed, the patient should be instructed to keep it perfectly still for a few seconds or the sensation of heat may become unbearable. It is withdrawn and

immersed repeatedly, the wax being allowed to solidify on the limb after each immersion, until five or six coats of wax have been applied. The part is then wrapped up in jaconet and cotton-wool for 20 to 30 minutes. At the end of the treatment the wax is easily peeled off. The wax can be used again and again. This method is very valuable in the treatment of hands and feet of those affected by rheumatoid arthritis. When the affected joint cannot be immersed in the wax (knee, shoulder, etc.), several coats of hot wax are applied by means of a large paint brush, jaconet and cotton-wool being used to retain the heat as before.

All the methods outlined can be used in the home and are comparatively cheap. Those described above are efficient and the average patient or his friends can readily be instructed in their effective use.

Manufacture of Plaster Splints

Wrist splint. Soak a plaster of Paris bandage 3 yd. long and 4 in. wide in luke-warm water to which a little salt has been added (one to two teaspoonsful to a basin of water). On a smooth surface (a sheet of thick plate-glass is perhaps the best) make a slab 14 to 16 in. long by rolling the bandage backwards and forwards upon itself. As each successive layer of bandage is added it is rubbed smooth with the palm of the hand in order to get rid of air bubbles. When the slab is complete it is grasped firmly with the finger and thumb about 6 in. from one end and compressed into a bar (Fig. 9), which is then placed between the first finger and thumb of the patient's hand, the shorter end of the slab being on the palmar aspect. This end is moulded across the patient's palm just proximal to the metacarpo-phalangeal joints and round on to the dorsal aspect of the hand and wrist. The other end of the slab is moulded across the dorsum of the hand and up the forearm (Fig. 10). A plaster bandage is now applied to the forearm and wrist, which is held slightly in dorsiflexion and the transverse palmar arch maintained by pressure of the operator's thumb (Fig. 11) until the plaster has firmly set. The plaster on the anterior aspect of the forearm and wrist is now cut away (Fig. 11) and the splint slipped off. The splint is allowed to dry for 12 hours, after which it can be readily slipped on and off and when in use kept in place by a bandage (preferably crêpe) applied to the forearm. In the acute stage its function is to prevent deformity and secure absolute rest to the joint. In the subacute and chronic stages, where flexion deformity of the wrist already exists, a series of these plasters may be used for its correction, according to the technique described for the knee (p. 468).

Hand and wrist splint. Make a short slab of plaster bandage 3 to 4 in. wide and 6 to 8 in. long, consisting of six thicknesses of bandage. It is moulded around the fingers and hand. Make a second slab 10 to 12 in. long and 4 in. wide, consisting of six to eight thicknesses of bandage. Apply it along the forearm, hand and fingers, overlapping the first slab (Fig. 12). The two slabs are now fixed together with a plaster bandage. While the plaster is still soft, ulnar deviation is corrected, the wrist dorsiflexed, and the palmar arch restored. When the plaster is firm, the splint is slipped

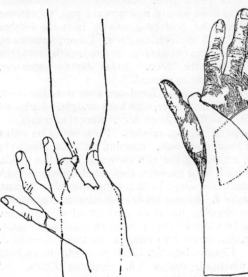

Fig. 9.—Showing how plaster slab is compressed to form a bar by the fore-finger and thumb.

Fig. 10.—Showing the slab moulded into position, short end across the palm and over the dorsum of the hand and up the forearm.

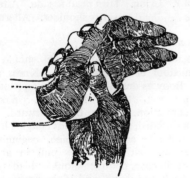

Fig. 11.—Showing how the splint is moulded to hold the wrist in dorsi-flexion. Dotted lines on the anterior aspect of the wrist indicate where plaster is to be cut.

off and trimmed in order to ensure its easy application and removal. When in use it is held in place by a forearm bandage, as shown in Figs. 12 and 13. The splint is used for rest in the acute stage and correction of ulnar deviation and flexion deformity of wrist in the subacute and chronic stages.

Rest splint for use in the acute stage of rheumatoid arthritis. For the manufacture of this type of splint a mould is required, consisting of a length of aluminium 4 in. wide and about 18 in. long. It is bent at one end

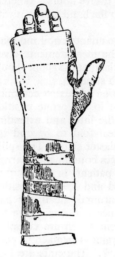
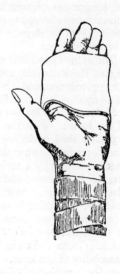

Fig. 12.—Hand and wrist splint—posterior aspect.

Fig. 13.—Hand and wrist splint—anterior aspect.

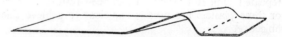

Fig. 14—Aluminium mould used in manufacture of rest splint for hand and wrist.

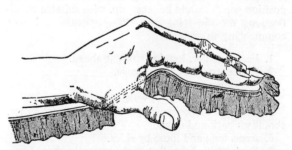

Fig. 15.—The mould (shown by dotted lines) has been covered with stockinet. The hand is resting on the plaster slab. The stockinet is used to mould the slab to the hand and wrist as described.

so as to form an eminence upon which the hand rests (Fig. 14).

The mould is covered with a single layer of stockinet and a plaster slab is made and placed upon the mould. The slab should overlap slightly around the edges of the aluminium. The patient's hand and forearm are then pressed on the slab (Fig. 15) and the stockinet pulled tight over them, the thumb being left free. This has the effect of moulding the plaster firmly to the limb. When the plaster has become set, the splint is removed and trimmed and allowed to dry for twelve hours. When in use it is kept bandaged firmly to the hand and arm with a crêpe bandage.

The splints described must be adapted and modified to suit the individual case. The measurements given are approximate, and it is essential that the splint should be as light as is compatible with strength.

Serial plasters for the correction of flexion deformity of the knees. With the patient in the prone position a plaster shell encircling half the limb and extending from one inch below the gluteal fold to beyond the toes is built up by a series of plaster slabs. The splint is removed, trimmed and the edges bound with a narrow plaster bandage. With the patient in the supine position, the splint is reapplied and fixed in position with three plaster cuffs, one around the upper part of the thigh, one below the knee and one above the ankle. These cuffs are sufficient to ensure complete immobility of the knee. The splint is retained in position for a minimum of one week. The cuffs are then readily removed with a knife or plaster shears without discomfort to the patient. As a rule a useful gain in extension will be possible and a second plaster is applied in the improved position. The procedure is repeated until full extension has been restored. Two or three plasters are usually sufficient to achieve this objective.

Postural, Breathing and Re-educational Exercises

For the useful execution of any exercise, correct posture is imperative. The following is the correct standing position which should be taken up, with suitable modifications for the lying and sitting positions, before commencing an exercise:

1. Feet together, looking straight ahead.
2. Knees straight but not tense.
3. Abdomen in, seat down.
4. Rib cage lifted out of waist-line.
5. Shoulder blades pulled gently towards each other, shoulders back and down.
6. Arms long and loose by sides.
7. Neck and head pulled back, ears over shoulders.
8. Body weight slightly forward over toes and outer borders of feet.

The body should feel relaxed. To relax does not mean to collapse, but to maintain an effortless balance without strain.

The correct postural position must be checked, and readjusted if necessary, after the performance of each exercise, whether in lying, sitting or standing.

EXERCISES IN LYING

Lying position: On firm support, head, pelvis and feet in line, back flat, hands by sides, feet dorsiflexed.

ABDOMINAL AND BREATHING EXERCISES. *Exercise 1.* Lying with knees bent. Contract lower abdominal muscles with an inward and upward pull, tighten the buttock muscles, and progressively raise the lumbar then the dorsal spine off the floor. Lower, vertebra by vertebra from the dorsal spine downwards flattening the back against the floor. Relax before repeating. Breathing should be normal.

Exercise 2. Lying. Bend one knee over the chest, straighten leg and lower, with knee straight. Back, and other leg, should be flat on floor. Repeat alternate.

Exercise 3. Lying, relaxed. Place hands on either side of lower chest wall. Keeping back flat, breathe in slowly, expanding the ribs outwards into the hands. Hold breath for a moment, then exhale slowly through the mouth, allowing ribs to collapse inwards. Repeat.

Exercise 4. Repeat above, but reinforce the expiration by drawing the abdominal muscles in and up. Relax all muscles and tension before breathing in again.

ARM, SHOULDER AND NECK EXERCISES. *Exercise 5.* Lying. Lightly clasp the hands in front. Raise both arms overhead, stretch tall. Separate hands, and pulling shoulder blades firmly together, lower arms sideways against the floor, completing a circle. Repeat.

Exercise 6. Lying. Raise arms sideways to shoulder level, palms upward. Press arms and head firmly against floor, chin in, and raise upper back off floor. Relax and lower arms to sides. Repeat.

Exercise 7. Lying. Turn head to side. Alternate.

Exercise 8. Bend towards shoulder. Alternate.

EXERCISES IN SITTING

Sitting posture: Thighs and buttocks should be supported on stool of correct height. Knees and feet together. Body as described for standing posture.

SHOULDER AND TRUNK EXERCISES. *Exercise 9.* Postural correction. Relax body forward, chin on chest, back rounded, arms and hands hanging heavy and loose. Gradually straighten spine, beginning from lumbar region. At same time pull in abdominal muscles, lift rib cage, contract shoulder blades and pull shoulders back and down, and lastly stretch neck and head. The feeling of relaxation should still be present with the arms long and loose. Repeat between exercises.

Exercise 10. Repeat exercise 5 in the sitting position.

Exercise 11. Swing arms loosely forwards and upwards, then back. Repeat.

Exercise 12. Clap hands sideways overhead, and drop to sides again. Repeat.

Exercise 13. Using ball or other object, pass this from the right hand behind the neck to the left hand, and then behind back to the right hand. Repeat and alternate.

Exercise 14. Sitting, feet and knees apart, hands on hips. Bend upper part of trunk to side; alternate.

Exercise 15. Position as above. Turn trunk to side; alternate.

EXERCISES IN STANDING

Exercise 16. Postural correction. Stand against wall, head, shoulders and hips against wall, chin and abdomen in. Stretch tall without strain. Walk forward retaining correct posture. Repeat.

Exercise 17. Following above exercise, walk along a straight line keeping feet straight, and using heel-to-toe leverage.

Exercise 18. Standing, feet straight and 4 to 6 in. apart, hands on hips. Repeat exercises 14 and 15. Avoid sway of pelvis or ankles.

Exercise 19. Standing. Inhale, raising arms sideways and upwards, rise on toes and stretch tall. As heels sink, lower arms to sides and exhale, drawing abdomen in.

FOOT EXERCISES

Exercises to correct faulty body mechanics should always include training in the proper use of the feet. It should be remembered that when a muscle is used in the right way it becomes stronger, and therefore before any foot exercises are given the patient should be shown how to use the feet properly. The correct standing position must begin with the position of the feet in weight-bearing. The feet should be comfortably straight ahead with the weight on the outer border, toes on the ground. Use of the feet in this position means correct use of all the foot muscles.

Exercise 1. Sitting, cross knees. Make half circle with foot, down, in and up. The inward, upward pull is the important result.

Exercise 2. Same position, turn foot in slightly. Pull foot up and push down, using ankle joint.

Exercise 3. Same position. Turn foot in, curl toes under hand. Pull foot up when toes are curled.

Exercise 4. Standing, weight well forward, body in good line, hands on hips. Lift inner borders of feet, relax half-way and repeat. Toes cling to floor.

Exercise 5. Same position. Lift inner borders of feet, rock from heel to toe. Do not let inner borders of feet down.

Exercise 6. Heel-and-toe walk on line. Described in previous list.

Exercise 7. Sitting. Pick up marbles with toes, turn foot up, and transfer marbles to your hand.

Exercise 8. Sitting. Place bath towel, folded full length, on floor; using toes and outer border of foot, draw whole length of the towel towards you. Do not let heel move out of position or rest on towel.

HAND EXERCISES (*Active*)

STARTING POSITION. Sitting at a table with the forearm at a right angle and supinated to mid-position.

EXERCISES TO ENABLE PATIENT TO FLEX FINGERS. 1. Flexion of each joint of the fingers separately into the palm of the hand, assisted by other hand or operator.

2. Place a small rubber ball into the palm and tell patient to alternately 'squeeze and release'. This may be made more difficult by using a soft piece of sponge.

EXERCISES TO OVERCOME FLEXION DEFORMITY. 1. Placing the hand as flat as possible on the table and with the forearm fixed stretch the fingers forward as far as possible.

2. Stretching fingers and lifting each up off the table separately.

EXERCISES TO OBTAIN EXTENSION OF WRIST. 1*. Forearm supinated, hand over edge of table, wrist extension.

Same exercise may be performed with gravity eliminated, i.e. with forearm in mid-position; or gravity resisting, i.e. forearm pronated.

2. Place forearm on table, palm downwards; raise forearm up, keeping hand fixed.

3. Wringing a duster.

4. Climbing up the wall bars.

EXERCISES TO OBTAIN FLEXION OF WRIST. Same as 1*, except the arm is pronated in the first part of exercise and the wrist is moved to the flexed position.

OTHER EXERCISES

1. Stretching the fingers upon the table, separate them as far as possible. If adduction is limited, adduct each finger separately to the middle line of the hand.

2. Forearm supinated, flex the thumb into the palm of the hand.

3. In same position oppose thumb to little finger.

4. With wrists extended and resting on edge of table, perform movements with fingers as if playing piano, taking care not to produce ulnar deviation.

5. Picking up objects (large ones to commence with) such as a reel of cotton with the thumb and each finger separately. This may be progressed by picking up large pins, needles and small pins.

6. Writing with pencil.

19. Some Common Disorders in Infancy and Early Childhood

J. H. HUTCHISON

INTRODUCTION

In no field of medical practice have the therapeutic advances of the past 25 years made a greater impact than in paediatrics. This is reflected in the large fall in the infant mortality rate in Britain during those years. It is also shown in the fact that during childhood (after the first year of life) the most common causes of death are now accidental violence (including poisoning) and malignant disease. In particular, the severe bacterial infections, including tuberculosis, no longer head the list of the common causes of death. On the other hand, the many potent drugs have greatly increased the responsibility of the physician, because all pharmacologically effective preparations may be toxic to some individuals. This is more likely if their use is injudicious or haphazard.

That diagnosis must precede treatment is a platitude. Yet, this basic rule of therapeutics is, perhaps, more often broken in the case of young children than other age-groups, particularly in the prescribing of antibacterial drugs—for example, their use in the case of an ill, fevered child in whom a pyogenic meningitis has not yet been clearly diagnosed. When so used (sometimes in inadequate dosage) they may save the child's life but at the expense of permanent hydrocephalus, spastic palsy or mental retardation. It is certain also that some cases of chronic pyelonephritis and renal failure in adult life have resulted from inadequate drug treatment of acute pyelonephritis during infancy or childhood when fever and toxaemia may be marked but urinary symptoms absent. The prescription of sulphonamides and antibiotics is also very common in upper respiratory infections of childhood although most of these are due to viruses which are not susceptible to this form of treatment. It is, moreover, important to remember that during the neonatal period (first 28 days of life) some drugs of proven value can have serious toxic effects which are not encountered in older patients. It is, therefore, incumbent on the physician to use these powerful therapeutic weapons accurately, and only when there are clear indications for them.

Drugs. In children and infants drugs are best administered in liquid form or as powders suspended in honey, rose-hip syrup or jam. Under the age of 5 years, tablets, pills and capsules are potentially dangerous because they may be inhaled. There have also been many tragic episodes because children have mistaken coloured tablets for sweets. Indeed, the incidence of children admitted to British hospitals with drug poisoning has risen considerably since the advent of the National Health Service.

A suitable method of giving an unpalatable medicine to an infant is to wrap him firmly in a blanket and to place him in a semi-erect position. The mouth is opened by pressure on the cheeks with the thumb and forefinger of the left hand, and the medicine is poured from a teaspoon or medicine dropper on to the back of his tongue with the right hand. So long as the mouth is held open he must then swallow before he can take his next breath.

Various formulae have been devised to estimate the doses of drugs for infants and children. Some are based on age, some on weight, and others on surface area. A full-term infant weighing 7 lb. (3·2 kg.) requires 12·5 per cent. of the average adult dose; a 12-month-old infant weighing 22 lb. (10 kg.) requires 25 per cent.; a 7-year-old child weighing 50 lb. (23 kg.) requires 50 per cent.; and a 12-year-old child weighing 88 lb. (40 kg.) requires 75 per cent. of the average adult dose. This method is less open to objection than the others, all of which are valueless in practice. None the less, the percentage method must not be used for premature infants or those of low birth weight in whom immature hepatic and renal function make special consideration necessary in the case of certain drugs, e.g. sulphafurazole, chloramphenicol, streptomycin, novobiocin, kanamycin and vitamin K analogue (menaphthone). Even in older children the percentage method can lead to the prescribing of suboptimal doses of some drugs such as prednisone, thyroxine and ferrous salts. In the author's opinion the only really satisfactory solution is for the physician to familiarize himself with the individual dosage of the commonly used drugs and to consult the relevant literature when he is in any doubt.

The particular vulnerability of the foetus and newborn infant to certain drugs has become increasingly obvious within recent years. The most dramatic example was the somewhat delayed discovery that an apparently safe sedative, thalidomide, when taken during pregnancy could result in gross foetal abnormalities such as phocomelia, haemangioma, microtia, atresia of the gut, and congenital heart disease. This drug has, of course, been withdrawn from the market, but other commonly used drugs may have severe toxic effects in the newborn. Thus, the risk of kernicterus (cerebral nuclear jaundice) developing in premature infants is greatly increased by vitamin K analogue (menaphthone), salicylates, sulphafurazole and novobiocin. The liability of chloramphenicol to cause blood dyscrasia in the adult is well recognized. It is less well known that when it is given to the newborn in the dosage customarily employed in older infants (100 mg. per kg. per day) death may result. The infant suddenly becomes ashen-grey and flaccid with abdominal distension, diarrhoea and cardiovascular collapse—'the grey baby syndrome'. This disastrous effect is due to the fact that chloramphenicol has to be excreted by the liver after conjugation with glucuronic acid. In the newborn infant the enzyme system responsible for this reaction is immature and highly toxic blood levels of the drug may develop. Even the tetracyclines, commonly regarded as one of the safest groups of antibiotics, carry unexpected effects in the perinatal period. When given to the newborn infant or to an expectant mother during the last six months of pregnancy the drug may be deposited in the tooth buds and bones. This is because the tetracyclines act as chelating agents which bind bivalent metal ions. When calcium is so bound in the body fluids the complex may be deposited in the teeth and bones which are growing rapidly in the foetus and newborn. High concentrations of the calcium-antibiotic complex can retard the growth of these structures; lower concentrations lead to yellow discolouration alone. However, after the teeth erupt and are exposed to the light the yellow colour darkens to brown. Teeth so discoloured also fluoresce in ultraviolet light. It appears that oxytetracycline is the least likely to produce these effects. The fact that high concentrations of oxygen (above 40 per cent.), when given over long periods, can produce retrolental fibroplasia and blindness in premature infants is well known.

It has become very clear that drugs of any sort should only be prescribed for pregnant women and young infants when there are imperative indications. The wise physician will, moreover, keep accurate records of all drugs and doses administered.

Fluid intake. The fluid balance of the young infant and toddler is much more precarious than in the older patient. When he is ill and fevered he is prone to develop dehydration due to a combination of diminished intake, excess loss of water from sweating, and increased insensible loss of water from the lungs if there is tachypnoea. Unlike the adult he cannot ask for fluids. Indeed, in the very young infant diminished fluid intake due to reluctance to feed, combined with vomiting and fever, can result in hypertonic dehydration with greatly raised levels of serum sodium and chloride. This can be caused by many infections, and the hypernatraemia in particular can lead to convulsions and permanent damage to the brain. The doctor should advise the early admission to hospital for intravenous fluid therapy of any infant whose fluid intake is greatly reduced as a consequence of anorexia or persistent vomiting. On the other hand, when the loss of body water is associated with a severe loss of electrolytes (sodium, potassium, chloride) as in diarrhoea, pyloric stenosis, intestinal obstruction or adrenal failure, a different type—the hypotonic type—of dehydration results, in which the osmotic pressure of the plasma can only be maintained by a considerable diminution in plasma volume. This oligaemia results in peripheral circulatory failure and pre-renal uraemia. While hypertonic dehydration requires dilute solutions such as one-quarter or one-fifth strength physiological saline, the treatment of hypotonic dehydration demands larger concentrations of electrolytes, and sometimes intravenous plasma. Mild degrees of dehydration in the young infant can be treated at home with oral half-strength saline, but more severe cases demand parenteral fluid therapy under laboratory control. *The vulnerability of the infant, especially during the first 12 weeks of life, to severe disturbances of body water and electrolytes cannot be overstressed. Unless an adequate fluid intake can be assured the infant should be referred to a paediatric unit early in his illness.* The older child is only rarely in danger of severe dehydration. During most acute illnesses it is sufficient to ensure that water in the form of sweet drinks, rich in glucose, are offered to him at frequent intervals during the day.

Diet. The safest food for the young infant is human milk but, unfortunately, few infants are breastfed for long in the Great Britain of today.

Q

Liquid cow's milk is too readily infected to be regarded as a safe substitute. The best form of food for young infants whose mothers do not breast-feed them is one of the dried or evaporated milks. The former is probably safer in the average household which does not possess a refrigerator. There is no advantage in one proprietary brand over another and the wise mother will choose the cheapest. During illness outside the gastro-intestinal tract there is rarely any need to change an infant's feeding formula, although extra fluid in the form of glucose in quarter strength physiological saline should be offered between feeds.

In the case of the older child suffering from acute illness the important consideration is a good intake of fluids and glucose. It matters little if he eats only small quantities of easily digestible but palatable food for some days. In chronic illness a high intake of protein is important and this can be remarkably encouraged by serving suitable foods in attractive forms.

Neonatal Conditions

Low birth weight. About 70 per cent. of newborn infants whose birth weights are 2·5 kg. or less are prematurely born. It is now recognized, however, that in the remaining 30 per cent., the low birth weight is related to intrauterine malnutrition. These infants, who are usually born *after* the 36th week of gestation, are usually referred to as 'dysmature' or 'light-for-dates'. The distinction between prematurity and dysmaturity is important because the complications which may arise are different and require different management.

Prematurity. A premature infant (low birth weight, short gestation) suffers from many disadvantages in comparison to the full-term baby. These include vulnerability to birth injury, hypoxia, unstable temperature control, inadequate respiratory function, immature sucking, swallowing and cough reflexes and extreme susceptibility to infection. This is reflected in the fact that in Britain today about 70 per cent. of all neonatal deaths occur in premature infants. In about one-half of all cases of prematurity the immediate cause of premature birth is to be found in maternal factors such as toxaemia, antepartum haemorrhage, diabetes mellitus, chronic renal disease and heart disease. In the remaining cases there is no obvious cause, but it is significant that the incidence of premature birth is considerably higher among the lower social grades of the community who too often fail to avail themselves of the regular antenatal care which is freely available in this country.

The problems which face the physician during and after the birth of a premature baby at home can be so difficult that he should ensure, whenever it is foreseeable, that a premature delivery is conducted in hospital where full facilities are available for both mother and infant. However, when a premature infant is born in a private house the first decision must be whether to keep him there or arrange his transfer to hospital. A delayed transfer usually indicates a mistaken initial assessment and too often involves a hypothermic and gravely ill infant. The decision will obviously depend upon a variety of factors such as the presence of a good home with satisfactory heating arrangements, on reasonable domestic and nursing assistance and particularly upon the state of the infant. Strong indications for immediate transfer of the baby to hospital are a birth weight below 1·8 kg., a rectal temperature which remains below 35° C. for longer than six hours after birth, respiratory difficulty of any degree and signs of cerebral involvement such as failure to suck after 24 hours, shrill crying, apnoeic attacks with cyanosis or convulsive twitching. When a premature infant is to be transferred to the neonatal paediatric unit of a hospital it is imperative to avoid dangerous chilling before and during the journey (p. 473). The baby should be transported in a specially heated 'carry-cot' or, preferably, in a portable incubator which can be operated by a 12-volt battery (Vickers, Ltd.). In some areas the hospital neonatal unit on the request of the family physician will send out such an incubator equipped with an oxygen supply under the supervision of a trained nurse to collect a premature or ill baby.

Whether the premature infant is to be cared for in hospital or at home, the objects to be achieved are the same: (1) the maintenance of body temperature which must never fall below 36° C. per rectum; (2) a food intake which will ensure rapid growth without causing vomiting or abdominal distension; (3) the prevention of infection; (4) protection from later iron and vitamin deficiencies. The hospital has, of course, many advantages and especially the skilled nurses who can supervise incubator care when this is required, who can tube-feed the most immature infants through in-dwelling nasal polyvinyl tubes and who can report to the medical attendants any sudden changes in the infant's respiration, colour or movements. The smallest premature infants are liable to develop dangerously high levels of serum bilirubin due to hepatic immaturity. In hospital it is possible to make frequent estimations in visibly jaundiced babies so that replacement transfusion can be undertaken if the level rises above 24 mg. per 100 ml. to obviate the risk of kernicterus.

The maintenance of body temperature in the home requires that the room temperature must never fall below 18° C. and is preferably at 21° C. In winter this can only be ensured with gas or electric fires in the absence of central heating. The coal fire is too apt to permit a dangerous fall in room temperature during the night. The cot temperature should be 32° C. This can be obtained with hot-water bottles, but the strictest precautions must be taken to avoid burning the infant by covering the bottles and separating them from him with several layers of blankets. Alternatively the bottles may be placed in pockets in the lining of the cot. A small electric blanket may also be used, but this should be placed over, never under, the infant. A bowl of water in front of the fire or a moist blanket over a central-heating radiator will ensure reasonable humidity. Although it is now customary to nurse premature infants unclothed in thermostatically controlled hospital nurseries, in the home loose, non-restrictive and heat-retaining clothing is essential. Bathing is a dangerous source of chilling and should be foregone in the case of the premature baby until he is old enough to maintain his own body temperature. A suitable method of cleaning the very soiled infant after the first day or two have elapsed is to lather him, area by area without full exposure, with hexachlorophene skin cleanser.

In hospital the maintenance of body temperature of a feeble premature baby will be ensured in an incubator where he can be placed in an ambient temperature of 32° to 35° C., and a humidity of at least 80 per cent. Oxygen should be given only if there is respiratory distress. It is a general rule in special care units for the newborn that the oxygen concentration in incubators must not be permitted to rise above 35 per cent. save on the precise instructions of the paediatrician, to minimise the risk of producing retrolental fibroplasia.

Feeding is frequently a difficult problem in premature infants, who require a high protein intake (over 5 g. per kg.) and extra carbohydrate as cane-sugar or lactose. On the other hand, they tolerate fat poorly. When the infant is vigorous and can suck well he should be put to the breast after 12 to 24 hours. His ability to suck should first have been tested with a glucose-water feed. Indeed, it is a good plan to start by aspirating the gastric contents of every premature infant using a sterile soft rubber catheter (English No. 8) and a 20-ml. syringe. This rids the stomach of fluids swallowed by the infant in the birth canal and confirms that there is no oesophageal atresia. The small feeble infant will be unable to obtain milk direct from his mother. Until recently the accepted practice in most neonatal units was to leave such babies unfed for 36 to 48 hours to minimize the risk of aspiration of gastric contents into the lungs. Many now doubt the wisdom of this practice and it has been suggested that it increases the incidence of the respiratory distress syndrome and of hyperbilirubinaemia. It is probably wise to start feeds not later than 24 hours after birth. If milk from a breast milk bank is available, this can be obtained and given to the infant from an ordinary small feeding bottle using a soft teat with a fairly large hole. The infant can be assisted in sucking by applying gentle rhythmic upward pressure on his chin with a forefinger. He should be propped up with head raised during, and for 15 minutes after, each feed to lessen the risk of regurgitation and aspiration of gastric contents into the trachea. Failing breast milk, one of the modified dried milks may be used. A suitable formula for a half-cream dried milk is three measures of milk powder made up to 3 fluid ounces with boiled water plus one rounded-off teaspoonful of sugar (21 Cal. per fl. oz.). To begin with, small volumes of this formula are given frequently. Most premature infants can tolerate 8 ml. every three hours at the start of feeding. The feeds are increased as rapidly as possible short of causing digestive upset. By the age of three weeks a daily fluid intake of 180 ml. per kg. is satisfactory. The premature infant requires at least 120 Cal. per kg. per day for satisfactory growth. When a premature infant is so small and feeble as to be unable to suck he is best fed through an indwelling polyvinyl catheter. This is passed into the stomach through the nose and can safely be left in situ for five days. The feeds are then administered accurately by syringe. It is rarely wise to keep such a feeble infant at home. Feeding by means of pipette, Belcroy apparatus or spoon all carry great risk of aspiration pneumonia and should at all costs be avoided.

The prevention of infection is a problem in the home and in hospital. Attendants must always wash their hands before and after handling the infant. All utensils, bottles and teats used for feeding must be thoroughly cleaned, first in cold and then in hot water, using a bottle brush. They should then be sterilized either by boiling for 10 minutes or by immersing them for at least four hours in 1 : 80 solution of sodium hypochlorite. Visitors should be restricted to the minimum, preferably only the father, and no person with any infection, however trivial, should be permitted to enter the infant's room.

In the premature infant the intake of vitamin D should not be less than 800 International Units daily. This can be supplied from the third week as one of the proprietary concentrates of vitamins A and D. The drops should be given to the infant by spoon which is wiped on his tongue. They should not be put into the feeds because they tend to get left behind in the teat. Iron should be given from the sixth week of life. A suitable prescription in which the oxidation of ferrous sulphate to the nonabsorbed ferric sulphate is largely prevented is:

Ferrous sulphate . . .	30 mg.
Dilute hypophosphorous acid	0·03 ml.
Dextrose	1 g.
Chloroform water to . .	5 ml.

Label: 5 ml. thrice daily.

This should be continued throughout the first year. Alternatively, one of the proprietary forms of ferrous succinate or iron chelate may be used. From the age of 4 months a mixed diet of iron-containing foods such as oatflour porridge, pre-cooked infant cereals, vegetables and egg yolk should be introduced. Vitamin C should also be given from the age of 1 month in the form of 5 ml. daily of rose hip syrup or concentrated orange juice diluted with water and sweetened. This is unnecessary, however, if one of the proprietary infant milks already fortified with ascorbic acid is being fed.

Complications of prematurity. Between the years 1947 and 1951 many premature infants who survived in Great Britain as a result of modern incubator care were found subsequently to be blind as the result of retrolental fibroplasia. Once it has developed, this disease is irreversible, but it can be prevented by ensuring that the oxygen concentration in incubators is not allowed to rise above 35 per cent. This rule must occasionally be broken in severe cases of respiratory distress, but this should

only be done under the guidance of an experienced paediatrician.

Kernicterus may develop when the serum bilirubin level rises above 24 mg. per 100 ml. The only effective treatment for hyperbilirubinaemia once it develops is replacement transfusion, often a difficult and dangerous procedure in the small premature infant. Drugs known to increase the risk of kernicterus in the newborn (p. 471) should not be prescribed. The value of intramuscular phenobarbitone as an 'enzyme inducer', and of exposure of the infant to blue light in reducing bilirubin levels has yet to be reliably assessed.

Hyaline membrane disease or the respiratory distress syndrome is the most common cause of death in premature infants. Treatment includes incubator care. A high concentration of oxygen may be required to abolish cyanosis. This must be regularly controlled with an electromagnetic oximeter, and the concentration of oxygen in the incubator reduced as rapidly as practicable. It is increasingly the practice to catheterize an umbilical artery and also to monitor the infant's arterial PO_2 at regular intervals. The level should not be allowed to rise above 150 mm. Hg. but, if possible, raised above 70 mm. Hg. The humidity in the incubator should not fall below 80 per cent. A broad spectrum antibiotic should be given intramuscularly to combat secondary infection of the atelectatic lungs. This routine care does not prevent a high mortality rate. Recently in Glasgow a greatly reduced mortality rate has followed the use of intravenous injections of 8·4 per cent. sodium bicarbonate solution (1 ml. = 1 mEq.) and of 20 per cent. fructose. The object of this treatment is to correct the severe acidosis which affected infants show, and it can only be carried out with safety under frequent biochemical control which involves estimations of the blood pH, PCO_2, plasma standard bicarbonate, and base excess on arterialized capillary blood by means of the Astrup microapparatus. In the most severely affected infants with falling PO_2 and rising PCO_2 levels, and having apnoeic attacks, assisted ventilation by intermittent positive or negative pressure respirators may be employed. Unfortunately, this demanding type of therapy has had only a marginal influence on the mortality rate.

Some premature babies develop the early anaemia of prematurity. This is to be distinguished from the later iron-deficiency anaemia (see above) and it cannot be prevented with iron. If the haemoglobin level falls below 7·5 g. per 100 ml. a blood transfusion of 30 ml. per kg. should be given into a scalp vein.

Intraventricular haemorrhage is an invariably fatal complication seen only in the premature. It is frequently difficult to diagnose with assurance during life but there is no effective treatment.

Dysmaturity. The dysmature infant (low birth weight, gestation usually over 36 weeks) is long, thin and scraggy with dry cracked skin and, frequently, meconium staining of the nails and umbilical cord. His appearance contrasts with the shiny oedematous look of the true premature baby. So does his eagerness to suck and he should be fed not later than eight hours after birth in order to replenish his poor glycogen stores. Although the dysmature infant is unduly light for the length of gestation there is as yet no generally agreed definition of dysmaturity or 'light for dates'.

The most common complication of dysmaturity is 'idiopathic symptomatic hypoglycaemia' which may develop from six hours to a few days after birth with 'jitteriness', apnoeic spells, lethargy or generalized twitching. Untreated it results in permanent brain damage. It has become the practice of the author to monitor the blood glucose levels of all dysmature infants every six hours with Dextrostix strips (Ames & Co.). If the Dextrostix fails to record a colour change (lowest reading 45 mg. per 100 ml.) the blood glucose level must be estimated in the laboratory. A value below 20 mg. per 100 ml. in the newborn demands immediate treatment as follows. An intravenous injection of 50 per cent. dextrose in water, 2 ml. per kg., by scalp vein. Thereafter, a continuous intravenous infusion of 10 per cent. dextrose in water (after 24 hours in quarter-strength saline) is given at a rate of 60 to 75 ml. per kg. per 24 hours. It is possible with this routine to prevent the development of hypoglycaemic manifestations and, it is believed, to prevent brain damage.

Neonatal infections. Although the death rate from neonatal sepsis has fallen markedly in recent years the best hospitals still make elaborate arrangements to reduce the risks of infection. These include the use of cubicles, a strict discipline involving good hand-washing techniques, masks and sterile clothing, and frequent bacteriological studies of the routes whereby infection may spread.

The biggest problem is presented by the *Staphylococcus aureus* which, as it occurs in maternity hospitals, is almost always penicillin-resistant and increasingly frequently resistant also to streptomycin and the tetracyclines, but still sensitive to methicillin and cloxacillin. Fortunately, the widespread use of hexachlorophane and the strict anti-infection disciplines now used in our maternity hospitals have greatly reduced the incidence of staphylococcal sepsis. Most infections are relatively minor in nature such as septic spots, conjunctivitis and umbilical sepsis. Systemic antibiotics should not then be used with the attendant possibility of further increasing the antibiotic-resistant staphylococcal population. In septic conditions of the skin good results are obtainable by topical application of antibiotics which are too toxic for systemic use, such as 1 per cent. neomycin or bacitracin ointments and powders. In 'sticky eye' 0·5 per cent. neomycin or bacitracin ointment can be applied to the palpebral conjunctiva several times each day. Subcutaneous abscesses are incised and drained. Any infant with even minor sepsis must, of course, be removed immediately from the neonatal to an isolation unit. Outbreaks of severe staphylococcal sepsis due to certain notorious phage types such as 80/81, and which cause deaths from pneumonia, septicaemia, or acute osteitis, have almost disappeared in recent years. When such infections are known to be staphylococcal in origin they are best treated with intramuscular cloxacillin (50 mg. per kg. per day) given in four divided doses. On the other hand, when the severity of an infection in the newborn infant demands treatment before the results of bacteriological investigations are known it is wise to cover a wider range of bacteria with a combination of cloxacillin and ampicillin, each given intramuscularly in a dosage of 50 mg. per kg. per day. Erythromycin (25 to 50 mg. per kg. per day) is also useful although more likely to lead to the emergence of resistant staphylococci. Cephaloridine, 20-40 mg. per kg. per day, may be valuable as it is effective against both gram-positive and gram-negative bacteria. It should be a rule that antibiotics are only prescribed after the relevant laboratory investigations have been arranged. These may include urine analysis and culture, blood culture, and culture of the cerebrospinal fluid.

The marked reduction of staphylococcal infections in the newborn seems to have been accompanied by an increase, of modest dimensions, in the incidence of infections by gram-negative bacteria such as *E. coli, Proteus* and *Pseudomonas aeruginosa*.

Most common is *E. coli* which frequently causes pyogenic meningitis or acute pyelonephritis. In neither case is diagnosis easy. The prognosis of coliform meningitis is grave. Treatment is best given as a combination of chloramphenicol (25 mg. per kg. per day) and sulphadiazine 125 mg. every four hours. Both drugs may have to be given intramuscularly initially. Colistin, given intramuscularly, may also be added in a dose of 150,000 units per kg. daily. The author has found that a reduced incidence of permanent sequelae such as hydrocephalus can be achieved by adding prednisolone to the treatment, 5 mg. four times daily for seven days, 5 mg. twice daily for seven days, and 2·5 mg. twice daily for seven days. In acute pyelonephritis, sulphadimidine, 125 mg. every six hours, is often effective. When urine culture reveals the *E. coli* to be sulphonamide-resistant a change can be made to ampicillin (50 mg. per kg. per day), or to kanamycin (15 mg. per kg. per day) given intramuscularly. Epidemic diarrhoea of the newborn is due to various specific types of enteropathogenic *E. coli*. It seems to have become rare in recent years. Treatment is along the same lines as that recommended for gastroenteritis in older infants (p. 485).

Cold injury of the newborn. Every winter in Great Britain a considerable number of newborn infants die from the effects of cold. This condition is entirely preventable. Premature and ill infants are at special risk. Sometimes the chilling takes place during the first bath after birth in a cold room. More often the infant becomes hypothermic later because the room temperature is allowed to fall below 18° C., especially during the night. Cold injury is by no means confined to poorer homes and the danger is insufficiently recognized by both physicians and midwives. The rectal temperature of the newborn must never be allowed to fall below 35° C. In the day-to-day care of the newborn the ordinary clinical thermometer with its lowest reading at 35° C. is valueless. All family physicians and midwives should equip themselves with low reading thermometers (29·5° to 43° C.). Only the rectal temperature is reliable in the newborn.

The first essential in the prevention of cold injury is a room temperature of at least 18° C. If this is impracticable the mother should be confined in hospital. The ritual of the daily bath is unnecessary, and it can be very dangerous in a cold room. If a newborn infant has to be transferred to hospital he should travel in a portable incubator or specially warmed cot. Once cold injury has developed a mortality rate of 25 per cent. can be expected. Rapid re-warming is dangerous because the increased metabolic activity of the warmed superficial tissues cannot be sustained by the still hypothermic viscera. The infant's rectal temperature should be slowly raised to 36° C. over a period of 36 to 48 hours. This can best be done in an incubator which is initially set at a temperature approximating to that of the patient. Feeds should be withheld until the infant is normothermic and able to suck. If the blood glucose falls below 20 mg. per 100 ml., a continuous infusion of 10 per cent. dextrose in water should be set up, 60 to 75 ml. per kg. per day. In the meantime, he should be protected against bacterial infection, to which the devitalized tissues are very prone, by a broad spectrum antibiotic given intramuscularly.

Birth injuries. Birth injuries are less common in modern obstetric practice than formerly but anoxic damage is still a major problem. The less severe injuries also deserve careful attention by the physician.

CEPHALHAEMATOMA is the effusion of blood between one or more of the bones of the vault of the skull and the pericranium. The resultant soft fluctuant swelling should be left severely alone; it will then organize and disappear in a few months. At this stage its hard edge must not lead to a mistaken diagnosis of depressed fracture. Aspiration of the blood in the cephalhaematoma carries the distinct risk of introducing infection without conferring any benefit to the child.

FRACTURES are seen commonly in the clavicle, femur, humerus and skull. Fracture of the clavicle requires no treatment but the mother should be warned and reassured about the lump of callus which will become visible and palpable in 10 days' time. The fractured femur is best treated by suspending the infant by both ankles from a bar placed across the top rail of the cot so that the buttocks are raised off the mattress. This form of extension should be maintained for 14 to 21 days. The fracture of humerus is 'splinted' by strapping the arm to the chest wall for 14 days. In all these cases the ultimate result is excellent and no great orthopaedic skill is required. Fractures of the skull may be spoon-shaped or linear grooves. In our opinion surgical elevation is rarely, if ever, necessary. The prognosis is excellent provided there is no underlying intracranial injury.

CEREBRAL BIRTH TRAUMA is due to one or more of three factors—asphyxia, prematurity and obstetric trauma. When asphyxia is the principal factor the clinical signs may be due to cerebral congestion, oedema or subarachnoid bleeding. Precise diagnosis is usually impossible and it is, in any event mainly of academic interest. In the premature infant massive haemorrhage frequently occurs into one or both lateral ventricles. This is invariably associated with the respiratory distress syndrome and is fatal. Traumatic haemorrhage, on the other hand, is usually subdural. When the blood tracks above the tentorium a somewhat characteristic clinical picture develops with convulsions (often unilateral), extreme irritability, and on the side of the haemorrhage there is ptosis and dilatation of the pupil.

The basic treatment for all these cases is temperature control, preferably in an incubator with the head raised, high humidity, periodic aspiration of excess mucus from the pharynx and, when there are apnoeic attacks, oxygen up to 35 per cent. concentration. Undue irritability, constant whimpering, or convulsive movements should be controlled with chloral hydrate 60 to 120 mg. every four hours. Tube-feeding, preferably through an in-dwelling polyvinyl tube, may be necessary until the sucking reflex returns. The exposure and handling of the infant which is required for successful lumbar puncture outweighs any possible benefit which might accrue. On the other hand, when there are localizing signs of subdural haemorrhage, and especially if the anterior fontanelle is tense and bulging, subdural taps and drainage of the blood from the subdural space are clearly indicated. A short large-bore needle with a short bevel should be introduced through the coronal suture just outside the lateral angle of the fontanelle. If fresh blood is present in the subdural space it will drip freely from the end of the needle. This procedure should be carried out on both sides and it can be repeated on several occasions until the fontanelle has become soft. The importance of an immaculate aseptic technique is obvious.

SUBDURAL HAEMATOMA must be distinguished from the acute subdural haemorrhage described above. The chronic haematoma (or hygroma) contains dark-brown altered blood, or a serum-like fluid at a later stage. Symptoms are rare before the age of 16 weeks. The diagnosis is confirmed by subdural tapping as described above.

In early stages complete recovery frequently follows repeated subdural taps during which not more than 15 ml. of fluid should be removed at one time because of the dangers of an unduly sudden reduction in intracranial pressure. In the case of longer duration the protein-rich xanthochromic fluid in the hygroma continues to accumulate in spite of repeated tapping. In these circumstances the neurosurgeon will require to remove as much of the enveloping membrane of the hygroma as possible. Before operation the infant's general condition must be made as satisfactory as possible, and anaemia may need to be corrected by blood transfusion. It should not be forgotten that subdural haematoma is frequently bilateral.

PERIPHERAL NERVE INJURIES. The facial nerve is frequently contused by a forceps blade as it runs forwards across the ramus of the mandible. No treatment is required and spontaneous recovery is usual in a few weeks.

The upper part of the brachial plexus may be torn giving rise to Erb's palsy. The treatment is to put the limb in a position of abduction and external rotation at the shoulder, flexion of the elbow and supination of the hand. This can be achieved immediately by pinning the baby's sleeve to the pillow alongside his head. Meantime, a suitable splint should be made of light material for longer treatment lasting some months. Infrequently the radial nerve is damaged as it winds round the outer aspect of the humerus. There is often an overlying area of palpable subcutaneous fat necrosis at the site of injury. The resultant wrist-drop should be corrected by a light cock-up splint. The prognosis in most nerve injuries is good, but not when the whole arm is paralysed as the result of extensive tearing of the brachial plexus. This degree of injury should never occur in modern obstetric practice.

Haemorrhagic disease of the newborn. In this disease spontaneous bleeding appears between the second and fifth days of life, most often including melaena. Deficiencies can be demonstrated in several of the clotting factors including factor VII (Proconvertin), Christmas factor (factor IX) and the Stuart Prower factor (factor X). Although the condition has often been called 'hypoprothrombin-aemia' there is, in fact, no certainty that the blood prothrombin level is greatly reduced. The incidence of the disease is about 1 in 800 births. In most instances of haemorrhagic disease of the newborn the loss of blood is quite moderate and spontaneous recovery takes place in a day or two.

It is, however, wise to administer vitamin K_1, which is now available for intramuscular injection (phytomenadione), in a dose of 2 to 5 mg. Vitamin K_1, unlike the older water-soluble analogue menaphthone, does not increase the risk of kernicterus. When the infant is breastfed it is important to confirm that melaena is not due to maternal blood ingested from a cracked nipple. This is easily done by a simple chemical test which can distinguish foetal from adult type haemoglobin. Infrequently, there may be very severe haemorrhage in this disease, signs such as extreme pallor, restlessness and shock developing with alarming speed. This situation calls for an emergency blood transfusion (30 ml. per kg.), via the umbilical vein.

Haemolytic disease of the newborn (erythroblastosis foetalis). The most severe cases are those due to blood group incompatibility between a rhesus-negative mother and a rhesus-positive foetus. The disease may also occur from ABO blood group incompatibility but is then rarely an emergency. In the common rhesus (Rh) cases it is almost always possible to predict the disease during pregnancy, and an affected infant should rarely, if ever, be born outside hospital. The blood group of every pregnant woman should be determined as early as possible. In the case of Rh-negative women, the serum should be tested for antibodies periodically throughout pregnancy. The presence of antibody, especially in rising titre, is a strong indication that the infant will be affected. When a woman has previously had an affected infant, and when her husband is heterozygous for the Rh factor, it is still possible for an Rh-negative and, therefore, unaffected baby to be born from a future pregnancy. In such an event there may be a deceptive rise of Rh antibodies during the pregnancy. None the less, it is still safer to advise that the confinement should be in hospital.

It is now possible to predict the probable severity of haemolytic disease due to rhesus incompatibility with an accuracy of above 95 per cent. by spectrophotometric examination of the amniotic fluid obtained by amniocentesis from about the 28th week of pregnancy. The indications for amniocentesis, which carries a small risk, are (i) a history of a previous stillbirth or severely affected infant, and (ii) an indirect Coombs' antibody titre which exceeds 1 in 8 at 32 weeks gestation in a first sensitized pregnancy. The procedure must never be performed after 36 weeks. By means of serial amniocenteses the progress of the disease in the foetus can

be followed and three groups can be defined. In the first, the infant will be unaffected or only mildly affected and the pregnancy is allowed to go to term. In the second, the infant has a significant anaemia and premature induction of labour between 34 and 36 weeks can obviate stillbirth or the birth of a moribund infant while still permitting the best possible maturity in the individual case. In the third group, containing only a small percentage of cases, foetal death or hydrops foetalis is almost certain before 34 weeks' gestation. It is for babies in this latter group that the technique of intra-uterine transfusion may sometimes be life-saving. This is, of course, a procedure for the obstetrician, after consultation with the haematologist and the paediatrician.

The correct use of replacement (exchange) transfusion is the only means at present available whereby death, from cardiac failure or kernicterus, can be prevented in severely affected infants. Confirmation of the diagnosis should be made at the time of birth by finding a positive Coombs' test in blood taken from the maternal end of the umbilical cord. This should be taken into a convenient anticoagulant. Positive indications for early exchange transfusion exist when the infant is also premature, or if the mother gives a history of having had a severely affected infant previously. Of the other cases, some are mild and will not require replacement therapy. The indications for those infants who do, vary somewhat among different paediatricians. The criteria which the author uses are a haemoglobin level in the cord blood below 15 g. per 100 ml. and/or a serum bilirubin level in the cord blood above 5 mg. per 100 ml. The donor blood should be Rh-negative, preferably of the same ABO group as the infant, and it should also be compatible with the mother's serum by the indirect antiglobulin technique. It should not be more than five days old. Replacement transfusions may have to be repeated on two or three occasions if the serum bilirubin level subsequently rises above 20 mg. per 100 ml. The same indication applies to late transfusion in cases of ABO incompatibility in which emergency treatment is never required.

TECHNIQUE OF REPLACEMENT TRANSFUSION. The umbilical cord is cut about 1 cm. from the abdominal wall. A polyvinyl catheter (gamma ray sterilized) is passed along the umbilical vein into the ductus venosus until a free return flow of blood occurs. A syringe connected to two three-way stop-cocks in series is then used to withdraw blood from the infant. This blood is discarded. The syringe is then refilled with donor blood for injection into the baby. The amount withdrawn, in volumes of 20 ml., is usually about 170 ml. per kg. The amount of blood replaced, also in volumes of 20 ml., is in the region of 30 ml. less than that withdrawn because many of the severely affected infants are in the high output type of cardiac failure. It is also common to inject 1 ml. of 8·4 per cent. sodium bicarbonate and 1 ml. of 10 per cent. calcium gluconate with each 100 ml. of blood to correct metabolic acidosis and hypocalcaemia respectively. Sodium bicarbonate is, however, only required in the initial transfusion. It must be stressed that although exchange transfusion is a life-saving technique its dangers—citrate tetany, sepsis, cardiac failure, air-embolism—are much greater in inexperienced hands, and in small units where suitable cases are too few to give the medical staff enough experience.

Prevention of haemolytic disease. The need for the procedures just described for the treatment of haemolytic disease of the newborn will diminish progressively as new methods aimed at its prevention are put into practice. These are based upon evidence that the 'bleed' of Rh(D)-positive foetal cells into the Rh(D)-negative mother takes place late in pregnancy or during labour, and that the consequent development of Rh antibodies does not occur for some weeks. There is strong evidence that a high degree of prevention can be achieved by the intramuscular injection of anti-D immunoglobulin into the Rh-negative mother soon after the birth of her Rh-positive baby. The supply of anti-D immunoglobulin is at present dependent on plasma from naturally sensitized Rh(D)-negative women. However, the policy of deliberate immunization of Rh(D)-negative male volunteers has now been approved in the United Kingdom. The present practice in Scotland is to offer protection with anti-D immunoglobulin to all Rh(D)-negative primiparae recently delivered of Rh(D)-positive ABO compatible infants, and also to Rh(D)-negative mothers having one previous child who give birth to ABO compatible Rh(D)-positive infants. In other words such mothers can be assured of having three infants unaffected by the disease.

Cardiac Failure in Infancy

There are many causes of this common emergency of the early weeks and months of life. The most frequent are paroxysmal tachycardia, endocardial

fibroelastosis and anatomical anomalies such as complete transposition of the great vessels, ventricular septal defect with pulmonary hypertension, and patent ductus arteriosus with or without coarctation of the aorta. Diagnosis is not difficult if it is recognized that undue breathlessness on exertion presents in an infant as difficulty in feeding, that hepatomegaly is prominent whereas jugular over-filling is not, and that oedema often first appears in the face and external genitalia.

The infant should be placed with head raised above the level of the feet, and then rapidly digitalized. The initial dose of digoxin, oral or intramuscular, is 0·1 mg. per kg. per day in four divided doses for 24 to 36 hours. The subsequent maintenance dose varies from 0·02 to 0·04 mg. per kg. per day as determined by clinical and electrocardiographic supervision. A convenient oral preparation of digoxin for infants is Lanoxin Paediatric Elixir (B. W. & Co.), of which 1 ml. contains 0·05 mg. digoxin. If the oedema is not removed by digitalization, chlorothiazide should be given orally in a total daily dose of 25 mg. per kg. The serum potassium level must be determined every few days. Hypokalaemia should be corrected with oral potassium chloride 500 mg. twice daily. Severe dyspnoea at rest is an indication for oxygen given in an incubator, oxygen box or oxygen tent according to the size of the baby. In the most severe cases the cow's milk formula (30 ml. = 14·2 mg. sodium) may be replaced by Edosol milk manufactured by Trufood Ltd. (30 ml. = 1 mg. sodium).

In cases of paroxysmal tachycardia an excellent prognosis can be given, but digoxin therapy should be continued for six months in view of the considerable tendency to relapse. In cases of congenital heart disease the infant should be transferred to a centre specializing in these problems as soon as the cardiac failure has been controlled. The cardiac surgery of infancy is fraught with difficulties and disappointments but some gratifying results can now be obtained. Endocardial fibroelastosis unfortunately carries a poor prognosis.

Diseases of the Repiratory System

Viral infections of the upper respiratory tract, which not infrequently spread to the lower respiratory passages, account for more illnesses during infancy and childhood than any other infective agents. These infections are droplet-spread and adults with head colds should, as far as possible, avoid coming in contact with young infants. It is important that the physician in this antibiotic era should realize that most respiratory infections will in fact recover spontaneously, and that the majority, being caused by viruses, will not be influenced beneficially by any of the presently available sulphonamides or antibiotics. The nomenclature of the inflammatory conditions of the respiratory tract, which is, of course, continuous from the nasal passages to the alveoli, is apt to be confusing because the areas of involvement vary from one case to another. The actual diagnostic name rarely describes the full extent of the disease, only its point of maximum impact.

Upper Respiratory Infections.

The vast majority of cases are due to viruses. Even in follicular tonsillitis only a minority of cases will be found to be due to beta-haemolytic streptococci. The clinical signs may vary from nasal obstruction due to rhinitis (which can be quite serious in young infants) to croup or cough due to laryngitis or tracheitis. Constitutional upset with fever, possibly an initial convulsion, or abdominal pain and vomiting may or may not be prominent.

In most cases only conservative methods of treatment are required. Rest in bed in a light airy room at a temperature of 18° C., and an adequate intake of fluids and glucose may be all that is necessary. High fever can be reduced by tepid sponging. Sleeplessness in an infant is best relieved with chloral hydrate, 200 to 300 mg. or elixir of methyl-pentynol, 2·5 to 5 ml. A suitable sedative for the toddler is quinalbarbitone 50 to 100 mg. If nasal catarrh interferes with feeding in an infant a few drops of 1 per cent. ephedrine in physiological saline instilled up each nostril before feeds relieves the obstruction temporarily. Oily nasal drops should not be prescribed as they may be aspirated into the lungs and produce a lipoid pneumonia. In cases of typical acute tonsillitis a throat swab should be sent to the laboratory for culture. Intramuscular benzylpenicillin, 500,000 units twice daily, is indicated only when beta-haemolytic streptococci have been isolated. The common practice of many physicians who prescribe sulphonamides or antibiotics for every fevered child is to be deplored, not only because it is bad clinical practice but because it can be dangerous. Secondary bacterial complications of upper respiratory infection, such as otitis media, can be treated energetically with intramuscular penicillin if they develop. In most children kept under adequate supervision, there is an uneventful recovery within seven to 10 days.

Acute bronchitis. This develops as an extension downwards of an upper respiratory infection. Many children with bronchitis are not seriously ill and the simple measures described above are sufficient treatment. There is little evidence that the so-called expectorant mixtures have any value. When a child with bronchitis is severely fevered, toxic and dyspnoeic it is probably wise to prescribe an antibiotic on the assumption that secondary bacterial infection has become superimposed. It is usually impracticable to obtain sputum for culture in the case of a young child, and a broad spectrum drug is preferable. A suitable preparation is oxytetracycline, 25 mg. per kg. per day, or ampicillin, 50 mg. per kg. per day in three or four divided doses. Oxygen is infrequently required in bronchitis.

Acute bronchiolitis of infancy. This is a severe viral infection seen only during the first year of life. A few days after the onset of mild upper respiratory catarrh the infant becomes severely distressed with dyspnoea, subcostal inspiratory recession, grunting, marked restlessness, and ashen-grey cyanosis. Severe spasms of coughing may cause vomiting and so interfere with feeding as to lead to dehydration. There may be crepitations or rhonchi over the lungs, but neither clinical nor radiographic evidence of pneumonic consolidation is present. Fever is usually less than 101° F. (38·3°C).

The urgent therapeutic need of these dangerously ill infants is oxygen. Indeed, the relief of hypoxia frequently results in dramatic relief of the restlessness, and even induces natural sleep. Humidity is also effective in relieving the respiratory distress. These conditions can best be obtained in a special type of oxygen tent fitted with a humidifier such as the Humidair (Vickers, Ltd.) or the Croupette (Air Shields, Inc.). An oxygen concentration of at least 40 per cent. is required to achieve a satisfactory arterial PO_2 in many infants with bronchiolitis or bronchopneumonia. The oxygen concentration in the tent should be monitored hourly with a paramagnetic oximeter because it is easy to allow the oxygen concentration to fall to low levels whenever the tent is opened for nursing measures. Regular recording by an oximeter reminds both doctor and nurse of the need to use the oxygen tent efficiently. It is the author's practice also to measure the PO_2 of arterialized capillary blood at intervals, the object of oxygen therapy being to maintain this above 70 mm. Hg. In a few cases where safe levels of PO_2 cannot be achieved and when the PCO_2 rises to 70 mm. Hg. or higher, tracheal intubation and intermittent positive pressure breathing may be necessary to save the infant's life. Feeding may prove difficult but it is only infrequently necessary to resort to intravenous fluids. It is customary to administer a broad spectrum antibiotic to these babies who are in danger of their lives, but it is doubtful if this does much good. The prime requirement, in addition to oxygen and humidity, is skilled nursing.

Pneumonia in infants. In this country today bacterial pneumonia during the first year of life is due to the *Staphylococcus aureus* in about 80 per cent. of cases. This seems to have supplanted the pneumococcal bronchopneumonia which was so common and lethal in the past. It is probable that the pathogenic staphylococci colonize the infants' noses in the maternity units soon after birth and that some intercurrent virus infection opens the way for the bacteria to penetrate the respiratory mucous membrane at a later date. This explanation is necessary to allow of rational treatment, because in most cases of pneumonia in infancy it is impossible to culture the causal organism early in the disease.

Staphylococcal pneumonia in infancy is almost always resistant to penicillin, and frequently also to tetracycline. Drug treatment must also be designed to deal with those cases due to bacteria other than staphylococci. A suitable combination is cloxacillin and ampicillin each in a dosage of 50 mg. per kg. per day in three or four divided doses, given intramuscularly or orally, according to the infant's condition and the presence or absence of vomiting. If the causal organism can be cultured from the throat or laryngeal swabs, the antibiotic can be more accurately chosen. In any event, if the infant is not markedly improved within 72 hours a change should be made. Suitable drugs are cephaloridine, 20-40 mg. per kg. per day, fucidin, 20 mg. per kg. per day or erythromycin, 50 mg. per kg. per day, the first being given intramuscularly, the others by the oral route. Dyspnoea and cyanosis must be relieved with oxygen given in an incubator or tent (Vickers, Ltd.). Nasal catheters and masks are not tolerated by children. Sleeplessness may require sedation with chloral hydrate 200 to 300 mg. The possibility of underlying fibrocystic disease of the pancreas should always be considered when a case of pneumonia in an infant fails to respond quickly to the antibiotics advised above.

Pneumonia in children. In older children staphylococcal pneumonia is quite rare, and the usual causal pneumococci are invariably sensitive to benzylpenicillin. Treatment should be started with 500,000 units given intramuscularly two or four times daily for three or four days. This can then be changed to oral phenoxymethylpenicillin, 250 mg. every six hours for another three or four days. If sputum can be obtained the physician can, of course, in the atypical case obtain considerable help from the bacterial sensitivities. The older child with pneumonia is seldom dangerously ill and oxygen therapy is rarely required. Thus treatment at home is usually quite practicable.

Empyema. In older children empyema has become very rare since the advent of penicillin. The occasional case is usually due to delay in starting treatment and the causal organism is most often the pneumococcus. Benzylpenicillin should be given both intramuscularly, 500,000 units two to four times daily, and intrapleurally in 100,000 unit doses to replace the pus aspirated from the pleural cavity. In many cases repeated aspirations with penicillin instillations will prove sufficient, but when the pus is too thick to come easily through a needle surgical drainage is required.

In infants empyema is still a fairly common condition and it is, nowadays, almost always due to the *Staphylococcus aureus*. Repeated aspiration with replacement by a suitable antibiotic is usually effective in bringing about resolution. Systemic antibiotic treatment should also be instituted. In empyema it is, of course, possible to determine the bacterial sensitivities rapidly from the first specimen of pleural pus obtained, and the antibiotic can be accurately chosen. The organism is rarely if ever penicillin-sensitive but methicillin is most valuable when given both intramuscularly, 100 mg. per kg. per day, and intrapleurally in 100 mg. doses. Alternatively, cloxacillin may be given, either orally or intramuscularly, in a dosage of 50 mg. per kg. per day, while methicillin is given intrapleurally. If the empyema does not quickly respond to conservative treatment, closed underwater drainage of the pleural cavity will be required, using a plastic catheter of the Malecot type which should be placed in the optimal position by a thoracic surgeon. Anaemia commonly develops in cases of empyema. It will not respond to iron, and blood transfusion is indicated if the haemoglobin level falls below 9 g. per 100 ml.

Bronchiectasis. This has become a relatively uncommon sequel to acute respiratory infections today, and most of the affected children come from the poorer sections of the community. None the less, if carefully supervised they do remarkably well on medical treatment.

General measures, such as an adequate dietary intake of protein and plenty of fresh air, should be carefully detailed to the parents, many of whom require education in these matters. Sepsis in the paranasal sinuses and teeth is common and merits attention. Postural drainage must be carried out twice daily. The child should be placed over the side of the bed with head hanging down and instructed to cough up as much sputum as possible. Percussion over the affected lung helps to dislodge pus from the dilated bronchi. Following this the child should be encouraged to breathe slowly and as deeply as possible for a period of 5 to 10 minutes. Intercurrent respiratory infections or febrile episodes due to the retention of secretions in the bronchiectatic area should be treated energetically with a broad spectrum antibiotic which is potent against the most common organism, namely *Haemophilus influenzae*. Suitable drugs are oxytetracycline, 25 mg. per kg. per day or ampicillin, 50 mg. per kg. per day.

When sputum cultures grow staphylococci as the predominant organism it is always possible that the bronchiectasis is secondary to fibrocystic disease of the pancreas. It is also worth while testing the serum of boys with bronchiectasis for its gamma globulin content because congenital hypogammaglobulinaemia, which like haemophilia is inherited as a sex-linked recessive, may present in this form. Boys so affected can be kept much more free of intercurrent infections if they are given a weekly intramuscular injection of pooled gamma globulin, 50 mg. per kg.

Resection of the diseased part of the lung should rarely be contemplated unless medical treatment has failed after at least a two years' trial. Even when the bronchiectatic tissue has been completely removed some cough and sputum tend to persist because of bronchitis in other parts of the bronchial tree. Thoracotomy should be undertaken only after extensive investigations such as bronchography and bronchoscopy. The most definite indication for resection is bronchiectasis which is confined to one lobe in a child who has been unable to lead a more or less normal life on medical treatment.

Diseases of the Digestive System

Disorders of the digestive system are notoriously common in infancy and childhood. Many are relatively trivial and due to incorrect or unwise feeding. Others are psychogenic and transient. Some, however, can be extremely dangerous such as appendicitis and intestinal obstruction. The physician must, therefore, make an unhurried and thoughtful examination of any child who complains of digestive symptoms. In the acute emergencies prompt diagnosis may be life-saving. In the chronic conditions accurate diagnosis must obviously precede the planning of treatment. One of the most satisfactory developments of the past 20 years has been the disappearance of the devastating epidemics of infantile gastroenteritis which used to cause so many deaths every autumn. This is attributable to the introduction of dried and evaporated milks and to improving standards of home hygiene. The sporadic cases of gastroenteritis today are, however, seen only in bottlefed babies. The breastfed infant has always been safe from this serious infection.

Thrush (*Monilial stomatitis*). This disease of the newborn is due to the fungus *Candida albicans*. The inflammation frequently extends from the mouth down to the cardiac end of the stomach. Rarely it may become blood-borne. The sources of infection are the mother's vagina at term or the mouths of healthy adults. In either case spread is via the hands to the breasts or feeding utensils.

Thrush can be effectively treated by placing 1 ml. of 0·5 per cent. aqueous solution of gentian violet into the infant's mouth thrice daily for three days. The solution must always be freshly prepared for each case, and unduly prolonged treatment can damage the baby's delicate buccal mucous membrane. A rather less reliable but also less messy treatment is with the antibiotic nystatin, 100,000 units orally every four hours for 10 days. Nystatin is poorly absorbed but it is effective against surface infections. Thrush can occur in children who are receiving broad spectrum antibiotics or corticosteroids and the physician should be vigilant in these circumstances.

Herpetic stomatitis. Most cases of aphthous and ulcerative stomatitis in young children are caused by a primary infection with the virus of herpes simplex. It may cause a most unpleasant illness which interferes with the intake of fluids and food. Spontaneous recovery takes place after 7 to

10 days and it is doubtful if any form of treatment influences the outcome. Symptomatic treatment with mouth washes may help to relieve discomfort.

Dental caries. This has become less common than formerly but it is still far too prevalent among the poorer sections of the community. The most effective measure lies in regular visits to the dentist during school holidays. A correct attitude towards the care of the teeth should be inculcated in childhood, but this becomes impossible in families where the parents lack it themselves. It may even involve the preservation of life itself in the case of children with congenital deficiencies of the blood-clotting mechanism, such as haemophilia. Even in this situation some parents show a remarkable resistance towards accepting advice which seems so obvious.

As dental caries is believed to result from the action of acids on poorly calcified teeth, carbohydrate fermentation should be discouraged by limitation of chocolates and sweets between meals, and the diet should contain calcium in the form of milk, vitamin D, and hard food like toast, rusks and apples. It has been shown that fluoridation of public water supplies (1 p.p.m.) significantly reduces the incidence of dental caries. This measure is now being employed in some areas of Britain, but in others it has met with much ill-informed and prejudiced resistance.

Vomiting in infancy. The most common cause of vomiting in infancy is underfeeding, which causes the swallowing of too much air. This may also result when the hole in the teat is too small. Diagnosis is based on a careful feeding history, and personal observation of the infant during a feed. A gratifying recovery is obtained simply by increasing the infant's intake of milk, or by enlarging the hole in the teat with a red-hot sewing needle.

It is always a mistake to dilute the milk under the misapprehension that it is 'too strong' for the infant. A few infants vomit persistently without obvious cause, and in spite of a correct feeding regimen. They are often the babies of overanxious parents who prove difficult to reassure. This type of 'habitual vomiting' must only be diagnosed when the various organic causes of vomiting have been excluded. Most of these cases undergo spontaneous recovery after mixed feeding has been established, and this should be encouraged from the age of 3 months with cereals, sieved vegetables, fruits as purées, potatoes and gravy and egg-yolk. When the infant is hyperkinetic or restless, chloral hydrate

200 mg. or phenobarbitone 8 mg. may be given four-hourly before feeds.

A more severe type of non-organic vomiting in infancy is *rumination* in which the infant can be seen to make purposeful attempts to regurgitate stomach contents. Unlike habitual vomiting this psychoneurosis of infancy may interfere with nutrition. Feeds should be thickened with a cereal, the baby should be propped up for an hour after each feed, and it is helpful to try to distract his attention when he is seen to be indulging in this form of oral self-gratification. Spontaneous recovery is the rule about the time the infant learns to stand unsupported.

There are, however, several much more serious causes of vomiting in infancy in which death or permanent disability can only be prevented by timely diagnosis and treatment.

Intestinal obstruction. There are various causes of intestinal obstruction, complete or partial, in the newborn. These include duodenal atresia, malrotation of the gut, meconium ileus due to fibrocystic disease of the pancreas, intestinal atresia, annular pancreas and Hirschsprung's disease. The most significant sign is the presence of bile in the vomitus which in the newborn must always indicate the need for immediate transfer to hospital, preferably in a portable incubator. The treatment is always surgical and expert supervision of fluid and electrolyte balance is essential before and after operation.

Pyloric stenosis. In our opinion the treatment of choice in hypertrophic pyloric stenosis is Ramstedt's operation, provided the services of an experienced surgeon are available. Within a few days this operation puts an end to the infant's projectile vomiting and failure to thrive, and the mortality rate should be virtually nil. On the other hand, the alternative medical treatment, which is based on the fact that spontaneous recovery occurs ultimately in pyloric stenosis, involves weeks of parental anxiety while vomiting continues to a varying degree, during which time there is always the danger of intercurrent infection. Medical treatment should, however, be considered in those relatively mild cases in which the diagnosis is delayed until after the age of 10 weeks. Whichever method of treatment is decided upon it is best that it be supervised by the physician as he is generally more familiar with the problems of feeding and fluid balance in young infants.

It is desirable that the infant's stay in hospital

should be kept to the minimum to obviate the dangers of ward infection. He should be nursed in a cubicle and protected from other children and unnecessary adult contacts. The operation should be performed within 24 hours of diagnosis unless the infant is manifestly dehydrated and marasmic. When there is clinical evidence of dehydration a serious loss of chloride, as well as water, has occurred from the extracellular fluid compartment. The excessive loss of this anion into the stomach also causes a metabolic alkalosis. In these circumstances 5 per cent. dextrose in half-strength physiological saline should be given by continuous intravenous infusion, 150 ml. per kg. for 24 hours before operation. It is helpful if this replacement therapy can be controlled by periodic estimations of the blood pH, plasma bicarbonate, PCO_2 and serum electrolytes. Gastric lavage with half-strength physiological saline should always be performed four hours before operation.

Oral fluids should be started four hours after operation with half-strength physiological saline, followed two hours later by 15 ml. of breast milk or half-cream dried milk. This regimen of alternating saline and milk feeds every two hours is continued for the next 48 hours, the volume of the milk feeds being increased by 15 ml. per feed every 24 hours. At this time the infant may be sent home to breast feeding; or if bottlefed he can go home on feeds of 60 ml. plus sugar every four hours with water given between feeds. Within a few days he should be receiving his full caloric requirements.

Medical treatment. The infant should be offered his full requirements at every feed. When a feed is vomited he should immediately be offered another, which is frequently retained. Gastric lavage with physiological saline should be carried out once or twice daily. Between feeds half-strength physiological saline should be offered freely. A spasmolytic drug should also be given 15 to 30 minutes before every feed. Suitable preparations and individual doses are atropine methyl nitrate, 1 to 2 drops of a 0·6 per cent. alcoholic solution, or scopolamine methyl nitrate, 1 to 2 drops of a 0·1 per cent. solution. This regimen is usually required for two or even three months before symptomatic recovery is complete.

Hiatus hernia. This congenital anomaly is always accompanied by incompetence of the sphincteric mechanism at the cardia (chalasia). It is characterized by vomiting from the early weeks of life, and by the presence of excess mucus and altered blood in the vomitus. The diagnosis must be confirmed by means of a barium swallow under the observation of a radiologist experienced in dealing with young infants. The most important therapeutic measure is that the infant be maintained in an upright position day and night. This can be most easily achieved in a specially constructed box of suitable size, and made of padded wood or plastic. Suitable plastic supports which achieve the same purpose are commercially available. When the infant is bottlefed the feeds should be thickened with one of the pre-cooked cereals, but the advantages of this measure do not justify the discontinuance of breast feeding. Aluminium hydroxide mixture B.N.F., 2·5 to 5 ml., may be given with each feed. When there is a hypochromic anaemia from chronic loss of blood the following prescription is useful:

Ferrous sulphate . . .	200 mg.
Dilute hypophosphorous acid	0·03 ml.
Dextrose	1 g.
Chloroform water to . .	5 ml.

    Label: 5 ml. three times daily.

In about 70 per cent. of cases functional recovery takes place on this regimen. Persistent vomiting and haematemesis indicate severe peptic ulceration of the oesophagus and oesophageal stricture may result. In such failures of medical treatment surgery must be carefully considered although, unfortunately, none of the operations employed in this disease gives consistently satisfactory results.

Constipation. Mothers of young babies frequently 'diagnose' constipation and resort to medication without seeking medical advice. In most instances inspection of the stools will, in fact, show them to be normal in consistence. It is quite common for healthy infants to have infrequent bowel movements and this does not constitute constipation. In true constipation the stools are small and hard; indeed, the hard faecal masses are readily palpable through the lower abdominal wall. The most common cause is underfeeding, which is easily enough corrected by increasing the milk intake. Apart from underfeeding, true constipation in a young infant invariably has an organic cause such as cretinism, idiopathic hypercalcaemia, renal tubular disorders, pyloric stenosis or Hirschsprung's disease. The treatment must be directed towards the primary cause after accurate diagnosis. Indeed, the occasions on which the use of laxatives alone is justifiable or beneficial in infancy must be very infrequent.

In older children constipation is frequently a symptom of organic disease such as infection, raised intracranial pressure or anal fissure. More often, however, it has a non-organic basis. The most common is the prolonged misuse of laxatives. In other cases, toilet training has been so much enforced that the child has from an early age related the act of defaecation to an unhappy battle of wills. This finally results in a strong disinclination to empty the rectum, and it may go on to acquired (terminal reservoir) megacolon. Sometimes the impacted faeces so irritate the mucous membrane as to cause spurious diarrhoea with faecal soiling of pants (encopresis). A severe psychological disturbance of later onset can also cause this distressing and very difficult problem of encopresis.

The first therapeutic requirement is an accurate understanding of the basis of the constipation in each case. Perhaps most frequently the correct procedure is the withdrawal of laxatives combined with a firm reassurance to the parents of a good prognosis. The use of saline rectal wash-outs or of bisacodyl suppositories often allows the bowel to regain a normal rhythm. Some disturbed children also require child guidance treatment. Laxatives are useful to empty a constipated lower bowel during illness, or as an initial measure in chronic constipation, but their prolonged use is to be deprecated. Suitable laxatives for children are the standardized total active principle of senna pod (Senokot) in the form of granules, 4 g., and liquid paraffin and magnesium hydroxide emulsion B.P.C., 5 to 10 ml. When there is an anal fissure the stools should be rendered soft with laxatives, and 1 per cent. amethocaine ointment can be applied locally on a pledglet of cotton-wool inserted into the anus.

Gastroenteritis. Diarrhoea and vomiting in a young infant may be due to parenteral infections such as pyelonephritis, acute otitis media and osteitis which should, of course, receive suitable treatment. Much more frequently the cause is infection of the bowel itself by one of the enteropathogenic strains of *Escherichia coli*, or other intestinal pathogens like the *Salmonella* group. The real danger of gastroenteritis lies in the rapid loss of body water and electrolytes with resultant oligaemia, renal failure, metabolic acidosis and final peripheral circulatory failure. The aims of treatment are to rest the diseased bowel, to correct the loss of fluid and electrolytes and to eradicate the causal organism. When the dehydration is mild these aims can be quite well achieved in the home. Indications for admission to hospital are severe vomiting or dehydration.

Milk feeds should be completely withdrawn for 24 hours. They should be replaced by half-strength physiological saline, 180 ml. per kg. per day, given in small volumes every two hours during the day and every four hours during the night. This usually results in quick relief from diarrhoea and vomiting. It must be stressed that water alone cannot correct dehydration of this type and it can in fact be dangerous by producing water intoxication. After 24 hours milk feeds are reintroduced in small but increasing quantities. A start may be made with 15 ml. feeds of one of the half-cream or 'humanized' dried milks every four hours, and increasing by 15 ml. per feed per day until the infant's full caloric requirements, 110 Cal. per kg., are met. As the feeds are increased in volume the half-strength saline between feeds should be correspondingly reduced; it should be replaced after two or three days by water between feeds because an excess of sodium chloride can cause oedema. Sugar should be added to the feeds only when the stools regain their normal consistence.

From the start of treatment an oral antibiotic should be prescribed and its suitability confirmed by bacteriological examination of a rectal swab. Most enteropathogenic strains of *E. coli* are sensitive to neomycin (50 mg. per kg. per day), polymyxin B (100,000 units per kg. per day), and colistin (150,000 units per kg. per day), each given in four divided doses in solution. These drugs being poorly absorbed from the gastrointestinal tract are preferable to the tetracyclines or chloramphenicol. Purgatives and laxatives must never be prescribed as they obviously aggravate the loss of fluids and solutes from the bowel.

In the severely dehydrated infants admitted to hospital intravenous fluid replacement is frequently required using various dilutions and mixtures of glucose-saline, citrated plasma, sodium lactate and sodium bicarbonate. After the initial dehydration has been corrected a serious deficit of body potassium may be reflected in hypokalaemia and require the use of intravenous or oral potassium chloride. This type of emergency treatment demands expert handling by an experienced paediatrician and should never be undertaken by those unfamiliar with the problems of fluid balance in young infants.

It is also very helpful although not essential to have the facilities of a modern biochemical laboratory.

A distinction must be made between gastro-enteritis, which is a disease of the first year, and bacillary dysentery due to one of the Shigella group of bacteria, which may affect children of all ages. In the latter, the stools usually contain blood, mucus and pus. The treatment of bacillary dysentery in the child is on the same lines as in adults although the infant's susceptibility to dehydration is frequently a more serious problem (pp. 33, 253).

Coeliac disease. The most common causes of steatorrhoea during infancy and childhood are coeliac disease and fibrocystic disease of the pancreas (p. 487). There are, however, other rare causes such as abdominal tuberculosis, giardiasis, regional ileitis, congenital absence of bile salts, hypogammaglobulinaemia and α-betalipoprotein-aemia. Obviously, treatment designed for coeliac disease will be ineffectual in these conditions and accurate diagnosis must always precede treatment. This often demands exhaustive investigations such as faecal fat output, xylose and glucose absorption tests, barium studies and jejunal biopsy. The serum iron and whole blood folate levels are also low in coeliac disease. True coeliac disease is to be regarded as a gluten-induced enteropathy and, when the diagnosis is correct, an excellent response to treatment may be confidently predicted.

Gluten is a protein contained in wheat flour and rye flour. It is not present in pure wheat or rye starch. Its presence in the diet of children with coeliac disease interferes with the intestinal absorption of neutral fat, carbohydrate, fat-soluble vitamin D, and sometimes of iron, folic acid, vitamin B complex and protein. The basis of the treatment is, therefore, a gluten-free diet plus certain supplements. In Britain a gluten-free diet means, in effect, one from which wheat flour has been completely excluded. At the start of treatment, if diarrhoea is severe and abdominal distension gross, the diet may have to be restricted to 1·2 litres (2 pints) of skimmed milk daily. As the stools improve the diet can be rapidly increased to that of a normal child *except* for the exclusion of wheat flour. A list is given below of foods containing gluten which should be forbidden:

All bran and bran flakes	Cream of wheat
Bread ⎫	Diabetic rolls
Biscuits ⎪ Unless made with	Doughnuts
Cakes ⎬ pure wheat starch	Energen rolls
Scones ⎪	Ice cream (only those makes
Toast ⎭	listed below allowed)

Breakfast cereals (only those listed below allowed)	Macaroni
Noodles	Malted milk
Ovaltine	Sausages
Procea bread	Semolina
Proferin rolls	Sister Laura's Food
Packet and pudding mixtures	Shredded Wheat and Shreddies
Pastry mixtures	Spaghetti
Patent foods (Farex, Farola, etc.)	Sugar Smacks
Pie meat	Tinned soups, meats (only those listed below allowed)
Puffed Wheat and Sugar Puffs	Vermicelli
Rusks	Vita Wheat
Ryvita	Weetabix
	Wheat flakes

The following foods, being free of gluten, can be included daily as in a normal diet:

Baked beans	Jams
Bisto	Marmalade
Boiled sweets	Meat, fresh—all kinds
Breakfast cereals—Corn-flakes, Post Toasties, Puffed Rice, Rice Krispies, Sugar Ricicles	Milk
	Oatmeal (in moderation)
	Oatcakes (if made from pure oatmeal)
Butter	Porridge oats
Cheese	Poultry
Chocolate, plain or milk	Rice
Cornflour	Rice flour
Custard powder	Sago
Eggs	Soya flour
Fish, fresh—all kinds	Sugar
Fruits, all kinds	Tapioca
Fruit juices and squashes	Vegetables (all kinds, including potatoes)
Honey	
Ice cream (made by Walls, Lyons, Eldorado or Hoods)	

Tinned soups and meats as follows:

Fray Bentos: Brisket, corned beef, ox tongue, cream of tomato soup.
H. P. Ltd.: Baked beans, tomato soup.
H. J. Heinz: Cream of celery, green pea, tomato and onion soups.

Bread made from pure wheat starch and gluten-free biscuits can be purchased from several commercial sources in this country. It is also possible to obtain pure wheat starch for baking loaves, scones and cakes in the home. Milk may, of course, be given freely.

An adequate intake of vitamins is also important. Calciferol (vitamin D_2), 800 to 1,600 units daily, should be given in every case, and probably also vitamin A, 1,500 to 2,500 units daily. This can be given as one of the proprietary preparations in which vitamins A and D are presented in water miscible form. Ascorbic acid, 50 mg. daily, can best be given in the form of fresh fruit or as tablets. Compound vitamin B preparations need be added to a gluten-free diet only when there is clinical evidence of deficiency such as angular stomatitis or glossitis. Iron-deficiency anaemia is common and should be treated with oral ferrous sulphate, 200 mg. thrice daily. If the haemoglobin level fails to rise rapidly, iron-dextran complex can be given intramuscularly. Megaloblastic anaemia due to folic-acid deficiency is rare in childhood. However, in most cases the presence of folic-acid deficiency is reflected in a low whole blood folate level. It should be treated with folic acid, 5 mg. orally daily.

There is room for difference of opinion as to whether the coeliac patient should ever return to an ordinary gluten-containing diet. It is not uncommon to encounter a young adult, who having been successfully treated for coeliac disease in childhood, again suffers from all the manifestations of the disease some years after returning to a normal diet. The stress of pregnancy is particularly likely to precipitate such a relapse. Others appear to have 'outgrown' the disease and to remain healthy on an ordinary diet. However, Sheldon has shown that some of these apparently healthy individuals have abnormally low levels of serum folate or iron. On the other hand, it is probably unrealistic to expect an adolescent or young adult who feels well, and who only vaguely recalls his earlier stay in a paediatric ward, to adhere indefinitely to a gluten-free diet. Certainly the diet should be enforced until after the period of most rapid growth (post-puberty). Thereafter, in the absence of symptoms, gluten may be gradually reintroduced but the patient should preferably remain under medical supervision.

Cystic fibrosis of the pancreas. This is a genetically determined disorder which, in fact, involves all the exocrine glands—pancreas, liver, sweat, mucous and salivary glands. Although steatorrhoea arises from pancreatic insufficiency, the most serious feature of the disease is the invariable development of staphylococcal bronchiolitis and generalized obstructive emphysema. In many cases death takes place in infancy from pulmonary sepsis, and the prognosis is directly influenced by the success with which this infection can be controlled. Unfortunately, it can never be completely eradicated, and death is common about the time of puberty from cor pulmonale. In some cases portal hypertension secondary to biliary cirrhosis complicates the picture. None the less, more and more of these patients are now living into adult life as treatment becomes more effective. It has now been recognized that the male survivors are all sterile due to absence or obliteration of the vasa deferentia.

Most affected children must be maintained permanently on antibiotic therapy to control the respiratory infection. Unfortunately, the staphylococcus tends to develop resistance to one antibiotic after another, and regular sputum cultures with bacterial sensitivity tests are essential to treatment. Benzylpenicillin is rarely useful and resort must be had to a series of oral antibiotics over long periods. The most useful antibiotic for long-term use is cloxacillin, 50 mg. per kg. per day. The author now believes that this should be started as soon as the diagnosis has been confirmed, and whether there is obvious lung infection or not. In acute exacerbations of pulmonary infection a change of antibiotic, chosen on the basis of sensitivity tests, is often effective. Suitable oral drugs are erythromycin (50 mg. per kg. per day) or fucidin (20 mg. per kg. per day). In some children with cystic fibrosis who have been on prolonged antibiotic therapy, sputum cultures yield gram-negative bacteria such as *H. influenzae*, *E. coli* or *Proteus mirabilis*. They may then require the intramuscular administration of drugs such as cephaloridine (20-40 mg. per kg. per day) or kanamycin (15 mg. per kg. per day). If sputum culture yields *Pseudomonas aeruginosa* in the child who has already had much antibiotic therapy the drug of choice is usually gentamicin given intramuscularly in a dose of 2·5 mg. per kg. per day. Antibiotics may also be given by inhalation in aerosol form and streptomycin 250 mg. or neomycin 250 mg. five times daily have sometimes proved valuable. When the sputum is viscid the child suffers from distressing spasms of coughing. Relief may be obtained by the use of a Humidair (Vickers, Ltd.) or Croupette (Air Shields, Inc.) into the humidity chambers in which are put 10 per cent. propylene glycol in 3 per cent. sodium chloride. The patient can frequently spend the night in such a special atmosphere which can be arranged to contain air or oxygen. After 10 or 12 days the sodium chloride begins to irritate the respiratory mucous membrane and should be withdrawn from the aerosol. Postural drainage (p. 210) and physiotherapy regularly supervised are also of considerable value, and should be instituted as soon as the child is old enough to co-operate. These measures can be combined with aerosol therapy using an electrically operated pump, aerolyser and face mask for home treatment.

The diet should be rich in protein (at least 6 g. per kg.), and low in fat. It should be liberally salted in view of the excessive loss of sodium chloride in the sweat in this disease. In hot climates an additional 2 to 3 g. of salt should be given daily. Some advantage is obtainable from the administration of pancreatin before or with each feed or meal. This may be given in the form of pancreatin, 1 g. per dose, or as a more concentrated proprietary preparation like Pancrex V (Paines and Byrne), 1 to 3 g. per dose. A vitamin mixture should be prescribed, preferably in water-miscible form such as Abidec (Parke Davis & Co.), 1 ml. daily.

As children with cystic fibrosis live longer a few begin to suffer from attacks of severe abdominal colic, probably due to inspissated bowel contents. This can be treated with n-acetylcysteine (Airbron), 20 per cent. solution diluted to twice its original volume with distilled water. The dosage is 5 ml. four times daily for 1 to 2 weeks; thrice daily for 1 to 2 weeks; twice daily for 1 to 2 weeks; and then once daily. Unfortunately, this preparation has a foul smell, and must be prepared fresh every few days. Occasionally such a child develops intestinal obstruction demanding surgery.

The services of a surgeon may be required under several circumstances in the course of this protean disease. Thus, intestinal obstruction from meconium ileus may occur soon after birth; rarely, lobectomy may be necessary for bronchiectasis; portal hypertension may necessitate a porto-caval anastomosis.

Disaccharide and monosaccharide intolerance. In recent years it has been recognized that the absence of the enzymes lactase or sucrase from the intestinal mucosa can lead to lactose or sucrose intolerance respectively. This results in diarrhoea as soon as these carbohydrates are ingested by the infant. The stools are loose, frothy and highly acid. The infant fails to thrive and has abdominal distension. Exclusion of the offending sugar from the diet relieves the symptoms completely. The diagnosis is highly probable if the stool pH is below 5·5 and if an emulsion of the stool gives a positive reaction with Clinitest tablets. Final confirmation rests upon the results of sugar-loading tests and enzyme assay of the jejunal mucosal biopsy. These tests require admission to hospital, which should be advised in every suspected case. Most cases are congenital and present in early infancy, but sometimes the condition is secondary to coeliac disease or infections of the small bowel.

Failure to absorb monosaccharides—glucose and galactose—is much less common although producing similar manifestations from the early weeks of life. Diagnosis again requires investigation in hospital, and treatment demands the exclusion of milk and its replacement with a synthetic diet. In monosaccharide intolerance the absorption of fructose proceeds normally.

Diseases of the Nervous System
Convulsions. A convulsion is one of the commonest emergencies in paediatric practice. During infancy convulsions are most often caused by cerebral birth trauma, hypoglycaemia and hypocalcaemia, or they fall into the group called 'idiopathic convulsions of infancy'. When they are related to birth trauma or asphyxia they are best controlled with chloral hydrate, 60 to 120 mg four-hourly. The administration of oxygen in a concentration not exceeding 35 per cent. may also be necessary if the infant is in respiratory distress. Lumbar puncture is best avoided and is unlikely to relieve the situation.

Hypocalcaemic tetany during the newborn period frequently occurs some days after an uneventful birth; it is rare in breastfed babies. The serum calcium level is below 8 mg. per 100 ml., whereas the phosphate level is raised. It can be treated with oral calcium chloride, 300 mg. four-hourly for three days, which abolishes the tetany by producing a metabolic acidosis, or by an intramuscular injection of 10 per cent. calcium gluconate, 3 ml. of which abolishes the tetany by raising the total serum calcium. Tetany is now rarely seen in older infants, thanks to the abolition of rickets. It can be treated along the same lines with larger doses of calcium gluconate while the rickets is cured with calciferol. The management of hypoglycaemia in the newborn has been discussed on p. 475. In older infants, idiopathic convulsions should be controlled with chloral hydrate, 300 mg. four-hourly, or phenobarbitone, 8 mg. four-hourly. When fits persist in spite of sedation the possibility of pyridoxine-dependent convulsions should be considered. These are characteristically associated with marked hyperacusis, extreme irritability and a peculiarly rapid fluttering of the eyelids. In this rare inborn error of cerebral metabolism larger amounts of pyridoxine are required than are available in a normal diet. Confirmation of the diagnosis can be obtained by the fact that convulsions due to this cause will stop immediately after 10 mg. of pyridoxine hydrochloride are given intramuscularly. The disordered electroencephalograph also reverts to normal. Subsequent biochemical studies are required to determine the infant's permanent daily requirement of pyridoxine.

Another type of convulsive disorder peculiar to infancy is called 'infantile spasms'. These are almost invariably accompanied by mental deficiency and they consist of numerous myoclonic jerks of the trunk, head and limbs. Infantile spasms are associated with gross abnormalities on the E.E.G. and do not respond to anti-convulsants. They frequently cease on treatment with intramuscular corticotrophin, 40 mg. daily, or with oral prednisone, 20 mg. daily. The mental deficiency is usually irreversible, but hormone treatment may have to be continued for some weeks or months before the infantile spasms finally cease.

In older children the most common type of convulsion is that provoked by fever at the onset of an acute infection, although this explanation should not be accepted after the age of 5 years. It is only acceptable, moreover, after careful examination has excluded intracranial organic disease such as meningitis, encephalitis or tumour. A convulsion occurring after the age of 5 years, or one of long duration always arouses the suspicion of epilepsy, and in these circumstances the prognosis should be somewhat guarded. Whatever the cause, if a convulsion does not stop within a few minutes an intramuscular injection of paraldehyde 0·15 ml. per kg., should be given. Paraldehyde for injection must always come from a sealed ampoule because it may undergo dangerous decomposition when kept in a bottle, and it must not be given with a disposable syringe. Alternative drugs with a smaller safety margin when given intramuscularly are sodium phenobarbitone (5 mg. per kg.), and phenytoin sodium, 50 to 100 mg. In status epilepticus these drugs may be given in repeated doses or in combination. The use of general anaesthesia, although popular in the past, is fraught with risks—aspiration of gastric contents, pulmonary oedema, rise in intracranial pressure—and is best avoided. The value of diazepam in status epilepticus has recently been recognized, given in a dose of 2 to 10 mg. by slow intravenous or by intramuscular injection. It is important, also, to maintain a clear airway and to abolish cyanosis with oxygen. The time-honoured mustard bath is to be condemned. It can only raise the fevered child's temperature still more. Tepid sponging is more rational and will give anxious parents something to do. After the convulsion the physician must carefully review the case in an effort to reach a firm diagnosis. In some cases this may require several specialized methods of investigation.

In established 'idiopathic' epilepsy of the grand mal type a wide range of anti-convulsants is now available. These must be tried singly or in combination until the best possible control of the fits has been obtained. Phenobarbitone in a dosage of 30 to 60 mg. twice or thrice daily is commonly the initial treatment, but this frequently causes restlessness and hyperkinetic behaviour in some young children and the author now prefers to start treatment with phenytoin sodium, 50 mg. twice daily. Other drugs which may be used singly or in combination in difficult cases are primidone, 125 to 250 mg. twice or thrice daily, carbamazepine, 100 to 200 mg. twice to four times daily, and sulthiame, 50 to 200 mg. twice or thrice daily. The last is especially valuable in cases of temporal lobe epilepsy. In petit mal the most useful drugs are ethosuximide, 125 to 250 mg. thrice daily or, if this fails, troxidone, 150 to 300 mg. thrice daily. It is important that the physician makes himself familiar with the possible toxic effects of the drugs which he prescribes (p. 552).

Mental deficiency. There is a multitude of causes of mental deficiency, some due to chromosomal abnormalities like mongolism, some due to single gene defects such as phenylketonuria and galactosaemia, and many due to intra- or extra-uterine environmental influences which include rubella virus, toxoplasmosis, intrapartum anoxia, kernicterus, pyogenic meningitis and head injury. Prevention is possible in relation to some of these causes such as the better practice of obstetrics and paediatrics in preventing foetal anoxia, the use of replacement transfusion in hyperbilirubinaemia, and the prompt correction of neonatal hypoglycaemia. It is, however, possible to offer specific curative treatment in only a very few of the conditions in which mental deficiency is a feature and then only at an effective level when diagnosis is made early and before irreversible damage to the actively growing brain of the baby has occurred This is, of course, the purpose of the screening programmes for diseases such as phenylketonuria, galactosaemia, homocystinuria, etc. and which are now established for all newborn infants in many areas of the United Kingdom. It is, therefore, important that each child receives full investigation. Indeed, the general public nowadays are remarkably well informed on such problems, and modern parents rightly demand that each retarded child is given the opportunity to develop his potential. In most instances this starts when the physician, who must be sure of his ground, tells the parents that their child is mentally handicapped. This is an unpleasant but essential duty which the physician should not delegate to anybody else, and which he must discharge at the earliest opportunity after the diagnosis has been established. The term 'mental deficiency' should be avoided, but the parents can be given the facts by explaining to them that the child is slow to develop, that he will to some degree be backward, but that their efforts guided by the physician, the educationist and others can ensure that his progress is the best of which he is capable. Parents of a mentally handicapped child should be encouraged to join one of the admirable voluntary societies for mentally retarded children in which they are assured of the friendly and informed help of other parents with similar problems. Some of these societies run short-stay homes in which the retarded child can spend a pleasant holiday, while the mother has another baby or recovers from illness. Mentally retarded children frequently have physical disabilities such as partial deafness, refractive errors, and cerebral palsy which must be recognized and treated. Formal intelligence testing by a psychologist will help the education authority to place the educable child in a special school or occupational centre suitable to his capacity. He should not be sent to an ordinary school where his inability to cope with work or normal children can lead to behaviour problems and needless unhappiness. The most severely retarded children frequently require long-term institutional care. This decision will obviously depend on many factors additional to the presence of low-grade mental deficiency, such as the home conditions, the parents' competence and wishes, the effect on other children in the family, and the child's own personality and capacity for affection. In most cases drugs have no place unless to control convulsions or undue restlessness. It is, of course, particularly important to detect those children who can be helped by drugs or dietetic measures.

CRETINISM. The treatment is discussed on page 290.

PHENYLKETONURIA. By the time this inborn metabolic error causes obvious signs of mental deficiency treatment cannot return the brain to normal activity, although it can occasionally greatly improve the child's behaviour and intellectual state.

The brains of these infants are not, however, damaged at birth and they will develop normally if a diet sufficiently low in phenylalanine content is started early. In Scotland all newborn infants are now screened for this disease between the 5th and 14th days of life. The Guthrie bacterial inhibition test is a reliable technique for revealing an abnormally high serum phenylalanine level. There are, however, other screening techniques of equal sensitivity such as spectrofluorimetry of the blood, or chromatography of blood or urine. In every infant with a positive test the final diagnosis must be confirmed by biochemical estimations of the serum phenylalanine and tyrosine levels, and by chromatography of the urine for ortho-hydroxyphenylacetic acid. It has now been recognized that not every case of hyperphenylalaninaemia is due to classical phenylketonuria requiring treatment. It should also be stressed that screening for phenylketonuria by Phenistix has been shown to fail to detect at least 40 per cent. of cases in the newborn and should be discontinued.

The aim of treatment is to maintain a serum phenylalanine level of about 4 mg. per 100 ml. A level below 2 mg. per 100 ml. is undesirable and one above 8 mg. per 100 ml. is also unacceptable, as in both cases there is a risk of brain damage. This requires hospital supervision and expert dietetic management. Treatment is started on a phenylalanine-free food which is, in effect, a casein hydrolysate which has been freed of phenylalanine and to which has been added certain amino acids, fats, minerals, carbohydrates and vitamins.

When the serum phenylalanine level has come down to normal some phenylalanine-containing foods are carefully added to the diet, such as milk, cornflour, vegetables, fruit, potato, gluten-free bread, and butter. The phenylalanine content of the diet should be so controlled that the serum phenylalanine level is maintained below 5 mg. per 100 ml. as far as possible. During infancy the most useful phenylalanine-free preparation is Minafen (Tru-food). About the age of a year this is usually changed to Cymogran (Allen & Hanbury) or Lofenalac (Mead Johnson). This treatment is extremely expensive. It requires the utmost co-operation from intelligent parents, and this is not always available. However, under optimal environmental conditions, and provided treatment is started in the early days of life, the results are often most gratifying. In Britain the special phenylalanine-free preparations, although foods, may be prescribed on National Health Service prescription forms. It is only rarely that this arduous and expensive regimen is worth starting in children over the age of 3 years.

Galactosaemia. In this disease the inability of the body to convert galactose to glucose results in the accumulation in the tissues of a toxic intermediate, galactose-1-phosphate. This results in damage to the brain, liver, lens of the eye and kidneys. A reducing substance is found in the urine and can be shown to be galactose. It is possible, however, to make the diagnosis in the umbilical cord blood of the newborn infant, tested because of a previous case in the family, before he has ingested his first lactose-containing milk feed. All the manifestations of the disease, including cerebral damage, can be prevented or reversed in many of the affected infants provided diagnosis is made soon after birth. In some areas the Guthrie test has been modified to screen for galactosaemia (and other metabolic errors) in addition to phenylketonuria. The treatment consists of a lactose-free diet, and is achieved by substituting for milk a special preparation such as Low-Lactose Food (Cow and Gate) or Nutramigen (Mead Johnson). As the child gets older and on to a more varied diet these expensive artificial foods become less essential. There is evidence, also, that the older child develops the ability to tolerate some lactose in his diet. This treatment obviously requires hospital supervision and regular biochemical control.

Other inborn errors of metabolism causing cerebral damage have been recognized in recent years, mostly with the help of modern chromatographic techniques. Several of these are now treatable by special diets, e.g. maple syrup urine disease, homocystinuria, tyrosinosis, etc.

Enuresis

This diagnosis must never be made until an organic basis for the bed-wetting has been excluded. This symptom can, of course, be due to the polyuria of chronic pyelonephritis or renal failure, to diabetes mellitus or to diabetes insipidus. It may also be due to pyuria in the presence of good renal function, to an aberrant ureter, or to a defect in the nerve supply to the bladder. In most cases organic disease can be excluded on the basis of a careful history, clinical examination and urine analysis which must include microscopy.

The treatment of enuresis is unsatisfactory. This is, in part, due to our poor understanding of its causes. While some cases are due to obvious psychological disturbances few paediatricians or urologists would accept such a basis in the great majority. Routine practice is to advise fluid restriction after 5 p.m., to make the child empty his bladder just before going to bed, to awaken him some hours later again to empty the bladder and to repeat this once more during the night. Those who believe that enuretics have a small bladder capacity also encourage the child to hold his urine for longer and longer periods during the day. In some cases these measures are successful; more often they fail. Success is more likely if the child receives constant parental encouragement and understanding. Some advise that a calendar be kept on which the child proudly marks his or her 'dry' nights. Scolding and punishment, on the other hand, can only aggravate the situation and surround it with tension and anxiety. Some excellent functional results can be obtained by the use of an electrical device incorporated in a small sheet placed in the bed under the child's buttocks. The first drop of urine completes an electrical circuit and causes a bell to ring, and the child awakens to empty his bladder. This is really the production of a conditioned reflex which is usually established in a few weeks if the treatment is going to be successful. When there are obvious psychological disturbances every effort should be made to relieve them. These include disharmony in the home and difficulties at school. Very few of these children require Child Guidance treatment and the psychiatrist has met with no more success in this problem than the paediatrician or the urologist.

The relative inefficacy of drugs is shown by the numbers and variety which have been tried at one time and another. These include ephedrine, 30 to 60 mg. thrice daily, amphetamine, 5 to 10 mg. at night to lighten sleep, and propantheline bromide 15 mg. thrice daily, with sometimes another 30 mg. at the parents' bed-time. The latest is imipramine, 25 to 50 mg. at bed-time.

Many paediatricians have formed the impression that enuresis is more common in children whose parents have made over-enthusiastic attempts at toilet training in early infancy when bladder control is physiologically impossible. This is only developed about the age of 15 to 18 months. It is very doubtful if toilet training is advisable in infancy although modern mothers trained in 'cleanliness' are frequently difficult to convince in this respect. There is a good deal of evidence to indicate that children from stable homes who have not received any formal toilet training as infants develop normal bladder control at the same age as those who have been so 'trained'.

The Periodic Syndrome (*Cyclical Vomiting*)

Cyclical vomiting is the best recognized form of a rather mysterious symptom-complex in which recurrences are periodic. Although the condition often presents as periodic episodes of severe vomiting, each of a few days' duration, in other children vomiting is a minor feature and abdominal pain is the principal complaint. In either event, headache is a fairly frequent accompaniment. There is often a family history of migraine, and in some cases the periodic syndrome of childhood is replaced by migraine in adolescence or adult life. Sufferers from this complaint are usually highly strung, thin children and they are frequently highly intelligent. Individual attacks seem often to be precipitated by minor infections or emotional upsets. Acetonuria is a constant finding, but the term 'acidosis' is to be avoided; not only are there many unrelated causes of acidosis but in the periodic syndrome acidosis is, in fact, the exception and not the rule.

In attacks characterized by intractable vomiting, glucose-containing fluids should be given frequently by mouth in small volumes. One or two injections of chlorpromazine, 25 mg., may stop the vomiting, after which it may be continued by mouth, 25 mg. thrice daily for a few days. When dehydration is severe it is sometimes necessary to administer 5 per cent. glucose in half-strength physiological saline by continuous intravenous infusion. Recovery is usually rapid after the vomiting ceases and a light semi-solid diet can be increased to a normal one in a few days. When attacks are very severe the possibility of high intestinal obstruction should be remembered. In these cases, usually associated with malrotation of the bowel, there will be a metabolic alkalosis as reflected in a high plasma bicarbonate level, and a straight radiograph of the abdomen may be helpful. They must, of course, be relieved by operation.

When the periodic syndrome takes the form of recurrent abdominal pain, propantheline bromide, 15 mg. thrice daily, is sometimes effective.

Between attacks it is best to allow the child an ordinary diet. There is no evidence that fat limitation and extra glucose diminish their frequency. The parents often require repeated reassurance to prevent their anxiety transferring to the child. Attempts to 'fatten him up' by giving large quantities of cream and vitamin preparations are undesirable. Although we do not believe that this recurrent illness is an epileptic variant, the regular administration of phenobarbitone, 30 mg. twice daily, is sometimes effective in reducing the frequency of attacks.

References

ADAMSON, T. M., COLLINS, L. M., HAWKER, J. M., REYNOLDS, E. O. R. & STRANG, L. B. (1968). Mechanical ventilation in newborn infants with respiratory failure. *Lancet*, **2**, 227.

BOWMAN, J. M. & POLLOCK, J. M. (1965). Amniotic fluid spectrophotometry and early delivery in the management of erythroblastosis foetalis. *Pediatrics*, **35**, 815.

CAMPBELL, M. A., FERGUSON, I. C., HUTCHISON, J. H. & KERR, M. M. (1967). Diagnosis and treatment of hypoglycaemia in the newborn. *Arch. Dis. Childh.* **42**, 353.

CATZEL, P. (1963). *Paediatric Prescriber*, 2nd Ed. Oxford: Blackwell.

CLARKE, C. A. (1967). Prevention of Rh-haemolytic disease. *Br. med. J.* **4**, 7.

CORNBLATH, M. & SCHWARTZ, R. (1966). *Disorders of Carbohydrate Metabolism in Infancy*. London: Saunders.

GUTHRIE, R. & SUSI, A. (1963). A simple phenylalanine method for detecting phenylketonuria in large populations of newborn infants. *Pediatrics*, **32**, 338.

HUTCHISON, J. H. (1967). *Practical Paediatric Problems*, 2nd Ed. London: Lloyd-Luke.

KOMROWER, G. (1969). Metabolic abnormalities and mental retardation. *Br. J. hosp. Med.* **2**, 840.

LILEY, A. W. (1965). The use of amniocentesis and fetal transfusion in erythroblastosis fetalis. *Pediatrics*, **35**, 836.

SHELDON, Sir W. (1969). Prognosis in early adult life of coeliac children. *Br. med. J.* **2**, 401.

SIMPSON, H. & FLENLEY, D. C. (1967). Arterial blood-gas tensions and *p*H in acute lower-respiratory-tract infections in infancy and childhood. *Lancet*, **1**, 7.

SMALLPIECE, V. & DAVIES, P. A. (1964). Immediate feeding of premature infants with undiluted breast-milk. *Lancet*, **2**, 1349.

TANNER, J. M. (1970). Standards for birth weight or intrauterine growth. *Pediatrics*, **46**, 1.

20. The Care of Old People

S. ALSTEAD and W. F. ANDERSON

ATTITUDE OF THE DOCTOR

The sense of well-being, reflecting the composite character of health, is not the prerogative of the young and robust. It is conspicuous in the prime of life; and though the pattern derived from its component parts changes with advancing years it is not extinguished by the gradual onset of the physiological state of senescence. The doctor should, therefore, impress on the relatives that changes in the health of old people must be regarded as the result of disease and not dismissed as 'signs of old age'. Further, when this outlook is genuinely accepted and implemented by the doctor, he becomes increasingly aware that medical practice among old people does not differ essentially from practice among other patients. The efficiency of the geriatrician is primarily determined by his skill in diagnosis and treatment; and by applying conventional methods he can expect outright cure in a substantial proportion of his older patients. In the practice of medicine complete objectivity on the part of the doctor is rarely possible, and perhaps even more rarely is it desirable. Those who take care of old people are under a special obligation to identify themselves with the problems inseparable from illness in the later decades of life. Treatment on conventional lines must be amplified: it includes appropriate instruction to patients on how to adapt themselves to the limitations imposed on their physical and mental activities by the degenerative processes of senescence; and it is inevitable that stress should be placed on the *prevention* of physical deterioration, accidents and illness. Such work is exacting. It is seldom enlivened by the results so often achieved in other branches of therapy such as operative surgery, but it calls for a good deal of forbearance and resourcefulness. The intelligent anticipation of individual requirements is often rewarding. In the five years that precede retirement many people benefit greatly by deliberate planning and by availing themselves of instruction in the subject at lectures and by reading. Part-time work undertaken by elderly people after retirement—if employment is desired—undoubtedly contributes to the maintenance of physical and mental health.

The aged person, when sick, often presents a double challenge to the doctor: in addition to the disabilities of senescence there may be an independent disease with a pathological basis in no way different from that occurring in younger people. There is a much greater likelihood that physical examination will reveal unsuspected abnormalities —findings which may or may not have a bearing on the patient's complaint. It is, therefore, imperative to make a full and comprehensive examination on seeing a new patient, and in addition rectal examination and gynaecological assessment should be matters of routine. At the same time diagnosis must be realistic. The physician should record his considered opinion regarding the significance of any abnormality in terms of disability. A woman suffering from scirrhous cancer of the breast may in fact have become a permanent resident in hospital because she has painful feet caused by corns. In deciding on the kind of management needed, the numerical age of the patient is not infrequently the least important guide. The restoration of health and independence is the objective to be kept clearly in view, and the fullest use should be made of all the faculties that remain.

THE NATURAL HISTORY OF AGEING

Some knowledge of the range of the normal bodily functions in the last decades of life is obviously necessary for the physician who undertakes the care of the aged. The subject, however, has until recently received comparatively little attention from clinicians. The classic descriptions of the physical and mental changes that accompany old age have been written by laymen, among whom Shakespeare and Cicero are pre-eminent. Little is known of the physiological processes of aging. Haranghy has investigated the physical and mental condition of 23 centenarians: six were bedridden; the others were apparently healthy, apart from involutional changes and some decrease in the function of the sense organs. It has been claimed that ageing is associated with progressive loss of cells in many of the viscera; and atrophy is attributed to inadequacy of blood supply or to impairment of specific enzyme systems. In addition to tissue ischaemia other mechanisms have been proposed to account for ageing; they include auto-immune disease, radiation, mutational events and other conditions. Daily experience in the post-mortem room suffices to show that these concepts are seldom relevant to the problem in hand. The difficulty does not lie in demonstrating degenerative disease, but rather in determining why one or other of the lesions should suddenly have precipitated the patient's death. It would appear that the solution of the mystery of death in old age will come from a fuller understanding of the biochemical mechanism of cellular metabolism rather than from histological study.

Survival to advanced old age does, of course, increase the chance of developing more than one type of pathological abnormality. This is often apparent at autopsies. Lesions may be discovered which are gross in character and of different aetiologies; and some of these may have gone undetected while the patient was alive. Such experience serves to remind the physician of the special importance of careful and systematic examination of old people in order to avoid overlooking pathological conditions which may be clinically 'silent'. It has been well said that more mistakes are made by not looking than by not knowing. Sometimes diseases are easily diagnosed because they are rare and create a clinical picture that is consistent from one case to another. On the other hand, in elderly patients common ailments often present with atypical symptoms and lead to misdiagnosis.

Again, after long experience of this kind of work, the physician and the pathologist tend to share the view that while it is not surprising that people die of their diseases, it is astonishing that they are able to live for months or even years despite the presence of advanced disease.

Excessive dyspnoea on exertion in old people is attributable to a reduction in the vital capacity of the lungs brought about by increasing rigidity of the thoracic cage; but the results of tests of respiratory function in some old people may be of doubtful value. Contributing factors in the cardiovascular system are progressive loss of elastic tissue in the blood vessels and deterioration in capillary function resulting in impairment of the peripheral circulation. If other abnormalities supervene such as pulmonary infection or emphysema, there is likely to be a disproportionate increase in the severity of dyspnoea and distress. Anderson and Cowan reporting on arterial pressure in symptomless old people studied 306 men and 240 women. They

concluded that mean systolic and diastolic pressures increase with age and that this change is greater in the systolic readings. In the ninth decade of life systolic pressures as high as 220 mm. in men and 230 mm. in women, and diastolic pressures of up to 105 mm. were found; but it is also emphasized that there is a wide range of blood pressure in healthy old people. From what has been said above it is not surprising that in old age the heart is often found to be enlarged; this may be obvious on clinical or radiological examination, but due regard must be paid to the effects of kyphoscoliosis, chest deformity and emphysema on apparent heart size. Cardiac failure in old people is commonly associated with progressive coronary artery occlusion and consequent myocardial ischaemia. Another precipitating factor is coronary thrombosis. This occurs more frequently than is commonly supposed as many cases are 'silent' and are identified only by full investigation. Again, it is by no means rare to find in the last decades of life the typical signs of rheumatic valvular disease (with or without cardiac decompensation) dating from an infection some 50 years previously. Pomerance found cardiac amyloidosis at necropsy in 10 per cent. of subjects aged over 80 years and in 50 per cent. of those over 90. Congestive cardiac failure had been recorded in 5 out of 21 of the cases described, and presumably amyloidosis had caused or aggravated the disability during life. It is also possible that unsuspected amyloid degeneration of the myocardium accounts for excessive sensitivity to digoxin.

Physical examination of the nervous system in apparently healthy old people by different observers has revealed considerable discrepancies. W. F. Anderson and his colleagues in Glasgow surveyed 592 people over 60 years of age. Abnormalities were found in only a small minority. Five per cent. had loss of one or more tendon reflexes. There was complete loss of vibration sense at the malleoli and knees in only 2 per cent., and in a further 2 per cent. there was partial loss at these sites; but none had lost vibration sense at the elbows and wrists. Again, in this series, none showed abnormal pupillary reactions that could be attributed to senescence. Nisbet's observations made on the pupillary reflex in patients over the age of 80 at Foresthall Hospital, Glasgow, showed that only 30 per cent. failed to react. A much higher incidence of neurological abnormalities had been recorded some 10 years earlier by Howell, but here the subjects were a fairly homogeneous social group—

340 Chelsea Pensioners. Muscle power, assessed by the hand-grip, decreases with age. Anderson and Cowan found that in men and women hand-grip pressure is significantly related to body weight and age.

Obvious involvement of the kidneys by arteriosclerosis as seen at autopsy is compatible with a clinical record which reveals no evidence of florid impairment of renal function (de Wardener; Strauss and Welt).

In the lungs, rhonchi are fairly common. These signs must have significance in terms of infection or other pathological states, but it is often true that they are not accompanied by pulmonary symptoms. A more serious view should be taken of crepitations—which may, of course, be part of a clinical picture of pneumonia or the heralds of approaching cardiac failure. Increased pigmentation of the skin is common and is most marked in those who have lived in dirty and verminous conditions. Ecchymoses are often found on the wrists and the back of the hands; the exposed extremities may well be more liable to trauma on account of the thin, inelastic skin and the loss of subcutaneous tissue which are characteristic of advanced old age. Deafness, defective vision and occasional incontinence of urine are also noted in surveys of the health of the aged. At rest in bed the normal body temperature is about 36° C., and therefore a temperature at or below the conventional normal of 37° C. may in fact be a sign of low-grade fever; this conclusion can, of course, be reached only in retrospect. The physiological reaction of the body to a cold environment is often defective in old people. In consequence they may be the victims of accidental hypothermia. If the body temperature is below 35° C., a firm diagnosis of hypothermia can be made (p. 505). A low-reading thermometer should always be available to doctors and nurses who look after old people.

Many observers have commented on the frequency of progressive decalcification of the skeleton. Thus among old people, minor injuries may cause fractures; and it is important to remember that in contrast to the clinical picture in middle age, even a fractured femur may be accompanied by symptoms that are trifling. The patient may complain chiefly of loss of power in the affected limb, and in fracture of the femur pain may be referred to the knee. The process of decalcification is accelerated by prolonged rest in bed and by immobilization of limbs. Foods rich in available calcium must be given (one pint of milk daily and green vegetables)—even though radiological evidence of response to therapy is slow to appear. Osteoporosis of uncertain origin is particularly common among elderly women. Nurses who look after them should be warned that sudden or forceful movements of the limbs may easily fracture them. Diminished glucose tolerance is often demonstrable and glycosuria is not uncommon (2 per cent. in Anderson's series). The obese patient with mild diabetes responds well to dietetic management aimed at weight reduction (p. 319). In aged diabetics hyperosmolar coma (without ketosis) is an occasional occurrence. Ketonuria without glycosuria is usually due to starvation. Achlorhydria is common but the view that it may be a cause of diarrhoea among the aged is no longer widely held; the usual causes of enteritis—especially contaminated food—are certainly more important. Treatment should not begin until a rectal examination has been carried out. Not infrequently old people are stated to be suffering from 'enteritis' or 'achlorhydric diarrhoea' when digital examination of the rectum reveals that the essential abnormality is impaction of scybala and a recurring overflow of liquid faeces (p. 501). This type of diarrhoea may recur unless the patient's diet is adjusted by including fresh food (raw fruit and green vegetables), thus ensuring the daily evacuation of a normal stool.

MANAGEMENT OF OLD PEOPLE IN THEIR OWN HOMES

Except in special circumstances, the fewer old people who live in institutions the better for all concerned; and it is significant that more than 95 per cent. of old people live in their own homes. The importance of the family doctor's rôle in preventive medicine, as this bears on the management of the aged, can scarcely be exaggerated; his courteous and considerate attitude to the older members of the family encourages the others to discharge their obligations with good grace. Sound advice offered by relatives is often ignored by old folk until the same guidance comes from the doctor—when it is regarded as treatment and accepted without demur. Thus the general practitioner can do a great deal to maintain old people's activities and hobbies and their interest in local affairs. He can foster a wider appreciation of the dignity of old age; he can strengthen self-respect in old people, and he has unrivalled opportunities to defend them against ridicule and humiliation. He should emphasize to the household the importance of safeguarding the aged from infection by relatives and others suffering from the common cold. Steps should be taken to ensure that food is protected against fly-borne infections.

The doctor's chief aim should be to prevent the bedfast state, notwithstanding the timidity and even the opposition of the old person and the family. Men who retire should be warned of the danger they run in abandoning *routine*; too great an attachment for the dressing-gown and soft slippers, an unkempt appearance and a perpetual vagueness about the day's arrangements are grave prognostic signs. Such simple activities as getting up betimes and dressing properly, taking a modest part in the household duties, going out for walks, attending church service and visiting the bowling green or club are all valuable in preventing boredom and lethargy which predispose to physical deterioration. The whole policy should be directed towards creating independence.

Education

The great majority of industrial workers are compulsorily retired at 60 to 65. It has consequently become apparent that many people need lectures on the art of enjoying their enforced leisure and in avoiding the perils of too much idleness. Courses of instruction organized by local authorities and other bodies are often invaluable. In some districts there are also centres where hobbies and crafts are taught to classes of retired persons. Retired employees' associations are also helpful in maintaining continuity of relationship between former members of a firm. Some industrial concerns now have re-employment schemes under which a retired employee can work for one day a week and receive for this a full day's pay. This is excellent for morale. In some parts of the country voluntary organizations run agencies which help retired workers to find part-time employment if they desire this.

The Active Life

The relatives should refrain from doing too much for the old person. These varied activities and gentle exercise out of doors promote sound sleep at night. Outdoor shoes must be checked periodically (say at the end of each month) to see that footwear is serviceable and comfortable. It has been established beyond question that the most

important single measure in preventing incontinence and many other disabilities is to keep the patient on his feet. Another major disaster which is liable to overtake the neglected bedridden patient is contracture deformity of the legs. The limbs ultimately become fully flexed at the knees and the thighs are brought up towards the abdomen. This complication adds to the patient's misery and greatly increases the difficulty of nursing. Fortunately, in many parts of the world where geriatric medicine has become established, these appalling sequelae to the bedridden state are largely prevented.

The gospel of mobility should not, of course, be carried to extremes. Like most other people the elderly need periods of peace and quiet; and with a little forethought this should not be difficult to arrange, even in a large and busy household. A rest, lying down, in the middle of the day is preferable to going to bed too early at night. On the other hand, too much sleep during the day is a common cause of insomnia at night, and in these circumstances hypnotics may be used unnecessarily. The old person should, therefore, set a limit to the afternoon rest period. This can be done by making a routine of re-joining the household for tea—say at 4 p.m.; and if he can take outdoor exercise thereafter so much the better. The domestic arrangements should be reviewed, and some attention should be give to minor structural alterations which can often make life easier and safer for old people. For example, it is a great advantage to have the bedroom near the bathroom and on the same floor. Suitable handrails can be put up in difficult places. Local authorities are now permitted to adapt houses to suit a disabled elderly person by installing handrails, adjusting the height of a kitchen sink or providing rails round a W.C. Highly polished floors, especially if they have loose rugs on them, should not be tolerated. Where the gas or electricity supply is controlled by a slot-meter this should be easily accessible. Sometimes the tenant has to stand on a chair or mount a ladder in order to insert a coin in the meter. This practice creates a serious hazard for old people. The appropriate authority is usually willing to consider a doctor's recommendation that a badly sited meter should be made accesible. The need for adequate lighting on stairs is often overlooked. Similarly, a light should be provided near the old person's coat peg and cupboard—so often relegated to dark corners and hence common sites for accidents. The use of high shelves should be forbidden as the reaching up—accompanied by hyperextension of the cervical spine—may aggravate vertebral artery insufficiency and cause a syncopal attack.

Amenities

Attention to minor amenities pays handsome dividends: a comfortable armchair suited to the patient's particular needs; a book-rest that lies across the arms of the chair; a convenient cupboard for his exclusive use where books, papers and other personal belongings can be kept; easy access to an extra blanket during the night; a bedside commode; a rubber-ferruled walking-stick or, for greater stability, the three- or four-legged walking-stick; and when a radio loudspeaker would cause inconvenience to others, the use of light-weight headphones, an ear-piece or the pillow-phone may prove acceptable. The same principle can be applied to television. These are some of the special requirements of older people, but it is scarcely necessary to add that individual needs vary. Apparatus such as a commode, bedpans or rubber sheets can be obtained on loan from the district nursing association. In suitable circumstances the domiciliary services of the local authority should be used. In discussing amenities, vague generalizations are reprehensible. There is a place for two or three short conferences between doctor, patient and a sensible relative who is genuinely interested. The outcome should be a concise memorandum written by the doctor, listing the items that apply to the particular patient.

Health Propaganda

Doctors can also perform a useful service as citizens by drawing the attention of town councillors to the medical aspects of house construction. For example, in some new houses the staircase is excessively steep. This alone can result in hardship for tenants when they are old and perhaps suffering from physical disabilities. A great deal of practical help and advice is available to the family doctor through the Director of Social Work, the Hospital Service (especially if there is an active geriatric department), and through voluntary organizations such as the Old People's Welfare Committee. Such matters are of great importance, but further discussion would be out of place in this book.

Common Complaints

Stiffness and slowness of movement are common, especially for the first hour or two of the day. The disability is attributable to the replacement of elastic tissue by fibrous tissue in the structures around the joints, and this is a characteristic of senescence. No special treatment is called for, as the symptoms are usually alleviated by gentle excercise. If, however, stiffness persists it may lead to an excessive limitation of movement, in which case a short course of physiotherapy is indicated: exercises are most important; massage is sometimes helpful; and local heat (radiant heat, wax baths) is of some value—though a few patients obtain more relief from cold compresses to the affected joint. Painful feet often result from callosities and other minor abnormalities which are amenable to treatment by the chiropodist. Peripheral vascular disease is sometimes accompanied by troublesome paraesthesia in the feet, and patients may complain bitterly of a burning sensation and of 'pins and needles' which are most severe at night when the feet are warm in bed. Some relief may be obtained from keeping the feet exposed to the cool air. Local applications are useless, but washing the feet in tepid water before retiring and on rising in the morning is helpful. Footwear should not be too heavy, and tight lacing of the shoes or boots should be avoided. In this condition leather soles are recommended rather than rubber ones. Drugs are of limited value. Nicotinic acid in doses of 50 to 100 mg. twice or three times daily may be tried as a means of causing vasodilatation. Excessive sympathomimetic activity of smooth muscle (in blood vessels) can sometimes be reduced by means of tolazoline hydrochloride. The first dose should be 25 mg. by mouth after food, but up to 200 mg. may be given daily in divided doses. If tolazoline hydrochloride causes gastric irritation and nausea, nicotinyl alcohol may be tried as an alternative; it is available as an injection (100 to 200 mg. in ampoules containing 50 mg. per ml.). In severe cases, and where the general condition of the patient warrants it, lumbar sympathectomy should be considered (p. 140).

Muscular cramps, especially in calf muscles, are common in old people and are sometimes relieved by tolazoline hydrochloride—which is more effective than quinine. The normal hygiene of the skin, hair and nails should be maintained. Particular attention should be paid to cleanliness of the genitalia and perineum, and the routine of thorough washing with soap and warm water after defaecation should be urged. The cationic germicides such as benzalkonium chloride inhibit the growth of ammonia-producing bacteria in the urine and can therefore be used as a wash (1 : 5,000 to 1 : 1,000) to relieve dermatitis of the perineum and buttocks. The daily use of dusting-powder to prevent intertrigo is important especially in obese subjects and in women with pendulous breasts. The use of lamb's wool is highly effective in keeping the epidermis dry and wholesome where skin surfaces are in apposition; cotton—in the form of 'cotton-wool'—quickly becomes soggy and should not be used. Calamine lotion and methylated spirit in equal parts is an effective remedy for intertrigo. In resistant cases crystal violet should be ordered as crystal violet paint B.N.F. This should be used only under the direction of the district nurse; it is a messy preparation and when it is used for the treatment of old people firm supervision is necessary to prevent disagreeable complications.

Dizziness is a fairly common and distressing symptom, especially in advanced old age. It alarms the relatives no less than the patient and is often urged as a reason for transfer to hospital. The word 'dizziness' is used by old people to describe the effects of different clinical syndromes. Rarely it means true rotational vertigo; more commonly it is the light-headedness of postural hypotension resulting from delayed vasomotor adjustment to standing up suddenly; and ' dizziness' may also be mentioned when the patient really means the sense of insecurity and instability that result from weakness of the leg muscles. The disability may be aggravated by continuous cerebral ischaemia which is the consequence of partial occlusion of the main cerebral arteries and the basilar artery. There is also the possibility that 'dizziness' may be the consequence of drug therapy, for example following the administration of barbiturates and antihypertensive preparations. Johnson and colleagues have shown that in some old people postural hypotension accompanies cerebrovascular disease. The patients are thought to be suffering from the effects of blocking of baroreceptor reflexes. Many of them benefit from graduated exercises involving changes of posture. Elastic stockings may be helpful. The blood pressure should always be recorded in the standing position and while recumbent. Dehydration in such patients must be avoided and drugs such as chlorpromazine used with extreme care.

It appears also that in many cases 'dizziness' is the result of lack of concentration on the business of purposive bodily movement, and this can some-

times be remedied by firm and explicit instructions from the doctor. Again, it is well known that an old person while reading or even while at table may 'nod off to sleep' for half a minute or so. If, on wakening, he immediately tries to stand and to walk (often merely in an attempt to cover his embarrassment) there may be marked unsteadiness which is inaccurately described as 'dizziness'.

The effects of dizziness are aggravated in an old person because after stumbling he lacks the agility to respond rapidly enough to postural reflexes. He must learn to avoid sudden changes of posture. Severe exacerbations call for a couple of days' rest in bed and then gradual rehabilitation. Dimenhydrinate appears to be of no value in this condition. Reasonable precautions should be taken to minimize the danger of falling. For example, the constant use of a fireguard is imperative. At the same time, the doctor should urge the relatives not to make too much of this handicap. The patient may be reassured by recalling that many energetic and distinguished men have continued to live (and work) to a ripe old age despite the inconvenience of such bouts of dizziness. No active treatment of any value is known, but the Cawthorne-Cooksey exercises used in the management of Ménière's syndrome for the improvement of labyrinthine function are worthy of trial. This regimen is indicated only when true vertigo is present.

Deafness and defective vision call for thorough examination on conventional lines. As remedial measures—such as removal of wax from the ears—may confer untold benefits on the aged, relatives and doctors should not dismiss these disabilities as the incurable stigmata of senility without giving the matter careful consideration.

The onset of *mental confusion* in an old person creates a problem in differential diagnosis. It may be due to senile dementia, cerebral arteriosclerosis, but it may also occur as one manifestation of a cerebrovascular catastrophe. Mental confusion therefore warrants immediate examination of the central nervous system. Strachan and Henderson described a broad spectrum of mental abnormality due to vitamin B_{12} deficiency in the absence of anaemia, megaloblastic erythropoiesis or any clinical evidence of subacute combined degeneration. The incipient toxaemia of undiagnosed infection (pneumonia, pyelonephritis, deep-seated abscess, etc.) may also precipitate mental confusion. Hypothyroidism is an occasional cause and, in an old person, it is easily overlooked. Nisbet has noticed that mental confusion may occur in old people when they experience the physical discomfort of a distended bladder, and that this precedes any rise in blood urea. Distress associated with abnormalities of other viscera may present as a state of mental confusion—for example, a loaded rectum, severe tympanites, gross effusions into the serous sacs, etc. The misinterpretation of mental confusion associated with visceral abnormalities may lead to a catastrophe for the patient and humiliation for the doctor. The only safeguard is repeated and careful physical examination and adequate documentation. The unskilful use of drugs is a fairly common cause of mental confusion in old people. Hyoscine, bromides and barbiturates are best avoided, as they are more likely to aggravate than to relieve the symptoms. If hypnotics must be used, chloral hydrate (1·5 g.) or glutethimide (500 mg.) are to be preferred. Chloral hydrate should be well diluted and flavoured with syrup of ginger. Newer preparations which have now become established as hypnotics and which can be used for old people include dichloralphenazone (500 mg. to 2 g.) and triclofos (500 mg. to 2 g.). There is also a syrup of triclofos which is useful for elderly people. For confusion with agitation thioridazine, 10 to 50 mg. thrice daily, is usually effective. It is conveniently given as a syrup. If an immediate action is required the Injection of Chlorpromazine Hydrochloride should be used: it is given intramuscularly or intravenously—not subcutaneously. This is preferable to the intramuscular injection of paraldehyde—often a very painful experience for the conscious patient.

Depression. Progressive cerebrovascular disease may be accompanied by depression and the risk of suicide. These circumstances warrant consultation with a psychiatrist. If depression is a conspicuous symptom an appreciation of adverse circumstances (for example, in the home) may be far more important than drug therapy. A diagnosis of depression sometimes presents difficulties: a patient may be well aware of his plight and may strive to disguise the true position by assuming a mask of cheerfulness and optimism when in the company of friends or when he is visited by his doctor. In general the anti-depressive drugs—such as imipramine hydrochloride (p. 425)—are prescribed only for the management of exacerbations of symptoms. The monoamine oxidase inhibitors are best reserved for the treatment of patients in hospital. Occasionally thioridazine in doses of 10 mg.

three times daily is useful for patients suffering from depression accompanied by agitation; it should not be used for the withdrawn and apathetic depressive.

Cardiac failure, usually associated with hypertension or with progressive occlusion of the coronary arteries, is a common cause of restlessness and persistent attempts to get out of bed. In such cases it is also necessary to remember that drugs of the digitalis group, if given in excess, readily cause mental confusion in old people. It is commonly noted that the elderly become mentally confused on transfer from familiar surroundings to the hospital ward; but in some cases they are simply bewildered. Not every patient who is apparently restless is abnormal; an old person may be convinced with good reason that he should visit the bathroom. A patient's behaviour when overtaken by cerebral softening probably reflects somewhat on the skill of the physician and nurses who have cared for him. Excessively rigorous suppression of the restless patient is often followed by violent resistance. In these matters judgment and experience count greatly, but the Shakespearian injunction is worth remembering:

> Fetter strong madness in a silken thread,
> Charm ache with air, and agony with words.

In old people the beneficial effects of the digitalis glycosides (p. 85) can be produced by relatively small doses. After the initial loading dose of digoxin aimed at abolishing gross cardiac failure, a maintenance dose of 0·25 mg. once daily for three to five days per week may suffice. If more is needed the drug should be given every day; and an additional dose of 0·25 mg. can be ordered on alternate days. As in younger patients, the most striking effects are seen in patients with cardiac failure accompanied by atrial fibrillation. If the heart is in sinus rhythm the therapeutic effect is usually less dramatic and the benefits less obvious. In such circumstances the physician must decide in the course of a few days whether it is worth while to continue the treatment. In old people the toxic effects of the digitalis group of drugs (p. 87) are commonly overlooked; their effects have been studied by Dall. Powerful diuretics such as mersalyl, the thiazides and frusemide are of great value in the management of cardiac insufficiency in old people; and the skilful use of these drugs may prevent nocturnal dyspnoea and other distressing manifestations of left ventricular failure. The danger of causing hypokalaemia by this type of treatment is a special hazard among old people. Many old people with a history of several episodes of congestive failure are more likely to respond to diuretics than to digitalis glycosides.

Patients who develop cerebrovascular catastrophes (other than minor lesions with fleeting symptoms) should be admitted to hospital as medical emergencies. They require continuous expert nursing and orthopaedic management to prevent overstretching and damage to paralysed muscles; and the first phase of physiotherapy should be started at once (p. 373). The hygiene and feeding of the helpless patient, who is often unconscious and incontinent, can rarely be undertaken satisfactorily in a private house. Depletion of the patient's tissue fluids can often be corrected by giving physiological saline by subcutaneous drip with hyaluronidase. Failure to admit such patients to hospital prejudices the patient's chances of recovery and diminishes the effectiveness of a course of rehabilitation.

Anticoagulant drugs have been used in the hope of preventing the extension of thrombosis in the cerebral vessels. However, this form of treatment is potentially dangerous in these circumstances: it may convert a self-limiting thrombosis into a fatal cerebral haemorrhage. In practice it is wise to restrict anticoagulant therapy to cases of undoubted cerebral embolism and to those patients in whom cerebral thrombosis is characterized by a 'stuttering onset' (Barham Carter).

Sensitivity to cold. Old people are usually very sensitive to cold and draughts, and this is explained partly by their relative inactivity and partly because of the alterations in their cutaneous vasomotor responses. Adequate and suitable clothing is therefore essential, but a regimen which includes gentle exercise in the fresh air should be encouraged rather than the practice of seeking comfort in an excessive amount of clothing and a stuffy room. One of the peculiar things about the behaviour of old people is that they are very fond of an open coal fire, but they often find it too warm to sit in the sun. Many old people who complain excessively about feeling cold are inviting attention to the fact that they are suffering from myxoedema or anaemia. Characteristically these diseases advance so insidiously that the patient's relatives may fail to notice any change, or having observed some deterioration they dismiss it as being mere evidence of senility.

Malnutrition. The dietetic habits of old people vary widely. In institutions they often eat voraciously—perhaps because they have little else to interest them—but in general they eat sparingly. Lack of outdoor exercise contributes to this. Another factor in many instances is the reluctance of the old, in their own homes, to go to the necessary trouble to obtain varied and well-cooked meals, thus gradually eliminating most fresh foods from their diet. On inquiry it is often found that old people (and especially the edentulous) have eaten no apples, pears or citrus fruits for years. This may be a serious matter, especially among old men who live by themselves or in lodging houses, for after a year or two they may develop scurvy with gross anaemia, oedema and sheet haemorrhages in the legs. In the 15-year period 1940-54 there were at least 100 cases of frank scurvy admitted to one general hospital in Glasgow (Thomson). The use of daily vitamin supplements (see B.N.F.) is often justified because of the reluctance of such people to change their eating habits, and because—in Great Britain at least—the price of fresh fruit is almost prohibitive; and in institutions diets tend to contain too little vitamin C. Osteomalacia also occurs and is thought to be due to deficiency of vitamin D in the diet and lack of exposure to sunlight (Anderson and colleagues). There is also evidence that folic acid deficiency is not uncommon (Read and colleagues).

Recent work (Judge) suggests that many elderly people have an inadequate dietary intake of potassium with consequent muscle weakness, apathy, and impaired intellectual function; such individuals are unduly sensitive to digitalis preparations and are easily precipitated into frank hypokalaemia by diuretics. Some loss of weight occurs in the majority of old people, but sudden or marked loss of weight calls for careful investigation. Chronic alcoholism in the elderly is often associated with marked loss of weight as the victim prefers to spend money on alcohol rather than on food. Obesity in old age is rare among men—probably because it is a liability which seriously reduces the chances of survival among those who have hard work to do. On the other hand, if women lapse into a vegetative existence as their domestic responsibilities diminish they are likely to become obese—especially if they fall into the common habit of eating large amounts of bread and butter, jam and cakes. Anderson and Cowan, who studied obesity in older women, concluded that when the body weight is more than 24 per cent. above the ideal weight (judged by height and weight), the blood pressure is significantly higher than that of women of normal weight. Most old people are well advised to make breakfast and a midday dinner their main meals. They usually sleep better at night if they go to bed after a light carbohydrate meal. In the daily dietary it is important to maintain an adequate intake of protein in the form of meat, fish or eggs and to eat fats sparingly, but for some old people lack of money may make this advice difficult to follow. Further support for these views has been provided by Exton-Smith and Stanton. In old people, fluid intake is often grossly inadequate and this may partly explain the frequent occurrence of constipation and faecal impaction. Tea and coffee and large volumes of fluid are, of course, to be avoided after about 6 o'clock in the evening to reduce nocturnal frequency of micturition. This is particularly important in old age in view of the tendency to a diminishing bladder capacity in the later decades of life.

The management of *constipation* is dealt with elsewhere (pp. 247, 504). Old people usually have a fixed habit in this matter of bowel movements, and if they are accustomed to taking a laxative regularly it is usually unwise to interfere with the ritual. When a patient comes under medical care on account of 'constipation' he should be investigated fully and a rectal examination made before purgatives are ordered. Liquid paraffin has been incriminated as an occasional cause of malnutrition and colitis when taken daily over a long period of years, but this does not preclude its occasional use. It is best taken in doses of a teaspoonful four times a day after food, as large single doses are liable to result in leakage through the anus. In debilitated old people there is a danger that this bland oil may be aspirated from the pharynx into the respiratory tract and accumulate at the bases of the lungs. The anthracenes are probably the most satisfactory purgatives for regular use by the old, and the preparation Senokot is widely regarded as effective and reliable; alternatively magnesium hydroxide mixture may be used. On occasion, glycerin suppositories may be tried, as their irritant action is restricted to the rectum and the risk of causing diarrhoea is reduced. Beogex is a suppository which, in the presence of moisture in the rectum, releases carbon dioxide and precipitates immediate evacuation in mild cases of faecal impaction. As an alternative to anthracene laxatives, acetphenolisatin and related compounds are in common use. They are oxyphenisatin acetate

(10 mg. orally) and bisacodyl (10 mg. orally); the suppositories of bisacodyl contain 5 or 10 mg. In general practice the use of 'disposable enemata' is often a time-saving aid to the district nurse; they are available as a retention enema (arachis oil 130 ml.) or an evacuant enema (sodium diphosphate 10 g. and sodium phosphate 8 g.). The doctor must be alert to recognize cases of spurious diarrhoea caused by faecal impaction. The rectum may be loaded with scybalous masses and the irritation set up causes the patient to pass frequent liquid motions. It is usually necessary to remove these masses digitally after lubrication with liquid paraffin. Thereafter, neostigmine, 15 mg. by mouth, twice daily after meals for a few days is useful in preventing recurrence: this type of constipation scarcely warrants the use of irritant purgatives.

The *onset of actual illness* is a signal for immediate investigation and treatment. One of the hazards to which the aged are exposed is the practice among the laity to attribute all ill-health to the patient's advanced age and to defer seeking medical help. Old people are, of course, susceptible to most of the diseases that afflict those of middle age, such as pneumonia, cholecystitis, hypertensive heart failure, infection of the urinary tract, arthritis, etc., and appropriate treatment for such conditions is described elsewhere in this book. The early use of antibiotics, e.g. penicillin, in the first few hours of respiratory tract infections is often valuable, even though it may only prevent the spread of secondary invaders. Elderly men, thought to be suffering from chronic bronchitis, are sometimes found to have pulmonary tuberculosis.

Radiological examination of the chest as a routine procedure in the first clinical assessment of all old people is the best safeguard against this serious error. If symptoms persist the X-ray examination of the chest should be repeated. Miliary tuberculosis in the elderly commonly presents as pyrexia of unknown origin accompanied by restlessness and loss of weight (Proudfoot and colleagues).

In the care of old people in their homes experience teaches the importance of rapid assessment in cases of mental confusion, incontinence, inability to walk, and when there are complaints (even of a minor character) following falls and other injuries. A fall may be the prelude to a wide variety of illnesses in elderly people. It warrants making a careful examination for evidence of an underlying cause such as infection, toxaemia, cardiovascular disease or even the presence of a malignant tumour. The onset of depression calls for the expert guidance of a psychiatrist (p. 425).

The care of the dying often provides a searching test not only of the physician's professional skill but also of his personal qualities. It has been well said that 'a painful death-bed is a reproach to the doctor'. Periodic re-examination is often more rewarding than might be expected. Minor complications and disabilities may be discovered. When effective treatment can be given these patients are often profoundly grateful, though realizing that the therapy is purely palliative. And even when nothing new is found, the ritual of physical examination may itself bring consolation to incurables. Perhaps it serves to confirm that the doctor possesses special knowledge and techniques and that these are always at the disposal of the patient.

MANAGEMENT OF OLD PEOPLE IN HOSPITAL

Geriatrics and general medicine. Much that has been said about the attitude of the practitioner toward the aged (p. 493) applies also to the relationship between doctor and patient in hospital. There are illnesses which, among the aged and younger people, run much the same course and call for the facilities that are available only in hospitals. In such circumstances it is illogical to deprive the older person of the benefits of treatment in a medical or surgical ward. It is not practicable to discuss here the functions of general hospitals in this context: suffice it to say that prejudice dies hard. There is, however, a growing realization of the need for a positive and constructive policy to deal with the disabilities of old people, and a wider appreciation of some of the difficulties of medical practice among patients who no longer enjoy a sense of security within the social structure of the community. Such considerations have also affected profoundly current medical and administrative policy which seeks the best way of treating the increasing numbers of aged infirm people. It is generally agreed that the medical care of old people should fall within the scope of every practitioner; but it must also be conceded that if the great majority of general physicians find it irksome to look after the aged and the long-term sick, there is much to be said for segregating the aged in our hospitals so that they may benefit from the attention of doctors who display a sustained and lively interest in their welfare. Something of this attitude has been increasingly apparent in the changing structure of the medical services of the United Kingdom since 1948. Many general hospitals now make provision for geriatric units which specialize in the assessment and management of the disabilities of older people—disabilities that are often defined in terminology which is medico-social as well as pathological. The rise of geriatrics as a specialty has provided a notable chapter in the history of medicine. Not the least important aspect of geriatric medicine is the composite character of the subject; inevitably it cuts across the conventional lines of classification which originate in pathology or in techniques.

Progressive patient care. The hospital physician who is responsible for the care of a large number of people who are both old and ill, often finds it helpful to classify them into fairly homogeneous groups. It is desirable to have wards reserved for new admissions where diagnostic work and careful assessments can be made prior to prescribing courses of treatment. In geriatric hospital practice the concept of *progressive patient care* is being applied: after initial diagnosis and therapy, the patient may be transferred to another unit for rehabilitation and continuing treatment. If long-term hospital care is required—shown by the results of an adequate trial period—the patient is sent to a long-stay annexe. Patients who are ambulant but show mental impairment should share a ward, because elsewhere they are liable to upset sensible patients—though they do not worry one another. The psycho-geriatric group of patients deserves to be carefully surveyed by the hospital psychiatrist. This ensures that good judgment and long experience will be brought to bear on problems related to the best use of accommodation. Many of these ambulant but confused old people are now transferred from general hospitals or mental hospitals to purpose-built homes provided by forward-looking local authorities.

One result of the successful practice of geriatric medicine is that patients formerly known as 'bed-ridden/mentally normal' are now comparatively rare. The bed-ridden still exist, but they comprise largely those who are obviously dying, and those who are so grossly deranged through confusion or profound apathy (accompanied usually by incontinence) that they are out of touch with their surroundings and their attendants. Local authorities are playing a vital rôle in the care of the elderly by building homes specifically designed for frail old people.

Principles of management. There are few indications for modifying the general management of a patient in hospital merely on the grounds of old age. If the doctor's approach to diagnosis and treatment is the same as that adopted for patients in younger age-groups, he will seldom be far wrong in his handling of the case. This is merely a restatement of general policy as it bears on the practice of geriatrics in hospitals: the various techniques available to physicians and surgeons should be fully exploited for the benefit of the patient, irrespective of his age. Admission to hospital with a disabling illness often makes the old person acutely aware of the element of insecurity in his way of living. For the inmate of a lodging house a few weeks in hospital may prove on the whole a pleasant interlude in his primitive and drab existence; but when he is discharged from the ward as a convalescent he is apt to find himself more sensitive to the rigours of his normal surroundings and less able to fend for himself. Again the old person, living with his married son and his grandchildren, may for a long time remain oblivious to the problems that face the young parents committed to the responsibilities of raising a family. Illness, transfer to hospital, and recovery retarded by residual disability, may suddenly reveal to him that it is neither practicable nor fair to return 'home'—where his needs would place an intolerable burden on a family already embarrassed by inadequacy of accommodation. Thus it often happens that in the hospital ward the patient's problems (personal, domestic and social) rapidly crystallize out. The clinician is therefore obliged to look to the Medical Officer of Health, the Director of Social Work, the medical social worker, the priest or minister, and many others to help in meeting difficulties which may be complex.

As compared with a general medical or surgical unit, a geriatric ward is run on more informal lines; and this is appropriate to the outlook of patients who are advanced in years. In general, therapy proceeds at a slower tempo, but there is a good deal of activity in a geriatric ward; patients are encouraged to be up and about. The safety of all patients while in hospital has become a matter of considerable medico-legal importance, but there is clearly an obligation to take special precautions in the case of old people. For example, there is now no justification for exposing patients and their visitors to the hazards of slippery floors. In geriatric units to which acutely ill patients are admitted, it is highly desirable that there should be continuing treatment at a long-term annexe. Further, in these circumstances the services of physiotherapists, occupational therapists, speech therapists and medical social workers are indispensable. Geriatric physicians attach great importance to visits made to a patient's home before his admission to hospital and to follow-up visits after he has been discharged. The value of day hospitals and day centres as part of the total geriatric service is now established.

The diseases and disabilities most commonly encountered among the aged in hospital are: *degenerative diseases of the cardiovascular system* resulting in cardiac insufficiency, cerebrovascular catastrophes with paralysis, progressive arteriosclerotic dementia, and senile gangrene; *arthritis of various kinds*; *malignant disease*; and ill-health arising from *inadequate personal hygiene* and *faulty nutrition*. The immediate treatment of all these conditions will be found in the appropriate sections of this book. Certain problems, however, call for special comment:

Incontinence. The onset of intractable incontinence provides a strong indication for transferring a patient from his home to hospital. Few households can cope with the problems inherent in this situation. As already stated, when a patient is allowed to become bedridden, incontinence often follows sooner or later. A high proportion of patients who have developed this complication recover normal control of the sphincters when they have been taught to walk again; and some patients show improvement even at the stage of sitting in a chair for part of the day. During this phase of re-education the patient should wear protective clothing. The importance of this observation in relation to the prevention and treatment of incontinence is obvious. Further it should be noted that well-meaning but misguided relatives often keep old people in bed as part of the treatment of the incontinent state.

The following are common causes of urinary incontinence and call for appropriate treatment as an essential preliminary to re-education: (a) The most important cause of urinary incontinence is impairment of cerebral cortical control of the bladder resulting from organic cerebral disease, the toxaemia of acute illness, or psychological factors. The disability is associated with a diminished bladder

R

capacity. Isaacs and Walkey found that 80 per cent. of 118 doubly incontinent patients had brain damage, and 73 per cent. of 175 patients without brain damage were fully continent. (*b*) Gynaecological abnormalities including uterine prolapse and urethral caruncle. (*c*) Obstruction to outflow of urine due to prostatic hypertrophy in men, or overdistension of bladder with overflow incontinence in women; the bladder wall may be so thin and flabby that the distended bladder cannot be felt during routine palpation of the abdomen. In women carbachol orally 1 mg. daily increasing slowly to a maximum of 2 mg. three times per day may be effective in promoting emptying of the distended bladder. (*d*) If infection in the urinary tract is persistent it is wise to consider mechanical defects which cause partial obstruction to the flow of urine. Stones in the urinary tract are an occasional cause of intractable infection. Many elderly men are reported to be incontinent when in fact they are simply clumsy in handling the urinal and therefore soil the bed. Soiling of the skin with urine and faeces necessitates prompt and frequent attention from the nursing staff, not only for the immediate comfort of the patient but also to prevent maceration of the skin, infection and the development of pressure sores.

Many patients are classed as incontinent of faeces who have not in fact lost control of the sphincter but who have become unable to empty the rectum completely unless they are allowed an adequate amount of time. They should devote half an hour or so every day to the task of emptying the lower bowel completely, but at first it may be necessary to resort to the occasional use of a simple enema. They should be provided with a bedside commode and a screen, care being taken to ensure comfort and warmth, and the patient should be encouraged to read and smoke a pipe if he so desires. The McCullagh commode has proved to be satisfactory. Much can be done to prevent the inconvenience of incontinence by instituting in the ward a two-hourly round of urinals and bedpans, but this regimen depends on adequate staffing.

A common cause of faecal incontinence is loading of the rectum—faecal impaction. This is often revealed by the patients contaminating their hands with excreta. The importance of preliminary rectal examination must be emphasized. Incontinence pads and protective plastic clothing are available.

Hemiplegia. The first phase of treatment may be that of the unconscious patient (p. 385).

In any patient in whom difficulty in swallowing is suspected, it is essential that the first drink of water should be given by a doctor. Direct assessment of the patient's disability enables the doctor to give firm instructions about fluid therapy.

When the patient is sufficiently well to co-operate and when the pulse-rate and the temperature have settled, the procedures listed below are adopted step by step. The general principles of this treatment consist in preventing damage to paralysed muscles and maintaining the functional efficiency of all joints. Practical details should be obtained from manuals of orthopaedics and physiotherapy.

1. The immediate institution of *passive movement*, all joints being put through a full range of movement twice daily.
2. The use of the Balkan beam or the Guthrie-Smith frame to permit of suspension and extension of the affected limbs.
3. The encouragement of *active movement* as recovery occurs, and the maintenance of power in all other muscles of locomotion, including those of the trunk.
4. Transfer of the patient from bed to a chair for treatment as soon as it is feasible.
5. The use of exercises designed to teach the patient to raise himself from the sitting to the standing position (bed-end exercises).
6. Instruction by graduated exercises in walking, first with human assistance, then with mechanical aids and finally without help of any kind.

Graduated therapy of this kind is the key-note to policy in a geriatric unit. The theme is developed in various ways according to the needs of individual patients. When the skill and resourcefulness of the doctor are matched by the patient's character and doggedness, therapeutic results can indeed be remarkable. In adjusting themselves to a variety of disabilities there are matters of common interest to old people. Sessions of physiotherapy and re-education are necessarily brief, and, therefore, patients must be encouraged to practise their exercises in the wards and elsewhere. All who are concerned with the management of the patient regard it as a continuing responsibility to assess his progress and to decide how much of the day he can spend up and about in the ward. It is imperative that the old person should have serviceable shoes which are correct for size and fitting; many patients do not realize that though they are living in a hospital, bedroom slippers are not an adequate alternative to shoes. Appropriate footwear is indispensable if the patient is to reap the benefits of physiotherapy including bed-end exercises. There is a variety of appliances to facilitate walking—the Zimmer walk-aid, tripod and quadruped sticks, calipers, toe-springs, arm slings (for a paralysed limb that is an encumbrance). Great ingenuity has been exercised in devising equipment for the use of patients in geriatric wards and to facilitate the work of the staff who look after old people. A selection of these items is included as an Appendix to this chapter; this apparatus has become part of the standard equipment in the geriatric unit at Stobhill General Hospital, Glasgow. Publications devoted to geriatric practice are to be found in the medical libraries of most general hospitals. Some of these books can be recommended to the patients themselves or to members of the patient's household. They are listed on p. 508. They provide invaluable reference literature for the use of disabled but intelligent people—both at home and in hospital. There are sections which deal concisely with mobility, lifting, dressing, eating and drinking, recreation, domestic work, transport and the planning of accommodation in the home; advice is offered on alterations and appliances suitable for the bathroom, and the needs of the incontinent patient receive detailed consideration.

Contracture deformities. Contracture deformity is one of the complications of the bedfast state. The patient who is kept in bed for months or years usually becomes apathetic and morose. In this state he spends an increasing proportion of his time curled up, assuming a posture recalling that of the foetus *in utero*. Even in the absence of organic disease of the locomotor or nervous systems, such patients are liable to develop contractures by spontaneous shortening of muscles and tendons. The only rational approach to this problem is preventive; the bedfast state must be avoided at all costs. Remedial surgical and orthopaedic measures are of limited value. It is a relatively simple matter to straighten limbs and perform arthrodesis, but the patient is still left with severely wasted muscles. In the orthopaedic management of contractures, the effect of gravity should be fully exploited. For example, contractures of the knees may be corrected simply by suspending the limbs by the ankles in a Guthrie-Smith frame. Surprising success has often been achieved in this way.

When muscle spasm is an aggravating factor, and especially when pain is troublesome, diazepam may be given; 10 mg. per day is enough for an elderly patient and it should be given late in the day, for example 6 p.m. and 10 p.m. Persistent pain in hemiplegic limbs is occasionally attributable to the co-existence of latent epilepsy (Fine). If the pain is accompanied by involuntary twitchings in the hemiplegic limbs, anticonvulsant therapy should be started; phenytoin (p. 381) is the drug of choice.

It must be admitted that even with the most enlightened management of patients with paralysis, arthritis and other locomotor disabilities, it is likely that a time will come when attempts to walk or to use a wheelchair must be abandoned. Such patients have reached the bedfast state and are liable to develop contracture deformities. The onset of these disabilities can, however, be delayed by continuing physiotherapy; active and passive movement of the joints should still be carried out, and massage often prevents and relieves painful muscle spasm.

Accidental hypothermia. Accidental hypothermia in the elderly is caused by exogenous and endogenous factors and in most cases both are present. The exogenous factor is exposure to cold, and endogenous factors include endocrine disorders such as myxoedema, neurological disorders (for example, a cerebrovascular incident and confusional states), myocardial infarction, severe infections and the toxic effects of drugs such as the phenothiazine derivatives. This state is said to exist when the body temperature is below 35° C. and the history is usually one of progressive confusion, slurred speech, involuntary movements and ataxia. Even those parts of the body that are protected by clothing feel cold to the touch; placing a hand on the patient's abdomen is the most useful diagnostic test.

The treatment of this condition includes the care of the unconscious patient, the discovery and treatment of predisposing conditions, passive re-warming and general supportive measures. Passive re-warming is achieved by placing the patient in a room heated to 30° C. and preventing further heat loss. General supportive measures consist in the administration of a broad spectrum antibiotic such as cephaloridine (p. 16) or ampicillin (p. 15), parenteral fluids (a warm solution of 5 per cent. glucose or a plasma-expander of low molecular weight such as dextran), corticosteroids (hydrocortisone intravenously, 100 mg. six to eight hourly), oxygen, and—in cases of myxoedema only —triiodothyronine (p. 292).

WARD HYGIENE AND GENERAL WELFARE OF OLD PEOPLE IN HOSPITAL

Careful attention to every aspect of ward hygiene is particularly important when the great majority of the patients are long-term cases. High standards should not, however, be achieved at the expense of comfort and by sacrificing the general atmosphere of homeliness so much desired by old people. A day-hall is invaluable because it allows patients to escape from the all too familiar surroundings of the ward; there must be adequate space for walking and provision should be made for occupational therapy. It is now the usual practice to have two day-spaces and each is provided with wash-basins and W.C.s. One of these day-spaces is reserved for patients who are at the earliest stages of rehabilitation; the other is for those who have reached a more advanced stage of independence. The skilful use of colour for interior decoration has transformed many wards and day-rooms where formerly drabness was absolute. Armchairs are now available which are comfortable and also well designed for the special needs of old people. Hand-rails at strategic points in the ward and annexes are a boon to many patients. Doors should be wide and their potential danger to the infirm is diminished if they are fitted with a transparent glass panel. Old people usually lack the self-confidence and the agility to deal with swing doors and may therefore be seriously injured by them. Although immediate responsibility for these arrangements devolves upon the nursing staff, the ultimate responsibility is the doctor's, and he can help his nursing colleagues by showing a practical interest in their work and their problems. In a geriatric ward it is particularly important that drudgery and excessively strenuous work should be eliminated. This policy gives the nurse more time to look after her patients—who need unremitting care and encouragement.

It is important to seize every opportunity to apply advances in medicine, in hygiene and in other fields to the welfare of the aged. The use of deodorants in wards occupied by incontinent patients is one example; and in suitable cases the charcoal blanket is a boon not only to the patient but indirectly to patients in neighbouring beds. Incontinence pads are readily available. The old-fashioned sputum mug has been banished; even the washing of such receptacles was an appalling imposition on the nursing staff. Cups made of waxed cardboard and provided with lids are readily available, they can be collected by an orderly several times daily and destroyed in the incinerator. Disposable urinals and bedpans are now manufactured. Soiled linen should not be slunged by ward staff but should be promptly despatched in suitable containers to the laundry. The adequacy of methods and appliances in the ward kitchen and in the sanitary annexes should be reviewed jointly by the physician and the ward sister from time to time with special regard to the number of patients in the ward.

THERAPEUTICS AND THE DYING

Inevitably the time comes when it is obvious that the patient, afflicted by a lethal disease, is in fact dying. Ominous changes occur in his appearance and demeanour in a period of hours or days. At this time there may be little or nothing to be done in terms of active intervention by the doctor. His rôle may be to hold a watching brief, but this is often a phase which taxes to the utmost the skill and resourcefulness of the nurse. The patient himself is likely to sense the crisis. He should be supported by those who can face the situation with equanimity. Loneliness may be far more upsetting than pain; and so long as he knows that his own people are near him, he is unlikely to lapse into panic.

If the doctor is sure that death is inevitable he should not interfere with the natural course of events without careful consideration. In such circumstances drugs such as analeptics are contraindicated; they do not prolong life but merely postpone death. It is clearly unethical for a doctor to do anything that would cause his patient to die; but it may also be culpable to allow the dying patient to endure unnecessary suffering of mind or body. Many patients prefer to retain their mental faculties unclouded by sedatives and hypnotics in the daytime. In others the state of misery and anxiety clearly calls for symptomatic relief; and here a mixture of heroin (5 mg.) and cocaine (5 mg.) made up with gin and a sweet vermouth is often highly effective. Insomnia calls for the bold use of hypnotics: chloral hydrate or a similar preparation (p. 446) followed by brandy (30 ml.) with soda water is usually effective. Dyspnoea may cause considerable alarm for the patient and his attendants. Nocturnal dyspnoea is often due to left ventricular failure. It may be prevented by using a diuretic in the late afternoon—for example, frusemide 40 mg. at 4 p.m. The diuretic action is complete by 10 p.m.—when the patient can be settled for the night. If, despite preventive measures, dyspnoea occurs morphine must be given at once; 5 mg. can be injected intravenously and then 10 mg. intramuscularly. A troublesome dry cough should be suppressed promptly with heroin (5 mg. intramuscularly). Hiccough may yield to the usual manœuvres—breath-holding, or snuff to promote sneezing. Inhalations of CO_2 are often effective, and this treatment merely entails re-breathing of expired air, using a polythene bag of about 2 litres capacity; the procedure is continued until it induces tachypnoea—about a minute.

When a dying patient lapses into coma respiration often becomes stertorous. The noise can be minimized by placing the head in the lateral position and by using an airway to prevent obstruction of the fauces by the tongue. Other kinds of noisy breathing ('the death rattle') are due to the accumulation of mucus in the trachea and large bronchi. This may persist for many hours and is a source of distress to the relatives. It can be abolished by injecting hyoscine hydrobromide 0·4 mg. intravenously; within half an hour this greatly reduces the volume of secretion produced by the bronchial mucosa.

These patients should not be regarded as an anonymous group—'the dying'; they die as they lived—within the perpetual miracle of individuality, and they look to doctors, to nurses and to the priest to preserve for them in this, their greatest extremity, the dignity of man. In Henley's words:

So be my passing!
My task accomplished and the long day done,
My wages taken, and in my heart
Some late lark singing,
Let me be gather'd to the quiet west,
The sundown splendid and serene,
Death.

References

ANDERSON, I., CAMPBELL, A. E. R., DUNN, A. & RUNCIMAN J. B. M. (1966). *Scott. med. J.* **11**, 429.
ANDERSON, W. F. & COWAN, N. R. (1966). *Br. J. prev. soc. Med.* **20**, 141.
CARTER, A. B. (1960.) *Lancet*, **1**, 345.
DALL, J. L. C. (1965). *Lancet*, **1**, 194.
DE WARDENER, H. E. (1961). *The Kidney*, 2nd Ed., pp. 76-77. London: Churchill.
EXTON-SMITH, A. N. & STANTON, B. R. (1965). *Report of an Investigation into the Dietary of Elderly Women Living Alone*. London: King Edward's Fund.
FINE, W. (1966). *Geront. clin.* **8**, 121.
FINE, W. (1967). *Br. med. J.* **1**, 199.
HARANGHY, L. (1965). *Gerontological Studies in Hungarian Centenarians*. Budapest.
JOHNSON, R. H., SMITH, A. G., SPALDING, J. M. K. & WOLLNER, L. (1965). *Lancet*, **1**, 731.
JUDGE, T. G., in *Proceedings of the Fifth European Meeting of Clinical Gerontology*; p. 295. Brussels, 1968.
POMERANCE, A. (1965). *Br. Heart J.* **27**, 711.
PROUDFOOT, A. T., AKHTAR, A. J., DOUGLAS, A. C. & HORNE, N. W. (1969). *Br. med. J.* **2**, 273.
READ, A. E., GOUGH, K. R., PARDOE, J. L. & NICHOLAS, A. (1965). *Br. med. J.* **2**, 843.
STRACHAN, R. W. & HENDERSON, J. G. (1965). *Q. Jl. Med.*, **34**, 303.
STRAUSS, M. B. & WELT, L. G. (1963). *Diseases of the Kidney*, p. 502. London: Churchill.
THOMSON, T. J. (1954). *Glasg. med. J.* **35**, 363.

APPENDIX

Selection of Items used in a Geriatric Unit

WALKING AIDS

Warrals (tripod sticks) in 3 sizes.
  Remploy Ltd., Queensway, Croydon, Surrey, or Queen Elizabeth Avenue, Hillington, Glasgow, S.W.2. Distributors: Macarthy's Ltd., Balmore Industrial Estate, Glasgow, N.2.
  Can also be hired from Queen's Nurses in some areas. (Remploy will also supply 4-legged wooden sticks —not adjustable; state height required.)
Zimmer Walking aid.
Zimmer quadruped (adjustable).
  Zimmer Orthopaedic Ltd., George Street, Industrial Estate, Bridgend, Glamorgan, or through Hogg & Ross Ltd., Dunsinane Avenue, Dundee, or 106 Bath Street, Glasgow, C.2., or at 37 George IV Bridge, Edinburgh 1.
Metcalfe walking sledge.
  M. Masters & Sons Ltd., 240 New Kent Road, London, S.E.1.
Fordham walking-machine with 3 wheels and a brake.
  Fordham Pressings Ltd., Melbourne Works, Dudley Road, Wolverhampton.

HEARING AIDS

Communicator.
  House of Hearing Centre Ltd., 75 Renfield Street, Glasgow, C.2.

CHAIRS

Junior and Senior Travaux wheel-chairs.
  Richards Son & Allwin Ltd., Great Bridge, Tipton, Staffs. (Wheel-chairs must have two back wheels and a hand-brake.)
Pel Geriatric Chairs with drop arms—canvas or padded.
  Pel Ltd., Oldbury, Birmingham, or 50 Wellington Street, Glasgow, C.2.
High-backed padded chair C57/HB.

Steel style chairs.
   New Equipment Ltd., Croxdale, Co. Durham, or at
   395 Sauchiehall Street, Glasgow.
Sanichair.
   G. McLoughlin & Co., Victoria Works, Oldham
   Road, Rochdale, Lancs.

FRAMES AND HOISTS

Guthrie-Smith equipment and parallel bars.
   Stanley Cox Ltd., Electrin House, 93 New Cavendish
   Street, London, W.1.
Hoyer hoist—with adjustable base, nylon slings.
   John Bell & Croyden, 50 Wigmore Street, London,
   W.1.
Ambulift.
   Mecanaids, Mercia Road, Gloucester.

BED AND BEDSIDE EQUIPMENT

Dunlopillo adjustable bed cushions (3 ft.)—useful as
   leg-rest in bed.
   Dunlop Rubber Co. Ltd., (Dunlopillo Division), 209
   St. George's Road, Glasgow, C.3., or Bintex Ltd.,
   Harrogate, Yorks.
The ripple bed—useful in the prevention of pressure
   sores.
   Talley Surgical Instruments Ltd., 47 Theobold
   Street, Borehamwood, Herts.
   The equipment is available at a rental of 52½p. a
   week.
McCullagh commode.
   Chas. F. Thackray Ltd., Park Street, Leeds, or 1-2
   Queen Margaret Road, Glasgow, W.2.
Urinal trolley.
   Albert Brown Ltd., Chancery Street, Leicester.
Charcoal Blanket.
   Sutcliffe, Speakman & Co., Leigh, Lancs.

EQUIPMENT FOR INCONTINENT PATIENTS
Incontinence pads.
   Smith and Nephew-Southalls Ltd., Bessemer Road,
   Welwyn Garden City, Herts.
   Can be prescribed by general practitioners in Scot-
   land.
Simplic bed incontinence appliance (1176).
   J. G. Franklin & Sons Ltd., Birbeck Works, Col-
   vestone Crescent, Dalston, London, E.8., or from
   Remploy or other surgical fitters.
Hilliard 'Ybwet' bags.
   W. B. Hilliard & Son Ltd., 123 Douglas Street,
   Glasgow, C.2.
Clinimatic disposal unit: Mark III.
   Vernon & Co. Ltd. (Pulp Products), Slater Street,
   Bolton.

Further Reading

ANDERSON, W. F. (1967). *Practical Management of the
   Elderly.* Oxford: Blackwell.
ISAACS, B. (1965). *An Introduction to Geriatrics.* London:
   Baillière, Tindall and Cassell.
THOMPSON, M. K. (1969). *Geriatrics and the General
   Practitioner Team.* London: Baillière, Tindall and
   Cassell.
Handbook of Information on Old People's Welfare in Scotland.
   Edinburgh: Pergamon Press.
Practical Aids for the Disabled (1964). British Red Cross
   Society.
Gadgets for the Disabled. Booklet obtainable from The
   National Association for the Paralysed, 1 York Street,
   Baker Street, London, W.1.
Aids for Disabled. Down Bros. & Mayer & Phelps Ltd.,
   32 New Cavendish Street, London, W.1.
Equipment for the Disabled. 4 volumes. Published by The
   National Fund for Research into Poliomyelitis and
   Other Crippling Diseases, Vincent House, Vincent
   Square, London, S.W.1.
HUGHES, H. L. GLYN (1960). *Peace at the Last.* London:
   UK and British Commonwealth Branch Gulbenkian
   Foundation.

21. Common Tropical Diseases and Helminthic Infections

F. J. WRIGHT

INTRODUCTION

The selection of subjects for this section was made primarily to meet the requirements of students and practitioners in countries with temperate climates. The large number of people coming or returning from the tropics makes it desirable for information on tropical diseases to be readily available. The treatment of some of the cosmopolitan diseases, such as bacillary dysentery, which are, nevertheless, commoner in the tropics, is described in other sections. Some of the tropical diseases may run an acute course and end fatally if not diagnosed early and promptly treated. It is therefore most important that medical practitioners in non-tropical countries should be able to recognize these diseases and know how to treat them. Malaria and amoebic dysentery are the two tropical diseases most commonly seen in this country, hence their treatment has been dealt with in detail.

Travellers to the tropics should be instructed not only as to those vaccinations which are obligatory but also in the available methods for protection against endemic disease. Information as to the vaccination certificates required by health authorities can usually be obtained from travel agents. Vaccination may be required against yellow fever, smallpox and cholera, while protection against poliomyelitis and enteric fever (TAB) is usually advisable. Diphtheria, tetanus and tuberculosis also present risks for those who have not been adequately immunized. If vaccination against both yellow fever (certificate valid for 10 years) and smallpox (certificate valid for three years) is required, then vaccination against yellow fever (p. 527) should be obtained first. Visitors to a malarious area must be instructed in the correct use of antimalarial drugs (see below). Methods of prevention of disease are described in each section, but it is convenient to have ready a summary of advice. This is available as a brochure, *Notes on the Preservation of Personal Health in Warm Climates*, published by The Ross Institute of Tropical Hygiene, London, price 25p. (5 shillings).

MALARIA

CYCLE OF THE DEVELOPMENT OF THE PLASMODIUM. To have a proper appreciation of the therapeutics of malaria, it is necessary to understand the life cycle of the malaria parasites. There are four species which cause malaria in man: *Plasmodium falciparum, P. vivax, P. malariae* and *P. ovale*. The infection is acquired when the parasites, in the stage of sporozoites, are injected into man by the biting of infected female mosquitoes of the genus *Anopheles*. The sporozoites leave the circulation within half an hour and the pre-erythrocytic stage of development takes place in parenchymal liver cells without disturbing the host. At the end of six days the developing pre-erythrocytic schizont of *P. falciparum* is mature and ruptures, liberating merozoites into the blood stream, where they invade erythrocytes, but no parasites remain in the liver. The pre-erythrocytic stages of *P. vivax* and *P. ovale* last eight days and that of *P. malariae* rather longer; and as well as invading erythrocytes, a persistent exo-erythrocytic cycle in liver cells may be maintained causing late relapses. The characteristic bouts of fever are caused by the liberation of merozoites from the malarial schizonts which have developed in red cells. This erythrocytic cycle takes 48 hours in the case of *P. vivax* and *P. ovale*, 72 hours by *P. malariae,* thus giving rise to tertian and quartan fevers respectively. The cycle is less well synchronized in *P. falciparum* infections and the fever is more insidious and irregular. To terminate fever, drugs must be effective in this stage. After a few days of fever some of the circulating parasites develop into sexual forms, gametocytes. These cause no symptoms but are infective for mosquitoes and are responsible for the spread of the disease to others by *Anopheles* mosquitoes.

ANTIMALARIAL DRUGS

Quinine. From the seventeenth century, cinchona bark, a traditional remedy of South America, and quinine, obtained from it in 1820, proved effective in combating malaria. Quinine acts on the erythrocytic stage and, except for certain strains of parasites, it rapidly controls an attack of malaria. It has the serious disadvantages of causing tinnitus and, if taken irregularly, it may precipitate blackwater fever. Its use is no longer generally recommended but it is still valuable for parenteral injection in the immediate treatment of severe falciparum malaria in small children. This also applies to adults if the parasite exhibits resistance to chloroquine and other antimalarials.

Mepacrine. This drug was introduced in 1932 under the name of Atebrin. It is a powerful drug with a similar action to quinine. It has now been superseded by newer drugs which less frequently provoke undesirable side-effects.

Chloroquine and amodiaquine. These two drugs are 4-aminoquinolines. Although chloroquine was synthesized in 1934, it and amodiaquine did not begin to come into general use until 1944. They are highly effective drugs acting in the same way as quinine and mepacrine but with few disadvantages. Strains of *P. falciparum* resistant to 4-aminoquinolines have become a problem in a few areas, especially where these drugs have been used on a large scale as prophylactics. There is so far no parenteral preparation of amodiaquine available but amopyroquin, a closely related compound, has recently been introduced for this purpose. With therapeutic doses, headache, mental excitement, pruritus and difficulty in focusing may be experienced. Chloroquine is, therefore, not recommended for aeroplane pilots. With prolonged use as a suppressant a dermatosis may arise; a greyish pigmentation has been reported after the prolonged use of amodiaquine. Chloroquine administered parenterally to small children is rapidly absorbed and may cause a rapidly fatal chemical encephalitis. For infants quinine should be substituted for chloroquine; for older children 5 mg. per kg. body weight should not be exceeded as a single dose.

Proguanil and pyrimethamine. Proguanil and chlorproguanil are biguanides and pyrimethamine is a diaminopyrimidine. Proguanil, introduced in 1945, was proved to stop the development of *P. falciparum* in the pre-erythrocytic stage and to have a slow action against the erythrocytic stage of all the malaria parasites. It also inhibits the further development of gametocytes of *P. falciparum* in the mosquito. Chlorproguanil and pyrimethamine have a similar action but can be administered at weekly intervals for prophylaxis.

The chief disadvantage of these three drugs is the occasional occurrence of a strain of *P. falciparum* exhibiting resistance to them. If resistant to proguanil, the strain is usually also resistant to pyrimethamine. They act too slowly to be used for the treatment of overt malaria in non-immunes.

Primaquine is an 8-aminoquinoline and appears to be the least toxic of this group of which the first, pamaquin, was introduced in 1925. These drugs destroy the gametocytes and it was hoped that they would be of public health value in preventing mosquitoes from becoming infected. Their toxicity, however, makes them unsuitable for the mass administration which would usually be necessary for this purpose. They are also effective against the pre-erythrocytic and exo-erythrocytic phases of the parasites. The main use of primaquine is to obtain radical cure of *P. vivax*, *P. malariae* and *P. ovale* infections by its action against the persistent exo-erythrocytic phases of these parasites in the liver.

GENERAL MANAGEMENT. The patient is nursed in bed and given treatment to relieve any troublesome symptoms. During the cold stage extra blankets and warmth will be required, but with the onset of the hot stage bed-clothing has to be reduced, and when the temperature is over 40·5° C. tepid sponging is needed. The patient should be encouraged to drink fluids freely, and aspirin or paracetamol may be given for the relief of headache. When vomiting is severe and dehydration develops, parenteral isotonic saline and glucose will have to be administered, but in severe infections, with much haemolysis, blood transfusion is preferable. As soon as the temperature has been controlled, a generous diet may be allowed and the patient permitted to get up. In convalescence, ferrous sulphate should be given for anaemia (p. 143).

Specific Treatment of a Clinical Attack

The initial objective in the treatment of an attack of malaria is to destroy the parasites which have invaded the erythrocytes. The drug of choice is chloroquine, or alternatively amodiaquine. If, however, there is a clear history that one of these drugs has been used regularly as a prophylactic in a correct dose, resistance must be assumed and quinine substituted. The initial adult dose of either chloroquine or amodiaquine is 600 mg. of the base followed in six hours by 300 mg. and subsequently 150 mg. twice daily for three further days. If the fever is not quickly controlled the diagnosis should be doubted or the possibility entertained of infection by a resistant strain of parasite necessitating the use of quinine as described below. Immediate administration of potent antimalarial drugs is required for all patients with *P. falciparum* malaria. The only possible exceptions to this rule are indigenous adults brought up in a hyperendemic zone who may exhibit a considerable tolerance to the infection.

Treatment of complicated falciparum malaria. When the attack is complicated by hyperpyrexia, vomiting, hypotension or coma, parenteral antimalarial treatment becomes a matter of great urgency. Chloroquine given intramuscularly is rapidly absorbed and is safe except for small children (p. 510). It is effective in all but the most fulminating infections unless the parasite is resistant to chloroquine. The dose is 200 to 300 mg. base for adults and followed by 200 mg. after four hours until oral treatment becomes possible. Ampoules are available containing 200 mg. of the base in 5 ml. of water. Amopyroquin, allied to amodiaquine, in a dose of 150 mg. base intramuscularly is an alternative to intramuscular chloroquine. When there are signs of a severe infection or when the general condition calls for intravenous fluids, chloroquine should be given slowly intravenously and may be conveniently given by injection into the delivery tube of the intravenous drip set. A grave infection may be associated with severe anaemia, which must also be combated at once by blood transfusion. When the patient is in a state of shock, the use of noradrenaline or better still, metaraminol has been recommended on the basis of its successful use in experimental infections. Dexamethasone 4 to 6 mg. intravenously every four to six hours has also been used with apparent success. If the patient remains in coma, lumbar puncture should be performed. The removal of cerebrospinal fluid may accelerate the recovery of consciousness by relief of increased intracranial pressure. It also serves to exclude concomitant pyogenic meningitis and viral encephalitis. Continuing fever with persistent parasitaemia would indicate resistance to 4-aminoquinolines.

As an alternative to parenteral chloroquine or amopyroquin, quinine may be administered intravenously, well diluted, through a fine-bore needle at a rate not exceeding 60 mg. per minute. A suitable initial adult dose is 500 mg. of quinine dihydrochloride, and if necessary this dose may be repeated in four to six hours. Not more than 2 g. should be given in 24 hours. Quinine administered in this way has saved many lives and is the drug of choice for small children when parenteral therapy is indicated. For adults, however, quinine is more toxic than chloroquine and, if given to a patient who has had recurrent falciparum malaria, it may precipitate blackwater fever. Intramuscular in-

jections of quinine, though effective, are liable to cause severe pain and local necrosis. Intravenous injection is, therefore, generally preferable. When chloroquine-resistant strains are prevalent a combination of sulfadoxine, 1 g. and pyrimethamine, 50 mg. given orally in a single dose has proved effective, particularly for partially immune patients. Sulphalene combined with trimethoprim is also effective. Dapsone, used for leprosy, also acts as an antimalarial.

Radical cure of malaria. All forms of malaria respond to suitable antimalarial treatment, but after treatment there may be recurrences except in *P. falciparum* infections. These relapses are due to the persistent exo-erythrocytic phase and may recur at intervals over a period of many months. The disease can, however, be eradicated by the administration of primaquine, 7·5 mg. base twice daily for 14 days. This treatment should follow the ordinary therapeutic course of chloroquine, amodiaquine or quinine, but primaquine should never be used in conjunction with mepacrine. Such a course gives a radical cure rate of about 95 per cent. While taking primaquine the patient often appears cyanosed due to the formation of methaemoglobin inside the red cells (methaemoglobincythaemia). This is not dangerous and the drug may be continued. All patients taking primaquine should, however, remain under close medical supervision as an unpredictable intravascular haemolysis may occur. The resulting anaemia necessitates an immediate cessation of the drug which is excreted in 24 hours. Sephardic Jews and coloured races are more liable to this complication owing to the incidence of an inherited abnormality in the erythrocytes of a deficiency of glucose-6-phosphate dehydrogenase. Alternatively, relapses may be prevented by the taking of 300 mg. chloroquine base plus 45 mg. primaquine base once a week for eight weeks after stopping the regular prophylactic drug. The only side-effect of note is diarrhoea.

Tables 13 and 14 give suitable curative and prophylactic courses of treatment for the various antimalarial drugs in different age-groups.

Blackwater fever. Since the introduction o the newer antimalarial suppressive drugs this serious and urgent complication of chronic *P. falciparum* infection has become rare. It may, however, still be seen even in Britain especially if someone suffering from chronic *P. falciparum* malaria is incorrectly given a large dose of quinine.

INITIAL TREATMENT. The patient is anxious

R*

TABLE 13

TREATMENT OF A CLINICAL ATTACK OF MALARIA

	Chloroquine (oral)	Inj. soluble chloro-quine I.M. or I.V.	Amodiaquine	Amopyroquin dihydrochloride	Inj. quinine dihydrochl. I.V.
Directions	Initial dose=twice the daily dose, followed in 6 hours by daily dose, then daily for 3 further days.	Give intramuscularly, or—for very urgent cases —intravenously, slowly; repeat in 4 or 6 hours.	On 1st day give 1½ × daily dose, then daily as below for 2 or 3 days.	Intramuscularly only.	For urgent cases only, dissolve dose in at least 10 ml. of isotonic saline, give slowly intravenously not more than 60 mg. per minute. If necessary repeat up to maximum of 1·8 g. in 24 hours.
Age in years	Daily dose of base	Dose of base	Daily dose of base	Dose of base	Dose of salt
Birth–1 1–4 5–8 9–15 Adult	50 mg. 50–100 mg. 100–150 mg. 150–300 mg. 300 mg.	} Contraindicated 5 mg./kg. body weight 200–300 mg.	50 mg. 50–100 mg. 100–150 mg. 150–400 mg. 400 mg.	3 mg./kg. body weight 150 mg.	Age in years / 20 × 600 mg. 600 mg.
Preparations available.	Tablets of 150 mg. and 50 mg. base.	Ampoules of 5 ml. containing 200 base.	Tablets of 200 mg. base and 150 mg. base.	Ampoules containing 150 mg. base.	Ampoules containing 600 mg. Further dilution required.

Parenteral quinine is usually advantageously followed by oral chloroquine or amodiaquine for three days. Where only oral quinine salts are available or the parasite is resistant to other drugs, quinine should be continued for a total of ten days. The dose of quinine dihydrochloride taken orally is 600 mg. three times daily.

TABLE 14

PROPHYLAXIS OF MALARIA

	Proguanil	Chlorproguanil	Chloroquine	Amodiaquine	Pyrimethamine
Directions	Daily	Weekly	Weekly, or ½ dose twice a week or ⅐ dose daily.	Weekly, or ½ dose twice a week.	Weekly. Contraindicated if strains resistant to proguanil or pyrimethamine are reported. (Keep bottle away from children.)
Age in years	Dose of salt	Dose of salt	Dose of base	Dose of base	Dose of base
Birth–1 1–4 5–8 9–15 Adults	25–50 mg. 50 mg. 50–100 mg. 100 mg. 200 mg.	5 mg. 10 mg. 10 mg. 20 mg. 20 mg.	37–50 mg. 50–100 mg. 100–150 mg. 150–300 mg. 300 mg.	50–100 mg. 100–133 mg. 133–200 mg. 200–400 mg. 400 mg.	6·25 mg. 6·25 mg. 6·25–12·5 mg. 12·5–25 mg. 25 mg.
Tablets available.	100 mg. salt (87 mg. base).	20 mg.	150 mg. and 50 mg. base.	200 mg. base and 150 mg. base.	25 mg. base.
		Combinations of chlorproguanil 20 mg. and chloroquine 150 mg. base and chloroquine and pyrimethamine are available for weekly administration.			

The drugs should be taken with complete regularity, beginning on the day of arrival in the malarious area and continued for four weeks after leaving. Proguanil or pyrimethamine may be combined with chloroquine or amodiaquine if the taking of either has been irregular or appears locally to be inadequate. Proguanil is the drug of choice unless there is local resistance to it.

and restless and benefits from 200 mg. soluble phenobarbitone by intramuscular injection. Skilled nursing with the minimum of disturbance is essential.

HAEMOLYSIS. Blackwater fever is the result of a sudden intravascular haemolysis. Although the cause is not fully understood, corticosteroids should be administered as they appear to prevent further waves of haemolysis.

ANAEMIA. The haemolysis may rapidly reduce the number of red cells to a dangerously low level and the anaemia and reduced renal blood flow are important factors in the causation of acute renal failure. The destroyed red cells should be replaced by carefully cross-matched blood transfusions. When the quantity required is great, packed cells may be used to avoid overloading the circulation with fluid.

ANURIA AND DEHYDRATION. As long as the patient is passing satisfactory quantities of urine, he should be encouraged to take liberal quantities of fluid by mouth. Dehydration should be corrected if necessary by intravenous salines (p. 627). Fever and perspiration in a hot climate increase the demands for fluids. The colour of the urine passed will indicate if haemolysis is still continuing and a decrease in its volume may herald anuria. Once anuria has become established the prognosis is grave and the treatment recommended on p. 273 should be started at once. Dialysis is of value in suitably selected cases (p. 277). Although unnecessary movement of patients is to be deprecated, in order to obtain skilled treatment it may be desirable to take advantage of air transport to convey them to a specialized centre.

SUBSEQUENT TREATMENT. When dehydration has been overcome and diuresis is satisfactory, chloroquine or amodiaquine (but not quinine) should be given to eliminate any persisting *P. falciparum* infection. Convalescence is usually uninterrupted, but ferrous sulphate should be given to combat any persisting anaemia (p. 143). One attack of blackwater fever seems to predispose to further attacks if a fresh infection with *P. falciparum* is acquired. Therefore, after recovery from blackwater fever the great importance of taking prophylactic antimalarial drugs with complete regularity must be impressed upon the patient if he proposes to remain in a malarious country.

Causal Prophylaxis and Suppression

The sporozoites introduced by the female *Anopheles* are not susceptible to any known antimalarial drug. Clinical attacks of malaria can, however, be prevented by drugs which affect the plasmodium either in its pre-erythrocytic forms (causal prophylaxis) or after it has entered the erythrocytes (suppression). Drugs used for the prevention of malaria, their sites of action and dosage are described on pp. 509–512. The drug must be started not later than the day of arrival in the endemic area and must be taken with complete regularity throughout the period of residence. After leaving the malarious country the drug should be continued for four weeks to ensure that no attack of falciparum malaria will occur. This will also delay and may prevent relapses of other forms of malaria. Failure to continue with anti-malarial drugs on leaving the tropics has been followed by severe or even fatal attacks of falciparum malaria. It should be noted that even when this advice is followed facliparum malaria may occur if the parasite is partly resistant to the drug used. Complete regularity rather than a particular choice of drug is the keynote of success. For this reason it may be unwise to recommend a change of programme to someone who has satisfactorily pursued one of the alternative regimens prescribed on p. 512. Some people find it easier to remember to take a drug daily than at weekly intervals. It will be noted that none of the recommended regimens necessarily prevent the acquisition of *P. vivax*, *P. malariae* or *P. ovale* which, after stopping the suppressant drug, may cause an attack of malaria necessitating radical cure by primaquine (p. 511). As resistance to chloroquine has arisen particularly in areas where there has been widespread use of it for prophylaxis, the 4-aminoquinolines (chloroquine, amodiaquine) are now only advised as suppressants if local strains of malarial parasites are known frequently to be resistant to proguanil and pyrimethamine but sensitive to chloroquine and amodiaquine.

Semi-immune persons brought up in a malarious country from birth may need only small doses of prophylactic antimalarial drugs.

Personal protection in malarious areas. Spraying the inside walls of houses with a residual insecticide, or the use of an aerosol 'bomb', will reduce the number of mosquitoes (p. 538) and has proved of immense value in the control and eradication of malaria. Nevertheless, the protection afforded by anti-malarial drugs is so great that they should always be taken.

SUMMARY

Drugs recommended: OVERT ATTACK. 4-aminoquinolines (chloroquine, amodiaquine, amopyro-

quin), quinine, sulfadoxine plus pyrimethamine.

PROPHYLAXIS AND SUPPRESSION. Proguanil,
pyrimethamine, chlorproguanil, 4-aminoquinolines.

RADICAL CURE (*P. vivax, P. malariae, P. ovale*).
Primaquine (8-aminoquinoline).

References

COVELL, G., COATNEY, G. R., FIELD, J. W. & SINGH, J.
    (1955). *Chemotherapy of Malaria.* Geneva: W.H.O.
PETERS, W. (1969). Drug Resistance in Malaria. *Trans.
    R. Soc. trop. Med. Hyg.* **63**, 25.

AMOEBIASIS

Intestinal Amoebiasis

SPECIFIC TREATMENT. When there are symptoms of active amoebic disease, treatment must be
started without delay, but when amoebic cysts only
are discovered in a person who has no clinical
symptoms of the disease, then the call for treatment
is not so clear. If cysts are found in a person who,
in the course of his work, is likely to contaminate
food, then treatment should be given unless the
cysts prove to be of the non-pathogenic minuta
strain. Otherwise each case must be decided
separately, the possibility of the later development
of a liver abscess being balanced against the time
and cost required to eradicate the infection, and the
likelihood of reinfection in an endemic area.

Emetine. It is advisable to start treatment with
a daily parenteral injection of emetine hydrochloride for a few days. The dose for an adult of
average weight is 60 mg. in 1 ml. of water daily
given intramuscularly and continued until the acute
symptoms have been controlled; this usually takes
three or four days. When the patient is underweight or very debilitated, the daily dose should be
reduced to 30 mg. Children receive doses proportionate to age; under three years 10 mg. should not
be exceeded, and from three to six years 20 mg.
Emetine hydrochloride should not be given continuously for more than seven days. During treatment with parenteral emetine the patient must be
confined strictly to bed, since the drug is toxic and
occasionally has serious effects, especially on the
heart muscle, producing a fall in blood pressure,
a rapid pulse and electrocardiographic changes.
Dehydroemetine hydrochloride is used in the same
dosage as for emetine hydrochloride. It appears to
be equally effective and is perhaps less toxic.

Emetine bismuth iodide. As soon as the acute

symptoms have subsided, oral treatment should be
started. There is a choice of three drugs. The most
effective, emetine bismuth iodide (EBI) is also the
most unpleasant. It is given as a fine powder in
gelatine capsules, 200 mg. in each. One capsule
(200 mg.) should be given daily, the patient being
allowed up to the bathroom. The gelatine covering
protects the stomach from the irritating effect of the
drug. It is best given at 10 p.m., four hours after
the last meal, with a large draught of water. If a
sedative such as sodium amytal, 200 mg., is
administered about 15 minutes before giving the
EBI, there will be much less risk of nausea and
vomiting. Nausea tends to become less troublesome as the treatment progresses but there is often
a recurrence of diarrhoea.

Diloxanide furoate, given orally in a daily dose of
20 mg. per kg. for 10 days is an attractive alternative
to EBI. It is much less toxic than EBI, the only
side-effect being flatulence. Reports as to its
efficacy vary, but as it can be taken while the patient
remains ambulant, it is being increasingly used and
the course can be repeated if necessary.

Metronidazole, used in the large dose of 40 mg.
per kg. body weight daily, in three divided doses,
for five days is about equally successful and may
also destroy amoebae that have invaded the liver.
When the disease has been long-standing, response
to the above drugs may be incomplete.

If chronic infection is combined with malnutrition, benefit may result from preliminary administration of an antibiotic such as tetracycline, but
to obtain a radical cure this must be followed by
specific anti-amoebic treatment as described above.

A month after completion of treatment, tests of
cure should be carried out, at least six stools being
examined for the presence of *E. histolytica* cysts
by an experienced worker and the examination
repeated later if symptoms recur. A sigmoido-
scopic examination may also provide useful
information. Should relapse occur or residual
infection be found, the full course of treatment
should be repeated.

TREATMENT OF INTESTINAL COMPLICA-
TIONS. A mass of granulomatous tissue containing
amoebae ('amoeboma') may simulate a carcinoma
of the colon or rectum. It usually responds well
to emetine hydrochloride. A daily intramuscular
injection of 60 mg. should be given for six to nine
days followed by diloxanide furoate or metronidazole or, after an interval of a week, by EBI. If
the mass does not resolve, the possibility of a con-

comitant carcinoma must be entertained. Rarely, surgical treatment is required to overcome residual narrowing of the intestinal lumen. Perforation of the caecum or colon also necessitates surgical intervention when emetine is required in addition. When surgery of an amoebic infection has been unwittingly undertaken and emetine not given, rapid amoebic ulceration of the skin around the wound has sometimes occurred. This is abruptly terminated by intramuscular emetine hydrochloride. Rarely haemorrhage from an amoebic ulcer of the bowel may make blood transfusion necessary.

GENERAL MANAGEMENT. During the acute stage of the disease, careful nursing, in pleasant surroundings if possible, is very important. Once the diarrhoea has been controlled, the patient, who is often poorly nourished, should be given a generous diet rich in protein and with a high vitamin content. He should be encouraged to take liberal quantities of fluids. Emetine is a toxic drug and when receiving treatment the patient must be kept strictly at rest, and any changes in the cardiovascular system carefully noted.

A person who has suffered from chronic amoebiasis is liable to become introspective and conscious of the bowels. Colicky pains, flatulence and occasional diarrhoea, due to residual non-specific changes in the bowel wall, are frequently experienced for some considerable time after the amoebic infection has been cleared. This should be explained to the patient and everything possible done in the way of reassurance. If the stools remain free from cysts the repeated taking of anti-amoebic drugs should be discouraged.

PERSONAL PROPHYLAXIS. The disease is caused by faecal contamination of food and drink conveyed either by the hands of cyst passers or by flies or other arthropods. Cysts can survive ordinary chlorination of water, and viable cysts have been found in the intestine of flies and cockroaches more than 24 hours after ingestion. In areas where the disease is prevalent, all water and milk should be boiled before use and uncooked vegetables and unskinned fruit avoided. Lettuce is a frequent vehicle of infection and the traditional application of potassium permanganate solution is useless. Only lettuce which has been very thoroughly washed or grown under controlled conditions can be eaten with impunity. Under ideal conditions all food handlers should be investigated before being given employment, to exclude those passing amoebic cysts, and examination of the stools

repeated at regular intervals. This, however, is rarely feasible in practice.

Hepatic Amoebiasis

Early recognition of hepatic amoebiasis before the formation of a large abscess is most important as a complete and rapid cure can be expected in all cases where treatment is given at this early stage.

SPECIFIC TREATMENT. Parenteral emetine and oral chloroquine are both highly effective in the treatment of hepatic amoebiasis. Metronidazole is under trial (p. 514). Emetine hydrochloride is given in the usual daily dosage (p. 514) over a period of nine consecutive days or for a shorter period followed by chloroquine. The patient must be kept at complete rest in bed during the period of administration of emetine and for three days after stopping it. In the absence of a large abscess or secondary infection, resolution usually commences in a few days, the temperature settles and the enlargement and tenderness of the liver soon subside. Dehydroemetine hydrochloride, 80 mg. daily by intramuscular injection, may be substituted for emetine hydrochloride. Similar results have been obtained with oral chloroquine. The adult dose is 600 mg. of base, daily for two days, followed by 300 mg. (base), daily for about 21 days. Chloroquine owes its curative effect to the thirty-fold concentration of the drug in the tissues, especially the liver and lungs, where amoebicidal levels are soon reached. It is less toxic than emetine, but with high dosage, insomnia, headaches, disturbances of vision, gastrointestinal upsets and pruritus may be experienced. If treatment is prolonged beyond 21 days the eyes should be repeatedly examined and if corneal or retinal opacities are detected chloroquine should be withheld. Chloroquine rivals emetine hydrochloride in efficacy and, as it is not toxic to the heart, it is especially indicated in a patient with myocardial damage where the use of emetine creates an additional risk. A combination of these two drugs may be employed in patients who have proved resistant to treatment with either drug when given separately.

When the response to treatment is unsatisfactory, the temperature not settling to normal or enlargement and tenderness of the liver persisting, the presence of an abscess requiring aspiration must be suspected or the diagnosis revised. Even though the diagnosis of a sizeable abscess is made at the onset, it is important, when the indications for aspirating it are not urgent, to give emetine or chloroquine for several days before aspiration. If the amoebic origin of a suspected abscess is in doubt or if a high neutrophil leucocytosis is present suggesting secondary pyogenic infection, then the addition of an antibiotic is desirable. If resolution is incomplete, aspiration of the liver must be undertaken. Even a persistently raised E.S.R. would suggest that aspiration is desirable. For exploration of the liver, a large-calibre needle fitted to a two-way 20 ml. syringe should be used. Unless the abscess is pointing, the site of maximum tenderness or oedema should be selected for exploration. Occasionally it may be necessary to perform a liver-scan, following the injection of a radioactive substance, to discover the site of the abscess. In the absence of localizing signs, the right anterior axillary line in the eighth or ninth intercostal space should be chosen. A local anaesthetic injected into the capsule of the liver is usually sufficient. The needle is inserted, where necessary, to a depth of 9 cm., suction being maintained all the time. If the abscess is not found at the first exploration, the point of the needle should be withdrawn to the interspace and re-inserted into the liver in a different direction. Three explorations through one skin puncture may thus be made. Where necessary, further exploration should be made in the posterior axillary line. Occasionally, especially when the abscess is in the left lobe of the liver, laparotomy may be necessary to locate it. The size of the abscess may vary from a few millilitres up to three litres. As much of the contents as possible should be aspirated from the cavity and the procedure should be repeated daily or on alternate days until little or no fluid is obtained. Nothing is to be gained by the introduction of emetine or chloroquine into the cavity as the amoebae are chiefly in the liver substance on the periphery of the abscess. The introduction of a small quantity of air assists in defining the abscess cavity radiologically but opaque solutions are unnecessary and usually best avoided. A specimen of the fluid withdrawn should be examined for amoebae (although these are usually absent) and cultured to exclude a persisting secondary bacterial infection. If the fluid has the typical anchovy sauce appearance, or is of a chocolate colour, it is almost certainly amoebic in origin but a yellow fluid forms in a chronic amoebic abscess, as well as in some which are secondarily infected.

If open surgery has been necessary to locate the abscess, under modern conditions aspiration is followed by the insertion of a drainage tube, using an antibiotic to check proliferation of any secondary bacterial invader.

In addition to the abscess being emptied, the course of emetine hydrochloride or chloroquine must be completed.

Where bacterial infection is present, sensitivity tests should be carried out on the infecting organism, but an antibiotic should be administered at once.

Occasionally more than one abscess may be present in the liver, and this makes the prognosis more serious. The presence of a second abscess should be suspected when clinical improvement is not maintained although the cavity has been emptied completely and has not refilled. Further exploratory punctures or laparotomy may then be required to discover and empty the remaining abscess. Following resolution of the liver abscess, it is advisable to give a course of treatment for intestinal amoebiasis even though amoebae are not found in the stools, otherwise re-infection of the liver from the bowel is likely. Even after a satisfactory response to treatment, hepatic amoebiasis may yet relapse, and then a further course of treatment will be required.

Pleuro-pulmonary amoebiasis. This is usually due to direct extension of the hepatic abscess through the diaphragm. The abscess may rupture into the base of the right lung or into the pleural cavity. With involvement of the lung parenchyma, a bronchial fistula may occur allowing the contents of the cavity to be coughed up. In such circumstances recovery often takes place with the administration of emetine or chloroquine and with postural drainage. If unsuccessful, surgical aid will be required. Where the pleural cavity has been invaded with material from a sterile abscess, conservative treatment with emetine or chloroquine and aspiration of the pleural cavity and liver may be all that is required, but if secondary bacterial infection is present, open drainage must be employed in addition to chemotherapy. Involvement of the peritoneal and pericardial cavities may occur very occasionally and should be similarly treated.

External rupture. An abscess may drain spontaneously by rupture into the colon or by penetrating the chest wall. Anti-amoebic treatment should then be given to prevent spreading ulceration of the colon or skin.

SUMMARY

Drugs recommended: FOR INTESTINAL AMOEBIASIS. Intramuscular emetine or dehydroemetine hydrochloride, followed by oral emetine bismuth iodide, diloxanide furoate or metronidazole.

FOR HEPATIC AMOEBIASIS. Parenteral emetine as above, oral chloroquine or metronidazole.

Reference

POWELL, S. J., WILMOT, A. J. & ELSON-DEW, R. (1968). Further trials of metronidazole in amoebic dysentery and amoebic liver abscess. *Trop. Dis. Bull.* **65**, 1118.

AFRICAN TRYPANOSOMIASIS
(AFRICAN SLEEPING SICKNESS)

It is important to make the diagnosis of trypanosomiasis as early as possible, since delay may lead to invasion of the brain, when effective treatment is more difficult.

SPECIFIC TREATMENT. Suramin and pentamidine give good results in early acute infections, but they cannot pass the blood–brain barrier and consequently are of little use by themselves when the central nervous system is invaded; at this stage the arsenicals are indicated—melarsoprol or the water-soluble melarsonyl potassium.

Suramin is a complex organic urea compound which is preferably given intravenously. If given intramuscularly it is painful and liable to cause necrosis, but these effects can be mitigated by the simultaneous administration of hyaluronidase. It is advisable to make the first dose a small one, 200 mg., to test for sensitivity, after which the dose can be increased to 1 g. dissolved in 10 ml. of distilled water and given at intervals of three or five days up to a total of from 5 to 10 g. Children tolerate the drug well; a safe single dose for a child under three years of age is 250 mg.; from 3 to 10 years 500 mg. and over 10 years 1 g. doses can be given. Early infections respond well to suramin. During treatment the urine should be examined before each injection and, if proteinuria has developed, the course may require modification; it should be discontinued if casts appear. Toxic effects also include nausea, vomiting, skin eruptions and polyneuritis.

Pentamidine isethionate, an aromatic diamidine compound, has trypanocidal properties, but it is recommended only for early infections by *T. gambiense*. The dose is 4 mg. per kg. body weight; in adults an initial dose of 25 mg. is followed by 200 mg. given intramuscularly or intravenously daily for 12 to 15 days. Intramuscular injections are painful. When the intravenous route is employed a fall of blood pressure is likely to occur; the injection should, therefore, be given slowly with the patient recumbent. To counteract hypotension a syringe loaded with noradrenaline should be ready for use if required.

Melarsoprol. When the nervous system is involved an arsenical is needed. The clinical state of the patient or an abnormal cerebrospinal fluid will indicate this requirement and it is to be expected as early as four weeks from the onset of symptoms in rhodesiense trypanosomiasis. Tryparsamide has been superseded by melarsoprol which is a chemical combination of melarsan oxide and dimercaprol. Although the toxicity is reduced by the persence of the latter, the drug still is toxic and requires to be used with caution. The main toxic effect is the production of coma. Formerly attributed to arsenical encephalopathy it is probably due to a Jarisch-Herxheimer reaction to the death of many trypanosomes. The initial dosage of melarsoprol should be based on clinical assessment of the general condition of the patient rather than on body weight. The more severely ill require small doses at first and may benefit from having a few injections of suramin beforehand. Melarsoprol is prepared as a 3·6 per cent. w/v solution in propylene glycol. It is given slowly intravenously through a fine needle, care being taken to prevent leakage. The following schedules have proved successful.

Schedule 1, for adults, weight 50 kg. or more, in a good condition with C.S.F. protein less than 40 mg. per 100 ml.

Days 1, 2, 3; 2, 2·5, 3 ml. respectively.
   10, 11, 12; 3·5, 4, 5 ml. respectively.
   19, 20, 21; 5 ml. on each day.

Schedule 2, for children, underweight adults or those with C.S.F. protein greater than 40 mg. per 100 ml. The maximum dose is calculated as 3·5 mg. per kg. body weight but never exceeding 5 ml. The calculated maximum dose for the body weight should be reduced by multiplying by the following decimals:

Days 1, 2, 3; 0·1, 0·2, 0·3 respectively.
   10, 11, 12; 0·5 on each day.
   19, 20, 21; 0·5, 0·5, 0·8 respectively.
   28, 29, 30; maximum dose on each day.

The first period of three days can be lengthened to five days if tolerance is poor. Melarsoprol has cured many late cases of *T. rhodesiense* infection which would otherwise have been fatal. Neurological sequelae in those surviving are uncommon but there have been occasional deaths from encephalopathy. These have become less frequent with increasing experience. Late cases of the more insidious gambiense trypanosomiasis also survive but permanent neurological sequelae may persist because of irreversible damage sustained by the brain prior to treatment.

Melarsonyl potassium, a water-soluble compound, has the advantage of being suitable for intramuscular administration and is less toxic than melarsoprol. It gives good results in *T. gambiense* infections but is less reliable against *T. rhodesiense*. The initial dose is 2 mg. per kg. body weight, followed by three daily doses, each of 4 mg. per kg. For intermediate and late cases, after a rest period of 7 to 10 days, a further four daily doses are given.

Nitrofurazone. The use of this drug is limited because of undesirable side-effects to patients relapsing after two courses of treatment with melarsoprol. The dose is 0·5 g. eight-hourly for one week, repeated three times at intervals of one week. This treatment has sometimes proved curative when all else has failed.

GENERAL MANAGEMENT. It is important that the patient should be treated for any other infection which he may have. Nursing in bed during the febrile stage is essential. The diet should be a generous and well-balanced one, which is especially important in those who are already undernourished. When treatment has been delayed, and the nervous system has been damaged, the patient may be completely bedridden and require to be fed.

PERSONAL PROPHYLAXIS. In endemic areas chemoprophylaxis can be achieved by the use of suramin or pentamidine isethionate, given intramuscularly, since their slow excretion results in the retention in the body of quantities that suffice to exert a suppressant effect. A single dose of 1 g. of suramin or pentamidine isethionate, 4 to 5 mg. per kg. body weight, gives protection for six months in *T. gambiense* infections, but for a shorter period against *T. rhodesiense*, where the protection is only for about two months. In *T. rhodesiense* areas the possibility of the infection being merely masked by suppression of its clinical features until a late stage has been reached is a real danger. Hence it is safer not to employ chemoprophylaxis in these areas but to examine the blood repeatedly and especially if fever occurs. Prompt treatment with suramin will

then be curative. If an attempt is made to eradicate *T. gambiense* from an area, employing mass chemoprophylaxis, a preliminary survey should be first carried out to enable adequate treatment to be given to those found to be already infected. Elimination of the tsetse fly from man's environment remains, however, of prime importance, particularly in *T. rhodesiense* areas where animal reservoirs of infection are believed to exist.

SUMMARY

Drugs recommended: FOR EARLY GAMBIENSE TRYPANOSOMIASIS: pentamidine, later melarsoprol or melarsonyl potassium.

FOR EARLY RHODESIENSE TRYPANOSOMIASIS: suramin, later melarsoprol.

Nitrofurazone is used only for relapsed patients.

Reference

ROBERTSON, D. H. H. (1962). Chemotherapy of African trypanosomiasis. *Practitioner*, **188**, 80.

LEISHMANIASIS

Visceral Leishmaniasis (*Kala azar*)

SPECIFIC TREATMENT. The response of visceral leishmaniasis to drug treatment varies according to the geographical area in which the disease has been acquired. In India and Pakistan the disease is readily controllable, but in the Sudan and East Africa response to specific treatment is less satisfactory. Consequently while one course of treatment usually cures visceral leishmaniasis contracted in Asia, in the African variety two or more courses are often required. Urea stibamine, a pentavalent antimony compound, is commonly used in India and Pakistan in the treatment of visceral leishmaniasis and gives satisfactory results. It is available in powder form in ampoules requiring the addition of sterile pyrogen-free distilled water before injection. Urea stibamine treatment is usually free from undesirable side-effects; it is given intravenously in the following daily doses for adults: initial dose 100 mg., second day 200 mg., subsequent doses 250 mg. Fifteen daily injections should be given and the course repeated after a month if necessary. Sodium stibogluconate has been used with success in many areas. A suitable course of treatment for an adult is 10 daily intravenous injections of 600 mg. repeated if necessary after an interval of 14 days up to a total dosage of 12 or even 18 g. Children tolerate a relatively larger dose of antimony than adults and indeed seem to require it. One-third of the adult dosage may be given to children from 5 to 10 years of age. Diethylamine *p*-aminophenylstibonate, another pentavalent antimony compound, is favoured in certain centres. The daily dose is 100 to 300 mg. in 5 per cent. solution intravenously or intramuscularly to a total of 3 g.

The diamidine compounds, pentamidine isethionate and 2-hydroxystilbamidine isethionate have also been used in areas where the disease is resistant to antimony treatment. Stilbamidine should never be used as it may be followed by irreparable neural, hepatic and renal damage: it has been replaced by 2-hydroxystilbamidine, which is much less toxic and can be given by the intravenous route in daily doses for an adult of 250 mg. for 10 days. The course may be repeated after intervals of 14 days up to a total of 7·5 g. given over a period of 58 days. Side-effects such as fever, rigors and headaches are not uncommon with 2-hydroxystilbamidine, but these can be relieved by the administration of 10 mg. mepyramine maleate three times a day during the course. If pentamidine is employed it is given as in the treatment of trypanosomiasis (p. 517). When the disease does not respond to a full course of one drug, then a second course or treatment with one of the other drugs must be undertaken. Some strains are resistant to 2-hydroxystilbamidine.

Cure of visceral leishmaniasis can only be accepted when the patient remains afebrile, the leucocyte count returns to normal, the enlargement of the spleen and liver disappears and when this state is maintained over a period of observation of at least 12 months.

The treatment of post kala azar dermal leishmaniasis is the same as for visceral leishmaniasis. Response to treatment is usually slow, but some patients respond well to pentamidine.

GENERAL MANAGEMENT. Treatment for other concomitant infections such as malaria, brucellosis, tuberculosis or ancylostomiasis may be necessary. In the presence of tuberculosis, pentamidine is less disturbing than antimonial drugs until the tuberculosis is under control. A generous, well-balanced diet is given along with plenty of fluid. The patient should rest in bed and be carefully nursed until the temperature has returned to normal and strength has been regained.

PROPHYLAXIS. In endemic areas infected dogs should be destroyed. Sandflies should be kept down by clearing up breeding-grounds and by the use of insecticides and repellents (p. 538). Attempts are being made to produce immunity by the use of a vaccine prepared from leishmaniae but its efficacy awaits evaluation.

SUMMARY

Drugs recommended: sodium stibogluconate, pentamidine.

Cutaneous Leishmaniasis (*Oriental Sore*)

An important part of the treatment in long-standing cases of cutaneous leishmaniasis is the cleansing of the sore. There is often a gross superadded infection with pyogenic organisms, and the sores do not respond well to specific treatment until this has been brought under control. The crust should first be removed by the application of moist dressings and the exposed surface then kept clean. Penicillin or other suitable antibiotics may also be required in addition.

SPECIFIC TREATMENT. Spontaneous healing usually occurs in from 12 to 18 months; a scar then forms and may be disfiguring. Healing may be expedited and scar formation minimized by the parenteral injection of pentavalent antimony compounds as described for visceral leishmaniasis. Alternatively, a solitary ulcer, not situated on the face, may be made to heal by exciting an inflammatory reaction after sepsis has been overcome. Unipolar coagulation diathermy has produced very good results. Unless leishmaniae are destroyed in the deeper tissue there is a possibility of a lingering infection manifested later as leishmaniasis recidiva.

Diffuse cutaneous leishmaniasis occurring in Ethiopia and Venezuela is treated by repeated courses of pentamidine isethionate (p. 517) but weekly glucose tolerance tests are required to detect the early signs of drug-induced diabetes.

PREVENTION. The deliberate production of an oriental sore at a site normally covered by clothing produces an active immunity and prevents the occurrence of a disfiguring ulcer. For this purpose 0·1 to 0·2 ml. of a culture of splenic emulsion from infected hamsters containing live leishmaniae is injected intradermally.

Reference

BRYCESON A. D. M. (1970). Diffuse cutaneous leishmaniasis in Ethiopia. *Trans. R. Soc. trop. Med. Hyg.* **64**, 369.

LEPTOSPIROSIS

SPECIFIC TREATMENT. *Penicillin.* Although a field trial of antibiotics yielded equivocal results, there are good reasons for believing that penicillin administered during the first four days of the illness destroys the leptospires and arrests the disease. The dosage employed is 600,000 units every four hours for six doses, followed by the same dose every six hours for four to six days. A brisk initial reaction is usually provoked and may be accompanied by hypotension necessitating urgent resuscitation (p. 643). If the patient is known to be allergic to penicillin, another effective antibiotic, such as tetracycline, should be used.

GENERAL MANAGEMENT. The patient should be kept at rest in bed on a low protein diet and encouraged to drink plenty of fluids containing glucose and orange juice. For severe vomiting, intravenous isotonic saline may be required, but care should be taken not to overload the circulation, especially when oliguria exists. When renal damage is severe and oliguria or anuria is present, treatment on the lines described on p. 273 should be started. The risk of haemorrhage, which is often associated with low levels of prothrombin in the blood, calls for the use of phytomenadione, 25 to 50 mg. daily.

PERSONAL PROPHYLAXIS. All food should be protected from contamination by rats, the carriers of the leptospira. The possibility of being infected by *L. canicola* from dogs or pigs should not be forgotten. The urine and faeces of the patient should be disinfected, and the attendants must disinfect their hands carefully and wear gloves if they have any abrasions of the skin. Anti-rat measures should be carried out where workers are likely to become infected. Sewer workers, miners and fish curers are particularly liable to this risk and should be instructed about personal protection. Bathing or swimming in canals or stagnant pools likely to be infected should be avoided. Swimming pools should be chlorinated and protected from rats.

References

MACKAY-DICK, J. & ROBINSON, J. F. (1959). Penicillin in leptospirosis. *Lancet*, **2**, 515.

MACKAY-DICK, J. & ROBINSON, J. F. (1959). Treatment of leptospirosis with oxytetracycline. *Lancet*, **1**, 100.

TYPHUS FEVERS
(RICKETTSIAL DISEASES)

SPECIFIC TREATMENT. The various fevers due to rickettsiae vary greatly in severity, but all respond to broad-spectrum antibiotics. Chloramphenicol was the first to be used and it is remarkably effective. The typhus fevers, however, respond very satisfactorily to tetracycline; and as pancytopenia is a rare but grave complication of chloramphenicol therapy, it is wiser to use tetracycline. The drug is used in the standard dose of 250 mg. four times daily, but for the first day double this dose may be employed. In severe infections the dose is 500 mg. four times daily for the first three days. The fever usually settles within two or three days. As the action of tetracycline is principally bacteriostatic there is some tendency to relapse and the drug should, therefore, be continued for five to seven days after the fever has subsided. Q fever rarely continues for long, but tetracycline reduces the incidence of complications and is of value in the more severe cases.

GENERAL MANAGEMENT. The patient suffering from louse-borne relapsing fever is a danger to others unless he has been thoroughly deloused. All highly febrile patients require the usual nursing for fever. Hot sponging gives great relief by the gentle perspiration which follows it; if hyperpyrexia is present (over 41° C.), cold sponging is required. If headache is intense, lumbar puncture should be performed to relieve the increased intracranial pressure and to exclude a concomitant pyogenic meningitis. Delirium may need to be controlled by sedatives before the specific chemotherapy takes effect. In mite-borne typhus serious pulmonary involvement may be a feature and there may be indications for oxygen therapy.

Convalescence is usually protracted—especially in older people—and evidence of impairment of the cardiac reserve justifies cautious management.

The local eschar and glandular enlargement commonly seen in tick-borne and mite-borne infections require no special measures other than the specific chemotherapy described above.

PREVENTION. *Louse-borne typhus.* This disease occurs in epidemics when the body louse *Pediculus humanus (corporis)* is being carried by man and becomes infected with *Rickettsia prowazeki.* The head louse, *P. humanus (capitis)*, is a relatively unimportant vector. Late relapses (Brill's disease) may occur after many years, in the absence of lice and when remote from the endemic area. This persistence in the human carrier may account for the beginning of a new outbreak although a reservoir among rodents has been postulated. Primarily, prevention of the disease demands the avoidance of overcrowding and poverty which predispose to bad hygiene and louse infestation in man. The organism is excreted in the faeces of the louse and gains entrance into the human body through the scratching and excoriation of the skin consequent upon the irritation caused by the louse bite. Inhalation of dust contaminated by infected louse faeces is another way in which infection may occur. Louse-borne typhus is chiefly a disease of colder climates and especially follows wars and the crowding together of refugees. Nevertheless, no community which harbours lice is free from the danger that infection may be introduced. Infestation by lice may now be effectively controlled by the liberal use of insecticides (p. 538). At the time of his admission to hospital the patient should be attended by nursing staff wearing louse-proof clothing. The patient is shaved to get rid of all infested hair; he is thoroughly washed and his clothing is carefully disinfested before it is returned to him. As louse faeces contain rickettsiae, steps must be taken to diminish the risk of spread of epidemic typhus by infected dust; dry sweeping and dusting of wards must be forbidden. It should be noted that a patient may be infested with lice but be suffering from some other rickettsial disease such as flea-borne typhus. A diagnosis of trench fever also makes it imperative to destroy all body lice.

Tick-borne typhus. In endemic areas dogs should be regularly disinfested of ticks and should not be allowed to sleep in bedrooms. When walking through scrub country protection of the legs may reduce the risk of picking up an infected tick from cattle or game. It should be noted that, although a household dog is the usual offender in introducing and feeding the vector tick, the rickettsiae are not responsible for the tick fever of dogs which is a protozoal infection not transmissible to man.

Rocky Mountain spotted fever. This is also a tick-borne rickettsial infection acquired in the Americas.

Flea-borne typhus (Murine typhus). Except in the aged this is usually a mild disease conveyed to man from fleas which normally live on small rodents. The measures employed in the prevention of plague are indicated, and grain stores should be protected from invasion by rodents.

Mite-borne typhus (Scrub typhus). This infection is acquired when man disturbs the scrub country in endemic areas. Infected larval mites are the vectors. Protection is afforded by treating clothing with insect repellents (p. 538).

Q fever. This infection, caused by *Coxiella burneti* is acquired by inhalation of particles of dust, straw, hair or wool contaminated by infected animals, particularly sheep. It can also be conveyed by unpasteurized milk and by the placentae of infected cows.

ACTIVE IMMUNIZATION. Vaccines have been prepared from rickettsiae cultivated in eggs. Cox's vaccine containing killed *R. prowazeki*, *R. mooseri* or *R. rickettsi* are effective in preventing louse-borne typhus, flea-borne typhus or Rocky Mountain spotted fever respectively. Three doses, each of 1 ml., are given at intervals of 7 to 10 days and, where the risk is great, booster doses of 1 ml. should be given at three-monthly intervals. Vaccines against other rickettsiae are less readily available, and the effectiveness of a short course of tetracycline on the appearance of an eschar following a tick or mite bite in an endemic area, or the prompt treatment of an attack, makes active immunization less important. A vaccine containing killed *Coxiella burneti* is useful for administration to laboratory workers.

BRUCELLOSIS
(UNDULANT FEVER)

SPECIFIC TREATMENT. The severity of symptoms and the duration of fever in untreated brucellosis vary greatly. The employment of antibiotics has completely altered the outlook in this infection. Relief of fever and arthritic pain can now be confidently predicted. Recently acquired and mild infections frequently terminate if the patient is treated with tetracycline alone. To effect a more certain resolution of the disease and to make relapse less likely a combination of tetracycline (2 g. daily) and streptomycin (1 to 1·5 g. daily) is employed over a period of two to three weeks. Particularly in chronic or relapsing infections a sulphonamide, such as sulphadimidine (4 g. daily) should be given in addition. In the older age-group streptomycin should be used with caution owing to the possibility of damaging the auditory nerve. In malnourished patients administration of vitamin B complex is desirable to avoid precipitating avitaminosis. Although the initial response is excellent some cases become chronic and it may be difficult to distinguish a continuing infection from its sequelae or a reinfection.

PERSONAL PROPHYLAXIS. Brucella infection is mainly contracted by contamination with infected animal discharges and by drinking unpasteurized milk, but cream cheeses may also harbour the organism for up to two months. It is important to remember that milk from tuberculin-tested cattle may not be pasteurized. Laboratory personnel, veterinary surgeons, cowherds, slaughter-house workers and others may acquire infection in the course of their daily work. The organism is easily destroyed by heating the milk to boiling-point or by pasteurization. The immunization of calves with S.19 vaccine and improved hygienic measures have proved to be reasonably effective in the control of the disease in cattle. Vaccines for the control of *Br. melitensis* infection in sheep and goats have recently been prepared.

Ordinary precautions as for typhoid fever should be observed by those nursing a case, and care should be taken to disinfect the patient's urine, although spread from a human infection is very rare. In bacteriological laboratories infections are readily acquired, especially through the conjunctiva and by inhalation.

CHOLERA

Cholera formerly was caused chiefly by the Inaba, Ogawa or Hikojima strains of *Vibrio cholerae*, but since 1961 infections due to *V. eltor* have become widespread, penetrating from the Far East to the Middle East and Africa. Originally *V. eltor* appeared to be of low pathogenicity, but recent outbreaks have been of increased severity.

SPECIFIC TREATMENT. Tetracycline, 250 mg. six-hourly for three days or furazolidone in single doses of 400 mg. daily reduces the length of time the dejecta contain vibrios but a favourable outcome depends chiefly on adequate hydration.

NON-SPECIFIC TREATMENT. During an epidemic of cholera, people should be encouraged to seek advice at the first appearance of gastro-intestinal disturbance. The majority of cases are first seen in the stage of copious evacuation and in a condition of dehydration and circulatory col-
lapse. The urgent need is very rapid replacement of the lost water and electrolytes by the intravenous route so as to restore the general and renal circulation and prevent tissue anoxia. In practice it is always necessary to make a clinical assessment of the severity of the state of dehydration and thus to estimate approximately a patient's needs in terms of water and electrolytes. At the bedside the physician's opinion is based on the general appearance of the patient, the pulse and blood pressure, the output of urine, and information regarding the volume of fluid lost by vomiting and by diarrhoea.

INTRAVENOUS INFUSIONS. It is usually necessary to give 2 litres of fluid by the intravenous route in the first hour and 1 litre in the second and third hours. Subsequently fluid is given as indicated by the condition of the patient. The bulk of the fluid should be isotonic saline or isotonic sodium bicarbonate solution (14 g. per litre) prepared by special modern sterilization techniques. Where the necessary apparatus is not available for its correct preparation one-sixth molar (18·7 g. per litre) sodium lactate solution is a substitute but has the disadvantage that lactic acid acidosis may develop. For every 2 litres of isotonic saline, 1 litre of sodium bicarbonate solution should be given. These patients are also depleted of water and require to be given additional water intravenously in the form of 5 per cent. dextrose solution. For every 3 litres of fluid containing sodium chloride or sodium bicarbonate, 1 litre of 5 per cent. dextrose solution should be given in addition. For further details see p. 253. The intravenous fluid is not warmed above room temperature for fear of inducing hyperpyrexia in the reaction stage of the disease. Should hyperpyrexia occur, cold sponging in addition to corticosteroids may be of value. Hydrocortisone hemisuccinate (50 mg.) should then be added to the infusion fluid. Rectal temperatures should be taken at frequent intervals throughout the illness and the urine output recorded. While fluid is being given, an indication of the patient's further needs is usually apparent from the clinical appearance. If, however, there is room for doubt, the degree of haemoconcentration may be estimated from the patient's whole blood, using the copper sulphate drop method of Phillips and Van Slyke. Once a free flow of urine is established, intravenous fluid is needed only if the patient is unable to take sufficient fluid by mouth. Fluid should be taken orally as soon as it can be retained and may be administered by an intragastric drip, if necessary.

No attempt should be made to replace the potassium loss until the kidneys have started to function freely. If facilities are available for the determination of serum potassium and if the concentration is found to be reduced to 3 mEq/l. or less, intravenous potassium should be given (p. 257). In the absence of laboratory facilities it is safer to give potassium by mouth in a dose of 2 g. potassium chloride four times daily. In the field, good results have, however, been obtained by the intravenous infusion of an aqueous solution containing in each litre sodium chloride, 5 g., sodium bicarbonate, 4 g. and potassium chloride, 1 g. Children require especial care and Ringer lactate (B.P.) with pH adjusted to 7 is the intravenous fluid of choice. If anuria occurs, the prognosis is very grave and the treatment recommended for its relief should be instituted (p. 273).

GENERAL MANAGEMENT. During the acute phase of cholera, everything possible should be done to conserve the patient's strength. When the urinary output is satisfactory, milk and other bland foods may be added as desired by the patient. Convalescence is usually rapid and satisfactory if the acute stage has not been complicated by renal damage. The chronic carrier state does not usually occur, as convalescent patients do not continue to pass vibrios in the stool for longer than one month except in the case of *V. eltor*, which may continue to be excreted for years.

PERSONAL PROPHYLAXIS. All discharge from the patient must be disinfected; the same applies to soiled articles of clothing. The hands of the attendants must be carefully cleansed and disinfected after tending the patient and before eating. Preferably, gloves should be worn while on nursing duty. All drinking water and milk must be boiled, food must be protected from flies, and uncooked vegetables as well as raw and unripe fruit should be avoided.

VACCINATION. Vaccination with a killed suspension of selected smooth strains of *V. cholerae* or *V. eltor* should be given in two doses, 0·5 and 1 ml. representing 4,000 and 8,000 million organisms respectively, at an interval of one to four weeks to all persons at risk. Immune bodies can be detected in the blood by the fourth day and remain up to six months. The international certificate becomes valid six days after the first injection. Vaccination, combined with improved hygiene due to an awareness of cholera, may arrest an outbreak. Controlled observations indicate, however, that vaccination alone may reduce the expected incidence of cholera by only 25 per cent. and perhaps by less if the prevalent strain is not included in the vaccine.

References

CARPENTER, C. C. J., MITRA, P. P., SACK, R. B., DANS, P. E., WELLS, S. A. & CHAUDHURI, R. N. (1965). Clinical evaluation of fluid requirements in Asiatic cholera. *Lancet*, **1**, 726.

CHAUDHURI, R. N., NEOGY, K. N., SANYAL, S. N., GUPTA, R. K. & MANJI, R. (1968). Furazolidone in the treatment of cholera. *Lancet*, **1**, 332.

NALIN, D. R., CASH, R. A., ISLAM, R., MOLLA, M. & PHILLIPS, R. A. (1969). Oral maintenance therapy for cholera in adults. *Lancet*, **2**, 370.

PHILLIPS R. A. (1964). Water and electrolyte losses in cholera. *Federation Proc., Wash.* **23**, 705.

GIARDIASIS

Giardia intestinalis is a flagellate and its presence in the intestine is frequently associated with diarrhoea and abdominal symptoms. Outbreaks of diarrhoea associated with heavy infections of giardia are by no means uncommon in children's nurseries in Great Britain.

Metronidazole in doses of 200 mg. three times a day for up to 10 consecutive days in an adult, and a proportionately smaller dose for children, may get rid of this infection, but even repeated treatments fail on occasions. Children under four years of age can be given one-quarter of the adult dose, and from four to eight years half the adult dose of the drug. The infection tends to lessen when the stools become more solid, and this may follow the administration of bismuth salicylate given in 3 g. doses three times a day.

TROPICAL SPRUE

The aetiology of tropical sprue is unknown but the term is applied to a form of malabsorption, resembling wheat-gluten sensitivity, but not due to this, that arises during or after residence in certain tropical countries. A few apparently typical cases have been reported from Rhodesia, but it arises very rarely, if ever, in other parts of Africa. No causative agent has been identified, hence there is no specific treatment.

For the dehydrated, wasted or severely anaemic patient complete rest in bed is essential. Dehydration must be combated, if necessary by infusions of isotonic saline, and potassium salts must be supplied if the plasma is deficient in potassium (p. 257).

Severe diarrhoea should be checked by the administration of codeine (p. 444). Profound anaemia necessitates an immediate blood transfusion, and occasionally there is a place for intravenous nutrition using preparations such as Aminosol to provide amino acids and Intralipid as a source of calories.

All patients with recent acute disease should be given 10 mg. of folic acid intramuscularly daily for three days, followed by 5 mg. orally twice daily. Serum folate levels are low and the administration of folic acid produces a brisk response: megaloblastic bone marrow becomes normoblastic; there is a reticulocytosis followed by an improved blood count and the symptoms, including glossitis, stomatitis, steatorrhoea and flatulence are ameliorated. If serial jejunal biopsies are done, the atrophic villi are seen to be rapidly replaced by normal villi. Although this disease is not necessarily associated with deficiency of vitamin B_{12}, it is wise to give 1,000 mcg. of hydroxocobalamin intramuscularly when starting folic-acid therapy in case there is a concomitant deficiency of it—when folic-acid treatment might precipitate neurological complications.

If the anaemia is also hypochromic, ferrous sulphate should be administered (p. 143). Haemorrhages into the skin arise from deficiency of prothrombin; this is corrected by giving phytomenadione, 25 mg. intramuscularly daily until normal prothrombin levels are attained. Tetany, which may occur in severe cases from malabsorption of calcium, is controlled by the giving of intravenous calcium gluconate (p. 299) and calciferol. Evidence of multiple vitamin deficiency warrants giving a preparation containing thiamine 10 mg., riboflavine 5 mg. and nicotinamide 50 mg. twice daily for a few weeks. If the patient is seriously ill, treatment with corticosteroids is sometimes life saving.

At first, fats and carbohydrates in the diet should be limited, but they can gradually be increased as recovery sets in, although some degree of intolerance of fat may be a feature for a few months. Following a good response, a patient may return to the tropics after six months of freedom from marked symptoms, with little risk of a recurrence. It has not been established whether it is necessary for a small dose of folic acid to be taken regularly after recovery, but provided the subject does not exhibit histamine-fast achlorhydria, this may be a wise precaution, especially in the tropics. If not taken regularly, it should certainly be taken during pregnancy or restarted at the first indication of a recurrence of symptoms.

It now appears clear that if treatment for tropical sprue has not been started within six months of onset, the response to the treatment outlined above is unsatisfactory in about a quarter of the patients. Such patients are usually helped by a course of antibiotics, presumably by an alteration taking place in the intestinal bacterial flora. Various courses have been tried such as tetracycline, 1 g. daily for 7 to 14 days.

Patients require reassurance and encouragement but it is also necessary to make sure, particularly if the response is imperfect, that the diagnosis, which rests on rather indefinite grounds, is correct by taking steps to exclude malignant disease, wheat-gluten enteropathy and other conditions which may cause or simulate malabsorption syndromes.

References

MATHAN, V. I., JOSEPH, S. & BAKER, S. J. (1969). Tropical sprue in children. *Gastroenterology*, **56**, 556.
O'BRIEN, W. (1968). The diagnosis and treatment of tropical sprue. *Trans. R. Soc. trop. Med. Hyg.* **62**, 148.

LEPROSY

The infectivity of leprosy is slight, but susceptibility to the infection is variable. In Britain the Medical Officer of Health for the area must be notified when it is diagnosed. Strict segregation is undesirable and quite unnecessary in tuberculoid and neural leprosy when smears made from scrapings from cut dermis do not reveal the causative organism, *Mycobacterium leprae*. It is prudent to obtain the advice of a specialist to ensure that an accurate assessment is made before treatment is started.

Specific Treatment

To enable specific treatment to be carried out successfully it is important to obtain the confidence and collaboration of the patient. It is essential to allay the misplaced fear which is often associated with this disease but yet to prepare the patient for a prolonged course of treatment.

Dapsone. This drug (di(*p*-aminophenyl) sulphone) is generally to be recommended. To avoid toxic effects the dose is initially small and is only very slowly increased. The following course should be followed unless intolerance of the drug becomes evident. Initially, for an adult, dapsone is given in a dose of 25 mg. weekly increasing this by 25 mg. weekly until a dose of 50 mg. twice weekly is reached. For patients with lepromatous leprosy double this dose may be required to maintain a satisfactory response. For children under five years, one-fifth of the adult dose and from 5 to 12 years one-half of the adult dose should be dispensed.

If possible, treatment with dapsone should be delayed until the haemoglobin level has reached 10 g. per cent. Anaemia before and during treatment is combated by oral iron (p. 143), except where it results from haemolysis (p. 158). Lepromatous leprosy may be responsible for an anaemia which will not improve until after dapsone treatment has begun to be effective.

Given in the small doses recommended, reactions to the drug are rare. In tuberculoid leprosy, there is a pronounced cellular reaction on the part of the host tending to arrest the disease. Chemotherapy hastens cure and, if started in time, prevents neural damage which would lead to deformities. Drug treatment for tuberculoid leprosy should be continued for a minimum of two years and for not less than twelve months after signs of activity of the disease have ceased. The clinical manifestations of lepromatous leprosy may be dramatically affected or respond only extremely slowly, but treatment must be continued for at least 12 months after *Myco. leprae* showing a normal structure have been found in smears from the dermis. Recent observations have confirmed that *Myco. leprae* having a beaded appearance are dead and can be ignored. Nevertheless, as undamaged organisms may persist in deeper tissues, especially nerves, patients usually continue treatment for many years. Since relapses may occur after apparent cure, re-examination at intervals is essential.

When regular treatment can be ensured only by parenteral injections, dapsone suspended in a suitable vegetable oil can be used in a strength of 200 mg. per ml. The following dose schedule is recommended: first month, 1 ml. weekly; second month, 2 ml. once in two weeks; third month, 4 ml. once a month; and thereafter 6 ml. monthly. The injection should be given deeply intramuscularly, and not more than 3 ml. in one site at a time. Dapsone acetaldehyde bisulphite is presented in a 20 per cent. w/v solution, the equivalent of 200 mg. dapsone being contained in 1 ml., and is administered intramuscularly. Dosage is as indicated in the directions which accompany the ampoules.

Toxic effects are rare if the doses recommended are not exceeded. Larger doses may cause a dermatosis, neuritis, hepatitis or a psychosis. A reactional state may be precipitated by chemotherapy although such a reaction is not solely or necessarily due to the drug. The treatment of reactions is considered below.

Thiambutosine (a diphenyl-thiourea compound) is a useful alternative to dapsone for oral administration. The daily dose is 1 g. increased by 500 mg. at fortnightly intervals to a standard maximum dose of 3 g. daily. After 18 months of its use resistance to the drug may develop.

Clofazimine (see below) and **rifampicin** (p. 72) are also proving to be useful in the treatment of leprosy.

Isoniazid and streptomycin are active against *Myco. leprae*. This combination is particularly useful for a time if the patient also has tuberculosis.

Sulphonamides. Long-acting sulphonamides such as sulfadoxine are widely used in some countries.

TREATMENT OF REACTIONAL STATES. If the patient is exhibiting an allergic dermatosis, psychosis or hepatitis attributable to dapsone this drug should be stopped. In other patients with active leprosy for whom the dose of dapsone has been as advised above, it or an alternative antileprosy drug should be continued.

Clofazimine, 100 mg. three times daily, is of great value in reactional states as it exerts an antiinflammatory effect and is at the same time bacteriostatic. It does, however, produce a ruddy complexion and may cause dark pigmentation in skin already affected by leprosy. This makes the drug unacceptable, on cosmetic grounds, to some people. If clofazimine is declined, older methods should be attempted, such as oral chloroquine 150 mg. (base) three times daily for two weeks, or if there is no response, stibophen injection (B.P.) 2 ml. intramuscularly on alternate days for six doses. If dapsone has been stopped, thiambutosine may be substituted temporarily.

A complication frequently seen in reactional states in tuberculoid leprosy is agonizing pain arising from swollen nerves constricted by the epineurium. This responds well to clofazimine. Alternatively, great relief can be obtained by the intraneural injection of hyaluronidase (1,500 units) dissolved in 1 ml. of 2 per cent. procaine solution mixed with 1 ml. of hydrocortisone suspension (25 mg. per ml.). A reaction in the eyes calls for the use of 1 per cent. atropine sulphate drops or ointment for full mydriasis, and the application of 1 per cent. cortisone ointment. If necessary, mydricaine (a solution of atropine, cocaine and adrenaline) and cortisone can be injected beneath the conjunctiva. Corticosteroids should be used only if other methods fail, as subsequent withdrawal is liable to be followed by an exacerbation.

GENERAL MANAGEMENT. A very important part of treatment is a regimen of good food, regular exercise and the treatment of any intercurrent disease such as dysentery, tuberculosis, malaria, kala azar and ancylostomiasis. The morale of the patient should also be kept up by agreeable occupation and, if possible, gainful employment.

Early attention should be paid to the possible effects of neural damage. Much can be done to protect an anaesthetic limb from injury, and by physiotherapy and orthopaedic measures to prevent and correct deformities. Even patients who are severely mutilated may be rehabilitated. In lepromatous leprosy close observation of the eyes is essential.

PERSONAL PROPHYLAXIS. In countries where the disease is endemic, leprosy is usually acquired early in life, probably because close contact with infective relatives occurs mostly in childhood. There is substantial evidence that BCG vaccination (p. 66) under certain environmental conditions reduces the risk of acquiring leprosy. Adults should take reasonable precautions and children should be removed from lepromatous parents until they are no longer infective. A child who has lived for some time in contact with an untreated lepromatous patient can advantageously be given oral dapsone for two years as a prophylactic. Particular care should be taken to disinfect the nasal discharges of patients with lepromatous leprosy and also their eating and drinking utensils. Medical and nursing staff treating lepromatous patients should use protective clothing and rubber gloves or wash frequently with soap and water.

SUMMARY

Drugs recommended: Dapsone, thiambutosine, clofazimine, rifampicin.

References

BROWN, S. G. (1967). The drug treatment of leprosy. *Trans. R. Soc. trop. Med. Hyg.* **61**, 265.

REES, R. J. W., PEARSON, J. M. H., & WATERS, M. F. R. (1970). Experimental and clinical studies on rifampicin in treatment of leprosy. *Br. med. J.* **1**, 89.

WATERS, M. F. R. (1969). *Lepr. Rev.* **40**, 21.

DENGUE

SPECIFIC TREATMENT. Dengue is a fever of short duration due to several strains of an arbovirus of Group B, conveyed to man by the bites of infected mosquitoes of the species *Aedes aegypti*. There is no specific treatment.

NON-SPECIFIC TREATMENT. The chief symptoms are very severe pain in bones and, after the fever is over, a degree of mental depression. Relief of pain should be attempted by the administration of aspirin or paracetamol and codeine in full doses. If these prove inadequate, stronger analgesics such as pethidine, methadone or dihydrocodeine bitartrate should be administered (pp. 443–445). Although the disease is of short duration, there is a danger that drug addiction may occur in association with the depression during convalescence, which makes caution necessary in the prescription of those analgesics which may be habit forming.

Recently some outbreaks of dengue in South-East Asia have been accompanied by haemorrhagic rashes and severe toxicity. For such, corticosteroids should be employed. Other dengue-like viral diseases require similar treatment but convalescence may be more protracted.

PREVENTION. There is no vaccine against the virus of dengue. The abolition of favoured breeding places of the *Aedes*, chiefly small collections of water in containers and coconut shells near to houses, and the use of insecticides and mosquito repellents (p. 538) are essential measures in prevention.

SANDFLY FEVER

SPECIFIC TREATMENT. This disease is very similar to dengue but is caused by a small group of closely related arboviruses conveyed by bites of species of *Phlebotomus* ('sandflies'). There is no specific treatment.

NON-SPECIFIC TREATMENT. This is the same as for dengue.

PREVENTION. The breeding places of sandflies, chiefly cracks and crevices, should be filled in or old crumbling houses replaced. Personal protection can be obtained by the application of insect repellents to exposed parts (p. 538). The mesh of a mosquito-net is too wide to prevent the entrance of sandflies but if the net is sprayed with an insecticide (p. 538) it acts as an effective barrier. A net with a smaller mesh cannot be tolerated in the tropics. No vaccine is available.

RELAPSING FEVER

SPECIFIC TREATMENT. The object of treatment is to cut short the febrile illness and to prevent subsequent relapses. The causative organisms, *Borrelia recurrentis* and *Bor. duttoni*, are inhibited by tetracycline, which is the drug of choice, although subsequent relapses of tick-borne relapsing fever due to *Bor. duttoni* may be experienced. The daily dose for an adult should not exceed 1 g. in four divided doses. If a larger dose is given dangerous hypotension is more likely to result from a Jarisch-Herxheimer reaction to the death of the organisms. Treatment should be continued for seven days and after a week's interval this course should be repeated.

GENERAL MANAGEMENT. The usual management of a febrile patient should be undertaken, i.e. nursing in bed, sponging with hot or tepid water, aspirin or paracetamol for the relief of headache, and the maintenance of an adequate fluid intake.

If there are signs of meningitis, lumbar puncture should be performed. Jaundice due to hepatitis is a well-recognized complication and is relieved by the specific treatment. Palsies are infrequent except after recurrent bouts of tick-borne fever, when physiotherapy may be required.

PERSONAL PROPHYLAXIS. The prevention of louse-borne relapsing fever is dependent on the destruction of lice (p. 538). The ticks which act as vectors of relapsing fever are soft ticks of the genus *Ornithodorus* which become active in the dark. They live chiefly under the surface and in cracks of primitive houses plastered with mud. Avoidance of sleeping in such houses, the spraying of them with benzene hexachloride (BHC) or applying a 5 per cent. mixture in sawdust prevents transmission.

Reference

BRYCESON, A. D. M., PARRY, E. H. O., PERINE, P. L., WARRELL, D. A., VUKOTICH, D. & LEITHEAD, C. S. (1970). Louse-borne relapsing fever. *Quart. J. Med.* 39 N.S., 129.

YELLOW FEVER

SPECIFIC THERAPY. There is no specific treatment for this disease, and serum from convalescents, even if available, is of no value after symptoms have developed.

NON-SPECIFIC THERAPY. The disease varies greatly in severity, from a mild attack with no recognizable symptoms to a very severe and rapidly fatal disease with classic symptoms and signs. In severe cases, careful nursing of the patient at complete rest in bed is essential. The room should be mosquito proofed as the virus is in the blood in the early stages and is transmitted by *Aedes* mosquitoes.

As much fluid as possible should be taken containing the juice of citrus fruits and glucose. When vomiting is troublesome, 5 per cent. glucose solution should be given intravenously, alternating with isotonic saline solution. To combat acidosis, 10 to 15 g. sodium bicarbonate can be given daily by mouth in divided doses. If there is much vomiting isotonic sodium bicarbonate solution (14 g. per litre) or one-sixth molar (1·87 per cent.) sodium lactate solution can be given intravenously as required (p. 253). Anuria is a very serious complication, for which the treatment recommended on p. 273 should be employed. The application of an ice-bag to the head or lumbar puncture may give welcome relief when headache is severe. If the temperature rises unduly, cold sponging should be employed.

PERSONAL PROPHYLAXIS. Immunization with yellow fever vaccine is the most important method of personal prophylaxis. As it is essential that yellow fever vaccination should confer a reliable immunity, valid international certificates of vaccination can only be issued at approved centres. A list of the centres in Britain is issued by the Ministry of Health and the Scottish Home and Health Department and is available at most travel agencies. Strict immigration regulations, supported by control of *Aedes* mosquito breeding around international airports, prevents the introduction of this disease to new 'receptor' areas, i.e. countries where *Aedes aegypti* are present but the virus of yellow fever has not been introduced. These regulations prohibit the entrance of a traveller (over the age of 1 year) from an endemic zone unless in possession of a valid certificate of vaccination. The vaccine used in Britain is the 17D strain of attenuated virus maintained in chick embryos. The vaccine is issued dry in ampoules and must be kept cold until used when it is dissolved in sterile isotonic saline and injected subcutaneously. Immunity develops within 10 days after a single injection and lasts for at least 10 years, the period of validity of the certificate. Neither local nor general reactions occur in the vast majority of cases, but allergic reactions may result in subjects hypersensitive to egg or chicken protein. These can usually be minimized by giving the vaccine in divided and gradually increasing doses; symptoms during an attack are controlled by injecting adrenaline. There is a remote risk of encephalitis if the vaccination is carried out under the age of nine months. It is also thought that the giving of yellow fever vaccination within 21 days of a preceding primary smallpox vaccination increases the risk of encephalitis. For these reasons when both vaccinations are required within a short time, that for yellow fever should be given first. If at all possible children under nine months should not be taken to endemic areas although some temporary immunity may be inherited from an immune mother. After the age of nine months an interval of a clear week should elapse following yellow fever vaccination, before a primary vaccination against smallpox or vaccination against poliomyelitis is carried out. Even for an adult, if a primary vaccination against smallpox has been inadvertently carried out first, 21 days should elapse before that for yellow fever is given. The interval is less important with revaccination against smallpox. Travellers may present themselves to general practitioners prior to receiving yellow fever vaccination requesting vaccination against smallpox and, if it is given, may have to cancel travelling arrangements. It may be advisable to withhold yellow fever vaccination during pregnancy.

There is no specific treatment for encephalitis following yellow fever vaccination, but so far as is known, the rare cases following 17D virus have all made a complete recovery.

RABIES

Once established, this disease is believed to be invariably fatal. It is, therefore, of the greatest importance to take all necessary steps in the prevention of the disease after exposure to infection.

TREATMENT OF THE ESTABLISHED CASE. A patient with rabies should be nursed in a quiet room with subdued light. Muscular spasms can be relieved by chlorpromazine given intramuscularly, 100 mg. for an adult, repeated as required and, if necessary, combined with intramuscular paraldehyde 3 to 6 ml. When spasms are violent, control can be obtained by inhalation of chloroform.

Bromethol gives relief by keeping the patient just unconscious. This may be administered by a continuous intravenous drip, but the better way in such a case would be by slow continuous rectal infusion in a sufficient dose to produce narcosis for several hours at a time. The dose of bromethol is 0·1 ml. per kg. of body weight, administered rectally as a 2·5 per cent. solution in distilled water. The solution should be tested by means of congo red or Universal Indicator in order to detect the presence of hydrobromic acid. This breakdown product is highly irritating to the mucosa of the bowel. Occasionally encephalitis due to other causes may simulate rabies. The possibility of recovery in suspected rabies should, therefore, be entertained, and by resorting to tracheostomy, as in the management of tetanus (p. 53), the lives of some patients suffering from rabies may in the future be saved. There is little danger to the nursing staff as the human salivary glands are rarely infected; nevertheless, reasonable care should be taken as human bites can convey the disease.

TREATMENT OF THOSE WHO HAVE BEEN EXPOSED TO INFECTION. Careful local treatment of a bite by a suspected animal is very important. The wound should be thoroughly washed immediately with soap and water, if necessary opening it up. Lacerated wounds, particularly on the face, should not be tightly stitched. When preliminary cleansing is efficiently done within 30 minutes of the bite, some infections are prevented and in others the incubation period is prolonged, enabling immunization to become effective.

A dog which has caused a bite and is suspected of being rabid should not be killed but be kept securely tied up with two collars and chains, and observed. If it survives for 10 days then it was almost certainly not infective at the time of tying up. Should it develop an illness during this period and die, or have to be killed, two portions of the brain from the region of the corpus callosum, one in formol saline and the other in glycerin, should be sent to an experienced pathologist for examination for Negri bodies and isolation of the virus, but in an endemic area negative pathological findings do not exclude rabies. In specialized centres a rapid immunofluorescent technique is now employed in diagnosis. In Britain, except in quarantine kennels, it is most unlikely that an infected dog will be found. Nevertheless, whenever the suspicion is strong, the Veterinary Authorities should be informed, either directly or through the police. The same rules apply to bites by cats and other animals in or from endemic areas.

After the local treatment has been applied, if there is any likelihood of the animal having been infective, prophylactic treatment must be given without delay. Contact of the unbroken skin with saliva of a rabid animal does not constitute an exposure.

Risks are classified as follows:

Class I. Slight risk: licks on abrasions, bites or scratches that have not drawn blood, on any part of the body except the head, face, neck or fingers. Licks on the intact mucous membrane.

Class II. Moderate risk: licks on cuts or abrasions on fingers. Bites or scratches on the fingers less than 0·5 cm. long and not penetrating the skin. Bites and scratches on all parts of the body, excluding the head, face, neck or fingers, that have drawn blood but are less than 13 cm. long and are without any extensive laceration.

Class III. Severe risk: licks on abrasions and all bites and scratches on head, face or neck. Severe bites or scratches on fingers. Five or more bites drawing blood anywhere. All extensive lacerations. All jackal and wolf bites. All cases in Class II where treatment has been delayed over 14 days.

In view of the rare occurrence of neuroparalytic accidents following anti-rabies vaccination, people in Class I should await the death of a confined suspected dog before commencing treatment.

Hyperimmune serum. In addition to a course of vaccine, patients in Class III, where the risk is great and the incubation period liable to be short, should be given an initial dose of hyperimmune anti-rabic serum to produce temporary passive immunity. A single dose of 75 International Units per kg. body weight is given intramuscularly and, if possible, an equal quantity is infiltrated around the wound.

Vaccines. A great variety of anti-rabic vaccines are used in different countries. The virus may be either attenuated or killed. The latter is used in the Semple-type vaccines which are in general use, but both the method of preparation and the dosage recommended vary considerably. Detailed instructions are issued with every ampoule of the vaccine issued. The recommended course varies with the degree of risk but lasts from 7 to 14 days.

The vaccine is given subcutaneously into a different area of the abdominal wall each day. If the dose is more than 5 ml. for an adult or 2 ml. for a child, it is given in divided doses in two areas.

For patients in Class III the course is supplemented 10 and 20 days after the last usual dose by injections of a vaccine prepared from duck embryo. During treatment the patient should live quietly and avoid alcohol. The immunity conferred lasts only three months.

Local allergic reactions may be alleviated by antihistamines. Neurological complications including polyneuritis, Landry's paralysis and encephalitis have been experienced. They usually appear within a few days of completing the course of vaccination. The severity of polyneuritis, at least, may be diminished by corticosteroid treatment. These untoward results are serious but rare, and should not deter the physician from using vaccine therapy in order to protect a patient when there is an appreciable risk of such a serious disease as rabies. Nevertheless, it was hoped that a vaccine containing a virus grown in embryonate ducks' eggs would be less likely to be followed by neuroparalytic disorders, although it does contain embryonic neural tissue. As this vaccine does not appear to be as potent as the Semple type, it is advocated only for booster doses as above or where the risk of having been infected is minimal.

PERSONAL PROPHYLAXIS. In a country where rabies is a risk, all suspected animals should be avoided. Dogs showing signs of choking should be handled with great care, as this is often the first sign of rabies. The fingers should never be put into a dog's mouth. Dogs may be protected by a single injection of living chick embryo vaccine (Flury) once a year and it is important that this should be done. Wolves, jackals and other infected animals should be destroyed. Where the vampire bat is the vector, these creatures must be destroyed, and cattle protected by chick embryo vaccine.

The incubation period in dogs is long and variable. Animals imported from endemic countries must be kept in effective quarantine. The length of quarantine enforced in Great Britain is 6 months with strict isolation, and vaccination.

SUMMARY

In preventive inoculation hyperimmune serum is used, followed by a vaccine of Semple type or vaccine from duck eggs if the risk is minimal and for reinforcing doses.

Reference

W.H.O. EXPERT COMMITTEE ON RABIES (1966). *Tech. Rep. Ser. No.* 321, 5th Report.

EFFECTS OF HEAT

ACCLIMATIZATION to heat is an essential preparation for workers in certain industries in cool climates as well as for people who go to live in the tropics. It can be achieved by exercise daily under artificially produced or natural hot weather conditions for two or three weeks, by the end of which time metabolism will have become adjusted. This adjustment includes an increase in the total circulating fluid volume of the body to compensate for the expanded vascular bed. The salt loss in the sweat also decreases although the total secretion of sweat is increased. This conservation of salt is brought about mainly by increased activity of the adrenal glands with enhanced production of aldosterone but also probably by the action of the antidiuretic hormone on the renal tubules and the sweat glands. As a physiological process, when the body temperature rises above 37·7° C. the rate of sweating begins to decrease, and by the time a body temperature of 40·5° or 41° C. is reached, sweating may have ceased altogether. After acclimatization there is only a small rise of body temperature above normal during hard manual work. Consequently evaporation of the ordinary output of sweat helps to maintain a normal body temperature. This response to acclimatization is important in the prevention of heat hyperpyrexia. The mechanisms underlying disturbance in water and electrolyte balance and acid base equilibrium are discussed on pp. 253–264.

HEAT SYNCOPE or fainting is a common cause of incapacity in warm conditions. It may occur with exercise, sudden change of posture, standing still for a long time, or even at rest—when unsuitably clothed—in a warm atmosphere with a poor circulation of air. Fainting is then due to an expanded vascular bed with an inadequate compensatory increase in blood volume. When, following acclimatization, the blood volume has increased, heat syncope is less likely. The treatment is simple: unnecessary clothing is removed and the patient is rested in a cool atmosphere, recumbent, with the head low and the feet raised.

HEAT EXHAUSTION produces distress, with a pale sweating skin, increased pulse rate and often a raised rectal temperature (a cold moist man). Dehydration is usually marked, and no chlorides can be found in the highly coloured scanty urine, indicating that there is depletion of both salt and water. Heat exhaustion is often brought on by unusual heat or by extra effort in hot conditions when the patient has not taken enough fluid and salt to balance the increased loss by sweating. When dehydration is limited to loss of the extracellular fluid, there will be no thirst. Consequently water depletion up to as much as 2 litres may be present without producing any symptoms.

The importance of water depletion as the primary cause of heat exhaustion needs to be stressed. Adequate salt replacement, however, is also essential (pp. 253–257).

Early symptoms of heat exhaustion may be loss of appetite, nausea, muscular cramps, and changes in personality. At this stage removal into a cool atmosphere and enough cool water to drink, with salt as required, will soon restore the patient. If, however, the disorder is not recognized in the early stages and treatment is delayed, the results are often poor. In such cases intravenous infusions of saline are indicated, the quantity depending upon the patient's condition as in cholera (p. 522). Useful guidance can also be obtained from measuring the output of chloride in the urine. When patients suffering from heat exhaustion are neglected they may develop hyperpyrexia.

TROPICAL ANHIDROTIC ASTHENIA develops towards the end of the seasonal spell of hot weather. The majority of patients with this disorder have suffered from prickly heat which has left extensive areas of lichen tropicalis with consequent impairment of sweating. The condition develops insidiously with the following symptoms—lack of energy, diminished sweating, and marked polyuria (the dilute urine containing chloride). A rise of temperature is common and occasionally hyperpyrexia occurs. The plasma chlorides are usually slightly decreased.

Prolonged treatment is required. The patient must live in a cool climate (for example at a hill station) until the skin has recovered and sweating has returned to normal: this may take up to two months.

HEAT HYPERPYREXIA may begin dramatically without any previous warning symptoms or signs in a person who appears to be neither dehydrated nor deficient in salt. He may have retired to rest feeling quite well and be found in coma a few hours later, but more characteristically loss of consciousness is preceded by prodromal signs typical of cerebral irritation. On examination a dry burning skin is very characteristic (the hot dry man). When the temperature reaches between

40·5° and 41·5° C., unconsciousness supervenes. In cases of secondary heat hyperpyrexia, however, the early symptoms are those of heat exhaustion or tropical anhidrotic asthenia.

Treatment of heat hyperpyrexia aims at reducing the temperature as quickly as possible to prevent permanent injury to vital structures. This is best achieved by covering the stripped patient with a cool wet sheet and promoting evaporation by fanning. As the temperature falls, provided the brain has not been irreparably damaged, consciousness returns. Cooling should be stopped when the rectal temperature has fallen to around 38·5° C., otherwise the temperature, which continues to fall, may reach excessively low levels. As anoxia is often present, oxygen should be administered. Chlorpromazine should be given (100 mg. intramuscularly) and an adequate airway maintained. If return to consciousness is delayed, lumbar puncture and removal of excess cerebrospinal fluid is indicated. Intravenous hydrocortisone hemisuccinate (100 mg.) should be given if there is circulatory failure. Renal or hepatic failure require appropriate treatment (pp. 273, 249). During convalescence there may be evidence of unstable control of body temperature.

When hyperpyrexia is secondary to heat exhaustion, dehydration is usually severe. Therefore, in addition to treatment for reduction of the high temperature, adequate water and salt replacement is essential. Depending on the duration and degree of hyperpyrexia, the patient may recover completely or be left with residual brain damage. In a malarious area the possibility that cerebral malaria is the cause of hyperpyrexia should be entertained and treatment given accordingly (p. 511).

PREVENTION OF ILL-EFFECTS OF HEAT. Careful selection should be made of those required to work under hot atmospheric conditions. General physical fitness and mental stability are important; people in the younger age-groups are, as a rule, more suitable for such employment. Febrile conditions, gastrointestinal upsets, alcoholic excess and lack of sleep all predispose to the ill-effects of heat. It is highly important that the skin should be healthy and that sweating should occur normally.

Where the atmospheric temperature is very high leading to excessive sweating, even those fully acclimatized will require to take additional fluid and salt. A daily intake of up to as much as 15 litres of cool drinking water and 30 g. of sodium chloride per person may then be needed to prevent water and salt depletion. The extra salt, three level teaspoonfuls, is usually taken with food and in the drinking water, but when necessary it can be made available in enteric coated tablets each containing 650 mg. of sodium chloride.

In addition, everything possible should be done to improve working conditions; and, for indoor work, arrangements should be made to encourage evaporation of sweat by free circulation of the air and by reduction of high temperatures and excessive atmospheric humidity by means of air-conditioning. Clothing should be light and loose fitting. Hard or prolonged manual work should not be undertaken when atmospheric conditions are exceptionally unfavourable. A wet-bulb temperature around 26·5° C. with an air temperature of 32° C. should indicate the need for special care on the part of those in charge of workers. Off-duty living conditions should be made as cool and comfortable as possible.

PRICKLY HEAT. Prickly heat arises from blockage of sweat ducts within the prickle cell layer of the epidermis. Sweat is thus secreted into the epidermis and causes severe irritation. Clinically the condition is called miliaria rubra or miliaria pustulosa. The latter is nearly always the result of irritation in the tissues which converts the vesicular fluid into sterile pus; these minute pustules are rarely infective in origin. It follows that the principles of treatment are to minimize sweating and to relieve the blockage.

If sweating can be reduced by transferring the sufferer into an air-conditioned room or other cool environment, the effects of blockage of the sweat ducts gradually subside in a week or two. The procedures recommended under prevention should be adopted as far as possible. Washing should be gentle and the sparing use of hexachlorophane soap appears to be beneficial. In severe cases the application of anhydrous lanoline will restore sweating and it is worth while to use this method when artificial cooling is difficult to arrange. A sedative (phenobarbitone, 30 mg. six-hourly) may be required when irritation is intense.

Prevention. Any process which damages the skin is liable to lead to plugging of the orifices of sweat ducts. Therefore, maceration of the skin by sweat or liquid applications, irritation from clothing (whether from friction or a chemical), and excessive washing should be avoided. Soap should be of good quality and used sparingly. Hexachlorophane soap is refreshing. After bathing a light application of a fine dusting powder is helpful. It is important to wear loose-fitting clothing which must be changed frequently. If possible, sudden exposure to heat must be avoided and diets which are known to promote excessive sweating are obviously undesirable. Curries and alcohol should be taken in moderation, if at all.

Reference

LEITHEAD, C. S. & LIND, A. R. (1964). *Heat Stress and Heat Disorders.* London: Cassell.

HELMINTHIC INFECTIONS

Schistosomiasis (*Bilharziasis*)

SPECIFIC TREATMENT. Trivalent antimony compounds exert a specific lethal effect on the adult schistosome and destroy the larva inside the ovum. Sodium antimony tartrate is of known efficacy, so is still employed in spite of its disadvantageous side-effects. The patient should be lying down and fasting when the treatment is given. Starting with 30 mg., the dose is increased by 30 mg. until a maximum of 120 mg. is reached. A total of at least 2 g. is required to cure an adult. The dose is dissolved in 5 or 10 ml. of sterile pyrogen-free distilled water and given daily or on alternate days intravenously. In endemic areas weekly injections are sometimes employed. For relapses the course should be repeated after an interval of not less than six weeks. Cough, vomiting and lumbar pains commonly occur soon after each of the larger doses and pain in the shoulders or other joints may be troublesome, but apart from these inconveniences the drug is usually well tolerated, provided the liver and kidneys are healthy. The effect on the heart should be assessed clinically and, if indicated, by serial E.C.G. determinations. During the administration of sodium antimony tartrate, care must be taken to ensure that none escapes into the tissues, otherwise there will be a very severe and painful local reaction. A newer trivalent antimonial, stibocaptate, incorporates dimercaprol and is administered intramuscularly in a course of four to five injections on alternate days or as tolerated. The maximum total adult dose is 2·5 g. Side-effects are less than those produced by sodium antimony tartrate and the rate of cure is similar.

Lucanthone. Oral treatment with lucanthone hydrochloride (a thioxanthone derivative) can be used. The recommended daily dose is 60 mg. per kg. body weight for six days. The results are not very good, but urinary infections appear to respond best; when parenteral treatment is difficult to arrange, it has a field of use. Toxic effects such as nausea, anorexia, headache, dizziness and epigastric and abdominal pains may be experienced.

Hycanthone. Recently, another thioxanthone derivative, hycanthone, has been introduced. It is administered intramuscularly in a single dose of 3 mg. per kg. body weight, and it is claimed to produce a high percentage of cures. It is contra-indicated if phenothiazines have been taken and its safety in pregnancy has not yet been established.

Niridazole. This drug has been used successfully. A dose of 25 mg. per kg. body weight is given orally for seven days. The chief toxic effect is the occasional production of a temporary psychosis. The drug is detoxicated in the liver and should not be used in the presence of hepatic disorders. Another drug under investigation for oral administration is *trichlorophon.*

LOCAL TREATMENT. With a long-standing haematobium infection marked changes may be produced in the urinary tract. Pyogenic infection and calculus formation may occur and carcinoma of the bladder is a recognized complication in areas of high endemicity. Fibrosis around the ureteric orifice into the bladder may produce back pressure and hydronephrosis. These complications require appropriate local measures in addition to specific treatment. In chronic *S. mansoni* and *S. japonicum* infections, involvement of the liver may lead to cirrhosis with resulting portal hypertension and associated splenomegaly. For such patients splenectomy and portal-caval anastomosis may be considered; the removal of a large spleen gives relief to the patient and there are indications that those so treated are not so liable to develop ascites and haemorrhages. Splenectomy also reduces the incidence and severity of changes in the blood due to hypersplenism. When there is extensive disease of the rectum and sigmoid colon, surgical treatment may be required. The removal of large papillomata through the sigmoidoscope gives considerable relief. Involvement of the central nervous system is a rare complication met with especially in *S. japonicum* infection; the resulting granuloma may cause pressure symptoms. In these cases intensive and repeated courses of antimony are required and occasionally surgical intervention.

PERSONAL PROPHYLAXIS. In areas where schistosomiasis is prevalent, bathing or wading in irrigation ditches, canals or pools should be avoided. Ordinary clothing gives no protection in infected waters; rubber thigh-boots and rubber gloves are essential when working in these waters. In such areas drinking water must first be filtered, sterilized by boiling or stored out of contact with snails for two days. Concentrations of chlorine suitable for dealing effectively with the usual bacterial contamination of water are insufficient to kill the cercariae, which are, however, killed by Halazone in a dilution of one part in a million.

SUMMARY

Drugs recommended: Intravenously, sodium antimony tartrate; intramuscularly, stibocaptate or hycanthone; orally, niridazole.

References

FORSYTH, D. M. & RASHID, C. (1967). Treatment of urinary schistosomiasis. *Lancet*, **1**, 130.
MCMAHON, J. E. & KILALA, C. P. (1966). Clinical trial with Ambilhar in *Schistosoma mansoni* infections in Tanzania. *Br. med. J.* **2**, 1047.
WOLFE, H. L. (1967). Treatment of urinary schistosomiasis with niridazole. *Lancet*, **1**, 350.

Cestodiasis (*Tapeworm Infection*)

Taenia saginata (*beef tapeworm*). The only type of taeniasis which occurs in Britain is caused by *T. saginata*. The infective larval stage 'cysticercus bovis' may be present in beef which, if ingested without adequate cooking, leads to the development of the adult worm in man, but *T. saginata* does not cause cysticercosis in man. Many vermifuges are available, but the least disturbing effective anthelmintic for *T. saginata* is niclosamide [5-chloro-*N*-(2-chloro-4-nitrophenyl) salicylamide]. Apart from ensuring that the bowels have been opened normally, no preparation is required. Before breakfast two tablets, each of 500 mg., are chewed to produce an emulsion which is then swallowed with a few sips of water and one hour later a further dose of 1 g. is similarly taken. The tablets have a pleasant taste and do not cause vomiting. The direct effect of niclosamide is to cause disintegration of the tapeworm. The patient should be informed that if segments do not reappear within 15 weeks cure can be presumed. The scolex can be detected only if purgatives are given following the administration of the anthelmintic; and this is disagreeable and unnecessary.

Taenia solium (*pork tapeworm*). On theoretical grounds disintegration of a mature segment of *Taenia solium* during treatment with the drug described above, might lead to the disaster of cysticercosis. It is, therefore, probably wiser to treat *T. solium* with the old-fashioned remedy, filix mas (male fern), although niclosamide has been used with success. To ensure cure when filix mas is used the patient requires 48 hours' preparation, during which time only fruit drinks are given and saline aperients are administered daily. On the third morning, for an adult, 2·5 ml. of a fresh extract of filix mas in capsules or in a suspension is given at 6 a.m. and again at 6.15 a.m. and 6.30 a.m. The patient takes only sips of water until 7 a.m. when 60 ml. of saturated sodium sulphate solution are given. For children appropriately smaller doses are used. If the scolex is not passed by 9 a.m., an enema is administered. Food may be given as soon as the scolex has been seen or in any case by 9.30 a.m. Before and during treatment the patient should be isolated to prevent cysticercosis being acquired by others.

PERSONAL PROPHYLAXIS. Meat should be inspected for cysticerci and infected meat avoided. This is particularly important in areas endemic for *T. solium* where uninspected pork should not be eaten. Thorough cooking of meat will kill the larvae and this should be practised where meat inspection is not carried out. In some underdeveloped countries where nutritious foods are in short supply the rejection of all beef infected with cysticerci is impracticable and would deny the people a valuable source of protein.

Cysticercosis

Normally the cysticercus stage of *T. solium* takes place in the pig, but sometimes this stage occurs in man and causes serious trouble. When ova gain access to the stomach of man, the shells are digested away and the liberated larvae penetrate the intestinal mucosa and are carried to many parts of the body, where they develop into cysticerci. The most common locations are the subcutaneous tissue and skeletal muscles. Here they cause few or no symptoms; however, cysts may develop in the brain. About five years later the larvae die. In muscles calcification of the cyst wall ensues, but in the brain disintegration of the cyst and local oedema are liable to produce irritative symptoms, causing epileptic fits and personality changes. The cysticerci are uninfluenced by treatment but fits can usually be controlled by phenobarbitone and, if necessary, phenytoin as used for idiopathic epilepsy (p. 381). Later it may be possible to discontinue the drugs. Most patients so treated ultimately make a good recovery. Surgical treatment is only required exceptionally to overcome persistent or recurrent internal hydrocephalus or to remove cysts from special sites such as the optic chiasma and trigeminal ganglion.

PERSONAL PROPHYLAXIS. This is very important, especially in parts of the world where infection of the pig with cysts of *T. solium* is common. A patient harbouring *T. solium* in his intestine should be treated as soon as possible, to prevent cysticercosis following the regurgitation of a gravid segment or the ingestion of ova contaminating the hands. Nurses and attendants should handle with great care all dejecta, especially faeces containing the mature segments of *T. solium*, and take every precaution to avoid contamination of their hands and food. In endemic areas raw vegetables should be avoided, as they may have been contaminated with ova or segments of *T. solium* from a man harbouring this worm.

Hydatid cyst. This condition represents the larval stage of the small tapeworm, *Echinococcus granulosus*, which lives in dogs and foxes as the definitive host: the usual intermediate hosts are sheep and cattle, but man may also be one and in him the larvae form large cysts in various organs, particularly the liver and lungs. Aspiration of a cyst should not be attempted either for diagnosis or treatment, as the fluid, besides being toxic, contains scolices which may escape into the tissue and so disseminate the disease widely.

Hydatid disease is rare in Britain. It is common in Iraq, Australia and some other countries. Many years may elapse between the time of the original infection and the onset of clinical signs of hydatid disease.

There is no specific drug therapy, but when it is causing pressure symptoms surgical removal of the cyst and its laminated membrane may be required. Care must then be taken during the operation to prevent the implantation of scolices leading to the development of further cysts. Scolices can be destroyed by washing out the hydatid cavity with 1 : 200 formalin solution. The residual cavity may have to be marsupialized. Pulmonary cysts, being specially liable to rupture, should be removed. If a cyst is fully calcified it can usually be left with impunity. Cysts in a long bone usually call for amputation. Antibiotics are useful in the control of secondary pyogenic infection.

PERSONAL PROPHYLAXIS. Close contact with dogs (especially sheep-dogs), the hosts of the adult worms, must be avoided. An uninfected dog may acquire ova on its fur by rolling on ground contaminated by infected faeces. Also, after handling sheep whose wool may be infected from the faeces of dogs, the hands should be carefully washed especially before eating.

Filariasis

SPECIFIC TREATMENT. Diethylcarbamazine has been shown to be effective in the treatment of filariasis. This drug has a destructive action on the microfilariae, probably by facilitating phagocytosis. In the case of *Dipetalonema perstans*, which fortunately is largely non-pathogenic, the blood is less easily freed of microfilariae. The adult worms of most species are also killed by diethylcarbamazine, but less readily than the microfilariae. This is especially the case in infections with *Onchocerca volvulus*, where the microfilariae not infrequently reappear some time after treatment has been completed. The usual course of treatment with diethylcarbamazine is 6 to 12 mg. per kg. body weight daily, given orally in three divided doses after food, for a period of three weeks.

It is advisable to start with a small initial dose, as this diminishes the tendency to allergic reactions which result from destruction of the microfilariae. The dose is then gradually increased as the drug is tolerated. Even with this precaution, however, fever, pruritus, headache, arthralgia, malaise or nausea may be very troublesome. Relief of these symptoms is afforded by the use of the antihistamines, but exceptionally corticosteroids may be required. In rare instances serious cerebral allergic reactions have been reported in loiasis treated with diethylcarbamazine due, it was thought, to the destruction of microfilariae in the brain. Such a reaction is unlikely if the initial dose is small but when headache is severe or there is other evidence of an adult *Loa loa* near the orbit, extra care is advisable.

In *Wuchereria bancrofti* and *Brugia malayi* infections the most satisfactory results are achieved when treatment with diethylcarbamazine has been started early before obstructive lesions in the lymphatics have occurred; even in the late cases, however, improvement may result. Antibiotics are useful in combating the pyogenic infections which probably play a part in some of the attacks of

.

lymphangitis that often precede permanent lymphatic obstruction. In long-standing elephantiasis surgical measures are required to improve the lymph drainage and remove redundant tissue. Preliminary radiographic demonstration of available lymphatic channels is of assistance in planning the operation. In loiasis an adult worm occasionally passes under the conjunctiva; if it lingers it can be removed, after instilling cocaine, by using a curved needle. Though a worm may similarly be plucked from the skin, removal is scarcely necessary now that there is an effective treatment for loiasis.

Onchocerca volvulus often causes intense itching and produces a thickening and infiltration of the skin with loss of elasticity. Small subcutaneous nodules may also be found in various parts of the body, particularly around the pelvis. These nodules should be removed for they contain adult worms which may resist chemotherapy and cause reinfection of the skin with microfilariae. Ocular complications in heavy infections give it the name, African River Blindness.

The administration of diethylcarbamazine characteristically causes an initial increase in the dermatosis and, if the eyes are affected, may cause an acute and harmful ocular reaction. For these reasons the initial dose should be only 50 mg. and, if necessary, the reaction modified by the use of antihistamines. If the drug is well tolerated, the dose is doubled, usually on consecutive days, until a maximum of 9 to 12 mg. per kg. body weight daily is reached, this quantity being divided into three doses per day. If the reaction is severe, corticosteroids should be substituted for antihistamines. When lesions of the eye are present corticosteroids should be administered from two days before the onset of treatment and 5 per cent. hydrocortisone eye drops instilled into the eyes if increased inflammation occurs. When treatment is successful there is improvement in vision (if it was previously impaired) and relief from the dermatosis. Suramin, given intravenously, is more rapidly lethal to the adult *O. volvulus* than diethylcarbamazine, but because of its toxicity it is usually reserved for infections which have persisted in spite of adequate treatment with diethylcarbamazine. Suramin is liable to cause renal damage, with the appearance of casts and protein in the urine; polyneuritis and urticaria are other occasional complications. As the infection itself is not dangerous to life, treatment by suramin should not be lightly undertaken. The course of treatment for an adult consists of an initial test dose of 200 mg. followed by five weekly doses each of 1 g.

Tropical pulmonary eosinophilia. This syndrome is now usually believed to be an allergic reaction in the lungs to dead microfilariae perhaps of a species for which man is an unusual host. The serum of such patients gives a positive filarial complement fixation test. The condition responds to diethylcarbamazine in doses of 12 mg. per kg. body weight given in three divided doses daily for five days. A few patients relapse and require a further course of treatment.

PERSONAL PROPHYLAXIS. This consists in measures against the vector of the particular filarial worm. Certain species of mosquitoes are responsible for the spread of *W. bancrofti* and *B. malayi*, and may be combated by insecticides. The vectors of *Loa loa* are various species of mango-fly, including *Chrysops dimidiata* and *C. silacea*, which bite mainly in the daytime. In endemic areas the dwelling should, therefore, be protected by gauze, and insecticides should be used. *Onchocerca volvulus* is transmitted by several different species of *Simulium*. Measures on the lines employed against mosquitoes are of value against this vector and the vicinity of fast running streams where simulia breed should be avoided as far as possible.

Guinea Worm

Dracunculosis or dracontiasis is an infection by *Dracunculus medinensis* or guinea worm. The adult female emerges from the subcutaneous tissue, generally of the leg. The treatment of dracunculosis has been greatly improved by the introduction of niridazole (p. 532). The drug is taken orally, 25 mg. per kg. body weight daily in two divided doses for 10 days. Ulcers are dressed with calcium hypochlorite solution. Niridazole facilitates the removal of the extruding worm which is wound out around a sterile orange-stick during a period of several days. Following the use of niridazole, inadvertent rupture of the worm is less dangerous, pain is relieved and ulcers heal quickly. Nausea caused by the drug, may be controlled by promethazine, 25 mg. each morning. In late cases, with abscess formation, antibiotics and prophylaxis of tetanus may still be required.

Infection is contracted from drinking water containing infected cyclops (water flea), the intermediate host; filtering the water removes the cyclops; they are also readily killed by boiling the water. Wells should be covered by lids. Further,

S

the shaft should be so constructed that its wall projects above the level of the adjacent ground. Water should be drawn only from above so that the risk of contamination of the well by discharges from affected people is greatly reduced. After infection diethylcarbamazine may kill larvae before symptoms arise.

Reference

ODUNTAN, S. O., LUCAS, A. O. & GILLES, H. M. (1967). Treatment of dracontiasis with niridazole. *Lancet*, **2**, 73.

Ancylostomiasis (*Hookworm Infection*)

SPECIFIC TREATMENT. Profound anaemia should be corrected before the patient is given specific treatment. The most commonly used and cheapest drug is tetrachloroethylene. The dose is 0·1 ml. per kg. body weight to a maximum dose of 4 ml. The drug should be administered when there is no food in the stomach but purgation is not necessary. Two or more courses of treatment are usually required, but these should not be given until 10 days have elapsed. Tetrachloroethylene rapidly deteriorates in warm climates and must be stored in a cool dark place. It should not be given during pregnancy or if the liver is diseased.

Bephenium hydroxynaphthoate, a quaternary ammonium compound is proving effective in the removal of *Ancylostoma duodenale* but is less successful against *Necator americanus*. It is also effective in removing *Ascaris lumbricoides*. It is given before breakfast as a single dose of 5 g. of dispersible granules (containing 2·5 g. base) in a cup of water. No preparation or purgation is necessary.

NON-SPECIFIC TREATMENT. The irritation of ground itch caused by infecting larvae can be relieved by the application of an ointment containing zinc oxide and salicylic acid or a steroid cream under an occlusive dressing. Anaemia associated with a hookworm infection responds well to treatment with iron in adequate doses. A well-balanced diet containing meat and vegetables is desirable. Where the anaemia is severe, it should be treated by ferrous sulphate (p. 143) before giving the anthelmintic. A blood transfusion may be desirable, but grave anaemia due to ancylostomiasis is frequently associated with oedema. Care must, therefore, be taken to avoid overloading the circulation, and the use of packed cells is preferable. A further safeguard is to give a few doses of frusemide (p. 89) to promote diuresis and reduce the blood volume.

PERSONAL PROPHYLAXIS. The infection is acquired by walking barefoot over soil harbouring infective larvae. These do not travel appreciably laterally and only develop readily in warm moist soil. The use of latrines to avoid fouling the ground is to be advocated, but unless the latrine is used properly the surrounding soil may become contaminated and highly infective. The provision of footwear should be encouraged in endemic areas. A foreshore which is washed by the sea at high tide remains uninfected.

Ascariasis (*Roundworm Infection*)

Ascaris lumbricoides is the nematode commonly known as the roundworm. *Toxocara canis*, the common roundworm of dogs, does not usually progress beyond the larval stage in man, giving rise to 'visceral larva migrans', but occasionally mature *Toxocara canis* develop in the human intestine.

SPECIFIC TREATMENT. Piperazine is the drug of choice; it gives excellent results and is not toxic to the host. Various preparations are available, but the most palatable is Piperazine Citrate Elixir (B.P.C.) which is particularly suitable for administration to children. The doses recommended (B.N.F.) are for adults, 30 ml., and proportionately less for children. An alternative preparation is a combination of piperazine phosphate and senna. A single dose of 10 g. of the mixture is administered. To those under six years of age, 5 to 7 g. should be given. In heavy infections a tangled mass of worms may cause intestinal obstruction necessitating surgical intervention. As treatment with piperazine causes so little disturbance, it may be employed as a diagnostic test for ascariasis: it may cause the expulsion of a solitary male *Ascaris* which would not have been revealed by prior examination of the stool.

PERSONAL PROPHYLAXIS. In areas where infection is common, uncooked vegetables and other raw food should be avoided. The hands should be thoroughly washed before meals.

Strongyloidiasis

Infection with *Strongyloides stercoralis* is common in the tropics and sub-tropics and is especially prevalent in the Far East. It may produce chronic diarrhoea and occasionally very trying 'creeping eruptions' in the skin.

SPECIFIC TREATMENT. The most successful treatment is thiabendazole, given in a dose of 25 mg. per kg. body weight twice daily on two to four successive days.

PERSONAL PROPHYLAXIS. As for ancylostomiasis.

Enterobiasis (*Threadworm Infection*)

If one member of a family is infected with *Enterobius* (Oxyuris) *vermicularis* it is safest to assume that the rest of the family and associates are also infected with threadworms and all should be treated simultaneously.

SPECIFIC TREATMENT. Piperazine salts administered as a single dose as described for ascariasis are effective in a high percentage of cases, but it is wise to repeat the treatment after one week. As it is often difficult to exclude re-infection, further treatments may be necessary. Viprynium embonate is also highly effective and now rivals piperazine. It is given in a single dose of 5 mg. per kg. body weight. The drug colours the stools red.

GENERAL MANAGEMENT AND PERSONAL PROPHYLAXIS. It is very important to prevent re-infection with ova; nails should be kept short and the hands of the infant or child washed carefully, especially before meals. Nail-biting must be discouraged. Prior to cure an antihistamine cream applied around the anus relieves itching. Effective anthelmintics have removed the necessity for further local measures and in institutions the use of vacuum cleaners minimizes the spread of ova in dust.

Trichuriasis (*Whipworm Infection*)

Trichuris trichiura, the whipworm, does not usually cause appreciable trouble except perhaps in heavily infected young children. Thiabendazole can be used as advised for strongyloidiasis.

Trichiniasis

In the early stages when, however, the infection is rarely suspected, tetrachloroethylene followed by a vigorous purge may reduce the number of maturing *Trichinella spiralis* in the bowel. Later, corticosteroids are of considerable value in controlling the acute and dangerous systemic disturbances which are due to the dissemination of the larvae.

Thiabendazole given in the dosage indicated above may later be administered to afford relief from continuing symptoms attributable to the cysts in muscle.

PERSONAL PROPHYLAXIS. Since rats can carry the infection to pigs, access of rats to pigsties should be prevented. Although gross infection of pork should be obvious if proper examination of meat is undertaken in the slaughterhouses, infected carcasses do escape detection. It is essential, therefore, that all pork should be more thoroughly cooked than other carcass meat and this applies especially to pork sausages. Outbreaks of trichiniasis have frequently been traced to the consumption of partially cooked pork sausages. Wild pig, walrus and polar bear are also sources of infection.

22. Pesticides and Repellents

A. R. Mills

Pesticides

A wide range of chemicals is used against arthropod pests in agriculture as well as against those of medical importance. This chapter provides a short account of some of the pesticides in common use. A comprehensive survey of this vast and continually developing subject would be out of place.

In their general mode of action and their relation to insect resistance, the chlorinated hydrocarbon pesticides are at present divided into two groups. One group comprises DDT and chemically related compounds such as methoxychlor and DDD; the other group includes BHC and the cyclodiene-derived compounds such as dieldrin and chlordane.

Because of their chemical stability and low vapour pressure, these residual pesticides remain active for many months when they are sprayed on a surface. Arthropods resting on the sprayed surface pick up particles of the pesticide which eventually kill them. A few anopheles, however, rest only out of doors consequently spraying of houses will not affect these mosquitoes. Also the irritant effect of the residual pesticide causes some insects to be repelled from the treated surface, an effect most marked with DDT. A further difficulty is that certain arthropods become resistant to pesticides.

DDT[1] [OMS–16][2] [(Dicophane, 1,1,1,-trichloro-2, 2-di(p-chlorophenyl) ethane] is specifically toxic to arthropods while having only slight toxicity to vertebrates. It is usually prepared as a water-dispersible powder but dissolves easily in a variety of solvents including kerosene. It is non-volatile at atmospheric temperatures and is unaffected by light, air or water.

DDT in minute concentrations is lethal to larval and adult mosquitoes, to the non-resistant adult housefly, to larval and adult lice and to many other arthropod vectors of disease. It is cheap, almost universally available and is effective under a wide range of conditions. In vector control programmes DDT has been used in very large quantities and continues to be used and no reports of any harmful effects have been recorded among the thousands of people who use it daily in malaria eradication campaigns. The record of safety of DDT to man has been outstanding during the past twenty years and its low cost makes it irreplaceable in public health at the present time. Limitations in its use would give rise to grave health problems in the majority of the developing countries. The exact mode of action of DDT is not known, but when it comes in contact with an arthropod it penetrates the cuticle, diffusing in the lipoids of the nervous system. This results in paralysis which gradually becomes widespread and this is the cause of death. The action of the poison is slow and arthropods sometimes recover if they have received only a very small dose. If handled with reasonable care, DDT is innocuous to human beings, but precautions should be taken to avoid contaminating food and to avoid spilling concentrated solutions on the skin. While impregnating clothing or blankets with DDT, the air of the room may become heavily contaminated with DDT dust and prolonged inhalation may produce toxic effects, including severe general malaise and ataxia.

Recent studies on the amount of p,p'-DDT and p,p'-DDE (the principle metabolite of DDT) measured on whole blood samples by gas chromatography in 94 men occupationally exposed to pesticides in Florida, USA, showed that DDT levels were transient and related to the recency of exposure of the worker. Sequential sampling could be a tool for surveillance of persons occupationally exposed to DDT and the results could be related to the efficiency of measures taken to avoid its absorption over prolonged periods.

DDT is an effective application against rat fleas in the control of plague. Indoor residual spraying with DDT at a dosage of 2 g. per sq. m. will bring about a marked reduction in flea density. 'Patch dusting' with DDT (10 per cent.) powder is easy and cheap. The dusting powder, which can be given to each householder with instructions for use, is deposited in small quantities under grain bins, on rat runs and in other places where it is not likely to be disturbed. With this method DDT gave an index of 0·3 four months after application, dieldrin (1·5 per cent.) and aldrin (2 per cent.) dusting

[1] Name recommended by the International Organization for Standardization (ISO).
[2] Designation in OMS (WHO) index of pesticidal compounds.

538

powders gave zero flea indices. In some localities rat fleas have also become resistant to DDT.

Where DDT-resistant lice are not encountered, a powder containing 10 per cent. of DDT is the preferred treatment for human infestation. It can be distributed in sifter-top cans (about 50 g. capacity) for individual use, or applied to large groups with compressed air dusters. The powder is applied over the inner surface of the underwear, with special attention to the seams and is spread individually by hand. Mass treatment using hand-operated dusters or motor-driven air compressors have given good control of louse infestation and/or typhus in large groups of people. The clothing is not removed, the powder is blown down the neck of the shirt, up the sleeves, into the loosened trousers from several angles at front and back. In delousing women an extra quantity may be blown down the neck of the dress and application at the waistline omitted. In all cases the hair, the head covering, extra clothing and bedding should be treated. A single application will eradicate infestation. Although DDT is not ovicidal, its long residual action will kill nymphs that hatch from eggs, usually in about two weeks. DDT-resistant lice are destroyed by a powder containing 1 per cent. of lindane or malathion, but a second application within one week or three to four weeks respectively, may be necessary. A pesticide emulsion designated NBIN (68 per cent. benzyl benzoate, 6 per cent. DDT, 12 per cent. benzocaine, 14 per cent. Tween 80) can be used for head and crab lice. When pesticidal powder is used on the head, people are naturally inclined to wash the hair because of its dusty appearance. If the hair is washed after treatment, the powder should be applied at weekly intervals.

When DDT in a suitable formulation (solution, emulsion or water dispersible powder) is applied to a surface, the solvent evaporates and leaves a fine film of DDT crystals. A surface so treated remains lethal to insects alighting on it or moving over it for a considerable time afterwards. The nature of the surface to which a residual film is to be applied is of great importance. Solutions and emulsions may be unsuitable for application to absorbent areas such as mud walls. The pesticide is absorbed with the solvent and does not remain on the surface. With suspension, on the other hand, only water is absorbed and the suspended matter is left on the surface.

Dosages of residual pesticides, which vary with the concentration of the preparation, the rate of application and the nature of the surface, are generally given in grams per square metre, the spray mixture being so diluted as to require a universal application rate of 4 litres of prepared spray per 100 sq. metres. The persistence of a residual pesticide varies so much on different surfaces, in different weather and against different insects that it is not possible to give a general figure for this. These sprays are applied to the walls, ceilings and other surfaces to a point just short of run-off; in some cases spraying of outside eaves may be useful. A rate of application of 4 litres of finished spray per 100 sq. metres is equivalent to spraying to a point of run-off in most cases. The control of adult anopheline mosquitoes by application in this way is the principal measure employed in anti-malaria programmes. Windows and doors should be kept closed during spraying; foodstuffs should be protected, but furniture should not be removed.

This residual spraying is effective against susceptible houseflies, fleas, bed bugs, sand flies and mosquitoes. Larval control in anti-malaria campaigns has limited application at present. For control of anopheline larvae, DDT can be used in a solution containing 6 g. of DDT per litre of fuel oil, hand sprayed at the rate of 9·4 litres per hectare. It may be sprayed from aircraft as a 20 per cent. solution in methylated naphthaline at the rate of 56 to 112 g. of DDT per hectare.

To penetrate heavy vegetative growth over water courses, granular or pellet preparations of the toxicant are recommended. Dieldrin cement pellets have kept artificial water containers, crab holes and tree holes free of culicine larvae for one year. Smokes and fogs containing DDT may be dispersed by smoke bombs, smoke candles or fog generators. These may be used in bush, forest or in high buildings where spraying is difficult. Aerosol dispensers containing mixtures of pyrethrins and residual pesticides are used as knock-down sprays for enclosed spaces such as aircraft. A Standard Reference Aerosol has been formulated and is used in aircraft for 'Blocks-away' destruction of insects in the control of *Aedes aegypti* and yellow fever. This compound sometimes produces mild toxicity in some passengers and members of the crew as evidenced by coughing and by irritation of the eyes, nose and throat.

DDT is used against susceptible houseflies, tsetse, blackflies, sandflies and midges, mosquitoes, ticks, chiggers (mites), fleas and bedbugs.

Dieldrin [OMS–18].   Use of dieldrin has been limited because of a significant risk of toxicity to man and animals and its potentiality for the production of a rapid selection of resistant vector strains. Nevertheless it has a more rapid action than DDT and is the most persistent of the three chlorinated hydrocarbons.   Dieldrin is effective against a wider range of arthropods than DDT and has been used successfully against ticks, fleas, cockroaches, bedbugs, mosquitoes and other pests.   It is, however, toxic to humans and precautions are necessary when using it.   Serious poisoning by chlorinated-hydrocarbon pesticide is characterized by incoordination, hyperirritability, intermittent clonic-tonic convulsions and, finally, respiratory failure or ventricular fibrillation or arrest.   It should be emphasized that the earliest signs of poisoning both by the chlorinated-hydrocarbon group and the organo-phosphorus group of pesticides are essentially mundane in character, such as headache, fatigue and mild indigestion which might reasonably be attributed to the effects of long hours of work under trying conditions.

The precautions to be taken should include the following as a minimum.   All operators should be instructed about the risks involved in the use of the toxicants and receive directions for handling them safely.   They should have adequate technical and medical supervision together with the provision of facilities for the treatment of any casualties. Operators applying pesticides of all types should wear some form of impervious head-covering which should be regularly cleaned, a short cape of impervious material and chemically resistant waterproof gauntlet gloves, aprons, rubber boots and, when necessary, face masks or respirators.   Facilities for washing the skin or clothing in case of spillage or splashing should be provided.   Operators should not work more than an eight-hour day.   Separate working clothes should be used; they must be changed and washed frequently.   Workers should not smoke or eat without first washing their hands. Handling of concentrates, the equipment used and the precise labelling in a form comprehensible to the operator are important and should follow standard procedures.

Organophosphorous and carbamate compounds. Organophosphorous compounds such as malathion [OMS–1], fenthion [OMS–2], fenitrothion (OMS –43) and others have been developed as pesticides. As a group they are extremely toxic to arthropods and vertebrates, inactivating cholinesterase.   Be-

cause of this toxicity they should be used only where it has been proved that DDT and dieldrin are ineffective as treatments.   Organophosphorous compounds such as malathion [OMS–1] and diazinon have been used against cockroaches, fleas, mosquitoes (adults and larvae), sandflies and midges and houseflies.   They can be sprayed as surface applications but their residual effect is short. Carbamates such as carbaryl [OMS–29] and Baygon [OMS–33] and others are being tested for efficiency and toxicity. WHO have a programme for testing and evaluating new insecticides in seven stages of increasing magnitude and complexity and for concurrent investigations of the hazards. Five relatively new compounds, Baygon [OMS–33] Carbamult [OMS–716] fenitrothion [OMS–43] dicapthon [OMS–214] and bromophos [OMS–658] have shown promise as residual adulticides against malaria vectors.

Resistance to these new insecticides is developing in various species.   The selection of the best one to use against any particular species in any particular place requires a knowledge of the presence or absence of resistance and the relative economy of the available effective compounds.

Toxicity.   The effects of both organophosphorous compounds and the carbamates have been related to the inhibition of tissue cholinesterases (ChE) at synaptic sites and to an accumulation of excessive amounts of acetyl-choline in effector organs.   The symptoms are mostly, if not exclusively, of a cholinergic nature.   A diagnosis of anticholinesterase poisoning can be made from a history of exposure followed by the onset of all or some of the signs and symptoms, depending on whether exposure to the toxicant was local or whether through systemic absorption.   Local signs may be marked miosis, sometimes unequal, frontal headache, dimness of vision, pain on focusing, occasional nausea and vomiting, hyperaemia of conjunctivae, rhinorrhoea, tightness in chest with wheezing, sweating at site of exposure and fasciculation of striated muscle at site of exposure to the liquid.

In systemic absorption, in addition to the above symptoms, anorexia, nausea, vomiting, abdominal cramps, epigastric and substernal tightness, diarrhoea, tenesmus and involuntary defaecation may occur.   There is increased sweating, salivation and lachrymation.   There is frequent or involuntary micturition, the subject is easily fatigued with mild weakness, muscular twitching, fasciculations, cramps dyspnoea and cyanosis. Blood pressure may be raised and giddiness, tension, anxiety, restlessness and emotional lability may occur. This may be followed by drowsiness, confusion, slurred speech, ataxia and coma with the absence of reflexes, convulsion, depression of the respiratory and circulatory centres with dyspnoea, cyanosis and fall in blood pressure. Death appears to be primarily asphyxial in some instances and cardiovascular in others. After exposure to organophosphorous pesticides, the first symptoms may not occur until after the individual has left work. In some instances illness may develop at night, and its association with occupational poisoning may not be recognized immediately. In the case of over-exposure to a pesticidal carbamate the signs of poisoning develop rapidly, during or immediately after exposure, with incapacitating symptoms which prevent further exposure, making the operator stop work long before a dangerous dose can be absorbed. Recovery is rapid and complete and chronic or cumulative effects are extremely improbable. Owing to these characteristics there have been no cases of severe poisoning after occupational exposure to carbamates.

Several methods are available for determining ChE activity and it is recommended that the activities of blood cholinesterases be determined regularly in operators exposed to the organophosphorous compounds of intermediate or greater toxicity because operators may have to be withdrawn from exposure if the activity of their blood ChE decreases significantly from a well-established pre-exposure value. The choice of method to be used will depend on the nature of the compound and the laboratory facilities available.

The therapy of anticholinesterase poisoning includes, in addition to the use of drugs, removal of the toxic agent and decontamination of exposed skin with an alkaline solution of soap and water. Suction of the airways, tracheostomy and positive pressure respiration may be necessary at a later stage. Atropine sulphate is recommended as first aid in the case of poisoning. It should be injected immediately after the appearance of any local pulmonary or systemic signs of anticholinesterase poisoning in doses larger than those used for other purposes. When signs and symptoms are mild, 1 to 2 mg. of atropine should be injected intramuscularly and the injection repeated, if necessary, at intervals of 30 minutes until symptoms are relieved. Any patient sick enough to receive even one dose of atropine should be under medical observation for at least 24 hours because symptoms may reappear. Mild symptoms due to carbamate compounds have been known to respond to the administration of atropine by mouth or to remit spontaneously. When symptoms of poisoning are severe, 4 to 6 mg. of atropine should be injected intravenously, or, if this is not feasible, intramuscularly. Repeated doses of 2 mg. at 5 to 10-minute intervals should be given until symptoms are relieved. In severe anticholinesterase poisoning, the effect of each injection of atropine may be transient lasting only 10 to 30 minutes. The patient must, therefore, be observed as closely as possible for recurrence of signs of poisoning and atropine must be repeated at appropriate intervals for at least 48 hours if his clinical condition requires it. In severe poisoning as much as 50 mg. of atropine may be required on the first day.

Atropine may reduce heat loss by inhibition of sweating and under hot environmental conditions this may be dangerous, particularly in young children. It is, therefore, important that the patient be kept cool and quiet. In no circumstances must a patient who has received even one dose of atropine be allowed to perform muscular work; and he must be kept under observation for at least 24 hours or until he is fully recovered. Automatic injectors and other injection devices of reliable construction for the administration of atropine and other drugs should be at hand during spraying operations. Although some atropine analogues may be superior to atropine for treating poisoning by specific compounds, none has been found that is better in all respects. In recent years it has been demonstrated that certain oximes, when used in combination with atropine, provide more effective therapy than atropine alone in poisoning with some anticholinesterases. According to present knowledge, oximes should never be given to people intoxicated with carbamates. Pralidoxine and toxogonin have been used successfully. The following drugs must not be given to persons poisoned with anticholinesterases: morphine, barbiturates and tranquillizers.

RESISTANCE. The greatest hindrance to chemical control of certain arthropod species is the occurrence, through chemical selection, of changes in the genetic composition of their populations. These changes may cause increased general tolerance or specific resistance to certain pesticides through the ability of the arthropod to detoxicate the chemical and this results in failure of control operations in the field. Many species which are important in public health work, including mosquitoes, flies, cockroaches, bedbugs, lice, ticks, fleas and midges, have been reported in certain parts of the world to be physiologically resistant to one or more of the insecticides commonly employed in their control. In a number of areas pesticide resistance developed by anophelines appeared to be due mainly, if not entirely, to selection pressure resulting from the use of agricultural pesticides or of mosquito larvicides containing DDT, gamma BHC or dieldrin. The detection of resistance should be an integral part of control operations, since this is the only way to establish that failure is, in fact, the result of resistance and is not due to other factors. The need for a different pesticide is thus confirmed. Kits for measuring susceptibility levels of adults and larvae for a number of vectors are available from the Vector Control Unit, Division of Environmental Health, World Health Organization, Geneva, Switzerland.

Pesticides should be employed only when necessary, their use being carefully planned.

The maximum success in control operations can be achieved only if competent personnel direct their attention to the efficiency of the equipment used for spraying or dusting, the formulation and application of the pesticide, the nature of the surface to which the formulation is applied and its absorption in the material, the stability and potency of the pesticide and the inherent powers of survival of the species. To achieve maximum success in control operations, full recognition must be given to these aspects in the field evaluation of any control programme. In addition, it is emphasized that all control procedures must be adequately supervised by competent personnel if they are to be successful.

Despite remarkable advances in the development of pesticides, it would be wrong to assume that procedures based solely on pesticides are the only techniques used in operational programmes. In any such programme, environmental sanitation may be the key to successful control. The basic tenets for accomplishing control consist in the adoption of such measures as the reduction of mosquito sites by draining, flooding or filling, or the reduction of fly breeding through proper storage and disposal of manure, vegetable refuse and garbage. While pesticide measures are subordinate to adequate sanitation, maximum control cannot usually be achieved without chemical aids, either as

a supplementary or an emergency phase. Although this is true for arthropod and rodent control, it does not apply to disease control. This has been accomplished in some species with pesticides alone, for example, by measures directed at only a part of the insect population, such as mosquitoes entering habitations. Some control measures may be specific only in certain territories with a peculiarity of climate, or because the local strain of vector displays certain physiological or behavioristic qualities. Thus measures effective in one country may be of less value in another.

There is at the present time considerable concern at the contamination of the environment with pesticides. Residues of DDT, dieldrin and gamma BHC are found in samples of rain water from the Outer Hebrides, Cornwall and Central London. The present findings suggest that the atmosphere carries small amounts of these pesticides in common use either as vapour or by adhesion to dust particles and that they are 'scrubbed-out' by rain or snow.

In the United Kingdom, USA, France, India and in other countries, the chlorinated pesticides have been identified in the body fat of people whose work does not involve the use of these chemicals. Similar deposits have been reported in animals, birds, sea birds, eggs and fish. In the case of the Bermuda petrel, various considerations implicate contamination by pesticides as a probable major cause of the reproduction decline. Reports of the finding of deposits of DDT in Adélie penguins and a crab-eating seal from Antarctica shows how far this contamination through the food chain has progressed.

Pesticides are known to leave residues in food, even when used in accordance with good agricultural practice. A joint FAO/WHO committee has studied the pertinent data in order to evaluate the consumer hazard arising from the use of pesticides. The joint committee based its recommendations on a high rate of food consumption being the ninth decile of consumption derived from consumer intake studies in the USA. This figure could be exceeded by only about 15 per cent. of the population. 'Tolerances' defined as 'the permitted concentration of residue actually remaining when the food is first offered for consumption'—have been recommended for a range of pesticides. Since preparation of foods and cooking decreases the residue a considerable safety factor is incorporated.

BIOLOGICAL CONTROL. Faced with this

contamination of the environment, the results of which cannot be foreseen, great efforts are being made to replace methods using insecticides by biological and other methods of control. A search is going on for naturally occurring poisons and disease organisms that might in turn control or eliminate the vectors of human disease. It is important to bear in mind, however, that a biological agent or toxic product of an organism will not necessarily present either a greater or lesser health hazard than a synthetic material. All the most poisonous materials so far known are, in fact, of natural origin. Therefore any material, living or dead, proposed as a pest control agent should be subjected to the same searching examination for potential toxicity to man as is applied to synthetic pesticides. Particular attention to hazards may be needed in the case of fungi. These can produce not only a variety of potentially toxic metabolites, including carcinogens, but a number of them can become established in mammalian tissues and give rise to granulomata. Others seem able to induce hypersensitivity reactions leading, for example, to progressive tissue damage in the lungs which may be fatal.

GENETIC CONTROL of certain insect pests has been used successfully. Harmful genetic factors and mechanisms which may be useful for control and eradication of pests include cytoplasmic incompatibility, hybrid sterility, artificial sterilization, translocations, inversions and deleterious genes. Induced sterility is a method of proved effectiveness against a few species, while translocation and cytoplasmic incompatibility hold promise for the control of others.

Repellents

Diethyltoluamide (DET) has proved to be the outstanding all-purpose repellent. Chlordiethyl benzamide is also highly effective against a wide range of species, and ethylhexanediol, dimethylphthalate (DMP), dimethylcarbate and indalone are all good general repellents that are outstanding against certain species. They are colourless liquids and may be applied repreatedly to the human skin without causing ill effects other than smarting of delicate areas such as the lips and eyes. They damage plastics, watch crystals and fountain-pens, and some kinds of rayon, but not nylon, cotton or wool. If applied to the skin, protection against bites from arthropods will last about two to four hours. DET and chlordiethylbenzamide feel less oily on the skin than the other repellents; and DET is sufficiently effective to permit some dilution with alcohol, which increases its cosmetic acceptability still more. It may also be combined in a cream. For protection against chiggers (the larvae of mites of trombicula and related genera) the clothing should be impregnated with benzyl benzoate which withstands washing, or with DET which is less durable. The repellent can be applied to the inside of the clothing by hand, by spray or by impregnation of the outer clothing using the repellent in a volatile solvent.

The Expert Committee on Insecticides of the World Health Organization frequently reviews the recommended methods for vector control, pesticide resistance and the toxic hazards of pesticides to man. The *World Health Organization's Technical Report Series* should be referred to for details regarding the control of any specific vector.

Reference

WORLD HEALTH ORGANISATION (1970). *Tech. Rep. Ser. Wld Hlth Org*. No. 443.

23. Acute Poisoning

HENRY MATTHEW

This chapter is concerned only with the treatment of acute poisoning in general and in hospital practice. The treatment of poisoning occurring as an industrial hazard is discussed on pp. 556–566.

Information Service

The frequency of poisoning, accidental and self-administered, is steadily increasing. Further, in recent years the public have had access to a rapidly increasing number of new chemical compounds used as drugs or for domestic purposes. The fact that many of these preparations are extremely poisonous is not widely known. It follows that the doctor, confronted by a patient suffering from poisoning, will often lack information indispensable to his proper management. To meet this difficulty a Poisons Information Service has been set up in Britain, and a doctor may obtain help, day or night by telephoning one of the following numbers:

Belfast:	Royal Victoria Hospital.	Tel. 0232—40503
Cardiff:	Royal Infirmary.	Tel. 0222—33101
Edinburgh:	Royal Infirmary.	Tel. 031—229 2477
London:	Guy's Hospital.	Tel. 01 407 7600
Leeds:	General Infirmary.	Tel. 0532—32799
Newcastle:	Royal Victoria Infirmary.	Tel. 0632—25131
Eire:		Tel. Dublin 45588

At these centres information is available as to whether the substance is known to be poisonous and treatment can also be discussed with a doctor. The value of this service has been fully established; and not the least important part of its work consists in providing reassurance, when this is justified by the circumstances, that the patient is unlikely to suffer any harmful effects.

Incidence of Poisoning

With the increase in prescriptions for antidepressants, tranquillizers and non-barbiturate hypnotics there has been a change in recent years in the incidence of poisoning by various drugs. Four years ago poisoning by barbiturates accounted for 60 per cent. of poisoned patients admitted to hospital, but now only 30 per cent. of patients entering hospital for this reason have taken this type of drug. There has been a corresponding rise in incidence of poisoning by methaqualone (occasionally alone, but more commonly in combination with an antihistamine as Mandrax or Paldona), benzodiazepines such as chlordiazepoxide, diazepam or nitrazepam and tricyclic antidepressants including amitriptyline and imipramine. Salicylates still account for about 15 per cent. With the substitution of natural gas for coal gas there has been a fall in admission of patients suffering from poisoning by carbon monoxide. It should be remembered that there is a definite trend for several drugs to be taken simultaneously and that alcohol, which promotes absorption and enhances the effect of certain drugs, is also frequently taken with them.

Principles of treatment

In the vast majority of instances of poisoning a specific antidote does not exist. It follows that successful treatment depends on observing basic therapeutic principles rather than by consulting a list of antidotes. Poisons enter the body by ingestion, by inhalation or by absorption through the skin. In treatment, appropriate steps must immediately be taken to limit further entry of poison into the body. This is achieved by considering whether absorption from the alimentary tract can be limited by causing vomiting or by resorting to gastric aspiration and lavage; by removing the patient into fresh air; and by cleansing the skin after the removal of contaminated clothing. It is impossible to exaggerate the importance of acting with the utmost speed to prevent further inhalation of a poison or its absorption through the skin.

Gastric lavage. Should the doctor promote vomiting and undertake gastric aspiration and lavage? The answer will depend on three factors: (a) the substance ingested; (b) the patient's state of consciousness; and (c) the length of time that has elapsed since the poison was ingested. If the patient has swallowed paraffin oil (kerosene) or other petroleum distillates, emetics should not be used, neither should gastric lavage be performed. This firm contraindication is based on the fact that the entry of even a small quantity of these substances into the lungs causes severe pneumonitis. Great care must be exercised in passing a stomach tube in corrosive poisoning, in alcoholics, in patients who have had surgical operations on the stomach, and in the very young and elderly; but the benefits from the procedure outweigh the potential dangers of perforating the oesophagus or stomach.

The fully conscious patient should be made to vomit by putting one's finger into his throat; if initially unsuccessful this can be repeated after giving a tumblerful of tepid water containing a dessertspoonful of common salt. Apomorphine hydrochloride, even though its effects can be neutralized by nalorphine, may produce hypotension, collapse and persistent vomiting and is best avoided. Gastric irritants such as ipecacuanha or copper are slow in action and unreliable. Even when vomiting has been produced, it may still be essential to carry out gastric aspiration and lavage.

In the drowsy patient (semiconscious) emetics are to be avoided in view of the danger of aspiration pneumonitis, but provided the gag and cough reflexes are still present, gastric aspiration and lavage can be employed. In the deeply unconscious patient these reflexes are in abeyance, and therefore the procedure is undertaken *only if the lungs can be protected by the insertion of a cuffed endotracheal tube.*

If four hours have elapsed since the poison was taken, very little of it will be recovered by the use of emetics and by gastric lavage. If it is known that the poison was taken less than four hours previously, aspiration and lavage may be helpful. In salicylate poisoning, persistent pylorospasm almost invariably develops and this retards the passage of the drug from the stomach. It is, therefore, virtually never too late to evacuate the stomach. The patient is conscious and large amounts of salicylate can be recovered up to 20 hours after ingestion.

It is important that a stomach tube of adequate bore should be used. A Jacques rubber tube (English gauge 30) should be passed, with the foot of the bed raised some 18 inches and the patient lying on his left side. A gag may be necessary to prevent biting on the tube. When the tube has been passed, its position in the stomach is verified by aspiration of gastric contents or by blowing a little air through it while auscultating over the abdomen—when a bubbling sound will be heard. Aspiration should then be carried out by lowering the funnel to which the stomach tube is attached, to a level well below the patient's head. Dakin's syringe and Senoran's evacuator are of much less value in acute poisoning than in pyloric stenosis. Aspiration must be attempted prior to lavage, as the initial lavage inevitably drives some of the stomach contents into the duodenum and promotes absorption. When no further material can be aspirated, repeated careful lavage with tepid water should be undertaken using no more than 300 ml. each time. This procedure is continued until the returning fluid is clear. Except in the specific instances of opiate, cyanide or iron poisoning, there is little to be gained by using lavage fluid other than water.

If an opiate has been ingested, lavage should be undertaken with a very dilute solution of potassium permanganate, using one solution-tablet (B.P.C.) dissolved in $3\frac{1}{2}$ litres (6 pints) of tepid water and ensuring that this fluid is itself washed out with water prior to withdrawing the tube. If cyanide has been ingested, the stomach should be washed out with 25 per cent. sodium thiosulphate; in acute iron poisoning appropriate amounts of a solution of desferrioxamine, 2 g. in 1 litre of warm water, should be used. Following lavage, 10 g. of desferrioxamine in 50 ml. of water should be left in the stomach.

In salicylate poisoning haemorrhage from the stomach is such a rare occurrence that it is unnecessary to use sodium bicarbonate to protect the gastric mucosa.

Barbiturate Poisoning

Much of the advice advocated for barbiturate poisoning is applicable to poisoning by other hypnotics, sedatives, tranquillizers and antidepressants.

Removal to hospital. A patient suffering from barbiturate poisoning and showing impairment of consciousness should be removed to hospital. Respiratory depression, shock and coma, occurring together or separately, call for appropriate treatment; and measures to promote removal of the poison from the body may have to be considered. Before sending the patient to hospital certain precautions should be taken: (*a*) removal of all debris, dentures and excess secretion from the mouth and nose; (*b*) maintenance of free airway by laying the patient on his side and keeping him in this position during the journey with an oropharyngeal or cuffed endotracheal tube inserted; (*c*) artificial respiration, if there is severe respiratory depression (a properly equipped ambulance carries a Stephenson Minuteman resuscitator and suction apparatus); (*d*) if there is significant hypotension (systolic pressure less than 90 mm. Hg.), metaraminol should be given intramuscularly (2 to 5 mg.).

It is very important that a doctor sending a poisoned patient into hospital should provide a note naming, if possible, the poisons taken, the time of ingestion, and the probable amounts. If he has no precise information, he should supply a list of the poisons (tablets, etc.) to which the patient had access. On arrival in hospital, in addition to the above measures, the severity of the illness must be dully assessed by attention to the following:

Respiratory failure. The respiratory minute volume should be measured using the simple spirometer (Wright). If this is less than 4 litres it is likely that mechanical means of assisted respiration will be required (p. 652) and in such circumstances an anaesthetist's help is essential.

Shock. Shock should be treated by elevation of the foot of the bed followed, if necessary, by the administration of the vasopressor drug, metaraminol. It should be given intramuscularly in a dose of 2 to 5 mg. The effect develops in about ten minutes and will usually last for one hour. When an immediate response is required up to 5 mg. should be injected *slowly* intravenously. If two or at most three intramuscular or intravenous injections of metaraminol fail to raise the pressure to 90 mm. Hg., it is necessary to resort to the supplementary measure of plasma transfusion—or alternatively the use of whole blood, dextran or rheomacrodex. These infusions are best controlled by monitoring the central venous pressure.

Hypothermia may aggravate hypotension and may be overlooked unless a low reading thermometer is used. If the temperature be below 95° F., some form of gentle heating is indicated.

Coma. The management of coma is inseparable from the treatment of shock and the maintenance of an adequate respiratory exchange. A high standard of nursing care is essential as the patient may be unconscious for several days. Prophylactic antibiotics are not indicated unless the patient shows evidence of respiratory infection on admission (p. 201), or has aspirated vomitus possibly as the result of injudicious gastric lavage. Intravenous infusions (p. 253) will be required, with careful recording of fluid balance, if the patient has been unconscious for more than 12 hours. Bullous lesions (which occur in 6 to 8 per cent. of patients in barbiturate poisoning) usually develop within 24 hours following ingestion. The occurrence of these bullae provides a valuable aid in the differential diagnosis of the cause of coma. They should be treated in the same way as burns.

Gastric lavage. *see above.*

Laboratory findings. In a deeply unconscious patient the serum barbiturate level and the type of barbiturate (long- medium- or short-acting) should be determined. A common mistake, however, is to assess the severity of poisoning by the blood level alone. The assessment must be on a basis of the clinical features, for many patients are habituated and their tissues tolerant to the drug. Thus, an epileptic who has taken an overdose of phenobarbitone may have a blood level of 10 mg. per 100 ml. and be merely drowsy, whereas a patient unused to phenobarbitone would be deeply unconscious and dangerously ill with such a concentration in the blood.

Augmented elimination. Measures designed to augment elimination of barbiturate are required in less than 5 per cent. of patients suffering from barbiturate poisoning; hence the temptation to employ such measures must be avoided except in severely ill patients poisoned by long-acting barbiturates, in whom the intensive supportive therapy already described fails to cause improvement. Enhanced excretion may be attempted by extra-corporeal haemodialysis (p. 278), peritoneal dialysis (p. 643), forced osmotic alkaline diuresis or passage of blood over ion exchange resins. The choice of method will usually be governed by the availability of apparatus.

HAEMODIALYSIS. There can be no doubt that haemodialysis is at least twice as effective as the other methods in removing the long acting barbiturates.

PERITONEAL DIALYSIS. The longer-acting barbiturates can be removed by peritoneal dialysis, but this procedure is now seldom used. The medium- and short-acting barbiturates unless present at very high blood levels will not be removed in worthwhile amounts by either haemodialysis or peritoneal dialysis.

FORCED DIURESIS. Forced osmotic diuresis, using urea and alkalinization of the urine, is greatly favoured by the Scandinavian school in cases of poisoning with long acting barbiturates. Very careful assessment regarding pre-existing renal or cardiac disease is essential if complications such as pulmonary congestion are to be avoided. The employment of urea as a diuretic is open to some criticism and mannitol is now generally favoured, If forced diuresis is indicated, the following regimen is advocated.

1. Insert urinary catheter.
2. Intravenous infusion of:

500 ml. 1·26 per cent. sodium bicarbonate ⎫
500 ml. 5 per cent. laevulose   ⎪
500 ml. 0·9 per cent. saline   ⎬ in rotation.
500 ml. 5 per cent. laevulose   ⎪
500 ml. 5 per cent. mannitol   ⎭
10 ml. of 10 per cent. calcium gluconate eight-hourly.

These fluids must be given at a rate of 1 litre in the first hour and 500 ml. hourly thereafter. Frusemide may be added. Adjustments in the regimen may have to be made according to the patient's response and fluid and electrolyte balance. Careful biochemical monitoring is essential.

The urinary pH should be measured hourly and, if below 7·5, substitute 1·26 per cent. sodium bicarbonate for 0·9 per cent. saline in the above regime.

A very careful maintenance of fluid and electrolyte balance is essential. The amount of barbiturate removed by forced osmotic alkaline diuresis and peritoneal dialysis is approximately the same.

It is worth repeating that such methods which attempt to enhance elimination should be used only when intensive supportive therapy fails to prevent deterioration; and it is only with long-acting barbiturates that a worthwhile recovery of drug is likely to be achieved.

Withdrawal fits and disorientation may be encountered when barbiturate therapy is stopped abruptly in patients habituated to the drug or when large amounts are removed rapidly from the body.

BEMEGRIDE. It is now clearly established that although bemegride is a reasonably potent analeptic, it is not a specific barbiturate antagonist. Intravenous infusion of this drug which aimed at bringing the patient up to and maintaining him at a safe level of unconsciousness has been abandoned, as it did not result in an improvement in overall mortality but was followed by an increase in morbidity.

Salicylate Poisoning

Salicylates, next to barbiturates, are the drugs most commonly taken in deliberate overdose. The ingested salicylate is usually in the form of aspirin but it should be remembered that one teaspoonful (4 ml.) of methyl salicylate (oil of wintergreen) contains the equivalent of twelve tablets of aspirin (4 g.). Salicylate may also be taken in compound tablets with such substances as phenacetin and codeine but it is the salicylate in these compounds which produces the serious acute toxic effects.

Assessment. Treatment naturally varies with the severity of the poisoning. This is often difficult to assess for the following reasons: (a) although the patient is conscious, unless he is desperately ill, the number of tablets taken may be deliberately misstated; (b) vomiting almost always occurs soon after ingestion, and the amount retained is therefore uncertain; and (c) the symptoms of salicylism may all occur at the plasma level of 32 mg. per 100 ml. (the concentration often aimed at in treatment) and as they may not increase in intensity at higher plasma levels they provide no indication of the severity of the poisoning. The plasma salicylate level is a reliable measure of the severity of poisoning, with the important reservation that when the drug has been taken more than 12 hours previously the plasma level may be deceptively low. Twelve hours after ingestion the disturbance of acid-base metabolism will more accurately reflect the severity of poisoning than the plasma salicylate level; at this stage in these patients there may be impairment of consciousness. These circumstances apart, it may be said that moderate to severe salcylate poisoning exists in an adult if the level is over 50 mg. per 100 ml. This results from taking about 50 ordinary (300 mg.) tablets of aspirin. It must be remembered, however, that absorption of the drug varies greatly. Infants are especially susceptible to the serious acid-base derangements of salicylate intoxication, and severe poisoning may exist despite a plasma level as low as 30 mg. per 100 ml.

Treatment. As already stated, it is never too late to aspirate and wash out the stomach. If there be any doubt on clinical grounds about the severity of poisoning a blood specimen must be taken for immediate estimation of the salicylate level. While awaiting this result full therapy is started. Immediately following gastric lavage forced alkaline intravenous therapy is begun with the following mixture given at a rate of 2 litres per hour for three hours and thereafter 1 litre per hour until the serum salicylate is less than 35 mg. per cent. when the drip may be stopped.

Saline	0·9 per cent.	—0·5 litre
Laevulose	5 per cent.	—1 litre
Sodium bicarbonate	1·26 per cent.	—0·5 litre
Potassium chloride		3 g.

The rate of infusion is most important. Fortunately, as salicylate is very frequently the poison chosen by young persons with healthy renal and cardiovascular systems, there are few contraindications to intravenous therapy. The result of the initial serum salicylate level is usually available within an hour, and further treatment will be governed by the report. If it is less than 50 mg. per 100 ml. the intravenous therapy can be discontinued and the patient simply encouraged to drink plenty of fluid. If the level is greater than 50 mg. per 100 ml. the intravenous therapy must be maintained for the period already advocated. Diuresis may be facilitated with frusemide, 40 mg. intravenously, but this is not usually required. Severe dehydration may exist initially as the result of hyperventilation, vomiting and profuse sweating; hence a high urinary output is not to be expected until after at least two hours of intravenous therapy. As the patient is conscious, fluids must be forced by mouth and catheterization is unnecessary. Although it is rare in practice to encounter a bleeding tendency resulting from salicylate poisoning, it is wise to give vitamin K_1 (phytomenadione), 15 mg. intramuscularly, to all patients with moderate or severe poisoning.

The rare contraindications to forced alkaline diuretic therapy are persistent hypotension and impaired renal function. In such circumstances peritoneal dialysis will effect satisfactory removal of salicylate, especially if the dialysing fluid is rendered alkaline or if albumin is added. Haemodialysis, if readily available, might be undertaken if the serum salicylate level exceeds 100 mg. per 100 ml. Nevertheless, in a condition in which immediate treatment is of the utmost importance, the delay occasioned by preparation of the apparatus severely limits its value; but this method must be seriously considered when there is failure to respond to adequate forced alkaline diuresis.

In infants and young children exchange transfusion, if it can be undertaken promptly, is a satisfactory substitute for forced alkaline diuresis or peritoneal dialysis, but haemodialysis has great technical disadvantages.

Carbon Monoxide

Treatment is a matter of urgency, starting with removal of the victim from the poisonous atmosphere. The basic principles of intensive supportive therapy already described for ingestants apply equally to poisoning due to carbon monoxide. Particular attention, however, must be paid to patency of the airway and the respiratory function.

The decision to give 100 per cent. oxygen or a mixture of 95 per cent. oxygen and 5 per cent. carbon dioxide is best made on the results of arterial blood-gas analysis. However, in practice it is highly improbable that any harm will result from giving 100 per cent. oxygen.

Cerebral oedema frequently occurs in poisoning of any degree of severity. It is readily diagnosed by the discovery of papilloedema. If there be any suspicion of cerebral oedema rapid reduction of intracranial tension is a matter of urgency. This is achieved by the intravenous infusion of 500 ml. of 20 per cent. mannitol over a period of 20 minutes followed by 500 ml. of 5 per cent. dextrose over the next four hours.

The administration of oxygen at a pressure of 2 atmospheres markedly increases the amount of oxygen carried in the blood, and promotes the dissociation of carboxyhaemoglobin. This therapy is very effective during the first half-hour after removal from exposure, but when given after the delay inevitable in reaching hospital it is very much less effective both as a life-saving measure and in preventing complications. The provision of hyperbaric chambers mounted in a vehicle which could be rushed to the scene of the poisoning would, therefore, be of great value.

Carbon monoxide poisoning is most frequently seen in the elderly and a degree of myocardial ischaemia or actual infarction is almost inevitable in poisoning of any severity. Every patient who has suffered other than a mild degree of exposure to carbon monoxide must be kept at rest for three days pending assessment of damage to the cardiovascular system. Treatment of any myocardial damage, arrythmias or congestive heart failure is on conventional lines (p. 81).

Tranquillizers

It is evident that this group of drugs is being used with increasing frequency as a means of self-poisoning. The effects vary considerably—depending on the place occupied in the scale between tranquillizers and tranquillo-sedatives, i.e. from chlorpromazine to benzodiazepines. In overdose from chlorpromazine and closely related compounds, before the patient lapses into coma there may be disorientation, ataxia and slurred speech, Parkinsonian rigidity and tremor, and involuntary movements leading to the muscular spasm of torticollis. Hypotension, hypothermia and shallow respiration may develop but the increased tendon reflexes and tachycardia may help to differentiate the condition from barbiturate poisoning. Coma

TABLE 15

Poison	'Antidote'	Administration	Remarks
Cyanides and Hydrocyanic Acid.	(1) Amyl Nitrite followed by (3)	Inhalation. Up to 6 perles being broken in series.	An acute medical emergency. Produces cellular asphyxia.
	(2) Sodium Nitrite followed by (4)	3% sol. 10 ml. i.v. over 3 min.	Sets containing syringes already loaded with antidotes (2) and (3) should be available in any working place where cyanide is used. Also should be available in hospitals serving industrial areas.
	(3) Sodium Thiosulphate.	50% sol. 25 ml. i.v. very slowly.	
	(4) Sodium Thiosulphate.	Gastric lavage with 25% solution.	If poison has been swallowed.
Organophosphorous compounds.	Atropine Sulphate.	2 mg. i.v. repeat 1 mg. every 10 minutes till signs of atropinization occur.	Blood sample for cholinesterase level. Atropine blocks peripheral actions of excessive acetylcholine.
	Pralidoxime (P$_2$S).	2 g. in 5 ml. water i.v. slowly; repeat in 3 hours.	Regenerates cholinesterase.
Opiates.	Nalorphine.	10 mg. i.v. and repeat every 15 minutes till adequate ventilation is achieved.	Competes with opiate for attachment on cells as has similar structure.
Domestic Bleach.	Sodium Thiosulphate.	Gastric lavage. 0·1% solution.	Commonly imbibed by children. Not very harmful.
Amphetamine.	Chlorpromazine.	100 mg. i.m.	If severe will require forced diuresis rendering urine acid to promote excretion.
Paraffin and Kerosene.	None.	N.A.	Commonly drunk by children. Initial symptoms are gastro-intestinal but danger lies in pulmonary oedema. Do NOT wash out stomach. If respiratory complications present give steroids and antibiotics.
Lysergic Acid	Chlorpromazine	100 mg. i.m.	May have to be repeated in 20 minutes if 'trip' especially bad.

is not usually as deep as that occurring in severe barbiturate poisoning

With the benzodiazepines the effects listed above are seen infrequently, but there is usually drowsiness and occasionally hypotension of mild degree.

Treatment is entirely symptomatic and is to be found under that described for barbiturates (p. 545). The methods already mentioned to enhance elimination (p. 546) are of no avail in this type of poisoning.

Acute Iron Poisoning
This is the most serious type of acute poisoning seen in children. It is common because most iron tablets are attractively coloured, and they are often left in medicine cupboards and elsewhere within easy reach of children. In the moderate to severe form the prostrate, shocked child with severe haemorrhagic gastroenteritis needs to have the remaining iron in the gut rendered non-absorbable and the free iron in the circulation inactive.

Fortunately the potent chelating agent desferrioxamine is available and should be used as follows, speed being absolutely essential:

(1) Inject 2 g. intramuscularly. (2) After gastric lavage using a solution of desferrioxamine 2 g. in 1 litre of warm water, leave 10 g. desferrioxamine in 50 ml. of fluid in the stomach. (3) Set up an intravenous drip to infuse desferrioxamine at a rate of not more than 15 mg. per kg. of body weight per hour to a maximum dosage of 80 mg. per kg. of body weight in 24 hours. For the purpose of infusion the drug may be added to whole blood, normal saline or dextrose solution. (4) Give 2 g. intramuscularly 12-hourly until the clinical condition is satisfactory and the serum iron has fallen to less than 500 mcg. per 100 ml. It should be noted that improvement occurring during the first 12 hours after ingestion may not be maintained, as iron—initially taken up by the reticuloendothelial system—is released 12 hours later and this results in worsening of the condition. (5) Carry out full supporting therapy for shock, acidosis, electrolyte disturbance and blood loss. Treat convulsions with barbiturates or paraldehyde.

Antidepressants

The effects of overdosage of the tricyclic group are especially severe in children. Twitching and convulsions are best controlled by phenobarbitone intramuscularly (300 mg. in adults) whilst shock usually responds to raising the foot of the bed and giving metaraminol 2·5 mg. intramuscularly if necessary. Tachycardia is best treated by propranalol or practolol, and the dangerous bizarre cardiac arrhythmias by lignocaine (p. 121) or the insertion of a cardiac pacemaker. Fortunately the acute effects wear off within about 16 hours. However, hallucinations and disturbance of sleep may be evident for up to 72 hours, and these are best treated with chlorpromazine.

Methaqualone

This drug is usually taken in the combined form with the antihistamine diphenhydramine as Mandrax or Paldona. The effects of overdosage are similar to those seen in barbiturate poisoning except that the level of unconsciousness is seldom so deep. However, a tendency to pulmonary oedema, increased capillary permeability and direct myocardial damage makes for increased difficulty in management as compared with barbiturate poisoning. Except at very high con-

centrations in the blood, haemodialysis is of no avail in promoting removal. Forced diuresis, necessitating the administration of large volumes of fluid, is dangerous when there is already a risk of pulmonary oedema attributable to the toxic effect of the drug.

Paracetamol

Following the ill-advised encouragement to replace aspirin with paracetamol in the home medicine cupboard, paracetamol and preparations containing it, are encountered with increasing frequency in self-poisoning. The initial effects are on the upper alimentary tract with nausea and vomiting. There then may be a latent period during which the patient feels reasonably well but two to three days after ingestion acute liver failure may set in. There is no known way of preventing his complication which carries a high mortality and which may occur following the ingestion of 10 g. of paracetamol, that is 20 tablets of the more popular preparations.

Paraquat

Weed-killers are described on p. 568, but this particular substance is included here as it may be taken accidentally. In the granular form for domestic use, the effects, although sometimes severe, are not usually fatal. However, the liquid concentrate supplied to farmers and horticulturists is sometimes left in lemonade bottles by those who have obtained it from professional users. Even a mouthful of the concentrate may prove fatal. The initial effects are on the liver, kidneys and brain. After a latent period of some 10 days, involvement of the lungs may become apparent clinically and radiologically. With the exception of the effects in the lungs, the changes in the tissues—although on occasion severe—are reversible. In the lungs, a proliferative terminal bronchiolitis and alveolitis, once started, is progressive, and there is no known way of arresting the process. Management, therefore, consists simply in supporting the vital functions in the hope that the lungs have been spared. The effects of early forced diuresis whilst preparing for haemodialysis have not yet been assessed, but if urine analysis shows that paraquat has been absorbed these measures should be used.

Other Poisonous Agents

Table 15 gives the management of the less common but important agents encountered in poisoning for which an 'antidote' is available.

Psychiatric Assessment

Self-poisoning in adults is nearly always deliberate and not accidental. Most patients intend only to make themselves ill—not to kill themselves; and their motive is to create a new kind of crisis which will provide an escape from personal problems which have become intolerable. It is wrong to describe such an act as 'attempted suicide'. In the majority of instances, irrespective of whether the patient has thought in the past about taking an overdose, when he actually poisons himself he does so impulsively. Self-poisoning is frequently an important symptom of psychological disorder; and

even when it is not, the techniques of psychiatry are most suited to discovering the truth. The dose taken does not, of course, reflect the severity of the underlying psychiatric condition; the swallowing of five aspirin tablets may be symptomatic of a far more serious situation than the ingestion of 50 tablets. It is imperative that the message which the patient is trying to convey by the act of self-poisoning should be correctly interpreted. If the practitioner is unable to comprehend the message or is in doubt regarding the underlying psychological disorder he should promptly seek expert psychiatric help.

24. Ill-health due to Drugs

G. M. WILSON

NATURE OF DRUG THERAPY

Drugs used in the treatment of disease may show a wide variety of pharmacological actions but they fall roughly into two broad categories.

In the first they replace a substance essential for health which is not otherwise available as a result of dietary deficiency, malabsorption or loss of secretion by an organ. Examples are the use of ascorbic acid in scurvy, hydroxocobalamin in pernicious anaemia and thyroxine in hypothyroidism. In the first example, no hazard is likely to arise; and in the second, the only risk is that associated with a parenteral injection: excess of the agents causes no harm. In the third, the dose of the drug must be carefully regulated as ill-health may result if the correct amount is not given. In general, when drugs are used as physiological replacements in correct dosage ill-effects do not usually occur provided that no other defects are present and left uncorrected.

In the second category, the therapeutic effect is due to interference with biochemical processes either in the patient or in invading organisms. This pharmacological action is essentially a toxic process which must be strictly limited to the system whose function is to be altered in order to avoid widespread ill-effects. This is the basis of most drug therapy and success depends on precision of dosage and a high degree of selectivity in the site of action. These are not often attained, and so some undesirable effects occur with most potent drugs. The mechanism of their development may be explicable but is often complex and ill understood. As the variety of toxic reactions is very large some provisional form of classification must be attempted.

UNDESIRABLE EFFECTS FROM DRUGS

Errors in dose. An overdose may be due to a misunderstanding on the part of the doctor, nurse, pharmacist or patient. Increasing attention has been paid to errors of this sort in hospital, and improved schemes for ordering and administration of drugs have recently been proposed and should contribute towards the elimination of these faults. They occur more frequently when drugs are taken at home or at work and are most difficult to check.

Clear instructions are a pre-requisite whenever potent drugs are prescribed.

An overdose due to self-poisoning is now one of the commonest medical emergencies and the drug has usually been prescribed by the patient's own doctor. The prevention and management of self-poisoning is described on pp. 544-551.

Overdosage is not necessarily immediately apparent. Slow cumulation of some drugs in the body may not be recognized until an untoward feature appears such as a haemorrhage during treatment with anticoagulants.

Delayed excretion or metabolism. Renal or hepatic insufficiency may increase the retention of a drug in the body. Unduly high blood levels of streptomycin may occur in patients with diminished renal capacity, for example in the elderly who are particularly prone to show toxic effects from this drug. At the other extreme, in the very young the hepatic metabolism of several drugs is defective owing to immaturity of the enzyme systems, particularly glucuronyl transferase. An example is the slow metabolism of chloramphenicol in babies which leads to extremely high blood levels of the drug and the onset of the 'grey syndrome' (p. 471).

The demonstration of inherited deficiencies in enzyme activity which may decrease the rate of inactivation of drugs has been a particularly interesting advance in our understanding of drug toxicity. Slow inactivators of isoniazid and of suxamethonium can be picked out as more liable to experience untoward effects from these agents. Such studies in pharmacogenetics constitute one of the important growing-points in the understanding of ill-health due to drugs.

Interaction of drugs. Interference with metabolism may also be caused by the administration of drugs which have enzyme-inhibiting properties. This is a noticeable feature of the monoamine oxidase inhibitors which have complex effects on the actions of many drugs including sympathomimetics, other antidepressants, central nervous system depressants particularly pethidine, and antihypertensives. They may also interact with sympathomimetic substances present in certain foods—principally tyramine found in cheese, yoghurt, meat and yeast extracts, wines and beers. The effect of monoamine oxidase inhibitors may persist for two or three weeks after their administration has been stopped.

Some drugs have enzyme-inducing properties and may speed the inactivation of certain other drugs in the liver. Phenobarbitone acts in this way and during its administration the hepatic metabolism of warfarin is enhanced. After stopping phenobarbitone the microsomal enzyme activity usually returns to normal within two to three weeks but if warfarin is continued in the same dose its plasma concentration may rise to a dangerous height. Metabolic interactions between drugs are being increasingly recognized as an important cause of fluctuations in plasma concentrations which may lead either to a decrease in therapeutic efficacy or to precipitation of toxic effects.

The action of a drug in the body usually depends on the concentration of the fraction that is not bound to plasma protein and is free to diffuse. Displacement of a drug from the protein by another agent with a higher affinity for the binding site enhances its free level and thus its pharmacological activity. In this way the effects produced are those of overdosage. For example, haemorrhage may occur in a patient being treated with warfarin if phenylbutazone is given in addition.

Side-effects due to widespread pharmacological action. A few potent drugs are highly selective in their site of action. Penicillin is remarkable in this respect; it is lethal in low concentration to certain invading bacteria but does not interfere with human cellular metabolism even when given in massive dosage. At the other extreme, the effect of cortisone and allied steroids in pharmacological dosage is extremely widespread and far exceeds the therapeutic action desired in a particular structure. In general, the wider the range of action of a drug the greater is the liability to side-effects and it is hardly surprising that corticosteroids may produce unwanted reactions in practically every system of the body.

The side-effects of many drugs can often be predicted from their known pharmacological action. This is well illustrated by the numerous agents acting on the autonomic nervous system and used in the treatment of hypertension. The only desired action is blocking of the sympathetic vasomotor nerves; the many actions elsewhere are side-effects. The extent to which these undesirable reactions may be anticipated depends on the knowledge of the pharmacology of the drug and of the function of the structure on which it acts. An unsuspected pharmacological action of a drug may first become apparent when it is revealed as an undesirable effect in a patient. Then it may subsequently be reproduced by appropriate experiments in animals. As it is impossible at present to forecast all the actions of a drug from its chemical structure and as the amount of preclinical testing is necessarily limited, unexpected pharmacological actions will continue to come to light when new drugs are employed in man.

The central nervous system is the site of many unwanted side-effects. Psychotropic drugs frequently possess a wide range of actions in the brain, many of which constitute undesirable side-effects. Ataxia is a common complication following treatment with most cerebral depressants and can be particularly troublesome in the elderly. Little is known about the biochemical processes responsible for normal functioning of the cells of the central nervous system. Even less is known about the abnormalities at cellular level that manifest themselves as psychiatric illness. Moreover, the development of symptomatic remedies endowed with a selective pharmacological action is made difficult by the occurrence of serious side-effects such as anxiety and depression.

Secondary effects of drugs. These are usually most evident in relation to the control of infections. Corticosteroids, by interfering with the natural defence mechanisms, may lead to the spread of infections otherwise localized. Broad-spectrum antibiotics such as the tetracyclines, by eliminating many sensitive bacteria, may leave the way open to overgrowth of other organisms such as resistant staphylococci and monilia.

Hypersensitivity reactions. These can take many different forms and may constitute some of the most dangerous toxic effects of drugs. The basis is sometimes a well-established antigen-antibody reaction which may follow injection of a foreign protein such as tetanus antitoxin of equine origin or exposure to penicillin. The severity of the response varies widely from an erythematous or urticarial skin eruption to anaphylactic shock. In other instances the mechanism is ill-understood. This applies particularly to the development of agranulocytosis, aplastic anaemia and the different types of jaundice that may occasionally follow the administration of certain drugs. Sensitization probably plays a part as the reaction develops only after the drug has been given for a week or more on a first occasion or on exposure to a second course.

Psychological factors. The importance of suggestion in producing beneficial responses to treatment has long been recognized; similarly some of the reported ill-effects of drugs may be due to psychological factors rather than pharmacological actions. In many clinical trials inert tablets have produced as many reports of side-effects as the active agent. A slight change in the appearance of a preparation that has acquired an unfortunate reputation may lessen considerably the incidence of supposed ill-effects. It is important to be equally critical in claiming both benefit and harm from drugs.

Recognition of ill-health due to drugs

The side-effects of drugs may resemble features developing in naturally occurring disease and the actions of drugs may obscure the interpretation of laboratory investigations. It is therefore essential to obtain a full account of recent drug therapy and of any toxic reactions to drugs that may have occurred in the past. Unfortunately this is difficult to achieve and inquiries may be delayed until suspicion has been aroused that the disorder may be drug-induced—often only after the patient has had numerous and uncomfortable investigations of an obscure illness. As so many new and potent drugs are being introduced, inquiries should not be delayed until this stage has been reached. New and unsuspected toxic reactions can only be revealed if a drug history is taken *as a routine*.

Reporting of toxic reactions. A procedure for the reporting of suspected adverse reactions to drugs has been established in Britain. Reports should be sent to the Medical Assessor, Committee on Safety of Medicines, Queen Anne's Mansions, Queen Anne's Gate, London, S.W.1. Thus, any harm being caused by a drug may be promptly recognized and an early warning given. There is already considerable international co-operation in the exchange of such information. The success of the reporting scheme depends on the co-operation of all doctors who prescribe drugs.

Studies on the toxicity of drugs, particularly the incidence of dangerous reactions, should be on a sound epidemiological basis. With modern computing techniques the number of patients exposed to a drug and the amount prescribed can be ascertained; the main difficulty lies in ensuring adequate reporting. Though a drug may be recognized as occasionally causing some serious toxic effect

such as agranulocytosis, the frequency of the event is rarely known. Information on a sound quantitative basis is essential for the future assessment of the value of drug therapy.

PREVENTIVE ASPECTS

When potent drugs are used in the treatment of disease there is always the danger that harm may result. No amount of toxicity testing in animals can eliminate this risk though it may prevent some of the more toxic compounds coming to clinical trial and may direct the attention of the clinical investigator to possible dangers. The limitations of studies in animals must be recognized. Many human reactions to drugs cannot be reproduced in the experimental animal. Some toxic effects of a new drug may not be described until after several thousand patients have received it. This is particularly the case if the toxic effect is novel and unexpected and if it appears only some time after the course of treatment has been completed or after prolonged administration.

The difficulty of predicting the toxicity of drugs in man throws a considerable burden on the clinician. Before any drug is prescribed he should always inquire whether the patient has previously been treated with it and experienced any untoward effects. Closely related drugs usually produce similar toxic effects and also cross-sensitization. The multitude of unrelated proprietary names which may disguise similar or closely related drugs or a compound mixture may trap the unwary into prescribing a preparation known to have caused trouble previously. There is a strong case for the general use of approved names in the interests of safety and the quicker recognition of toxic effects. The latter is particularly important to ensure that the offending drug is promptly withdrawn and any appropriate treatment started. In general, the length of time that a drug is given without realizing that it is producing harm is directly related to the duration and seriousness of subsequent morbidity from the toxic effects.

There is inevitably greater uncertainty in employing a new drug than in using an established one whose harmful effects have been fully recognized. The value of a new drug can be ascertained only by extensive use, and no progress would be achieved if only the older remedies were employed. When a relatively untried drug is prescribed, the doctor must ensure that the patient is fully safeguarded and that the effect, whether beneficial or harmful, can be clearly ascertained. The new drug should not be administered along with a multiplicity of other agents.

Adequate records must be kept. Whenever toxic effects are encountered they should be noted at the time. The patient himself or a responsible relative should be informed of the name of the drug or the nature of the treatment that has caused the reaction. This will ensure as far as possible that he is not again exposed to the same hazard.

Treatment of Side-effects and Toxic Effects

When a harmful reaction to a drug is observed a decision has to be made on a continuation, modification or abandonment of the treatment, and this will depend largely on the circumstances. Account must be taken of the gravity of the illness being treated, the severity of the disturbance produced by the drug and the availability of alternative therapy. The simplest procedure is to stop the drug, but this may not always be possible or desirable.

In cases where difficulties arise from unwanted pharmacological actions of a drug, a reduction in dose and the prescription of an additional drug may enable treatment to be continued—for example in the management of high blood pressure the dose of guanethidine may be reduced if a thiazide diuretic is given at the same time (pp. 112-117). In the treatment of myasthenia gravis atropine given along with neostigmine will antagonize the unwanted parasympathomimetic actions but leave intact the desired action at the skeletal neuromuscular junctions. However, the possibilities of counteracting side-effects are limited and successful arrangement of appropriate doses is usually difficult. It is easy to arrive at a situation where a summation rather than antagonism of side-effects is all that is achieved.

The effects of an excess of some drugs may be partially overcome by the administration of a competitive inhibitor; for example, nalorphine in morphine or pethidine overdosage and vitamin K in treating haemorrhage due to a coumarin anticoagulant. The acceleration of elimination is sometimes possible. This is discussed in the sections on poisoning and renal dialysis (pp. 546, 277).

Most difficulty is caused by severe hypersensitivity reactions occurring during the treatment of a serious disease; for example, skin eruptions due to penicillin in a patient suffering from bacterial endocarditis or to streptomycin in tuberculosis. The first choice is to switch to another drug, but if this is impracticable, desensitization may be attempted, but this is seldom practicable. More dangerous manifestations of drug toxicity such as blood dyscrasias or jaundice are a clear indication for immediate and permanent withdrawal of the drug. The treatment of these complications is discussed elsewhere (pp. 172, 173).

Conclusion

Occasional toxic effects are unavoidable when potent drugs are employed in the treatment of disease. The safety of a drug is thus always a relative matter and must be assessed in relation to the seriousness of the clinical condition, the efficacy of the agent in curing the illness or in relieving symptoms and its liability to cause adverse reactions. Though much attention has rightly been paid in recent years to harmful effects, it is most important that a proper sense of proportion be preserved. Many serious conditions which previously exacted a heavy toll in mortality and morbidity can now be relieved by drugs which may occasionally cause some dangerous toxic reactions. In these cases there is no doubt that the overall benefit greatly exceeds the harm. On the other hand, serious toxic effects, even if they occur only rarely, are not acceptable from drugs used for the alleviation of trivial conditions. Discrimination in the selection of drugs by the prescriber is a most important safeguard in reducing the incidence of ill-effects

25. Industrial Diseases

A. T. DOIG and S. ALSTEAD

INTRODUCTION

'When a Handicrafts-man is taken ill, he must be cur'd by Vomiting, or Purging, or Searing, or Incision; for if a Physician tells him of a long Diet, and Bolstering up his Head, and the like, he presently replies, That he has not leisure to lie by it, and that it will be of no use to him to lead an idle crazy Life, and neglect his Business. Upon this he takes leave of the Physician, and returns to his usual way of living.'—PLATO, quoted by RAMAZZINI in 1705.

The difficulties that beset the physician of Plato's Republic in the treatment of the diseases of tradesmen have persisted through the ages. Industrial disease may be well established before advice is sought and often, as in silicosis and occupational cancer, is progressive in nature. The patient's financial resources may be small and his family anxieties great. His desire to return to work is offset by the knowledge that the job which awaits him is the one which was responsible for, or contributed to, his illness. All these factors operate against the prospect of cure. The circumstances serve to underline the importance of prevention of industrial diseases; this is far more rewarding than making elaborate provision for sick and demoralized workmen and searching for antidotes to industrial poisons. In recent years a considerable sense of communal responsibility for these matters has arisen, and is reflected in the literature—which encroaches more and more on architecture, engineering, education and law. Periodical examinations of workmen in certain trades (whether conducted voluntarily or required by statute) are now leading to the discovery of an increasingly high proportion of cases of industrial disease in the early stages—sometimes even before symptoms are present. Such examinations include radiological investigation of persons exposed to the risk of inhaling dust and biochemical testing of the blood and urine in those who work with lead and mercury.

Many conditions quite outside the scope of factory control may influence the susceptibility of workers to industrial disease, and there is need for increasingly close co-operation between general practitioners and their professional colleagues charged with the more technical surveillance of conditions inside the factory that may affect health. It cannot be too strongly emphasized that health is affected by the sum of all the factors operating on the body, from within and from without. These are hereditary influences, the domestic setting with its components such as housing, diet, personal habits and the use of leisure, and—not least—the environment at the place of employment, with all the physical and psychological accompaniments. These circumstances must be kept in mind by those who seek to promote the health of the industrial worker.

The practitioner renders an important service to his patient and to the community by promptly discharging his statutory duty to inform H.M. Chief Inspector of Factories[1] of all cases of notifiable industrial disease contracted in premises subject to the Factories Act. These diseases are poisoning by lead, arsenic, mercury (including their organic compounds), beryllium, cadmium, manganese, phosphorus (including tricresyl or triphenyl phosphate or due to the anticholesterinase action of any organic phosphorus compound), aniline (including nitro- or amide derivatives of benzene or chlorobenzene or their homologues), and carbon bisulphide; chronic benzene poisoning, toxic jaundice, toxic anaemia, anthrax, chrome and epitheliomatous ulceration, and decompression sickness (caisson disease or compressed air illness). Their occurrence indicates some fault in working methods or environment, and notification leads not only to an investigation of the case specified and of fellow-workers similarly exposed, but to consideration of improvements to prevent the occurrence of further cases.

The Factory Inspectorate are of course interested not only in the notifiable diseases listed above but in any others that are considered to be attributable to occupation in premises under the Factories Act (which includes building operations, works of engineering construction, docks, etc.); and under the Offices, Shops and Railway Premises Act the Medical Inspectors of Factories (telephone numbers under Factory Inspector) are ready to advise and help in regard to suspect cases.

In the case of many industrial diseases due to poisons of a non-cumulative nature, cure rapidly follows withdrawal from exposure, and treatment may be unnecessary or purely symptomatic. There is a very large number of toxic chemical substances and also many other kinds of potential hazard in industry. In this

[1] Department of Employment, Baynards House, 1–13 Chepstow Place, London, W.2.

556

chapter reference is made only to the more important industrial diseases and to those conditions calling for specific treatment.

Effects of High Temperatures

Diseases due to heat may be classified into three clinical types: (1) heat exhaustion; (2) heat cramps; and (3) heat retention. Owing to improved measures affecting ventilation, and the wider use of oil instead of coal for heating boilers, serious effects are practically unknown in British workplaces. Some acclimatization occurs in people persistently exposed to high temperatures: the salt content of the sweat progressively diminishes—revealing a mechanism for its conservation.

There is no doubt about the efficacy of sodium chloride in the prevention and treatment of disabilities caused by excessive sweating. As a preventive measure it is usually given as saline drinks containing 0·1 to 0·25 per cent. salt. Milk drunk freely is helpful as it contains 0·3 per cent. salt. Effervescent drinks with lemon or other flavouring can be made with prepared tablets containing sodium chloride, 300 mg., compounded with sodium bicarbonate and citric acid. Preparations of this kind should be available for workers exposed to excessive heat. They should be warned against drinking plain water during or after severe sweating.

Heat exhaustion. In slight cases the sufferer should be laid flat in a cool place and his clothing should be loosened. Cool saline drinks should be administered. In severe cases there is considerable dehydration with haemoconcentration and low urinary output. The patient must be nursed in bed. The aim of treatment is to restore the blood volume to normal, to correct salt and water depletion, and to prevent circulatory failure. Intravenous injections of physiological saline may be necessary. It is advisable to keep a fluid balance chart. If possible estimations of the chloride content of the plasma should be made and the output of salt in the urine should be recorded.

Heat cramps. Saline drinks usually give prompt relief: these contain 2 to 4 g. of salt per litre—a solution two or three times stronger than that used in drinks given to prevent heat exhaustion. In severe cases the pain is agonizing and calls for intravenous injection of 500 ml. of normal saline to accelerate recovery. If severe pain persists despite intravenous infusion of saline, a small dose of morphine hydrochloride (5 mg.) should be injected slowly intravenously.

Heat retention (*Heat stroke: Heat hyperpyrexia*). In addition to salt depletion there is oedema of the brain with derangement of the heat-regulating centre. The essentials of treatment are (1) the immediate reduction of fever; (2) rest in the recumbent position; and (3) administration of fluids; (4) the need for elaborate and prolonged management may be diminished by giving a small dose of chlorpromazine by slow intravenous infusion (25 mg. in 300 ml. normal saline in 20 minutes).

Increase of heat loss by evaporation is more effective than cooling by application of ice. The patient should be stripped and placed on a bedstead with a fenestrated mattress to allow free circulation of air around him. Cool water should be sprayed or sponged over him. Evaporation may be aided by the use of hand or electric fans. Alternatively he may be placed in a bath of cold water. Massage or friction may help appreciably to maintain the circulation in the skin and thus increase heat loss. Rectal temperature readings and the heart rate should be charted every 15 minutes and the blood pressure recorded half-hourly. Unless there is renal failure fluids should be given freely: if the patient is co-operative, half-strength saline flavoured with fruit juice should be given by mouth; but if he resists feeding, an intragastric drip should set up. In addition, normal saline should be given intravenously: 600 ml. is infused in the course of about 30 minutes, and thereafter the rate of administration is adjusted according to the requirements of the individual patient. Rectal administration of saline is feasible, but somewhat uncertain regarding the quantity of fluid actually absorbed. When the temperature falls to 39·5° C., vigorous measures can be eased, the patient being placed in blankets with ice-packs to his head. If there are signs of respiratory depression, artificial respiration should be started and the effect of oxygen therapy noted (pp. 652, 646). Cardiac failure is likely to be associated with oligaemia, and peripheral circulatory collapse, and is remedied by measures aimed at restoring the normal blood volume and electrolyte levels (pp. 628, 253). As hepatic damage is a common occurrence, the clinical findings and the blood chemistry should be checked frequently (pp. 249, 253).

If there is evidence of cerebral oedema (as shown by retinal congestion and papilloedema) and convulsions supervene, an attempt may be made to reduce the intracranial pressure (p. 400). If convulsions persist, paraldehyde should be given: 3 ml. should be injected into the upper and outer quadrant of each buttock and the area massaged briskly to accelerate absorption. Lumbar puncture for the relief of symptoms due to increased intracranial pressure is potentially the most effective method; but it is not without hazards (p. 400) and cannot be undertaken until the convulsive state has been controlled by a general anaesthetic.

A prolonged and quiet convalescence lasting several weeks is necessary, and special care must be taken to avoid any possibility of another attack.

Decompression Sickness

The Work in Compressed Air Special Regulations 1958 (and the Amendment Regulations 1960) impose requirements for the health, safety and welfare of persons employed in compressed air in premises to which the Factories Acts apply. These include works of engineering construction such as tunnelling, bridge building, and excavations for docks. The various health requirements include medical supervision of the workers following a thorough initial examination, the keeping of a personal health register for each worker and of detailed records of each compression and decompression. New workers must be educated in regard to the risks inherent to the work and provided with a leaflet containing advice as to the precautions to be taken. Where pressures greater than 18 pounds per square inch (p.s.i.) exist, medical examinations must be repeated monthly, and a medical lock must be provided for the treatment of any cases of decompression sickness which may occur. Further, because workers may be taken ill (caisson disease) after leaving work, they must wear labels (provided for them) indicating that they work in compressed air and giving information about the site of the medical lock provided for treatment. Hospitals in the district must be informed that such work is being undertaken. A Schedule to the Regulations contains rules relating to the compression and decompression of workers, and includes a table which lays down the minimum times to be taken in reducing the pressure to atmospheric pressure. Decompression sickness rarely occurs in persons who have been subjected to less than 18 p.s.i. working pressure and therefore the Schedule to the Regulations lays down times to be observed only in regard to decompression from pressures exceeding 18 p.s.i.

These compressions and decompressions of normal healthy workers usually take place in locks provided at the entrance to the shafts, tunnels or chambers in which the work is being carried out. In the case of divers, decompression is accomplished by raising the worker to various levels in stages and letting him remain at each stage for longer periods as the surface is approached. The Admiralty have a Code of Rules controlling Naval practice.

Where a case of decompression sickness occurs far from a medical lock, as in deep-sea diving, every effort must be made to transport the patient as quickly as possible to a recompression chamber. The Admiralty maintain medical locks at two stations in Scotland, H.M. Dockyard, Rosyth (Telephone No. 038-34 2121) and Clyde Submarine Base, Faslane (Telephone No. 0436 4321). In addition to making its medical locks and experienced personnel available for civilian cases, the Royal Navy may also help with transport, including the use of a helicopter.

Apart from high-altitude decompression sickness which may be met with in flying above 20,000 feet in non-pressurized cabins, and which is generally relieved rapidly and completely by descent to lower levels, treatment must in all cases be by recompression of the affected worker so as to redissolve the bubbles of nitrogen in the body fluids. Thereafter decompression aims at returning the worker to atmospheric pressure without the formation of fresh bubbles. Decompression sickness occurs in two types.

Type 1 cases, characterized only by joint pains and known as "the bends", are usually amenable to fairly simple treatment, but there are varying opinions as to how this should be accomplished. Two main methods are in use: one is to compress the patient to the pressure at which he was working —or two or three pounds higher—and then to decompress him in a manner similar to that laid down in the Schedule to the Code of Regulations, the slow phase, however, being extended according to the severity of the case; the other method— usually considered the better in this country—is to compress the patient only to the pressure required to relieve the pain which is usually found to be about 8 p.s.i. below the working pressure level and after 10 to 15 minutes at this pressure the normal process of decompression is completed. It seems that fewer patients require further treatment with this second method. The first has the disadvantage that more nitrogen will be taken up by the tissues when they are exposed to the higher pressure required. Frequently patients complain of residual soreness in the affected joints after treatment, but usually have no difficulty in distinguishing clearly between this and the pains of persisting or recurring bends. Domestic remedies such as simple analgesics and liniments may give temporary relief of pain but this response does not warrant delaying the patient's return to the medical lock, for neglect of proper treatment may well be a factor in the subsequent development of avascular necrosis of bone. In general, bends will be minimized by anything increasing the flow of blood in the limbs. Hence warmth in the decompression chamber and hot drinks should be provided, as well as dry clothing when necessary. The value of exercise during decompression is uncertain; it appears to predispose to bends in high altitude flying and has never been clearly proved to be useful in tunnellers and caisson workers when leaving high pressures. During decompression after treatment the patient should be encouraged to exercise his limbs gently and to move at intervals.

Type 2 cases are those exhibiting serious symptoms indicating involvement of brain, spinal cord, heart, lungs, bones or other important tissues. Those most frequently encountered are paresis ('divers' palsy'), vertigo ('the staggers'), fits, unconsciousness and dyspnoea ('the chokes'). No time must be lost in recompressing such patients to the working pressure, or higher if necessary, to relieve symptoms. This effective pressure should be maintained for at least half an hour; thereafter there should follow slow decompression with mild temporary recompression if symptoms reappear. A rate frequently employed is 15 minutes per pound down to a pressure of 12 p.s.i. This pressure is then maintained without any further decompression for a period of four hours (spoken of as a 'soaking period'). Thereafter the pressure is reduced by 1 lb. every 30 minutes to atmospheric level with soaking periods at 8, 4 and 2 p.s.i. Decompression over the last few pounds is just as important as at the higher pressures, and a tendency to shorten the time must be resisted. Even with such slow decompression some patients redevelop symptoms and must be recompressed for further periods followed by even slower decompression. The treatment sometimes lasts into the second or third day and one successful case has been described requiring over nine days' continuous treatment under pressure in the medical lock. During the treatment of type 2 cases, medical attendance is necessary. After decompression patients who have had a severe attack of type 2 disease should be transferred to hospital for a period of observation and to ensure full recuperation. Most of these patients should be forbidden to work again in compressed air, although in some of

the slighter cases work at strictly limited pressures or for limited periods may be allowed.

In specially deep diving, a mixture of oxygen and helium is used instead of air. This avoids the danger of nitrogen narcosis caused by dissolved nitrogen on cell function. The substitution of helium for nitrogen is less likely to produce symptoms because the solubility of helium in body fat and fluids is lower than that of nitrogen. Also, decompression can be effected in a shorter time. On the other hand, at high pressures, because of the increased partial pressure of oxygen, symptoms of oxygen poisoning may occur. All divers using oxygen apparatus must be warned about the early symptoms of oxygen poisoning and of the need to come up immediately if such effects are noted. On breathing fresh air the symptoms gradually subside; the patient usually falls asleep and awakes with no more than a temporary headache.

Poisoning by Metals

Lead. Lead poisoning is treated by giving chelating agents. The preparations used are either sodium calciumedetate or D-penicillamine. Both are effective in promoting the excretion of lead and both are available for oral and intravenous administration; but while sodium calciumedetate given intravenously is slightly more effective than oral or intravenous penicillamine, it is much less effective when given by mouth. In mild or moderate cases penicillamine given by mouth is the usual method employed.

SODIUM CALCIUMEDETATE acts through its powerful affinity for lead. The calcium ion is displaced from the complex molecule to accommodate the lead ion. Thus a non-ionizable and non-toxic compound of lead is produced and this is safely and rapidly excreted by the kidney. Other metals which normally occur in the tissues such as iron, cobalt and copper are unaffected because they are strongly bound to tissue proteins; sodium calciumedetate therefore acts selectively on the available lead ions.

A convenient preparation for intravenous administration is sodium calciumedetate injection (B.P.). The dose is 0·2 ml. per kg. body weight twice daily (morning and evening) for up to five days according to the patient's needs. The solution containing each dose is added to 500 ml. of 5 per cent. dextrose solution and is given by intravenous drip over a period of one hour. Thrombophlebitis is common at the site of injection. Nausea and diarrhoea may be troublesome. The symptoms of overdose are drowsiness, fatigue and shivering.

Sodium calciumedetate is virtually non-toxic when given carefully for therapeutic purposes; there may be a temporary fall of blood pressure, but this is not important. Nevertheless, if large quantities of this compound are excreted in the urine during intensive or prolonged treatment, damage to the renal tubules is likely to occur—heralded by proteinuria and aminoaciduria; and casts may also be found in the urine. Thus the continuing risk of lead nephropathy may be temporarily increased by the injudicious use of a chelating agent which is itself potentially nephrotoxic. A course of de-leading treatment should not exceed five days, but two or three courses may be given separated by periods of one week. Although intravenous administration gives quicker and better results than the oral route, sodium calciumedetate is effective by mouth in doses of 1 g. four times daily. If there is a large quantity of lead in the bowel, however, sodium calciumedetate given by mouth may hasten absorption and intensify the symptoms of lead poisoning. The excess of lead should therefore be removed from the intestine by gentle purgation (Elixir of Cascara, 4 ml. in the evening) and simple enemata for three days before de-leading begins, but it is important to avoid causing diarrhoea by giving excessive doses of irritant purgatives.

Oral administration of sodium calciumedetate has been used as a prophylactic measure for workers exposed to lead, but the writers consider that this is rarely justifiable. Symptoms or signs indicating excessive lead absorption should be dealt with by a proper course of treatment and the working environment should be inspected in order to determine the source of the exposure and to control it. If treatment is given while exposure continues, symptoms are masked, and this creates a false sense of security. Abuse of the drug may result in improper dosage and creates new hazards.

DIMERCAPROL (BAL) is not used in lead poisoning.

PENICILLAMINE, a metabolite of penicillin, is a valuable antidote for use in poisoning due to lead, copper and mercury. The preparation used is D-penicillamine; this is more effective and less toxic than L-penicillamine or DL-penicillamine. Chemically it is D-3-Mercaptovaline, and its chelating action derives from its possessing a sulphydryl

group (cf. dimercaprol, p. 561). It was principally used for the elimination of copper from the tissues in hepatolenticular degeneration (p. 406) and for cystinuria, but in the past few years penicillamine has been employed increasingly in subacute and chronic lead poisoning in preference to sodium calciumedetate. The advantage claimed for penicillamine is that the treatment does not call for the close supervision that is needed when sodium calciumedetate is administered orally; this applies particularly to the treatment of lead poisoning in children. Penicillamine is given in doses of 600 mg. to 1·5 g. daily; it can also be given intravenously but this is rarely necessary. It results in a reduced output of urinary coproporphyria, and a fall in the lead and δ-aminolaevulic acid levels in the blood. The lead is excreted entirely in the urine. Patients under treatment should, of course, be removed from the environment in which they contracted poisoning. Penicillamine administration may be continued for up to four weeks. Treatment is still fairly expensive —about £3 a week. It is possible to treat a patient simultaneously with oral penicillamine and sodium calciumedetate intravenously, thus producing a summation of effect. Toxic effects reported from D-penicillamine include depression of haemopoiesis and prolonged therapy may produce a nephrotic syndrome. The risk of toxic effects is reduced by giving pyridoxine daily in doses of 50 mg. DL-penicillamine and L-penicillamine are much more toxic and are not recommended. As with sodium calciumedetate, penicillamine should not be used prophylactically for workmen exposed to the risk of lead poisoning.

Chelating agents give prompt relief in lead poisoning and they should be given at once to bring acute or subacute symptoms under control. Occasionally, however, they are not immediately available. In these circumstances calcium gluconate, 10 ml. of 10 per cent. solution, should be given slowly intravenously. The patient should also be given a diet rich in calcium (a supplement of 3 pints of milk daily) and the urine should be kept alkaline by means of a mixture containing potassium citrate and sodium citrate. This regimen causes the lead in the blood to move into the bones and muscles. The need for de-leading at a later date should be explained to the patient.

Peripheral neuritis with paralysis calls for the co-operation of an orthopaedic surgeon. Iron-deficiency anaemia is corrected on conventional lines (p. 143). Attention should be paid to the patient's physique and the need for physiotherapy and rehabilitation should be considered.

In lead encephalopathy, sodium calciumedetate is the treatment of choice; it is well tolerated by children. Restlessness can be controlled by the intramuscular injection of 200 mg. of sodium phenobarbitone. Further symptomatic improvement is sometimes obtained from lumbar puncture.

Poisoning by tetra-ethyl-lead. In poisoning by organic lead compounds the use of chelating agents may result in an increased excretion of lead in the urine. Their use is, therefore, to be recommended although the patient is usually acutely ill because of the widespread action of the organic lead compound on the central nervous system: restlessness, excitement and convulsions may occur. Thus sedatives are usually needed, and the best is phenobarbitone sodium: if immediate control is needed 200 mg. should be injected intravenously; if the need for sedative action is less urgent, 200 mg. should be given intramuscularly and then 100 to 200 mg. intramuscularly every four hours according to the individual patient's requirements. Morphine should not be used. In a toxaemic state it may cause dangerous depression of the respiratory centre.

General management and nursing are on the lines adopted for the unconscious patient (p. 385). Parenteral infusion of glucose-saline and feeding by intragastric drip are necessary, and a fluid balance chart is indispensable to the proper management of the patient. When it is necessary to empty the lower bowel suppositories of bisacodyl should be tried. If these fail to cause evacuation, the use of a simple enema is recommended.

Arsenic. Industrial arsenic poisoning is uncommon today. There are three main forms: that produced by the absorption (usually by inhalation) of inorganic arsenic compounds, poisoning by arseniuretted hydrogen gas, and the effects of exposure to organic arsenicals.

In subacute or chronic poisoning due to inorganic compounds, in addition to removing the patient from exposure and promoting elimination through the kidneys and bowels, the specific treatment by dimercaprol (BAL) should be employed. Its action and dosage are discussed below. Dimercaprol is also used as an antidote in poisoning due to mercury, gold and bismuth, but it is of no therapeutic value in lead, cadmium and iron poisoning.

DIMERCAPROL (BRITISH ANTI-LEWISITE). This compound, 2, 3-dimercaptopropanol, was developed during the Second World War as an antidote

to arsenical gases such as Lewisite. Fortunately it was not needed for this purpose, but its applications in the treatment of heavy-metal poisoning were explored with interesting results bearing on the practice of medicine. The toxic effects of heavy metals are attributable to their interference with the sulphydryl enzyme systems of cell proteins. It follows that any substance which 'offers' a large number of sulphydryl groups is potentially of therapeutic value. If it can diffuse into the body tissues, it may satisfy the affinity of a heavy metal for sulphydryl and thus safeguard this grouping in certain enzymes which are indispensable for normal metabolism. The complex formed by the interaction of a heavy metal and a dithiol is relatively stable and in this form it may be excreted harmlessly. There is, however, some tendency to dissociation and a risk of recurring toxaemia. It is, therefore, important to ensure that the dithiol available is always considerably in excess of immediate requirements. This is achieved by adequate dosage and repeated administration.

Dimercaprol is administered by intramuscular injection as a 5 per cent. solution in arachis oil with benzyl benzoate. Skin lesions are no longer treated by inunction, but contamination of the eyes with arsenical vesicants can be treated with a 5 per cent. oily solution instilled into the conjunctival sac; complete recovery follows prompt treatment. With the exception of irreversible changes, such as aplastic anaemia and hepatocellular jaundice, all the toxic effects of severe arsenical poisoning can be relieved, but success depends largely on early treatment and especially on giving adequate doses in the first 48 hours. The following dose schedules incorporate recommendations set out in the B.P.C. 1968 for the treatment of arsenical poisoning with dimercaprol:

	(a) Severe Poisoning Dose 3 mg. per kg. body weight	(b) Mild Poisoning Dose 2·5mg. per kg. body weight
Day		
First	6 doses	6 doses
Second	6 doses	6 doses
Third	4 doses	2 doses
Fourth–tenth	2 doses daily	1 or 2 doses daily

In acute and subacute mercurial poisoning, doses should be generous (scheme (a)), but the toxic effects of gold yield to smaller doses (scheme (*b*)). In chronic mercury poisoning doses according to scheme (*b*) should be used and careful watch kept for evidence of kidney damage.

Various side-effects following the administration of dimercaprol have been observed, namely nausea, vomiting, a burning sensation in the mouth, throat and eyes, pain in the teeth, lachrymation, salivation and elevation of the blood pressure. They generally develop rapidly, within 15 to 20 minutes after each injection, and subside within a few hours.

Poisoning by arseniuretted hydrogen (arsine), though relatively rare, is one of the commonest causes of occupational toxic jaundice. In spite of the typical clinical picture it is probable that many cases go unrecognized. The sudden occurrence of severe illness with gastric upset and haemoglobinuria in an industrial worker or chemist should suggest the diagnosis; and rapidly developing jaundice, anaemia, and evidence of renal damage would greatly strengthen the suspicion.

Symptoms usually develop some hours after exposure has taken place, probably when the patient is at home. If, while at work, he becomes ill or is known to have been exposed to this gas, he must immediately be withdrawn from exposure, and any clothing contaminated with the chemicals he has been using should be removed. Prompt removal to hospital is essential, and general measures should be instituted forthwith to deal with pain and anxiety and to minimize shock. Early deaths are often due to pulmonary oedema. When this is present, oxygen—preferably under pressure—offers most hope.

Dimercaprol has been used in most of the recently published cases, but the results are not entirely convincing. Locket and his colleagues say that it should be given if the patient is seen within the first 24 hours; after that it is more likely to do harm. Dextrose and saline, with or without calcium gluconate, should be given intravenously, but the co-operation of the hospital biochemist is imperative in order to avoid such hazards as hyperpotassaemia and overloading the circulation in patients with renal damage and oliguria. The prognosis has been much improved by using the artificial kidney (p. 277), as renal failure is the main cause of death in patients who survive earlier complications. Intrathecal injection of 2 ml. of heavy cinchocaine to produce high spinal anaesthesia may be tried as a means of improving renal circulation. Blood transfusion is undoubtedly helpful, especially if there is severe anaemia. Recently, total replacement blood transfusion has been advocated. The treatment is logical because it greatly diminishes the amount of arsenic in the blood and almost eliminates reduced haemoglobin and cellular debris. Thus total replacement blood transfusion reduces the risk of damage to the renal glomeruli and tubules, but this procedure must be carried out *as soon as the diagnosis of arsine poisoning is made.*

Arsenic trichloride and some of the organic arsenical compounds, particularly the dichlorarsines, are extremely powerful irritants and act as vesicants, lachrymators, sternutators and lung irritants. They may readily pass through the skin and give rise to systemic poisoning. Death may occur after apparently trivial contamination such as a splash of arsenic trichloride on the skin. A person who is splashed or otherwise contaminated by any of these compounds must have all the soiled clothing stripped off *immediately* and the skin cleansed by continuous irrigation with cold water from a running tap. As soon as possible dimercaprol should be administered intramuscularly as discussed on p. 561. Inunction is no longer considered necessary for the treatment of skin lesions; in fact, it has been shown that the action of an ointment containing 5 per cent. dimercaprol is likely to be systemic rather than local for, applied elsewhere than to the affected skin, the eruption clears just as rapidly and the arsenic excretion in the urine increases during this treatment. For pulmonary irritation caused by arsenic trichloride and the organic arsenicals oxygen therapy may be required, and the treatment recommended for gassing with nitric oxides (p. 566) should be given. Dimercaprol, 3 to 5 per cent. in aqueous solution or as an ointment, gives excellent results in the treatment of burns of the eyes with irritant arsenical compounds *if used within five or ten minutes.*

It has been stated that in precancerous and cancerous skin lesions due to arsenic compounds, the arsenic content of the lesions is high and is reduced almost to nil by dimercaprol therapy. The lesions themselves, however, are unaffected.

Mercury. The treatment of chronic poisoning from inorganic mercury compounds consists mainly in removing the patient from exposure to mercury, in attention to his general health, and in promoting elimination by the bowels and kidneys by giving fluids and saline aperients. The disability is likely to be extremely tedious; it may last for years and in some cases never completely disappears. Symptomatic measures should not be under-rated. Sialorrhoea may be relieved by small doses of belladonna, such as Belladonna Dry Extract B.P., 30 mg. twice or thrice daily. Opium has been used for over a century (as by Thackrah), but on general grounds this is a less desirable drug for long-term treatment. Stomatitis should be treated with mouth-washes with appropriate dental supervision and extractions if necessary.

Dimercaprol (BAL) is of great value in acute mercury poisoning (as from mercuric chloride) if administered early enough to prevent toxic effects on the renal tubules. It has generally given disappointing results in chronic mercury poisoning though some authors have found it of value even in cases where sodium calciumedetate failed to give benefit. Prolonged courses are indicated using relatively small single doses. The majority of reports, however, suggest that sodium calciumedetate is more efficient than dimercaprol. Opportunities for clinical trials are infrequent, because this kind of poisoning is now uncommon, but N acetyl DL-penicillamine has been used with success in a few recent cases. Bidstrup (1964), summarizing reports on treatment, states that N acetyl DL-penicillamine appears to be the most effective method available and to be without side-effects in chronic mercury poisoning. She advocates the administration of doses of 250 mg. four times daily for 10 days, repeated as indicated by the patient's condition after an interval of two to three weeks.

Poisoning by organic mercury compounds leads to severe and permanent involvement of the central nervous system. This results in ataxia, dysarthria, and constriction of the visual fields, but memory and intelligence are unaffected. Dimercaprol has been tried in many patients but has not proved effective in the disease in its common form. When, however, poisoning has resulted from ingestion or absorption from the skin over a short period, it may be of value and should be tried. The dose is 2 ml. of a 5 per cent. solution (arachis oil is used as a solvent). It is injected intramuscularly 4-hourly during the first day, then twice daily until the fourth day, and a single dose on the fifth and sixth days. If the skin has recently been contaminated, it should be cleansed to prevent chemical burns and blistering, and if the poison has been swallowed the stomach should be washed out with a protein-containing fluid such as egg-white in water.

When there has been damage to the central nervous system, physiotherapy, massage and re-educative movements for the limbs are necessary. The patient will require much encouragement in his efforts to learn to walk again and in the use of common articles such as pencil, knife and fork. Speech therapy may result at length in considerable improvement and a measure of independence.

Fulminate of mercury is mainly used in factories for the manufacture of detonators and percussion caps. Very few systemic effects have occurred from its use, but cases of dermatitis, with occasional ulceration (principally of the face, neck, hands and forearms), conjunctivitis, and inflammation of nasal and buccal mucous membranes were extremely numerous during the Second World War. Preventive measures included the use of 10 per cent. aqueous solution of sodium thiosulphate as a wash before and after work and before meals. A 2 per cent. solution was useful in the prevention and treatment of the conjunctivitis.

Urine analysis for mercury content is valuable in the management and control of cases of inorganic and organic mercury poisoning, as well as in prophylaxis.

BERYLLIUM. Although the industrial uses of beryllium and its alloys are increasing, beryllium disease is still rare. Its most usual manifestations are skin lesions which include dermatitis, ulcers and granulomata; acute pneumonitis or 'chemical pneumonia'; and chronic or delayed pneumonitis, often termed berylliosis.

Most cases of dermatitis are regarded as being due to the development of hypersensitivity to beryllium salts, not to primary irritation. Complete removal from contact should be effected; thereafter treatment on symptomatic lines is usually sufficient. Ulcers and granulomata follow lodgement of beryllium compounds or particles of metal in the dermis and healing does not take place until these are removed either in the natural discharges from the lesions or therapeutically by curettage or excision. The suggestion that pulmonary lesions may occur in cases of beryllium disease of the skin without inhalation of beryllium compounds needs confirmation, but radiological investigation of the lungs in cases with lesions of the skin would appear to be worth while.

Acute beryllium pneumonitis is a serious disease which necessitates the patient's spending many weeks resting in bed. Relapses, sometimes with the onset of pulmonary oedema, have followed premature resumption of activity. There is no specific therapy. Attempts to eliminate beryllium by the use of dimercaprol and solubilizing agents have been disappointing and the inhalation of phosphate buffer (pH 7·4) in an attempt to reduce the rate of release from the lungs has been without effect. Penicillin-streptomycin aerosol therapy may be used to control secondary bacterial infection. Such infection is, however, rare. Sedatives and cough suppressants (p. 440) may be required for severe coughing and to obtain sleep. Oxygen may be required. There have been comparatively few opportunities for a trial of corticosteroids in acute beryllium pneumonitis, but most experienced observers believe that their use, early in the disease, often produces striking benefit.

Of the treatment of chronic berylliosis, Hunter says that attempts to increase the rate of elimination of beryllium with injections of dimercaprol have not been successful. Most writers have found that corticosteroid therapy has been well worth a trial on the basis of its reducing the cellular and fibrous tissue reactions; and also on the assumption that sensitization plays a part in the aetiology of the disease. In many cases great symptomatic relief has been reported, particularly of the dyspnoea. In some there has also been a temporary improvement in the physical signs and even in the radio-logical picture. These signs and the symptoms usually reappear if the treatment is discontinued too abruptly. Formerly corticosteroid therapy was advocated only in severe berylliosis, when necessary to prolong life and relieve respiratory and cardiac distress. This view is no longer held and at the 1958 Symposium on Beryllium Disease in Boston, early treatment with doses as large as the patient can tolerate were advised, continuing until there was no further improvement, using pulmonary function tests to check the response. Thereafter the maintenance dose should be adjusted to control the pulmonary diffusion defect. The dose of prednisolone recommended for initial treatment is 30 to 60 mg. daily, and for maintenance 5 to 20 mg.

As in acute beryllium pneumonitis, most reports on the use of chelating agents in the chronic form of the disease are disappointing. Cash and his fellow workers, however, state that they obtained a definite increase in the renal excretion of beryllium using sodium calcium edetate, 500 mg. to 1 g. given intravenously in 1,000 ml. of 5 per cent. dextrose in water. Administration was over a three- or four-day period. They suggest that long-term intermittent therapy might favourably affect progress. It may be that this is so when the patient is currently or has been recently exposed to beryllium, but many patients suffering from chronic beryllium disease develop symptoms only many years after ex-posure has ceased.

Oxygen therapy, by nasal catheter or by intermittent positive pressure, may give considerable relief. Some-times its benefit may be partly psychological, as in those who seem to be able to go for short walks between periods of therapy. If signs of cardiac failure develop, appropriate measures should be taken, including the use of digoxin and diuretics. The need for parenteral administration of water and electrolytes is determined after plasma analysis. While the use of antibiotics does not influence the disease itself, the lungs damaged by beryllium disease are more prone to infection, especially in winter, and the use of tetracycline in prophylaxis and treatment usually requires consideration.

Cadmium. Chronic cadmium poisoning is an in-dustrial hazard of increasing importance. It is usually the sequel to the inhalation of cadmium fumes or dust for long periods, usually five years or more. The characteristic symptoms include dysp-noea on exertion, discolouration of the teeth (yellow ring), anaemia and 'cadmium sniffles'. The organs chiefly affected are the lungs which become the seat of emphysema, and the kidneys, where the tubules are damaged, resulting in the presence in the urine of a protein of a special type. Although there is evidence to show that dimercaprol increases the excretion of cadmium in animals under experimental conditions, this treatment also increases the toxic effect of the metal on renal tubules. Experimental work has indicated that the use of sodium calciumedetate should also be used with caution for the same reason; and as this preparation given in excessive doses may itself cause renal damage (p. 273), careful supervision of treatment is essential. Recently, however, three cases of chronic cadmium poisoning, with respira-tory symptoms and proteinuria, have been success-fully treated with sodium calciumedetate given orally, 500 mg. every two hours, with complete recovery in two to three weeks.

Acute poisoning is due to inhalation of cadmium dust or fume, usually the latter arising from opera-tions where cadmium has been subjected to high temperatures as in welding, burning, spraying, brazing or casting metal. It takes the form of severe pulmonary irritation developing within a few hours of exposure, and may end fatally from pul-monary oedema or infection. Treatment is on lines similar to that for gassing by nitric oxides (p. 566).

Poisonous Fumes, Gases and Organic Compounds

Carbon Monoxide. The immediate treatment of carbon monoxide poisoning is directed to (1) restoration of normal breathing, and (2) abate-ment of shock. If breathing has ceased, artificial respiration should be started immediately the patient has been carried into fresh air. The first few moments after the discovery of a gassed patient are vitally important and no time must be wasted. The techniques used are described in detail else-where (p. 548).

Cyanogen compounds, Hydrocyanic acid and cyanides should be used only with meticulous care. Poisoning in industry has occurred in their manu-facture and from their use particularly in the disin-festation of ships and premises. Accidents have occurred in heat treatment departments, chemical laboratories, electroplating shops and during photographic processing.

Many cases of cyanide poisoning will inevitably be fatal; death occurs at once from large doses, and even after exposure to small quantities much depends on the speed with which specific treatment is made available. Cyanide prevents cellular metabolism dependent on cytochrome oxidase. The complex which is formed with the oxidizing enzyme, however, is dissociable: thiocyanate is formed in the tissues and enzyme activity is restored. Immobilization of cytochrome oxidase can be prevented by 'offering' methaemoglobin to the cyanide ion. Cyanmethaemoglobin is thus formed. Sodium thiosulphate is then given to combine with cyanide released from the cyanmethaemoglobin and to fix it as thiocyanate. The formation of methaemoglobin in the patient's circulating blood is achieved by *slowly* injecting sodium nitrite intravenously, 500 mg. dissolved in 10 to 15 ml. of water over a 10-minute period. Some delay is almost inevitable while the injection is being prepared, and during this time amyl nitrite should be given by inhalation —the contents of one capsule every few minutes. Following the administration of sodium nitrite, slow intravenous injection of sodium thiosulphate should be started, 50 ml. of a 10 per cent. solution being given over a period of 10 to 15 minutes. Wherever there is a risk of cyanide poisoning these materials should be kept readily available. While pursuing this programme of treatment immediate attention must be given to oxygen therapy, for it is imperative that the body tissues should be rapidly and completely oxygenated: artificial respiration may be required. If necessary, a respiratory stimulant such as the Nikethamide Injection (B.P.), 5 to 10 ml. should be given slowly intravenously. If the systolic blood pressure falls below 100 mm. Hg., pressor agents should be given such as metaraminol acid tartrate, 0·5 to 5 mg. intravenously, followed by 2 to 10 mg. intramuscularly.

As an alternative to treatment with sodium nitrite and thiosulphate, methylene blue can be used, 5 to 50 ml. of 1 per cent. solution, by slow intravenous injection but it is much less effective. If the response is unsatisfactory, the treatment should be repeated, and if a relapse occurs after partial recovery, smaller doses may be used the second time. If the poison has been swallowed, the stomach should be washed out, using sodium thiosulphate (25 per cent.), or potassium permanganate (1 in 7,000 solution), or hydrogen peroxide (60 ml. of 3 per cent. H_2O_2 in 600 ml. water).

Recently hydroxocobalamin has been successfully used in the treatment of animals poisoned with two or three lethal doses of hydrogen cyanide, and it is suggested that a massive dose (1·5 to 2 g.) of this substance combined in aqueous solution with sodium thiosulphate, 400 mg. per kg. given intravenously, would be justifiable in the treatment of cyanide poisoning in human subjects. Rapidly successful treatment of a severe case in a 61-year-old man by cobalt ethylendeiamine tetra-acetate, 300 mg. in two equal doses of 10 ml. spaced by a 10-minute interval is reported by Bain and Knowles (1967).

If cardiac arrest occurs, external cardiac massage (p. 643) must be started at once. Naturally no other treatment can be of value until the circulation has been restored. When the heart begins to beat, nitrite/thiosulphate and oxygen therapies are started or resumed; and it is particularly important to take steps to ensure rapid and complete oxygenation of the tissues (p. 647).

Sulphuretted hydrogen. Hydrogen sulphide has an irritant action on the conjunctiva and mucous membranes in low concentrations, but in high concentrations its powerful action on the nervous system causes immediate respiratory paralysis, the affected person falling as if pole-axed. There is also an asphyxiant action by inhibition of cell respiration. The patient must be removed immediately from the contaminated area into the fresh air, and artificial respiration and oxygen therapy started at once. He must be kept warm. General symptomatic treatment and after-care are as for other poisonous gases. Careful watch must be kept for signs of lung irritation or oedema, or bronchopneumonia, and appropriate treatment instituted if they occur. Sulphacetamide drops or ointment to the eyes and bland applications to mucous membranes are indicated for local irritation.

Irritant gases. It is convenient to consider the irritant gases in two groups, those with an immediately irritant action and those whose action is delayed.

In industry the common irritants with an immediate action are sulphur dioxide, chlorine and ammonia. Coughing, sneezing, lachrymation and respiratory embarrassment occur at once, and the danger and discomfort are so obvious that exposed workers retreat hastily from the source of gas. Sudden overwhelming exposure may, however, cause collapse with asphyxia and death unless rescue is prompt. After removal from the contaminated atmosphere the affected person must be ordered to rest until he has fully recovered. He must be kept warm and should be encouraged to sip fluids such as fruit drinks or tea. Artificial respiration is sometimes required. Oxygen should be administered adequately in all moderate or severe cases. Cough is usually troublesome and, if not relieved by oxygen, a small dose of morphine (5 mg.) should be given intramuscularly. In this kind of poisoning patients may prove excessively sensitive to morphine (depression of respiration) and the physician should be ready to give nalorphine hydrobromide (10 mg.) intravenously as an antidote. If there is bronchospasm, aminophylline, 250 mg., may be injected slowly intravenously. When bronchial irritation is only slight, inhalations of steam (with or without friar's balsam) may prove helpful. Restlessness may be the result of dyspnoea and there may be mental confusion or excitement associated with cerebral anoxia. The symptoms are relieved by giving oxygen. A small dose of hyoscine hydrobromide (0·2 mg.) injected intravenously is valuable as a cerebral sedative: its central action facilitates the general management of the patient and in the respiratory tract a spasmolytic action and reduction of bronchial secretion are also helpful. If venous engorgement of the head and neck persist even when the air-way is clear and oxygen therapy adequate, venesection should be performed to relieve the right heart; 300 to 600 ml. of blood should be removed.

Ammonia causes particularly severe irritation in the upper respiratory passages and the eyes; and the skin may have been splashed with ammonia liquor. Lesions of the skin and mucous membrane should be irrigated or sprayed with water or weak acetic acid: vinegar (1 part of vinegar in 4 of warm water) is usually available. The eyes should be washed out with milk or water. If there is much ensuing pain, cocaine drops should be instilled and atropine drops used to ensure full dilatation of the pupils for the protection of the iris. For less severe irritation to the eyes, olive oil or castor oil drops may be used. Lesions of the skin and mucosae should be covered with saline soaks (cotton gauze) pending the patient's transfer to hospital. Severe irritation in the upper respiratory tract may result in oedema of the larynx and necessitate tracheotomy; and during the first week signs of bronchiolitis or other types of pulmonary infection are likely to appear. Darke and Warrack recommend that one of the tetracyclines should be given for the prevention and treatment of these conditions, 500 mg. six-hourly for five days and then twice daily for one week.

The *industrial gases* which are likely to cause delayed irritation are mainly nitric oxides (nitric oxide, nitrogen dioxide, and nitrogen peroxide; 'nitrous fumes'), and phosgene. Their action is very insidious, as there may be little or no irritation at the time of exposure. When the work has entailed pickling metals with nitric acid or dealing with a spillage of such acid, or handling phosgene, there may be little difficulty in attributing subsequent symptoms to the correct cause. Sometimes, however, neither the patient nor his employer may be aware of the exposure. Such a situation may arise if welders, burners or others are working in a confined space where one or more oxyacetylene or similar torches are being used. Dangerous concentrations of nitric oxides may be formed in as short a time as 15 minutes from the combination of atmospheric oxygen and nitrogen by the heat of the flame. The use of halogenated hydrocarbons as fire extinguishers is a well-known source of phosgene.

Treatment in general follows that described for combating the effects of immediate gaseous irritants. Persons known to be exposed should be kept under observation for 48 hours. The delayed onset explains why the illness seldom starts at work, but when it does the workman must be placed at absolute rest and in spite of his protestations he must be forbidden to walk. Oxygen without carbon dioxide should be administered, and he should be removed by stretcher and ambulance to hospital where continuous oxygen therapy (3 to 10 litres per minute, with only short breaks to observe progress) should be given. In hospital the management of the case should be shared by the anaesthetist and the physician. Atrophine sulphate, 1 mg. intravenously, should be given to diminish secretion in the respiratory tract. When this is copious, raising the foot of the bed on a chair may help but for most patients postural drainage is too strenuous to be permitted. Secretions may be aspirated from the bronchial tract by catheter attached to a mechanical sucker. Signs of overloading of the right heart call for venesection. Nikethamide, 5 ml. intravenously every one to two hours, is a powerful stimulant. Morphine is contraindicated. The prevention and treatment of infective complications, using a tetracycline, is the same as that given above. Prolonged rest is required in convalescence especially if there is persistent tachycardia or dyspnoea on effort.

Organic compounds. Many organic compounds used in industry, aromatic and aliphatic, are volatile and most of them are readily absorbed through the skin. Exposure to the concentrated vapour, for example in enclosed spaces due to overspilling of vessels or bursting of pipes, leads to intoxication which may be quickly followed by narcosis and death. Prompt removal from the contaminated atmosphere into the fresh air and artificial respiration are immediately essential if the patient is unconscious, and oxygen should be administered as soon as it is available.

Injections of nikethamide (5 ml. intravenously) as a respiratory stimulant may be indicated. The patient should be kept warm and completely at rest. Complications such as pulmonary oedema or infection are to be expected and are treated with a full dose of atropine and an antibiotic as described above.

Cases of chronic poisoning from long-continued exposure are rare, and specific therapeutic measures are usually neither available nor necessary. Treatment should be directed to whatever condition is produced, for example, aplastic anaemia from chronic benzene exposure, toxic jaundice from chlorinated naphthalenes, or nephrosis from carbon tetrachloride.

Chronic benzene poisoning. Benzene or benzol, C_6H_6, must not be confused with benzine which is 'gasoline' or 'petrol'. Chronic poisoning may result from exposure usually over a period of several years to materials containing benzene. The characteristic effect of long-continued benzene exposure is depression of all haemopoietic tissue resulting in aplastic anaemia and agranulocytosis. This may occur without any previous symptoms suggestive of over-exposure. So insidious is this action that an advanced degree of dyshaemopoiesis may be found to exist in a person who denies all symptoms of ill-health. It may follow some years after exposure to benzene has ceased and the breakdown may be precipitated rather suddenly by a special call on the blood-forming tissues such as occurs during pregnancy or with the onset of infection. In the slightest cases, discovered for example in symptomless workers by routine blood examination, improvement may follow withdrawal from exposure aided perhaps by general measures such as a holiday in the open air. In most cases, however, treatment is disappointing. Repeated blood transfusions over a period of three to six months offer the best chance of recovery by trying to keep the patient alive in the hope that the bone marrow will regenerate. General management and symptomatic measures are described on p. 159 and p. 628.

Aniline poisoning. This term refers not only to poisoning by aniline itself but to acute, subacute or chronic disease of any organ due to poisoning by a nitro- or amino-derivative of benzene, chlorbenzene or their homologues. In addition to aniline, which is amino-benzene, the substances which most frequently cause it in industry include nitrobenzene (oil of mirbane), dinitrobenzene, mono, di- and tri-nitrotoluene, nitrophenols, dimethyl aniline, para-nitraniline, paraphenylene diamine, phenyl hydrazine, and toluidines. These substances are volatile and absorption may be by inhalation, but the most important route of entry is by the skin. It follows, therefore, that the first essential in cases of splashing of skin or clothing with any of these compounds is immediate removal of all contaminated clothing and cleansing of the skin, preferably using cool or tepid water with a spirit soap if it is available. Absorption through the skin is rapid, and severe and even fatal poisoning may follow within an hour if cleansing is neglected.

Symptoms are due to the methaemoglobinaemia, and anoxia and cyanosis develop quickly with associated headache, dizziness, nausea, weakness and dyspnoea, the syndrome being often called 'anilism'. After removal of clothing and cleansing of the skin, oxygen should be administered until the cyanosis has cleared. The patient should be kept warm and at rest, and given hot sweet coffee; and, if a respiratory stimulant is required, an injection of nikethamide 5 ml. may be given slowly intravenously as often as may be necessary. Alcohol increases the toxic effect and is contraindicated. Intravenous injection of methylene blue, 1 to 1·5 mg. per kg. body weight as a 1 per cent. aqueous solution, may be given for its reducing effect on methaemoglobin —10 ml. is a usual dose for a man of average weight. In convalescence there may be an indication for treatment with iron if the blood picture reveals hypochromic anaemia.

Exposure to some of these compounds over a period of several months may result in chronic poisoning; the poisons are usually inhaled. Symptoms may appear as general malaise with anorexia, indigestion, lassitude and dyspnoea; and blood examination may show a mild hypochromic anaemia. Much more serious is toxic jaundice

T

which may be met with particularly in workers with trinitrotoluene. The patient should be treated in hospital where thorough cleansing of the skin should be carried out. There is no specific therapy. Fluids and glucose are given freely by mouth. Dextrose in 5 per cent. solution may be infused intravenously, giving up to 3 litres per day to ensure a urinary output of 1,500 to 2,000 ml. daily. A bland diet without much fat but with plenty fruit and vegetables should be given. If hepatic failure occurs the measures outlined on p. 249 should be used. After recovery, further work in contact with nitro-compounds should be prohibited.

Aplastic anaemia is occasionally seen as a result of poisoning by trinitrotoluene, more rarely by dinitrophenol, the onset sometimes being long after exposure has ceased. The treatment is described on p. 160.

Weed Killers, Insecticides and Fungicides

Over 150 different chemicals are currently available for the control of pests and diseases of growing crops, excluding those such as fumigants and rodenticides used for their protection during storage. Many are of low toxicity but the Agriculture (Poisonous Substances) Regulations (1966 to 1969) specify 40 individual substances or related groups for which protective measures are laid down. These include certain dinitro, organo-phosphorus, organo-chlorine, organo-mercury and organo-tin compounds, arsenites, endothal, fluorocetamide and nicotine. Additions will no doubt be made to this list from time to time.

Many substances which create poisoning hazards in industry are also occasional causes of severe illness in the home. This is particularly true of weed-killers and pesticides, and some of these are dealt with in the chapter on Acute Poisoning (p. 550). Containers such as metal or plastic drums disposed of as refuse may still contain enough poison to be lethal; and children may suffer from severe poisoning after drinking from or playing with such containers.

Dinitro compounds. Dinitro-orthocresol (DNOC, DNC); Dinitro-butyl phenol (Dinoseb, DNBP). Both compounds increase the oxidative metabolism and thus produce symptoms of fatigue, excessive sweating, thirst and loss of weight; and both can readily be absorbed through the skin as well as by inhalation and ingestion. The earliest evidence of absorption may be a sense of euphoria. This occurs when the concentration in the blood

is approximately 20 mcg. per gramme. As they are intense yellow dyes, contamination of the skin can readily be recognized.

There is no specific treatment. The illness may progress rapidly and death may occur in a few hours after the onset of symptoms. Absolute rest is essential, and admission to hospital should be arranged unless the journey from a remote country district would be dangerously fatiguing. Contaminated clothing should be removed and the skin cleansed with soap and water. If the poison has been swallowed, the stomach should be washed out. Cold sponging or an ice bath is used to reduce the temperature, and large quantities of isotonic saline are given by mouth if the patient can swallow, or parenterally to replace fluid and electrolytes lost by sweating. Oxygen may be required. A sedative such as sodium phenobarbitone, 90 mg. intravenously, repeated if necessary, should be given if the patient is restless or apprehensive. Once recovery starts, it is usually rapid.

If possible, blood for analysis should be removed at the beginning of treatment. Certain laboratories in the United Kingdom are equipped to carry out determinations of the dinitro content of the blood. Their names may be obtained from the Poisons Information Service (Telephone Nos. p. 544). Blood examinations are of great use to indicate excessive absorption in suspected or asymptomatic cases. Any worker with a concentration of 10 to 20 mcg. per ml. of whole blood (or 20 to 40 mcg. per ml. of serum) should be carefully supervised to ensure that all precautions are being taken. If it is over 20 mcg. per ml. of whole blood, he should be removed from the work because at this figure further absorption of even small amounts may lead to a very rapid increase in the blood level and the onset of illness.

Organo-phosphorus compounds. The most toxic members which are at present in use are dimefox, disulfoton, mevinphos, parathion, phorate, schradan, TEPP and thionazin. Somewhat less toxic are azinphos-ethyl, azinphos-methyl, chlorfenvimphos, demeton-methyl, demeton S-methyl, dichlorvos, oxydemeton-methyl, phosphamidon and vamidothion. These are sold under a large number of trade names, but the chemical name must appear on the label of the proprietary product. They act as cholinesterase inhibitors thus allowing the accumulation of large amounts of acetylcholine. Cholinesterase levels may be lowered considerably —to about 30 per cent. in the brain—without seriously affecting normal function, but further reduction rapidly produces grave symptoms. Anorexia, nausea and confusion are followed by vomiting, cramp-like pains, salivation and twitchings, and these progress to convulsions, diarrhoea, pulmonary oedema, respiratory depression, coma and death.

The antidote is atropine sulphate and it is imperative that it be given without delay in large and repeated doses until the patient is fully atropinized and this condition maintained until recovery ensues. The first dose should be 2 mg. given intravenously. Further injections, usually of 1 mg. given subcutaneously or intramuscularly, may be required hourly, half-hourly or—especially in the early stages—more frequently. When, however, the patient is cyanosed there is a danger that atropine may produce ventricular fibrillation and an attempt must, therefore, be made to relieve the cyanosis by artificial respiration and oxygen. As the skin is the most important route of absorption, all clothing that might be contaminated should be removed and the skin thoroughly cleansed with soap and water. Oximes with a special cholinesterase reactivating action are now available and if procurable in time should be given. There are two products of equal effectiveness, P2S (pyridine-2-aldoxime methanesulphonate) and P2AM (PAM)—the methiodide. P2S has the advantage of being the more soluble in water. It is dispensed in ampoules and the drug is available at all hours from certain hospitals listed by the Scottish Home and Health Department and the Ministry of Health, the names of which can be obtained from the Regional Hospital Boards. The recommended initial dose is 1 g. dissolved in 6 ml. of water intramuscularly or by slow intravenous injection. Further doses may be necessary at intervals of three to four hours. Atropine should also be given in order to block the muscarine-like action of the poison and should be continued until the pupils begin to dilate and the mouth becomes dry. Large doses of atropine are well tolerated by patients suffering from poisoning by organophosphorus compounds. A mild degree of atropinization should be maintained for 24 hours after recovery.

Pulmonary oedema may occur in severe cases and should be treated by propping the patient up, giving oxygen preferably under slight pressure and frusemide 80 mg. intravenously. Aspiration of bronchial secretion may be required, and it may be necessary to pass an endotracheal tube or to perform tracheotomy. In respiratory depression some method of artificial respiration, preferably mechanical, will usually be necessary.

If possible, a sample of blood should be removed early in the illness for the determination of cholinesterase activity. Such examinations, of great value in prophylaxis and in the diagnosis of suspicious cases, are also helpful in management during recovery.

Organo-chlorine compounds. Endrin appears to be the most toxic, although aldrin, dieldrin and endosulfan have similar effects. However, following the reports of the Advisory Committee on Pesticides and other Toxic Chemicals, their use has been severely restricted. Industrial absorption is commonly through the skin, but accidental ingestion has not been infrequent. Giddiness, headache, nausea and twitchings which become epileptiform convulsions are the usual disturbances. Treatment consists in removal of contaminated clothing, thorough cleansing of the skin, and the administration of barbiturates to control the fits; intravenous injection of quick-acting preparation such as sodium thiopentone may be needed at the outset. If ingestion has taken place, gastric lavage and saline laxatives should be used (a tablespoonful of magnesium sulphate in warm water.) There are no specific chemical tests to confirm the diagnosis, nor are antidotes available.

Fluoracetic acid and derivatives. Nausea, and mental apprehension followed by twitchings and epileptiform convulsions, associated with lowered blood pressure and cardiac arrhythmias, are the usual symptoms. Depending on the route of absorption, cleansing of the skin and removal of contaminated clothing, or gastric lavage followed by magnesium sulphate administration, should be carried out. Barbiturates have been disappointing in treatment and must be used cautiously on account of the danger of depressing the respiratory centre.

Ionizing Radiations

Industry, lagging some 50 years behind medicine in the use of X-rays, has benefited by the melancholy example of the effects of overdosage to pioneers in this field. Severe effects from industrial exposure are extremely rare in this country. The hazard, however, is now widespread. Although radium is employed only on a small scale, X-rays have found increasing application in industry, and the development of atomic stations for power and research has made available a very large number of radioactive isotopes for which new uses are continually being found.

The type of radiation encountered (alpha, beta, gamma, X-rays, neutrons, etc.), the dose, the period of exposure, the site of the body receiving irradiation and many other factors influence the effects produced. These include conjunctivitis and cataract, erythema, dermatitis, necrosis, scarring, telangiectases and malignant ulceration of the skin. Radiation sickness and severe constitutional symptoms may also occur; and specialized tissues may be affected with resulting blood dyscrasias, tumour formation (especially in bone), fibrosis in viscera, sterility and genetic effects. The treatment of many of these conditions is governed by general principles. For example carcinoma caused by X-rays, should be treated by surgical removal and skin grafting, while aplastic anaemia should be treated by repeated blood transfusions and by the measures described on p. 160.

When it is known or suspected that there has been overexposure to radioactivity, the person should be kept at rest and admitted to hospital for observation. Certain hospitals throughout the country have been nominated as being suitably equipped to deal with radiation casualties, including the carrying out of any necessary decontamination. Their names may be obtained from the Regional Hospital Boards. The immediate lethal whole body dose of medium kV X-rays and gamma rays for man is about 500 r, and 150 r will cause acute radiation sickness in half of those exposed. It is seldom that the exact dosage received is known at the time of the exposure. Careful notes must, therefore, be made of the times of onset of any symptoms which appear as these will give some indication of the severity of the injury. A cytogenetic method of estimating radiation by the examination of chromosome aberrations has been developed. Five to 10 ml. of blood should be placed in a heparinized tube and sent without delay to Dr. G. W. Dolphin, UKAEA, Radiological Protection Division, Harwell, Berks. If it is unlikely that a lethal or near lethal dose has been sustained, a conservative regimen should be followed. The patient must be kept warm to counteract shock, and sedatives given for restless-less or apprehension. Patients who are allowed to choose their own diet prefer fluids or semi-solid easily digested food in the early days, and a low residue intake is probably to be preferred because of the possibility of radiation damage to the intestinal mucosa. The urine excretion should be kept greater than one litre daily and if fluids are not tolerated orally, they must be given per rectum or intravenously. Special precautions must be taken to guard against infection. Attendants should be masked and gowned and free from respiratory or other infections. It is better to refrain from giving antibiotics or blood or platelet transfusions unless these are clinically indicated. Strict asepsis must be observed and injections given as infrequently as possible.

Numerous preparations have been used with varied success for controlling sickness. The most effective appear to be pyridoxine hydrochloride, 10 mg. four times daily by mouth, and anti-emetics such as cyclizine, 50 mg. two or three times daily.

Careful haematological observation must be maintained, particularly on the platelet count which is considered to be a good prognostic indicator: a fall below 100,000 per cu. mm. should be viewed with concern. Toluidine blue or protamine have been used to control the haemorrhagic tendency—both in daily doses of 2 to 3 mg. per kg. body weight intravenously, but never exceeding 5 mg. per kg. body weight. In severe cases marrow transfusions may be indicated if donor material is available. If the patient recovers he should be kept under surveillance for the remainder of his life.

When radioactive material has been spilt or scattered by breakage of containers, emergency measures include evacuation and sealing of the room. No attempts should be made to clean up until the arrival of trained and competent persons. The occupants of the room should not be allowed to leave the premises until they have been monitored. Contaminated clothing should be removed and placed in disposable containers, and all persons affected should wash with soap and detergents in baths with several changes of water or under showers. Particular attention must be paid to the nails. Abbatt and his colleagues recommend the use of EDTA/soap mixture. The di-sodium compound is the most efficient of the ethylene diamine tetra acetic acid compounds, forming a complex with the active isotope so as to make it no longer ionizable and so preventing its reattachment to the skin. Immersion of contaminated parts in potassium permanganate solution is also recommended, staining being later removed by 5 per cent. bisulphite. Cleaning should not be so vigorous that the parts are chafed or roughened. This treatment should be repeated on the following day, its efficiency being checked by monitoring.

If there is any possibility that radioactive material has been inhaled or ingested, arrangements should be made for the carrying out of tests to ascertain the body burden. These tests, carried out singly or in combination, include: estimation of radon in expired air, estimation of body gamma activity measured externally, tissue biopsy (particularly of bone, as many products of uranium fission are bone-seekers), and radiochemical analysis of excreta. A complete blood examination should also be made. Elimination by chelation should be attempted, but so far little has been published to indicate the effectiveness of such agents vis-à-vis the various radioactive isotopes.

Pneumoconiosis

When inhaled, some dusts lie in the lung tissues for long periods without provoking permanent histological changes such as fibrosis; symptoms are absent and there is no disability. The best known of these 'benign pneumoconioses' are siderosis, stannosis and baritosis caused by iron, tin and barium respectively; the dust particles are usually either the metal or metallic oxides in the case of iron and tin, and the sulphate (barytes) in the case of barium. In these conditions the abnormality is restricted to the radiograph which discloses bilateral discrete opacities in the lungs. The appearance may be identical with that of simple pneumoconiosis of a fibrotic type, and great psychological trauma may result if a patient suffering from one of these benign conditions is mistakenly told that he has silicosis. No treatment is required for these conditions beyond explanation and reassurance. Working conditions in which the patient has been exposed to excessive dust or fumes should be reviewed. Cases are known in which the radiological findings have returned to normal when exposure to the causal dust has ceased, the discrete radiological opacities having slowly disappeared.

On the other hand, because the fibrosis in silicosis and the other fibrotic pneumoconioses is permanent and does not respond to any known drug therapy, treatment of these conditions has been largely neglected. This is unfortunate. Nothing is calculated to depress the patient more than hearing his doctor say, 'I am sorry there is nothing I can do for you'. There are in fact many things to be done to help these patients. They are: (1) treatment of the pneumoconiosis itself; (2) treatment of complications such as chronic bronchitis and emphysema; (3) treatment and prevention of tuberculosis; (4) general management and advice, including provision of occupation.

1. As has been stated, there is no effective therapy for established fibrotic lesions, but it is claimed that in cases of *acute* silicosis accompanied by bronchiolitis and dyspnoea corticosteroid therapy (p. 216) sometimes gives relief. In such cases the lesions are very cellular, and collagenous fibrosis is not extensive because the illness is of short duration. Treatment with preparations of metallic aluminium and aluminium hydroxide have not proved to be of benefit despite initial encouraging results. The Report of the Third International Conference of Experts on Pneumoconiosis held in Sydney in 1950 stated that 'the Conference had no evidence that aluminium powder is of value as a therapeutic agent in human silicosis'.

In all cases, however, attention should be devoted to maintaining and if possible improving the patient's general health; when weather permits he should take daily exercise within his tolerance. Carefully controlled breathing exercises may help to improve the vital capacity and prevent wasting of the muscles of respiration. A thorough general examination of the patient should be made because it may disclose the presence of conditions which, untreated, interfere with his comfort or restrict his exercise. Abnormalities of the nose and throat may embarrass respiration, causing discomfort during the day and restlessness at night. The presence of a hernia interferes with coughing; varicose veins and abnormalities of the feet may be the reason for the patient's failure to take exercise. Obesity may seriously aggravate the disability, and reduction of weight will then produce conspicuous improvement, subjectively and objectively.

2. Concomitant respiratory diseases such as chronic bronchitis (p. 194), bronchiectasis (p. 209), emphysema (p. 197), tuberculosis (p. 75) and bronchospasm (p. 215) should be treated just as vigorously as in the non-silicotic patient.

Once cor pulmonale (p. 93) has developed, the prognosis is very poor. The skilful and early use of specific therapy to terminate infection in the respiratory tract is of the utmost importance; and the prophylactic use of the appropriate antibiotics during fog or inclement weather may also be helpful in delaying the onset of cardiac complications. When there are asthmatic symptoms the use of spasmolytics may also be beneficial (p. 215).

3. The prevention of tuberculosis must be regarded from two points of view—safeguarding the pneumoconiotic patient from tuberculosis, and safeguarding others from the tuberculous pneumo-

coniotic patient. These objectives can be achieved only by studying the circumstances of the individual patient in his home, at work and elsewhere. Every effort should be made to treat adequately any tuberculous patient with whom he is in contact (p. 67).

If a patient suffering from pneumoconiosis develops tuberculosis he may have to give up work because he becomes a source of danger to fellow-workers who are continuing to work in a dust-laden atmosphere. Pneumoconiosis Medical Boards have power to reject applicants for work in certain processes in factories, sandstone, potteries, and asbestos industries if they are found to be suffering from tuberculosis; similarly at their statutory periodical examinations in these industries they have power to suspend workers who have developed tuberculosis. When they examine applicants for certificates of disablement on account of pneumoconiosis, they have power to suspend—on account of active pulmonary tuberculosis—a worker in any of the industries scheduled for disablement benefit purposes; and this includes mining.

4. Too often the workman whose illness is diagnosed as pneumoconiosis is advised to give up his job. On occasion this is the worst advice that could be given. The elderly workman, especially when skilled, has little prospect of securing alternative employment, and such advice virtually means that he is being urged to cast himself on the human scrap-heap. Mental and physical deterioration rapidly follow cessation of work if there is no hope of re-employment; and in their own words these men 'have nothing to do but wait for the undertaker'. It follows that *one of the most important aims of treatment must be to keep the patient employed up to his capacity.* If an elderly workman after spending most of his working life in a dusty job develops pneumoconiosis, it is unlikely that remaining in this work for a few more years will significantly aggravate the disease. The position is different in the case of a younger man who has developed the disease after a comparatively short exposure. Such a man is either unduly susceptible to dust disease or his occupation has been especially hazardous. He must be advised to seek dust-free, or at least less dusty, employment. Schemes exist at Ministry of Labour Training Centres for training such men in new trades, engineering, painting, bricklaying, plastering, woodwork, etc. Disability in cases of simple pneumoconiosis is often slight and the writers have seen many pneumoconiotic ex-

miners working happily and competently for years at new jobs, often involving fairly arduous work. Many of these men had almost forgotten that they were 'chest cases'. In fact even pneumoconiosis of moderate or great severity may be compatible with work entailing considerable physical exertion. The doctor need not be too insistent on advising a light job. As in the management of many patients with heart disease the assessment of *function* is of far greater practical importance than a detailed knowledge of the pathological consequences of the lesion.

When a patient's disability is first diagnosed as pneumoconiosis he is faced with many problems and he must try to find the answers to them. It is the doctor's duty to explain the position to him and offer him guidance. Meiklejohn has prepared a most useful leaflet for this purpose which is reproduced in Merewether's *Industrial Medicine and Hygiene*, 1956, **3**, 71–72. The general features of the disease are briefly described. There is also a discussion on the important question of what the affected worker should do about his job. The decision is one which the workman must make for himself, as he alone knows all his circumstances. With advice from various sources (for instance his own doctor, and the local Disablement Resettlement Officer of the Department of Employment), he can decide whether he should continue at his present work, seek alternative employment—which almost certainly means receiving a smaller wage—or choose to undergo a period of training or rehabilitation.

Pneumoconiosis Medical Boards have limited powers of suspension of workmen who have pneumoconiosis without tuberculosis. In most industries they cannot suspend workmen who have reached 45 years of age and who have had 20 or more years' exposure to a fibrinogenic dust, unless the workman requests a certificate of suspension. In the coal mining industry they have no power to suspend no matter what the age or experience of the workman or the degree of his disease. In all industries, however, they may send the workman a letter advising him whether he can reasonably continue to work in the industry. In the coal mining industry the letter may advise the workman to work in 'approved dust conditions'. These are conditions in which the concentration of dust particles does not rise above certain prescribed maximum levels. The workman is asked to give the Board permission to inform his employer of its findings and recommendations in order that he may be placed in suitable working conditions.

A claim for disablement benefit in respect of pneumoconiosis or byssinosis is initiated by application (usually supported by a medical certificate) at any office of the Department of Health and Social Security, where a series of leaflets can be obtained explaining the various benefits and allowances available.

References

ABBATT, J. D., LAKEY, J. R. A. & MATHIAS, D. J. (1961). *Protection against Radiation. A Practical Handbook.* London: Cassell.

BAIN, J. T. B. & KNOWLES, E. L. (1967). *Br. med. J.* **2**, 763.

BIDSTRUP, P. J. (1964). *Toxicity of Mercury and its Compounds.* London: Elsevier.

BROWNING, E. (1961). *Toxicity of Industrial Metals.* London: Butterworth.

BUCHANAN, W. D. (1962). *Toxicity of Arsenic Compounds.* London: Elsevier.

CASH, R., SHAPIRO, R. I., LEVY, S. H. & HOPKINS, S. M. (1959). *New Engl. J. Med.* **260**, 683.

DAVIES, T. A. LLOYD (1957). *The Practice of Industrial Medicine,* 2nd ed. London: Churchill.

GOLDBERG, A., SMITH, J. A. & LOCHHEAD, A. C. (1963). *Br. med. J.* **1**, 1270.

HUNTER, D. (1957). *The Diseases of Occupations,* 2nd ed. London: English Universities Press.

LOCKET, S., GRIEVE, W. S. M. & PHILLIPS, L. (1952). *Trans. Ass. ind. med. Offs.* **2**, 14.

MEREWETHER, E. R. A. (1956). *Industrial Medicine and Hygiene.* London: Butterworth.

WOODCOCK, S. M. (1958). *Br. J. ind. Med.* **15**, 207.

26. Common Diseases of the Skin

ALAN LYELL

'Thou art all fair my love; there is no spot in thee.'

The Song of Solomon

INTRODUCTION

Skin diseases tend to dismay or to bore the doctor, but neither response is appropriate if one is to help such patients. These are numerous, often obsessed by the visible burden of their illness, occasionally shunned by their fellows, and tend to be resentful at the apparent impotence or indifference of the profession. This tense situation, inflated and distorted by ignorance on both sides, will often yield to commonsense measures allied to the minimum of specialized knowledge of a kind that is well within the competence of the general practitioner.

The skin, being the rind of man, is subject to influences arising from within him and from outside. Endogenous precipitating factors may be physical and emotional. The environmental inquiry should include the patient's home, his work and his hobbies. Skin disease provides an excellent example of the way in which many factors combine to upset the balance that we call 'normal health', and perhaps the greatest bar to understanding dermatology is to assume that each named disease has one single cause. It is more profitable to regard skin diseases as reactions to a variety of stimuli, acting singly or in combination. Looked at in this way, the diagnosis of the eruption, a matter of visual recognition, is the key that gives direction to the search for precipitating factors. In *erythema nodosum*, for example, tuberculosis, streptococcal infection, rheumatic fever, sarcoidosis or certain drugs may be responsible, although any discovered abnormality might be aetiologically significant and should be considered. In other parts of the world the list could well be different. In *eczema* the eruption may result from several factors acting in concert, such as infection, emotion, trauma and sensitization. The full explanation of the disease is seldom clear, but it is important to make the best use of such knowledge that we do possess. The possibility of contact irritation is often overlooked but is preventable. Contact irritants may fail to arouse suspicion because they include such 'harmless' things as clothing, shoes, cosmetics, soaps and medicaments, and because they may have been used or worn for some time without any obvious harm resulting. Industrial contact irritants are often blamed by the patient because of their financial implications, and one has to guard against undue scepticism if this possibility is to receive open-minded consideration.

Any correctable abnormality should be treated, for example anaemia, urinary infection or depression, even though it may appear to be unconnected with the dermatosis. Rashes are a common toxic effect of most drugs and the medicaments that the patient is receiving should be reviewed, remembering that these can be given by many routes. It is very seldom easy to discover all the drugs that a patient is taking, and one has to consider sometimes whether a drug is being taken unknowingly in food or drink, e.g. penicillin in milk or quinine in tonic water.

TOPICAL THERAPY: GENERAL PRINCIPLES

Having looked at the patient broadly, one can then afford to let one's attention contract to consider the skin itself and to decide how disease can be modified by local treatment. Traditional dermatological therapy, if burdened by the obscurity of empiricism, has the practical virtue of comforting the patient and healing his skin, if skilfully administered. Specific measures are available for infections and infestations, but most local treatment is non-specific and is designed to soothe or to stimulate the skin. Above all else it should do no harm, but this is not always easy to realize and some people prove allergic to apparently harmless preparations. The blandest ointment will upset the grease-sensitive skin. Certain drugs, such as antihistamines, the benzocaine group of local anaesthetics, sulphonamides, acriflavine, penicillin, neomycin, chloramphenicol and streptomycin, should be avoided externally because of their ability to sensitize. With neomycin the symptoms can resemble an insidious recrudescence of the original eruption rather than the florid reaction usually taken to be typical of contact dermatitis. Combination of the sensitizer with a corticosteroid does not prevent the reaction occurring, but may delay recognition of the part played by the sensitizer.

In general the fewer and simpler the constituents of an external application the better. Turner's famous cerate contained only four ingredients— butter, wax, olive oil and calamine, and it represents a type of protective application that has been the basis of sensible dermatological treatment. The use of compound applications introduces an appreciably increased risk of sensitization.

To stimulate the skin it is necessary to find a concentration of medicament that will prove effective without irritating. With dithranol it is usual to begin with 0·1 per cent., and increase this as necessary, whereas tar and sulphur may begin at 1 per cent. It is also wise to start to use any new preparation on a small area of skin, in order to limit the extent of any adverse reaction. The fair skinned and freckled, who burn rather than pigment in the sun, often prove to have rather sensitive skins. While it is necessary to reach an appropriate concentration of the medicament to produce a result, the time at which this is attempted must be carefully chosen. It is unwise to stimulate a skin that is already much inflamed or erupting, as this may result in a further extension of the eruption, or cause an erythrodermia, and stimulation is reserved for chronic, recalcitrant dermatoses.

The form of the application chosen depends on the nature of the reaction. Weeping eruptions require wet applications, whereas dry eruptions are treated by ointments. Pastes protect the skin well but cannot be used on hairy areas, unless the hair is shaved. The simplest dermatological pharmacopoeia might consist of calamine liniment (or plain corticosteroid lotion) for wet eruptions, plain corticosteroid ointment (or zinc ointment) for dry ones. Calamine lotion is drying and is best reserved for treating irritation in the absence of marked alterations in the skin. For the grease sensitive, lead and zinc lotion and Lassar's paste are appropriate for wet and dry stages respectively. Non-greasy creams have a cosmetic but not a therapeutic advantage over ointments. The effect of corticosteroid applications can be enhanced by occluding the treated area with polythene film, or it can be localized by injecting the corticosteroid into the lesion.

The amount of application required depends upon the area to be covered. Corticosteroids and antibiotics are effective when used sparingly, and it is desirable that they should be so used in the interests of economy, and of limiting their absorption. Nevertheless there is a practical limit to frugality if a satisfactory result is to be obtained, and the patient will need about 15 g. of ointment for one application to the whole body surface. There is no doubt that some 'failures of treatment' occur because too little drug is used.

The patient can apply medicaments himself up to a point, but when large areas are involved or many dressings are needed, particularly if his hands are affected, he requires some help. Few district nurses have the time or inclination to deal with this problem, but most skin departments provide facilities for out-patient dressings, which can be a means of avoiding admission to hospital in such cases. On the other hand it is often better to regard admission as a rapid means of returning the patient to his normal life, rather than as a last resort in a difficult case.

Frequent changes of treatment are undesirable, since they increase the risk of sensitization. The desire to change often results from a failure to appreciate the likely course of the dermatosis. Genuine failure to respond should be met by a review of the patient as a whole rather than by an unwise attempt to apply a new preparation. Contact and infective factors that have been overlooked will prevent a response, even to corticosteroids. A familiar example is the failure of the infective eczema accompanying scabies to respond to local treatment until the infestation has been dealt with.

The emotions are important in skin disease and require special consideration. They are concerned as one of the primary provocative factors, though they are seldom if ever solely responsible, but they are also involved secondarily in the alarm and despondency that can result from developing a skin disease. It is difficult for the immaculate to understand this form of anguish, but it is a real affliction, and its existence requires to be acknowledged by the doctor as a first step towards reassuring the patient. The patient should be told if the malady is not infectious, as he may feel morally unclean. Sometimes the patient will require psychiatric help in this predicament, but treatment of emotional factors by psychotherapy is often disappointing. The patient's insistence that he is disfigured or incapacitated by a dermatosis that the doctor can barely see is a different problem, suggesting a psychosis or malingering.

T*

Systemic Therapy

Systemic treatment is indicated for any reason suggested by the general medical examination. Occasionally, however, specific effects of systemic treatment will be successful, such as corticosteroids in acute drug reactions and pemphigus, antibiotics in erysipelas, antihistamines in urticaria, dapsone or sulphapyridine in dermatitis herpetiformis and methotrexate in selected cases of psoriasis.

Prognosis

There is an adage that skin diseases never get better. In fact they improve as often as do general medical diseases. Dermatology has its recalcitrant cases of eczema and psoriasis, while medicine has peptic ulceration, rheumatoid arthritis and ulcerative colitis, not to mention chronic bronchitis and emphysema. A successful eventual outcome will depend upon either spontaneous remission or the correction of precipitating factors, but the immediate result can owe much to skilful symptomatic treatment.

The importance of the diagnosis lies not in the name itself, although to the patient this may have a magic significance, but in the clue that it gives to understanding the nature of the disease. Useful as local treatment of the skin may be it is, with the exception of some conditions for which specific therapy exists, of less fundamental importance than the elimination of precipitating factors. Of these, contact irritants are particularly important because they are common, easily overlooked and their removal is effective. Local treatment plays an important part in symptomatic relief and it is suggested that the medicaments prescribed should be as bland as possible, unless stimulation of the skin is specifically required, and that the common sensitizers should be avoided for external use. It is unwise to allow concern for the skin to divert attention from care of the whole man.

Acne Rosacea

This embarrassing disease affecting the face consists of an abnormally active flushing reflex which is stimulated by trifling thermal or emotional stimuli, or by reflex action from the stomach in response to hot, spicy food or drink. Sulphur preparations used locally are effective. Oral tetracycline is very helpful given in courses, combined with local treatment with hydrocortisone and vioform, but fluorinade steroid applications are contraindicated.

Acne Vulgaris

The fundamental stimulus provoking the onset of acne vulgaris is probably androgenic. Acne may develop during treatment with corticosteroids and it is also an accompaniment of acromegaly. Oestrogen given by mouth or by subcutaneous implantation undoubtedly controls acne. Nevertheless, except in severe cystic cases, this is not recommended because the large doses that are necessary may have undesirable effects, such as interference with testicular activity, permanent gynaecomastia and disturbance of the menstrual rhythm. Most cases occur after puberty, at an age when people are sensitive about their appearance, and when they are usually impatient of delay in obtaining a cure. It must be stressed that the benefits of treatment appear only slowly, and that persistence with treatment is the best means of avoiding eventual scarring, which, especially in untreated or partially treated cases may be severe enough to require plastic surgery.

The routine treatment is to peel the skin. Sulphur, resorcin and salicylic acid (4 per cent. of each) and zinc oxide (24 per cent.) in a soft yellow paraffin base is applied to the affected areas at night and washed off in the morning. In order to achieve an effect it is sometimes necessary to increase the strength of the sulphur to 8 or even 12 per cent. and, in very tough skins, to use a strong peeling paste such as resorcin and camphor (10 per cent. of each), precipitated sulphur 30 per cent., anhydrous lanoline 15 per cent. and soft yellow paraffin 35 per cent. Some skins which will not tolerate these strong substances (particularly the sulphur) have to be treated with ultraviolet light, applied in a dose to produce a good peel, once weekly. An alternative is an abrasive but chemically inert paste called Brasivol which is prepared to contain particles which are fine, medium or coarse: the pastes are used in that order for a month at a time.

Oral treatment with antibiotics is applicable to severe cases which cannot be satisfactorily controlled with local treatment; oxytetracycline can be given by mouth, 1 g. daily for two to three weeks followed by 500 mg. daily for a further two or three weeks. Local antiseptics are also useful, and the skin can be washed with surgical spirit or hexachlorophene.

Diet has little to offer as a rule, but occasionally the avoidance of chocolate, or of foods containing lard or of some other foodstuff, is dramatically successful.

In severe cases cysts develop; they are very liable to secondary infection for which antibiotics may be required orally. Cysts may be punctured with the electrocautery and the cavity painted with pure phenol.

Alopecia

The *premature loss of hair*, which affects the crown of the head and the temporo-frontal regions in men and in women only the crown, is not amenable to treatment.

Alopecia areata is due to inactivity of the hair follicles, usually temporary, which may have an auto-immune basis. There is no means of knowing how long the disturbance will last in any individual patient. Bad prognostic signs are onset before puberty, a family history of total alopecia, and dystrophy of the nails. The immediate prognosis can be determined by pulling the hair at the edge of the patches; if it comes away easily and painlessly the process is spreading. No treatment has any regularly predictable effect, except the systemic use of corticosteroids (p. 589) which is rarely justified. Injections into the lesions are useful when the disease is localized. The application of betamethasone valerate or fluocinolone acetonide ointment combined with polythene occlusion can be helpful occasionally. It is probable that improvement, occurring during any kind of treatment is merely incidental; the natural history of the disease is usually towards resolution. When indicated by the emotional state of the patient a sedative such as phenobarbitone 30 mg. twice daily should be given.

The hair may fall out—a *defluvium* of hair—following some toxic illnesses (especially pneumonia and influenza), in thyrotoxicosis, during the use of certain drugs such as heparin and cyclophosphamide and after parturition. This does not require treatment; the hair can be expected to grow again completely. In myxoedema and anaemia the growth of hair may be diminished but this does not justify the administration of thyroxin or iron to everybody who complains of loss of hair.

The preceding forms of alopecia must be distinguished from the rarer ones in which there is *scarring* of the scalp. Here there is destruction of the hair follicles and there is no hope of any regrowth. Reference to a dermatologist is desirable, however, as it may be possible to arrest the disease. It is also important to remember that alopecia areata can be closely imitated by *secondary syphilis*, and that alopecia with scaling and pustulation may be due to *ringworm*.

Trauma can cause alopecia, whether from pulling at the hair as a nervous habit, from the prolonged tension on the hair induced by certain hairstyles or from sustained pressure on the scalp in the unconscious patient. In any form of loss of hair it is advisable to avoid unnecessary brushing and combing and to prohibit massage, since these measures in themselves can cause considerable loss if carried to excess. Hairbrushes with natural bristles are less traumatic than those with nylon bristles particularly the square-ended variety, the sharp angles of which tear the hair in brushing. If dandruff is present, the scalp should be shampooed once or twice weekly using cetrimide solution or soap spirit B.P.C. to which has been added 2 per cent. of oil of cade. For local application betamethasone valerate lotion can be applied by rubbing in gently (making partings with a comb for the purpose if the hair is thick).

Ano-Genital Pruritus

This condition results when any potentially pruritic eruption affects the ano-genital region. It is aggravated and prolonged by the process of lichenification (p. 584). Pruritus has a pleasurable component, especially when it has this distribution. In sexual frigidity ano-genital pruritus may serve to rationalize the psychological disability. In some patients these attitudes towards pruritus greatly increase the difficulty in finding effective treatment.

Diabetes, threadworms and tinea must first be excluded. Local abnormalities causing vaginal discharge and secondary dermatitis are fairly easily diagnosed from the history and a careful physical examination.

For the symptomatic relief of the irritation the corticosteroid ointments have proved invaluable, but a missed tinea infection can become much worse. They should be combined with anti-infective agents to deal with the mixed flora of micro-organisms found in this region, including nystatin to deal with yeasts. Yeast infections of the bowel resulting from oral antibiotic therapy can precipitate anal pruritus. The bowel flora usually reverts to normal spontaneously when antibiotic therapy is stopped, and the pruritus subsides so that oral nystatin is seldom required.

Chilblains (p. 140)

Chilblains are due to an abnormal reaction of the skin vessels to cold. The constitutional factors that produce this state are not understood. Those who are subject to chilblains must take an intelligent interest in the technique of preventing chilling of the affected areas of skin.

Large doses of ultraviolet light, by temporarily damaging the skin vessels, make them unable to shrink with cold for some months after treatment. Three to four times the erythema dose is given to the area of skin expected to be involved just before the time of the usual onset of chilblains, and this treatment is repeated twice at weekly intervals. For established chilblains 5 per cent. compound tincture of benzoin in hydrous wool fat ointment is a soothing application. Some cases are so severe as to warrant sympathectomy.

Dermatitis Herpetiformis

The lesions cause a great deal of irritation and this is a source of misery to the patient. The sulphone, dapsone, is specific; it is given in a dose of 50 to 150 mg. daily. This drug, however, is not free from toxic effects: it may cause anaemia with Heinz body formation in the red cells, and should be given in the minimal effective dose as its use has to be continued for many years while the disease remains active. The majority of patients suffer from intestinal malabsorption which may require a gluten-free diet.

Drug Eruptions

The treatment of drug eruptions is simply to stop the offending drug, and to treat the eruption symptomatically until it disappears. If the patient is very ill, intravenous or oral corticosteroid treatment may be required (p. 589). The difficulty is in knowing which eruptions are due to drugs. Vivid widespread erythemas will be recognized easily, but there are many occasions when the eruption mimics or produces a commonplace dermatosis such as the urticaria caused by acetylsalicylic acid, erythema multiforme due to barbiturates, erythema nodosum due to sulphonamides and acneiform eruptions due to bromides or iodides. There are also patterns of eruption which are familiar to the dermatologist but not generally known, such as the bizarre purpura which shows a dependent distribution that is characteristic of carbromal sensitivity. Again there is the curious phenomenon of the fixed drug erup-

tion. An erythematous or somewhat livid patch recurs intermittently in the same piece of skin over a period of many months. It is usually caused by taking phenolphthalein but sometimes other drugs such as quinine, barbiturates, analgesics and antibiotics are responsible. There are other occasions when an eruption is accompanied by a severe toxic illness perhaps with fever, lymphadenopathy or changes in the peripheral blood reminiscent of glandular fever.

Eczema

Eczema is an inflammation of the epidermis brought about by a variety of factors, not all of which are understood, having acute, subacute and chronic stages. The acute stage is characterized by epidermal vesicles. Except on the palms and soles, these break readily, giving rise to exudation of serum. The vesicular appearance is responsible for the name, derived from a Greek word meaning 'to boil'. A subacute stage, depending upon exfoliation of the horny layer of the epidermis and vasodilatation, presents a reddened moist appearance. The chronic stage, in which the skin is regenerating an abnormal (parakeratotic) horny layer is characterized by scaling and cracking, as well as by a thickening of the skin referable to cellular infiltration in the dermis. The healing process may be developed indefinitely either by recrudescences of acute eczema or by the process of lichenification, a leathery thickening resulting from compulsive rubbing of the itchy skin. For medical purposes eczema and dermatitis are synonymous, but one should remember that the lay mind looks upon dermatitis as having an occupational cause. For practical purposes eczema is synonymous with dermatitis though the latter is used in a general way to describe dermal as well as epidermal inflammation, as in dermatitis herpetiformis. Eczema is to be preferred when a specifically *epidermal* reaction is implied.

Eczema is a reaction pattern of the skin rather than a disease entity. With the exception of contact eczema the mechanism leading to attacks is poorly understood, but it is likely that infections, contact factors, the emotions and the state of the general health combine to produce the reaction. In some cases hereditary factors predominate, the family pattern of disease comprising infantile eczema, atopic eczema, asthma, migraine, hay fever and urticaria.

The healing power of nature can be aided in a

number of ways. *Symptomatic treatment* of the eczematous skin provide the rest and protection necessary for healing, while the anti-inflammatory action of the corticosteroid drugs is useful in controlling the reaction. However, the eczema is likely to recur when treatment is stopped unless any *precipitating and perpetuating factors* have been sought and eliminated. Consequently the management of the patient must include consideration of these factors.

SYMPTOMATIC TREATMENT

Acute eczema is best treated by using wet dressings of ichtho-calamine liniment (ichthammol 1 per cent., calamine 8 per cent., lanoline 6 per cent. in equal parts of linseed oil and lime water) or of $\frac{1}{2}$ per cent. silver nitrate in water. Severe acute eczema of the hands requires in-patient treatment or dressing in a dermatological out-patient department. Soaking the hands in a dilute solution of iodine (dilute solution of iodine B.P., 1 in 50 in water) before dressing is useful in the presence of infection. Antibiotics systematically administered may also be necessary. Corticosteroid applications have little place in the treatment of acute eczema, except when it is of very small extent, when a lotion should be used rather than an ointment.

Subacute and chronic eczema. There comes a point in the treatment of acute eczema at which the skin begins to crack and to become uncomfortable. At this stage, ointment or paste applications are necessary. Satisfactory results are possible with old-fashioned applications, such as ichthammol paste (ichthammol 1 per cent., zinc oxide 15 per cent. in soft yellow paraffin), preceded by crystal violet paint B.P.C., if necessary, to control infection, but the availability, ease of application and effectiveness of corticosteroid applications has made them now the first choice. The corticosteroid used is largely a matter of individual preference and expense. The quickest results are obtained with the fluorinated steroids, such as betamethasone valerate and fluocinolone acetonide, and the safest anti-bacterial is chlortetracycline (3 per cent.). Neomycin and soframcyin containing applications should not be used because of their sensitizing potential. This is not prevented by the corticosteroid part of the application.

The healing effect of crude coal tar in chronic eczema is still useful. The risk of malignancy in the skin therapeutic application is minute, although prolonged occupational contact may be carcinogenic. Crude coal tar, 2 per cent. in zinc paste, is the usual preparation. It is particularly useful in treating nummular eczema.

An unexpectedly poor result is sometimes obtained from the application of ointment. Such patients may be sensitive, reacting either to the lanoline or the mineral grease of the base. The precise cause can be sought by patch testing, when it may be possible to find an application free from the offending substance. They tolerate pastes better than ointments, and in this situation Lassar's paste is useful.

The natural response to the irritation caused by eczema is to scratch, which leads to the inoculation of organisms as well as the lichenification of the eruption. A vicious circle of itching leading to scratching and to further itching and further scratching is readily established. To break this cycle it may be necessary to occlude the affected part, for which purpose zinc-gelatine bandages are useful. While Unna's paste may be the best application for routine use in a dermatological department there are more easily applied proprietary bandages available for use outside hospital, some of which contain added corticosteroid. The confirmed scratcher may feel miserable when he can no longer get at his itch, and sedation, for example with a systemic antihistamine preparation, is useful. Localized chronic patches of lichenification that resist treatment may yield to the application of corticosteroids under polythene occlusion, to the high strength fluorinated applications that are now available, or to the local injection of corticosteroid.

There is still a small but definite place for superficial X-ray therapy in intractable eczema, especially of the hands, provided that the treatment is given by a skilled operator who is aware of the hazards of overdosage. It should be reserved for patients whose eczema has resisted an adequate course of conventional treatment.

The deep cracks that can open up in the skin in chronic eczema respond well to the dental preparation orabase, which can be moulded into them. Cobbler's wax used to be found useful for the same purpose.

PRECIPITATING AND PERPETUATING FACTORS

The ide phenomenon. Any patch of localized eczema can lead after a time, presumably by a humoral mechanism, to a symmetrical eczematous eruption that may be of small or large extent, and may completely overshadow the primary patch. This phenomenon can be precipitated by, for example, a patch of contact eczema, a fungus infection or a 'varicose' eczema. Therefore, in symmetrical eczematous eruptions including eczema of the fingers, one may be observing the ide reaction to a white metal dermatitis, a tinea pedis or any other patch of primary eczema. The primary patch is not necessarily very prominent and may therefore escape casual observation, but upon its successful treatment will depend the cure of the ide eruption.

The infective element. Eczematous skin always becomes secondarily infected and in some cases the infection will cause the eczema to persist. Seborrhoeic (flexural infective) eczema appears to be directly associated with infection; and this calls for appropriate treatment. The flexures, where the skin is warm and moist, are the sites mainly affected; and this is an additional reason for controlling obesity in such patients. Scratching of the itchy skin gives rise to infection by inoculation and may result in folliculitis, abscesses or even cellulitis. Infections with fungi, yeasts and viruses also occur. Corticosteroid preparations may cause exacerbation of a fungus infection. Yeast infections, which cause many cases of flexural eruption (intertrigo) are particularly common in diabetics. The viruses of vaccinia and herpes simplex can infect eczematous skin, the resulting illness often being severe or even lethal. Consequently, it is unwise to vaccinate patients who have active eczema particularly those suffering from atopic eczema. Such patients should also be kept out of contact with the recently vaccinated and those suffering from active herpes simplex infections.

The control of bacterial infection may be by local or systemic means. Lymphangitis, cellulitis and abscess formation require systemic antibiotics. Unless a resistant organism is likely, in which case cloxacillin should be chosen, the usual choice is penicillin, until the organism is identified. Local applications usually suffice. The effective but messy dyes such as crystal violet paint B.P.C. and magenta paint B.P.C. diluted in three parts of water have been largely replaced by cleaner preparations, except for flexural eruptions, where they are the treatment of choice. Among antibiotic applications 3 per cent. chlortetracycline ointment

is recommended for its comparative freedom from the risk of sensitizing the patient. Among non-antibiotic applications iodochlorhydroxquinoline ointment is useful. In some individuals it causes irritation, but this is immediately obvious, whereas with neomycin the onset of irritation may be so insidious that it can be missed by the unwary. The choice of a non-antibiotic application also has the theoretical advantage that there is no risk of sensitizing the patient to an antibiotic that might be needed subsequently to save his life. Sulphonamides are not recommended for local application. In yeast infections, nystatin ointment offers a cleaner, but no more effective, alternative to crystal violet paint B.P.C. The infection may prove impossible to clear without treating any underlying diabetes mellitus. Infection may enter the skin through chapping in cold weather, for which a good prophylactic application is equal parts of salicylic acid ointment B.P. and glycerin of starch.

Contact eczema. A common cause of failing to control eczema is having missed a contact allergen. The effects of primary irritants and degreasers are less easily overlooked. Contact eczema is a large subject in its own right and cannot be discussed in detail here, but there is need for a high index of suspicion. Hazards exist at work, at play, from clothing, cosmetics, from hobbies and from medicaments. The environment is filled with an ever-increasing number of potential allergens. The history is useful, the eruption having started on the area of skin that would have come into contact with the allergen, although it may have spread subsequently to other areas. Where contact is intermittent, remissions and exacerbations alternate at an appropriate interval. The skin of the eyelids and of the genitalia is thin and sensitive and may react by transfer of the allergen on the fingers before the fingers themselves are affected. This confusing state of affairs is usual in primula eczema and nail varnish eczema. The action to be taken is to separate the patient from the allergen, which may imply a change of work unless contact can be prevented by a physical barrier such as impervious gloves (with cotton ones underneath), or by attention to working technique.

The possibility of contributing to this hazard by local medication is considerable: antihistamines, surface anaesthetics, penicillin, neomycin, soframycin, sulphonamides and flavine for local application should all be avoided. It is not correct to suppose that corticosteroid applications used simultaneously will protect against sensitizing local applications, and most applications carry some risk of sensitization, which must be accepted and watched for. The danger lies not only in the active medicaments but in the bases and preservatives used.

The possibility of a contact eczema can be investigated by patch testing, not only against any allergens that are suspected from the history, but also against a battery of the commonly encountered agents. This service is available in some dermatological clinics.

Genetic predisposition. The suspicion that a tendency exists in some patients to develop eczema is difficult to prove and has been disputed, even where the influence of heredity seems most obvious, in atopic eczema (the asthma-eczema syndrome). Nothing can be done to eliminate this hypothetical influence, but the possibility that it exists helps in understanding the prolonged course of the eczema and in sympathizing with its victims who may be reduced to a state of misery. The problem is rather akin to the management of asthma and, in exceptional cases, may justify the use of long-term systemic corticosteroid therapy, as discussed at the end of this chapter.

Emotional aspects. The notion that eczema is basically a psychosomatic phenomenon is obviously too facile, but it is true that the emotional state of the patient can influence the eruption markedly, and it is possible for nervous influences to be the predominant stimulus (neurodermatitis). The treatment of the itch—scratch—further itch cycle has been discussed already under the symptomatic treatment of eczema. Sedation is important in these patients and commonsense readjustment of the patient's life and habits can be helpful in lowering emotional tension. It is occasionally possible to divert into other channels the energy expended on scratching, as in one patient who was encouraged to take up cycling, a sport at which she became very successful. Itching is one of the many symptoms that may betray depression, and if this is suspected the help of a psychiatrist is required. On the other hand a reactive depression is a common sequel to a prolonged skin disease.

The state of general health. It is important to correct such disorders as anaemia, carious teeth, unbalanced diet or occult infection, for example in the urinary tract. An occasional patient with an eczema that is resistant to treatment will be found to be suffering from malabsorption and will be helped by a gluten-free diet. The only unusual feature about the appearance of the eruption in such cases is its occasional tendency to become pigmented. The inhalation or ingestion of allergens to which the patient is sensitive may occasionally produce an eczema, in which case testing may prove helpful. Venous stasis in the legs, often associated with varicose veins, is the basis of 'varicose' eczema. It is to be controlled either by the application of pressure by bandaging (from toes to knee) or surgically, by treatment of varicose veins, and especially by tying the perforating veins that connect the deep and superficial venous systems. These measures are more important than external applications designed to control the eczema or the complicating infection.

Erysipelas

Erysipelas, called 'la rose' in France and still called rose in Scotland, is due to an infection of the skin with haemolytic streptococci. It will respond to systemic penicillin and sulphonamides given in full doses as for an acute infection (pp. 3, 43). Search should be made for any crack in the skin through which infection could have entered, for example at the angle of the nostril, the junction of the ear with the skin of the scalp or at the outer canthus of the eye. Any such lesion should be treated with an antiseptic ointment such as clioquinol, not only until the crack has healed but for several months afterwards to try to prevent a recurrence. Repeated attacks of erysipelas are likely to lead to lymphatic damage with consequent chronic oedema of the tissues and, since it is impossible to restore the normal lymphatic drainage, it is important to treat recurrences of erysipelas promptly and vigorously.

Fungus Infections

The introduction of griseofulvin has provided an effective means of treating ringworm of the scalp, including favus, and is an improvement in the treatment of ringworm of the nails. Nevertheless, it is not very effective in ringworm of the feet (athlete's foot) nor is it effective against yeasts; thus monilial paronychia and systemic monilial infections are not helped by it. Griseofulvin is taken by mouth and it becomes loosely incorporated in skin, hair and nails during their growth, making them unacceptable to the fungi which thus find themselves deprived of their usual food—freshly formed keratin—and they are cast off as the keratin-containing tissues undergo normal wastage by desquamation, etc. The recommended dose is 0·5 g. daily of the finely divided form taken in divided doses after meals. Reduction of the dose below the recommended level is likely to prove unsatisfactory. In treating ringworm of the scalp a course lasting six weeks is necessary, and it should be combined with the local use of Whitfield's ointment and clipping the hair short. The proper duration of treatment is very difficult to assess even with full mycological control, and it is possible that further experience will modify current views on this dosage. In ringworm of the nails the treatment will have to be continued for nine months or more until the last traces of the diseased nail have disappeared. The local use of fungicides is recommended, for example magenta paint B.P.C., and removal of the diseased, friable nail is desirable. This can be done by using a piece of broken glass or sandpaper as a scraper; all the scrapings should be burnt. Very few toxic effects have resulted from treatment with griseofulvin apart from mild gastro-intestinal upset; disturbance of porphyrin metabolism has also been reported.

Two new fungicides for topical application, pecilocin and tolnaftate, are promising, but neither will deal with infection due to yeasts.

Tinea pedis. This extremely chronic infection usually takes the form of macerated skin between the toes which causes little trouble until the feet get very hot when there is liable to be an explosive outbreak of an acute eczema with vesiculation due to the fungus growing vigorously in the skin under the warm, moist conditions. Should this exacerbation provoke an ide eruption, it is important to realize that the ide does not contain active fungus elements and it is, therefore, appropriate to treat it as an eczema without using fungicides. The active fungus infection should be treated initially as an acute eczema, using soaks or wet dressings. The patient should be kept in bed and give an oral antibiotic if there is lymphangitis. Fungicides such as Whitfield's ointment (benzoic acid compound ointment B.P.C.) and Castellani's paint (magenta paint B.P.C.) are used when the acute stage has passed.

In the resting phase the disease is sometimes intractable. If an attempt is made to eradicate the disease, it is essential to keep the skin as clean, dry and cool as possible, to destroy fungus present on the footwear, to prevent re-infection and to continue using fungicides. In order to comply with this advice, the patient needs to adhere to a very exacting programme of personal hygiene. He should wash his feet twice daily in soap and water and dry the skin very carefully afterwards, using a towel kept exclusively for his use. Dead skin should be removed with forceps, not the finger nails; and Whitfield's ointment should be rubbed thoroughly into the webs between the toes, after which the feet and the socks should be dusted with zinc undecenoate dusting powder B.P.C. He should wear a thin pair of white cotton socks next to the skin, putting on a clean pair after every washing and having the dirty pair boiled. His oversocks should be thin and—in order to minimize sweating—not made of synthetic fibre. He should wear thin, leather-soled shoes or sandals. The shoes should be treated with formalin vapour by sealing them in a tin containing a saucer of liquid formaldehyde for 24 hours. If he perseveres with these instructions for some months he may be cured, but if he is, he will have to continue taking precautions against re-infection for the rest of his life by refusing to walk anywhere in bare feet (except on his own bath mat) and by continuing to take particular care of his feet, using zinc undecenoate ointment B.P. prophylactically.

Cattle ringworm. In farming areas ringworm derived from farm animals causes severely inflamed lesions (kerion). They are self-limited because the severity of the reaction casts the fungus off the skin. The pustulation that occurs is not due to secondary infection so much as to hypersensitivity developed against the causative fungus, so that oral corticosteroid therapy has a place in very severe infections. To allow the disease to take its course may involve an illness of 8 to 16 weeks, but its duration can be reduced by giving griseofulvin by mouth for two or three weeks early in the course of the infection. After having removed the debris by gentle washing or with starch poultices and having clipped the surrounding hair short, local dressings are applied: they consist of 5 per cent. ichthammol in water used as wet dressings under oiled silk. Later an ointment, containing equal parts of a corticosteroid ointment and Whitfield's ointment, should be rubbed in thoroughly twice daily until all pustulation has ceased. The remaining lumpiness can then be left to settle spontaneously. It should be noted that although large lesions are tumid and studded with pustules, no benefit is obtained by incision because the pus is contained within the individual hair follicles.

Tinea circinata. Ringed lesions of the open skin usually respond quickly to Castellani's paint or to Whitfield's ointment. Infections due to *Tricho-phyton rubrum* may prove resistant (onychia is almost certain to co-exist) and then griseofulvin by mouth is necessary. The diagnosis of tinea circinata calls for consideration of the origin of the infection; the scalp should be examined for the scaly, bald patches of ringworm, and inquiry should be made about possible animal sources—particularly contact with kittens and puppies.

Scalp ringworm. Griseofulvin is the treatment of choice. It is very desirable that the public health and school medical authorities should be informed of cases so that they can take steps to trace the source of infection and to find all the cases in order to prevent epidemic spread of the disease.

Groin infections. The infection often stems from the feet, which should be treated simultanously. If the skin is acutely inflamed, treatment should first be that used in acute eczema. When the angry phase has subsided fungicides may be applied, for example, Whitfield's ointment or Castellani's paint. When the infection appears to have been cured the patient should still take the precaution of drying himself thoroughly after his bath, and should dust the skin with zinc undecenoate powder B.P.C.

Nail infections. Formerly, infection of the nails with fungus was often incurable even though the affected nails were avulsed and fungicides applied during their subsequent growth. With griseofulvin the results are sometimes good and permanent cure can occur.

Furunculosis

Recurrent boils can be a symptom of a systemic disorder such as diabetes mellitus, and they call for thorough medical examination. They may also complicate scabies. The staphylococci which cause the lesions are harboured in the nose, throat, perianal skin or other focus, from which they are disseminated over the general surface of the skin. The skin should be washed daily in a bath using hexachlorophene, special attention being paid to the possible primary foci. An appropriate antibiotic cream (determined by sensitivity tests) should be applied to the boils and to the skin immediately surrounding them, and also to the nostrils. In a severe case the patient should take sulphafurazole tablets by mouth, 500 mg. three times daily for the first month, twice daily for the second and once daily for the third month.

Herpes Simplex

Herpes simplex usually presents as a patch of blisters that recur repeatedly on the same piece of skin, often near the mouth but sometimes on the genital region or on a finger. It results from a latent cellular virus infection subject to repeated reactivation and beyond the reach of the circulating antibodies that can be demonstrated in the blood. The recurrences are determined by a variety of stimuli such as exposure to the sun, the common cold, menstruation and emotional stress; and particularly severe attacks can be precipitated by severe infections. An antibiotic corticosteroid ointment may help to abort the attack and diminishes the chance of scarring from secondary infection. No certain method of treatment exists for preventing recurrences and the reputedly successful ones are so diverse and bizarre that one is tempted to think that the power of suggestion is the common factor. It is important that patients with active lesions should not come into close contact with those suffering from eczema, since, if infected with the virus of herpes simplex, the resulting illness can be very severe or even fatal.

Herpes Zoster

The natural variability of the disease makes it impossible to assess the results of early treatment in individual cases and attacks cannot be aborted. The objects of treatment are to relieve pain (which can be extremely severe), to protect the affected skin from friction, to prevent secondary infection and—if the eye is involved—to prescribe mydriatics and seek the help of an ophthalmologist as soon as possible. The pain is best treated by keeping the patient warm in bed, by painting the skin with flexible collodion B.P., and thereafter powdering it with zinc, starch and talc dusting powder B.P.C., by protecting it from friction by a thick layer of cotton-wool and by giving oral analgesics. The local or systemic use of antibiotics is indicated only in severe attacks or if the eye is involved (p. 610). It has been suggested recently that systemic corticosteroid treatment will diminish the severity of an attack and lessen the chances of post-herpetic pain.

Post-herpetic pain can be a grievous problem and is liable to occur in elderly patients. Analgesics (aspirin or paracetamol) are used and their effect can be enhanced by giving promazine hydrochloride. There is a tendency for improvement to occur up to six months after the attack. In the intractable case the problems are similar to those found in the management of trigeminal neuralgia and may require to be reviewed by a neurosurgeon.

Impetigo Contagiosa

Impetigo contagiosa and its more serious variant, pemphigus neonatorum, are due to superficial infection of the epidermis with pathogenic staphylococci or streptococci. It is a common sequel to chicken-pox. Not infrequently pediculosis capitis or scabies is the underlying disease; if present these conditions should be treated first. For localized outbreaks the application of chlortetracycline ointment is suitable, after having removed the crusts by bathing or with starch poultices. A swab should be taken before starting treatment so that, in the event of the disease failing to respond, no time will be lost in prescribing an appropriate alternative. When the lesions are extensive it is more satisfactory to give full doses of oxytetracycline by mouth, as for an acute infection. The cure of the impetigo often reveals an unsuspected eczema requiring treatment. Failure of the impetigo to respond calls for a review of the diagnosis; in particular the possibility of underlying ringworm should be considered. The occurrence of a case of pemphigus neonatorum in a maternity unit calls for an urgent bacteriological survey of the patients and staff.

Insect Bites

People who say that insects like biting them base their belief on the fact that their skins are severely affected, whereas their more fortunate neighbours appear to escape. It is more true to say that all are bitten but only the hypersensitive ones react badly to the bites. Those who are susceptible should certainly use insect repellents (dibutylphthallate cream), and experience may justify the taking of antihistamines in anticipation of exposure to attack by insects. Established bites should be treated with calamine lotion or corticosteroid applications as well as by any measures required to deal with secondary infection. *Papular urticaria* of children is usually due to insect bites; but the mother will seldom countenance this explanation because it is regarded as an implied criticism of the standard of hygiene in her household. The local use of crotamiton cream B.N.F. and an antihistamine elixir by mouth is usually effective. If this fails, the child should be admitted to hospital; here cure takes place spontaneously but when the child goes home a relapse is only too likely to occur.

Lichen Planus

Lichen planus causes unbearable irritation. It should probably be regarded as a special form of neurodermatitis since most patients have a background of emotional difficulty. There are some cases, however, which result from a physical cause such as a reaction to anti-malarial drugs or to gold therapy. The eruption is self-limiting; it lasts for a period of months or years; the more acute the onset the more rapid is the course, and disappearance of the lesions is heralded by their intense pigmentation. Isoniazid aminosalicylate tablets, one tablet (100 mg.) per 20 lb. body weight, have been recommended, but the natural tendency for the disease to regress makes their true worth difficult to assess. An investigation of the circumstances of the patient's emotional life may suggest practical means of alleviating difficulties at home or at work. There may be an indication for a radical change in the patient's way of life since some patients are shouldering an unmanageable burden of responsibility or are burning the candle at both ends for financial or other reasons. Betamethasone valerate and fluocinolone acetonide under polythene film occlusion are effective, but it should be emphasized that considerable corticosteroid absorption can result from this method. In very severe generalized eruptions there is a place for a limited course of oral corticosteroid therapy. Chronic localized patches—especially of the warty variety—are best treated by injecting corticosteroids into the lesions (p. 589).

Lupus Erythematosus

Chronic discoid lupus erythematosus is believed to be due to a localized auto-antibody phenomenon. It responds to anti-malarial drugs given by mouth and to inunction with betamethasone valerate and fluocinolone acetonide. Local injection of triamcinolone is used for stubborn lesions. Mepacrine was the first anti-malarial to be used but stains the skin yellow and chloroquine is now preferred. Chloroquine phosphate, 500 mg. daily, is given initially and when the eruption has been brought under control, the smallest effective dose is given for maintenance—usually between 1 and 2 g. per week. It is convenient to reduce the dose by omitting certain days from treatment, since this will give some relief from gastric irritation which is a common side-effect of chloroquine. The most serious toxic effects concern the eye. The patient complains of blurred vision which is caused by interference with accommodation. This disorder may cause inconvenience (reading, driving a car, etc.), but it is not in itself of grave significance. Serious ocular complications, however, include damage to the cornea, the retina and the optic nerve. Symptoms develop insidiously: complaints of coloured halos around lights are significant, and may herald serious impairment of vision. It is, therefore, most desirable that patients receiving prolonged courses of chloroquine should be seen regularly by an ophthalmologist. The affected skin should be protected from direct sunlight (these patients should never sunbathe) and from cold wind. Cosmetic preparations that hide the scars should be used.

Acute disseminated lupus erythematosous requires long-term systemic corticosteroid therapy under proper supervision. It is usual to maintain patients on this treatment for the rest of their lives. Immunosuppressive agents are also used.

Lupus Vulgaris

Lupus vulgaris is due to tuberculous infection of the skin. The diagnosis makes it essential to examine the patient for evidence of other active foci of the disease. Lupus vulgaris was formerly one of the dermatological horrors; it caused appalling scarring because of the relentless spread of the disease. Nowadays, however, it is justifiable to regard the disease as 'benign' because of the excellent results which are readily obtained from antituberculous drugs. Dermatologists have not been troubled by resistant organisms in the skin, but it is well to remember that this problem does face the chest physician and that, if a pulmonary focus is present, full combined treatment should be given to minimize the chance of resistance developing. A suitable regimen is to give streptomycin by injection, 1 g. twice weekly, and 300 mg. of isoniazid daily by mouth in divided doses. Ulceration of old lesions of lupus vulgaris should arouse the suspicion of malignancy. The best means of settling this question is to carry out a biopsy and to seek the help of an experienced pathologist.

Paronychia

Chronic paronychia due to yeast or staphylococcal infection is a troublesome disease in housewives and others whose occupations require repeated immersion of the hands in water. The first essential is to enforce dryness, and unless this can be done the chance of cure is small. Nystatin ointment can be applied at night and worked into the nail fold. During the day the patient should use a preparation which will readily seep into the nail fold, such as Castellani's paint or hydrargaphen. The usual sources of infection are the garden, the kitchen sink and the bowel. When the condition has healed, special care should be taken to avoid trauma to the hands through working in the garden or in the kitchen since these forms of injury open the way for further infection.

Pediculosis

Infestation with *head lice* is best treated by wetting the hair with paraffin (kerosene) and swathing the head in a towel for an hour. The paraffin must disperse widely in the hair down to the scalp but must not run into the eyes or down the neck. An alternative is dicophane application, B.P.C., but this does not destroy the fertile eggs and, therefore, the treatment should be repeated on three occasions at weekly intervals. After either application the hair is washed thoroughly. It is then combed with a fine-toothed comb moistened in vinegar to loosen the cement holding the eggs (nits) on to the hairs. Subsequently any impetiginous lesions should be treated (p. 584).

Body lice live in the seams of the clothing and are dealt with by steam disinfestation of the clothes. When this is not available, laundering and careful ironing of the seams, combined with a sprinkling of dicophane dusting powder will suffice. Crotamiton cream which will help to relieve the intense itch produced by the disease will also kill any parasites on the body.

Pubic lice (*crab lice*) live among stiff hairs holding on with either claw, and are found in the eyebrows, eyelashes, axillary and pubic hair. In the pubic region they are easily dealt with by shaving, but around the eyes they should be treated with mercuric oxide eye ointment and removed by gentle washing with liquid paraffin. The shaved areas can be treated with dilute ammoniated mercury ointment.

Pemphigus

Pemphigus vulgaris was formerly fatal, but corticosteroids given by mouth will usually suppress the eruption and permit a normal life. A few patients have apparently recovered and have been able to dispense with the treatment, but the majority need treatment for life and the smallest dose which will effectually keep the condition under control should be sought. *Pemphigus neonatorum* is a form of impetigo and requires antibiotic therapy as for an acute infection.

Pityriasis Rosea

This common condition is sometimes confused with secondary syphilis—but this, by comparison, is a rarity. If the diagnosis is in doubt a full clinical survey and serological tests for syphilis must be carried out. Pityriasis rosea is not obviously infective but in other respects it behaves like an infection. There is a primary lesion at onset followed by the ide eruption, with its resolution after a course of six to eight weeks and an immunity to further attacks. Emulsifying ointment B.P. is all that need be applied in the average episode, and in mild cases nothing is needed. When the disease is severe and the lesions become confluent in the flexures, the patient should be advised to stay in bed for a few days, and a corticosteroid ointment should be applied to the areas most severely affected.

Pruritus

Pruritus which is secondary to skin disease is controlled by treating the eczema, scales etc. which is producing it. It is tempting to apply local anaesthetic and antihistamine preparations to the skin, but this temptation should be resisted because these preparations are sensitizing agents. Sedatives are useful when given orally, and this applies also to antihistamines which are valuable for their sedative and tranquillizing properties. A combination of promethazine hydrochloride 12·5 mg. and amylobarbitone 50 mg. is useful; but if promethazine causes undue drowsiness it can be replaced by triprolidine hydrochloride. In the elderly, however, barbiturates are often poorly tolerated; they may produce a state of confusion and then the itch plays a disturbing and demoralizing rôle. In these circumstances chloral hydrate is the best drug to use, after allowing a few days to elapse without the use of any cerebral depressant drugs. For local treatment one should be content with simple applications of low sensitizing potential such as a mixture of equal parts of linseed oil and lime water, or liquefied phenol 1 ml., zinc oxide 2 g., calamine 1 g., glycerin 2 ml., magnesium hydroxide mixture B.P., to 30 ml. These preparations may be either painted on frequently or used as wet compresses.

A separate problem arises when, in spite of the patient's complaint of intense irritation, nothing abnormal is visible except the marks that he has made by scratching himself. There are many possible explanations: scabies, in a person who is so clean that few lesions develop; pediculosis corporis, recognized by examining the seams of the underclothing; senile change in the skin; a side-effect of certain drugs such as morphine or carbromal (neither of which should be used by patients liable to pruritus or actually suffering from the condition); psychoses, when the patient usually presents the doctor with a folded piece of paper stated to contain 'the insects'; a manifestation of renal or hepatic disease; a symptom heralding a metabolic disorder such as diabetes mellitus; an accompaniment of blood dyscrasias including the leukaemia and polycythaemia vera; and, fairly commonly, lymphadenoma. This differential diagnosis, by no means exhaustive, may serve to emphasize the need for taking a detailed history and making a thorough physical examination.

Psoriasis

It is rarely gratifying to undertake the treatment of chronic psoriasis unless the patient is prepared to spend a lot of time on it. On the other hand the average patient is inconvenienced rather than incapacitated: he is embarrassed by visits to the barber and the swimming-pool, for example. Many decide wisely to live with their spots.

The severest manifestations of the disease, the generalized pustular and exfoliative varieties, may threaten life, and require treatment in hospital. The pustular form of psoriasis is becoming much more common, largely due to the effect of corticosteroid drugs, and these should probably never be used systemically and as seldom as possible locally. The exfoliative variety can be precipitated by injudicious treatment with older remedies, tar and dithranol, that are returning to favour as the mainstay of treatment.

An eruption entering an active phase must be treated gently, for example by the application of soft paraffin and by sedatives given by mouth. Active treatment is reserved for eruptions that are static. Tar and dithranol are messy to use, and dithranol stains clothing indelibly. Decolourized proprietary preparations of these substances, although more acceptable cosmetically, are less active therapeutically. Sizeable discrete patches are best treated with crude coal tar incorporated in zinc paste and applied accurately to the lesion. Multiple small lesions are best treated with ointments which have a basis of soft yellow paraffin.

Tar is a sensitizer and photosensitizer so must be used cautiously, after enquiry about previous reactions, and applied initially to a limited area in a strength of 1 per cent. which can be raised gradually to 10 per cent. as necessary. Ultraviolet light therapy may be combined with tar to advantage, but this treatment should be given, in a physiotherapy department rather than at home, where it cannot be controlled properly. The tar is best applied at night and removed in the morning (using olive-oil if necessary to soften the paste) with soap and water. During the day soft yellow paraffin is applied. Fluorinated corticosteroid ointments, for example betamethasone valerate and fluocinolone acetonide will accelerate the initial resolution of lesions and may be used in certain circumstances where a rapid result is desirable; but their routine application to large areas and over long periods is undesirable. Folliculitis, is a complication of tar therapy that sometimes limits its usefulness and requires anti-infective measures and temporary abandonment of tar therapy. Dithranol is an irritant substance that must be used carefully and kept away from the eyes, which it can damage. It is applied in zinc paste accurately to the lesions, starting at 0·1 per cent. and working up gradually to 2 per cent. as necessary. It must be used cautiously in flexural eruptions, which are best treated initially as an intertrigo (p. 580). Scalp lesions are treated by an oil of cade ointment (oil of cade 12 per cent., yellow oxide of mercury and camphor of each 4 per cent., aqueous emulsifying ointment to 100 per cent.), shampooing with oil of cade 10 per cent. in spirit soap and applying fluocinolone acetonide and liquid paraffin equal parts during the day.

Acute guttate psoriasis is usually related to haemolytic streptococcal infection in the throat. Repeated attacks call for long-term penicillin treatment, as in rheumatic fever, and possibly tonsillectomy.

There are a few patients whose lives are severely hampered by psoriasis, some of whom also have psoriatic arthropathy. They present a most difficult problem which is properly the province of the dermatologist. He may consider it justifiable to treat them with one of the anti-mitotic agents such as methotrexate, in spite of its potential hazards to the liver and bone marrow. Such treatment is not suitable for routine use and requires close supervision. Systemic corticosteroid treatment creates more problems than it solves and should not be used.

Scabies

Scabies is due to a mite, *Acarus scabiei*. The female burrows superficially in the skin to lay her eggs. The infestation is derived from close contact with another person suffering from the disease, and in families it spreads readily. Animal scabies causes only a transient eruption in humans. The prominent part of the eruption, which is very itchy, is an ide resulting from the development of hypersensitivity to the products of infestation but it is necessary to treat the whole body surface—excluding the head—to be certain of a cure. The whole household must be treated simultaneously. Sulphur ointment B.P., or gamma-benzene hexachloride (which is less messy), is applied to the whole surface of the body below the chin on three occasions at 12-hour intervals. Twelve hours after the last application the patients should have a bath, put on clean underclothes and change their sheets. Benzyl benzoate application B.P. is less effective than these two preparations. They should now be cured of the infestation. Continuing irritation should be treated as an eczema but in no circumstances should the anti-scabetic treatment be continued. Children should be treated with half-strength, and babies (whose heads must also be treated) with quarter-strength sulphur ointment B.P. ($2\frac{1}{2}$ per cent. of sulphur). Any accompanying sepsis of the skin must wait until the anti-scabetic treatment has been applied. Gamma-benzene hexachloride lotion is an effective alternative treatment.

Sunburn

Burning of the skin as a result of excessive exposure to the sun is best treated with calamine lotion, lead and zinc lotion or a local corticosteroid preparation. Local use of antihistamines is contraindicated because of the risk of sensitization. It should be noted that cosmetic lotions, designed to imitate the colour of sunburn, offer little or no pretection.

Adverse reactions to an apparently small dose of sunlight suggest that the skin has become photosensitive. This may be a drug reaction (antibiotics, phenothiazines, sulphonamides), contact with certain plants (such as hogweed), with a cosmetic (such as lipstick), with a local application (such as tar or oil of bergamot) or with soap. Alternatively there may be an inherent state of photosensitivity; this is often idiopathic but is sometimes associated with abnormalities of porphyrin metabolism. Apart from the removal of any causative stimulus and avoidance of the sun, the application of a 'light screen' such as mexenone cream corticosteroids locally and chloroquine by mouth may be helpful. The toxic effects of chloroquine are mentioned on page 452.

Sycosis Barbae

This form of chronic folliculitis of the beard region has become much less common since the days of antibiotics. The causative organism, usually staphylococcus aureus, lurks in the depths of the follicles and is not readily accessible to local applications. Local preparations should therefore be massaged well into the skin, night and morning. Experience has shown that it is best to prescribe a succession of different antibacterial applications rather than to continue with the same one: thus, chlortetracycline ointment could be followed by quinolor compound ointment, iodochlorhydroxy-quinoline ointment, etc. A small amount should also be applied inside the nostrils. If such treatment gives rise to discomfort it can be combined with local corticosteroid therapy. The shaving tackle should be cleaned carefully and if possible sterilized after every use; and when shaving the strokes should be made only with the grain of the hair.

Urticaria

Urticaria is the result of localized oedema in the skin produced by leakage of fluid without red cells from the blood. The transient increased permeability of the vessels is usually brought about through the release of histamine (or histamine-like substances), by a variety of stimuli including injury, and the occurrence of antigen–antibody reactions. Some skins weal abnormally with injury (dermographism). Urticaria is a common disability, but it is often of limited duration.

Provocative stimuli. In cases that defy antihistamines and persist, a search for provocative stimuli is the only rational method of precedure.

The diet. Two days of starvation, except for water to drink, should result in the clearance of a food urticaria. The food responsible may be identified by adding foodstuffs one by one to the diet, or, less satisfactorily, by a food diary.

Of *drugs*, penicillin and aspirin are said to be the commonest causes of chronic urticaria. The eruption can outlast the giving of penicillin by many months. This is possibly due to the ingestion of traces of penicillin in milk and partly by inhalation, for example, in hospitals. Aspirin often acts as a non-specific stimulus by aggravating urticaria due to other causes.

Inhalants, such as mould spores, dusts and pollens, which do not necessarily cause sneezing or ocular discomfort, produce a seasonal or intermittent pattern of attack according to the climatic conditions under which they are produced or their location. Skin testing facilitates precise identification, but specific desensitization may not be practicable.

The hollow viscera, such as the gut and gall-bladder can contain organisms or products of their activity which are absorbed and act as antigens. Yeast infection of the bowel or of diverticulae of the bowel (including blind loops left by surgery often) causes urticaria.

The patient's tissues may harbour infections, parasites or a tumour which is breaking down rapidly, and these can act as antigens. The auto-immune disease, disseminated lupus erythematosus can present as urticaria, and so can the vascular disease, polyarteritis nodosa.

Emotional stimuli can be entertained as factors only when, in addition to a lack of physical causes, there are positive psychological ones. Suppressed anger at some intolerable but apparently irremediable situation is a potent stimulus.

Symptomatic treatment. The antihistamine drugs, taken by mouth, are often effective but it may be necessary to find by trial and error which drug suits the individual patient. Resistance can develop to a particular antihistamine in a week or two, necessitating a change. The intramuscular injection of an antihistamine is worthy of trial if the response to oral treatment is poor. One of the chief anxieties about antihistamine treatment in the ambulant patient is the possible effect on the ability to handle machinery, particularly motor cars and aeroplanes, for even if antihistamines do not cause drowsiness they may impair judgment. Children tolerate these drugs well and for them elixirs are very acceptable. Corticosteroids usually control urticaria but their use is justifiable only to tide the patient over an acute attack. In fulminating attacks or when the airway is threatened by oedema, adrenaline hydrochloride solution, 1 ml. (1 in 1,000), should be given subcutaneously, and hydrocortisone hemisuccinate intravenously.

The Corticosteroids in Skin Disease

Local Application. Betamethasone valerate and fluocinolone acetonide, are so much better than their predecessors that the need to use other routes of administration is diminishing. Lichen planus, lichen simplex and chronic discoid lupus erythematous respond to them, particularly if penetration of the drug is assisted by the technique of occluding the anointed area with an impervious layer of material such as polythene sheeting or if the greater strength applications now available are used. The possibility of systemic absorption must always be remembered. Atrophy of the skin may result from continual application.

Intra-cutaneous injection. Injection of corticosteroid into resistant lesions, for example of discoid lupus erythematosis and lichen planus may succeed where local application fails.

Systemic treatment. Costicosteroids are needed as a life-saving measure in fulminating illness associated with drug eruptions, urticaria and erythema multiforme of the Stevens–Johnson type. The treatment should be started by giving 100 mg. of hydrocortisone sodium succinate intravenously and 40 mg. of prednisone in divided doses by mouth, during the first 24 hours. The dose is adjusted thereafter according to the patient's response; the daily dose should be tailed off and eventually stopped as soon as the activity of the disease has abated—which will probably be within three weeks.

Long-term corticosteroid treatment is required in exfoliative dermatitis, the pemphigus group of diseases, mycosis fungoides, the cutaneous reticuloses and disseminated lupus erythematosus. Because these are mortal diseases or at least endanger life, such treatment is obviously justifiable. After initial high dosage of the order of 60 mg. of prednisone daily to achieve control, a maintenance dose as low as 10 to 15 mg. of prednisone daily is often possible.

Difficulty arises in deciding whether to use systemic corticosteroid treatment in chronic non-fatal dermatoses, for if such treatment is begun it may have to be continued indefinitely. It is established practice to use oral treatment to tide a patient over a severe attack of urticaria, erythema multiforme or a drug eruption, since these are likely to be self-limiting. A severe attack of eczema which is attributable to some remediable stimulus, such as contact with a known irritant, can reasonably be suppressed during the period of its activity with the prospect of being able to stop the treatment within a few weeks. The management of lichen planus is more debatable, since local application of the newer corticosteroids under occlusion is so effective. Most debatable of all are cases of obstinate and disabling dermatosis when there is some prospect of being able to effect material improvement there is the risk of the patient permenently requiring corticosteroid treatment. Many dermatologists regard the risk as too great to contemplate in any circumstances; but this is perhaps a somewhat extreme view. It seems probable that if the maintenance dose can be kept at or below 10 mg. of prednisolone daily, and never exceeding 15 mg. daily (except under conditions of stress as mentioned below), the risks are very much reduced and may be acceptable for the few patients who would fall within the terms of the following conditions:

1. The dermatosis is so severe as to interfere seriously with the patient's life and ability to work.
2. A carefully supervised and adequately prolonged period of treatment (say one year) by other means has failed to bring substantial relief.
3. There is no history suggesting peptic ulceration, psychosis, diabetes mellitus, significant hypertension or severe osteoporosis.
4. There is no active focus of tuberculosis. A past history of this disease requires that antituberculous drugs should be given concurrently with corticosteroids. A close watch should be kept during treatment in all cases, irrespective of a known history of tuberculosis, for signs of this disease.
5. The patient is intelligent and co-operative. He should understand the nature of the risk involved in the treatment and accept it. He should be prepared to attend regularly for follow-up, and should carry a corticosteroid treatment card which should be kept up to date.

It is recommended that the initial daily dose of prednisolone should be 15 mg., that, except as mentioned below, this dose should never be exceeded, and that the maintenance dose should be kept at or below 10 mg. daily at a level at which the disease is just active. If worthwhile improvement has not occurred within 12 weeks, the treatment should be abandoned by gradually tailing off the dose.

An increased dose must be given in the presence of infection or if the patient is anaesthetized.

Skin Diseases of the Ear and Nose

The principles of treating skin disease in these sites are the same as for the skin in general. Eczema, psoriasis and staphylococcal folliculitis are the commonest diseases. The narrow external auditory meatus readily becomes blocked by scales or crusts and it must be cleaned out both for the purpose of treatment and in order to examine the drum to ensure that it is normal. This toilet is best done by using cotton-wool on an applicator rather than by syringing. The technique is not easy and the more severe cases should be dealt with by Ear, Nose and Throat specialists. The clean external auditory canal is then packed with gauze impregnated with the appropriate medicament. Most of the eczema in this site is complicated by infection—sometimes by yeasts; it calls for a combination of corticosteroid with an antibacterial agent and, if necessary, nystatin. Particular attention is drawn to the section on eczema dealing with the contact element and listing kinds of application that are undesirable for fear of causing sensitization. They include neomycin, soframycin, antihistamines and surface anaesthetics, and they cause sensitization as readily if applied to the ear as to the open skin. It is justifiable to use corticosteroid applications for treating psoriasis of the external auditory canal.

Lichenification (localized neurodermatitis) is very common in the region of the external auditory meatus. These patients may have an obsession about wax in their ears, or may have developed an irritation in response to a crack or minor injury. Whatever the reason, obsessive rubbing and poking with their fingers may defeat all attempts to cure the condition. The local sedative effect of a corticosteroid application or of crude coal tar is helpful.

Acute staphylococcal folliculitis may supervene from inoculation of organisms by rubbing or it may be of a general staphylococcal infection of the skin. The disease is painful in the acute stage. A useful application is 10 per cent. ichthammol in glycerine.

Both the ear and the nose are prone to develop cracks in the skin through which haemolytic streptococci can enter the tissues, producing erysipelas. It is important not only to give a systemic antibiotic in this infection (pp. 12-13) but also to treat the cracks for some months afterwards with an antibacterial agent, in order to prevent the recurrences that are prone to occur.

Lupus vulgaris is now a rare disease in the United Kingdom, but for that reason the diagnosis is often missed. The nose and ear are common sites. The infection progresses relentlessly unless specific treatment is given (p. 78), and leads to destruction of tissue.

Further Reading

Acne Rosacea

SNEDDON, I. B. (1969). Adverse effect of topical fluorinated corticosteroids in rosacea. *Br. med. J.* **1,** 671.

Acne Vulgaris

BEVERIDGE, G. W. & POWELL, E. W. (1970). The problem of acne. *Practitioner,* **204,** 635.

Antihistamines

Today's Drugs Editorial (1970). *Br. med. J.* **1,** 217.

Contact Eczema

FISHER, A. A. (1967). *Contact Dermatitis.* London: Kimpton.

Fungus infections

IVE, F. A. & MARKS, R. (1968). Tinea incognito. *Br. med. J.* **3,** 149.

Herpes Zoster

ASHTON, H., BEVERIDGE, G. W. & STEVENSON, C. J. (1969). The management of herpes zoster. *Br. J. Derm.* **81,** 874.

Psoriasis

STANKLER, L. (1970). The problem of psoriasis. *Practitioner,* **204,** 625.

Scabies

ALEXANDER, J. O'D. (1968). Scabies and pediculosis. *Practitioner,* **200,** 632.

Zinc

HUSAIN, S. L. (1969). Oral zinc sulphate in leg ulcers. *Lancet,* **1,** 1069.

27. Venereal Diseases

R. Lees

Incidence

Early experience of penicillin therapy in venereal diseases created the widespread belief that these infections had been conquered. It is now realized that this is not true. In the past decade there has been a notable increase in venereal disease in almost every country in the world. This is especially true of gonorrhoea as many strains of the gonococcus are now resistant to penicillin and other antibiotics. Some patients become unwitting carriers of the infection either because of the low virulence of some strains of gonococci or because of inadequate initial treatment. There are numerous factors—medical, social and moral—to explain this disquieting increasing incidence of venereal disease and the difficulties attending its diagnosis and cure. In recent years treatment and tests of cure have often tended to be slipshod and the search for the hidden cases and sources of infection to be neglected. Stricter application of the principles of control will almost certainly solve this problem. More attention is being paid to its moral, psychological and social aspects, especially in adolescents in whom an increased incidence of sexual promiscuity is causing widespread concern. Other factors are homosexuality and a high incidence in immigrants.

Prevention

An adequate discussion of the prevention of venereal disease would include a survey of many aspects of biology, sociology and moral philosophy. It would hardly be appropriate, however, to attempt to deal at length with such matters in this textbook. On the other hand, the family doctor will almost certainly fail to do justice to his responsibilities if he does not recognize two trends of thought on this subject. First, there are limitations to the effectiveness of drugs, for even the antibiotics cannot—without reservations—be classed as specific remedies. Secondly, the ubiquity of venereal disease underlines the fact that the health of the individual and the health of the community cannot always be considered separately. Hence its prevention is bound to be affected by the attitude of people towards promiscuity, prostitution and the sanctity of marriage; and broadly this attitude is determined by the ethos displayed in a community. The doctor who maintains an intelligent interest in these matters is the better equipped to advise those who seek guidance on how to avoid venereal infections; and it would be difficult to exaggerate the importance of this professional responsibility in relation to the prevention of physical disease and the relief of unnecessary anxiety.

The doctor may be consulted by a man (or a woman) recently exposed to the risk of infection. If a man reports within a few hours—not more than 24—after coitus with a woman suspected of suffering from venereal disease he should be advised to wash his genitals, thighs and lower abdomen with soap and warm water. The application of antiseptic lotions or ointments is of little value, and strong preparations may be positively harmful if they excite a chemical inflammation. The injection of 2·4 g. of procaine penicillin will certainly prevent gonorrhoea and will almost certainly prevent syphilis. Such treatment should not be given frequently. Observation and also serological tests should be made during the following three months. The chances of successful prophylaxis are less certain in the female than the male. A woman or girl recently exposed to infection (by sexual assault or otherwise) should have the vulva gently but thoroughly cleansed and be given an antiseptic douche (e.g. irrigation of chloroxylenol B.N.F.). An injection of 2·4 g. of procaine penicillin should be administered intramuscularly if such treatment can be undertaken within 24 hours of coitus.

If a nurse or doctor has pricked or scratched the skin while attending to a patient with contagious syphilis, the area should be cleansed and disinfected and 1 mega unit of penicillin given at once, and then procaine penicillin, 600 mg. daily for seven days. Serological tests for syphilis should be carried out every four weeks for four months.

If prophylaxis by early treatment cannot be undertaken within 24 hours it is better to give no treatment but to keep the patient under observation. Instructions should be given to watch for the development of signs and symptoms of disease and appropriate tests should be undertaken, the patient being kept under observation for four months.

GONORRHOEA

The natural history of gonorrhoea has changed in the past 30 years. Formerly the patient experienced characteristic symptoms and signs within a few days of infection. Today many patients experience little disturbance and may be unaware that they have acquired the disease. It follows that people who have exposed themselves to infection should be fully examined. There are also many instances where the unskilled use of specific remedies has created 'latent cases': the patient is symptom free but is nevertheless contagious. Whatever the circumstances, the 'missed case' of gonorrhoea presents special hazards to the individual, his family and the community. It is, therefore, obvious that the management of a case of gonorrhoea, irrespective of its apparent severity, calls for: (1) immediate bacteriological confirmation of the diagnosis; (ii) thorough treatment with specific remedies; (iii) clinical and bacteriological follow-up in convalescence; and (iv) accurate documentation.

The diagnosis is established by the examination of smears and cultures taken from the urethra, cervix and other areas liable to be infected. The use of cultures on an appropriate medium is essential in all cases in which the diagnosis may have to be substantiated in a court of law. If the technique for collecting specimens is sound, cultures in addition to smears give a much higher number of positive results than the examination of stained smears alone. Cultures should be employed in female cases both for diagnosis and as tests of cure. The use of Stuart's medium enables swabs to be sent to a distant laboratory even if 48 hours elapse before the specimen can be examined by the bacteriologist. Special methods are used for rectal examination.

ACUTE GONORRHOEA IN MEN

In the majority of cases the finding of typical gram-negative diplococci intracellularly in a smear of urethral discharge establishes the diagnosis, but in addition to smears, reliance is placed increasingly on cultures and the laboratory will determine the antibiotic sensitivity of the strain of organism isolated. The patient should be given an injection of penicillin at once, provided there is no history of sensitivity to this drug. The dose still in use in many hospitals is 600 mg. of procaine penicillin. It is recommended, however, that in addition 300 mg. of benzyl-penicillin should be given intramuscularly. This combined penicillin therapy should be repeated after 24 hours. If gonococci are still found in the secretions or if the bacteriologist reports that the organism shows resistance to penicillin, drugs of the tetracycline group or erythromycin should be given, 250 mg. four times a day for five days. Formerly, injections of streptomycin were advocated, but the gonococcus is often resistant to this drug and toxic effects frequently occur. The gonococcus can be killed by almost any of the antibiotics in common use, but penicillin is the cheapest, and it is still the most effective provided it is given in adequate doses. Certain proprietary mixtures of benzylpenicillin and procaine penicillin giving a total daily dose of 1 g. have proved satisfactory. A few strains of gonococcus will be killed most easily by high concentrations of penicillin induced by dosage such as 2 g. three times a day. Erythromycin, 250 mg. four times a day for five days, gives a high proportion of cures. Kanamycin, 1 g. injected on two successive days, is also advocated.

Treatment by an oral penicillin (p. 5) is effective in gonorrhoea, but it is not recommended unless the patient can be trusted to take the drug regularly and for the time advised. A dose of 250 mg. phenoxymethylpenicillin four times a day for three days will prove effective in about 90 per cent. of cases.

When there is a recurrence of symptoms this is due to reinfection in many cases, but if this can be excluded a search should be made for a focus of persistent infection and intensive treatment given, using the same drug or another antibiotic such as tetracycline or erythromycin in doses of 1 g. daily for five days.

Persistence of the symptoms but without the presence of organisms may be due to a coincident infection with *Trichomonas vaginalis*, or due to abacterial urethritis. For such cases appropriate treatment is described later (p. 605).

The patient should be advised to avoid alcoholic drinks for two weeks, and to abstain from sexual intercourse until cure is established. As the discharge diminishes rapidly it is seldom necessary to advise special precautions against soiling of clothing and bed linen. The simplest protection is a square of lint pinned inside the pants; clothing or linen which has been soiled by discharge can be sterilized by soaking for some hours in a weak chloroxylenol solution and then laundered in the usual way. The patient should take baths daily. After using the bath it may be rendered safe for others by swabbing immediately after use with chloroxylenol and finally ensuring that it is left dry. Care must be taken to avoid the use of towels which may be used by others, especially by young girls.

ACUTE GONORRHOEA IN WOMEN

It is much more difficult to establish the diagnosis in women than men, and repeated tests using both smears and cultures from the urethra, vagina, cervix and Bartholin's glands may be necessary. The continued high incidence of gonorrhoea is due, in part, to inefficient methods of diagnosis. The disease is more difficult to cure in women, and the use of antibiotics for leucorrhoea without exact diagnosis and bacteriological control is a great disservice to the patient and to the community. Tests conducted immediately after a menstrual period may prove positive though previous tests have been negative. Rectal infection is not rare.

The treatment advised for an uncomplicated case is the intramuscular injection of 300 mg. of benzylpenicillin plus 600 mg. of procaine penicillin. This therapy should be repeated after 24 and 48 hours. If there is any complication the dosage should be higher—such as 300 mg. benzylpenicillin twice daily supplemented by 600 mg. of procaine penicillin once daily, continued for five to seven days according to the clinical response. In cases of penicillin resistance a drug of the tetracycline group should be prescribed—for example, chlortetracycline, 250 mg. four times daily for one week. Erythromycin, 250 mg. four times a day for five days, is equally effective and kanamycin, 1 g. injected on two successive days, gives almost a 100 per cent. cure.

The same general principles apply to women as to men. Sexual intercourse must be avoided and patients should be warned that in the acute and subacute phases of the infection vigorous exercise during menstrual periods is likely to cause pelvic infection. A woman may use a sanitary pad as protection against soiling, but vaginal tampons are not recommended.

Serological and Bacteriological Tests

At the outset the blood should be tested to exclude syphilis by sensitive and specific tests. While the Wassermann and Khan tests are quite reliable the best results are now obtained by the V.D.R.L. (Venereal Disease Reference Laboratory) and R.P.C.F.T. (Reiter's Protein Complement Fixation Test). Little reliance can be put on the gonococcus complement fixation test. The tests for syphilis should be repeated at intervals of four weeks until four months after the end of treatment.

Tests of the secretions collected from the genito-urinary tract should be made at the end of the first, second and third weeks, and then at the end of two and three months after treatment. In women the specimens should be obtained immediately after menstruation. A man should have the secretion expressed from the prostate and seminal vesicles by prostatic massage examined on at least two occasions during tests of cure. If all tests remain negative, and there is no coincident infection, the patient can be assured of cure. It is important to be emphatic about cure when this is justified as otherwise many patients have secret fears for years, causing much unhappiness.

Local Complications of Gonorrhoea in Men

These are now rare in this country; the commonest are prostatitis and epididymo-orchitis.

Acute prostatitis. The patient should be kept in bed and the pain relieved by appropriate sedatives; some patients require injections of morphine and atropine. Hot baths often relieve difficulty with micturition, and even though retention of urine threatens, it is seldom necessary to catheterize, and this should be avoided if possible. The acute symptoms and signs generally subside within 48 hours of treatment with penicillin unless an abscess has formed. Benzylpenicillin should be given in large amounts—at least 1·2 g. per day—and continued for five to seven days. If an abscess has formed it may point into the urethra, and when rupture occurs there is a profuse discharge of pus and rapid relief ensues. In exceptional cases it may be necessary to drain a prostatic abscess by perineal incision, which is a major operation of considerable technical difficulty.

Subacute or chronic prostatitis. This often occurs in the course of gonorrhoea and is easily overlooked. Treatment by prostatic massage twice weekly, and several courses of antibiotics should be continued until the fluid obtained by prostatic massage is free from excess of pus and organisms.

Epididymitis. Precipitating factors are sexual excitement or coitus, heavy manual work or occasionally very active exercise. The pain may be severe for a few days, but is generally relieved by hot kaolin poultices, a supporting bandage and pad, and if necessary analgesic drugs. Rest in bed is

generally necessary for a few days. Benzylpenicillin in doses of 600 mg. thrice daily should be
given for three to five days; rapid relief of pain and
urinary symptoms follows. The swelling of the
epididymis subsides more slowly and may not be
complete for two or three weeks. Most cases
resolve completely without permanent damage, but
a few may have residual fibrosis of the lower pole,
and if bilateral epididymitis has occurred sterility
may result.

Patients who have epididymitis have in addition
infection of the prostate and seminal vesicles, and
after the acute phase the latter should be given the
treatment advised for subacute or chronic prostatitis.

Epididymitis due to organisms other than the
gonococcus is not uncommon, and may be due to
infection of the bladder, prostate and urethra with
E. coli, staphylococcus, *B. proteus* and rarely
Trichomonas vaginalis. There is also a type of
non-specific epididymitis which does not appear to
be associated with urinary infection but causes
severe epididymo-orchitis, often followed by testicular atrophy. The cause is unknown, and no
specific treatment is likely to be effective. Tuberculous epididymitis is occasionally mistaken for
venereal infection, and in those who have lived in
tropical countries filarial infection has to be considered. In older men suffering from epididymitis a
complete genito-urinary investigation should be
carried out to exclude stricture of the urethra,
enlarged prostate or the presence of calculi and
chronic infection.

Epididymitis associated with staphylococcal or
coliform infections may lead to suppuration and
rupture of the abscess into the scrotal sac. The
scrotum becomes distended with pus which must be
evacuated surgically and in addition active treatment must be given with the antibiotic to which the
organism is sensitive.

Balanitis. Phimosis and superficial erosion of
the glans penis and inner surface of the prepuce are
often encountered in gonorrhoea. Syphilis and
chancroid must be excluded. Healing is rapid if the
gonorrhoea is treated with streptomycin, 1 g. daily
for three days and 1 g. of sulphadimidine is given
four times a day for five days. The tissues should
be kept clean by saline dressings or by syringing
below the prepuce. Such treatment does not hinder
the diagnosis of syphilis by dark-field examination
of exudate from the abraded area. Serological
tests for syphilis must be continued for four
months.

Peri-urethral abscess. This complication of
gonorrhoea is now rare and is found mainly in
relation to a stricture of the urethra. If the abscess
points externally it should be aspirated and penicillin solution (1 ml. containing 150 mg.) injected
into the abscess cavity. At the same time active
treatment of the infected urethra is continued.
Dilatation of the urethra by bougies is subsequently
necessary to prevent stricture, but this should be
delayed until the inflammation has subsided completely.

Conjunctivitis. Gonococcal infection of the
conjunctiva of an adult is rare in Britain but not
uncommon in primitive peoples. A very severe
inflammation occurs, often causing damage to the
cornea and thus impairment of vision. Treatment
consists of parenteral administration of penicillin—
for example 1·2 g. at once, followed by procaine
penicillin, 600 mg. once daily for three to five
days. (Injection of procaine penicillin B.P. 2 ml.
contains 600 mg.). This should be supplemented
by irrigation of the conjunctival sac with 1 per
cent. saline at blood temperature and the instillation every hour of drops of penicillin solution (6 mg.
per ml.) for 24 hours. After the first day drops of
10 per cent. solution of sodium sulphacetamide
may be instilled every four hours. If treatment is
given without delay early complete recovery is to
be expected.

Infections of the skin. Gonorrhoea seldom
causes infection of the skin but, occasionally, small
abscesses occur, especially in the skin of the penis,
or a small sinus develops. Infected parameatal
glands, or infection of the small glands at the
frenum may occur. If a collection of pus forms
this should be aspirated or drained, and a permanent cure is achieved by destroying the infected
duct or sinus by the use of an electric cautery
needle.

The lesions associated with keratoderma blen-
norrhagica (pustules and hypertrophic papules on
the soles and palms, and the characteristic balanitis)
are regarded now as non-gonococcal, and part of
Reiter's syndrome (p. 597). They need no special
treatment apart from protection.

Local Complications of Gonorrhoea in Women
Urethritis. In women this is seldom troublesome.
Infection of the parameatal ducts (Skene's tubules)
is best treated by obliteration by electric cautery.

Bartholinian abscess. This may be treated by aspiration and injection of penicillin solution. If the abscess has burst leaving a sinus, it is often necessary to drain it more completely by incision, followed by packing the cavity. Chronic infections may require operative removal of the gland.

Vaginitis. This is generally due to coincident infection by *Trichomonas vaginalis*, yeasts or fungi and the treatment is described on p. 605.

Cervical erosion. The acute erosion associated with gonococcal infection of the cervix heals rapidly under specific treatment, but chronic erosions, due to chronic infection by a variety of organisms and damage to the external os, generally require treatment by cauterization or excision.

Metritis. This is very frequently associated with salpingitis. The patient should be confined to bed for three to seven days; sedatives and analgesics are given to relieve pain, and penicillin is injected in doses of 300 mg. four times a day for three to five days. This treatment usually gives rapid relief. Pessaries and tampons are useless, and douching is harmful. If the vagina is heavily infected it may be treated once daily by swabbing with a dilute antiseptic, using a bivalve speculum, and the patient should be nursed in the semi-recumbent position. If there is a mixed infection tetracycline or erythromycin should be given (500 mg. four times daily).

Salpingitis (*and salpingo-oophoritis*). This may occur as an acute abdominal emergency and present a difficult diagnostic problem. When the diagnosis of gonococcal infection can be established the treatment is chemotherapeutic rather than surgical and the prognosis is good unless a pyosalpinx develops.

Pain is relieved by analgesics: paracetamol in doses of 1 g. four-hourly may be tried, but in severe cases it may be necessary to give several doses of morphine (15 mg.) and atropine (1 mg.). Some relief may be obtained by hot applications to the lower abdomen. Douching or any form of vaginal treatment is likely to make the patient worse.

The patient should be nursed propped up in a semi-recumbent position and penicillin should be given in doses of 300 mg. four times a day and continued until the temperature falls to normal. It is advisable to give erythromycin or tetracycline in addition, especially in cases which occur in the puerperium or after a miscarriage.

If the condition has progressed to pyosalpinx the affected tube and ovary will remain palpable *per vaginam* as a mass in the pelvis, often with wide-spread adhesions. Surgical removal can be undertaken with greater safety and ease after adequate chemotherapy for two to three weeks.

In many cases the tubal infection is never acute: it presents as a subacute or chronic inflammation, often with extensive adhesions and inflammation in the pelvis, causing recurrent backache, menstrual pain and irregularity, urinary infection and general ill-health. Several examinations may be required before the nature of the infection becomes clear.

Treatment consists in (*a*) giving penicillin or erythromycin for five to ten days—treatment which may be repeated with advantage during the next menstrual period; (*b*) diathermy directed to the pelvic organs, given daily at first and later on alternate days for a month; (*c*) in a few instances benefit may follow dilatation of the cervix and uterine curettage, but this should not be undertaken till adequate trial has been made of chemotherapy and short-wave diathermy. If extensive damage has occurred, a total hysterectomy and salpingectomy should be performed.

Proctitis. This occurs in both men and women, usually as the result of unnatural sexual acts. It may be a sequel to a prostatic abscess.

Treatment by injections of penicillin daily for five days (p. 597) may be supplemented by rectal irrigations or the use of suppositories containing proflavine. These are required only when there are extensive areas of infiltration and superficial ulceration, and this is exceptional. Proctoscopic examination will indicate how long treatment has to be continued. Special media are used for tests of cure.

Metastatic Complications of Gonorrhoea

These are now uncommon and occur mainly in chronic or neglected cases or when inadequate treatment has left an unsuspected focus of infection. Many of these complications, formerly attributed to gonorrhoea, are now regarded as being due to Reiter's syndrome or to non-specific urethral infections (p. 596).

Arthritis. Acute gonococcal arthritis involves a large joint as a rule, and is similar to acute infective arthritis due to other organisms. There is acute pain and limitation of movement with swelling, redness and severe fever. If the joint is aspirated or explored surgically, it is found to contain a purulent exudate, and often the synovial membrane and the articular surface are eroded. Pus taken from the joint may contain gonococci, but it is often difficult to find the organism and negative reports by the bacteriologist do not preclude the diagnosis.

Acute gonococcal arthritis requires vigorous treatment with penicillin: the dose is 300 mg. four times daily for five to ten days. It is often advantageous to inject it into the joint after aspiration of the pus, and for this purpose 1 ml. of the injection of penicillin B.P. (containing 150 mg. per ml.) is satisfactory. The joint should be partially immobilized, but plaster fixation is seldom advisable. In addition to penicillin it may be necessary to give appropriate antibiotic therapy for the control of other organisms present in the genital tract. The usual measures for relief of pain are adopted. In gonococcal arthritis it is wise to start passive and active movements as soon as the pain abates, and diathermy is sometimes helpful. At a later stage massage and exercises will contribute to full recovery of function.

Chronic arthritis associated with gonorrhoea is often difficult to diagnose and may simulate closely other types of chronic infective or rheumatoid arthritis; a strongly positive G.C.F.T. along with a history suggesting previous gonorrhoea and the presence of a focus of infection in the pelvic organs helps to confirm the diagnosis. Such patients benefit relatively little from sulphonamides, penicillin or other antibiotics. The most valuable measures are those designed to secure drainage of any enclosed focus of infection. Diathermy to the pelvic organs is helpful; prostatic massage will be necessary in males and treatment (or removal) of chronically infected pelvic organs in females.

Iritis (*and iridocyclitis*). This can be present as an acute condition with much pain, exudate and adhesions in the anterior chamber and subsequent deterioration of vision. A few patients have attacks recurring at intervals of several months or even years. Chronic cases tend to be associated with considerable adhesions and corneal opacity.

Acute cases require rest in bed, full dilatation of the pupil by atropine, application of heat to the eye, and large doses of penicillin. When the ocular inflammation has subsided any foci of infection in the genital tract should receive appropriate treatment. Steroids locally help to preserve vision.

Chronic iritis responds to treatment similar to that described above for acute iritis. In resistant cases hydrocortisone eye drops should be instilled three or four times a day. There is a frequent association with chronic prostatitis; if this is present it also requires treatment (p. 593).

NON-GONOCOCCAL URETHRITIS IN MEN

This condition has become very common; many cases are trivial, but others are as severe as gonorrhoea and much more difficult to treat. There are many possible causes, and it is particularly important to carry out tests which will exclude gonorrhoea and identify the causal organisms. Therefore, before any treatment is given, smears of the urethral discharge should be prepared for examination and cultures inoculated—using either the discharge or the deposit from the centrifuged urine. In many cases, although the smear may show numerous pus cells, no growth is obtained on culture. Some cases are due to infestation with *Trichomonas vaginalis*. A few are attributable to fungus infection, and virus infection has been suspected but not proved.

Subacute urethritis is often part of a widespread infection of the urinary tract associated with pyelonephritis or cystitis, enlarged prostate, urethral stricture, calculus, neoplasm or a combination of two or more of these conditions. It is important to establish a complete diagnosis and not to be content to treat the one sign—urethritis—of a more generalized disease. Some cases of severe and recurrent urethritis are due to active homosexual practices, and treatment is futile while sodomy continues.

Any series of cases of non-gonococcal urethritis is made up of a variety of infections, and indeed there are patients in whom bacterial invasion has not been confirmed. It is therefore impossible to visualize 'specific treatment' in the usual sense. Nevertheless, the use of certain antibiotics results in clinical cure in a high proportion of cases. The most effective preparation is tetracycline, 500 mg. four times daily for five days. Alternatively, erythromycin can be used, 250 mg. four times daily for five days; or streptomycin, 1 g. injected intramuscularly daily for three to five days. Penicillin is seldom effective and should not be used. The sulphonamides are often curative (sulphadimidine 2 g. followed by 1 g. four times daily for 10 days), but this therapy is less reliable than treatment with the tetracyclines.

Many cases of non-specific urethritis are associated with subacute or chronic prostatitis, and failure to eradicate infection from this focus may explain recurrences.

Residual urethritis, often obstinately resistant to treatment, may follow gonorrhoea, or may be due to a supervening 'virus' type of infection or to stricture of the urethra developing earlier than usual. If there are no obstructive complications and if the invading organisms are accessible to antiseptics, final recovery often follows urethral irrigations twice daily with solutions such as oxychloride of mercury 1 : 6,000 solution ; chloramine T, 1 : 5,000 solution; or potassium permanganate, 1 : 8,000 solution. Chronic prostatitis or stricture of the urethra calls for appropriate treatment.

Urethritis associated with *Trichomonas vaginalis* infection usually subsides rapidly following treatment with metronidazole which is very effective (p. 606). The main difficulty arises from reinfection, and simultaneous treatment of the sexual partner is important. Where symptoms persist, urethral irrigations twice daily (see above) and prostatic massage should be employed.

Reiter's syndrome. The full syndrome comprises non-gonococcal urethritis, arthritis, conjunctivitis, iritis and skin lesions; and there is usually irregular fever, increased blood sedimentation rate, and, occasionally, an abnormal electrocardiographic record. In many cases the syndrome is incomplete, and symptoms referable to the genito-urinary or intestinal tracts may be present.

The condition is not relieved by sulphonamides, penicillin, streptomycin or chloramphenicol but about 30 per cent. of cases appear to benefit from oxytetracycline in doses of 2 g. per day for five days. Repeated courses may be given. The urethritis is amenable to urethral irrigations of 1 : 6,000 solution of oxycyanide of mercury. Sulphacetamide eyedrops (B.P.C.) instilled two-hourly give relief from conjunctivitis. If iritis occurs, the pupil should be kept fully dilated (1 per cent. atropine sulphate locally) and Hydrocortisone Eye-Drops, B.P.C., instilled every four hours.

Painful joints call for the following palliative therapy: aspirin, 1 g. four-hourly; light splints (not plaster) for affected joints, and radiant heat or diathermy if pain persists and is troublesome; corticosteroids are effective but are seldom necessary; phenylbutazone may be used if aspirin does not give relief (p. 450).

The skin lesions require no special treatment except protection, and as the crusts of keratodermia begin to separate the process can be assisted by soaking with arachis oil or by the application of elastoplast.

In addition to the symptomatic measures described above, it has been found that some patients benefit from fever therapy—though this is an empirical form of treatment. Febrile reactions are induced by injecting TAB vaccine intravenously. The first dose should be small (not over 25 million organisms) and subsequent doses at intervals of two or three days should be increased according to the fever induced by previous doses. Three to six doses may be needed.

Reiter's syndrome has a tendency to recur even after apparent recovery and without reinfection. The probability of recurrence, however, is even greater if the patient acquires a gonorrhoeal or a non-specific urethritis.

Permanent damage to the joints is an occasional sequel. Physiotherapy (heat, massage, movement, exercises) may be needed for several months.

Stricture of the urethra. In all patients who have had severe or prolonged urethritis, routine urethroscopic examination during convalescence may enable the physician to make a diagnosis of stricture in its earliest stages, and appropriate treatment may ensure permanent relief. First, chemotherapy is required in order to suppress the urinary infection which is almost invariably present, and then progressive dilatation of the stricture is carried out by bougies and sounds. Instrumental treatment calls for strict asepsis. In a few instances excision of the stricture is possible. The treatment of most of the complications of stricture of the urethra is surgical.

SYPHILIS

In the United Kingdom and most European countries there has been an increase in early contagious syphilis. Though not yet alarming, it indicates the need to search for and discover the sources of infection and contacts. Many cases are due to male homosexual practices or are 'imports' from tropical and other countries where there is a high incidence of the disease. Cases of inherited syphilis are now very rarely seen. There has been a moderate increase in the number of patients with late syphilis, and some bizarre forms are encountered. Recent improvements in serological diagnosis have aided the detection of late syphilis.

DRUG TREATMENT
Penicillin

This is still the most effective drug, and procaine penicillin in aqueous suspension with aluminium monostearate is the preparation of choice. The arsenical compounds and bismuth have been discarded. There is no evidence that syphilis has become penicillin-resistant, or that cases of early syphilis are being masked by the use of penicillin and other antibiotics given for gonorrhoea and other infections. The concentration of penicillin required for efficient treatment is not high, but it must be maintained almost constantly for a considerable period—for example 10 days in early syphilis and not less than 20 days in late syphilis. There is little or no benefit to be derived from high concentrations of penicillin except in a few cases of syphilis of the central nervous system or the eye. A more troublesome problem now is the increasing number of people who are sensitized to penicillin and in whom an injection of the drug may produce signs and symptoms varying from a mild skin eruption to a dangerous (or even fatal) syncope. Oral treatment of syphilis with penicillin has not been widely used, but there is scope for this method in children. Again, when prolonged courses are given to combat the effects of syphilis on the cardiovascular and nervous systems oral preparations are to be preferred because patients find a protracted series of injections very irksome. There is some place for the use of penicillins with a more sustained action than that of procaine penicillin: benzathine penicillin has been employed effectively in late syphilis, but it should not be used in early syphilis as the blood levels attained with this preparation are inadequate for the needs of such patients.

The amounts of penicillin required in the treatment of syphilis in an adult are:

Early syphilis (sero-negative)—6 g. in 10 days.

Early syphilis (sero-positive) and secondary syphilis within five years of onset—12 to 20 g. in 20 days.

Late syphilis—12 to 20 g. in 20 days, and several courses may be required.

The doses given above are average and are based on current clinical experience. In late syphilis the effects on symptoms and signs and the patient's general condition provide the best guide to general management rather than a rigid observance of a particular scheme of dosage. Heroic attempts to reverse 'positive' reactions in the blood or cerebrospinal fluid are to be deprecated.

Other antibiotics. Many antibiotics have some effect in syphilis, but the tetracyclines or erythro-

mycin are the only practical alternatives to penicillin. The dose advised is 30 to 40 g. over a period of 14 to 20 days. The results are not as good as with penicillin; side-effects are common and prolonged supervision and testing are essential.

BISMUTH. Most physicians have abandoned the use of bismuth in the treatment of syphilis, and it is certainly not required in the early stages of the disease. Nevertheless we believe it is still valuable in late syphilis. Bismuth oxychloride can be given as the B.P.C. injection which is a sterile suspension containing 10 per cent. of the bismuth salt. This preparation is given intramuscularly, usually at intervals of five to seven days, and a series of injections is given for 10 to 12 weeks. The precautions necessary prior to each injection are to test the urine for protein, to record the weight and to examine the condition of the teeth and gums. This drug may cause stomatitis and a blue line of bismuth sulphide on the gums (if the patient is not edentulous); these toxic effects can be avoided by insisting on careful hygiene of the mouth and teeth.

Bismuth therapy is a valuable prelude to treatment with penicillin in late syphilis; it supplants penicillin in chronic or relapsing cases; and it is used as a supplement to erythromycin in those unfortunate patients who cannot tolerate penicillin because of sensitivity reactions.

ORGANIC ARSENICALS. These drugs have been supplanted by penicillin in the treatment of all types of syphilis. They are now seldom used. If, however, a patient is intolerant of penicillin, the organic arsenicals may be given, and the best for this purpose is oxophenarsine hydrochloride.

HERXHEIMER REACTIONS. The reaction of Jarisch–Herxheimer may result from the treatment of syphilis by any specific drug which acts quickly. The main features occur within 12 to 48 hours of giving an effective dose of the drug and consist of a rise in temperature up to 40° C., a rapid pulse and a general constitutional upset. At the same time the signs of the disease are temporarily aggravated—the skin eruption becomes more intense, the primary lesions larger and more oedematous, and the lymph glands more swollen and tender. This reaction is most pronounced in early syphilis, in which it is of little consequence apart from the discomfort which is experienced by the patient. In late syphilis the Herxheimer reaction may be more serious and may constitute a danger to life, especially if there is ulceration of the larynx or coronary arterial disease. Neurological signs may be seriously aggravated especially in dementia paralytica when maniacal outbursts may develop, or in optic atrophy when a rapid contraction of the visual field may occur.

It has been demonstrated that the Herxheimer reaction is an 'all or none' phenomenon, and that the practice of starting treatment with minute doses of the drug is futile. Small doses have no therapeutic value; as soon as they reach a sufficient size to have any curative effect they may cause reactions which tend to be prolonged. Whenever it is particularly important to avoid Herxheimer reactions (e.g. in cardiac cases) a short preliminary course of bismuth injections should be given (three or four weeks); penicillin may then be used with safety. If there is no contraindication the Herxheimer reaction may be suppressed by giving 40 mg. of prednisone daily in divided doses for four or five days.

In early syphilis there is no danger from the Herxheimer reaction; the infection must be controlled and the patient made non-contagious by the immediate use of penicillin in adequate doses. The onset of a febrile reaction, a skin rash and general malaise must not be confused with the hypersensitivity reactions which occur not uncommonly during the course of penicillin therapy. When the clinical disturbances are attributable to the Herxheimer reaction, recovery is rapid and treatment with penicillin must be continued.

Early Syphilis

Treatment must be prompt, vigorous and sustained. For a case of sero-negative primary syphilis it suffices to give 600 mg. of procaine penicillin daily on 10 consecutive days. The patient becomes non-contagious in 24 to 48 hours, so that isolation in hospital is unnecessary. The local lesion requires only a bland dressing and healing occurs within 7 to 10 days.

Serological tests should be performed after the first, second and third months subsequent to treatment and thereafter every three months for a total period of two years. Sexual intercourse should be forbidden during the first six months as relapse, though uncommon, may occur within this period and will be accompanied by positive serological tests. It is unnecessary to forbid alcohol.

Sero-positive and Secondary Syphilis

Sero-positive cases within one year of infection and secondary syphilis require double the amount of penicillin advised for early syphilis. The daily dose should be increased to 600 mg. benzylpenicillin twice daily for 20 days. Herxheimer reactions are usual in the first 24 hours. The titre of the serological tests should be noted each month following treatment and a rapid decline to a negative test should occur, usually within three months. If the titre remains high, or if it declines and then rises appreciably, a relapse is imminent and further treatment should be undertaken. Relapsed patients are often contagious even though there may be no obvious lesions of the skin or mucous membranes. Relapse of this type is uncommon, but it may be overlooked unless regular serological control is maintained. More frequent is an alleged relapse which is in reality a reinfection, the patient acquiring a fresh inoculation of organisms at a new site, and the blood reactions slowly becoming 'positive'. Such reinfections are as readily cured by penicillin as the original one. Patients who relapse after apparent recovery develop positive serological tests for syphilis in a high titre; they may have small ulcers and fissures at the muco-cutaneous junctions, and *Treponema pallidum* may be identified in the exudate from these lesions.

Occasionally, at this stage of the infection there are clear indications of involvement of the central nervous system and meninges—such as headache and paresis of one or more of the cranial nerves, usually the 3rd, 4th or 6th nerve. Additional evidence is obtained from examination of the cerebrospinal fluid: the cell count is high (20 to 100 per ml.) and the total protein may be increased (60 to 100 mg. per 100 ml.); the Wassermann reaction is usually positive and the Lange gold sol test gives a maximum change in the third zone, but occasionally figures of the 'paretic' type are recorded (5554210000). Such meningeal infections respond rapidly, and usually completely, to treatment with penicillin. The amount advised is 1 g. daily for 21 days. One month after this course the CSF should be re-examined, and if the cell count and protein content are normal no more treatment is required. Nevertheless, prolonged observation is essential and lumbar puncture should be repeated after six months. If the CSF is still markedly abnormal, repetition of the penicillin course totalling 20 to 30 g. is advocated, supplemented by an intramuscular injection of bismuth (200 mg.) weekly for 10 weeks. The ultimate prognosis is very good, complete recovery being almost invariable.

U

Gummatous Syphilis

The patient presents with a gumma of skin, bone or subcutaneous tissue. Effective treatment consists of penicillin, 20 g. in 21 days, followed by an intramuscular injection of bismuth oxychloride, 200 mg. weekly for 10 weeks. The courses of penicillin and bismuth may be repeated two or more times, but it is wise to remember that the positive serological tests in such cases are usually persistent, and more harm follows overdosage with specific remedies than is likely to ensue from the disease. It is important to ascertain whether the cardiovascular and nervous systems are also affected by active syphilitic disease. If these structures are involved treatment should be given on the lines described below. Prolonged observation of the patient is essential.

Cardiovascular Syphilis

This should be suspected in all syphilitic patients who have had the disease for 10 years or more. A meticulous examination at the outset for the earliest signs of aortitis should be repeated at intervals of 6 to 12 months.

In established cases the best that can be achieved is to arrest the syphilitic process and to help the patient to adjust his life to a regimen suitable for his age, disease and circumstances. In a few cases surgical measures may prolong life.

Treatment consists of general management (rest, diet, hygiene, etc.), special measures (digoxin and diuretics) if there is evidence of cardiac failure (p. 85) and specific treatment with penicillin and bismuth to bring the active syphilitic infection under control. It is essential that penicillin therapy should be prolonged, but it must not be too intensive. Reactions of the Herxheimer type must be avoided. Treatment which includes the immediate administration of large doses of penicillin is apt to lead to a 'therapeutic paradox', in which the patient makes a spectacular recovery for a period of weeks or months and then rapidly deteriorates as fibrosis occurs in the damaged tissues. If this misfortune develops the patient's chief requirement is relief of cardiac symptoms; little benefit can be expected from further treatment with penicillin.

Treatment of cardiovascular syphilis should begin with weekly injections of bismuth (injection of bismuth oxychloride B.P.C., 200 mg. intramuscularly for 5 to 10 weeks). The presence of slight proteinuria is not a contraindication to the use of bismuth injections, but the amount of protein in the urine should be estimated every week: it is likely to diminish as myocardial function improves. Penicillin has been given safely to many thousands of patients suffering from syphilitic involvement of the cardiovascular system. In a very small number untoward effects have been reported including angina, dyspnoea and death within 48 hours of starting treatment due to occlusion of a coronary artery or rupture of an aneurysm. If penicillin is given only after a five-week course of bismuth injections, the risk of serious reactions is greatly reduced. A dosage scheme based on 600 mg. of procaine penicillin daily is well tolerated and should be continued for three weeks and then, after an interval of about a month, the course should be repeated. Subsequent treatment is guided by clinical observation. Each patient must be considered as an individual problem; treatment by schedule is unwise. Even when the disease is severe, patients with cardiac and aortic syphilis may survive for many years if treatment is cautious at the start, and provided that they are carefully supervised during the subsequent long period of observation.

Syphilis of the peripheral vessels is a comparative rarity and reacts well to the type of treatment advised for gummatous lesions (see above).

Syphilis of the Central Nervous System

General paralysis of the insane (G.P.I.). Dementia paralytica is now generally diagnosed and treated at a relatively early stage and therefore complete or partial recovery is usual. This early stage is the phase usually characterized by disorders of conduct. The supervision and control of the patient has, therefore, to be seriously considered. Many require admission to hospital, and even there they may prove disturbing or dangerous unless special provision is made for their management. They may be uncooperative, noisy, or dirty in their habits rather than maniacal or suicidal. Initially treatment may aggravate the symptoms and a patient who is merely a talkative nuisance may be transformed into a dangerous maniac. Admission to a mental hospital may be the only way to ensure adequate treatment.

In the preliminary physical examination special attention should be paid to the nervous and cardiovascular systems. A lumbar puncture should then be carried out. General paralysis of the insane is not benefited initially by treatment with bismuth, so the risk of precipitating a Herxheimer reaction by penicillin therapy must be accepted. As a rule it is necessary to give it in full doses without delay of more than a few days—time that will necessarily be spent in examination, observation and sedative treatment. The aggravation of symptoms after penicillin may be associated with a febrile reaction and the patient should be confined to bed and receive sedatives as required. Benzylpenicillin, in doses of 300 mg. four times a day should be given for at least two weeks, supplemented by bismuth, 200 mg. intramuscularly once each week for 10 weeks.

By clinical observation and by periodic examination of the cerebrospinal fluid the patient's progress is assessed and his need for further treatment is determined. As a rule the cell count and protein content of the C.S.F. return to normal within six months, but the positive Wassermann reaction and the paretic gold sol curve remain unchanged for a long time. Some authorities consider it safe to stop treatment when the cell count and protein content of the C.S.F. are normal. In the writer's experience, however, it is wiser to secure appreciable improvement in the Wassermann reaction and gold sol test, and this may require two or three courses of penicillin and bismuth over a period of one to three years. When clinical recovery is complete and the C.S.F. is nearly normal a permanent recovery is probable. In a few patients, however, even when fully treated, the disease proves to be intractable: cerebral atrophy occurs with progressive dementia —often associated with epileptic seizures. These convulsions can be suppressed by symptomatic treatment, but the mental deterioration is incurable and usually progressive.

Fever therapy has been almost completely abandoned but is still beneficial for those patients who do not respond satisfactorily to penicillin. Pyrotherapy is carried out conveniently and effectively in a special fever cabinet, and this has supplanted the therapeutic induction of malaria—a form of treatment less easy to control and not without danger. The contraindications to fever treatment are an age over 55, maniacal excitement, nephritis, hypertension, severe cardiovascular disease, gross obesity and pregnancy.

Treatment by fever cabinet, though more efficient, is only available at a very few centres. Temperatures of 40·5° to 41° C. should be maintained for four to six hours and the sessions repeated on 8 to 12 occasions. The patient should be given 1·2 g. of benzylpenicillin just before entering the cabinet as there is some evidence that penicillin penetrates into brain tissue more readily during fever.

In G.P.I. the prognosis is favourable in about 30 per cent. if treatment can be given without delay; and this is true even when the severity of the symptoms causes concern. Maniacal or very depressed patients may recover completely. On the other hand, if mental deterioration has occurred, partial recovery or arrested progress of the disease is the best that can be expected. The value of partial success should not be underrated, for many of these patients live happier lives as a result of treatment and may also become easier to manage.

Tabes dorsalis. This condition responds moderately well to specific treatment. Some relief of symptoms may be expected, but the signs are unchanged.

The general treatment follows the lines advocated above, namely several courses of penicillin and bismuth, with assessment of clinical progress and tests of the cerebrospinal fluid as guides to the need for additional therapy. As a rule, established tabes dorsalis requires treatment for two years to ensure the maximum recovery. Fever therapy usually makes tabetics worse, but it may be tried if other remedies have failed in patients who have severe tabetic pains and crises. Fever therapy may also be indicated in rapidly progressing optic atrophy. It is most convenient to describe the treatment of tabes dorsalis under the headings of the commonest symptoms of the disease.

VISUAL FAILURE due to optic atrophy is often advanced before it is diagnosed and the response to treatment is very disappointing, but in about 30 per cent. of cases atrophy may be arrested. A short period of treatment with bismuth—e.g. two or three doses in 10 days—should be followed by penicillin (p. 598), and this should be continued for three weeks. The possible occurrence of a Herxheimer reaction should be prevented by corticosteroids. After an interval of four weeks a second course, which may be more intensive, should be given. Progress should be assessed by monthly measurement of the fields of vision. In cases where deterioration is rapid and is not slowed or arrested by two courses of treatment, fever therapy is indicated. A change of occupation is often necessary as a result of the disability. If there is severe loss of vision the patient should be registered as a 'blind person' and training carried out under the auspices of the various agencies who assist the blind. Such blind persons may acquire a high degree of skill and remain contented and useful citizens.

ATAXIA may diminish considerably following remedial exercises under the direction of a physiotherapist as described on p. 379. Tabetics employed among machinery or on dangerous sites should change their job. Ataxia is always worse after a period of confinement to bed and every effort should be made to prevent tabetics from becoming even partially bed-ridden. Whether the tabetic is fit to drive a motor vehicle has to be decided for the individual patient; it is generally unsafe for him to do so.

PAINS. The peculiar shooting pains of tabes dorsalis may vary from a mild nuisance ('the rheumatics') to agonizing bouts of pain that overwhelm even the most stoical. The pains generally diminish after treatment with penicillin and bismuth though they are often aggravated during the earlier stages of this treatment. For symptomatic relief moderate doses of mild analgesics should be tried (aspirin 1 g. or paracetamol 500 mg.), taken at the onset of a bout of pain and repeated within two hours if relief does not ensue. The doctor should guard against the patient becoming a drug addict, though potent analgesics (p. 440) may occasionally become necessary.

Chordotomy for relief of very severe pains is performed occasionally but is seldom advisable. It is attended by considerable risk and is not conspicuously successful.

INCONTINENCE OF URINE. This is usually associated with a chronically overdistended bladder and infection. It should be remembered that infection in the urinary tract shortens life in the majority of tabetics on account of pyelonephritis and renal failure.

This symptom should be prevented by teaching all tabetics to void urine at regular intervals, e.g. every two to three hours during the day rather than when they feel the desire to micturate. Indeed they often boast that they have a 'wonderful bladder' for they can go all day without passing water. This implies a serious stretching of the bladder muscle, with trabeculation and the formation of diverticula which predispose to infection. They must, therefore, empty the bladder completely as soon as possible after waking, at three-hour intervals during the day, and before retiring at night: this process may be assisted by squatting or by pressure on the abdomen. Catheterization of a tabetic should if possible be avoided.

Tabetics often come into hospital with overflow incontinence and chronic cystitis. The infection is treated by the appropriate drug or combination of drugs (pp. 281-84). The bladder may be emptied partially by suprapubic pressure or by the administration of carbachol (p. 504). In the worst cases (usually in the terminal stages of the illness) it may be necessary to insert a self-retaining catheter with strict asepsis and institute tidal drainage (p. 387).

ARTHROPATHIES. Charcot's disease of the large joints and perforating ulcer of the foot require orthopaedic treatment designed to restrict movement and relieve pressure or weight-bearing on the affected joint, but appliances must be designed so as to avoid excessive or abnormal strains on other joints. In a few early cases arthrodesis of a knee or ankle may give stability at the expense of mobility. In general, surgeons dislike performing operations on such joints as the results are bad. Immobilization of the tabetic in bed results in serious wasting and weakness of muscles, increased ataxia and difficulty in controlling bladder function.

GASTRIC CRISES. Gastric crises are very resistant to treatment, but tend to improve gradually after prolonged specific treatment.

In a crises the patient becomes exhausted and dehydrated and it is urgently necessary to stop retching and vomiting and to restore the depleted fluids of the body. Relief may follow administration of full doses of atropine, 0·5 to 1 mg. by hypodermic injection. Cyclizine hydrochloride, 100 mg. as a suppository, is worthy of trial as an antiemetic. Fluid, especially glucose saline, should be given intravenously until the patient can retain fluid taken by mouth. The most severe crises may be alarming but are practically never fatal; often the patient recovers suddenly, nausea ends and lost weight is regained rapidly if he can overcome his fear of taking food.

Syphilis during Pregnancy

Many cases of latent syphilis are discovered by routine antenatal tests. It is often necessary to confirm the diagnosis by using the most sensitive and specific serological tests. Adequate treatment of the woman will certainly prevent transmission of syphilis to the unborn child. The treatment is safe and rapid, so that if positive serological tests are found in the later months of pregnancy it is wise to start treatment with penicillin at once. Ideally this should begin before the fifth month and it has been established that 6 g. of procaine penicillin will safeguard the health of the child. It is often expedient to give more than this amount as pregnancy provides a favourable opportunity to cure the maternal infection and render further treatment unnecessary after delivery. If time permits it is desirable to give a course of 10 to 20 g. of penicillin.

The success of this treatment in preventing congenital syphilis is decided by clinical, radiological and serological examination of the child. At birth the child's blood may give positive tests for syphilis, but if the child is healthy the titre of the positive reactions will fall rapidly, and by the end of the sixth month the tests should have become negative and will remain so. It must be emphasized that if the mother has had adequate treatment during pregnancy a positive blood test in her infant in the first weeks of life does not justify a diagnosis of inherited syphilis. It is probable that if the woman is treated adequately in one pregnancy it is unnecessary to give her further treatment in subsequent pregnancies. However, in view of the simplicity and safety of the treatment, it is preferable to treat the woman in each pregnancy so long as positive serological tests are obtained.

Congenital Syphilis

Infancy. Young infants suffering from congenital syphilis must be regarded as being seriously ill: they are very susceptible to respiratory infections which may prove fatal; therefore it is wise to admit them to hospital. Specific treatment consists of penicillin, and as oral treatment is effective it is unnecessary to give it parenterally. The dosage should be approximately 60 mg. in Penicillin V Elixir, B.P.C. per day for an infant in the first three months of life. Treatment should be continued for three weeks. The child's progress should be checked by radiographs of the chest and the epiphyses of the long bones. Further courses of treatment are usually required. Children tolerate bismuth well and in order to measure the minute doses necessary a one in ten dilution of the injection of bismuth oxychloride B.P.C. should be made. As 1 ml. of this dilution contains 20 mg. of the bismuth salt it is easy to measure the usual dose for an infant, which is 10 mg.

Older children. Children of 7 to 12 years of age may be treated in much the same way as adults, the doses of penicillin and bismuth being adjusted according to body weight. Oral administration of phenoxymethylpenicillin in doses of 125 mg. up to 250 mg. three times a day, according to body weight, may be substituted for injections. In general they require about half the adult dose and tolerate therapy exceedingly well. The condition requires prolonged rather than very intensive treatment, and repeated courses of both penicillin and bismuth may be necessary over a period of one to two years. Some of the clinical manifestations of congenital syphilis appear to be resistant to specific treatment. Interstitial keratitis and bilateral hydrarthrosis of the knees (Clutton's joints) may get worse during active specific therapy. They are regarded by many as hypersensitivity phenomena rather than a syphilitic process, but they ultimately subside and the prognosis is much better if specific treatment is adequate. The serological tests are likely to remain positive, but this is unimportant.

Third generation syphilis. Contrary to popular belief it is now established that congenital syphilitic women almost invariably produce non-syphilitic children; and a congenital syphilitic husband does not infect his wife, and, therefore, his children will be healthy. This implies that there is no medical objection to the marriage of congenital syphilitics, though they should, of course, have adequate treatment to render them less likely to suffer from any disability from their inherited disease.

Interstitial keratitis. During the active inflammatory process the child should be kept in bed and provided with dark glasses. Atropine solution (1 per cent. eye-drops) should be instilled into the eyes twice daily and the child should not be allowed to read or to do anything requiring close vision because of the drug induced paralysis of accommodation. The active inflammatory process can be arrested by the use of hydrocortisone eye-drops twice daily—the treatment being continued for several months if necessary. For prolonged treatment it is easier to use an eye ointment containing 1 per cent. hydrocortisone.

It should be emphasized that hydrocortisone will only prove effective in abolishing the inflammatory changes—cellular infiltration, vascularization, and oedema of the tissues—but will not combat the underlying cause which is congenital syphilis. Moreover, it is valueless in the treatment of cases with scarring due to previous keratitis. The use of hydrocortisone, however, permits active treatment of congenital syphilis to be continued which may have to go on for many weeks or months. Interstitial keratitis is prone to relapse after an interval of months or even years. Relapse is often caused by an injury to the eye, by intercurrent illness, or stress of any type. The prognosis in relapsed cases is good, provided treatment is instituted early and the eyes are protected by the topical use of hydrocortisone.

Bone lesions. Lesions such as periosteitis of the tibia respond slowly but favourably to prolonged treatment with penicillin and bismuth. The dense bone and the deformity which may result will not disappear, but the bone itself is strong.

Dental deformities, such as Hutchinson's incisors and deformities of the nose, should receive appropriate cosmetic treatment from dental and plastic surgeons. Patients are naturally sensitive about deformities and their correction often alters their outlook on life.

Eighth nerve deafness. This usually develops rapidly and progresses to almost complete deafness. In the past treatment has proved valueless. Corticosteroids should be given in adequate doses to suppress a Herxheimer reaction, and penicillin administered in large doses (p. 597). Some patients appear to improve after prolonged treatment with corticosteroids.

Endemic Syphilis

Among many of the most primitive peoples of the world, especially in the tropics, syphilis occurs as a non-venereal disease of childhood. It is believed that though gummatous lesions of bone and skin are common the cardiac and central nervous systems are seldom affected, and inherited syphilis is rare. In such peoples treatment, much less than that advised for acquired syphilis, will suffice to render the patient non-contagious and may even cure the disease. It appears that one injection of 2·4 g. of procaine penicillin will prove sufficient, and millions of patients are being treated on this basis under the auspices of the World Health Organization. It is important to treat every patient and most of the contacts (e.g. family groups) and then to have regular surveys after several months to ensure that all contagious cases are controlled and relapsing or new cases treated. No attempt is made to produce serological cure. The lesions on the mouth and skin heal very rapidly, the health is greatly improved and even chronic late lesions heal.

The other treponematoses—yaws, bejel, pinta—described in standard texts on tropical diseases produce lesions which are similar to those of endemic syphilis.

CHANCROID
(SOFT SORE)

This disease is caused by the *Haemophilus ducreyi*, and is common in tropical and subtropical areas of the world and in large seaports. It is difficult to culture the organism. A specific skin test (Reenstierna's test) is used in chronic cases to prove the nature of the infection: 0·1 ml. of a vaccine of the organism is injected intradermally and if the reaction is positive a papule 10 mm. in diameter develops at the site of injection within 48 hours.

Chancroid is easily cured if sulphonamide treatment is begun before a suppurative bubo forms: indeed the success of such treatment may be used as a diagnostic test. While tests to exclude syphilis are being performed the patient should take 1 g. of sulphadimidine four times a day for seven days.

If a bubo has formed it requires no special treatment unless the pus threatens to point through the skin, in which case the abscess should be aspirated. Incision of the bubo is seldom required and should be avoided, for if extensive incisions are made, healing may be much delayed and lymph drainage obstructed. Penicillin is of no value in chancroid and will conceal coincident syphilis. Streptomycin is curative in doses of 1 g. intramuscularly twice daily for three to five days and it does not interfere with the diagnosis of syphilis. Tetracyclines are also curative in doses of 1 to 2 g. daily for seven days, but this treatment makes the early diagnosis of syphilis more difficult. There is no objection, however, to their use in chronic cases of suppurative bubo.

GRANULOMA INGUINALE

This granulomatous disease is generally a disorder of tropical countries and treatment was formerly very unsatisfactory. The infection responds well to antibiotics, especially the tetracyclines. Dosage with one or other of the tetracyclines should be 2 g. a day in divided doses for 14 days. In a few cases a second course of treatment with the same dose of a tetracycline is required. Streptomycin and chloramphenicol are less effective in this disease and more toxic. Attempts at surgical removal should be avoided. Prolonged supervision is advisable to detect relapse.

LYMPHOGRANULOMA VENEREUM

This virus infection is resistant to sulphonamides and penicillin, though these drugs may combat superimposed infection by other organisms. The tetracyclines or erythromycin, in divided doses of 2 g. daily for 10 to 15 days, provide the most effective treatment. It is important to test for coincident syphilis. Surgical treatment for ano-rectal stricture in late cases may prove necessary. If there is bubo formation with suppuration aspiration may be required but wide incision should be avoided.

'VENEREAL' WARTS

Warts on the genital area are due to a local virus infection without systemic effects and are not always venereal in origin. They grow rapidly in moist conditions and are inhibited by dryness. The most radical and often the easiest treatment is to infiltrate the wart-bearing area with 1 per cent. procaine and then to destroy the pedicle of the warts with the electric cautery. The cauterized area is kept dry by dusting with talc powder. If the warts have invaded the urethra, vagina or anus it may be necessary to cauterize under a general anaesthetic. It is important to destroy all the tiny warts as well as the large masses.

Podophyllin resin applied to the warts is often effective but is unsuitable for extensively affected areas. The skin surrounding the warts should be protected by soft paraffin and a 20 per cent. suspension of the resin in liquid paraffin should then be applied by means of a dressed probe or matchstick. This is allowed to dry for 10 minutes and the area should then be covered with dry gauze, the podophyllin being washed off after eight hours. 'Posalfilin' ointment, containing salicylic acid and podophyllin, is a convenient and effective preparation, though considerable irritation of skin and mucous membrane may result from podophyllin applications.

The local application of liquid nitrogen is a simple and very effective form of treatment.

TRICHOMONAS VAGINALIS INFECTIONS

This parasite is a common cause of vaginitis and other inflammations of the female genital tract; in addition it may cause urethritis, balanitis and pro-statitis in the male. In many men the parasite may cause no symptoms but exists in the genital tract for a short time after coitus. The man may thus be a carrier and may be responsible for repeated re-infections of his consort. The use of cultures will detect the parasite in a higher proportion of patients than the examination of wet smears, urine or stained specimens alone.

The treatment of *Trichomonas vaginalis* infection has been simplified and made much more effective by the introduction of metronidazole. For most patients a dose of 200 mg. by mouth three times a day for one week suffices. Treatment by pessaries may be used if vomiting prevents retention of the drug. When the drug is given by mouth some patients develop moniliasis and hence the simultaneous use of nystatin is justifiable. Metronidazole appears to be relatively non-toxic and can be used in pregnancy though it is probably wise to avoid its use in early pregnancy. Much higher dosage—e.g. 500 mg. four times a day for 10 days—may be administered but no great advantage seems to accrue and in general it seems preferable to give the drug in repeated courses of a week's duration.

Symptomatic relief and disappearance of *Trichomonas vaginalis* occur within 7 to 14 days in over 90 per cent. of patients. A second course may be administered to those not relieved, along with local treatment as outlined below. As reinfection from a sexual partner is very common it is wise to examine the husband (or wife) and treat both simultaneously. In view of the difficulty of demonstrating *Trichomonas vaginalis* in males it is permissible to treat the husband of a woman who has a chronic or relapsing *Trichomonas vaginalis* infection even though he appears healthy. Unless a condom is used sexual intercourse should be forbidden for about one month while tests for cure are being done. These should include culture of genital secretions for the parasite. Treatment during menstruation may be more effective than at other times.

Local treatment by antiseptic swabbing of the vagina, cervix and vulva may be used at the outset, but is seldom necessary after the first visit. The use of acetarsol or hydrargphen pessaries in women is now required only in resistant infections or when the patient is intolerant of metronidazole. In a few cases sickness occurs after each dose; more commonly there are complaints of nausea and a bad taste in the mouth but the course of treatment can be completed.

In men it is necessary to examine the urine and

the prostatic fluid on several occasions after treatment, culturing these materials in a special medium. Resistant infections in the male may need repeated massage of the prostate and seminal vesicles followed by urethral irrigation with 1 : 6,000 mercury oxycyanide lotion. The majority of such cases are examples of reinfection rather than true resistance.

Observations made during long-term treatment with metronidazole indicate that drug-resistant strains of the parasite are very rare. Failures are due to reinfection or very rarely to malabsorption of the drug, and this may be due to achlorhydria. The drug is present in human milk but does not appear to upset the baby.

FUNGUS INFECTIONS

Balanitis and urethritis due to fungus infections are usually associated with glycosuria (p. 316) or with fungus infection of the skin of the perineal area (p. 577).

Vaginitis due to *Candida albicans* (thrush) is common in pregnancy and is also found in associa-tion with glycosuria. In addition to treating associated diabetes, the vagina should be swabbed to remove the discharge and then painted through a speculum with 1 per cent. gentian violet. This may have to be repeated on several occasions at intervals of a few days. The antibiotic nystatin is effective when applied locally in pessaries or as a cream.

PARASITIC INFESTATIONS

Scabies. In many cases scabies may be acquired as a venereal infection and starting on the ano-genital region may be confined for a time to the genitals or buttocks. The treatment is described on p. 387.

Pediculosis pubis ('*Crabs*'). This is often a venereal infestation and is frequently overlooked. Its treatment is discussed on p. 585.

References

WILCOX, R. R. (1964). *Textbook of Venereal Diseases and Treponematosis*, 2nd ed. London: Heineman.
KING, A. (1964). *Recent Advances in Venereology*. London: Churchill.

28. Diseases of the Eye

W. S. FOULDS

General Considerations

In the eye, a relatively slight amount of damage which would be negligible elsewhere may lead to severe loss of function. Many of the ocular tissues are optically clear and following trauma or infection, the usual processes of repair involving vascularization and the formation of fibrous tissue, may lead to opacity in these tissues and serious loss of sight. The avascular vitreous cavity forms an ideal culture medium and once infection gains access to it, severe intra-ocular damage is inevitable. The neural tissues of the eye, the retina and optic nerve, are structurally and functionally part of the brain and share with the tissues of the brain an inability to regenerate if they are destroyed. Within a very small compass there are in the eye, a number of separate but mutually dependent structures and systems. Consequently, pathological changes in one part of the eye may have far-reaching effects on other eye structures. It is therefore important that eye diseases should be diagnosed early and treated vigorously and appropriately so that disability from the disease itself and from unchecked processes of repair can be minimized.

ROUTES OF ADMINISTRATION OF DRUGS TO THE EYE

Topical administration. Drugs may be administered to the eye topically as eye-drops, in ointments, in lotions or in water-soluble gelatin discs. The last two are not now in common use.

Topically administered drugs are effective in the treatment of superficial eye conditions and those drugs which are absorbed through the cornea may be used in this way in the treatment of intra-ocular disease. The intact corneal epithelium, however, is a barrier to the absorption of substances through the cornea, and such factors as lipid and water solubility are also important in this connection. In general, ointments give a more prolonged action than do drops but cause blurring of vision.

Subconjunctival injection. Because the sclera has no surface epithelium, drugs applied directly to its surface tend to diffuse readily through it to reach a high concentration in the intra-ocular tissues. Administration by subconjunctival injection is the most convenient way of achieving this. Subconjunctival injection of an antibiotic is commonly used in the treatment of intra-ocular infection, while substances such as corticosteroids and mydriatics may also be given by this route in the treatment of iridocyclitis.

Systemic administration. Drugs given orally or parenterally, reach the eye by way of the blood stream. To penetrate the intra-ocular tissues they must pass the blood/eye barriers which selectively influence the ease with which substances enter the eye from the blood stream. Of the antibiotics, the tetracyclines and penicillins penetrate poorly while chloramphenicol, streptomycin and sodium fucidate do so readily. Fortunately, the barriers break down when the eye is inflamed and under these conditions almost any antibiotic will penetrate the eye readily.

Systemically administered drugs have to be given in high dosage if effective levels are to be attained in the cornea and other non-vascular ocular structures. In treating ocular infections different routes of administration may have to be used simultaneously, and often it is advantageous to use a combination of different antibacterial drugs.

Techniques of administration of drugs to the eye. *Eye-drops.* The lower lid should be everted and the sterile dropper held so that a single drop can be expelled into the lower conjunctival fornix. Direct application to the cornea should be avoided and care should be taken to avoid contact of the dropper with the lashes and subsequent contamination of the drop container, unless a disposable single-dose applicator is being used. In babies, it may be necessary to apply pressure over the tear sac to prevent toxic systemic absorption by way of the naso-lacrimal duct.

Ointments. A sterile glass rod carrying a quantity of the ointment is inserted into the lower conjunctival fornix with the patient looking up. The patient closes the eye and the glass rod is withdrawn laterally, leaving the ointment in the conjunctival sac. Alternatively, the ointment is expressed from a collapsible tube directly into the lower conjunctival fornix. Contamination of the nozzle of the tube is inevitable with this method and it is important that the tube is kept exclusively for use by one patient. Single-dose applicators have much to commend them and may become standard.

Subconjunctival injection. Prior to subconjunctival injection, the conjunctival sac is anaesthetized by the

U*

instillation of a topical analgesic, such as amethocaine hydrochloride 1 per cent. at 5-minute intervals for half an hour. Between instillations, the eye is kept covered with an eye pad to prevent desiccation of the cornea. The injection is made with a number 20 hypodermic needle under the conjunctiva of the lower half of the globe with the eye elevated. Up to 1 ml. can be injected without undue chemosis.

Corticosteroids and the Eye

Because of their marked anti-inflammatory effect and because they reduce vascular proliferation during repair processes, corticosteroids have an important rôle in the treatment of eye disease. They may be used locally or systemically and these two routes of administration are often combined. Locally, corticosteroids are used as drops or by subconjunctival injection in the treatment of iritis and iridocyclitis and they are also valuable for such conditions as acne rosacea keratitis, spring catarrh and phlyctenular disease. Steroid preparations vary in solubility and in activity. In the eye, cortisone, hydrocortisone, prednisolone, betamethasone and dexamethasone are the more commonly used in order of increasing anti-inflammatory activity.

Dangers and side-effects. Local corticosteroids are contraindicated in corneal ulceration due to bacterial infection as they may increase the risk of corneal perforation. Corticosteroids are absolutely contraindicated in herpes simplex infections of the cornea because they facilitate widespread ocular involvement and this may be disastrous for sight. In general, corticosteroids should never be used in an inflamed eye if a definite diagnosis has not been made. About one-third of patients given local corticosteroids to the eyes develop a reversible elevation of intra-ocular pressure. This steroid reactivity is genetically determined. The prolonged use of corticosteroid eye-drops in a steroid reactor may lead to severe visual loss from glaucoma. It is important that patients using steroids locally for any length of time, be kept under adequate ophthalmic supervision.

Systemic and subconjunctival corticosteroids are used in the treatment of certain intra-ocular inflammations, especially choroiditis which is unaffected by locally instilled steroid. To be effective in the eye, fairly large doses are often necessary, a common regimen being 60 mg. of prednisolone daily for four days, reducing gradually to a maintenance level of 15 mg. daily, until the in-

flammation has settled. For subconjunctival injection, triamcinolone acetonide, 5 mg. in 0·5 ml. of water, may be used when a marked anti-inflammatory action in small bulk is required. In some cases of chronic uveitis a long-acting steroid preparation such as methyl prednisolone acetate, 40 mg. per ml., given by subconjunctival injection, may make it unnecessary to resort to systemic corticosteroid therapy.

OCULAR INFLAMMATION

Bacterial Infection of the Lids

Stye. Staphylococcal infection of a lash follicle results in the common condition of stye (hordeolum). The lid becomes swollen and painful and eventually pus discharges from the infected follicle. Infection may be transferred to a lash follicle in the opposing lid during blinking. Treatment consists of hot spoon bathing three to four times daily, together with the local use of an antibiotic ointment, such as chloramphenicol 0·5 per cent. If there is surrounding cellulitis, systemic penicillin usually induces rapid regression of the infection.

Blepharitis. A low-grade inflammation of the lid margins is relatively common and occurs in two forms, squamous blepharitis and ulcerative blepharitis. In patients with squamous blepharitis there is often an accompanying seborrhoea of the skin and scalp and secondary infection with staphylococci. The condition gives rise to redness and irritation of the lid margins but is not dangerous to sight. It has been suggested that a heavy infestation of the lash follicles with the sebaceous mite, *Demodex folliculorum hominis*, is an aetiological factor. Squamous blepharitis is resistant to treatment and subject to relapse. The scalp should be treated for dandruff (p. 580) and an antibiotic ointment, such as chloramphenicol 0·5 per cent. is massaged into the lid margins three times daily, to control secondary infection. Although combined antibiotic and steroid preparations, in general have little to commend them, this type of preparation is useful in the treatment of squamous blepharitis.

In ulcerative blepharitis there is widespread staphylococcal infection of the lash follicles. Loss of lashes due to destruction of the follicles occurs and distortion of the lid margin leading to trichiasis and corneal damage is relatively common. The condition is most usually seen in children who are poorly cared for. In treating the condition the general standard of hygiene must receive attention. Local treatment consists of removing crusts from the lid margins night and morning and the application of chloramphenicol 0·5 per cent. or framycetin 0·5 per cent. eye ointment to the lid margins.

Chalazion. This is a chronic granulomatous condition of a meibomian gland, secondary to obstruction of its duct and subsequent low-grade infection. The lesion is called a chalazion because it often resembles an ordinary hailstone in size and consistence. The treatment is surgical evacuation of the disorganized contents of the affected gland. Occasionally, an acute staphylococcal infection supervenes (internal hordeolum) in which case the treatment is as for stye. When the infection settles, incision and curettage may still be required.

Lid abscess. A widespread cellulitis of the lid may follow either a stye or an infected chalazion, particularly in infants. Gross swelling of the lid and a high fever results. Systemic penicillin leads to prompt improvement in most cases.

Orbital cellulitis. Orbital cellulitis may arise by the spread of infection from the accessory nasal sinuses or more rarely from infections of the lids or surrounding face being carried with the venous drainage into the orbit. The condition is differentiated from lid abscess by the gross restriction of ocular movement which occurs. Treatment is with massive doses of systemically administered antibiotics. Orbital cellulitis may be followed by cavernous sinus thrombosis; both eyes then become congested and proptosed, and the patient is acutely ill. Untreated, the condition is rapidly fatal, but it usually responds well to vigorous systemic antibiotic therapy.

Infection of Lacrimal Apparatus

In the infant, infection of the tear sac may follow a partial obstruction of the naso-lacrimal duct due to debris in the lumen. The tear sac should be expressed three times daily, with the tip of the little finger and this should be followed by instillation of a drop of chloramphenicol 0·5 per cent. into the conjunctival fornix. This treatment is effective in most cases. Occasionally, probing of the naso-lacrimal duct under general anaesthesia is required.

In adults, chronic infection of the tear sac arises as a sequel of obstruction of the naso-lacrimal duct and is a common cause of epiphora in the elderly. Treatment aims are relieving the obstruction and simple syringing of the tear passages with normal saline may be effective in mild cases. Usually,

however, surgical correction is required. Occasionally, an acute dacryocystitis may present with abscess formation over the tear sac and surrounding cellulitis. Treatment is with systemic penicillin and local hot bathing. If the abscess shows signs of pointing, pus is released through a skin incision over the tear sac. When the condition is quiescent, surgical relief of the underlying naso-lacrimal obstruction is necessary.

In some elderly patients, epiphora may occur without demonstrable obstruction in the lacrimal passages. Occasionally, slight displacement of the lower lacrimal punctum, due to a minimal ectropion of the lower lid, is the cause and this can be remedied surgically. Palliative treatment with zinc sulphate eye-drops 0·25 per cent. with or without the addition of sulphacetamide 5 per cent. may give relief.

Bacterial Infection of the External Eye

Conjunctivitis. Infection of the conjunctival sac with pyogenic bacteria is a common ocular condition. Usually, both eyes are affected and discharge from the inflamed eyes causes the eyelids to stick together. A conjunctival culture should be taken to establish the nature of the organism and its sensitivity to the commonly used antibiotics. Treatment, however, should not be delayed on this account. In children the most common organism causing conjunctivitis is the pneumococcus and in adults, the staphylococcus. The once common infection with the Koch-Week's bacillus (*Haemophilus aegyptius*) is now rarely seen. Infection with the gonococcus which was once a common cause of ophthalmia neonatorum, leading to blindness is now much less common than formerly. Gonococcal infection of the conjunctiva in the infant or in the adult leads to a markedly purulent conjunctivitis with gross chemosis of the conjunctiva and fairly rapid involvement of the cornea. In purulent conjunctivitis, systemic therapy with penicillin or tetracycline is a vital part of the treatment and is combined with repeated irrigation of the eyes with sterile saline and the frequent instillation of antibiotic drops (penicillin, chloramphenicol or framycetin). Initially, the drops should be used hourly in each eye and with systemic and local antibiotic therapy there should be a dramatic improvement in the ocular condition within a matter of hours. As in other types of conjunctivitis, local therapy with antibiotic drops should be continued for some days after the condition has apparently cleared. With the more common subacute types of conjunctivitis local therapy with chloramphenicol or framycetin eye-drops B.P.C. instilled into each eye two-hourly during the first day, and three times daily for a further three days or so, usually suffices to clear the condition. It is common to combine the use of antibiotic eye-drops during the day with the same antibiotic as an ointment at night. Outbreaks of conjunctivitis may spread through schools or similar institutions. Early diagnosis and treatment are essential and steps should be taken to prevent the spread of infection by way of face towels, and so on.

Corneal ulcer. If pathogenic bacteria gain access to the corneal stroma through a breach in the corneal epithelium, a corneal ulcer results. The infection may penetrate deeply into the cornea and pus may form in the anterior chamber. This commonly lies in the lower part of the anterior chamber with a fluid level and the condition is known as a hypopyon ulcer. If not treated adequately, perforation of the cornea follows and the eye is lost from widespread infection of the intra-ocular contents (panophthalmitis). A corneal ulcer may follow trauma, exposure of the eye due to facial palsy or unconsciousness, and sometimes arises without apparent preceding cause in the elderly and debilitated. The most common causative organisms are the staphylococcus, pneumococcus, and *Pseudomonas pyocyanea*. The latter organism penetrates the eye quickly and unless treatment is instituted promptly, the eye will be lost.

Gram-negative organisms such as *Pseudomonas pyocyanea* and *Bacillus proteus* are sensitive to a limited range of antibiotics only. In general, one should assume that any ocular infection may be due to a gram-negative organism and use an antibiotic active against both gram-positive and gram-negative organisms.

Treatment of corneal ulceration consists of the subconjunctival injection of 500 mg. of framycetin sulphate dissolved in 0·5 to 1 ml. of water, or of a mixture of 0·3 g. of soluble penicillin, together with 0·5 g. of streptomycin dissolved in a similar quantity of water. More recently fucidin or lincomycin have been found effective in this type of case. A mydriatic, such as atropine, is often included in the subconjunctival injection which is followed by the intensive use of local framycetin 0·5 per cent. eye-drops instilled at hourly intervals and the systemic administration of tetracycline or other antibiotics (p. 9). Atropine sulphate drops are used two to three times daily to combat the accompanying iridocyclitis. The patient should be seen by an opthalmologist as soon as possible. If a panophthalmitis develops, much visual loss results from the processes of repair, and the judicious use of systemic corticosteroids in combination with systemic and sub-conjunctival antibiotics, may save the eye in an otherwise hopeless case. The use of corticosteroids in this way must be supervised by an ophthalmologist.

Intra-ocular infections. Bacterial infection may gain entrance to the eye by way of a corneal ulcer, as the result of a penetrating wound or occasionally via the blood stream in the course of a systemic illness. In the latter instance the resulting panophthalmitis is seldom as severe as in the other two modes of infection. The treatment is as detailed for the treatment of a deep bacterial corneal ulcer. If treatment fails to control the infection quickly, evisceration of the eye may be required.

Virus Infections

The common virus infections affecting the eye are herpes zoster, herpes simplex, adenovirus infections and in some parts of the world, trachoma.

Herpes zoster ophthalmicus. This condition is characterized by a painful, vesicular eruption in the distribution of the first division of the fifth nerve on one side. Sometimes the second division is also affected when vesicles are found below the affected eye and in the mouth. The lids of the affected eye are swollen, the conjunctiva is congested and there is a variable degree of other ocular involvement. Keratitis accompanied by loss of corneal sensation may lead to permanent corneal opacity. A severe chronic anterior uveitis may permanently damage sight. Occasionally, a temporary paralysis of extra-ocular muscles is seen. The affected skin should be kept dry until the vesicles scab and separate. Secondary infection is best treated with tetracycline by mouth, 250 mg. six-hourly. If the eye itself is involved or if there is vesiculation on the nose in the distribution of the naso-ciliary branch of the fifth nerve, corticosteroid drops, together with atropine eye-drops 1 per cent. should be instilled three times daily, and an ophthalmic opinion should be sought. Post-herpetic pain may occur in the elderly or debilitated and is very intractable. Relief occasionally follows the use of carbamazepine, 100 mg. twice daily, but therapy is often without effect.

Herpes simplex. The vesicles of herpes simplex

may occur on the lids, and the virus commonly causes a recurrent follicular conjunctivitis. Its most serious ocular manifestation is dendritic ulceration of the cornea which may run a chronic relapsing course and lead to much corneal damage. In some cases, herpes simplex keratitis is followed by uveitis with secondary glaucoma and serious effects on vision.

Herpes simplex keratitis is one of the few conditions where a true antiviral agent can be used in therapy. Idoxuridine (I.D.U.) prevents replication of the virus by interfering with the synthesis of DNA. To treat uncomplicated dendritic ulceration I.D.U. is used in a 0·1 per cent. aqueous solution and is instilled hourly or two-hourly into the affected eye for 36 to 48 hours. The eye is covered with a pad and bandage and atropine eye-drops, 1 per cent., instilled every eight hours.

An alternative or additional treatment, is removal of the infected epithelium mechanically, chemically (using alcohol or a strong alcoholic solution of iodine) or by freezing, together with local antibiotic therapy to combat secondary infection and atropine eye-drops 1 per cent. three times daily, to control the accompanying reactive uveitis. *Local or general corticosteroids are contraindicated in herpes simplex infections of the eye.* These preparations may lead to widespread corneal involvement and sometimes perforation of the cornea and loss of the eye. It is important that the practitioner should recognize dendritic ulceration of the cornea, for complications and recurrences are common and an ophthalmic opinion should be obtained as soon as possible.

Adenovirus infections. Adenoviruses are responsible for many cases of kerato-conjunctivitis, characterized by follicular conjunctivitis, discrete superficial corneal infiltrates, pre-auricular adenitis and variable systemic malaise. The infection runs a self-limiting course and is unaffected by treatment although theoretically a response to local I.D.U. would be expected. Chloramphenicol eye-drops prevent secondary infection until healing occurs. Occasionally, widespread outbreaks of adenovirus keratitis have been traced to inadequate sterilization of eye instruments used in hospital out-patient departments.

Trachoma. Trachoma is still one of the commonest causes of blindness in the world. It is caused by a large virus-like agent. The ocular infection is characterized by a follicular conjunctivitis going on to scarring of the palpebral conjunctiva and a variable degree of corneal opacification and vascularization. Some of the changes may be due to secondary infection. A milder disease, Inclusion Conjunctivitis, is caused by a similar organism in areas where trachoma is rarely seen. The organism is present in the genito-urinary tract and infection of the eye may occur at birth or be acquired later.

Preventive treatment includes measures to improve hygiene and the use of active immunization. The organism is sensitive to antibiotics and therapy in an established case is by local and systemic tetracycline.

Vaccinia. Accidental infection of the eye with vaccinia occasionally occurs. The resulting keratitis may leave a permanently scarred cornea. The keratitis responds to treatment with I.D.U. as for dendritic ulceration. Locally applied gamma-globulin may be effective and systemic tetracycline to control secondary infection is a useful adjuvant.

Fungus Infections

Although uncommon in temperate climates, fungus infections of the eye are being increasingly recognized as important causes of severe and intractable ocular inflammation. Indolent corneal ulceration is the commonest manifestation but intra-ocular infection following trauma including ocular surgery also occurs. Diagnosis is by demonstration of the organisms in tissue scrapings or by culture. Therapy is unsatisfactory. Many anti-fungal drugs are at present being evaluated for their usefulness in the treatment of ocular mycosis. Infection of the lacrimal canaliculus with actinomyces is occasionally seen. There is epiphora and a creamy white discharge can be expressed from the obstructed canaliculus. Diagnosis is confirmed by microscopy of the expressed material. Mechanical removal of infected material from the canaliculus and the use of chloramphenicol 0·5 per cent. or penicillin 1 per cent. eye-drops for four to five days clears the infection.

Protozoal Infections

Toxoplasmosis is a relatively common cause of posterior and anterior uveitis. Usually, the infection is acquired in intra-uterine life and may give rise to extensive areas of choroidoretinal destruction and grossly impaired vision. The encysted organisms may become re-activated to give rise to an acute choroiditis in adolescence or early adult life. Diagnosis depends on the characteristic clinical appearance of healed toxoplasmic lesions and the presence of intra-cranial calcification, together with the demonstration of abnormal serum reactions to the complement fixation and cytoplasmic modifying dye tests. As these tests are commonly positive in the apparently unaffected population, a negative test may be of more clinical value than a positive result. In primary acquired toxoplasmosis, a very high and rising dye test titre is the rule.

Toxoplasma gondii is inactivated *in vitro* by pyrimethamine and by the sulphonamides. In active toxoplasmic uveitis, pyrimethamine 25 to 50 mg. daily, is given for four weeks, together with sulphadimidine 1 g. six-hourly. As pyrimethamine is a marrow depressant, a watch must be kept on the blood picture. It is usual to complement anti-protozoal therapy with systemic corticosteroids and local mydriatics (see treatment of uveitis below).

Metazoal Infections

The encysted larvae of the dog tapeworm, toxocara canis and the related toxocara cati may cause a severe endophthalmitis in children or give rise to a granulomatous mass in the retina. Other evidence of visceral larva migrans may be present and there is usually an eosinophilia. Treatment with diethyl-carbamazine 30 mg. three times daily, for one month has been suggested and should be combined with the standard therapy for non-specific uveitis.

Non-specific Inflammations

Allergic conjunctivitis. Acute allergic conjunctivitis is usually the result of sensitization to a locally applied medication. Atropine, penicillin and neomycin are common offenders but almost any eye preparation may cause an allergic reaction. Ointments are more prone to cause sensitization than drops. Allergic conjunctivitis may also arise from exposure to other allergens such as hair dyes, cosmetics and materials used in industrial processes. Hay fever is commonly accompanied by an allergic conjunctivitis. If contact with the allergen can be avoided, the condition settles spontaneously. In hay fever good results are obtained from local instillations of corticosteroid eye-drops, but antihistamines as eye-drops are less efficacious.

Spring catarrh and phlyctenular disease. Spring catarrh is a chronic conjunctivitis which affects adolescent boys and although it may last for many years, is self-limiting. It is characterized by proliferation and follicle formation in the palpebral and bulbar conjunctiva and may have an allergic basis as may phlyctenular conjunctivitis and keratitis. In these latter diseases poor social conditions and undernutrition are of undoubted aetiological importance. Phlyctenular conjunctivitis and keratitis which affect children and young adults were once common but the prevalance of each has shown a marked decrease with improved living standards. The diseases still occur in underdeveloped countries and their prevention is a problem in community medicine. The allergen may be tuberculo-protein. Chronic chest infection may be present and require suitable therapy. In all these types of chronic allergic conjunctivitis, local steroid eye-drops induce a rapid remission. In spring catarrh the frequency of instillation of steroid eye-drops is determined by the therapeutic response. Treatment may have to be continued for some years and the aim should be to achieve adequate control of symptoms with the minimum of topical therapy. When the cornea is involved local treatment with atropine 1 per cent. twice daily is required in addition until healing has taken place.

Uveitis. Inflammation of the vascular coat of the eye may occur as iritis, iridocyclitis or choroiditis, or the whole uveal tract may be affected simultaneously as uveitis. Inflammation of the uvea may complicate sarcoidosis and is seen in association with the connective tissue (collagen) diseases (p. 458). A particularly intractable uveitis known as sympathetic ophthalmia may affect both eyes after an injury to one. Sometimes in uveitis, a definite aetiological agent can be identified such as gonorrhoea, syphilis, toxoplasmosis or tuberculosis and treatment in these cases must be directed towards the underlying cause. Generally, however, the cause remains unknown and treatment is nonspecific, heavy reliance being placed on the corticosteroids given locally for anterior uveitis and systemically for posterior uveitis. In sympathetic ophthalmia and in the uveitis associated with sarcoid or auto-immune disease, systemic corticosteroid therapy is indicated.

Iridocyclitis. Attacks of iridocyclitis generally run a predetermined course and the aim of treatment is to prevent complications that might subsequently damage sight. The signs of iridocyclitis of diagnostic importance are ocular pain, circum-corneal congestion, a small pupil and a cellular deposit on the posterior corneal surface. The inflamed iris tends to adhere to the anterior lens capsule to form posterior synechiae. Dilatation of the pupil prevents contact between the iris and lens and lessens the risk of adhesion. Dilatation of the pupil is best achieved by the use of atropine eye-drops 1 per cent. three times daily, together with local heat usually as hot spoon bathing. Failure to prevent the formation of synechiae may lead to secondary glaucoma. If the pupil fails to dilate with locally instilled atropine, the mydriatic effect can be enhanced by the use of 1 per cent. adrenaline or 10 per cent. phenylephrine as eye-drops. In resistant cases the subconjunctival injection of mydricaine may be required (atropine, cocaine or procaine and adrenaline in saline). Other mydriatics which may be used are homatropine 2 per cent., hyoscine 0·5 per cent., lachesine 1 per cent., or cyclopentolate 1 per cent.

The anti-inflammatory action of the corticosteroids is useful in reducing the severity of an attack of iritis, although probably without effect on its duration. The decision as to whether systemic or local steroid should be used is one for the ophthalmologist. Pain may be a feature of iridocyclitis. It is usually relieved by adequate ocular therapy but analgesics may be required in the early stages of the disease (p. 440). Bed-rest is a useful adjunct in any severe case of uveitis and during the acute phase the affected eye should be covered with a pad and a bandage.

Choroiditis. The diagnosis of choroiditis is made on the basis of visual disturbance and the ophthalmoscopic finding of a hazy, oedematous area in the fundus. Specific aetiological agents are seldom identified although toxoplasmosis is a relatively common cause. Treatment consists of systemic corticosteroids, initially in high dosage to control the inflammation (prednisolone, 60 mg. daily) reducing to a maintenance dose (15 to 20 mg. prednisolone daily) until the choroiditis is inactive. The usual precautions in the use of systemic corticosteroids must be observed. The treatment of toxoplasmosis has already been described (p. 611).

Scleritis and episcleritis. Patches and nodules of inflammation may occur in the sclera or episcleral tissues. They may clear up spontaneously or be very resistant to treatment. The cause is seldom known but rheumatoid arthritis is the commonest associated disease. Episcleritis responds to local corticosteroids as drops, whereas the more deeply seated scleritis demands systemic corticosteroid therapy. Phenylbutazone or oxyphenbutazone 200 to 500 mg. daily, may be effective in the latter

condition but these drugs have important side-effects (p. 450).

Keratoconjunctivitis sicca. Rheumatoid arthritis is sometimes accompanied by destruction of the salivary and lacrimal glands leading to keratoconjunctivitis sicca (Sjögren's syndrome). The chronic irritation, photophobia and corneal damage may be relieved by local corticosteroid eye-drops or by artificial tears (e.g. 1 per cent. carboxymethyl cellulose or 1 per cent. gelatin in Ringer-Locke solution). These drops have to be used frequently and may be ineffective. Surgical occlusion of the lacrimal puncta is frequently followed by relief of symptoms. Other causes of dry eye are infiltration of the lacrimal gland in sarcoidosis and destruction of the gland as a result of X-ray therapy.

Retrobulbar neuritis. This localized inflammatory lesion of the optic nerve is commonly a manifestation of disseminated sclerosis. The onset is rapid with pain on movement of the eye and severe loss of central vision occurring during the course of three to four days. If the optic nerve head is involved the signs of papillitis are seen. Vision usually recovers spontaneously over a period of four to six weeks. Systemic ACTH (p. 453) is worthy of trial.

Trauma

The treatment of penetrating eye injuries is surgical. Blunt injuries to the eye often result in intra-ocular haemorrhage and reactive uveitis. Bed-rest is helpful and where uveitis is present, treatment with atropine eye-drops 1 per cent. three times daily, and a pad and bandage as for other types of uveitis should be instituted. Secondary glaucoma, dislocation of the lens or retinal detachment may result from a contusion and the patient should be seen by an ophthalmologist.

Chemical trauma. Chemical burns of the eye may cause immediate damage from tissue necrosis and late complications from uveitis, adhesion between the lids and the eye or from interference with the blood supply to the anterior segment of the eye.

Acids produce immediate damage and corneal opacification. Alkalis penetrate deeply into the eye and lead to long-lasting complications. Lime, as plaster, cement and similar compounds, is a common cause of alkali burns to the eye and recently, concentrated ammonia solutions used with criminal intent have led to severe ocular damage.

With all chemical injuries, prompt and copious irrigation with tap water is the most effective therapy. The patient's head should be held under a tap and the water made to run into the opened eye or the head should be immersed in a bucket of water and the patient instructed to blink the eyes under water. When lime has entered the eyes the upper lid should be everted and any particles of lime carefully sought and removed. With all chemical injuries, the patient should be referred to an ophthalmologist for specialist evaluation and further treatment.

Vascular Disease

Most manifestations of vascular disease in the eye, for example, hypertensive retinopathy, occlusion of the central retinal vein, and occlusion of the central retinal artery are an expression of an underlying systemic disorder and treatment should be directed to the general state of the patient. There is no conclusive evidence that anticoagulant therapy is of benefit in the treatment of either obstruction of the central retinal artery or of the central retinal vein. Occlusive vascular disease in the eye may be a manifestation of unrecognized glaucoma, which requires appropriate therapy (p. 615) Another important cause of retinal vascular insufficiency is giant-celled arteritis.

This type of arteritis may affect the central retinal artery leading to occlusion and permanent loss of sight in the affected eye or may affect the nutrient vessels to the optic nerve leading to ischaemic optic neuropathy and severe impairment of vision. The second eye is commonly affected after an interval of days or weeks. Systemic corticosteroid therapy, if instituted promptly, will protect the second eye from damage. On treatment with systemic steroid, some recovery in vision may occur in those cases affected by ischaemic neuropathy but no recovery of function is to be expected where occlusion of the central retinal artery has occurred. Typically, the E.S.R. is grossly elevated in giant-celled arteritis and the maintenance dose of steroid must be such that the E.S.R. is kept within normal limits. Commonly, it is necessary to continue corticosteroid therapy for a year or more. Occasionally, ischaemic optic neuropathy may result from degenerative vascular disease affecting nutrition of the optic nerve. There is evidence that systemic corticosteroid therapy may be of value in these cases also.

Metabolic Disease

Disorders of thyroid function. The exophthalmos associated with thyroid disease does not necessarily respond to treatment of the underlying dysthyroid state. In malignant exophthalmos there may be severe chemosis, venous stasis, exposure of the cornea and loss of the eye from corneal ulceration. Apart from surgical measures such as decompression of the orbits, massive doses of systemic corticosteroids (100 to 150 mg. prednisone daily) may be effective in reducing the condition to manageable proportions.

The upper lid retraction which is commonly seen in hyperthyroidism and sometimes persists when the patient is euthyroid causes ocular exposure and discomfort. It may be reduced by the local instillation of guanethidine eye-drops 5 per cent. once or twice daily.

Diabetes. There is as yet no effective therapy for diabetic retinopathy. Although the exudates in this type of retinopathy disappear on treatment with clofibrate 1 g. twice daily, there is no evidence that vision improves as a result of this therapy. The refractive state of the lens may be altered by changes in the blood sugar level. Temporary visual disturbances are common at the onset of diabetes and after the commencement of therapy.

Degenerative Diseases

One of the commonest causes of poor sight is senile macular degeneration. As yet there is no effective therapy for this condition. Claims that various dietary agents are useful are unsubstantiated.

Painful Blind Eye

When a blind eye becomes painful its removal is usually necessary. As a temporary measure pain may be relieved for some time (several weeks) by the retrobulbar injection of 1 ml. of 80 per cent. alcohol into the region of the ciliary ganglion. The injection of alcohol is preceded by an injection of 0·5 ml of lignocaine 2 per cent. The needle used for this injection is left *in situ* and the alcohol injected through the same needle after five minutes.

Toxic Conditions

The eye, and in particular the optic nerve, is peculiarly sensitive to a variety of toxic agents. Thus, severe ocular damage has been reported following exposure to lead, arsenic, insecticides, pesticides, industrial solvents, alcohol, methyl alcohol and many drugs used medically, including antibiotics, antimalarials and tranquillizers. Reference will be made to some of the commoner offenders.

Antimalarials. Chloroquin, hydroxychloroquin and similar antimalarials which are also used in the treatment of skin photosensitivity and of connective tissue (collagen) diseases may precipitate in the cornea to give reversible corneal opacities, or more seriously be taken up by the pigment epithelium of the retina to cause progressive and permanent visual loss. Patients on long-term therapy with these drugs should be kept under ophthalmic supervision.

Phenothiazines, This group of drugs including promazine, chlorpromazine and thioridazine may cause cataract or, like the antimalarials, permanently damage sight via their action on the pigment epithelium of the retina.

Methyl alcohol. This substance is usually taken in error for ethyl alcohol. It may cause blindness and in large doses, death. The general management of poisoning is described on p. 544.

Tobacco. A small proportion of elderly tobacco smokers develop a bilateral loss of central vision known as tobacco amblyopia. The visual effect is indistinguishable from the optic neuritis which occasionally occurs in patients with pernicious anaemia. There is evidence that both conditions are a manifestation of abnormal vitamin B_{12} metabolism. The visual defect in both responds to treatment with intramuscular *hydroxocobalamin* (1,000 mcg. three times weekly) but not as cyanocobalamin although both preparations promote normal haemopoiesis and other beneficial effects in pernicious anaemia (p. 151). In tobacco amblyopia complete cessation of smoking is followed by a recovery of vision in three to six months, but even if smoking is continued recovery follows the administration of adequate doses of hydroxocobalamin intramuscularly.

Concomitant Squint and Glaucoma

The treatment of concomitant squint and of glaucoma is largely the responsibility of the ophthalmologist, but the proper management of such cases requires the closest co-operation between the general practitioner and the specialist. It is therefore important to refer to certain general principles in the treatment of these diseases.

Concomitant squint. The development of bino-cular vision is nearly complete at the age of five but is not fully established until between 7 and 8 years of age. The four methods of treatment available are: the prescription of spectacles when these are required to correct an error of refraction; occlusion of the good eye when amblyopia has developed in the squinting eye; orthoptic treatment; and surgery. It is not the degree of squint that matters but whether it is constant or intermittent; if the squint is constantly present, or present for most of the day, the child should be referred for specialist examination without delay.

A child when only a year old will wear spectacles without distress, but a more important reason for insisting that a child with a noticeable squint should be examined at the tender age of one year is that a squint appearing at an early age may be due to a retinoblastoma. Although this most malignant form of neoplasm is relatively rare, early diagnosis may save not only the second eye but also the child's life.

Spectacles. If there is a moderately high error of refraction, as is so often the case in convergent squints, the provision of spectacles may be all that is required to bring the eyes into proper alignment and to allow Nature to take her normal course in the establishment of the reflexes governing binocular vision.

Occlusion. If the squint has existed long enough for the affected eye to become partially amblyopic from suppressive disuse, some form of occlusion of the 'good' eye should be advised. The child may resent this and the mother may be inclined to give in to the child and neglect this most essential part of treatment. The reason for occluding the 'good' eye must therefore be fully explained to the parent. The most effective form of occlusion is to cover the eye with elastoplast applied over a piece of white lint so as to prevent the plaster sticking to the eyebrows and eyelashes. Occlusion should be continued for three weeks in the first instance. Once the amblyopia has been largely overcome, some form of occluder which can be attached to the spectacles may be used in place of the elastoplast; but this clip-on type of occluder is useless in the treatment of amblyopia of any severe degree, since the child tends to peep around it in order to use his 'good' eye. The difficult time, for both child and parent, is the first three or four weeks while the 'good' eye is covered. This period requires the co-operation of the child, which is readily obtained if the doctor can make the parent understand the necessity of the procedure and encourage the child to make the 'lazy' eye work.

Orthoptics. Orthoptics is of value both in diagnosis and treatment. Trained medical auxiliaries should work in close collaboration with ophthalmic surgeons. It cannot, however, be used as a form of treatment until the child is nearly 4 years of age. The reason why some children are referred to orthoptic departments at an earlier age is to observe the effect of occlusion under skilled supervision.

Surgery. If a squint occurs during the first two years of life, if it is constantly present and not appreciably improved by spectacles, surgery should be advised after any amblyopia which may be present has been overcome by occlusion. By making the axes of the eyes parallel, the normal evolution of binocular function is assisted.

If the squint first appears when the child is $3\frac{1}{2}$ to 4 years of age, orthoptic treatment should be advised both before and after surgery.

Glaucoma. The maintenance of normal intra-ocular pressure depends upon an equilibrium between the inflow of aqueous from the ciliary body and its outflow through the tissues of the irido-corneal angle. In theory, raised intra-ocular pressure could result either from an increased inflow or a decreased outflow of aqueous. In practice, glaucoma, that is the condition of pathologically raised intra-ocular pressure, is nearly always due to an interference with the outflow of aqueous from the eye. The nature of the obstruction may be obvious, for example, blockage of the angle by inflammatory cells in uveitis. The treatment in these cases is directed at the underlying condition. More usually the cause is not readily apparent and the glaucoma is known as primary glaucoma.

Primary glaucoma is seen in three main forms, congenital glaucoma, closed-angle glaucoma and chronic simple glaucoma. Congenital glaucoma is rare and its treatment is surgical correction of the developmental abnormality of the irido-corneal angle which causes it.

Closed-angle glaucoma occurs in middle age onwards, in long-sighted eyes, due to a disproportion between the size of the lens and of the eye. It may present subacutely with recurrent attacks of misty vision, ocular discomfort and halos round lights or occasionally as the classical picture of acute congestive glaucoma. The obstruction to aqueous outflow in closed-angle glaucoma is mechanical blockage of the outflow channels in the angle by the root of the iris. This obstruction should be relieved surgically by peripheral iridectomy before permanent damage ensues. In acute closed-angle glaucoma the intra-ocular pressure may be lowered pre-operatively by reducing the rate of aqueous inflow by giving acetazolamide 500 mg. intravenously. Miotic drops such as pilocarpine 2 per cent. or eserine 1 per cent. should be instilled frequently into the affected eye to contract the pupil and draw the iris root out of the irido-corneal angle. Other ways of reducing a very high intra-ocular pressure pre-operatively are by giving urea or mannitol intravenously (p. 400). Medical therapy in closed-angle glaucoma is, however, only an adjunct to suitable surgical treatment.

In chronic simple glaucoma there is a moderate and variable elevation of intra-ocular pressure which eventually leads to cupping and atrophy of the optic disc and loss of vision. The condition is insidious in onset and symptomless. The nature of the obstruction to the outflow of aqueous in chronic simple glaucoma is not fully understood.

Treatment aims at keeping the intra-ocular pressure within normal limits all the time. The outflow of aqueous is influenced by the tonus of the ciliary muscle and can be increased by drugs which cause a contraction of this muscle. These drugs are usually given as eye-drops and the most commonly used are the parasympathomimetics such as pilocarpine 1 to 4 per cent. two or three times daily, and the anticholinesterases such as eserine $\frac{1}{4}$ to 1 per cent. two or three times daily, di-isopropylfluorophosphonate (DFP) 0·01 to 0·05 per cent. at night, demecarium bromide 0·25 to 0·5 per cent. once daily, echothiophate iodide 0·06 to 0·25 per cent. once daily. All of these drugs have the disadvantage that they constrict the pupil and so reduce the amount of light reaching the retina. Of these drugs the last three are synthetic preparations with a powerful and prolonged anticholinesterase action and this may not be limited to the eye. Further, they predispose to cataract and occasionally cause retinal detachment. Such preparations should be used only in close collaboration with an ophthalmologist.

Drugs increasing aqueous outflow may be combined with therapy to reduce aqueous inflow. The carbonic acid anhydrase inhibitors interfere with the ability of the ciliary epithelium to secrete sodium and water into the eye and effectively reduce aqueous inflow. For long-term use acetazolamide is given by mouth in a dose of 250 to 500 mg. daily. Sustained release preparations of 500 mg. daily, may produce fewer side-effects. Alternatively, dichlorphenamide may be given in a dose of 50 mg. two to three times daily. Common side-effects of the carbonic acid anhydrase inhibitors are gastric irritation, a reduction in plasma potassium level, and paraesthesia affecting the extremities. Occasionally, renal damage, marrow depression or exfoliative dermatitis occur. It is usual to give a potassium supplement with these drugs, commonly potassium chloride or potassium bicarbonate, 1 g. daily.

One or two per cent. adrenaline hydrochloride in a suitably buffered solution may be used as eye-drops once or twice daily, in the treatment of glaucoma. This drug reduces aqueous inflow and increases outflow but tends to cause rebound hyperaemia and ocular discomfort. Prolonged use may lead to ocular pigmentation and where there

is absence of the lens (aphakia), macular damage has been reported.

In general, treatment of chronic simple glaucoma is started with pilocarpine nitrate eye-drops 2 per cent. three times daily, and if this is insufficient to control the intra-ocular pressure, stronger concentrations or other drugs are tried until satisfactory control is attained. Only if medical therapy is ineffective is surgery indicated. The treatment of chronic simple glaucoma is time-consuming and demands the careful supervision of affected patients with measurement of the intra-ocular pressure, visual acuity and visual fields every few months for the rest of the patient's life. The treatment is best supervised in a properly organized glaucoma clinic.

Further Reading (ocular mycosis)
Trans. ophthal. Soc. U.K. 1969, **84**, 727.

29. Principles of Prescribing

A. G. MACGREGOR

The care of a sick person involves many procedures which do not necessarily include the administration of drugs or medicines. Throughout this volume emphasis is put upon the management and treatment of the patient as a whole, and drug administration for that patient may be of the least or of the greatest importance.

When drugs are used, therefore, the practitioner must be conversant with their pharmacological action and their expected effect upon the patient. Above all, he must know how best to assess and measure the effect of the drug, realizing that considerations not applicable in a laboratory have to be taken into account. The subjective appraisement by the patient of an effect has to be balanced against the objective evidence of measurable change, be it, for example, blood count, pulse rate, weight, or urine volume. The doctor treating the patient is equally liable to error, and he must ensure that bias, conscious or not, and possible anticipation of the expected effect do not influence the quality and value of his observations.

The physician, therefore, must always be critical in his use of drugs and of the results which it may be tempting to ascribe to them. Many important new remedies are subjected to properly controlled clinical trials before becoming generally available. Nevertheless, remedies are still used which have not been thus investigated, and when this is done the much publicized claims of the manufacturers or promoters may be discovered to be ill-founded.

Qualified practitioners are expected to conform to certain conventions when writing prescriptions: the pharmacist is instructed to supply the drug in a specified form and quantity for a particular patient. Adequate directions on the package, box or bottle should indicate the manner in which the drug is to be used. These directions should answer clearly four questions: how much, how often, when and in what manner is it to be taken or applied?

The distribution and use of certain drugs is limited by legal and statutory regulations; under the conditions applying to the National Health Service in the United Kingdom, further restrictions are applied to the content of a doctor's prescription.

The doctor is responsible for the accuracy of his prescription, and although it is customary for pharmacists in doubt about a script to confirm by direct reference to the doctor that the prescription does in fact represent his intention, this is only a courtesy and not an obligation.

The pharmacist's duty is to dispense the drugs which the doctor feels are the most suitable for his patient. He is rarely asked to dispense doses exceeding the maximum quantities recommended in the British Pharmacopoeia (B.P.). It is important that the doctor should discharge his duty scrupulously and exercise the utmost care in prescribing, always initialling doses which exceed those in the B.P. When this practice is adopted, the pharmacist recognizes that the dose represents the true intention of the doctor, and it is his duty to dispense that quantity of the drug.

Form of Prescription

The heading of the prescription should include the doctor's address (except in a National Health Service prescription on the official form), the date, and the patient's name and address. The main part of the script is preceded by the symbol 'Ŗ' which is an abbreviation for the Latin 'recipe' or 'take'.

The prescription then lists the drugs to be dispensed and the quantity of each to be taken by the patient in each dose. Then follow the instructions to the pharmacist regarding the total quantity of the drug or drugs to be dispensed, and the final section of the script specifies, under the heading 'Sig.' (an abbreviation for the Latin 'signetur', 'let it be labelled') the instructions to be given to the patient on the label of the box or bottle. Should the doctor wish the name of the drug to be included on the label of the bottle, or container, he should precede his labelling instructions with the letters N.P. (*nomen proprium*). This is a sensible practice which should be more widely adopted although it would be preferable for a container always to be labelled with the name of its contents unless otherwise specified by the doctor. This desirable convention has not yet been generally agreed by all the organisations concerned with the distribution of drugs. There are seldom occasions when it is undesirable that a patient should know the nature of his medicine.

It may seem unnecessary to stress the need for legibility in handwriting. Nevertheless, the prevalence of writing and signatures which cannot be deciphered still causes inconvenience and delay to pharmacists and patients. A prescription is only acceptable when signed by a doctor, and the pharmacist should be in a position to identify the writer and check the validity of a prescription by reference to the Medical Register, or to the doctor himself.

It is customary, although not legally obligatory, to add medical qualifications at the foot of a prescription, after the signature.

Legal Requirements in Prescribing

The nature and quantity of drugs that can be used in medicine are limited by certain legal qualifications. In the first place there are, of course, regulations that prevent potential poisons from being obtained by the public without due authorization, and further legislation specifies precautions to protect the patient and general community.

PHARMACY AND POISONS ACT, 1933. This Act and the consolidated regulations issued under the Poison Rules, 1964, and subsequent amendments, govern and control the sale and distribution of poisons throughout the country. The poisons list has two parts: those drugs in Part I can only be sold by pharmacists, but Part II poisons can also be sold by listed sellers of poisons. Most of the drugs of importance which are used in therapeutics are listed as Part I poisons.

The rules issued under the Act also include a number of Schedules specifying those drugs affected by further restrictions and exempted from certain provisions of the Act. Of these, Schedules I and IV are of interest to doctors: Schedule I poisons, most of which are in Part I of the Poisons List, can be sold without a prescription provided that the vendor knows the buyer, who must sign an appropriate entry in a poisons book; Schedule IV lists those drugs from Schedule I which require a signed medical prescription conforming to certain criteria, and Schedule IV is now subdivided into Parts I and II.

The purpose of the Schedule IV regulations, which are those which primarily affect medical practitioners, is to prevent the public having uncontrolled access to potentially dangerous substances such as sulphonamides, barbiturates or amphetamine. It is becoming customary for new drugs to be categorized in Schedule IV if risk accompanies their indiscriminate use, which applies particularly to drugs acting on the central nervous system. The prescription must include all the particulars specified earlier; and the total quantity of the active agent, or of the official preparation, to be dispensed must be stated. Private prescriptions may not be repeated unless specific instructions to the dispenser are given. A prescription on the National Health Service regulation form (E.C. 10) cannot be dispensed more than once.

THE DANGEROUS DRUGS ACTS (D.D.A. 1951) are concerned with the surveillance of the manufacture, importation and ultimate distribution of those drugs, the use of which is most likely to lead to addiction. Obvious examples are opium and many of its derivatives, cocaine, Indian hemp and synthetic analgesics like pethidine and methadone. Many of the regulations are designed to frustrate international trafficking in these drugs, and subsidiary legislation is from time to time introduced to supplement existing law. The Dangerous Drugs Act (1946) and the Consolidating Act (1965) have brought into operation measures for the control of narcotics in the United Kingdom which are consistent with the policies of the World Health Organization.

The Dangerous Drugs Acts lay down precise rules governing prescriptions for these drugs—rules similar in their scope to those affecting drugs listed in Schedule IV. Very detailed regulations ensure that supplies of dangerous drugs are controlled from the time of manufacture until used by the patient.

The Dangerous Drugs (*Notification of Addicts*) *Regulations*, 1968, provide that doctors notify known addicts to the authorities and require that treatment for narcotic addicts be given only in special centres.

THE DRUGS (PREVENTION OF MISUSE) ACT, 1964, gives certain power to the authorities to control and supervise the use of drugs such as the amphetamine derivatives.

THE PHARMACY AND MEDICINES ACT, 1941, specifies that drugs and preparations included in the British Pharmacopoeia and British Pharmaceutical Codex may only be supplied by registered medical practitioners, dentists and pharmacists, and by those persons licensed to do so before 1941. Further rules under this Act became operative in 1952. It is moreover made illegal to advertise a drug which claims to be a cure for certain diseases like diabetes, epilepsy, tuberculosis, venereal diseases and some other conditions.

A most important step to abolish secret and, usually, ineffective remedies was achieved by this Act, which also stipulates that any medicine must be suitably labelled on the container to indicate the names and quantities of its constituents. Unfortunately this does not apply to drugs dispensed from a prescription, and many boxes of tablets and bottles of medicine cannot be identified with certainty. In any such case of doubt, the drug should be discarded and destroyed.

THE PENICILLIN ACT, 1947, and its regulations ensure that penicillin and most other antibiotic substances can only be obtained by the public on the authority of a prescription.

THE THERAPEUTIC SUBSTANCES ACT, 1956, provides for official supervision of the manufacture, activity, sterility, etc., of a number of substances in which great care is required to ensure the production of reliable preparations. Subsequent amendments have included within the Act provisions which determine the conditions under which retail pharmacists may supply antibiotics.

The Medicines Act, 1968

This is a comprehensive measure which consolidates and rationalizes many of the licensing procedures that have accumulated piecemeal over the years in the United Kingdom. Among the many important provisions of the Act, the Minister of Health, the Secretary of State for Scotland, and the Minister of Health and Social Services for Northern Ireland, and the corresponding Ministers concerned with Agriculture, are designated either singly or jointly as the licensing authority with the responsibility for granting certificates and licences to market medicinal products for use in man or in animals.

The Act also establishes a *Medicines Commission* with membership drawn from the medical, veterinary, and pharmaceutical professions, and the pharmaceutical industry. The function of the Commission is to advise the Minister on the composition and terms of reference of advisory committees set up to consider, amongst many other things, the safety, quality and efficacy of drugs, the collection and dissemination of information about adverse reactions, the form and content of the British Pharmacopoeia, and the publication, for the information of the professions, of such compendia etc. as are thought to be appropriate. The Act also gives the Minister power to regulate and control the nature of advertisements about drugs, to ensure that

information contained in them conforms to the conditions under which a license for the product was authorised.

It is obvious that the powers vested in the Ministers, usually to be exercised on the advice of committees recommended by the Medicines Commission, are very extensive. The Act gives authority to a number of committees, such as the Committee on Safety of Drugs, which was established in 1963 and which functioned until superseded by the Medicines Act, by a purely voluntary non-statutory arrangement between the Goverment, the pharmaceutical industry, and the professions. Until the Medicines Commission was set up, the General Medical Council had the copyright, and published, the British Pharmacopoeia, and other committees of the Central and Scottish Health Services Councils helped doctors to decide which drugs to use in the treatment of their patients, and advised which were less likely to be effective or desirable. These functions may now be undertaken by appropriate committees established on the advice of the Medicines Commission.

Nomenclature of drugs. Drugs should always be described, if possible, by their official name, unless it is desired for a special reason that a particular proprietary preparation be dispensed. The 'official' name is that name applied to the drug in the British Pharmacopoeia (B.P.), the British Pharmaceutical Codex (B.P.C.), the British National Formulary (B.N.F.) or, if the drug is not included in such volumes, the approved name bestowed upon it by the Nomenclature Committee of the British Pharmacopoeia Commission. Lists of such approved names are periodically issued by the Commission, and a committee of the World Health Organization tries to ensure uniformity of nomenclature as between the different countries throughout the world.

Drugs should always be described in English and never by the Latin titles which used to be generally applicable.

NATIONAL HEALTH SERVICE PRESCRIBING. Prescriptions for patients being treated under the regulations of the National Health Service have to be written on the official forms (E.C. 10), which, however, cannot be used for private patients. Doctors are asked to use a separate prescription for each patient and not to include more than two items on any one form.

A doctor obtains his own personal requirements in Scotland by presenting a stock order form (E.C.

10A Scotland) to the pharmacist who supplies him and is reimbursed by the Executive Council. In England and Wales personal requirements are paid for from a fund based on the size of the doctor's list of patients. Somewhat different regulations apply to the provision of drugs in the relatively few remaining dispensing practices.

There is no absolute restriction on the prescribing of any drug which a doctor considers to be in the best interests of his patient, and doctors are not subject to any form of central direction as to what may or may not be prescribed. There are, however, certain relative restrictions qualifying prescribing habits. A doctor may be called upon to justify his prescribing to his colleagues on the Local Medical Committee if he appears to have prescribed excessively, or if he has prescribed substances which are not specified as drugs, which have not been shown to be of therapeutic value, or which have been advertised to the public.

The nature and quantity of the drugs prescribed by a doctor for the patients on his list are kept under review by the Executive Councils, and occasionally examples of what appear to be excessive and unjustifiable prescribing are referred to the Local Medical Committee. The latter may recommend, after inquiry, that a sum of money should be recovered by the Executive Council from the doctor concerned.

Drugs and preparations included in the British Pharmacopoeia (B.P.), British Pharmaceutical Codex (B.P.C.) and British National Formulary (B.N.F.) are freely prescribable (unless defined as foods, etc.). A committee appropriately constituted keeps under review the principles which determine whether a preparation should properly be regarded as a drug, food, toilet preparation or disinfectant.

Guidance to doctors regarding what should and, if possible, what should not be prescribed is given in a number of publications. A White Paper has defined those substances held to be foods, toilet preparations or disinfectants. Such reports have no statutory authority, but their existence is of assistance to Executive Councils, who may, after reference to the Local Medical Committee, recover from a doctor the cost of any substance which he has prescribed and which has been held not to be a drug. It can be well understood that it is frequently a matter of some difficulty to decide when, for example, a skin ointment becomes a toilet preparation and not a drug, or when certain 'invalid

foods' can be regarded as drugs that can be legitimately prescribed.

In many instances, however, although a drug may be given a standard specification and be included in the B.P. or B.N.F., it is only available on the market in the form of the proprietary preparations manufactured by individual pharmaceutical houses. In such circumstances pharmacists dispensing a prescription for the standard preparation have no alternative but to provide the proprietary drug. The latter is usually pharmacologically and chemically identical with the standard specification but may have, in addition, some colouring or flavouring agent which disqualifies it from being described as a standard preparation. A pharmacist is not permitted to dispense the equivalent standard official drug if presented with a prescription for the proprietary preparation, although such a procedure would often fulfil the doctor's therapeutic aims.

A great deal of helpful information is given to doctors in *The Prescribers' Journal*, issued every two months by the Ministry of Health and the Department of Home and Health for Scotland. Succinct and sensible advice is given on prescribing practice generally, on current costs of drugs and appliances, and regarding the introduction of new preparations as they become available for general prescription. The Consumers' Association publishes a fortnightly *Drug and Therapeutics Bulletin* to which doctors can subscribe and from which valuable information can be gathered.

Dosage and quantities of drugs to be prescribed. Dosage should always be specified in metric measures, as this is now generally applicable, and all new drugs are introduced and marked in metric quantities.

Young practitioners are often doubtful as to the quantities of a drug that should be prescribed. Several considerations govern this, including duration of the illness, the degree of danger attached to the use of the drug, and its cost. Usually tablets, capsules, and other dry preparations should be prescribed in quantities to cover the probable duration of the illness if this can be anticipated. Drugs which are to be used for long periods, for example, digoxin, iron or insulin, should be supplied in quantities sufficient for at least a month; shorter intervals involve increased costs due to dispensing charges, and inconvenience due to frequent visits to the doctor. Dangerous drugs such as barbiturates should be supplied in the smallest reasonable amount for the circumstances; and expensive drugs which are being used for the first time should also be ordered in small quantities.

When selecting the quantity of a liquid medicine to be supplied for a patient, it is convenient that the total quantity should be a multiple of the size of the dose. It is, therefore, desirable, for example, to prescribe the number of doses for liquid medicines in tens or multiples of ten. It is often convenient to prescribe for an adult 300 ml. of a mixture containing 20 doses each of 15 ml., and quantities of other preparations, in amounts related to 100 grammes or millilitres. The B.N.F. contains tables of recommended quantities and volumes.

Selection of preparation to be prescribed. A drug can usually be administered by mouth, and this should be the route of choice unless it is imperative that it be injected, either because it is unpalatable or inactive when taken orally, or because a different speed of action is required.

Such a medicine should, if possible, be given as a dry preparation, as a tablet or in a capsule, rather than as a mixture, tincture, elixir, etc. Tablets and capsules are far more convenient for both pharmacist and patient, they are a more accurate way of giving drugs, and are often cheaper with a lower dispensing fee. Only exceptionally is a mixture necessary; sometimes drugs cannot be dispensed as solids because of their physical properties; and drugs intended for infants have usually to be prescribed in a suitably flavoured liquid vehicle. Nevertheless, at least 25 per cent. of National Health Service prescriptions are still for mixtures, a percentage so high that it suggests the influence of outworn conventions.

The great majority of the drugs and preparations used nowadays are standardized and defined in the British Pharmacopoeia, but the British Pharmaceutical Codex and the British National Formulary list some substances and compound preparations not included in the B.P. Prescriptions specially written for individual patients are seldom justifiable. Standard preparations from the formularies should be prescribed whenever possible as they are readily available to the pharmacist, and much time, labour and expense are saved compared to that expended when non-standard mixtures, powders, ointments, etc., are prescribed.

There are few occasions when it becomes necessary to prescribe more than one drug at a time, and when it is necessary to do so, each drug is given for a specific purpose. The days of prescriptions containing a multiplicity of ingredients are ended, and

there is no justification for the perpetuation of polypharmacy.

Most of the really valuable drugs available have been developed by pharmaceutical manufacturing houses, and often they are distributed only in the proprietary form. They can usually be prescribed quite freely, and should be so prescribed when, as occasionally occurs, the proprietary preparation is cheaper than the official equivalent. Further, as new drugs become established there is inevitably an interval before they receive the recognition implied by inclusion in the British Pharmacopoeia or National Formulary. If shown to be of value, these proprietary preparations should naturally be freely used.

It is part of the pharmacist's business to make medicines palatable, but there is rarely any occasion to compete with the confectioner, though some latitude is desirable when he is dispensing for young children. A critical attitude should be maintained towards the prescribing of proprietary preparations. Many of the claims made in the advertisements distributed to members of the medical profession are not in fact justifiable, and the drugs may not be as useful or as therapeutically effective as the manufacturers would have the doctor believe, although the potential restraints upon advertising which are possible under the provisions of the Medicines Act, 1968, have curbed the more excessive claims There is often an acceptable and less expensive analogous standard preparation. The prescriber must always retain his critical faculties and should scrutinize carefully the evidence offered by manufacturers purporting to prove the therapeutic value of new preparations. A glossary on p. 654 lists the proprietary equivalents of drugs described in this book by their approved or official names and *vice versa*.

The Cost of Drugs and Prescriptions

Under present conditions in the National Health Service over £150,000,000 are spent annually on prescribed drugs—about 10 per cent. of the gross cost of the Service. A little over half of this sum covers the cost of the actual ingredients of the prescriptions issued, the balance representing dispensing fees, pharmacists' profit, allowance for containers, etc. It is, therefore, important to know how the costs of a prescription are calculated.

The pharmacist is repaid by the Health Service in respect of a prescription in the following way: he receives payment for the basic cost of the ingredients, which is the sum listed in the *Drug Tariff*. This publication issued by the Health Service authorities lists the cost of basic drugs, appliances, dressings, etc. It also details the procedure for the costing of proprietary preparations. These prices are increased by a percentage calculated on the total cost of ingredients due to the pharmacist at the end of each month, and this represents the oncost, or profit, to the pharmacist. The Drug Tariff applicable in England and Wales differs from that used in Scotland, and pharmacists north of the border are remunerated at a different rate. A container allowance is paid for each prescription; finally there is a dispensing charge, the size of which is calculated differently in England and in Scotland, and is dependent upon the type of preparation prescribed.

The total expense of a prescription to the Health Service can be several shillings, although the actual ingredients may cost only a few pence. A charge per item on each prescription, to be paid by the patient, has been introduced by the Minister of Health, certain specified groups, such as old age pensioners, children, and the chronic sick being exempted from such a direct charge. In the case of expensive drugs, the basic ingredient charge may completely swamp other charges, and the practitioner

should always be aware of the cost of such prescriptions and be discriminating in what he prescribes for his patients. It is uneconomic to prescribe inexpensive drugs in small quantities if they are to be taken for a prolonged period, as the overhead charges are so much in excess of the ingredient costs.

The Ministry of Health and the Department of Home and Health for Scotland publish for doctors histograms of comparative costs to the Health Service of many standard preparation contained in the British National Formulary and British Pharmaceutical Codex, and of comparable proprietary preparations. These publications provide invaluable safeguards against unnecessary and extravagant prescribing.

Undoubtedly the greatest economy in prescribing can be effected by really careful thought as to the necessity, in the first place, for any drug administration at all, the most suitable preparation to use, and the most sensible and economical quantity of the drug to order for the patient. Drugs should be, and usually are, solely prescribed so that the patient may benefit from their pharmacological effect. When a drug is prescribed purely as a placebo—often but not always an admission of professional failure—an inexpensive and innocuous preparation should be selected.

30. Technical Procedures

Sir JAMES FRASER and I. W. B. GRANT

INTRODUCTION

Before undertaking any of the procedures to be described in this chapter the doctor should ensure that he has four things: a good light, a comfortable stance or seat, a relaxed and co-operative patient adequately protected against bacterial infection. For most minor procedures a 'no touch' technique can be used in which the doctor works with clean dry hands and nothing which he has touched comes into contact with the patient; alternatively there is the full aseptic ritual in which the hands are not only cleaned but are also protected by gloves and the operation site is sterilized and isolated by towels. Carried to its logical conclusion this would imply the use of an operating theatre with proper disciplines, sterile air, freedom from dust and airborne particles and almost total isolation from the general environment. The peculiar hazards of infection in hospitals during the era of antibiotics are such that wherever possible such a theatre or specially equipped room should be used for all but the most trivial operations. However, regard to the appropriate techniques and a high standard of personal discipline are of the greatest value in preventing cross-infection and are sufficient for most of the procedures described in this chapter.

Preparation of the hands of the operator and of the patient's skin. The hands are washed with soap in running warm water. The use of the nail brush is confined to the nailfolds and nails; elsewhere it roughens the skin, which is potentially harmful. The duration of washing is a timed five minutes and the efficiency of bacterial removal is increased if a preparation which contains hexachlorophane is used routinely. The hands are then dried on a sterile towel. The skin of the patient is shaved if necessary and then washed with soap or hexachlorophane. For all minor procedures 2·5 per cent. iodine in spirit (weak iodine solution B.P.) is the best means of sterilizing the skin rapidly, but it must not be slopped over the area lest it should set up irritation in adjacent parts such as joint flexures. For sensitive areas such as the genital skin a 0·5 per cent. solution of chlorhexidine is less irritant and will provide adequate sterilization. The sterilized area is conveniently isolated by a towel,

50 cm. square, with a central hole 10 cm. square. The local anaesthetic (usually 2 per cent. lignocaine) should be ordered in small ampoules.

Sterilization of equipment. Complete destruction of all potentially harmful organisms cannot be achieved by the use of boiling water. Dry heat at 110° C. for one hour or steam at one atmosphere (121° C.) for 15 to 20 minutes is required to eliminate spore-forming bacteria. Thus, whenever possible, all equipment for even the most simple purpose should be sterilized by one or other of these measures, and most hospitals which maintain a central supply organization can supply prepacked, sterile equipment for dressings and minor procedures. The practitioner should avail himself of these or organize his own system if possible; small high-speed autoclaves which will sterilize packs and instruments are now readily available. Drums should not be used; towels, swabs and instruments are wrapped within a double thickness of linen or in a plastic envelope and will remain sterile after autoclaving for at least a year.

EMERGENCY STERILIZATION. In certain circumstances it may be necessary to rely either on boiling or chemical sterilization. These methods carry a significant risk but it can be minimized if syringes and instruments are scrupulously cleaned to remove all dirt that may be laden with spores.

STERILIZATION BY BOILING. A layer of lint is laid in a receptacle such as a sterilizer or saucepan and the instruments or syringes are placed upon it: needles are threaded through a separate piece of lint. Water is added, brought to the boil and kept boiling for not less than five minutes. After the instruments have been boiled, they should be allowed to cool with minimum exposure to air and are then removed with a sterile forceps.

DISINFECTION BY CHEMICALS. The only chemical disinfectant which is suitable for both instruments and syringes is 70 per cent. alcohol prepared by the dilution of industrial methylated spirit with sterile water. Its use for syringes is justified only when heat sterilization is quite impracticable. All-glass syringes should be used. Alcohol is used only rarely for instruments, but the same procedure can be followed.

Sterilization by boiling or by chemicals does not

624

meet contemporary bacteriological standards and as such the practice should be discouraged. Many commercial firms provide disposable instruments and equipment, including needles and plastic syringes of a very high standard, in pre-packed, pre-sterilized containers. Although slightly less satisfactory than a dry sterilized all-glass syringe, they are superior to those of glass construction with a metal plunger. They may be used in almost every situation and the ease with which they can be stored and carried makes them ideal for emergency use.

Mass injections. Particular danger of cross-infection with the virus of serum hepatitis occurs if mass inoculations or mass intravenous injections are performed. Whenever possible, dry-sterilized all-glass or plastic disposable syringes should be used. In such circumstances safe practice depends on the efficient organization of the routine to be employed so that sterile and used syringes are kept separate.

Venepuncture

Puncture of a vein may be necessary (1) for the intravenous injection of drugs or fluids or (2) for the withdrawal of blood to obtain a sample for analysis, to obtain blood for transfusion, or to reduce the volume of blood in the circulation as a therapeutic measure. For any of these purposes, a vein in one of the antecubital fossae is chosen. In an obese arm the antecubital veins may not be visible, but as a rule they are palpable when engorged. Care should be taken not to confuse a superficial brachial artery with a vein, particularly when intravenous medication is to be undertaken, because serious vascular complications may follow accidental intra-arterial injection. It is best to use one of the less movable veins situated laterally in the cubital fossae. Veins may be visible and prominent, but, particularly in the elderly, may slip from side to side under the skin. The vein is secured by stretching the skin distal to the point of puncture between the forefinger and thumb of the operator's free hand. Before it is punctured it should be made as prominent as possible: several manœuvres are available:

1. A tourniquet may be applied at the root of the limb, so as to obstruct the venous return without stopping the arterial inflow. This may be a turn of bandage twisted on itself; a piece of rubber tubing fastened by a forceps or by a half knot, or the cuff of a sphygmomano-

meter inflated to a pressure of about 30 mm. of mercury.
2. The limb may be allowed to hang over the edge of the bed for a few minutes before the puncture.
3. After the application of the tourniquet the patient may be directed to grasp a roller bandage firmly with his hand at intervals of 30 seconds.
4. A vein can frequently be made to dilate by tapping the skin over it. Applications of cold antiseptics cause the vein to contract.

Intravenous medication. A fine hypodermic needle[1] (26 s.w.g.) with a short bevel should be used. The fluid to be injected is drawn up out of its container, through the needle, into a syringe of appropriate size. The needle should not be passed to the bottom of the container, but the ampoule should be tilted to allow all the fluid to be drawn up with the needle resting on the wall. The syringe and needle are then inverted, the barrel is tapped to dislodge any bubbles of air, and the piston pushed upwards until fluid flows from the point of the needle. The skin is sterilized as already described. If a puncture of the skin is made while the surface is wet with spirit, some of the fluid is carried in on the needle point, thereby aggravating the pain. The needle is pushed through the stretched dry skin a little to one side of the selected vein, and then brought over it, with the bevel up ready to make the puncture; it is then pushed into the vein at an acute angle, and its position verified by gently withdrawing a little blood into the syringe. When the point is correctly placed, the obstruction to the venous return is removed and the contents of the syringe are slowly injected. *An injection should never be made unless blood has been withdrawn into the syringe, and after this has been done the position of the needle should not be altered until the injection has been completed.* The needle is then quickly withdrawn while the thumb of the left hand makes pressure upon the area of the puncture through a gauze swab or piece of sterile cotton-wool; if the patient flexes his elbow on this pad for a few minutes, a dressing is not required. Alternatively the patient may be asked to hold his arm upright for a few minutes, as extravasation may occur from a laterally placed vein if the elbow is flexed.

If the patient moves, there is a possibility that the

[1] There is an increasing tendency to standardize all syringes, needles and other equipment on Luer mounts.

needle will be dislodged from the vein, and its position must be verified again before the injection is begun or completed. If, during the injection, any swelling appears under the skin round the puncture, leakage has occurred: the injection should be stopped at once, the needle withdrawn and a vein in another limb used.

Withdrawal of blood. A short bevelled, disposable needle of No. 19 s.w.g. and an all-glass or a plastic disposable syringe of suitable size should be used. If possible, samples of blood for analysis should be taken from the patient at least eight hours after his last meal (e.g. in the morning before he takes breakfast). It should be remembered that certain measurements (e.g. calcium, bicarbonate and haematocrit) are altered by venous occlusion and that due precautions should be observed. Samples should be despatched as soon as possible after their withdrawal and the organization of laboratory analysis is greatly helped by the regular and prompt arrival of samples. Untreated, heparinized or oxalated blood may be collected in sterile test-tubes suitably prepared and having a rubber stopper. In most circumstances, however, it is preferable to use standard commercially available specimen tubes. These are accurately prepared with the correct additive and indicate by a line the exact quantity of blood to be added for each examination. These tubes are usually available through the laboratory or the central supply depot. The details of the nature of the samples required for the quantitative estimation of certain constituents of blood, and the normal range of these can be obtained from the laboratory that undertakes the investigation.

Therapeutic withdrawal of blood. The indications are cardiac failure with increased pressure in the systemic veins and polycythaemia. The technique is similar to that employed in the withdrawal of blood for transfusion and it may be possible, with appropriate arrangements, to use the blood for transfusion.

Intravenous Infusion

Fluid may be introduced into a vein through either a needle or a cannula. Administration is usually slow and intermittent—as by the drip technique— but circumstances may call for continuous and even rapid infusion of large volumes of fluid.

Apparatus. The administration of intravenous fluids, using a large glass container connected to a needle or cannula by a length of rubber tubing, may

occasionally be necessary in emergencies but its use is seldom justified in view of the risk of introducing pyrogens and infection even with careful sterilization. In practice this equipment has been replaced by pre-sterilized and disposable plastic units. These are both cheap and efficient and are available either as a giving-set alone or as a plastic bag containing the required infusion solution with tubing and needle combined. The latter units are easily and safely stored and are ideal for use in an emergency outside hospital practice.

Needles for intravenous infusion can be obtained in a variety of designs; they should be sharp, made of rustless material and have a short bevel. Fine needles may be used for the infusion of crystalloids, but when blood or plasma transfusions are to be made the standard needle of 16 s.w.g. is by far the best. Cannulae should also be rustless (they are sometimes supplied with a bulbous tip, but this makes their removal from the vein difficult, and this type should not be used). As an alternative to an indwelling needle, plastic intravenous cannulae are now readily available as pre-sterilized disposable packs. Of varying diameters and lengths, these can be inserted close to the elbow without the necessity of rigid immobilization of the joint. Apart from their technical convenience, they are more comfortable for the patient and greatly reduce the incidence of extravasation.

When the intravenous infusion is restricted to a small quantity of fluid or for a short period of time, the use of a needle is probably to be preferred. When the administration of fluids has to be continued for many days, for example, in hepatic or renal failure, and in the restless and unconscious patient, it is more satisfactory to make use of a cannula. In these circumstances, a long cannula is introduced into either the superior or inferior vena cava by way of the basilic or saphenous vein respectively. Fluid so introduced enters a large, rapidly flowing stream of blood and is immediately diluted. Solutions of a composition or concentration which would irritate the wall of a peripheral vein (e.g. hypertonic glucose or saline, protein hydrolysates) can safely be administered in this manner over a period of days or weeks. However, the most strict aseptic precautions must be observed at all times because of the risk of the introduction of virulent infection, usually staphylococcal. Caval infusions must only be undertaken by the expert and *never* in patients with severe sepsis. Pre-sterilized cannulae should always be used for this purpose.

For all intravenous infusions a head of pressure of about one metre is ample. If the patient's veins are in spasm, the reservoir may be raised higher; warming the limb with a hot-water bottle, electric blanket or fomentation may also help. In extreme cases, and if very rapid infusion is desired, fluid can be introduced under pressure with a rotary pump connected to the tubing of the giving set or by pumping air into the inlet tube of the bottle with a sphygmomanometer bulb; by this method up to 250 to 300 ml. of blood or other fluid can be given in one minute. When this is done, the infusion must be under the constant supervision of a doctor who must be aware of the danger of causing an air embolus. The air introduced is filtered through a cotton-wool plug in the inlet tube. Whenever it is expected that a pressure infusion may be required a pump or a sphygmomanometer bulb with an appropriate adaptor should be kept ready.

Fluids for intravenous use. These are prepared with great care from pure chemicals and distilled water, and thereafter sterilized. Unless every detail in their preparation receives scrupulous attention, pyrogenic reactions may occur. It is difficult and hazardous to prepare these solutions, and the doctor in general practice should procure them from firms which specialize in their production or from a hospital dispensary.

Methods of administration. Local complications are more prone to occur if the vein is exposed and cannulated for the intravenous administration of fluids, and, therefore, it is better to use a needle or percutaneous cannula when possible. When the veins are collapsed, as in shock, or if the patient is so fat that they cannot be identified under the skin, a suitable vein may have to be exposed and time should not be wasted in futile attempts to insert a needle. If the situation is urgent and particularly if a large volume of blood or other fluid must be administered quickly, the most prominent vein in one or other antecubital fossa is chosen. For ordinary infusions it is better to use a vein on the dorsum of the hand or of the forearm away from the flexures of wrist and elbow. If the needle or cannula is adequately secured by a turn of sterile elastic adhesive applied over a swab, it is unnecessary to splint the arm except in children or in delirious patients. Veins in the lower limb should *not* be used, because satisfactory flow through them cannot be assured, especially in shock; further, the patient is immobilized by the infusion and phlebo-thrombosis is more likely to occur.

'CUT DOWN' CANNULA METHOD. An intadermal weal of local anaesthetic (2 per cent. lignocaine) is made over the vein at the selected level, about 0·5 ml. of the solution is deposited in the tissues on each side of the vessel, and the area is compressed for a minute or two in order to distribute the anaesthetic. A tourniquet is applied to make the vein prominent and an incision about 1 cm. long is made at right angles to the vein while the skin is steadied by the fingers and thumb of the left hand. The wound is opened up and the vein cleared by inserting a closed small artery forceps on each side of the vessel in turn and opening the points of the forceps in a direction parallel to the vein. The closed artery forceps is then passed under the vein, and the tourniquet is released. A double strand of catgut is drawn under the vein by grasping its midpoint with the artery forceps, and the strand is divided so as to provide two ligatures of equal length. The distal of these is drawn to the distal part of the cleared vein and used to ligate it, the ends of the ligature being left long and secured by an artery forceps. The proximal ligature is drawn to the proximal end of the vein, and tied loosely as a half knot. Fluid is now allowed to flow through the infusion system and cannula until all air has been displaced. The flow is then stopped by clamping the tubing with an artery forceps about 15 cm. from the cannula. The cannula is laid on the sterile towel so that it can be picked up conveniently. A small cut is made in the distal skin flap about 0·75 cm. from the incision. The vein is now held by traction on the distal ligature and an oblique nick across half its circumference is made with fine blunt-pointed scissors. The insertion of one blade of the scissors into the nick allows the opening to be enlarged without any danger of completely dividing the vein. While the proximal lip of the opening is retracted, the cannula is inserted through the cut in the skin flap into the lumen of the vein; care must be taken to elevate the whole thickness of the wall of the vessel so that the glistening intima is displayed, otherwise it is possible for an inexperienced or careless operator to pass the cannula between the coats of the vein instead of into the lumen. The proximal catgut ligature is then tightened upon the cannula and the skin incision completely closed. The cannula is secured by passing a stitch through the skin to encircle its hilt and when the infusion has been completed it is easily removed by a sharp tug.

NEEDLE METHOD. The vein is made prominent

as already described. An intradermal weal of local anaesthetic is made to one side of the vein at a point slightly distal to the desired level of vene-puncture. A No. 16 s.w.g. needle is inserted through the weal and brought over the vein to make the puncture. After it has entered the vein, the needle should be passed upwards along the lumen for at least 1 cm. to ensure that it is lying correctly: if this is the case, a continuous free reflux of blood will occur. The infusion apparatus is connected to the needle by an adaptor and the fluid allowed to flow by unclamping the delivery tube. When the infusion is completed, the needle is withdrawn and a sterile dressing is applied.

The percutaneous technique for the insertion of an intravenous cannula is the same as that used for an intravenous needle. The vein is punctured by the wide-bore needle provided with each set. The cannula is passed into and along the vein as soon as blood can be seen within the lumen. The needle is now withdrawn and both it and the cannula are fixed to the skin with adhesive strapping. Sets of this type are available with the introducing needle within or outside the cannula. Those with the needle within are easier to manipulate and avoid damage to the plastic cannula by the sharp bevel of the needle. This may occur within the lumen of the vein during introduction with the consequent danger of a foreign body embolus.

Continuous fluid therapy. In all cases when intravenous therapy is to be continued for a number of days care must be taken to see that the fluid is accurately prescribed to meet the patient's needs and to avoid the dangers of under- or over-administration. For each 24 hours a careful record should be kept in which intake is charted against output. Output includes the urine, water lost from the lungs and skin (normally about 1 litre per 24 hours in temperate zones, but increased to 5 to 6 litres in hot climates or by high fever), by vomiting or by diarrhoea. The patient's weight is a further valuable guide to the administration of fluid, marked day-to-day fluctuations indicating excessive or inadequate infusion. The chart should always be totalled at the same time each day—preferably the early morning which is the usual time to review progress and arrange for the day's treatment. Fluid should be quantitatively and qualitatively prescribed *in writing* for the next 24 hours, just as with drugs.

Illustrative case. A middle-aged man who had begun to vomit from intestinal obstruction was admitted to hospital. During his first 24 hours 1,500 ml. of liquid were withdrawn from his stomach, and he took nothing by mouth. His urinary output was 800 ml. and his insensible loss 1,000 ml., resulting in a total fluid deficit of 3·3 litres. His vomit contained virtually no sodium, potassium at a concentration of 10 mEq./l. and chloride at a concentration of about 60 to 70 mEq./l. During the same period his total urinary potassium output was 60 mEq. and his urinary sodium output was 30 mEq. His replacement needs were consequently 3·3 litres of water, 90 mEq. of chloride, 30 mEq. of sodium and 75 mEq. of potassium. These were provided by 3 litres of 5 per cent. dextrose in water, to which were added in all 6 g. of potassium chloride (equivalent to 78 mEq. of potassium) and 300 ml. of normal saline. Slight over-replacement of chloride thus occurred but could be disregarded.

Duration of infusion. The period during which an infusion into a vein may be continued varies from patient to patient, with the type of fluid that is administered and with the equipment. For example, isotonic glucose (6 per cent.) is more irritant than saline, and rubber equipment more irritant than plastic. Using conventional methods of administration by needle or cannula the vein becomes within 24 hours the site of a non-infective phlebitis, ushered in by a feeling of local soreness; later the tissues in the immediate neighbourhood of the cannula become oedematous and the skin reddens, and if the infusion is continued, the redness and swelling spread along the vein. The appearance of any of these complications requires immediate withdrawal of the needle or cannula. If the infusion must be continued, another vein, preferably in the opposite arm, should be used.

The development of phlebitis can largely be prevented by strict aseptic precautions, by the use of plastic infusion sets and, as has been mentioned, by the use of cannulae discharging into the vena cava in carefully selected cases. When a caval catheter cannot be used it is usually preferable to give the daily fluid requirements over a short period in the morning, the infusion being taken down after the full amount has been given. The procedure is repeated each day.

Blood Transfusion

Blood is collected from a donor and mixed with a suitable anticoagulant; it may be infused immediately into a patient or it may be stored in hermetically sealed bottles in a refrigerator until required. Blood so stored should not be transfused after 14 days because by this time the cells are not only more prone to undergo lysis but the potassium concentration in the plasma has risen to dangerous levels by its release from the cells. Certain precautions must be taken to ensure that the transfusion is without danger to the patient, irrespective of whether fresh or stored blood is used.

General precautions. The persons from whom the blood is taken must be physically healthy; more particularly there should be no history or sign of any disease transmissible by blood (e.g. malaria, infective hepatitis, syphilis). The Wassermann reaction of a donor's blood should be proved to be negative.

At all times the blood must be protected by the most rigid aseptic technique from contamination by organisms. The sterilization of apparatus should be *by heat* (because antiseptics may spoil the blood), but the apparatus must not be hot when used and the blood must never be warmed above 40° C. For storage the temperature should be about 4° C. (the temperature of a domestic refrigerator) but should never be as low as 0° C., at which the cells are damaged. Blood removed from storage should be used within six hours and should be free from haemolysis, the presence of which is indicated by a red discolouration of the zone of plasma above the cell layer. Finally, blood must never be infused until it has been proved to be compatible with the blood of the patient.

Blood groups and compatibilities.[1] Many different blood groups have been distinguished and the number is steadily increasing, but transfusion practice is concerned mainly with the four chief groups (AB, A, B and O) and with the Rhesus factor. The four groups are so named because of the presence or absence of two agglutinogens named 'A' and 'B' in the red cells. Corresponding to these agglutinogens are their homologous antibodies or agglutinins named 'Anti-A' and 'Anti-B' respectively. The agglutinin is present in the serum of any blood in the cells of which the corresponding agglutinogen is absent. This reciprocal arrangement is shown in Table 16.

It will be seen that when any two whole bloods of different groups are mixed, some incompatibility

[1] For a full description of the blood groups see M.R.C. War Memorandum No. 9, 'The Determination of Blood Groups', and M.R.C. Memorandum No. 27, 'The Rh Blood Groups and their Clinical Effects'. H.M. Stationery Office. Also, Blood Groups in Man by Race, R. and Sanger, R., 4th Edit., 1967.

results: the red cells of at least one of the two samples contains an agglutinogen which corresponds to an agglutinin in the serum. Thus mixture

TABLE 16

Blood Group (and Agglutinogen in Cells)	Agglutinin in Serum
AB	None
A	Anti-B
B	Anti-A
O	Anti-A and Anti-B

of two whole blood samples results in some agglutination unless the bloods are of the same group. In giving blood transfusions it has been found that in routine practice the effect of the serum of the donor on the red cells of the recipient can be almost completely ignored; only the effect of the serum of the recipient on the corpuscles of the donor need be considered. This means that the blood infused does not always require to be of the same group as that of the patient; it must, however, be of a group the cells of which will not be agglutinated by the patient's serum. Reference to the Table will accordingly show that:

Group AB blood can be given only to a patient of Group AB.

Group A blood can be given to patients of Groups AB and A.

Group B blood can be given to patients of Groups AB and B.

Group O blood can be given to patients of any Group.

The Rhesus or Rh factors[2] are a group of antigens present in the red cells of about 85 per cent. of human beings. The remaining 15 per cent. are Rh-negative. In certain circumstances, Rh-negative individuals may develop in their sera homologous antibodies to Rh antigens and become 'Rh-sensitive'. This occurs when an Rh-negative patient is transfused with Rh-positive blood or when an Rh-negative mother becomes pregnant with an Rh-positive foetus, the Rh factor being inherited as a Mendelian dominant. If an Rh-negative woman is

[2] The name Rhesus is used because these antigens were first detected by the use of anti-Rhesus serum prepared by injecting the red cells of the Rhesus monkey into rabbits.

made Rh-sensitive either by transfusion or by her first pregnancy, any Rh-positive foetus which she subsequently conceives is affected by the Rh antibodies; in consequence the foetus may be stillborn or it may be born with a haemolytic anaemia, the condition of erythroblastosis foetalis. In the circumstances mentioned above, both mother and child must be regarded as 'Rh-sensitive', and if they are to be transfused, Rh-negative blood must be used. Similarly, if repeated transfusions are undertaken in Rh-negative patients, sensitization occurs unless Rh-negative blood only is used, and any subsequent transfusion of Rh-positive blood will result in a reaction and haemolysis of the donor's cells.

In practice, transfusion of Rh-positive blood to an Rh-negative patient must be avoided except when the urgency is such that life can be saved only by accepting the risk. Particular care must be taken to ensure that Rh sensitivity is not produced in any female child or any woman in the child-bearing period and that Rh positive blood is not given to a patient who may have previously been sensitized to the Rh factor. The possibility of such Rh sensitivity must always be considered in a person who has received previous blood transfusions or in any parous woman.

Stocks of Group O Rh-negative blood are maintained by Blood Transfusion Centres for use in emergencies when the administration of blood must precede the determination of group and Rhesus type. Fortunately, the rapid determination of Rhesus type is possible, and it should be unnecessary to use Group O Rh-negative blood without preliminary knowledge of the patient's group and Rhesus type.

Although several subgroups of the Rh factor exist, for practical purposes the Rh type of the recipient can be determined by testing his red cells for the presence of a single factor known as Factor D. The presence of this Factor indicates that the patient is clinically Rh-positive. The rarer subgroups are less likely to give rise to incompatibility between the bloods of donor and patient and this is avoided by a direct test of compatibility. All generalizations on the A, B, O or Rh groups must be qualified by the statement that such subgroups exist and may result in incompatibilities unless the donor blood is tested directly against that of the recipient. Consequently, a direct test of compatibility *must* be undertaken in every case to prove the suitability of blood for transfusion. The omission

of a direct test is not justifiable except in circumstances of extreme urgency and difficulty; under these conditions only Group O Rh-negative blood should be used.

Determination of blood group and rhesus type. A heavy responsibility rests upon the practitioner who undertakes the grouping and compatibility testing of blood for transfusion. Where possible this should be carried out by trained staff with adequate facilities. If this work must be undertaken it is necessary to adopt a technique devoid of the risks of clerical or technical error.

Blood Transfusion Centres carry out all procedures in test-tubes 5 cm. × 0·5 cm. in size, and this method of mixing blood and anti-serum should be adopted because it gives the most reliable results. If tubes are not available, the samples are mixed on a slide, agglutination being detected by examining the slide against a suitable white background.

Whether a 'tube' or 'slide' method is used, it is good practice to examine the blood not only for agglutinogen in the cells but also for agglutinins in the serum, because this double test prevents the occurrence of errors. Reference to Table 17 will

TABLE 17

Agglutination of unknown Cells by		Unknown belongs to
Anti-B Sera	Anti-A Sera	
+	+	Group AB
—	+	Group A
+	—	Group B
—	—	Group O

show that the group of any given blood can be determined by testing its corpuscles separately against two sera, one of which contains only Anti-A agglutinin, the other only Anti-B. Similarly, if cells of Groups A and B blood are available, they are used to test the serum of the unknown blood for the presence of Anti-A and Anti-B agglutinins. Anti-A and Anti-B grouping sera are obtained from bloods of Groups B and A respectively, and for the purpose of the test are provided in phials or capillary tubes. The high titre of the agglutinin required is best preserved by storing the serum in the frozen state in the ice compartment of a refrigerator.

Because it is suitable for emergency use, the rapid slide method will be described.

THE SLIDE TEST. Four millilitres of blood are withdrawn by venepuncture, carefully ejected into a glass tube and either centrifuged or allowed to stand for 30 minutes so that cells and serum may separate. The clot is then broken up with a fine pipette and four drops of it are suspended in 1 ml. of saline to give approximately a 5 per cent. concentration of red cells. One drop of this suspension is then added to a drop of Anti-A serum and to a drop of Anti-B serum placed at opposite ends of a glass slide appropriately marked on its under surface with a grease pencil: each suspension is stirred with a separate clean glass rod or with the separate halves of a new wooden match. If agglutination is going to occur, it usually does so rapidly, but an interval of 15 minutes should elapse before the results are finally read. During this time evaporation should be prevented by placing the slides on damp filter paper and covering them by inverted glass dishes. Agglutination is usually obvious to the naked eye, but in all cases the cells should be scrutinized under the low power of the microscope. According to the findings, the blood group of the person being tested can be determined thus:

The Rhesus group can be determined at the same time, but for this purpose an Anti-D serum that is potent *in saline* must be obtained. If only albumin Anti-D is available the test is incomplete and the help of an experienced blood transfusion officer should be sought or the risks accepted. One drop of the 5 per cent. cell suspension in saline is added to one drop of potent saline (agglutinating) Anti-D serum in a test-tube. The mixture is incubated at 37° C. for 10 to 15 minutes and centrifuged for 20 seconds. If agglutination has occurred, the sediment has a granular appearance, and this may be confirmed by transferring a sample to a slide and examining it under a microscope.[1] Agglutination indicates that the patient is Rh-positive.

Finally, the group of the unknown blood may be checked by testing its serum against known cells (Table 18). Serum is obtained by centrifuging the sample of blood; one drop is added to each of separate drops of Group A and Group B cells placed at opposite ends of a slide. This is examined after 10 minutes both by the naked eye and under the microscope. The serum test is read as follows:

[1] In certain circumstances the facilities for these procedures may not be available. The tube should then be placed in warm water at the temperature of the practitioner's hand, and after 15 minutes a drop is transferred to a slide and read directly under the microscope without attempting to observe the sediment.

X

TABLE 18

Unknown Agglutinates		Unknown belongs to
Group A Cells	Group B Cells	
+	+	Group O
−	+	Group A
+	−	Group B
−	−	Group AB

DIRECT TEST OF COMPATIBILITY. The direct test of compatibility must be made between the cells of the donor and the serum of the recipient. In addition, some of the Rh antigens in the serum of the recipient can be detected only if the cells of the donor are suspended in human albumen, and this is now an essential part of an adequate compatibility test. This test should be carried out as follows:

Two suspensions of cells from the donor are made by mixing one drop of blood obtained by finger prick with four drops of saline, and another drop of blood with four drops of 20 per cent. human serum albumen. If stored blood is to be used, cells for this test may be provided in a small test-tube attached to the blood bottle.

The serum of the patient may be obtained by withdrawing a few millilitres of blood from a vein and allowing it to clot in a test-tube, but is as easily obtained by drawing blood from a finger prick into a capillary glass tube. The tube is sealed at both ends in a flame and the serum given time to separate or obtained by centrifuging.[2]

Two drops of the recipient's serum are placed in two test-tubes, to each of which is added one drop of the saline and albumen suspensions of the donor's cells respectively. These tubes are then incubated for 10 to 15 minutes at 37° C. and centrifuged for 20 seconds. The sediment is transferred to a slide and examined under the microscope. If the blood is compatible, agglutination should not take place with either the saline- or albumen-suspended cells of the donor.

When several pints of blood are to be administered to the same patient they should be selected from the same group because bloods of different groups which are individually suitable for the patient may be incompatible with each other. If possible, cross-compatibility tests between bottles should be made.

[2] A centrifuge may be improvised by fastening the tube by sticking plaster to a blade of the fan of a motor-car or to the 'rim end' of a spoke of the back wheel of an upturned bicycle.

Technique for Emergency Blood Grouping and Compatibility Test

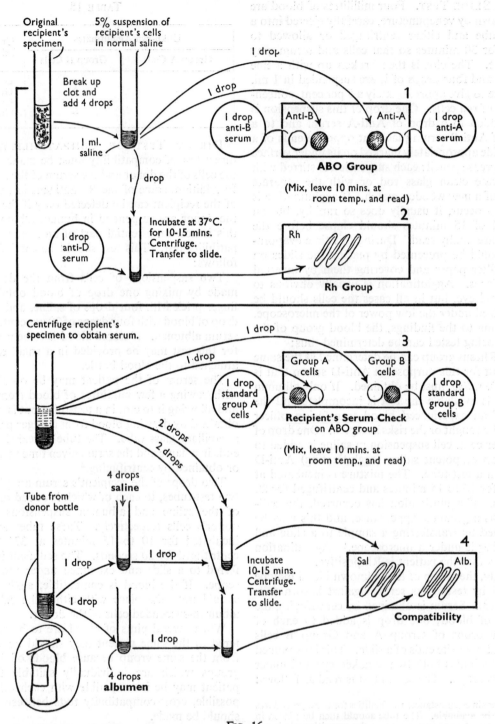

FIG. 16

With acknowledgments to Dr R. A. Cumming, Director of South-East Scotland Blood Transfusion Centre.

The procedures described here to determine the blood group and Rhesus factor and for establishing direct compatibility between donor and recipient are the simplest available and should be used in an emergency only. Whenever possible the blood of the recipient should be submitted to a Transfusion Centre where more complex tests can be applied and the possibility excluded of rare incompatibilities not revealed by the simple tests. The emergency methods available to the practitioner are summarized in Figure 16, which demonstrates a continuous technique for grouping and direct matching and which can be undertaken in the minimum of time with the maximum of safety.

Collection of blood for transfusion. When the indications are for the transfusion of *fresh blood* or in an emergency when blood is not available from a Transfusion Centre, the practitioner may have to select a suitable donor and withdraw the blood himself. The principle of the method does not differ from that used in Transfusion Centres, but the apparatus may have to be improvised.

The donor's physical health must satisfy the requirements already described (p. 629) and his blood must be proved compatible by grouping and by direct testing with the patient's serum. In emergency, or when grouping sera are not available, the direct compatiblity test must suffice.

TECHNIQUE. The donor should be recumbent. The cuff of a sphygmomanometer, or some other form of tourniquet, is placed round the arm to impede the venous return. Venepuncture, using a large-bore (14 s.w.g.) needle, is carried out into a distended vein in the ante-cubital fossa after the infiltration of a few drops of 2 per cent. lignocaine and the blood allowed to flow along about 25 cm. of 0·75 cm. tubing into a receiver. This may be any conveniently shaped bottle but the best type is the M.R.C. bottle from which air is released through a needle vent protected by a wool plug. Alternatively, and more elegantly, the blood may be collected into a plastic bag which facilitates its subsequent separation into plasma and red cells, should this be desired. The bottle or bag contains approximately 50 ml. of 3·8 per cent. sodium citrate which, like other solutions for intravenous use, has been prepared under strict chemical control. The addition of dextrose to this solution to produce acid-citrate dextrose B.P.C. prolongs the survival of red cells. To avoid clotting in the needle or tube during bleeding, the flow should be maintained at a steady rate by adjustment of the tourniquet and by directing the donor to clench and unclench his hand at intervals of about 10 seconds. The bottle is gently rotated to mix blood and citrate. When the required quantity of blood has been collected, the tourniquet is first released and the needle is then withdrawn. The puncture is covered by a sterile pad. The removal of 450 ml. of blood from a healthy adult is seldom attended by any unpleasant effects, but it is advisable to keep the donor recumbent for about a quarter of an hour.

Administration. In emergencies it may still be necessary to administer blood directly through an open system as described on p. 626 for the administration of fluids, but most practitioners faced with the occasional need for emergency transfusion should avail themselves of sealed M.R.C. bottles or plastic bags and one or other of the disposable plastic sets now available. One British pattern manufactured by Capon Heaton Ltd., Birmingham, is illustrated in Figure 17. Such sets have built-in air and blood filters and a heavy needle which perforates the rubber wad of the bottle. Detailed instructions for their use are supplied with them.

Blood may be stored at 4° C. for up to two weeks if dextrose has been added to the citrate. Stored blood should be inspected for evidence of haemolysis in the supernatant plasma and should be mixed only by gentle inversion of the bottle.

INFUSION OF CONCENTRATED RED CELLS. This raises the haemoglobin level with minimal addition to blood volume, and it is therefore, of value in the rapid correction of anaemia, in which plasma volume is not necessarily reduced. The red cells of one bottle of blood will usually increase the haematocrit from 3 to 5 per cent. Fresh blood not more than a week old is used, the supernatant plasma and white cells being withdrawn aseptically from two bottles of whole blood. The contents of the two bottles are then infused. Concentrated red cells deteriorate rapidly and should not be kept longer than two hours after 'packing'.

ADMINISTRATION OF PLASMA. All Blood Transfusion Centres prepare or provide bottles of liquid or dried blood plasma. Liquid plasma should be an absolutely clear solution and *must* be discarded if it shows any opacity or opalescence. Dry plasma is a yellow powder and is reconstituted for administration by the addition of pyrogen-free sterile distilled water; thereafter, *it should be used at once*. The quantity of distilled water which must be added is generally indicated by a mark on the bottle; about 400 ml. is required for 30 g. of the

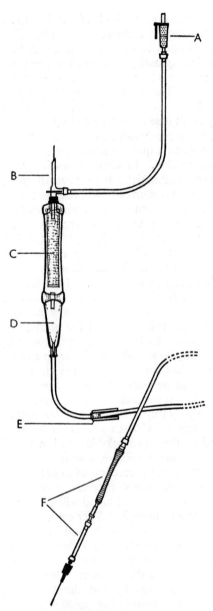

FIG. 17.—Plastic disposable set for blood transfusion: A=air filter; B=combined piercer and air inlet; C=filter; D=drip chamber; E=control clip; F=separate needle assembly with length of latex tubing for injection of drugs. Connections at A and F are Luer.

powder. To effect complete solution, the bottle must be shaken for about five minutes. The solution produced is opaque because of the presence of lipoid particles; nevertheless, it is safe to give it intravenously. Plasma is used in oligae-

mia when whole blood is not immediately available or when, as in severe burns and crush injuries, plasma alone is the predominant fluid lost. Tests of campatibility are not required.

Reactions to transfusion of blood or plasma. Minor reactions may occur during transfusion—usually shivering followed by fever and headache or nausea. They may be caused by impurities in the citrate solution or by lack of sterility of the apparatus. If the reaction is only slight, the transfusion may be continued, but the rate of delivery should be reduced; if the symptoms do not abate or pass off within five minutes, the transfusion should be stopped. If the reaction begins with a definite rigor, the flow should be stopped immediately.

Occasionally a reaction, possibly of an allergic type, occurs with pain in the chest, dyspnoea and circulatory collapse. An urticarial rash develops which may be widespread. Such reactions are not likely to occur if the same donor is used for a second transfusion to the same recipient. Although alarming, they are seldom serious, but if recognized while the transfusion is in progress, the flow should be stopped. Adrenaline, 0·5 ml. of 1:1,000 solution, is given subcutaneously and, in severe cases, an intravenous injection of 100 mg. of hydrocortisone hemisuccinate. If urticaria is severe and recurs when the effect of the adrenaline has worn off, antihistamines should also be given, such as 50 mg. of diphenhydramine four times daily.

Rarely, minor reactions which occur after completion of a transfusion are caused by the presence of an unusually high titre of agglutinins; this produces some agglutination of the recipient's cells if these belong to a group other than O. Such reactions are very seldom severe and are so rare that they are not usually considered in compatibility tests. They are treated by warmth, sedatives and adrenaline as described above.

Severe reactions are due to mistakes in cross-matching; this results in the rapid agglutination and haemolysis of the transfused red cells. Soon after the transfusion is begun, the patient becomes restless and complains of lumbar pain or pain in the chest and head. A rigor, severe dyspnoea and then respiratory and circulatory failure may follow rapidly. If the patient survives, fever follows and later jaundice. Haemoglobinuria is common and oliguria may indicate the development of renal tubular damage. The transfusion must be stopped at once and the urine made alkaline. If circulatory collapse is severe, it should be combated by transfusion of compatible blood, of plasma or of a plasma substitute. All urine passed by the patient should be measured and a record kept of fluid intake and output. If signs of renal failure appear, the treatment is as described on p. 273-278.

Whenever a reaction occurs during the transfusion of blood or plasma supplied by a Transfusion Centre, the remainder of the contents of the bottle should be preserved (with precautions against bacterial contamination) and returned with full particulars to the Blood Bank for examination.

Sometimes after the transfusion of several pints of stored blood without immediate incident, mild jaundice may develop within 24 to 48 hours. This is the result of haemolysis of a proportion of the transfused red cells which have become fragile after storage. The increasing use of very large quantities of blood by transfusion introduces other hazards in addition to the occasional occurrence of mild haemolytic jaundice. Bank blood is not exactly similar in chemical or physical properties to that normally circulating in the body. In particular, it contains considerable quantities of citrate ion and may be deficient in some factors concerned in clotting. Occasionally, if six bottles or more of blood are rapidly transfused, peripheral vasodilatation and poor cardiac action may persist in spite of a normal blood volume; this is probably—at least in part—a manifestation of citrate intoxication. The condition is prevented if during massive transfusion calcium gluconate is administered intravenously in the proportion of 20 ml. of 10 per cent. solution to every six bottles of blood. A similar amount or more should be given if the established condition is suspected after massive transfusion. The treatment of clotting defects is more difficult and less certain, and the help of a transfusion expert should be sought if possible. When he is not available, two pints of fresh blood should be rapidly transfused.

Serum hepatitis may occur up to 120 days after transfusion of either blood or plasma. The incidence of this complication varies widely and is never an indication to withhold transfusion. However, the use of plasma obtained from donor pools is justified only in an emergency.

Plasma substitutes. Solutions containing certain molecules of relatively large size may be used as substitutes for plasma in the treatment of conditions associated with shock and reduction of blood volume. Dextran (a complex carbohydrate) is the best; it is supplied in bottles similar to those of the standard blood transfusion equipment. Plasma substitutes are, like plasma itself, inferior to whole blood in the treatment of blood loss but have an effect comparable to that of plasma in restoring depleted plasma volume. They are valuable in maintaining blood volume in a patient suffering from shock during the time necessary to obtain compatible blood, but amounts of dextran greater than 2 to 2·5 litres should not be given unless absolutely necessary because haemodilution and disturbances in blood clotting may occur. Rheomacrodex, a form of dextran, with a low molecular weight, has the additional property of preventing sludging of the blood in the peripheral vessels and has specific indications in endotoxin shock and similar conditions. Additional advantages possessed by plasma substitutes are their low cost, their ease of storage and the absence of any risk of serum hepatitis. If blood transfusion is contemplated subsequent to the infusion of a plasma substitute, the blood for grouping and compatibility tests should be withdrawn before the infusion is begun, because rouleaux formation of the red cells, caused by plasma substitutes, may result in an inexperienced person making false readings.

Intradermal Injection

Occasionally it is necessary to introduce small amounts of fluid into the skin to test for the sensitivity on the part of the patient towards serum, bacterial products or extracts of certain animal and vegetable substances. The finest of needles should be employed, with a short bevel on its point. A small syringe containing the appropriate quantity of fluid is attached to the needle, and its contents are introduced into the skin where it is hairless, usually on the flexor surface of a forearm. The accurate placement of the fluid is secured by passing the needle, bevel downwards, at a very acute angle; if the point of the needle is correctly placed, the injection causes blanching of the skin over a small circular area.

Hypodermic Injection

By this route are administered (1) certain drugs, (2) vaccines and (3) certain hormones, e.g. insulin.

Drugs. These should be already in solution in ampoules. The primitive technique of making up a hypodermic injection from tablets of the drug should never be used as such a method is devoid of both elegance and safety. The needle should be the finest procurable and the ideal is to use a fresh one for each injection. Disposable needles for this purpose are available at a cost competitive with ordinary needles. Areas suitable for hypodermic injections are indicated in Figure 18. The skin at

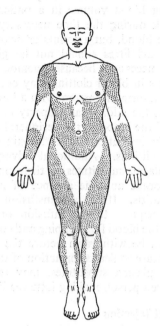

FIG. 18.—The stippled areas may be used for hypodermic injections.

the selected point is cleansed with spirit, a fold of it is picked up with the finger and thumb of the left hand, and the needle attached to the syringe is plunged into the *loose subcutaneous tissue* at the extremity of the fold. The piston is then gently withdrawn, to ensure that the point of the needle is not in a venule: if blood does not enter the syringe, the drug is injected, the needle withdrawn and the fluid evenly dispersed by massaging the area for a moment. Hypodermic injections should never be given into an inflamed area, or into one which may contain lymphatics draining such an area.

Vaccines. These are often supplied in bulk, in bottles with a thin rubber cap. The bottle is well shaken, and the cap is sterilized with spirit: if the bottle is new, a layer of paraffin wax may have to be removed from the rubber cap. The piston of the syringe is then withdrawn to the level of the dose desired; the needle is plunged through the rubber cap into the bottle, which is held *inverted*; air is

expelled into the bottle by pushing the piston 'home', and the equivalent dose of vaccine is then withdrawn into the syringe. A fresh needle and syringe *must* be used on each occasion if the transmission of hepatitis is to be avoided.

Insulin. See p. 323.

Intramuscular Injection

There are nearly 90 official injections and many more semi-official ones in common use. About a dozen of them are reserved for special purposes—for example, diagnostic tests, and to induce local anaesthesia. Of the remainder, about 50 are given intramuscularly; and a further 20 can be injected by this route, but are also well tolerated subcutaneously. Nearly all preparations for intramuscular injection are water soluble but a few, e.g. dapsone and bismuth salicylate, are suspended in oil and particular care must be taken to avoid their intravenous injection. Sera are usually given by intramuscular injection, but can also be given intravenously. A long needle (5 to 8 cm.) is used: the finer the bore, the less painful the injection, but it must be wide enough to allow for aspiration and expulsion of the material to be injected. Oily preparations are more easily drawn through the needle if they are warmed to about 40·5° C. Substances which would cause irritation in the subcutaneous tissues should be aspirated through the nozzle of a syringe, or if a needle is used for this purpose it should be replaced by a clean one before giving the injection.

Intramuscular injections can be made into the gluteal muscles, above a line joining the anterior superior iliac spine and the fold of the buttock at the natal cleft, or into the muscle mass on the lateral aspect of the thigh. Although it is more painful, the latter is preferred because the slight risk of damage to the sciatic nerve by an ill-directed needle is avoided. When a number of intramuscular injections are to be given, the site should be varied by using the limbs alternately or different zones previously mapped out on the sides of the thighs. The skin is sterilized and steadied by the forefinger and thumb of the left hand; the needle is held in the forefinger and thumb of the right hand, and is plunged through the skin perpendicularly, with a sharp stabbing movement, directly into the muscles. It is then held in position with the forefinger and thumb of the left hand, and the charged syringe is attached to it. Gentle suction is applied to ensure that the point of the needle is not in a blood vessel;

if it is correctly placed, the injection is slowly and steadily given and the needle withdrawn. Thereafter the area is massaged firmly to ensure even dispersion of the injected material.

Paracentesis of the Abdomen

This is indicated for diagnostic purposes and when ascites embarrasses movement, respiration or the action of the heart.

The point usually chosen for the puncture is either in the midline, equidistant from umbilicus and symphysis, or in either iliac fossa midway between umbilicus and anterior superior iliac spine. The bladder is emptied, and if the abdomen is hairy, it is shaved. The patient should be in a semi-reclining position, so that the fluid gravitates towards, and the intestines away from the lower abdomen; and before the abdomen is tapped a broad binder or roller towel should be placed round the upper part of the abdomen. This is tightened as the fluid escapes, and thus faintness from reduction of intra-abdominal content is prevented. Either of two methods may be employed for the withdrawal of fluid; a trocar and cannula may be used in order to drain the abdomen rapidly; or the ascitic fluid may be allowed to run continuously for 24 to 36 hours through a fine polyethylene tube.

Trocar and cannula. An ordinary trocar and cannula with a bore of about 12 s.w.g. is adequate. A scalpel with a narrow blade is required and a length of rubber tubing just wide enough to attach to the end of the cannula and long enough to reach a receptacle at the side of the bed. The abdomen is cleansed and sterile towels are placed around the selected point where an intradermal weal is raised with lignocaine solution. The deeper tissues are also infiltrated, but the stretched abdominal wall of the ascitic patient is usually very thin and only shallow infiltration is required. A small cut is made through the skin, of such a size that it will admit the point of the trocar and stretch to accommodate the cannula. The cannula with trocar in position is then pushed slowly through the abdominal wall; while doing this the right forefinger is kept firmly upon it to guard against its plunging too far into the peritoneal cavity. When resistance is overcome, the point of the instrument has reached the cavity. The trocar is withdrawn and fluid observed to flow before the cannula is connected to the rubber tubing. Not infrequently a loop of bowel floats up and obstructs the cannula so that the flow ceases. It can be restarted by moving the cannula up and down or from side to side. Occasionally a flake of lymph blocks the cannula and this can be dislodged by the cautious re-insertion of the trocar. As the abdominal swelling decreases the binder is tightened; but if the patient complains of faintness the flow is temporarily stopped until he recovers. When the flow finally ceases, the cannula is withdrawn and the tiny wound covered with a sterile pad.

Continuous drainage. Where the accumulation of fluid is large and gradual drainage is required, the most convenient method is to puncture the abdominal wall with a trocar and cannula, as already described, and to thread 2 mm. polyethylene tubing through the cannula into the peritoneal cavity. The cannula is then withdrawn and the tube connected to the receptacle at the bedside. As an alternative to the trocar and cannula, a convenient method, especially for continuous drainage, makes use of a pre-sterilized disposable intravenous cannula. The abdominal wall is punctured by the wide-bore intravenous needle after infiltration with local anaesthetic; the plastic cannula is passed into the peritoneal cavity and the needle withdrawn; the fluid is collected as usual. Often the flow of fluid will begin at once; if it fails to do so, a syringe may be attached to the external end of the tube, and gentle suction applied in order to establish syphon action.

Aspiration of the Pleural Cavity

This may be necessary either as a diagnostic procedure to determine the physical, cytological and bacteriological nature of a pleural effusion, to obtain a biopsy of the pleura or therapeutically to withdraw from the cavity a considerable amount of liquid (for example, pus in empyema, effusion in cardiac failure or blood in haemothorax).

Although it is occasionally necessary to choose an interspace which lies directly over the site of the effusion, as determined by clinical and especially radiological evidence, as a rule the puncture is made in the eighth intercostal space, 2 to 3 cm. behind the posterior axillary line, and nearer the ninth than the eighth rib in order to avoid the intercostal nerve and vessels. The patient may be either sitting with the shoulders thrown forward or propped up near the edge of the bed in a semi-reclining position with the arms folded. After the area has been prepared, an intradermal weal is raised with 2 per cent. lignocaine solution at the point selected for puncture and 2 ml. of the solution are then infiltrated into the tissues of the chest wall. It is essential to wait a few minutes to give the anaesthetic time to act and to reach the pleura.

Removal of a sample. A wide-bore (14 to 16 s.w.g.) short-bevelled needle is attached to a 5 ml. syringe and the needle is inserted through the weal of local anaesthetic into the pleural cavity. Negative pressure is maintained in the syringe so that liquid will flow at once when the cavity is reached. When the syringe is full, the needle is withdrawn and the sample transferred to a sterile test-tube with a closely fitting rubber stopper. The puncture is covered with a sterile swab.

Aspiration as a part of treatment. A large syringe (50 ml.) is used. This is connected to the aspirating needle by 12 cm. of stout rubber tubing. The aspirating needle is passed into the cavity as described and the syringe *slowly* filled; the tubing is then pinched or clamped with a spring clip or artery forceps and the syringe is disconnected and emptied. An alternative method is to use a syringe coupled to a three-way tap. The side channel of the adaptor is connected to a length of rubber tubing so that by turning the tap it is possible first to withdraw liquid from the chest and then to discharge it into a receptacle. With either method the accidental introduction of air into the pleural cavity should be avoided because pneumothorax induced accidentally is not invariably free from complications. Aspiration is continued until fluid is no longer obtained. If the patient complains of a feeling of tightness or actual pain in the chest, or develops a paroxysm of coughing, the symptoms may be due to mediastinal shift, and the operation should be stopped at once, the needle withdrawn and a small dressing applied to the site of puncture. In empyema, a test-tube of pus is saved from each aspiration; this is placed in a rack and the thickening of the pus can be followed by comparing the levels of cellular sediment in a series of specimens.

If the aspirated fluid is to be replaced by air, this should be done gradually: after the syringe is emptied it is filled with a slightly smaller quantity of air, which is introduced slowly into the pleural cavity. An alternative method is to insert the needle of an artificial pneumothorax machine through a separate puncture in the chest wall and to adjust the pressures so that air equal in volume to that of the liquid withdrawn is gradually introduced.

The introduction of air in this manner prevents sudden mediastinal shift.

Antibiotics or cytotoxic drugs may be introduced into the pleural cavity after aspiration has been completed. A separate clean syringe is charged with the relevant solution. After it has been confirmed that the needle point is still in the pleural space, the aspirating syringe is replaced by the second syringe and the fluid injected.

Pleural biopsy. A pleural biopsy may be obtained by using an Abram's biopsy needle. This instrument, which carries a sharp inner tube within the lumen of its needle, is inserted through the chest wall in the same way as the aspiration needle. The biopsy material is cut by the inner tube, the whole needle being thereafter removed and the specimen ejected.

Dangers of pleural aspiration. Very rarely puncture of the pleura is immediately followed by pleural shock, a condition characterized by extreme cardiac and respiratory failure. This is probably caused by air embolism, and if it occurs the needle must be withdrawn immediately. The treatment includes warmth, artificial respiration if necessary and the intravenous injection of 5 ml. of nikethamide over a period of a minute; this can be repeated if the response is considered inadequate.

Paracentesis of the Pericardium

The skin is cleansed, sterilized and then anaesthetized by intradermal and subcutaneous injection of procaine in the zone selected for puncture, as in performing a pleural paracentesis. When the presence of pus is suspected, a wide-bore needle (16 s.w.g.) may be necessary, but, in general, a medium bore will suffice (19 s.w.g.). The length of the needle required depends largely on the site of the puncture. The following sites are usually employed: (1) in the fifth left interspace, outside the apex beat but inside the limit of cardiac dullness; (2) in the fourth left interspace about 3 cm. from the sternal margin (far enough from the bone to avoid the internal mammary artery which descends in this region); (3) in the angle between the ensiform cartilage and the lowest ribs, the needle being directed upwards and backwards to reach the pericardial sac; (4) from the back, with abducted scapula, in the mid-scapular line in the seventh or eighth intercostal space. Of these, the first two are most generally used and appear to be devoid of risk. The penetration of the heart muscle by the needle is of no consequence provided that large coronary vessels are not punctured; this is an unlikely accident from a needle inserted outside the apex beat or over that part of the right ventricle which lies 3 cm. to the left of the sternum—a zone of the myocardium in which there are few large vessels. The epigastric and posterior routes are occasionally preferable when a loculated effusion has to be reached; the fluid is reached at a lower level than when an anterior puncture is performed, and therefore more complete drainage can be carried out. When large quantities of fluid are being removed, the rate of withdrawal should be slow to avoid the risk of dangerous pressure changes in the pericardium and the heart.

Lumbar Puncture

The introduction of a hollow needle into the subarachnoid space in the lumbar region is employed for both diagnostic and therapeutic purposes. Lumbar puncture is not a major or dangerous procedure, but, on the other hand, a casual attitude towards the technique is reprehensible and the procedure should not be allowed to become routine. Relative contraindications are the circumstances in which the chance of infection is high, such as in unsuitable surroundings, or when the patient's back is repeatedly soiled by faecal or urinary incontinence.

A lumbar puncture needle must be of fine bore, with a sharp, shortly bevelled point and a closely fitting stilette which locks in position so that stilette and bevel are aligned. Occasionally a needle of large bore is needed to withdraw thick exudate, but even viscous fluids (such as lipiodol) can be introduced through a fine needle if the ampoule containing the liquid is warmed in a bowl of hot sterile water to a temperature of 40° C. and the barrel of the syringe is kept warm by covering it repeatedly with gauze swabs soaked in hot water.

Technique. In most cases the puncture must be performed when the patient is in bed. It is more easily carried out if he lies on a firm mattress on his left side with a small pillow placed under his head in order to keep the cranial and spinal parts of the subarachnoid space at the same level. The patient then bends his head slightly forward and clasps his knees with his hands, so as to arch his back and thus open out the spaces between the spinous processes of the lumbar vertebrae (Fig. 19). Only in the most unruly or unco-operative of adults is a general anaesthetic needed, and usually a child can

X*

be gently but firmly held in the same position. Inhalation anaesthesia is undesirable because it interferes with the accurate measurement of cerebrospinal fluid pressure; if the pressure of the cerebrospinal fluid is to be measured premedication

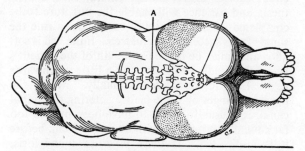

FIG. 19.—Patient in position for lumbar puncture. A, Site for lumbar puncture; B, Site for epidural injection. The stippled areas are suitable for intramuscular injections.

with chlorpromazine and pethidine should be ordered for adults but chloral hydrate usually suffices for children.

Usually the needle is inserted between the spines of the third and fourth lumbar vertebrae, a level which corresponds to the point where a line joining the highest points of the iliac crests crosses the spinal column. After the usual preparation of the skin, and with a towel in position, this point is identified with the left thumb and a weal is raised by intradermal injection of local anaesthetic in the midline with a fine hypodermic needle. A longer needle is used to infiltrate the deeper tissues in a forward and slightly cranial direction; *the needle should never be sunk to its full extent*, for needles tend to break at the junction of shaft and adaptor, and if the patient moves suddenly, a fully inserted needle may snap here and disappear below the skin.

The spinal needle is inserted through the same puncture in the skin, and with its bevel in the same plane as the spine[1]; it is then pushed slowly forward and cranially with the right hand while its direction is maintained by the forefinger of the left which rests on the skin. At a distance from the surface, which varies with age and build (in the average adult, 4 to 5 cm.) the needle is felt to overcome a certain resistance—that of the ligamentum subflavum between the laminae. If it is pushed on-

[1] Held thus it will separate, rather than sever, the longitudinally directed fibres of the dura. On its withdrawal, the small dural slit closes without leaking.

wards for 0·5 cm. it will have pierced the dura and entered the spinal subarachnoid space.

Difficulties in lumbar puncture. In adults lack of co-operation is likely only in those who are mentally confused or delirious; and even in these circumstances firm holding, careful local anaesthesia and patience will enable the puncture to be completed in the majority of cases. As a rule the same plan is successful in children. If the bed is soft allowance must be made for the tilt of the patient's body, the needle being directed a little downwards as well as forwards and cranially. When the needle impinges on bone before entering the spinal canal, it is usually found to have been pushed too far caudally; it must be withdrawn for 3 cm. before it is re-directed. If there is gross spondylosis, great patience may be required in searching for a gap between the laminae; another lumbar interspinous space may have to be explored—for example, between the second and third spinous processes. If fluid does not flow, and the operator is reasonably certain that the point of the needle is in the subarachnoid space, the needle should be slowly rotated, a manœuvre which is usually followed by a flow of fluid as a result of the clearing of a nerve root which previously blocked the aperture.

If the fluid which drops from the needle is blood-stained, a little should be allowed to run down the wall of a test-tube held on a background of white gauze. If the tint becomes progressively lighter, a small vessel has probably been opened by the needle. Readings of cerebrospinal fluid pressure are taken. Two or three samples are then collected in a series of tubes, and those that are clear (or only slightly tinted) used for investigation. When the cerebrospinal fluid already contains blood, the tinting persists and may be assumed to be of diagnostic importance. The significance of admixture of blood may then be assessed by allowing the sample to settle or by centrifuging it. When the blood results from local trauma, the supernatant fluid is clear; but when it has been derived from a previous subarachnoid haemorrhage with subsequent lysis of the red cells the supernatant fluid is yellowish (xanthochromia) or red. The fluid may show lysis of red cells if there is delay in making the examination, for example when the specimen is sent to the laboratory by post.

Cerebrospinal fluid pressure. Investigation of the pressure in the subarachnoid space is usually an important and sometimes an essential diagnostic procedure. It is estimated in terms of centimetres of cerebrospinal fluid, and the reading must, of course, be made before a sample is taken. The needle is connected by means of a three-way stopcock and adaptor and a short length of rubber tubing to a manometer made of glass and graduated in centimetres; the whole apparatus must be sterilized by autoclaving or boiling, but it should be remembered that pressures taken using a wet manometer may be inaccurate. The stopcock allows the operator (1) to close the lumen of the needle, (2) to allow cerebrospinal fluid into the manometer, or (3) to permit cerebrospinal fluid to flow directly into a sample tube. The manometer is held so that the zero mark is at the level of the needle. Pressure readings are useless unless the patient is relaxed and breathing quietly. Normally the fluid shows oscillations up to 0·5 cm. with each beat of the pulse and up to 1 cm. with each respiration; the mean is taken as the initial pressure.

If the subarachnoid space above the level of the needle is free from obstruction, variations in cerebrospinal fluid pressure will be indicated in the manometric levels. Rhythmic fluctuations of pressure with the arterial pulse and respiration is a sign of free communication, but further evidence can be obtained by the manœuvre of Queckenstedt. Compression of both jugular veins by an assistant for four seconds (the patient having been previously warned) normally leads to an increase in pressure in the intracranial veins of anything up to 30 cm. of water. If there is no obstruction to the free flow of cerebrospinal fluid, such venous compression is accompanied by a prompt rise in the level of the manometer; and the manometric pressure falls abruptly when the jugular compression is released. If obstruction of the subarachnoid space, for example by a spinal tumour, is present, then when jugular compression is applied, the manometric pressure may (1) remain stationary (complete block); (2) rise, but remain at a higher level when jugular compression is released (partial block); (3) rise or fall jerkily ('stair' response) when the jugular pressure is applied or released (partial block).

When block is present, the *initial pressure* is low; but manual compression of the abdomen will be followed by a rise in pressure, even when response to jugular compression is absent.

The information that may be obtained from investigation of the pressure of the cerebrospinal fluid is indicated in Figure 20.

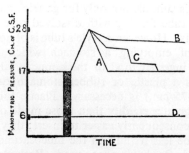

Fig. 20.—Diagrammatic representation of manometric response to jugular pressure. The black block represents compression of the internal jugular veins for four seconds. A, normal response; B, new higher level; C, 'stairway' fall; and D, lack of response (complete block).

The collection of samples. When manometric readings have been made, fluid is allowed to drip slowly into a tube or a series of tubes for further examination.

Tubes should be sterile, chemically clean and fitted with rubber stoppers. Fifteen millilitres of fluid are sufficient for all routine analysis, but when a space-occupying intracranial lesion is present, or is suspected, the withdrawal of fluid should be restricted to an amount which does not reduce the manometric pressure by more than one-third of the initial reading.

The number of tubes into which the sample is received depends on the type and number of tests which are desired and on the requirements of the laboratory or laboratories to which samples are to be sent. Thus, information may be desired on the (1) chemical, (2) cytological, (3) bacteriological and (4) immunological properties of the fluid. Three separate samples usually satisfy the requirements of most laboratories.

After the needle has been withdrawn, the skin puncture should be covered with a small dressing held in place by adhesive. The patient should be kept in the recumbent position and preferably prone rather than supine for 24 hours in order to avoid the unpleasant sequel of lumbar puncture headache.

Aspiration of Joints

Methods of puncturing the cavities of joints for diagnostic and therapeutic purposes are shown in Figures 21 to 26 and described in their accompanying legends.

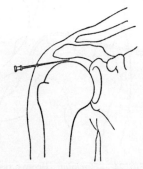

Fig. 21.—*Shoulder joint*. From immediately distal and somewhat posterior to the tip of the acromion process, the needle passes medially and a little cranially, over the humeral head.

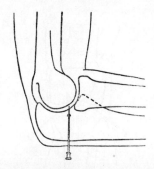

Fig. 22.—*Elbow joint*. With the forearm at right angles, and midway between pronation and supination, the needle passes anteriorly from a point immediately proximal to the head of the radius.

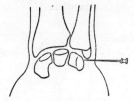

Fig. 23.—*Wrist joint*. From a point immediately distal to the styloid process of the ulna, the needle passes laterally.

Gastric Intubation

The passage of a tube into the stomach may be required either for diagnosis or for therapy. For diagnosis it is customary to use a fine tube (2 mm. internal diameter) of rubber or preferably of plastic, weighted at its end, and usually known as a Ryle's tube. This tube, or one of its numerous modifi-

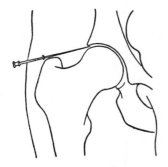

FIG. 24.—*Hip joint*. From a point immediately proximal to the mid-point of the upper border of the greater trochanter, the needle passes medially and slightly cranially, along the neck of the femur.

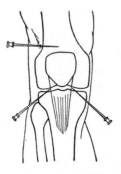

FIG. 25.—*Knee joint*. The needle may pass from either the medial or the lateral side (1) into the supra-patellar pouch, or (2) into the joint on either side of the ligamentum patellae.

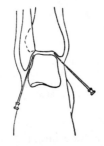

FIG. 26.—*Ankle joint*. From a point immediately distal to the tip of either malleolus, the needle passes cranially, and towards the median line of the tibia, between the malleolus and the talus.

cations, is suitable not only for gastric analysis but also for tube feeding with dissolved or emulsified foodstuffs. However, a Ryle's tube is of no use as a means of emptying a stomach which contains recently ingested food or thick mucus. For such purposes a plastic or rubber stomach tube (diameter 0·75 cm.) is necessary. Plastic tubes have slightly greater rigidity than those made of rubber and are consequently easier to insert; they are also said to be less irritant to the mucosa and can be discarded after having been used. Both plastic and rubber are available in radio-opaque forms.

Passage of a Ryle's tube. This tube is inserted through the nose. The patient is propped up on pillows and instructed to lean back. He is then examined to identify any deviation of the nasal septum. The anterior nares on the wider side is lightly anaesthetized with a pledglet of wool soaked in 5 per cent. lignocaine. The tube, lubricated with glycerin, is then inserted horizontally and gently pushed directly backwards until it touches the posterior wall of the nasopharynx. The slight overhang of this surface directs it downwards and as it slips over this wall the patient is told to swallow, so opening the entrance to the oesophagus and simultaneously closing the larynx. As the patient swallows, the tube is slipped down the gullet. Successive swallows will then propel the tube on into the stomach, or in the case of a plastic tube this can be gently pushed down without further aid from the patient. The tube is usually marked to show the approximate distance between the anterior nares and the cardia, but one can be certain that the tube has entered the stomach only when it is possible to withdraw gastric juice. Alternatively, the injection of 20 ml. of air down the tube while auscultating the abdomen below the left costal margin produces loud borborygmi if the tube is correctly placed. When it is essential to know the exact site of the end of the tube, radiological visualization of a radio-opaque tube makes this possible.

Passage of a stomach tube. Large tubes must be passed through the mouth. Often the patient is unconscious or unco-operative and in such cases a mouth gag is essential to protect the operator's fingers. A conscious patient may be positioned as for nasogastric intubation, but the unconscious patient is best laid on his side and facilities for raising the foot of the bed or couch should be available or improvised so that vomiting is not inevitably followed by inhalation. In the conscious patient the posterior third of the tongue and the soft palate may with advantage be sprayed with 2 per cent. lignocaine. This prevents the patient 'gagging' during the initial stages. The tube is lubricated with glycerin and the index and middle fingers of the operator's left hand are then passed backwards over the tongue depressing it slightly. The tube is slid into the hypopharynx between the two fingers and the patient is instructed to swallow. As the cricopharyngeal muscles relax the tube is pushed gently into the oesophagus and then firmly on into the stomach. A large aspirating syringe with a rubber bulb (a Dakin's syringe) is held ready and aspiration is begun the moment the tube has reached the stomach. In the unconscious patient swallowing cannot be induced at will and the initial entry of the tube into the oesophagus is achieved by inserting it very gently downwards along the posterior pharyngeal wall. Before aspiration or injection is begun the position of the tube in the stomach is checked by the method already described.

Peritoneal Dialysis

Peritoneal dialysis was originally introduced many years ago but was abandoned on account of a high incidence of infection. In recent years improvements in materials available for catheters have given rise to renewed interest in this method of treating renal failure. A nylon catheter is inserted into the peritoneal cavity by the technique of simple abdominal paracentesis (p. 637). This is connected to two bottles (2 litres), containing a suitable dialysate mixture suspended above the bed. The dialysate is run into the peritoneal cavity where it remains for 20 to 30 minutes; it is then allowed to drain away. The procedure is immediately repeated using a fresh supply of fluid. This cycle continues for 24 to 48 hours, by which time some control of the uraemia is usually achieved. Peritoneal dialysis is indicated when the rate of rise of blood urea is relatively slow, and in circumstances where extracorporeal dialysis is not available. It is less efficient than haemodialysis, and is frequently distressing to the patient. Peritonitis may also occur unless the procedure is carried out under strictly hygienic conditions.

External and Internal Cardiac Massage

The diagnosis of cardiac arrest, actual or impending, is assumed when in a collapsed patient no pulse can be felt and no heart sounds heard. A maximum of four minutes of complete arrest may be tolerated before irreparable damage occurs and lives may occasionally be saved by the prompt application of cardiac massage combined with the maintenance of an adequate airway within the safe period.

The essence of the successful management of this emergency is speed, which in turn means that the staff must be aware of the urgency of the situation, must be capable of reaching an accurate and immediate diagnosis and must be familiar with the equipment and procedure required for its treatment. Most hospitals and medical centres maintain a 'cardiac arrest trolley' which carries the equipment necessary for E.C.G. monitoring, defibrillation and endotracheal anaesthesia. This must always be available for immediate use and its location must be known to everyone concerned. The first steps will obviously be taken by the individual who is beside the patient, but both anaesthetist and surgeon will probably be required and it is important that an emergency call system is available whereby they can be informed of the incident, and where it has occurred, with the least possible delay.

External cardiac massage. This must be started as soon as possible in all patients in whom a diagnosis has been made or in circumstances of doubt, even if it is obvious that the arrest is not absolute and even if it is equally obvious that open massage will be needed. This may restart a heart which is in asystole and may maintain an adequate circulation during ventricular fibrillation pending the arrival of a defibrillator.

With the patient supine and on a rigid base, the flat of both hands, one on the top of the other, is placed over the mid and lower sternum which is rhythmically compressed directly backwards towards the dorsal spine at a rate of about 60 per minute. The force must be sufficient to produce a palpable carotid or radial pulse, but excessive force should be avoided since it may result in fractured ribs, damage to the liver or even rupture of the heart.

An adequate circulation may be maintained for long periods by this method but it must be remembered that a circulation without ventilation is ineffective in its main purpose, namely to avoid tissue anoxia.

External cardiac massage must, therefore, be combined with mouth-to-mouth respiration by an assistant or by the operator if he is alone. The direct technique is quite adequate but a Brook's airway is more hygienic and should be used if available (p. 652).

When the arrest occurs in the operating theatre or in a hospital ward, immediate steps should be taken to pass an endotracheal tube and maintain ventilation with the aid of an anaesthetic machine. In this way easy and effective ventilation may be maintained indefinitely, but if it is apparent that prolonged intubation will be necessary, it is advisable to perform a tracheostomy to avoid pressure necrosis within the larynx.

Failure to produce an adequate peripheral pulse or evidence of increasing cerebral anoxia such as increasing dilatation of the pupils, in spite of technically correct external massage, are immediate indications for thoracotomy and open massage. However, where an E.C.G. machine and equipment for defibrillation are available, an attempt should be made to confirm and correct ventricular fibrillation before resorting to the open method.

The open method. This is, of course, the method of choice when the arrest occurs during an abdominal or thoracic operation, but it is indicated as a primary procedure when external massage has proved to be ineffectual. It is carried out by making a bold incision through the fourth left intercostal space. The incision must be adequate in length and where a ribspreader is not available, it is usually necessary to stretch the incision, possibly fracturing the third or fourth ribs or both, to provide an exposure sufficient to enable the hand to enter the pleural space and to grasp the heart through the pericardium. It must be compressed between the fingers and thumb rhythmically and with sufficient force to provide an adequate pulse. If after a period of internal massage a co-ordinated and satisfactory contraction is still delayed, defibrillation should again be attempted.

Although the emergency thoracotomy requires no surgical skill and a minimum of instruments, the incision should subsequently be closed as if it were an elective procedure and preferably by someone familiar with the correct suture technique and using the appropriate equipment.

Whatever method is employed to restore cardiac action, it is impossible to estimate the time before normal activity will return. Regardless of the delay, however, it is important to presume that some degree of metabolic acidosis has occurred. In the majority of patients it is worth while anticipating this by setting up an intravenous infusion of $\frac{1}{6}$ M lactate or sodium bicarbonate, the amount being determined by the severity of the acidosis. The intravenous infusion of a hypertonic solution may

also be necessary to reduce the cerebral oedema which not infrequently follows prolonged cerebral anoxia.

Finally, the patient must be examined carefully for evidence of delayed cerebral, myocardial or renal damage, as the full extent of this may not become apparent for several days or even weeks after the cardiac arrest.

OXYGEN THERAPY

Oxygen supplied for medical use is specially prepared so as to be free of toxic constituents. In many hospitals nowadays pipe-lines from a central bank of cylinders or from a reservoir of liquid oxygen, carry the gas to the operating theatres and to individual beds in the wards. Each point is provided with a flow-meter, by which the rate of oxygen administration can be regulated. In less well equipped hospitals individual cylinders are used for supplying oxygen, but this is an inefficient and cumbersome practice which ought to be abandoned as soon as possible.

Arrangements can be made for oxygen therapy to be given in domiciliary practice, but the occasions on which this is indicated are relatively few. Because of difficulties in the supply and transport of cylinders it is seldom easy to maintain an adequate supply of oxygen in a private house, and when a patient is acutely ill, it is usually safer to move him to hospital, especially now that most ambulances are equipped with facilities for oxygen administration. Oxygen therapy can, however, be usefully employed in the home for the relief of intolerable dyspnoea, in patients with advanced chronic bronchitis and emphysema (pp. 195–198).

THEORETICAL CONSIDERATIONS

Oxygen lack or *hypoxia* is, of course, the prime indication for the administration of oxygen, but not all types of hypoxia respond equally well to this form of treatment. The excessive enrichment of inspired air with oxygen may in certain circumstances be dangerous. It is, therefore, necessary to review in some detail the mechanisms responsible for the production of hypoxia before presenting specific recommendations for its treatment.

Hypoxia can be defined as a state in which the amount of oxygen reaching the tissues is inadequate for their metabolic needs. The most serious clinical manifestations of hypoxia are due to a reduction of the partial pressure (or tension) of oxygen in specialized tissues such as the brain, heart, liver and kidneys. The level of oxygenation in these organs is, however, determined by the oxygen tension (Po_2) and the oxygen content of the blood perfusing them, and it is easier from the practical point of view to discuss the indications for oxygen therapy in terms of *hypoxaemia* (i.e. a reduction in the oxygen content of the blood) than of hypoxia. The oxygen content depends not only on the Po_2, but also on the oxygen capacity of the blood, which is directly related, except in conditions such as carbon monoxide poisoning, to the haemoglobin (Hb) concentration. The oxygen saturation (So_2) expresses the ratio of content to capacity as a percentage figure, and is related to the Po_2 in a complex way, determined by the oxyhaemoglobin dissociation curve, which in turn may be modified by the blood pH, and also by the body temperature. The oxygen content can be calculated from the So_2 and the Hb concentration, and the So_2 from the Po_2 and pH. Hypoxaemia can thus in practice be adequately investigated simply by measuring the Po_2, pH and Hb concentration.

Hypoxaemia has a variety of causes, which may be classified as follows:

1. Hypoxaemia caused by a reduction in the partial pressure of oxygen in the inspired air

This form of hypoxaemia, in which the arterial oxygen tension and content are reduced, is a potential hazard of mountain climbing and of high-altitude flying in unpressurized aircraft. It is relieved by breathing oxygen, provided the atmospheric pressure does not fall below one-fifth of normal.

2. Hypoxamia caused by incomplete oxygenation of the blood in the lungs

This type of hypoxaemia occurs whenever pulmonary ventilation is insufficient to maintain the alveolar oxygen tension at a normal level. It is associated with a reduction in arterial Po_2 and with an increase in the oxygen capacity of the blood if the condition is sufficiently chronic and severe to produce polycythaemia. The So_2 is, however, also reduced, and the oxygen content remains subnormal in spite of the increase in oxygen capacity. In some cases the alveolar Po_2 may be subnormal in spite of the fact that the minute volume of pulmonary ventilation is being maintained at a level which in healthy subjects would be regarded as normal or even above normal. This state of affairs usually results from inadequate ventilation of a proportion of the alveoli in relation to the blood flow through the adjacent pulmonary capillaries. In these circumstances overventilation of unaffected alveoli is usually sufficient to prevent any rise in the partial pressure of carbon dioxide (Pco_2) in the alveolar air and in the blood; indeed where alveolar ventilation is markedly increased, a mild degree of hypocapnia is not uncommon. Oxygen therapy in this type of hypoxaemia is unlikely to produce a significant increase in arterial Pco_2, and can be given without any special precautions. The conditions to which these considerations apply include acute pneumonia, acute pulmonary oedema, all forms of diffuse interstitial lung disease, massive pleural effusion and spontaneous pneumothorax.

An entirely different situation arises when alveolar ventilation is no longer sufficient to prevent an increase in the Pco_2 in the alveolar air and in the arterial blood. With increasing hypercapnia the respiratory centre becomes progressively more tolerant of carbon dioxide, and ultimately its activity is maintained almost solely by the stimulus of hypoxaemia. If this stimulus is reduced by the administration of oxygen, a further reduction of alveolar ventilation, with a consequent rise in arterial Pco_2 is inevitable. This situation is particularly liable to arise in patients with advanced chronic bronchitis and emphysema, and it may also develop in severe bronchial asthma, poliomyelitis with involvement of the respiratory muscles and central depression of respiration by opiate or barbiturate poisoning.

The practical implication of these theoretical considerations is that whereas all patients with hypoxaemia require oxygen, the concentration of this gas in the inspired air must, in patients with a raised arterial Pco_2 be carefully controlled so as to ensure that it does not precipitate a serious increase in the degree of hypercapnia. In most cases, provided suitable methods are used for giving oxygen, this hazard can readily be averted. In some patients with severe ventilatory failure, however, even a slight degree of oxygen enrichment of the inspired air may produce a sharp increase in the arterial Pco_2. Such patients are in a grave predicament, as they are desperately in need of oxygen, but cannot safely be given it for fear of aggravating an already serious degree of hypercapnia. The methods of dealing with this situation, which include the chemical stimulation of respiration and the use of artificial positive-pressure ventilation, are discussed on p. 652.

3. Hypoxaemia caused by right-to-left intra-cardiac or intrapulmonary vascular shunts

In this form of hypoxaemia the arterial Po_2 and oxygen content are reduced in spite of an increase in oxygen capacity caused by polycythaemia. The administration of oxygen in circumstances where a considerable proportion of the blood volume bypasses the lungs might not be expected to correct the hypoxaemia so produced. In actual practice a considerable increase in the Po_2 and oxygen content is often obtained, if oxygen is administered in a high concentration. The reason for this is that the excess of dissolved oxygen contained in the blood which has circulated through the pulmonary capillaries is taken up by the red cells and plasma which have bypassed the lungs.

Oxygen in high concentration can, therefore, relieve hypoxaemia in conditions such as Fallot's tetralogy. In practice, however, no attempt is made to administer oxygen continuously to these patients, as they become tolerant of severe chronic hypoxaemia. Nevertheless, oxygen may be of considerable value when the hypoxaemia is increased by complications such as respiratory infection or operation.

4. Hypoxaemia caused by a reduction in the oxygen capacity of the blood

In this type of hypoxaemia, which occurs in anaemia and in carbon monoxide poisoning, there is no significant reduction in the arterial Po_2 or So_2, and the hypoxaemia is due to a subnormal haemoglobin concentration, which is responsible for a reduction in oxygen capacity and content. For that reason the administration of oxygen to patients with anaemia cannot bring about any dramatic improvement in hypoxaemia. When the anaemia is very severe, however, the administration of oxygen in high concentration may, be increasing the amount of dissolved oxygen in the plasma, provide a small but vital extra supply of oxygen for the tissues.

In carbon monoxide poisoning oxygen therapy is indicated for a different reason, namely to accelerate the dissociation of carboxyhaemoglobin. In this condition efforts should be made to maintain a 100 per cent. concentration of oxygen in the inspired air. Hyperbaric oxygen therapy at 2 to 3 atmospheres (p. 650) is an even more rapid and effective method of dealing with carbon monoxide poisoning, but facilities for this treatment are available in only a few large centres.

5. Hypoxaemia caused by excessive extraction of oxygen from blood in the systemic capillaries

This type of hypoxaemia occurs in conditions such as cardiogenic shock following myocardial infarction, acute blood loss and peripheral circulatory failure, in which the rate of blood flow through the capillaries is seriously reduced and even the total extraction of oxygen from the blood passing through these capillaries may be insufficient to meet the needs of the tissues.

As there is no defect of oxygenation in the lungs, the arterial Po_2 and oxygen content are normal in this type of hypoxaemia, and the only effect of the administration of oxygen will be to produce an increase in the amount of dissolved oxygen in the plasma. In a critical situation, however, even this may be sufficient to tip the scales in the patient's favour. A high concentration of oxygen is, of course, essential for this purpose.

CLINICAL INDICATIONS FOR OXYGEN THERAPY

Although the administration of oxygen may under certain circumstances be of value in the treatment of disorders such as very severe anaemia, right-to-left cardiac or pulmonary vascular shunts, cardiogenic shock and peripheral circulatory failure, the conditions, apart from carbon monoxide poisoning (p. 548), in which it is most likely to exert a decisive effect are those in which there is incomplete oxygenation of the blood perfusing the lungs. Oxygen therapy is effective in all these conditions. In the more chronic diseases, however, hypoxaemia develops gradually, and the tissues have time to become adapted to the reduced oxygen tension. Although chronic hypoxaemia may give rise to serious ill-effects, including pulmonary hypertension, the continuous administration of oxygen to control it is impracticable. Oxygen therapy is thus indicated only in acute hypoxaemia and in exacerbations of chronic hypoxaemia. In the first category acute pneumonia and pulmonary oedema account for the bulk of the cases; the second is mainly composed of those patients with chronic bronchitis and severe emphysema who have

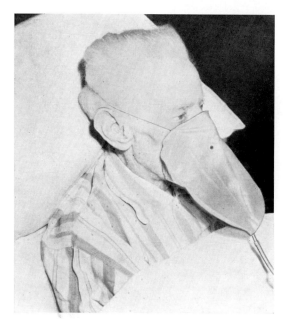

PLATE 1.—Polymask.
(*British Oxygen Company Ltd.*)

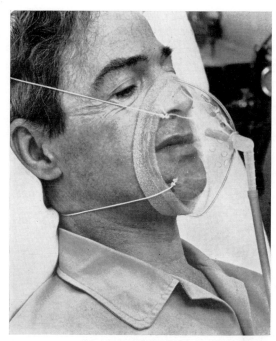

PLATE II.—M.C. mask.
(*Medical and Industrial Equipment Ltd.*)

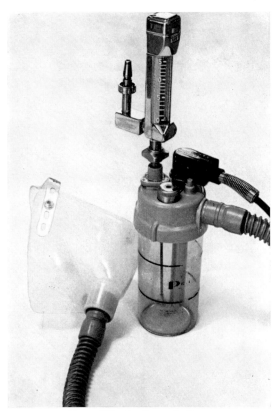

PLATE III.—Puritan nebulizer.
(*Vickers Limited Medical Group*)

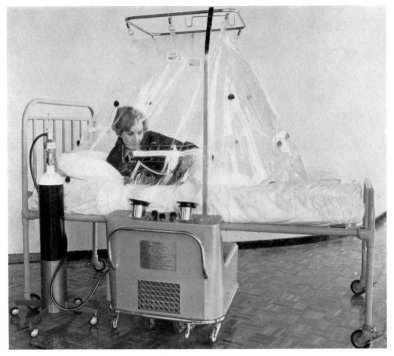

PLATE IV.—Refrigeration Oxygen Tent.
(*Vickers Limited Medical Group*)

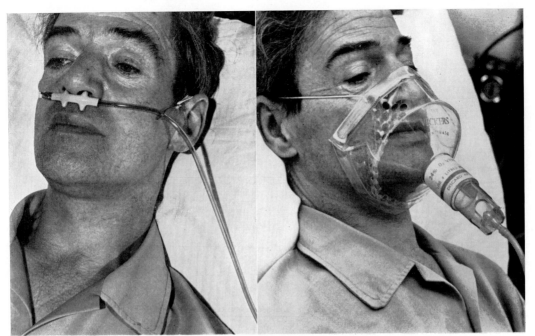

PLATE V.—Nasal cannulae

PLATE VI.—Ventimask
(*Vickers Limited Medical Group*)

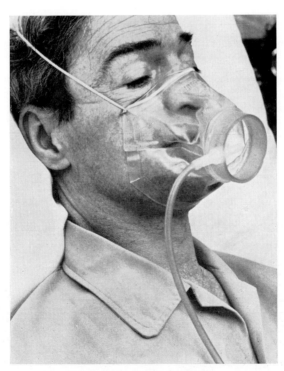

PLATE VII.—Edinburgh Mask.
(*British Oxygen Company Ltd.*)

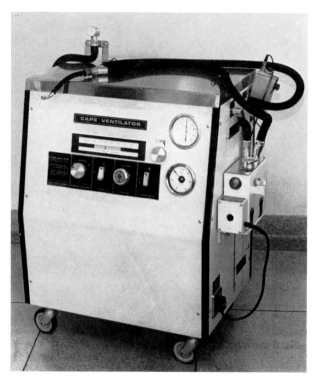

PLATE VIII.—The Cape Ventilator.
(*Cape Engineering Company Ltd.*)

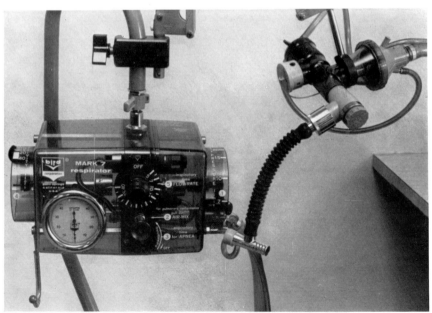

PLATE IX.—Bird positive pressure ventilator.
(*Bird Corporation British Oxygen Company Ltd.*)

developed increased hypoxaemia as the result of acute respiratory infection.

The clinical recognition of hypoxaemia usually presents no great difficulty. In a patient with acute pneumonia, for example, the development of central cyanosis is a reliable sign of oxygen lack, and a clear indication for oxygen therapy. Hypoxaemia is, however, much more difficult to detect in anaemic subjects, whose blood may contain insufficient haemoglobin for cyanosis to occur. It may also be difficult to recognize a significant increase in chronic hypoxaemia such as would warrant oxygen therapy. Cyanosis may have been present in this type of patient for months or years, and a slight increase in its degree can easily pass unnoticed. Where cyanosis is judged to be an unreliable index of hypoxaemia, the need for oxygen therapy must rest on other clinical manifestations, such as mental confusion, sweating, muscle twitching and, in chronic hypoxaemia of pulmonary origin, the development of pulmonary hypertension and cardiac failure.

Although clinical criteria are fairly reliable, it is essential for the degree of hypoxaemia to be determined with more scientific precision. Apparatus for estimating the Po_2 and/or So_2 of arterial blood samples is now available in most hospitals. These measurements, together with those of arterial Pco_2 and pH, are of considerable value in assessing the need for oxygen therapy, and in deciding how it should be given, particularly in patients with respiratory failure (p. 198). Oxygen is desirable for these patients whenever the Po_2 falls below 50 mm. Hg., or the So_2 below 85 per cent., and oxygen is essential when these figures are below 40 mg. Hg. or 75 per cent. respectively.

Some patients with severe emphysema and chronic hypoxaemia find that the inhalation of oxygen provides considerable temporary relief of intolerable dyspnoea. In such respiratory cripples the need for oxygen is particularly pressing after mild but necessary exertion such as bed-making, washing and defaecation. The provision of oxygen at the bedside, either in hospital or at home (p. 650), may spare these patients much respiratory distress. Portable oxygen equipment (p. 650) of the type used by mountaineers may permit a useful measure of physical activity in patients otherwise unable to move about because of shortness of breath. The apparatus is still expensive, cumbersome and unsightly, but may be of considerable value in selected cases.

Methods of administering Oxygen

Broadly speaking, two types of equipment are available for the administration of oxygen:

1. That which aims to secure the highest possible concentration of oxygen in the inspired air (high concentration oxygen therapy).

2. That which is designed to regulate the concentration of oxygen in the inspired air in such a way as to allow it to be maintained at a predetermined level between 24 per cent. and 35 per cent. (controlled oxygen therapy).

High-concentration oxygen therapy. This form of oxygen therapy is obligatory for all those conditions in which its effect depends on a very high Po_2 in the alveolar air, such as carbon monoxide poisoning and cardiogenic shock, but it can also be safely and effectively used for limited periods in the treatment of hypoxaemia of respiratory origin, provided that the level of alveolar ventilation is sufficiently well maintained to prevent hypercapnia.

In the first group of conditions the concentration of oxygen in the inspired air should be as near as possible to 100 per cent. For this purpose it is necessary to use a well-fitting oro-nasal mask with a non-return valve and either a reservoir bag or a demand-valve on the oxygen supply.

In the second group an inspired oxygen concentration of about 60 per cent. is usually adequate, and this can be provided by relatively inexpensive disposable polythene masks, such as the 'Polymask' (British Oxygen Company Ltd.) or the M.C. (Mary Catterall) mask (Medical and Industrial Equipment Ltd.), which are illustrated in Plates I and II, respectively. To achieve this concentration, the mask must fit the patient's face reasonably well and the rate of flow of oxygen into the mask must be at least 6 litres per minute. The Polymask incorporates a reservoir bag which conserves oxygen, but has the disadvantage of adding 1 to 2 per cent. of carbon dioxide to the inspired air. The same danger, to a lesser degree, arises with the M.C. mask if the oxygen flow is reduced to 1 to 2 litres per minute. These two masks should not be used in patients with hypercapnia, which will almost certainly be aggravated both by the respiratory depression caused by the inhalation of a high concentration of oxygen and by the rebreathing of carbon dioxide.

Whenever high-concentration oxygen therapy is

given, humidification is essential to prevent excessive drying of the respiratory mucosa. The old-fashioned method of bubbling the oxygen through a Wolff's bottle containing cold water is valueless. Adequate humidification can be achieved in two ways: (1) by passing the oxygen over water heated to the appropriate temperature in an East-Radcliffe humidifier, (2) by interposing a heated *nebulizer* of the conventional type between the flow-meter and the oxygen mask, or (3) by using an ultrasonic nebulizer. The second method is efficient and relatively inexpensive. A suitable apparatus is the Puritan nebulizer (Vickers Ltd. Medical Group), which is illustrated in Plate III.

An *oxygen tent* of conventional design, into which oxygen is delivered at a flow-rate of 8 litres per minute, provides an inspiratory oxygen concentration of between 50 and 60 per cent., but the patient's expired air raises the concentration of carbon dioxide within the tent to 1 to 2 per cent. This method of giving oxygen thus has the same theoretical disadvantages as masks incorporating rebreathing bags. In the Mark VI Refrigeration Oxygen Tent (Plate IV), however, a 'wash out' device permits the removal of a proportion of the carbon dioxide by the entrainment of ambient air, which simultaneously reduces the oxygen concentration. Modified in this way, the tent can be used for controlled oxygen therapy. A range of inspired oxygen concentrations of between 25 and 30 per cent. can be obtained by oxygen flow-rates of between 4 and 10 litres per minute, and the relatively rapid circulation of the oxygen/air mixture through the tent ensures that the carbon dioxide concentration is kept between 0·25 and 0·5 per cent., which in most cases is innocuous.

Although the oxygen tent may be of considerable value in the treatment of restless patients, particularly children (although some find the close confinement frightening at first), it is expensive to buy and is extravagant of oxygen. Its main disadvantage, however, is that it renders the patient relatively inaccessible to nursing and medical attention, almost every item of which necessitates opening a port in the tent, with a consequent reduction in the oxygen concentration. Patients with large amounts of sputum are particularly difficult to manage in an oxygen tent, and this is the main reason why it is seldom suitable for the treatment of patients with respiratory failure (p. 198).

Modern oxygen tents employ electrical refrigeration and are not difficult to maintain. Special precautions must, however, be taken to ensure that the internal temperature is maintained at the correct level (18·5° C.), particularly in unconscious patients, and that the hazard of fire is completely eliminated. Smoking must be prohibited in the vicinity, and nothing that might provoke spontaneous combustion—electric heating appliances, bell pushes, etc.—should be used inside the tent.

Controlled oxygen therapy. Because of the slope of the oxygen dissociation curve, a slight rise in alveolar Po_2 in patients with severe hypoxaemia of respiratory origin induces a relatively greater increase in arterial So_2, and thus of oxygen content, than in Po_2. As the degree of central depression of respiration caused by the administration of oxygen in hypercapnic patients is proportionate to the increase in arterial Po_2, slight oxygen enrichment of the inspired air in such patients may effect a significant improvement in arterial So_2 and oxygen content without provoking a dangerous increase in arterial Po_2. This observation provides the rationale for controlled oxygen therapy, which is the most valuable measure now available for the treatment of respiratory failure caused by alveolar hypoventilation.

The aim of controlled oxygen therapy is to administer the highest concentration of oxygen which will not initiate a progressive increase in arterial Pco_2. In patients with a severe degree of alveolar hypoventilation this may be as low as 24 per cent., only 3 per cent. above the concentration of oxygen in the atmosphere, while others may tolerate a concentration of 30 per cent. or even more. Facilities should be available for monitoring the Po_2 and/or So_2, the Pco_2 and the pH of arterial blood in every patient who is receiving oxygen for respiratory failure, in order to ensure that efforts to promote adequate oxygenation are not producing a dangerous degree of hypercapnia and respiratory acidosis. Many of these patients are still being treated without blood gas measurements, but such a practice amounts to little more than guesswork and in cases of severe respiratory failure it may have disastrous consequences.

With the introduction of the rebreathing technique for the estimation of arterial Pco_2 it is now possible without expensive equipment (1) to gauge the severity of respiratory failure when the patient is first seen, (2) to estimate the concentration of oxygen which can safely be given in the first instance, (3) to assess the patient's progress and (4) to determine whether the oxygen concentration in the inspired air at any particular juncture is producing a serious increase in hypercapnia. These matters and others related to the management of respiratory failure are discussed on p. 198.

When controlled oxygen therapy is given it is of course essential to be able to regulate within fairly narrow limits the concentration of oxygen in the inspired air. There is as yet no completely accurate method of doing this, but three devices are now commercially available by which the concentration can be maintained approximately at the desired level. These are:

(1) nasal cannulae (Plate V),
(2) the Ventimask (Plate VI) and
(3) the Edinburgh mask (Plate VII)

With *nasal cannulae* no precise control of the inspired oxygen concentration is possible, but it can be crudely regulated by adjusting the rate of flow. At 1 litre per minute the inspired oxygen concentration is between 25 and 30 per cent., and at 2 litres per minute it is between 30 and 35 per cent. Nasal cannulae are well tolerated by most patients, and have the advantage over masks of not having to be removed during meals, and of not interfering with the use of spectacles.

The *Ventimask* is available in three models designed to deliver oxygen at fixed concentrations of 24, 28 or 35 per cent. The basic component of the mask is a venturi tube through which oxygen is delivered at a rate of 4 litres per minute. This entrains a large volume of atmospheric air to produce a final oxygen concentration of 24, 28 or 35 per cent., according to the model used. It has been found by experience that the range of oxygen concentrations provided by these three masks is adequate for the treatment of most patients with respiratory failure. The entrainment of a large volume of ambient air virtually eliminates the rebreathing of carbon dioxide and dispenses with the need for humidification. Patients are able to tolerate Ventimasks for long periods, possibly because the pleasant breeze produced by the high rate of air flow eliminates the feeling of suffocation which many of them experience with other types of mask.

The *Edinburgh mask* consists of a loose-fitting plastic face-piece, with a 5 cm. diameter orifice open to the atmosphere. Into the centre of this orifice projects an oxygen delivery tube, which emits oxygen at the desired flow-rate into the mask at right angles to the air stream caused by the patient's ventilation. The inspired oxygen concentrations which are obtainable at various flow-rates when the minute volume of pulmonary ventilation is between 6 and 7 litres per minute are shown in Table 19, but it must be appreciated

TABLE 19

EDINBURGH MASK:
INSPIRED OXYGEN CONCENTRATIONS

Oxygen Flow (l./min.)	Inspired Oxygen (per cent.)	
	Mean	Standard Deviation
0·5	23·4	1·6
1·0	27·4	4·1
2·0	29·9	7·7
3·0	35·2	5·8

By kind permission of the *British Medical Journal*.

that with the Edinburgh mask the concentration at any given flow-rate may be considerably higher at lower levels of minute volume. This is however, probably not a serious disadvantage in practice, as the inspired oxygen concentration is unlikely to rise to a dangerously high level unless the minute volume is reduced to such a degree that artificial positive-pressure ventilation must be used to restore the situation. Nevertheless, it is clearly desirable, when using an Edinburgh mask, or indeed any other type of mask, in patients with severe respiratory failure, to estimate the arterial Pco_2 at regular intervals to ensure that the inspired oxygen concentration, whatever its actual level may be, is not depressing ventilation.

Duration of Oxygen Therapy

It is seldom difficult to decide when to terminate oxygen therapy in patients with acute hypoxaemia caused, for example, by pneumonia. In patients with chronic hypoxaemia, however, a rational decision on this point cannot be made without first estimating the arterial Po_2 or So_2. In general, treatment can safely be withdrawn if the arterial So_2 is still above 85 per cent. or the Po_2 above 50 mm. Hg. after the patient has been breathing air for 30 minutes, but many patients with advanced chronic respiratory disease can tolerate a more severe degree of hypoxaemia than this, and each case must, therefore, be judged on its merits. The development of mental confusion, sweating or a rise in blood pressure after oxygen therapy has been withdrawn is, however, an urgent indication for its resumption.

Equipment for Domiciliary Oxygen Therapy

Oxygen cylinders of 48 cu. ft. capacity, fitted with simple flow regulators, can be prescribed by general practitioners in the National Health Service. The original reason for providing this facility was to allow patients with pneumonia to be treated at home. In such patients oxygen is usually required for only a day or two, and can be administered safely and effectively by means of an inexpensive polythene mask, such as the Polymask or M.C. mask. In order to ensure adequate oxygenation and to prevent deflation of the reservoir bag, an oxygen flow-rate of 4 litres per minute (the 'high' setting on the regulator) is necessary, and two or more cylinders per day may be required. Humidification is probably not essential when oxygen is being given for short periods in this type of case.

At the present time, however, oxygen therapy in the home is being prescribed mainly for dyspnoea or hypoxaemia caused by chronic respiratory disease. Many such patients will require oxygen for several weeks at a time, either intermittently or continuously. In order to reduce transport costs it would clearly be more economical to provide larger cylinders (e.g. 120 cu. ft.) for some of these patients, but it may often be difficult or even impossible to carry such heavy and bulky containers up narrow flights of stairs in tenements or blocks of flats.

Many patients with chronic respiratory disease, however, require only intermittent slight oxygen enrichment of the inspired air for the relief of intolerable dyspnoea following exertion or bouts of coughing. This can be provided safely and economically by the use of a double nasal catheter, an Edinburgh mask or a Ventimask, used in conjunction with the standard domiciliary (48 cu. ft.) cylinder. These devices can now be prescribed on E.C. 10. For the sake of economy in the use of oxygen, a double nasal catheter or an Edinburgh mask should normally be prescribed. With an oxygen flow-rate of 2 litres per minute (the 'medium' setting on the N.H.S. regulator) these devices will usually produce an inspired oxygen concentration of between 25 and 35 per cent. and this should not be exceeded under uncontrolled conditions in view of the danger of inducing hypercapnia. *Oxygen therapy used intermittently in this way is not intended primarily to correct hypoxaemia, but to relieve dyspnoea*. Patients with severe hypoxaemia must be given controlled oxygen therapy *continuously*, but because of the amount of oxygen required, this form of treatment is seldom practicable in the home, and such patients should be admitted to hospital.

Portable oxygen equipment. The 'Portogen' apparatus (British Oxygen Company Ltd.) consists of a specially designed light-weight cylinder of 100 litres capacity, which can be recharged as often as necessary from a cylinder of standard size. It is provided with a regulator, control valve, gauge and carrying case, and the whole apparatus weighs less than 3 lb. It should be used in conjunction with a double nasal catheter or an Edinburgh mask at a flow-rate of 2 litres per minute (the 'medium' setting on the regulator).

Portable oxygen equipment is at present only available on loan from hospitals or by private purchase. It is expensive and its value is limited by the small capacity of the portable cylinder, which contains only sufficient oxygen to last for 50 minutes at 2 litres per minute. Judiciously used by intelligent patients, however, it can serve a useful purpose.

Hyperbaric Oxygenation

The administration of oxygen at a pressure of 2 to 3 atmospheres, which produces a considerable increase in the amount of oxygen dissolved in the plasma and extracellular fluid, is now being used with some success in the treatment of carbon monoxide poisoning (p. 548), ischaemia resulting from acute and chronic arterial insufficiency (p. 138), and anaerobic bacterial infections, such as those due to *Clostridium welchii*. It also seems to be of some value as an adjunct to the treatment of malignant tumours by deep X-rays, and as a means of reducing the risks of major cardiovascular surgery. The effects of hyperbaric oxygenation in myocardial infarction, shock and traumatic lesions of the brain are still under investigation, but this form of treatment is probably contraindicated in those forms of respiratory failure in which hypoxia is accompanied by hypercapnia.

Hyperbaric oxygenation can at present be undertaken only in a few medical centres and is extremely costly in terms both of equipment and personnel. Furthermore, it exposes the patient to the hazards of oxygen toxicity and otitic barotrauma, and medical personnel working in the pressure chamber to the hazards of nitrogen narcosis, air embolism and bone necrosis. The risk of fire is also considerable.

Although hyperbaric oxygenation may prove to be a major advance in the treatment of certain diseases, it is still in the early stages of development, and a final assessment of its value may not be possible for some years to come.

ARTIFICIAL PULMONARY VENTILATION

The resuscitation of victims of drowning, carbon monoxide poisoning or electrocution demands the immediate restoration of pulmonary ventilation by artificial means and its maintenance until spontaneous breathing returns. When the emergency occurs, as it generally does, in a situation where special apparatus for resuscitation is not available, it is essential that the person who has to deal with it, whether he be a doctor, an ambulance man or a member of the general public, should start artificial respiration immediately. It has now been generally accepted that manual methods of artificial respiration are inadequate and that *expired air resuscitation* by the mouth to mouth technique should be universally adopted. The theoretical objection to expired air resuscitation, namely that the patient is made to breathe air containing 4 to 5 per cent. of carbon dioxide (less if the operator is hyperventilating) does not appear to be of practical importance.

Before artificial respiration is begun the mouth and upper air passages must be cleared of secretions, water, etc. Children can be held up by the heels and heavy adults placed in the prone position for a few seconds—no longer, as time is precious in these emergencies. The victim is then laid on his back and the mouth quickly swabbed out with a handkerchief. Kneeling on one side the operator fully extends the victim's head, placing one hand on top of the head and the other below the neck to increase the tilt. The operator now inhales deeply and opens his mouth widely. He then places his mouth around the patient's mouth and having made an air-tight seal blows forcefully in adults, gently in infants and children.

When the chest is seen to expand, contact with the face is interrupted and the victim is allowed to exhale passively. The operator inhales deeply again and the inflation cycles are continued at a rate of about 15 per minute. During inflation and when the patient is exhaling the tilt of the head must be maintained. Any flexion of the neck will diminish the patency of the airway and part of the air may be blown into the victim's stomach.

If the abdomen is seen to bulge during inflation, a slight steady pressure should be exerted with one hand on the abdomen below the left costal margin while the tilt of the head is maintained with the other hand on top of the victim's head.

Cardiac arrest may have taken place at the same time as respiratory arrest (a common occurrence in electrocution), or may develop while artificial respiration is being performed. In these circumstances, closed cardiac massage (p. 643) must be started at once by a second operator, the efforts of the two being co-ordinated in such a way that one pulmonary inflation is interpolated between groups of four cardiac compressions. Artificial respiration may have to be maintained, if necessary by a team of operators, for several hours and should be abandoned only when spontaneous breathing returns or when irreversible cardiac arrest takes place.

Various methods have been devised for overcoming the aesthetic objections to expired air resuscitation. The simplest is to interpose a handkerchief between the mouth of the victim and that of the operator. There are, however, various types of tube which can be used to transmit air from the donor's mouth to the recipient's pharynx. The least complicated is an S-shaped plastic tube without valves; probably the best is the Brook Airway (Fig. 27), which incorporates a non-return valve and an expiration vent which effectively prevents the patient's expired air and pharyngeal secretions from entering the operator's mouth, while not impairing the efficiency of pulmonary ventilation.

If respiratory arrest occurs in a hospital with well-organized facilities for resuscitation, the situation is of course easier to handle. Nevertheless, there are occasions in which a period of expired air resuscitation may be vital to the patient's survival while special equipment is being brought to his bedside. All medical staff must therefore be fully conversant with this technique.

As soon as possible a cuffed endotracheal tube should be introduced, the air passages cleared of secretions by suction through a bronchial catheter, and positive pressure ventilation instituted by means of an Ambu Resuscitator (or similar device) connected to the endotracheal tube. Once adequate pulmonary ventilation has been re-established in this way the acute emergency is over and a considered decision can then be taken on further management which may involve the use of a mechanical respirator (p. 653), and possibly tracheostomy at a later stage.

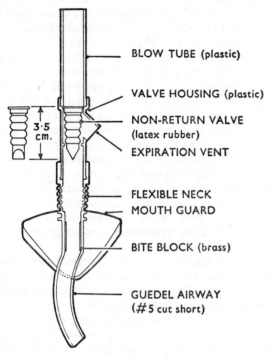

BLOW TUBE (plastic)

VALVE HOUSING (plastic)

NON-RETURN VALVE (latex rubber)

EXPIRATION VENT

3·5 cm.

FLEXIBLE NECK

MOUTH GUARD

BITE BLOCK (brass)

GUEDEL AIRWAY (#5 cut short)

FIG. 27.—Brook Airway (*Lancet*).

Mechanical Ventilators. A wide range of machines is now available for artificial ventilation. The negative pressure ('tank') ventilator has now been abandoned, and all the equipment in current use operates on the 'intermittent positive-pressure' principle, by means of which the lungs are inflated through a cuffed endotracheal tube inserted either through the mouth or via a tracheostomy. The indications for intermittent positive pressure ventilation include: (1) central depression of respiration caused by morphine or barbiturate poisoning, or by severe brain injuries; (2) interference with the nerve supply to the respiratory muscles, as may occur in conditions such as poliomyelitis, polyneuritis and myasthenia gravis; (3) inadequate pulmonary ventilation resulting from injuries causing instability and paradoxical movement of a portion of the chest wall ('stove-in chest'); (4) ventilatory failure supervening in patients with chronic bronchitis and emphysema (pp. 195–198) as a result of respiratory infection or following an operation on the chest or abdomen; (5) severe status asthmaticus; (6) tetanus,

in which the spasms are controlled by muscle-relaxant drugs while respiration is maintained by a mechanical ventilator.

The action of all positive pressure ventilators is to produce inflation of the lungs at a rate of 14 to 20 cycles per minute, expiration being allowed to occur passively between each phase of positive pressure. Some respirators are driven by an electric motor, others by compressed air or oxygen. In some models the change-over from the inspiratory to the expiratory phase is actuated merely by a timing mechanism; in others the change occurs when the pressure in the air passages exceeds a pre-set level or when a predetermined volume of air has been delivered. Some machines incorporate a mechanism which ensures that the application of positive pressure conforms with the rate and rhythm of whatever spontaneous breathing is still retained (patient-cycled ventilators).

The Cape ventilator (Plate VIII) is mechanically robust and reliable. This machine is suitable for most of the conditions in which intermittent positive pressure ventilation is required and is particularly useful when the lungs and/or chest wall are rigid and considerable force is required to produce adequate ventilation. The tidal volume and respiration rate can be adjusted to the patient's requirements, but the machine does not incorporate a 'patient-cycling' device. This means that the ventilator has to 'take over' the patient's respiration completely, and any spontaneous breathing must, if necessary, be suppressed by drugs such as morphine or suxamethonium, or by a period of manual ventilation sufficiently vigorous to reduce the arterial P_{CO_2}, and thus to diminish the patient's spontaneous respiratory drive. Most patients, however, adapt themselves remarkably quickly to positive-pressure ventilation, and these drugs are seldom required for more than 24 hours. Patient-cycling devices are indeed of doubtful value in the treatment of severe ventilatory failure, as the rate at which the patient 'triggers' the machine may fluctuate considerably, and this can lead to wide and unpredictable variations in the minute volume of pulmonary ventilation. They have, however, a useful place in the treatment of less advanced degrees of ventilatory failure, and are also of value during the stage of recovery, when the problem of 'weaning' a patient from artificial ventilation may present considerable difficulties.

The Bennett and Bird (Plate IX) types of positive-pressure ventilator are basically designed for patient-cycling, although they also provide for automatic cycling at a predetermined respiratory rate. They are not powerful enough to maintain an adequate level of ventilation in patients with 'stiff' lungs or a rigid chest wall, but are useful for 'assisted ventilation', i.e. for augmenting spontaneous breathing in patients with less severe degrees of respiratory insufficiency, and as they are driven by compressed air or oxygen, they have the advantage of not being dependent on an electricity supply.

Adequate pulmonary ventilation can be achieved by mechanical ventilators only if the positive pressure is applied below the glottis, i.e. through a cuffed tube placed in the trachea. An endotracheal tube passed through the mouth can safely be used for periods up to 48 hours, but may cause discomfort and ulceration of the vocal cords if left in position for a longer time. When necessary, tracheostomy must be performed and a cuffed tracheostomy tube inserted. Intermittent positive pressure ventilation can then be maintained indefinitely until adequate spontaneous pulmonary ventilation returns. The management of such patients requires the attention of a highly trained team of doctors and nurses, and should normally be undertaken in special units set up for the purpose. Adequate warming and humidification of the inspired air must be ensured in order to prevent damage to the tracheal and bronchial mucosa. The most careful precautions must be taken to avoid the introduction of infection and to prevent necrosis of the tracheal wall by pressure from the tracheostomy tube.

Recently, good results have been reported in bronchial asthma from the use of patient-triggered ventilation machines, such as the Bennett or the Bird, to deliver aerosols of bronchodilator drugs, e.g. 0·5 per cent. salbutamol, into the bronchi through a tightly fitting oro-nasal mask. Intermittent positive pressure ventilation of this type has also been used, without the addition of aerosols, in an attempt to improve pulmonary ventilation in patients with emphysema exhibiting 'air-trapping', but there is no evidence to suggest that this treatment is of any value.

Glossary

Preparations which have been mentioned in the text are listed alphabetically in the left-hand column, with their equivalent names opposite, in the right-hand column. Official or approved names are in roman and proprietary names in italic type.

Acetazolamide	*Diamox*
Acetohexamide	*Dimelor*
Acetphenolisatin acetate	*Bydolax; Cirotyl; Veripaque*
Acetylcystein	*Airbron*
Acetylsalicylic acid	*Angiers Junior Aspirin; Asagran; Aspro; Caprin; Genasprin*
Acetylsalicylic acid, enteric coated	*Nu-Seals Aspirin*
Acetylsalicylic acid, soluble	*Broprin; Disprin; Disprin Junior; Solprin*
Achromycin	tetracycline
Acthar	corticotrophin
Acth-Crookes	corticotrophin
Actidil	triprolidine hydrochloride
Actinomycin C	*Sanamycin*
Activated charcoal	*Darco G-60*
Adalin	carbromal
Adamantadine hydrochloride	*Symmetrel*
Adcortyl	triamcinolone
Adrenor	noradrenaline acid tartrate
Adreson	cortisone acetate
Adroyd	oxymetholone
Aerosol O.T.	dioctyl sodium sulphosuccinate
Aerosporin	polymyxin B
Airbron	acetylcysteine
Alavar P	alum precipitated pyridine extract
Albamycin	novobiocin
Albucid	sulphacetamide sodium
Alcopar	bephenium hydroxynaphthoate
Aldactone-A	spironolactone
Aldocorten	aldosterone
Aldomet	methyldopa
Aldosterone	*Aldocorten; Electrocortin*
Aleudrin	isoprenaline sulphate
Alficetyn	chloramphenicol
Alkeran	melphalan
Allopurinol	*Zyloric*
Allpyral G	alum precipitated pyridine extract
Alocol P	aluminium hydroxide
Aludrox	aluminium hydroxide
Aluminium hydroxide	*Alocol P; Aludrox; Collumina*
Alum precipitated pyridine extract	*Alavac P; Allpyral G*
Alupent	orciprenaline sulphate
Ambilhar	niridazole
Ambramycin	tetracycline
Amethocaine hydrochloride	*Anethaine; Decicain; Gingicain; Rexocain*
Amethopterin	methotrexate
Amicar	aminocaproic acid
Aminocaproic acid	*Amicar; Epsikapron*
Aminophylline	*Cardophylin; Diaphyllin; Phyldrox*
Aminophylline, enteric coated tablets	*Delaminoph*

654

Amitriptyline hydrochloride	*Laroxyl; Saroten; Tryptizol*
Ammonium chloride, enteric coated tablets .	*Nu-Seals Ammonium Chloride*
Amodiaquine dihydrochloride . . .	*Camoquin*
Amopyroquin hydrochloride	*Propoquin*
Amphetamine sulphate	*Benzedrine* .
Amphotericin B	*Fungilin; Fungizone*
Ampicillin	*Penbritin*
Amylobarbitone	*Amytal*
Amylobarbitone sodium	*Sodium Amytal*
Amytal	amylobarbitone
Anacordone	nikethamide
Anapolen	oxymetholone
Ancolan	meclozine hydrochloride
Ancrod	*Arvin*
Anethaine	amethocaine hydrochloride
Aneurine hydrochloride	*Benerva; Betavel*
Angiers Junior Aspirin	acetylsalicylic acid
Anisidione	*Miradon*
Ansolysen	pentolinium tartrate
Antabuse	disulfiram
Antazoline hydrochloride	*Antistin*
Antazoline mesylate	*Histostab*
Antepar	piperazine phosphate
Antepar Elixir	piperazine citrate
Anterior pituitary hormone . . .	*Gonadotrophon*
Antex Leo	Serum gonadotrophins
Anthisan	mepyramine maleate
Antiformin	sodium hypochlorite
Antipressan	glyceryl trinitrate
Antistin	antazoline hydrochloride
Antrypol	suramin
Antuitrin S	chorionic gonadotrophin
Anturan	sulphinpyrazone
Apresoline	hydrallazine hydrochloride
Aprinox	bendrofluazide
Apsin V.K.	phenoxymethylpenicillin
Aralen	chloroquine phosphate
Aramine	metaraminol acid tartrate
Arlef	flufenamic acid
Armyl	lymecycline
Artane	benzhexol hydrochloride
Artosin	tolbutamide
Arvin	ancrod
Arvynol	ethchlorovynol
Asagram	acetylsalicylic acid
Ascabiol	benzyl benzoate
Ascorbic acid	*Ascorvel; Redoxon*
Ascorvel	ascorbic acid
Aspro	acetylsalicylic acid
Astertit	chloroxylenol
A.T. 10	dihydrotachysterol
Atebrin	mepacrine methanesulphonate
Atromid S	clofibrate
Atropine methylnitrate	*Brovon; Eumydrin; Phylostropin*
Atropine sulphate	*Collyrium Atropine Chibret*
Aureomycin	chlortetracycline
Avertin	bromethol

Avloprocil A.S.	procaine benzylpenicillin
Avlosulphon	dapsone
Avoleum	vitamin A
Avomine	promethazine theoclate
Azathioprine	*Imuran*
B.A.L.	dimercaprol
Bactrim	trimethoprim with sulphamethoxazole
Barbenyl	phenobarbitone
B-Complex	vitamin B complex
Becomel	vitamin B complex
Becosym	vitamin B complex
Becovite	vitamin B complex
Beflavit	riboflavine
Befortiss	vitamin B complex
Belladonna alkaloids	*Bellafoline*
Bellafolline	belladonna alkaloids
Bemaphate	chloroquine phosphate
Bemegride	*Megimide*
Benadon	pyridoxine hydrochloride
Benadryl	diphenhydramine hydrochloride
Bendrofluazide	*Aprinox; Berkoside; Centyl; Neo-Naclex*
Benemid	probenecid
Benerva	aneurine hydrochloride
Benerva Compound	vitamin B complex
Benzalkonium chloride	*Calaxin; Drapolene; Empiquat B.A.C. Hyamine 3500; Marinol; P.R.Q. Antiseptic; Roccal; Zephiran*
Benzathine penicillin	*Dibencil; Neolin; Penidural; Permapen*
Benzedrine	amphetamine sulphate
Benzhexol hydrochloride . . .	*Artane; Pipanol*
Benzocaine compound lozenges . . .	*Menthesin*
Benztrone	oestradiol benzoate
Benzyl benzoate	*Ascabiol*
Benzylpenicillin	*Conspen; Crystapen; Eskacillin 100; Falapen; Hyasorb; Pondets Throat Lozenges; Solupen; Tabillin*
Bephenium hydroxynaphthoate . . .	*Alcopar*
Beplex	vitamin B complex
Berkmycen	oxytetracycline dihydrate
Berkfurin	nitrofurantoin
Berkomine	imipramine hydrochloride
Berkoside	bendrofluazide
Beta-Corlan	betamethasone sodium phosphate
Betamethasone	*Betnelan; Celestone*
Betamethasone sodium phosphate . .	*Betnesol: Beta-Corlan*
Betamethasone valerate	*Betnovate*
Betavel	aneurine hydrochloride
Bethanidine sulphate	*Esbatal*
Betnelan	betamethasone
Betnesol	betamethasone
Betnovate	betamethasone valerate
Betolvex	cyanocobalamin zinc tannate
Bidex	hexachlorophane
Bifacton	cyanocobalamin
Biocetab	cetrimide
Biogastrone	carbenoxolone sodium
Bioserpine	reserpine
Bisacodyl	*Dulcolax*

Bioserpine	reserpine
Bisacodyl	*Dulcolax*
Bitevan	cyanocobalamin
Brocadopa	dopa
Brocillin	propicillin potassium
Bromethol	avertin
Broprin	acetylsalicylic acid soluble
Brovon	atropine methyl nitrate
Broxil	phenethicillin potassium
Bucrol	carbutamide
Busulphan	*Myleran*
Butazolidin	phenylbutazone
Butazone	phenylbutazone
Butobarbitone	*Monodorm; Soneryl*
Bydolax	acetphenolisatin acetate
Calaxin	benzalkonium chloride
Calciferol	*Fortodyl; Radiostol; Sterogyl-15; Vitavel-D*
Calcium Disodium Versenate	sodium calciumedetate
Calcium gluconate effervescent tablets . .	*Calcium Sandoz*
Calcium Sandoz	calcium gluconate effervescent tablets
Calcitonin	*Thyrocalcitonin*
Calpol	paracetamol
Camoquin	amodiaquine hydrochloride
Capastat	capreomycin sulphate
Capreomycin sulphate	*Capastat*
Caprin	acetylsalicylic acid
Carbachol	*Chibret Carbachol Collyrium*
Carbamazepine	*Tegretol*
Carbenicillin	*Pyopen*
Carbenoxolone sodium	*Biogastrone*
Carbimazole	*Neo-Mercazole*
Carbromal	*Adalin*
Carbutamide	*Bucrol; B.2.55; Invenol; Nadisan*
Cardiacap	pentaerythritol tetranitrate
Cardophylin	aminophylline
Carisoma	carisoprodol
Carisoprodol	*Carisoma*
Cathomycin	novobiocin
Caved S	deglycyrrhizinised liquorice
Celacol M	methylcellulose
Celbenin	methicillin sodium
Celestone	betamethazone
Celevac	methylcellulose
Cellucon	methylcellulose
Cephalexin	*Ceporex; Keflex*
Cephaloridine	*Ceporin*
Cephalothin sodium	*Keflin*
Ceporex	cephalexin
Ceporin	cephaloridine
Cerevon	ferrous gluconate
Cetal	paracetamol
Cetavlex	cetrimide
Cetavlon	cetrimide
Cetrimide	*Biocetab; Cetavlon; Cetavlex; Morpan C.H.S.A.; Savlon; Vesagex*
Chloral hydrate	*Somnos*

Chlorambucil	*Leukeran*
Chloramine T	*Dygerma*
Chloramphenicol	*Alficetyn; Chloromycetin*
Chlordane	*Octachlor; Toxichlor; Velsicol 1068*
Chlordiazepoxide hydrochloride	*Librium*
Chlorhexidine gluconate	*Hibitane*
Chlormethine	mustine hydrochloride
Chlormethylencycline	*Megaclor*
Chloromycetin	chloramphenicol
Chloroquine phosphate	*Aralen; Avloclor; Bempahate; Resochin*
Chloroquine sulphate	*Nivaquine*
Chloros	sodium hypochlorite
Chlorothiazide	*Saluric*
Choledyl	choline theophyllinate
Chloroxylenol	*Astertit; CMX Antiseptic; Dettol*
Chlorpheniramine maleate	*Piriton*
Chlorphentermine hydrochloride	*Lucofen; Lucofen SA*
Chlorproguanil hydrochloride	*Lapudrine*
Chlorpropamazine hydrochloride	*Largactil*
Chlorpropamide	*Diabinese*
Chlortetracycline	*Aureomycin*
Chlorthalidone	*Hygroton*
Cholestyramine	*Cuemid*
Choline theophyllinate	*Choledyl*
Chorionic gonadotrophin	*Antuitrin S; Gonadotrophon L.H.; Physex Leo; Pregnyl*
Ciba 1906	thiambutosine
Cirotyl	acetphenolisatin acetate
Clinimycin	oxytetracycline dihydrate
Clofazimine	*Lamprene; B663; G.30 320*
Clofibrate	*Atromid-S*
Clomid	clomiphene citrate
Clomiphene citrate	*Clomid*
Cloxacillin	*Orbenin*
CMX Antiseptic	chloroxylenol
Cobadex	hydrocortisone
Cobalin	cyanocobalamin
Cobastab	cyanocobalamin
Codelcortone	prednisolone
Codelsol	prednisolone disodium phosphate
Cod liver oil	*Seven Seas Cod Liver Oil*
Cogentin	benztropine methanesulphonate
Colistin sulphomethate	*Colomycin*
Collumina	aluminium hydroxide
Collyrium atropine Chibret	atropine sulphate
Collyrium Carbachol Chibret	carbachol
Collyrium Eserine Chibret	physostigmine salicylate eye drops
Collyrium Sulphacetamide Chibret	sulphacetamide sodium
Cologel	methylcellulose
Colomycin	colistin sulphomethate
Complebin	vitamin B complex
Complebin Forte	vitamin B complex
Compocillin-VK	phenoxymethylpenicillin
Comprimettes Penicillin V	phenoxymethylpenicillin
Conspen	benzylpenicillin
Contax	acetphenolisatin acetate
Contrathion	pralidoxime mesylate
Coprola	dioctyl sodium sulphosuccinate

Coramine	nikethamide
Corlan	hydrocortisone sodium succinate
Cortef	hydrocortisone
Cortelan	cortisone acetate
Corticotrophin	*Acth-Crookes; Acthar; Cortrophin*
Cortistab	cortisone acetate
Cortril	hydrocortisone
Cortrizyl	cortisone acetate
Cortrophin	corticotrophin
Corvotone	nikethamide
Cremodiazine	sulphadiazine
Cronetal	disulfiram
Crystapen	benzylpenicillin
Crystalline penicillin (*see* Benzylpenicillin)	
Crystodigin	digitoxin
Cuemid	cholestyramine
Cumopyran	cyclocoumarol
Cyanocobalamin	*Bitevan; Cobalin; Cobatsab; Cytacon; Cytamen; Fermin*
Cyanocobalamin zinc tannate . . .	*Depinar*
Cyanocobalamin zinc tannate aluminium mono-stearate	*Betolvex; Genolvex*
Cyclizine hydrochloride	*Marzine; Sereen; Valoid*
Cyclobarbitone	*Phanodorm*
Cyclocoumarol	*Cumopyran*
Cyclogyl	cyclopentolate
Cyclopentolate	*Cyclogyl; Mydrilate*
Cyclophosphamide	*Endoxana*
Cycloserine	*Seromycin*
Cytacon	cyanocobalamin
Cytamen	cyanocobalamin
Daonil	glibenclamide
Dapsone	*Avlosulphon*
Daraclor	pyrimethamine with chloroquine sulphate
Daranide	dichlorphenamide
Daraprim	pyrimethamine
Darco G-60	activated charcoal
Dartalan	thiopropazate hydrochloride
D.B.I.	phenformin
D.D.T.	dicophane
Debrisoquine sulphate	*Declinax*
Decadron	dexamethasone
Deca-Durabolin	nandrolone decanoate
Decicain	amethocaine hydrochloride
Declinax	debrisoquine sulphate
Decortacete	deoxycortone acetate
Decortisyl	prednisone
Deglycirrhizinised liquorice . . .	*Caved S*
Dehydroemetine hydrochloride . .	*Mebadin*
Delaminoph	aminophylline (enteric coated)
Delta-Cortef	prednisolone
Delta-Cortelan	prednisone acetate
Deltacortone	prednisone
Deltacortril	prednisolone
Delta-Genacort	prednisolone
Deltstab	prednisolone

Demecarium bromide	Humorsol; Tosmilen
Demethylchlortetracycline hydrochloride	Ledermycin
Dendrid	idoxuridine (I.D.U.)
Deosan Green Label	sodium hypochlorite
Deoxycortone acetate	Doca; Decortacete
Dephraden	dexamethasone
Deseril	methysergide maleate
Desferal	desferrioxamine mesylate
Desferrioxamine mesylate	Desferal
Dettol	chloroxylenol
Dexacortisyl	dexamethasone
Dexamed	dexamphetamine sulphate
Dexamethasone	Decadron; Dexacortisyl; Oradexon
Dexamphetamine sulphate	Dephadren; Dexamed; Dexedrine; Dexten; Dextro-Amphe-tamine Sulphate-Dellipsoids D 24
Dexamphetamine sulphate spansules	Dexedrine Spansules
Dexedrine	dexamphetamine sulphate
Dexedrine Spansules	dexamphetamine sulphate spansules
Dexten	dexamphetamine sulphate
Dextran	Macrodex
Dextran 40-low molecular weight	Intraflodex; Lomodex; Rheomacrodex
Dextran 110	Dextraven 110; Intradex
Dextran 150	Dextraven 150
Dextraven 110	dextran 110
Dextraven 150	dextran 150
Dextroamphetamine Sulphate Dellipsoids D24	dexamphetamine sulphate
DF 118	dihydrocodeine acid tartrate
Diabinese	chlorpropamide
Di-Ademil	hydroflumethiazide
Di-Adreson	prednisone
Di-Adreson-F	prednisolone
Diamox	acetazolamide
Diaphyllin	aminophylline
Diazepam	Valium
Dibencil	benzathine penicillin
Dibenyline	phenoxybenzamine hydrochloride
Dibexin	vitamin B complex
Dibotin	phenformin
Dichloralphenazone	Welldorm
Dichlorphenamide	Daranide; Oratrol
Dicophane	D.D.T.
Dicyclomine hydrochloride	Merbentyl; Wyovin
Diethylcarbamazine citrate	Banocide; Ethodryl; Hetrazan
Diethylpropion hydrochloride	Tenuate; Tenuate Dospan
Diethyl toluamide	Mylol
Digitoxin	Crystodigin; Nativelle's Digitaline
Digoxin	Lanoxin
Dihydrocodeine acid tartrate	DF 118; Paracodin
Dihydrotachysterol	A.T. 10; Hytakerol
Dihydroxyphenylisatin	Veripaque
Diloxanide furoate	Furamide
Dimercaprol	B.A.L.
Dimelor	acetohexamide
Dimenformon	oestradiol benzoate
Dimethyl phthalate	Sketofax
Dioctyl Forte	dioctyl sodium sulphasuccinate
Dioctyl Medo	dioctyl sodium sulphasuccinate

Dioctyl sodium sulphosuccinate	*Aerosol O.T.; Coprola; Dioctyl Forte; Dioctyl Medo; Manoxol O.T.; Norval Siponol O 100*
Dipasic	isoniazid aminosalicylate
Dipaxin	diphenadione
Diphenadione	*Dipaxin*
Diphenhydramine hydrochloride . .	*Benadryl*
Direma	hydrochlorothiazide
Disipal	orphenadrine hydrochloride
Disipray	isoprenaline sulphate
Disodium cromoglycate	*Intal*
Disprin and Disprin Junior . . .	acetylsalicylic acid soluble
Distamine	penicillamine
Distaquaine G	procaine benzylpenicillin
Distaquaine V	phenoxymethylpenicillin
Disulfiram	*Antabuse; Cronetal*
Doca	deoxycortone acetate
Dopa	*Brocadopa; Larodopa*
Doriden	glutethimide
Drapolene	benzalkonium chloride
Dulcolax	bisacodyl
Duncaine	lignocaine hydrochloride
Duphalac	lactulose
Duracillin A.S.	procaine benzylpenicillin
Duromine	phentermine
Dygerma	chloramine T
Dytac	triamterene
Economycin	tetracycline
Edecrin	ethacrynic acid
Edrophonium chloride	*Tensilon*
Ef-Cortelan	hydrocortisone
Ef-Cortelan Soluble . . .	hydrocortisone sodium succinate
Effco Tonic	vitamin B complex
Electrocortin	aldosterone
Elixophyllin	theophylline
Eltroxin	thyroxine sodium
Emeside	ethosuximide
Emiquat B.A.C.	benzalkonium chloride
Endoxana	cyclophosphamide
Eneril	paracetamol
Entrosalyl	sodium salicylate
Epanutin	phenytoin sodium
Epsikapron	aminocaproic acid
Eptoin	phenytoin sodium
Eraldin	practolol
Ergometrine maleate	*Ergotrate*
Ergotamine Medihaler . . .	ergotamine tartrate spray
Ergotamine tartrate	*Femergin; Lingraine; Medihaler Ergotamine*
Ergotrate	ergometrine maleate
Erycin	erythromycin stearate
Erythrocin	erythromycin stearate
Erythromycin estolate . . .	*Ilosone*
Erythromycin ethyl succinate . . .	*Erythroped*
Erythromycin stearate . . .	*Erycin; Erythrocin; Ilotycin*
Erythroped	erythromycin ethyl succinate
Esbatal	bethanidine sulphate
Eserine Salicylate Minims . . .	physostigmine salicylate eye drops

Esidrex	hydrochlorothiazide
Eskacillin 100	benzylpenicillin
Eskacillin 200	procaine benzylpenicillin
Estigyn	ethinyloestradiol
Ethacrynic acid	*Edecrin*
Ethambutol dihydrochloride	*Myambutol*
Ethchlorvynol	*Arvynol; Serensil*
Ethinyloestradiol	*Estigyn; Lynoral; Primogyn C*
Ethionamide	*Trescatyl*
Ethisterone	*Gestone-Oral; Progestoral*
Ethnine	pholcodeine
Ethodryl	diethylcarbamazine citrate
Ethopropazine hydrochloride	*Lysivane*
Ethosuximide	*Emeside; Simatin; Zarontin*
Ethynodiol diacetate	present in *Demulen; Metrulen; Metrulen M; Ovulen*
Etrinol	lucanthone hydrochloride
Euglucon	glibenclamide
Eumydrin	atropine methyl nitrate
Falapen	benzylpenicillin
Fanasil	sulfadoxine
Febrilix	paracetamol
Femasc	testosterone propionate
Femergin	ergotamine tartrate
Fenfluramine hydrochloride	*Ponderax*
Fentazin	perphenazine
Fercuman	ferrous sulphate compound tablets
Fermin	cyanocobalamin
Ferrogradumet	ferrous sulphate slow release capsules
Ferromyn	ferrous succinate
Ferrous fumarate	*Fersamal*
Ferrous gluconate	*Cerevon; Fergon; Glistron*
Ferrous succinate	*Ferromyn*
Ferrous sulphate	*Ferrogradumet; Ferrous Sulphate; Emplets; Fersolate; Toniron*
Ferrous sulphate compound tablets	*Fercuman; Haemofax*
Ferrous Sulphate Emplets	ferrous sulphate
Fersamal	ferrous fumarate
Fersolate	ferrous sulphate
Flagyl	metronidazole
Florinef Acetate	fludrocortisone acetate
Floxapen	flucloxacillin
Flucloxacillin	*Floxapen*
Flufenamic acid	*Arlef*
Fluocinolone acetonide	*Synalar; Synandone*
Fluoxymesterone	*Ultandren*
Folcovin	pholcodeine
Folic acid	*Folvite*
Folvite	folic acid
Fortior	vitamin B complex
Fotrodyl	calciferol
Fouadin	stibophen
Framycetin sulphate	*Framygen; Soframycin*
Framygen	framycetin sulphate
Fructose	*Laevoral; Laevosan*
Frusemide	*Lasix*
Fucidin	fusidic acid (sodium salt)
Fulcin Forte	griseofulvin

Fungilin	amphotericin B
Fungizone	amphotericin B
Furacin	nitrofurazone
Furadantin	nitrofurantoin
Furamide	diloxanide furoate
Furan	nitrofurantoin
Furazolidine	*Furoxone*
Furoxone	furazolidine
Fusidic acid (sodium salts)	*Fucidin*
Gamma benzene hexachloride . . .	*Lorexane*
Gantanol	sulphamethoxazole
Gantrisin	sulphafurazole
Gardenal	phenobarbitone
Gardenal Sodium	phenobarbitone sodium
Genacort	hydrocortisone
Genasprin	acetylsalicylic acid
Geneserine	physostigmine
Genolvex	cyanocobalamin zinc tannate
Gentamicin sulphate	*Genticin*
Genticin	gentamicin sulphate
Gestyl	serum gonadotrophin
Gingicain	amethocaine hydrochloride
Glandubolin	oestrone
Glandubolin-Monobenz	oestradiol benzoate
Glibenclamide	*Daonil; Euglucon*
Glistron	ferrous gluconate
Glucophage	metformin hydrochloride
Glutethimide	*Doriden*
Glyceryl trinitrate	*Angised; Antipressan; Sustac*
Glycopyrronium bromide	*Robinul*
Glymidine	*Gondafon; Lycanol*
Gonadotrophin	anterior pituitary hormone
Gonadotrophins-chorionic	*Antuitrin S; Gonadotrophon L.H.; Physex Leo; Pregnyl*
Gonadotrophins-serum	*Antex Leo; Gestyl; Gonadotrophon F.S.D.*
Gonadotrophon F.S.H.	serum gonadotrophin
Gonadotrophon L.H.	chorionic gonadotrophin
Gondafon	glymidine
Gramophen	hexachlorophane
Griseofulvin	*Fulcin Forte; Grisovin Coarse Particle; Grisovin F.P.*
Grisovin Coarse Particle	griseofulvin coarse particle
Grisovin F.P.	griseofulvin fine particle
Guanethidine sulphate	*Ismelin*
Guanidine hydrochloride (moroxydine hydro-chloride)	*Virugon*
Haldrate	paramethasone acetate
Havapen	penamecillin
Helmezine	piperazine
Heparin	*Pularin*
Hermesetas	saccharin sodium
Hetrazan	diethylcarbamazine citrate
Hexabalm	hexachlorophane
Hexachlorophane	*Bidex; Cidal; Cramophen; Hexabalm; Phisohex; Pologol Hexachlor; Ster-Zac*
Hexamethonium bromide	*Vegolysen*
Hibitane	chlorhexidine gluconate

Y

Histostab	antazoline
Honvan	stilboestrol diphosphate
Humagon	human chorionic gonadotrophin
Human chorionic gonadotrophin	*Humagon; Pergonal*
Humatin	paromomycin sulphate
Humorsol	demecarium bromide
Hyalase	hyaluronidase
Hyaluronidase	*Hyalase; Rondase*
Hyamine 3500	benzalkonium chloride
Hyasorb	benzylpenicillin
Hycal	concentrated glucose drink
Hydrallazine hydrochloride	*Apresoline*
Hydrargaphen	*Penotrane*
Hydrenox	hydroflumethiazide
Hydro-Adreson	hydrocortisone
Hydrochlorothiazide	*Direma; Esidrex; Hydrosaluric*
Hydrocortisone and hydrocortisone acetate	*Cobadex; Cortef; Cortril; Efcortelan; Genacort; Hydro-Adreson; Hydrocortistab; Hydrocortone; Pabracort*
Hydrocortisone sodium succinate	*Corlan; Efcortelan Soluble; Solu-Cortef*
Hydrocortistab	hydrocortisone
Hydrocortone	hydrocortisone
Hydroflumethiazide	*Di-Ademil; Hydrenox; Naclex*
Hydrosaluric	hydrochlorothiazide
Hydroxocobalamin	*Neo-Cytamen*
Hydroxychloroquine sulphate	*Plaquenil*
Hydroxyprogesterone caproate	*Primolut-Depot*
Hygroton	chlorthalidone
Hyoscine hydrobromide	*Kwells*
Hyposan	sodium hypochlorite
Hytakerol	dihydrotachysterol
Ibuprofen	*Brufen*
Icipen	phenoxymethylpenicillin
Idoxuridine (IDU)	*Dendrid; Kerecid*
Ilosone	erythromycin estolate
Ilotycin	erythromycin stearate
Imferon	iron dextran complex
Imipramine hydrochloride	*Berkomine; Tofranil*
Imperacin	oxytetracycline hydrochloride
Imuran	azathioprine
Inderal	propranolol
Indocid	indomethacin
Indomethacin	*Indocid*
Insomnol	methylpentynol
Insulins:	
Insulin zinc suspension	*Insulin Novo Lente*
Insulin zinc suspension (amorphous)	*Insulin Novo Semilente*
Insulin zinc suspension (crystalline)	*Insulin Novo Ultralente*
Neutral soluble insulin	*Insulin Novo Actrapid; Nuso Neutral Insulin*
Insulin Novo Actrapid	neutral soluble insulin
Insulin Novo Lente	insulin zinc suspension
Insulin Novo Semilente	insulin zinc suspension (amorphous)
Insulin Novo Ultralente	insulin zinc suspension (crystalline)
Intal	disodium cromoglycate
Intradex	dextran 110
Intraflodex	dextran 40 (low molecular weight)
Intraval Sodium	thiopentone sodium

Invenol	carbutamide
Iodochlorhydroxyquinoline	*Vioform*
Iproniazid phosphate	*Marsilid*
Iron dextran complex	*Imferon*
Iron sorbitol injection	*Jectofer*
Ismelin	guanethidine sulphate
Isocarboxazid	*Marplan*
Isomist	isoprenaline sulphate
Isoniazid	*Mybasan; Neumandin; Nicetal; Pycazide; Rimifon*
Isoniazid aminosalicylate	*Dipasic*
Isoprenaline hydrochloride	*Saventrine*
Isoprenaline sulphate	*Aleudrin; Dispray; Isomist; Lomupren; Medihaler Iso; Meterdos-Iso; Neo-Epinine; Prenomiser*
Jectofer	iron sorbitol injection
Kabikinase	streptokinase
Kanamycin sulphate	*Kannasyn; Kantrex*
Kannasyn	kanamycin sulphate
Kantrex	kanamycin sulphate
Keflex	cephalexin
Keflin	cephalothin sodium
Kerecid	idoxuridine (I.D.U.)
Kinidin	quinidine sulphate
K Lens	methylcellulose eye drops
Kolpon	oestrone
Kwells	hyoscine hydrochloride
Lactulose	*Duphalac*
Laevoral	fructose
Laevosan	fructose
Lamprene	clofazimine
Lanoxin	digoxin
Lapaquin	chlorproguanil hydrochloride with chloroquine phosphate
Lapudrine	chlorproguanil hydrochloride
Largactil	chlorpromazine hydrochloride
Larodopa	dopa
Laroxyl	amitryptyline hydrochloride
Lasix	frusemide
Lederkyn	sulphamethoxypyridazinc
Ledermycin	demethychlortetracyline
Lederplex	vitamin B complex
Lenium	selenium sulphide
Lenticillin	procaine benzylpenicillin
Lergine	tricyclamol chloride
Lethidrone	nalorphine hydrobromide
Leukeran	chlorambucil
Levophed	noradrenaline acid tartrate
Librium	chlordiazepoxide hydrochloride
Lignocaine hydrochloride	*Duncaine; Lignostab; Xylocaine; Xylotox*
Lignostab	lignocaine hydrochloride
Limmisax	saccharin sodium
Lincocin	lincomycin hydrochloride
Lincomycin hydrochloride	*Lincocin; Mycivin*
Lindane (gamma benzene hexachloride)	*Lorexane*
Lingraine	ergotamine tratrate
Liothyronine sodium	*Tertroxin*

Lipoflavinoid	vitamin B complex
Lipotriad	vitamin B complex
Lomodex	dextran 40-low molecular weight
Lumopren	isoprenaline sulphate
Lorexane	lindane (gamma benzene hexachloride)
Low molecular weight dextran	*Intraflodex; Lomodex; Rheomacrodex*
Lucanthone hydrochloride	*Etrinol; Nilodin*
Lucofen	chlorphentermine hydrochloride
Lucofen S.A.	chlorphentermine hydrochloride
Luminal	phenobarbitone
Luminal Sodium	phenobarbitone sodium
Lycanol	glymidine
Lymecyline	*Armyl; Mucomycin; Tetralysal*
Lynoral	ethinyloestradiol
Lysivane	ethopropazine hydrochloride
Macrodex	dextran
Magnesium trisilicate	*Magsorbent; Trisillac*
Magsorbent	magnesium trisilicate
Mannitol	*Osmitrol*
Manoxol O.T.	dioctyl sodium sulphosuccinate
Mapharside	oxophenarsine hydrochloride
Marboran	methisazone
Marcoumar	phenprocoumon
Marevan	warfarin sodium
Marinol	benzalkonium chloride
Markacillin V-K	phenoxymethylpenicillin
Marplan	isocarboxazid
Marsolone	prednisolone
Marsone	prednisone
Marzine	cyclizine hydrochloride
Matromycin	oleandomycin
Mebadin	dehydroemetine hydrochloride
Meclozine hydrochloride	*Ancolan; Sea-Legs*
Medihaler Iso	isoprenaline sulphate spray
Medrone	methylprednisolone
Mefenamic acid	*Ponstan*
Megaclor	chlormethylenecycline
Megestrol acetate	present in *Nuvacon; Serial 28; Volidan*
Megimide	bemegride
Melarsonyl potassium	*Trimelarsan; Mel W*
Melarsoprol	*Mel B*
Mel B	melarsoprol
Melleril	thioridazine
Melphalan	*Alkeran*
Melsedin	methaqualone hydrochloride
Mel W	melarsonyl potassium
Menaphthone sodium bisulphite	*Vitavel K*
Menformon	oestrone
Menthesin	benzocaine compound lozenges
Mepacrine methanesulphonate	*Atebrin*
Mepavlon	meprobamate
Mephenesin	*Myanesin*
Mephenesin carbamate	*Tolseram*
Meprobamate	*Equanil; Mepavlon; Miltown; Pensive*
Mepyramine maleate	*Anthisan*
Merbentyl	dicyclomine hydrochloride

. . . . .	*Puri-Nethol*
. . . . .	mersalyl
. . . . .	*Merphyllin*
. . . . .	methoin
. . . . .	pyridostigmine bromide
. . . . .	present in *Conovid; Demulen; Feminor Sequential; Lyndiol; Norinyl-1; Orthonovin; Ovanon; Ovulen; Previson; Sequens; Sistometril*
ic	methylamphetamine hydrochloride
ol acid tartrate . . .	*Aramine*
. . . . .	methylprednisolone
s-Iso	isoprenaline sulphate
rmin hydrochloride . . .	*Glucophage*
thacycline hydrochloride . . .	*Rondomycin*
Methadone hydrochloride . . .	*Physeptone*
Methaqualone hydrochloride . . .	*Melsedin; Sedaquin*
Methedrine	methylamphetamine hydrochloride
Methicillin sodium	*Celbenin*
Methisazone	*Marboran*
Methoin	*Mesontoin*
Methotrexate	*Amethopterin*
Methylamphetamine hydrochloride . . .	*Metamsustac; Methedrine*
Methylcellulose	*Celacol M; Celevac; Cellucon; Cologel*
Methylcellulose eye drops . . .	*K Lens*
Methyldopa	*Aldomet*
Methylpentynol	*Insomnol; Oblivon*
Methylphenidate hydrochloride . . .	*Ritalin*
Methylphenobarbitone	*Prominal*
Methylprednisolone	*Medrone; Metastab*
Methyprylone	*Noludar*
Methysergide maleate	*Deseril*
Metilar	paramethasone acetate
Metronidazole	*Flagyl*
Mexenone cream	*Uvistat 22111*
Micryston Oestrone . . .	oestrone
Midicel	sulphamethoxypyridazine
Milton	sodium hypochlorite
Miltown	meprobamate
Minox	piperazine citrate
Mintezol	thiabendazole
Miocarpine S.M.P.	pilocarpine nitrate eye drops
Miradon	anisindione
Mogadon	nitrazepam
Monodorm	butobarbitone
Monodral	penthienate methobromide
Morpan C.H.S.A.	cetrimide
Mucomycin	lymecycline
Mustine hydrochloride	*Chlormethine*
Myambutol	ethambutol dihydrochloride
Myanesin	mephenesin
Mybasan	isoniazid
Mycardol	pentaerythritol tetranitrate
Mycifradin	neomycin sulphate
Myciguent	neomycin sulphate
Mycostatin	nystatin
Mycota	zinc undecenoate
Mydrilate	cyclopentolate

Myleran	busulphan
Mylipen	procaine benzylpenicillin
Mylol	diethyl toluamide
Myocrisin	sodium aurothiomalate
Mysoline	primidone
Naclex	hydroflumethiazide
Nadisan	carbutamide
Nalidixic acid	*Negram*
Nalorphine hydrobromide	*Lethidrone*
Nandrolone decanoate	*Deca-Durabolin*
Nandrolone phenylpropionate . . .	*Durabolin*
Nardil	phenelzine sulphate
Natamycin	*Pimafucin*
Nativelle's Digitaline	digitoxin
Natulan	procarbazine hydrochloride
Negram	nalidixic acid
Neoarsphenamine	*Novarsenobillon*
Neo-Cytamen	hydroxocobalamin
Neo-Epinine	isoprenaline sulphate
Neo-Hombreol	testosterone propionate
Neolate	neomycin sulphate
Neolin	benzathine penicillin
Neo-Mercazole	carbimazole
Neomin	neomycin sulphate
Neomycin sulphate	*Mycifradin; Myciguent; Neolate; Neomin; Nivemycin*
Neo-Naclex	bendrofluazide
Neostigmine	*Prostigmin*
Neumandin	isoniazid
Nialamide	*Niamid*
Niamid	nialamide
Nicetal	isoniazid
Nicotinamide	*Nicovel*
Nicotinic acid	*Nicovel*
Nicotinyl alcohol (tartrate) . . .	*Ronicol*
Nicoumalone	*Sinthrome*
Nicovel	nicotinamide
Nikethamide	*Anacordone; Coramine; Corvotone*
Nilevar	norethandrolone
Nilodin	lucanthone hydrochloride
Niridazole	*Ambilhar*
Nitoin	nitrofurantoin
Nitrazepam	*Mogadon*
Nitrofurantoin	*Berkfurin; Furadantin; Furan; Nitoin*
Nitrofurazone	*Furacin*
Nitroglycerin (*see* Glyceryl trinitrate)	
Nivaquine	chloroquine sulphate
Nivemycin	neomycin sulphate
N-methylisatin B-thiosemicarbazone (methisazone)	*Marboran*
Noludar	methyprylone
Noradrenaline acid tartrate . . .	*Adrenor; Levophed*
Norethandrolone	*Nilevar*
Norethisterone	*Primolut N*
Norethisterone acetate	*Norlutin-A; SH420*
Norethynodrel	present in *Conovid; Feminor Sequential; Previson*

Mercaptopurine	orphenadrine citrate
Merphyllin	norethisterone acetate
Mersalyl	dioctyl sodium sulphosuccinate
Mesontoin	neoarsphenamine
Mestinon	*Albamycin; Cathomycin*
Mestranol *monium Chloride*	ammonium chloride enteric coated tablets
pirin	acetylsalicylic acid enteric coated tablets
s	para-aminosalicylic acid enteric coated tablets
Metamsusto dium Salicylate	sodium salicylate enteric coated tablets
Metarami *ral Insulin*	neutral soluble insulin
Metastab	nystatin
Meterdo	*Mycostatin; Nystan*
Metfo	
Met	
Oblivon	methylpentynol
Octachlor	chlordane
Ocusol	sulphacetamide sodium
Oestradiol benzoate	*Benztrone; Dimenformon; Glandubolin-Monobenz: Oestro-form; Ovocyclin M Crystules*
Oestroform	oestrone
Oestrone	*Glandubolin; Kolpon; Menformon; Micryston Oestrone; Oestroform; Oestrosalve*
Oleandomycin	*Matromycin; Romicil*
Omnopon	papaveretum
Oncovin	vincristine sulphate
Opoidine	papaveretum
Oradexon	dexamethasone
Oratrol	dichlorphenamide
Orbenin	cloxacillin
Orciprenaline sulphate	*Alupent*
Orovite	vitamin B complex
Orphenadrine citrate	*Norflex*
Orphenadrine hydrochloride	*Disipal*
Osmitrol	mannitol
Ospolot	sulthiame
Ouabain	*Ouabaine Arnaud*
Ouabaine Arnaud	ouabain
Oxophenarsine hydrochloride	*Mapharside*
Oxymetholone	*Adroyd; Anapolen*
Oxymycin	oxytetracycline hydrochloride
Oxyphenbutazone	*Tanderil*
Oxyphenisatin acetate	*Bydolax; Cirotyl; Contax; Veripaque*
Oxytetracycline	*Oxydon; Terramycin*
Oxytetracycline dihydrate	*Berkemycin; Clinimycin*
Oxytetracycline hydrochloride	*Imperacin; Oxatets*
Oxytocin	*Pitocin; Syntocinon*
Pabestrol	stilboestrol
Pabracort	hydrocortisone
Pabrinex	vitamin B complex
Paludrine	proguanil hydrochloride
Panadol	paracetamol
Panar	pancreatin
Panasorb	paracetamol
Pancreatic extract	*Panar; Pancrex; Panteric; Trypsogen*
Pancrex	pancreatin
Panets	paracetamol
Panol	paracetamol

Panox	paracetamol
Panteric	pancreatin
Pantestin	testosterone propionate
Papaveretum	*Omnopon; Opoidine*
Para-amino salicyclic acid . . .	*Nu-Seals Pas*
Paracetamol	*Calpol; Cetal; Eneril; Febrilix; Panadol; Panasorb; Panets; Panol; Panox; P.C.M.; Tabalgin; Tetmal*
Paracodin	dihydrocodeine acid tartrate
Paradione	paramethadione
Paramethadione	*Paradione*
Paramethasone acetate	*Haldrate; Metilar*
Parentrovite	vitamin B complex
Parnate	tranylcypromine
Paromomycin sulphate	*Humatin*
P.C.M.	paracetamol
Penamecillin	*Havapen*
Penavlon	phenoxymethylpenicillin
Penbritin	ampicillin
Penicals	phenoxymethylpenicillin
Penicillamine	*Distamine*
Penicillin V-K	phenoxymethylpenicillin
Penidural	benzathine penicillin
Penotrane	hydrargaphen
Pensive	meprobamate
Penspek	phenbenicillin potassium
Pentaerythritol tetranitrate . . .	*Cardiacap; Mycardol; Pentral; Peritrate*
Pentazocine	*Fortral*
Pentobarbitone	*Nembutal*
Pentolinium tartrate . . .	*Ansolysen*
Pentostam	sodium stibogluconate
Pentothal	thiopentone sodium
Pentral	pentaerythritol tetranitrate
Perchlor	tetrachloroethylene
Pergonal	human chorionic gonadotrophin
Peritrate	pentaerythritol tetranitrate
Permapen	benzathine penicillin
Perolysen	pempidine tartrate
Perphenazine	*Fentazin*
Phanodorm	cyclobarbitone
Phenbenicillin potassium . . .	*Penspek*
Phenelzine sulphate . . .	*Nardil*
Phenergan	promethazine hydrochloride
Phenethicillin potassium . . .	*Broxil*
Phenformin	*D.B.I.; Dibotin*
Phenindione	*Dindevan; Theradione*
Phenmetrazine hydrochloride . . .	*Preludin*
Phenobarbitone	*Barbenyl; Gardenal; Luminal*
Phenobarbitone sodium . . .	*Gardenal Sodium; Luminal Sodium; Somnolens Elixir*
Phenoxybenzamine hydrochloride . .	*Dibenyline*
Phenoxymethylpenicillin . . .	*Apsin VK; Compocillin-VK; Comprimettes Penicillin V; Crystapen V; Distaquaine V; Econocil-VK; Econopen V; Icipen; Markacillin V-K; Penavlon; Penicals; Penicillin V-K; Stabillin V-K; Tonsillin; V-Cil-K*
Phenprocoumon	*Marcoumar*
Phentermine	*Duromine*
Phentolamine mesylate . . .	*Rogitine*
Phenylbutazone	*Butazolidin; Butazone*

Phenytoin sodium	*Epanutin; Eptoin*
Phisohex	hexachlorophane
Pholcodeine	*Ethnine; Folcovin; Pholox*
Pholox	pholcodeine
Phthalylsulphathiazole	*Sulfathalidine; Thalazole*
Phyldrox	aminophylline
Phylostropin	atropine methyl nitrate
Physeptone	methadone hydrochloride
Physex Leo	chorionic gonadotrophin
Physostigmine	*Geneserine*
Physostigmine salicylate eye drops	*Collyrium Eserine Chibret; Eserine Salicylate Minims*
Phytomenadione	*Aquamephyton; Konakion*
Pilocarpine nitrate eye drops	*Miocarpine S.M.P.*
Pimafucin	natamycin
Pipanol	benzhexol hydrochloride
Piperazine citrate	*Antepar; Helmezine; Minox*
Piperazine phosphate	*Antepar; Helmezine; Pripsen*
Piriton	chlorpheniramine maleate
Pitocin	oxytocin
Pitressin Tannate	vasopressin tannate
Plaquenil	hydroxychloroquine sulphate
Pologol-Hexachlor	hexachlorophane
Polymyxin B	*Aerosporin*
Polynoxylin	*Anaflex; Ponoxylan Gel; Salmocid*
Ponderax	fenfluramine hydrochloride
Pondets Throat Lozenges	benzylpenicillin lozenges
Ponoxylan Gel	polynoxylin
Ponstan	mefenamic acid
Potassium chloride	*Ruthmol*
Potassium chloride slow release tablets	*Slow-K*
Potassium perchlorate	*Peroidin*
Practolol	*Eraldin*
Pralidoxime mesylate	*Contrathion*
Pre Cortisyl	prednisolone
Prednesol	prednisolone disodium phosphate
Prednisolone	*Codelcortone; Delta-Cortef; Delta-Cortril; Delta-Genacort; Deltastab; Di-Adreson-F; Marsolone; Precortisyl*
Prednisolone disodium phosphate	*Codelsol; Prednesol; Predsol*
Prednisone	*Decortisyl; Deltacortone; Di-Adreson; Marsone*
Prednisone acetate	*Delta-Cortelan*
Prednisone sodium phosphate	*Predsol*
Predsol	prednisolone sodium phosphate
Pregnyl	chorionic gonadotrophin
Preludin	phenmetrazine hydrochloride
Prenomiser	isoprenaline sulphate
Prepalin	vitamin A
Primidone	*Mysoline*
Primogyn C	ethinyloestradiol
Primolut Depot	hydroxyprogesterone caproate
Primolut N	norethisterone
Pripsen	piperazine phosphate with senna
Pro-Banthine	propantheline bromide
Probenecid	*Benemid*
Procainamide hydrochloride	*Pronestyl*
Procaine benzylpenicillin	*Avloprocil A.S.; Distaquaine G; Duracillin A.S.; Eskacillin 200; Lenticillin; Mylopen; Pro-Stabilin*
Procarbazine hydrochloride	*Natulan*

Y*

Prochlorperazine maleate	*Stemetil*
Progestoral	ethisterone
Proguanil hydrochloride	*Paludrine*
Prolothan (A)	protamine sulphate
Promazine hydrochloride	*Sparine*
Promethazine hydrochloride	*Phenergan*
Promethazine theoclate	*Avomine*
Prominal	methylphenobarbitone
Propantheline bromide	*Pro-Banthine*
Propicillin potassium	*Brocillin; Ultrapen*
Propoquin	amopyroquin sulphate
Propranolol	*Inderal*
Pro-Stabilin	procaine benzylpenicillin
Prostigmin	neostigmine
Protamine sulphate	*Prolothan (A)*
Prothionamide	*Trevintix*
P.R.Q. Antiseptic	benzalkonium chloride
Pularin	heparin
Puri-Nethol	mercaptopurine
Pycazide	isoniazid
Pyopen	carbenicillin
Pyridostigmine bromide	*Mestinon*
Pyridoxine hydrochloride	*Benadon; Pyrivel*
Pyrimethamine	*Daraprim*
Pyrivel	pyridoxine hydrochloride
Quinalbarbitone sodium	*Quinalspan; Seconal Sodium*
Quinalspan	quinalbarbitone sodium
Quinicardine	quinidine sulphate
Quinidine sulphate	*Kinidin; Quinicardine*
Radiostol	calciferol
Rastinon	tolbutamide
Redoxon	ascorbic acid
Reserpine	*Bioserpine; Reserpine Dellipsoids D29; Serpasil*
Reserpine Dellipsoids D 29	reserpine
Resochin	chloroquine phosphate
Resonium A	sodium polystyrene sulphonate
Rheomacrodex	dextran 40-low molecular weight
Riboflavine	*Beflavit; Ribovel*
Riboral	riboflavin
Rifadin	rifampicin
Rifampicin	*Rifadin*
Rimiform	isoniazid
Ritalin	methyl phenidate hydrochloride
Robinul	glycopyrronium bromide
Roccal	benzalkonium chloride
Rogitine	phentolamine mesylate
Rolitetracycline	*Syntetrin*
Romicil	oleandomycin
Rondase	hyaluronidase
Rondomycin	methacycline hydrochloride
Ronicol	nicotinyl alcohol (tartrate)
Rovamycin	spiramycin
Russell's viper venom	*Stypven*
Ruthmol	potassium chloride

Saccharin sodium	*Hermesetas; Limmisax; Saxin*
Salazopyrin	sulphasalazine
Salbutamol	*Ventilon*
Salmocid	polynoxylin
Saluric	chlorothiazide
Sanamycin	actinomycin C
Saroten	amitryptyline hydrochloride
Saventrine	isoprenaline hydrochloride
Savlon	cetrimide
Saxin	saccharin sodium
Secona Sodium	quinalbarbitone sodium
Sedaquin	methaqualone hydrochloride
Sedormid	apronal
Selenium sulphide	*Lenium; Selsun*
Selsun	selenium sulphide
Septrin	trimethoprim with sulphamethoxazole
Sereen	cyclizine hydrochloride
Serensil	ethchlorvynol
Seromycin	cycloserine
Serpasil	reserpine
Seven Seas Cod Liver Oil	cod liver oil
SH 420	norethisterone acetate
Silcomplex	vitamin B complex
Sinthrome	nicoumalone
Siponol O 100	dioctyl sodium sulphosuccinate
Sketofax	dimethyl phthalate
Slow-K	potassium chloride slow release tablets
Sodium Amytal	amylobarbitone sodium
Sodium aurothiomalate	*Myocrisin*
Sodium calciumedetate	*Calcium Disodium Versenate*
Sodium hypochlorite	*Antiformin; Chloros; Deosan Green Label; Hyposan; Milton; Voxsan*
Sodium polystyrene sulphonate	*Resonium A*
Sodium salicylate	*Entrosalyl; Nu-Seals Sodium Salicylate*
Sodium stibogluconate	*Pentostam*
Sodium sulphomethyl polymyxin (sulphomyxin sodium	*Thiosporin*
Soframycin	framycetin sulphate
Solapsone	*Sulphetrone*
Solprin	acetylsalicylic acid, soluble
Solu-Cortef	hydrocortisone sodium succinate
Solupen	benzylpenicillin
Somnolents Elixir	phenobarbitone sodium
Somnos	chloral hydrate
Soneryl	butobarbitone
Sparine	promazine hydrochloride
Spiramycin	*Rovamycin*
Spironolactone	*Aldactone-A*
Stabilin V-K	phenoxymethylpenicillin
Steclin	tetracycline
Stelazine	trifluoperazine hydrochloride
Stemetil	prochlorperazine maleate
Sterogyl-15	calciferol
Stibophen	*Fouadin*
Stilboestrol	*Pabestrol; Stilboestrol Dellipsoids D.13*
Stilboestrol Dellipsoids D 13	stilboestrol
Stilboestrol diphosphate	*Honvan*

Stilboestrol dipropionate	*Stilbofax; Syntestrin*
Stilbofax	stilboestrol dipropionate
Strepolin	streptomycin sulphate
Streptaquaine	streptomycin sulphate
Streptokinase	*Kabikinase*
Streptomycin sulphate	*Strepolin; Streptaquaine*
Stypven	Russell's viper venom
Sulfadoxine	*Fanasil*
Sulfathalidine	phthalylsulphathiazole
Sulphacetamide sodium	*Albucid; Chibret Sulphacetamide Collyrium; Ocusol*
Sulphadiazine	*Cremodiazine*
Sulphadimidine	*Sulphamezathine*
Sulphafurazole	*Gantrisin*
Sulphamethoxypyridazine . . .	*Lederkyn; Midicel*
Sulphamethoxazole	*Gantanol.* Also present in *Bactrim; Septrin*
Sulphamezathine	sulphadimidine
Sulphasalazine	*Salazopyrin*
Sulphetrone	solapsone
Sulphinpyrazone	*Anturan*
Sulthiame	ospolot
Suramin	antrypol
Sustac	glyceryl trinitrate
Symmetrel	adamantadine hydrochloride
Synalar	fluocinolone acetonide
Synandone	fluocinolone acetonide
Syntestrin	stilboestrol dipropionate
Synthetic lysine vasopressin . . .	*Syntopressin*
Syntocinon	oxytocin
Syntopressin	synthetic lysine vasopressin
Tabalgin	paracetamol
Tabillin	benzylpenicillin
Tanderil	oxyphenbutazone hydrochloride
Tegretol	carabamazepine
Tenormal	pempidine tartrate
Tensilon	edrophonium chloride
Tenuate	diethylpropion hydrochloride
Terramycin	oxytetracycline hydrochloride
Tertroxin	triiodothyronine sodium
Testosterone propionate	*Femasc; Neo-Hombrol; Pantestin; Virormone*
Tetmal	paracetamol
Tetrachloroethylene	*Perchlor; Sd 2*
Tetracycline	*Achromycin; Ambramycin; Economycin; Steclin; Tetracyn; Totomycin*
Tetracycline phosphate complex . . .	*Tetrex*
Tetracocsactrin	*Cortosyn; Synacthen*
Tetracyn	tetracycline
Tetralysal	lymecycline
Tetrex	tetracycline phosphate complex
Thalazole	phthalylsulphathiazole
Theophylline	*Elixophyllin*
Theradione	phenindione
Thiabendazole	*Mintezol*
Thiacetazone	*Thioparamizine*
Thiambutosine	*Ciba 1906*
Thiamine hydrochloride	*Benerva; Betavel*
Thiampolex	vitamin B complex

Thioparamizone	thiacetazine
Thiopropazate hydrochloride	*Dartalan*
Thiopentone sodium	*Intraval Sodium; Pentothal*
Thioridazine	*Melleril*
Thiosporin	sulphomyxin sodium
Three-B	vitamin B complex
Thyrocalcitonin	calcitonin
Thyroxine sodium	*Eltroxin*
Tigloidine hydrobromide	*Tiglyssin*
Tiglyssin	tigloidine hydrobromide
Tineafax	zinc undecenoate
Tofranil	imipramine hydrochloride
Tolanase	tolazamide
Tolazamide	*Tolanase*
Tolbutamide	*Artosin; Rastinon*
Tolseram	mephenesin carbamate
Toniron	ferrous sulphate
Tonivitan B	phenoxymethylpenicillin
Tosmilen	demecarium bromide
Totomycin	tetracycline
Tranylcypromine sulphate	*Parnate*
Trescatyl	ethionamide
Trevintix	prothionamide
Triamcinolone	*Adcortyl; Ledercort*
Triamterene	*Dytac*
Triclofos	*Tricloryl*
Tricloryl	triclofos
Tricyclamol chloride	*Lergine*
Tridione	troxidone
Trifluoperazine hydrochloride	*Stelazine*
Triiodothyronine	*Tertroxin*
Trimelarsan	melarsonyl potassium
Trimethoprim	present in *Bactrim; Septrim*
Triprolidine hydrochloride	*Actidil*
Trisillac	magnesium trisilicate
Troxidone	*Tridione*
Trypsogen	pancreatin
Tryptizol	amitryptyline hydrochloride
Ultandren	fluoxymesterone
Ultrapen	propicillin potassium
Uniplex	vitamin B complex
Uvistat 22111	mexenone cream
Valium	diazepam
Valoid	cyclizine hydrochloride
Vanquin	viprynium embonate
Vasopressin tannate	*Pitressin Tannate*
V-Cil-K	phenoxymethylpenicillin
Vegolysen	hexamethonium bromide
Velbe	vinblastine sulphate
Velsicol 1068	chlordane
Veripaque	dihydroxyphenolisatin
Vesagex	cetrimide
Vibelan Forte	vitamin B complex
Vinblastine sulphate	*Velbe*
Vincristine sulphate	*Oncovin*

Viocin	viomycin
Vioform	iodochlorhydroxyquinolone
Viomycin	*Viocin; Viomycin P; Vionactane*
Viomycin P	viomycin
Vionactane	viomycin
Viprynium embonate . . .	*Vanquin*
Virormone	testosterone propionate
Virugon	guanidine hydrochloride (moroxydine hydrochloride)
Vitamin A	*Avoleum; Prepalin; Ro-A-Vit; Vitavel-A*
Vitamin B complex . . .	*B-Complex; Becomel; Becosym; Becovite; Befortiss; Benerva Compound; Beplex; Cobevit; Complegin; Complebin Forte; Dibexin; Effico Tonic; Fortior; Lederplex; Lipoflavinoid; Lipotriad; Orovite; Pabrinex; Parentrovite; Silcomplex; Thiamoplex; Three-B; Tonivitan B; Uniplex; Vibelan Forte; Vitaminum B Complex, Polfa*
Vitaminum B Complex, Polfa	vitamin B complex
Vitamin B$_{12}$	*Bifacton; Bitevan; Cobalin; Cobastab; Cytacon; Ctyamen; Fermin*
Vitamin K$_1$ (*see* Phytomenadione)	
Vitavel A	vitamin A
Vitavel D	califerol
Vitavel K	menaphthone sodium bisulphite
Voxsan	sodium hypochlorite
Warfarin sodium	*Marevan*
Welldorm	dichloralphenazone
Wyovin	dicyclomine hydrochloride
Xylocaine	lignocaine hydrochloride
Xylotox	lignocaine hydrochloride
Zarontin	ethosuximide
Zephiran	benzalkonium chloride
Zinamide	pyrazinamide
Zinc undecenoate	*Mycota; Tineafax*
Zyloric	allopurinol

Index

Printed by T. & A. CONSTABLE LTD., Edinburgh